Implantable Cardioverter-Defibrillators

FUNDAMENTAL AND CLINICAL CARDIOLOGY

Editor-in-Chief
Samuel Z. Goldhaber, M.D.
Harvard Medical School
and Brigham and Women's Hospital
Boston, Massachusetts

Associate Editor, Europe
Henri Bounameaux, M.D.
University Hospital of Geneva
Geneva, Switzerland

1. *Drug Treatment of Hyperlipidemia*, edited by Basil M. Rifkind
2. *Cardiotonic Drugs: A Clinical Review, Second Edition, Revised and Expanded*, edited by Carl V. Leier
3. *Complications of Coronary Angioplasty*, edited by Alexander J. R. Black, H. Vernon Anderson, and Stephen G. Ellis
4. *Unstable Angina*, edited by John D. Rutherford
5. *Beta-Blockers and Cardiac Arrhythmias*, edited by Prakash C. Deedwania
6. *Exercise and the Heart in Health and Disease*, edited by Roy J. Shephard and Henry S. Miller, Jr.
7. *Cardiopulmonary Physiology in Critical Care*, edited by Steven M. Scharf
8. *Atherosclerotic Cardiovascular Disease, Hemostasis, and Endothelial Function*, edited by Robert Boyer Francis, Jr.
9. *Coronary Heart Disease Prevention*, edited by Frank G. Yanowitz
10. *Thrombolysis and Adjunctive Therapy for Acute Myocardial Infarction*, edited by Eric R. Bates
11. *Stunned Myocardium: Properties, Mechanisms, and Clinical Manifestations*, edited by Robert A. Kloner and Karin Przyklenk
12. *Prevention of Venous Thromboembolism*, edited by Samuel Z. Goldhaber
13. *Silent Myocardial Ischemia and Infarction: Third Edition*, Peter F. Cohn
14. *Congestive Cardiac Failure: Pathophysiology and Treatment*, edited by David B. Barnett, Hubert Pouleur, and Gary S. Francis
15. *Heart Failure: Basic Science and Clinical Aspects*, edited by Judith K. Gwathmey, G. Maurice Briggs, and Paul D. Allen
16. *Coronary Thrombolysis in Perspective: Principles Underlying Conjunctive and Adjunctive Therapy*, edited by Burton E. Sobel and Désiré Collen
17. *Cardiovascular Disease in the Elderly Patient*, edited by Donald D. Tresch and Wilbert S. Aronow
18. *Systemic Cardiac Embolism*, edited by Michael D. Ezekowitz
19. *Low-Molecular-Weight Heparins in Prophylaxis and Therapy of Thromboembolic Diseases*, edited by Henri Bounameaux
20. *Valvular Heart Diseases*, edited by Muayed Al Zaibag and Carlos M. G. Duran
21. *Implantable Cardioverter-Defibrillators: A Comprehensive Textbook*, edited by N. A. Mark Estes III, Antonis S. Manolis, and Paul J. Wang

ADDITIONAL VOLUMES IN PREPARATION

Individualized Therapy of Hypertension, edited by Norman M. Kaplan and C. Venkata S. Ram

Atlas of Coronary Balloon Angioplasty, Bernhard Meier and Vivek Mehan

Implantable Cardioverter-Defibrillators
A Comprehensive Textbook

edited by

N. A. Mark Estes III
Antonis S. Manolis
Paul J. Wang

*Tufts University School of Medicine
and New England Medical Center
Boston, Massachusetts*

Marcel Dekker, Inc.   New York • Basel • Hong Kong

Library of Congress Cataloging-in-Publication Data

Implantable cardioverter-defibrillators : a comprehensive textbook / edited by N. A. Mark Estes III, Antonis S. Manolis, Paul J. Wang.
     p. cm. — (Fundamental and clinical cardiology; v. 21)
   Includes bibliographical references and index.
   ISBN 0-8247-9194-0 (alk. paper)
   1. Implantable cardioverter-defibrillators. I. Estes, N. A. Mark (Nathan Anthony Mark). II. Manolis, Antonis S. III. Wang, Paul J. IV. Series.
   [DNLM: 1. Tachycardia—therapy. 2. Arrhythmia—therapy. 3. Death, Sudden, Cardiac—prevention & control. 4. Defibrillators, Implantable. W1 FU538TD v. 21 1994 / WG 330 I344 1994]
RC684.E4I47 1994
617.4'120645—dc20
DNLM/DLC
for Library of Congress   94-13944
                                                                                                       CIP

The publisher offers discounts on this book when ordered in bulk quantities. For more information, write to Special Sales/Professional Marketing at the address below.

This book is printed on acid-free paper.

Copyright © 1994 by Marcel Dekker, Inc. All Rights Reserved.

Neither this book nor any part may be reproduced or transmitted in any form or by any means, electronic or mechanical, including photocopying, microfilming, and recording, or by any information storage and retrieval system, without permission in writing from the publisher.

Marcel Dekker, Inc.
270 Madison Avenue, New York, New York 10016

Current printing (last digit):
10 9 8 7 6 5 4 3 2 1

Printed in the United States of America

To Modestino G. Criscitiello, M.D., in recognition of his inspirational teaching of surface electrocardiography, electrophysiologic principles, cardiovascular physiology, and clinical cardiology at Tufts University School of Medicine and New England Medical Center

To my wife, Noël, and my children, Elise, Chace, and Katie

N. A. M. E. III

To my wife, Helen, and my children, Stavros, Theodora, and Anthony

A. S. M.

To my wife, Gloria, my children, Margaret and Catherine, my mother, Lillian L. Wang, and the memory of my father, Samuel S. M. Wang

P. J. W.

Series Introduction

During the past decade, Drs. N. A. Mark Estes III, Antonis S. Manolis, and Paul J. Wang built a center of excellence for electrophysiologic study at New England Medical Center. Their clinical research and teaching has been followed closely by investigators in the United States and in other countries where clinical electrophysiology has gained an increasingly important role.

Perhaps the most revolutionary advance in clinical electrophysiology is the advent of the implantable cardioverter-defibrillator. This "high-tech" device provides the promise for managing potentially lethal cardiac dysrhythmias with a "fail proof" mechanical approach devoid of the multitude of toxicities from antiarrhythmic pharmacological agents.

Most impressive is the comprehensive approach that Drs. Estes, Manolis, and Wang have taken in this outstanding book. Their text is written not only for the specialist but also to be clearly understood by the general clinical cardiologist, internist, cardiac surgeon, clinical nurse specialist, and health care administrator. This book will be particularly useful for trainees in cardiovascular medicine, as well as others who have completed their formal training but feel compelled to keep up with the important and astounding developments in this exciting field.

The editors have written many of the chapters themselves but have also relied upon their national and international connections to obtain the best possible contributions on every relevant aspect of the implantable cardioverter-defibrillator. With this text in hand I will be a more knowledgeable general clinical cardiologist. This text will help me participate in informed discussions regarding my individual patients and explain to my cardiac dysrhythmia patients the potential risks and benefits of this device.

Drs. Estes, Manolis, and Wang are to be congratulated for their important and unique contribution. Their timely book will be a most welcome contribution to the Fundamental and Clinical Cardiology series.

SAMUEL Z. GOLDHABER

Foreword

In 1994, implantable cardioverter-defibrillator (ICD) therapy has become the preferred treatment for cardiac arrest survivors. Tiered-therapy ICDs with antitachycardia pacing are frequently used to treat patients with recurrent sustained ventricular tachycardia (VT). The prevalence of ICD use has risen exponentially since 1994, most recently spurred by FDA approval of transvenous lead systems. Early clinical experience with ICD therapy soon led to "wish lists" of features for future ICDs. Industry has been responsive and more and more features from the "wish lists" have found their way into ICDs with each passing year. Even at this point in the development of ICD treatment, there is a broad spectrum of technologies, leads, and programmable features in devices approved for use in the United States and Europe.

Given the rapid development in ICD clinical use and technology, this comprehensive text edited by Drs. Estes, Manolis, and Wang provides a valuable summary of the dynamic ICD field. ICD therapy is viewed from many perspectives, including those of the physiologist, engineer, cardiologist, and clinical electrophysiologist, and from a European as well as American viewpoint. This book provides chapters on mechanisms of defibrillation, on indications for use of ICDs, on technical details of implantation and testing, and on dealing with technical, medical, and emotional problems during follow-up. The issue of cost-effectiveness is also addressed. Each of the ICDs available at the present time is described in detail.

The tough issues of adjunctive antiarrhythmic drug treatment in patients with ICDs are addressed. A thorough review of drug–device interactions and clinical drug experience is provided. The book describes a d-sotalol/ICD trial, the first of many studies, we hope, which will collect controlled data to evaluate the complex risk/benefit ratio of adjunctive antiarrhythmic drug treatment in ICD patients.

ICD treatment has achieved preeminence for treating malignant ventricular arrhythmias without scientific evidence for its advantage over alternative therapies. Some chapters review ongoing clinical trials that will scientifically examine the benefit/risk ratio of ICD treatment relative to alternative therapies and provide, at last, a scientific basis for ICD therapy. Some of these trials compare ICD treatment to drug therapy in patients who have already had cardiac arrest, while others examine the benefits and risks of ICD prophylaxis in patients who are at high risk of having cardiac arrest but have not yet had a malignant arrhythmic event. A stimulating and creative chapter on future directions of ICD therapy gives us an exciting glimpse of the future.

Implantable Cardioverter-Defibrillators: A Comprehensive Textbook achieves its goal of providing comprehensive and current information about ICDs for a broad spectrum of readers. This book will benefit all those who are interested in ICD therapy.

J. THOMAS BIGGER JR., M.D.
Professor of Medicine and Pharmacology
Columbia University
and Director, Arrhythmia Service
The Presbyterian Hospital in the City of New York
New York, New York

Preface

In the decade and a half since the introduction of the original version of the implantable cardioverter-defibrillator there has been a remarkable evolution in device technology and strategies for clinical use. The initial automatic implantable cardioverter-defibrillator required a thoracotomy for epicardial lead placement and was capable only of recognizing ventricular fibrillation and of treatment with a high-energy monophasic shock. Its clinical use was reserved for patients who had survived at least two episodes of cardiac arrest.

Current-generation devices incorporate tiered therapy for ventricular arrhythmias with antitachycardia pacing, low-energy cardioversion, and high-energy defibrillation with biphasic waveforms. Bradycardia pacing, data and electrogram storage, and nonthoracotomy lead systems, coupled with recognition of their effectiveness in preventing sudden arrhythmic death, have made device therapy the dominant strategy in treatment of survivors of cardiac arrest. Multiple trials currently in progress examining the role of implantable cardioverter-defibrillator in patients who are at high risk for but have not yet experienced sustained ventricular tachycardia or fibrillation will clarify the role of device therapy in this considerable patient population.

This book was conceived to fulfill the need for a text that would serve as an authoritative and scholarly yet practical reference for individuals involved in device design and for cardiologists, electrophysiologists, cardiac surgeons, internists, family practitioners, electrophysiology and cardiology fellows, nurses, and technicians involved in the care of the defibrillator patient. We have attempted to produce a comprehensive text that incorporates information relevant to the implantable cardioverter-defibrillator from the basic, engineering, and clinical sciences. To achieve this purpose we have included chapters discussing basic concepts of cardioversion, defibrillation, and antitachycardia pacing. Technical considerations, such as device design, energy storage, energy delivery, data storage, and effects of electrical magnetic interference (EMI) have been contributed by engineers experienced in device development. Experts in the clinical use of the implantable cardioverter-defibrillator have provided reviews on all aspects of preoperative evaluation, surgical and intraoperative assessment, and postoperative care. Separate chapters are devoted to the European experience with defibrillator therapy, the status of multiple trials in progress evaluating the role of device therapy in various patient populations, and consideration of the complex economic issues involving the implantable defibrillator. The clinical results with each device are reviewed in chapters on separate devices, and a detailed description of each device is provided in a comprehensive index. We have attempted to produce as complete a volume as possible and therefore have included information spanning work from the early laboratory observations of Mirowski, through all results with devices commercially approved and in clinical investigation, to considerations of future directions in device design and clinical use.

We would like to acknowledge with appreciation the many contributing authors who sent us excellent chapters and thereby made this volume possible. We would also like to gratefully recognize the superb organizational and secretarial skills of Denise Kirk and the helpful advice and assistance of Graham Garratt and the staff at Marcel Dekker, Inc. A special note of thanks is due our wives and children for their continued understanding and support of this and our other academic and medical endeavors. As editors, we have the sincere hope that this text will serve as a useful reference for students of arrhythmology, clinical practitioners, and investigators alike and contribute to the science and art of care of patients with the implantable cardioverter-defibrillator.

N. A. MARK ESTES III
ANTONIS S. MANOLIS
PAUL J. WANG

Contents

Series Introduction		*v*
Foreword		*vii*
Preface		*ix*
Contributors		*xi*

1 The Process of Defibrillation 1
Susan M. Blanchard and Raymond E. Ideker

2 The Defibrillation Threshold: A Reliable Method for Rapid Determination of Defibrillation Efficacy 29
Douglas L. Jones

3 Unipolar Defibrillation 55
Gust H. Bardy

4 Basic Concepts in Tachycardia Management by Pacing 61
James A. Roth and John D. Fisher

5 Low-Energy Cardioversion 89
Connor J. Haugh, Antonis S. Manolis, and N. A. Mark Estes III

6 Stored Ventricular Electrogram Analysis in the Management of Patients with Implantable Cardioverter-Defibrillators 99
Bruce G. Hook, David J. Callans, Henry H. Hsia, Raman L. Mitra, and Francis E. Marchlinski

7	Engineering Considerations in the Design of ICD Systems *Eliot L. Ostrow and Stephen J. Whistler*	113
8	Energy Storage and Delivery *Esther S. Takeuchi and William D. K. Clark*	123
9	The Effects of External Interference on ICDs and PMs *Walter H. Olson*	139
10	Data Storage *Richard Lu*	153
11	Historical Development of the AICD *Morton M. Mower and Robert G. Hauser*	173
12	Indications for the Implantable Cardioverter-Defibrillator *Arun Gadhoke, David S. Cannom, and N. A. Mark Estes III*	187
13	Survival of Patients with Implantable Cardioverter-Defibrillators *Richard N. Fogoros*	195
14	Implantable Cardioverter-Defibrillators in Children and Adolescents *Michael J. Silka, Jack Kron, and Paul C. Gillette*	205
15	Strategies for Management of Malignant Ventricular Arrhythmias: Role of Pharmacotherapy, Surgery, Ablation, and the Implantable Cardioverter-Defibrillator *N. A. Mark Estes III*	229
16	Preoperative Evaluation for Cardioverter-Defibrillator Implant *Joseph Zebede and Antonis S. Manolis*	257
17	Surgical Techniques for the Implantable Cardioverter-Defibrillator *Hassan Rastegar and Robert M. Bojar*	279
18	Intraoperative Testing *Kenneth A. Ellenbogen, Mark A. Wood, and Bruce S. Stambler*	295
19	Anesthesia for Surgical Placement of Automatic Internal Cardioverter-Defibrillators *George R. Gordon, William S. Panza, and Michael R. England*	319
20	Postoperative Care of the Implantable Cardioverter-Defibrillator Patient *David S. Cannom*	341
21	Surgical Complications of Defibrillator Implantation *Connor J. Haugh and Paul J. Wang*	353

Contents

22 Predischarge Testing of the Implantable Cardioverter-Defibrillator 367
Richard J. Lewis and Enrico P. Veltri

23 Antiarrhythmic Drug Use in the Implantable Cardioverter-Defibrillator Patient 371
Stephanie K. Stevens and N. A. Mark Estes III

24 Implantable Defibrillator Patient and Family Teaching 387
Laurie J. Butts, Carol D. Colburn, and Paul J. Wang

25 Psychiatric Aspects of the Implantable Cardioverter-Defibrillator 405
Gregory L. Fricchione and Stephen C. Vlay

26 Follow-up of Patients with Implantable Cardioverter-Defibrillator Devices 425
Lee A. Biblo, Mark D. Carlson, and Albert L. Waldo

27 Troubleshooting Implanted Devices 437
Richard J. Lewis and Enrico P. Veltri

28 Troubleshooting Antitachycardia Pacing in Patients with Implantable Defibrillators 445
Sergio L. Pinski, Tony W. Simmons, and James D. Maloney

29 Permanent Pacemakers and Implantable Cardioverter-Defibrillators: Potential Interactions 479
Andrew E. Epstein and Richard B. Shepard

30 Device Infection: Prevention and Treatment 495
Susan O'Donoghue and Edward V. Platia

31 Radiology of the Implantable Cardioverter-Defibrillator 505
Caroline Breckwoldt Foote and Antonis S. Manolis

32 Prediction and Prevention of Sudden Cardiac Death 557
J. Thomas Bigger Jr.

33 Use of the Implantable Cardioverter-Defibrillator in Patients Awaiting Heart Transplantation 585
John J. Smith, James E. Udelson, Marvin A. Konstam, and Deeb Salem

34 Analyzing the Costs and Cost Effectiveness of the Implantable Cardioverter-Defibrillator 595
Greg C. Larsen and Stephen G. Pauker

35 Implantable Cardioverter-Defibrillator Lead Systems 607
Antonis S. Manolis

36 Overview of the Implantable Cardioverter-Defibrillator 635
N. A. Mark Estes III

37	Automatic Implantable Cardioverter-Defibrillators: The Ventak Devices *Antonis S. Manolis*	655
38	The Telectronics Guardian 4202/4203 *Paul J. Wang*	675
39	The Medtronic PCD Pacemaker Cardioverter-Defibrillator *Raymond Yee, George J. Klein, and Kevin Wolfe*	683
40	The VENTAK PRx Implantable Cardioverter-Defibrillator *N. A. Mark Estes III*	695
41	The Telectronics Guardian 4210/4211 *Paul J. Wang*	713
42	Siecure: Tiered Antitachycardia Therapy with Bradycardia Support Pacing and Extensive Diagnostics *Asa Hedin, Martin Obel, and Paul A. Levine*	733
43	The AngeMed Sentinel Implantable Antitachycardia Pacer Cardioverter-Defibrillator *Patrick J. Tchou and Mark W. Kroll*	755
44	The Ventritex Cadence Tiered-Therapy Defibrillator: Device Description and Clinical Experience *Michael J. Reiter*	763
45	The CPI Endotak Nonthoracotomy Lead System *Ferdinand J. Venditti, Jr., David T. Martin, and David Shahian*	779
46	The DF Endocardial Defibrillation and Pacing Nonthoracotomy Lead System *N. A. Mark Estes III*	795
47	The Implantable Cardioverter-Defibrillators: European Clinical Experience *Werner Jung, Matthias Manz, and Berndt Lüderitz*	811
48	The Implantable Cardioverter-Defibrillator: Future Directions *Sanjeev Saksena*	845
	ICD Devices Index *Antonis S. Manolis*	871
	Index	915

Contributors

Gust H. Bardy, M.D.   Associate Professor of Medicine, University of Washington, Seattle, Washington

Lee A. Biblo, M.D.   Assistant Professor of Medicine and Staff Cardiologist, Case Western Reserve University, and University Hospitals of Cleveland, Cleveland, Ohio

J. Thomas Bigger Jr., M.D.   Professor of Medicine and Pharmacology, Columbia University, and Director, Arrhythmia Service, The Presbyterian Hospital in the City of New York, New York, New York

Susan M. Blanchard, Ph.D.   Associate Professor, North Carolina State University, Raleigh, North Carolina

Robert M. Bojar, M.D.   Associate Professor of Surgery, Tufts University School of Medicine, and Senior Surgeon, New England Medical Center, Boston, Massachusetts

Laurie J. Butts, B.S.N.   Pacemaker Nurse Coordinator, New England Medical Center, Boston, Massachusetts

David J. Callans, M.D.   Director, Electrocardiography, Philadelphia Heart Institute, Presbyterian Medical Center, Philadelphia, Pennsylvania

David S. Cannom, M.D.   Medical Director of Cardiology, Hospital of the Good Samaritan, and Clinical Professor of Medicine, UCLA School of Medicine, Los Angeles, California

Mark D. Carlson, M.D. Assistant Professor of Medicine, Case Western Reserve University, and Director, Cardiac Electrophysiology Laboratory, University Hospitals of Cleveland, Cleveland, Ohio

William D. K. Clark Director, Process and Product Quality, Wilson Greatbatch Ltd., Clarence, New York

Carol D. Colburn Implantable Cardiovecter Defibrillator Coordinator, New England Medical Center, Boston, Massachusetts

Kenneth A. Ellenbogen, M.D. Director, Clinical Electrophysiology Laboratory, and Associate Professor of Medicine, Medical College of Virginia, and McGuire Veterans Affairs Medical Center, Richmond, Virginia

Michael R. England, M.D. Assistant Professor of Anesthesiology, Tufts University School of Medicine, and Anesthetist, New England Medical Center, Boston, Massachusetts

Andrew E. Epstein, M.D. Professor of Medicine, Division of Cardiovascular Disease, University of Alabama at Birmingham, and University of Alabama Hospital, Birmingham, Alabama

N. A. Mark Estes III, M.D. Professor of Medicine, Tufts University School of Medicine, and Director, Cardiac Arrhythmia Service, New England Medical Center, Boston, Massachusetts

John D. Fisher, M.D., F.A.C.C. Director, Division of Cardiology, and Director, Arrhythmia Services, Montefiore Medical Center, Bronx, New York

Richard N. Fogoros, M.D. Associate Professor of Medicine, Medical College of Pennsylvania, and Director, Clinical Electrophysiology, Allegheny General Hospital, Pittsburgh, Pennsylvania

Caroline Breckwoldt Foote, M.D. Assistant Professor of Medicine, Tufts University School of Medicine, and Assistant Director, Cardiac Electrophysiology Laboratory, New England Medical Center, Boston, Massachusetts

Gregory L. Fricchione, M.D. Associate Professor of Psychiatry, Harvard Medical School, and Director, Consultation–Liaison Psychiatry Service, Brigham and Women's Hospital, Boston, Massachusetts

Arun Gadhoke, M.D. Assistant Professor of Medicine, Tufts University School of Medicine, New England Medical Center, Boston, Massachusetts

Paul C. Gillette, M.D. Director, Pediatric Cardiology, Medical University of South Carolina, Charleston, South Carolina

George R. Gordon, M.D. Assistant Professor of Anesthesiology, Tufts University School of Medicine, and Assistant Anesthetist, New England Medical Center, Boston, Massachusetts

Contributors

Connor J. Haugh, M.D.   Fellow, Division of Cardiology, Tufts University School of Medicine, and New England Medical Center, Boston, Massachusetts

Robert G. Hauser, M.D.   Cardiologist, Minneapolis Heart Institute, Minneapolis, Minnesota

Asa Hedin, M.S.E.E.   Manager, Antitachycardia Group, Siemens Elema AB, Solna, Sweden

Bruce G. Hook, M.D.   Director, Cardiac Electrophysiology Laboratory, Regional Cardiac Institute, Catholic Medical Center, Manchester, New Hampshire

Henry H. Hsia, M.D.   Assistant Professor of Medicine, Temple University School of Medicine, Philadelphia, Pennsylvania

Raymond E. Ideker, M.D., Ph.D.   Professor of Pathology and Biomedical Engineering, and Associate Professor of Medicine, Duke University Medical Center, Durham, North Carolina

Douglas L. Jones   University of Western Ontario and University Hospital, and John P. Robarts Research Institute, London, Ontario, Canada

Werner Jung, M.D.   Professor of Cardiology and Pulmonary Medicine, Friedrich-Wilhelm University, and University Hospital Bonn, Bonn, Germany

George J. Klein, M.D.   Professor of Medicine, University of Western Ontario, and Director, Arrhythmia Service, University Hospital, London, Ontario, Canada

Marvin A. Konstam, M.D.   Professor of Medicine, Tufts University School of Medicine, and Director, Cardiac Catheterization Laboratory, New England Medical Center, Boston, Massachusetts

Mark W. Kroll   AngeMed, Division of Angeion Corporation, Plymouth, Minnesota

Jack Kron, M.D.   Associate Professor of Medicine, Oregon Health Sciences University, Portland, Oregon

Greg C. Larsen, M.D.   Assistant Professor of Medicine, Oregon Health Sciences University, and Director, Cardiac Catheterization Laboratory, Portland Veterans Affairs Medical Center, Portland, Oregon

Richard J. Lewis, M.D., Ph.D.   Director, Clinical Arrhythmia Service, Sinai Hospital of Baltimore, Baltimore, Maryland

Paul A. Levine, M.D.   Vice President and Medical Director, Siemens Pacesetters, Inc., Sylmar, and Clinical Professor of Medicine, Loma Linda University Medical Center, Loma Linda, California

Richard Lu, M.Biomed.E.   Senior Research Scientist, Telectronics Pacing Systems, Englewood, Colorado

Berndt Lüderitz, M.D. Professor of Cardiology and Pulmonary Medicine, Friedrich-Wilhelm University, and Head, Department of Medicine and Cardiology, University Hospital Bonn, Bonn, Germany

James D. Maloney, M.D. Professor of Medicine, and Director, Center for Cardiac Arrhythmia Services and Electrophysiology, Baylor College of Medicine, Houston, Texas

Antonis S. Manolis, M.D., F.A.C.C., F.E.S.C. Associate Professor of Medicine, Tufts University School of Medicine and New England Medical Center, Boston, Massachusetts

Matthias Manz, M.D. Professor of Cardiology and Pulmonary Medicine, Friedrich-Wilhelm University, and University Hospital Bonn, Bonn, Germany

Francis E. Marchlinski, M.D. Director, Arrhythmia Services, Philadelphia Heart Institute, and Presbyterian Medical Center, Philadelphia, Pennsylvania

David T. Martin, M.B.B.S., M.P.C.P. Instructor in Medicine, Harvard Medical School, Boston, and Director, Cardiac Electrophysiology Laboratory, Lahey Clinic Medical Center, Burlington, Massachusetts

Raman L. Mitra, M.D. Assistant Professor of Medicine, and Director, Clinical Electrophysiology, Section of Cardiology, Rush-Presbyterian Medical Center, Chicago, Illinois

Morton M. Mower, M.D. Vice President of Medical Sciences, Cardiac Pacemakers, Inc., St. Paul, Minnesota

Martin Obel, M.S.E.E. Chief Engineer, Antitachycardia Group, Siemens Elema AB, Solna, Sweden

Susan O'Donoghue, M.D. Assistant Professor of Medicine, George Washington University School of Medicine, and Associate Director, Cardiac Arrhythmia Center, Washington Hospital Center, Washington, D.C.

Walter H. Olson, Ph.D. Senior Bakken Fellow, Tachyarrhythmia Research, Medtronic, Inc., Minneapolis, Minnesota

Eliot L. Ostrow Clinical Research Scientist, Tachycardia Projects, Intermedics, Inc., A Company of Sulzermedica, Angleton, Texas

William S. Panza, M.D. Assistant Professor of Anesthesiology, Tufts University School of Medicine, and Assistant Anesthetist, New England Medical Center, Boston, Massachusetts

Stephen G. Pauker, M.D. Professor of Medicine, Tufts University School of Medicine, and New England Medical Center, Boston, Massachusetts

Sergio L. Pinski, M.D. Staff Electrophysiologist, Cleveland Clinic Foundation, Cleveland, Ohio

Contributors

Edward V. Platia, M.D.   Professor of Medicine, George Washington University School of Medicine, and Director, Cardiac Arrhythmia Center, Washington Hospital Center, Washington, D.C.

Hassan Rastegar, M.D.   Associate Professor of Surgery, Tufts University School of Medicine, and Senior Surgeon, Cardiothoracic Surgery, New England Medical Center, Boston, Massachusetts

Michael J. Reiter, M.D., Ph.D.   Associate Professor of Medicine, University of Colorado Health Sciences Center, and Director, Arrhythmia Service, University Hospital, Denver, Colorado

James A. Roth, M.D., F.A.C.C.   Assistant Professor of Medicine, Montefiore Medical Center, Bronx, New York

Sanjeev Saksena, M.D.* Director, Arrhythmia and Pacemaker Service, Eastern Heart Institute, Passaic, and Clinical Associate Professor of Medicine and Pediatrics, UMD-NJ Medical School, Newark, New Jersey

Deeb Salem, M.D.   Professor of Medicine, Tufts University School of Medicine, and Chief of Cardiology, New England Medical Center, Boston, Massachusetts

David Shahian, M.D.   Assistant Clinical Professor of Surgery, Harvard Medical School, Boston, and Chairman, Department of Thoracic and Cardiovascular Surgery, Lahey Clinic Medical Center, Burlington, Massachusetts

Richard B. Shepard, M.D.   Professor of Surgery, University of Alabama at Birmingham and University of Alabama Hospital, Birmingham, Alabama

Michael J. Silka, M.D.   Associate Professor, Oregon Health Sciences University, Portland, Oregon

Tony W. Simmons, M.D.   Associate Professor of Medicine, and Director, Heart Station, Bowman Gray School of Medicine, Winston-Salem, North Carolina

John J. Smith, M.D., Ph.D.   Assistant Professor of Medicine, Tufts University School of Medicine, and Associate Director, Adult Cardiac Catheterization Laboratory, New England Medical Center, Boston, Massachusetts

Bruce S. Stambler, M.D.   Assistant Professor of Medicine, Medical College of Virginia and McGuire Veterans Affairs Medical Center, Richmond, Virginia

Stephanie K. Stevens, M.D.   Instructor in Medicine, Tufts University School of Medicine, and Research and Clinical Fellow in Cardiac Electrophysiology, New England Medical Center, Boston, Massachusetts

Esther S. Takeuchi, Ph.D.   Director, Electrochemical Research, Wilson Greatbatch Ltd., Clarence, New York

---

*Present affiliation: Private practice, Milburn, New Jersey.

Patrick J. Tchou, M.D.   Associate Professor of Medicine, University of Pittsburgh, and Director, Cardiac Electrophysiology, University of Pittsburgh Medical Center, Pittsburgh, Pennsylvania

James E. Udelson, M.D.   Assistant Professor of Medicine, Tufts University School of Medicine, and New England Medical Center, Boston, Massachusetts

Enrico P. Veltri, M.D.   Director, Division of Cardiology, Sinai Hospital of Baltimore, Baltimore, Maryland

Ferdinand J. Venditti, Jr., M.D.   Clinical Instructor, Harvard Medical School, Boston, and Chief, Cardiovascular Medicine, Lahey Clinic Medical Center, Burlington, Massachusetts

Stephen C. Vlay, M.D.   Professor of Medicine, State University of New York at Stony Brook, and Director, Coronary Care Unit and Arrhythmia Study Center, University Hospital, Stony Brook, New York

Albert L. Waldo, M.D.   The Walter H. Pritchard Professor of Cardiology and Professor of Medicine, Case Western Reserve University, and Director, Cardiac Arrhythmia Service, University Hospitals of Cleveland, Cleveland, Ohio

Paul J. Wang, M.D.   Director, Adult Heart Station, and Associate Director, Cardiac Electrophysiology and Pacemaker Laboratory, New England Medical Center, and Assistant Professor of Medicine, Tufts University School of Medicine, Boston, Massachusetts

Stephen J. Whistler, M.S.E.E.   Director, Design and Development Engineering, Intermedics, Inc., A Company of Sulzermedica, Angleton, Texas

Kevin Wolfe, M.D.   Lecturer, University of Manitoba, and Associate Staff, Health Sciences Centre, Winnepeg, Manitoba, Canada

Mark A. Wood, M.D.   Assistant Professor of Medicine, Medical College of Virginia and McGuire Veterans Affairs Medical Center, Richmond, Virginia

Raymond Yee, M.D.   Associate Professor, University of Western Ontario, and Director, Arrhythmia Monitoring Unit, University Hospital, London, Ontario, Canada

Joseph Zebede, M.D.   Instructor in Medicine, Tufts University School of Medicine, and Clinical and Research Fellow in Cardiac Electrophysiology, New England Medical Center, Boston, Massachusetts

1
The Process of Defibrillation

Susan M. Blanchard

North Carolina State University
Raleigh, North Carolina

Raymond E. Ideker

Duke University Medical Center
Durham, North Carolina

In 1940, Wiggers [1] described ventricular fibrillation (VF) as "an incoordinate type of contraction which, despite a high metabolic rate of the myocardium, produces no useful beats. As a result, the arterial pressure falls abruptly to very low levels, and death results within six to eight minutes from anemia of the brain and spinal cord." Defibrillation is the process that is used to interrupt fibrillatory activity in the heart, since spontaneous recovery from VF is rare other than in small animals [1]. During defibrillation, an electrical shock is applied transthoracically or directly to the heart. The strength of the shock must be sufficient to stop fibrillation yet not so strong that it causes damage to the myocardium. Recent advances in digital hardware [2,3], electrode construction [4], and identification of activations during VF [5] have made it possible to map activation sequences during fibrillation and immediately following defibrillation shocks. To understand how defibrillation works, it is first necessary to understand the mechanisms which underlie fibrillation.

I. INITIATION OF VENTRICULAR FIBRILLATION

A. Ventricular Fibrillation Induced by Ischemia and Reperfusion

An early study by Janse et al. [6] suggested that two mechanisms are responsible for ventricular arrhythmias during early ischemia: (1) a focal mechanism, possibly induced by injury currents across the border between normal tissue and the ischemic region; and (2) a reentrant mechanism involving reentry in the ischemic myocardium. To study excitation patterns and injury current flow in ischemic regions, Janse and colleagues simultaneously recorded electrograms from 60 extracellular epicardial and intramural sites in the left ventricles of isolated porcine and canine hearts during the first 15 min after occlusion and reperfusion of the left anterior descending artery (LAD). During the early ventricular arrhythmias that occurred after reperfusion, they observed fragmented wavefronts and multiple wandering wavelets which followed tortuous paths on the epicardial surface. They noted that circus movements were seldom complete and had small diameters (0.5 cm) when they were. Since mapping was limited to only a portion of the ventricles, a definitive assessment of the underlying mechanism could not be made.

Ideker's group [7] demonstrated a period of organized epicardial activation during the transition to VF. They induced VF in canine hearts by occlusion of the proximal circumflex artery for 15 min followed by reperfusion and recorded from 27 epicardial electrodes spaced over both ventricles. Analysis of the first 1.5–2.5 s of the transition from sinus rhythm or ventricular tachycardia (VT) to fibrillation revealed that ventricular activation occurred in an orderly, rapidly repeating sequence in all hearts. In each case, a single, organized wavefront broke through to the epicardium near the border of the ischemic-reperfused region and passed across the nonischemic portion of the ventricles to the opposite side of the heart. The decreasing time between successive activations indicated that the rate increased during the onset of fibrillation, while the decreasing distance between isochrones indicated that the duration of each cycle increased concurrently due to slowing conduction. As the conduction velocity slowed and the rate of activation increased, less time occurred between the end of one cycle of activation and the start of the next. The duration of each activation cycle soon grew longer than the interval between epicardial breakthroughs for consecutive cycles. When this occurred, the next activation front would break through to the epicardium in the ischemic-reperfused region before the previous activation front had terminated over the right ventricle. The overlap continued to increase during subsequent cycles and resulted in as many as three successive activation fronts being present on the epicardium simultaneously [8]. This is clearly demonstrated in Fig. 1, which shows that the 13th cycle in the transition from VT to VF began before cycle 12 terminated and ended after cycle 14 began. The overall duration of the 13th cycle over the entire heart was much longer than the time between cycles 12 and 13 or 13 and 14 at any given electrode site. Even though the body surface electrocardiogram appeared disorganized during this transition period, the experimental results demonstrated that the underlying cardiac activation sequence was actually organized and periodic. The actual mechanism by which activation was initiated during the transition to fibrillation could not be determined due to the limited number of electrodes, the wide spacing between the epicardial electrodes, and the lack of intramyocardial and subendocardial electrodes.

Pogwizd and Corr [9] used a computerized three-dimensional mapping system and recorded from 232 bipolar sites at eight transmural levels located throughout the feline heart to further delineate the electrophysiologic mechanisms responsible for malignant ventricular arrhythmias associated with reperfusion of ischemic myocardium. Regional ischemia was induced in six cats by a 10-min occlusion of the LAD followed by reperfusion. Prior to reperfusion, the total ventricular activation time during sinus rhythm was significantly delayed. VT occurred within 15 s after reperfusion in all size animals and progressed to VF in three. Both reentrant and nonreentrant mechanisms were responsible for nonsustained VT. In 75% of the cases of nonsustained VT, initial activation occurred at the border of the reperfused zone in the subendocardium and did not involve reentry. There was no association between intervening depolarizations and the time from the end of the last sinus beat to the beginning of VT, nor was there any evidence of continuous activity. The remaining 25% of the cases of nonsustained VT were reentrant in nature, with delayed midmyocardial activation from the preceding sinus beat reentering the adjacent subendocardium and resulting in a marked prolongation in activation. The delay was comparable to that produced during early ischemia without reperfusion and resulted in continuous activation that initiated the first beat of the VT in the subendocardium. VT which led to VF was usually initiated by a nonreentrant mechanism in the subendocardium at

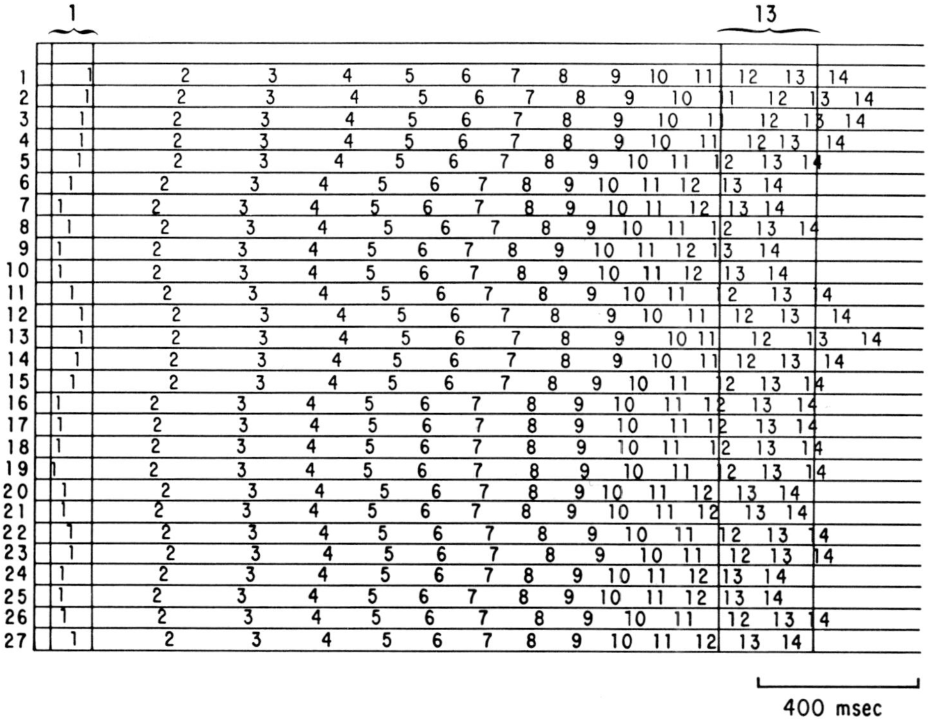

The Process of Defibrillation

Figure 1 Overlapping cycles during the transition to ventricular fibrillation. Electrodes are numbered along the ordinate, while the abscissa represents time. The times at which local activation occurred for each electrode are numbered consecutively. The time between activation fronts at an individual electrode site decreased as time progressed (e.g., the time between cycles 1 and 2 versus the time between cycles 13 and 14 at any electrode), while the time within an individual cycle throughout the heart increased (e.g., the duration of cycle 1 versus the duration of cycle 13 for all electrodes). Thus, activation occurred in repeating, overlapping cycles. (Reprinted from Ref. 7 by permission of The American Heart Association.)

the border of the reperfused zone (although intramural reentry contributed in some cases) and was maintained by both nonreentrant and reentrant mechanisms, which sometimes occurred in the same beat. Nonreentrant mechanisms arose from both the subendocardium and subepicardium, led to a very rapid acceleration of the tachycardia during the transition from VT to VF, and resulted in enhanced functional block and additional conduction delays. During nonreentrant VT, the total activation time of the transition beats exceeded the coupling interval and resulted in overlapping cycles of activation. The nature of this nonreentrant excitation was not determined but may have involved an abnormal form of automaticity or triggered activity.

The mechanisms underlying the development of VF during early myocardial ischemia that is not followed by reperfusion have also been studied by Pogwizd and Corr [10]. In four of 15 cats studied, occlusion of the proximal LAD led to VT, which then degenerated into VF in 1 to 5 min. In three of the four animals with VF, intramural reentry involving multiple activation sites in and around the border region of the ischemic zone was the primary factor in maintaining the VT that led to VF. The initiating mechanism could not be determined in the fourth animal. VT was also maintained by nonreentrant mechanisms which arose in the subendocardium and subepicardium. The transition from VT to VF was always the result of intramural reentry, with initiation of the reentrant beats occurring in the subendocardium and occasionally the subepicardium. During intramural reentry, acceleration of the VT resulted in increased functional block and conduction delay, as well as very rapid and inhomogeneous recovery of excitability. The total activation time for a given beat exceeded the coupling interval for that beat. Thus, the mechanism which underlies the transition from VT to VF during ischemia differs from the mechanism that is operational during subsequent reperfusion. The transition to VF after reperfusion is due to acceleration by nonreentrant mechanisms involving activation fronts which arise in both the subendocardium and the subepicardium, while nonreentrant mechanisms were not observed to contribute to VT acceleration in cases involving ischemia without reperfusion. Once VT acceleration occurred, subsequent development of VF was similar during ischemia and reperfusion.

B. Ventricular Fibrillation Induced by Electrical Stimulus

VF can also be induced by delivering a large electrical stimulus prematurely during the vulnerable period of the cardiac cycle. Such a stimulus was thought to result in an activation front that propagated away from the site of stimulation in all directions and then blocked unidirectionally when it reached regions that had not yet recovered excitability [11]. This nonuniform dispersion of refractoriness, which occurs when one site remains refractory long after an adjacent site has recovered, was thought to result in reentry. In this theory, activation continued to propagate through the adjacent regions that were more recovered and later circled back to excite the formerly blocked regions after recovery occurred. These later activation fronts then propagated back into the tissue that had been immediately excited after the premature stimulus and caused reentry and VF. While nonuniform dispersion of recovery probably plays a role in the initiation of VF during ischemia, investigators from Duke University [12–14] have demonstrated that it is not a requirement for inducing VF by electrical stimulation during the vulnerable period. They have shown that VF can be induced in some cases in which refractoriness changes uniformly, i.e., by approximately the same amount over a given distance throughout the region of interest.

Frazier et al. [12] recorded simultaneously from 117 epicardial electrodes covering a 30×30 mm region of the anterior right ventricle in 14 dogs. A train of 10 regularly spaced S1 stimuli (300–350 ms apart) was given simultaneously through a row of eight pacing wires on one side of the mapped region to create uniform, parallel activation fronts. The S2 stimulus was given through a mesh electrode that spanned one side of the mapped area and was adjacent to and at a right angle to the side at which the S1 was delivered. After the tenth S1, refractory periods were determined at 24 to 44 different sites and were found to be similar at all sites equidistant from the pacing electrodes. The shortest S1–S2 interval that produced a response that propagated to electrodes 3.8 mm away was taken as the recovery period duration for a given electrode site. This indicated that recovery was dispersed uniformly across the mapped region, with the earliest recovery occurring near the row of S1 pacing electrodes (Fig. 2). Both activation isochrones and isorecovery lines were found to be uniform and parallel. The recovery period was scanned using 25- to 250-V monophasic S2 shocks. The potential gradient electric field of the S2 shock was estimated by recording potentials from electrodes spaced known distances apart and then dividing the difference in potential at adjacent electrode sites by the distance between them and was used to indicate how rapidly the extracellular potential changed with distance. The S2 shocks were given at incremental or decremental S1–S2 intervals of 3 to 5 ms following the tenth S1 to span the recovery periods of the tissue under the plaque. Thus the lines of isopotential gradient were perpendicular to the isorecovery lines. Isogradient lines

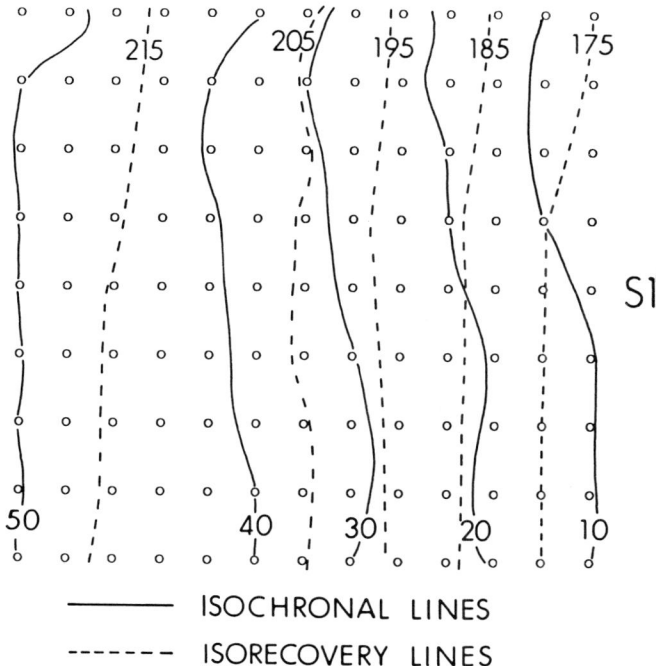

Figure 2 S1 activation and isorecovery patterns. Eight epicardial pacing wires were tied together as a single source (S1) and pulsed at 10 mA. Approximately parallel isochronal lines (solid lines) resulted from this S1 pacing. Conduction velocities between the isochrones were 0.5 to 0.7 m/s. In this example, recovery periods (dashed lines) were calculated at 32 electrode sites spaced evenly across the array. Refractoriness was essentially homogeneous, as indicated by the similar refractory periods at all electrode sites (166 ± 3 ms). The mean epicardial fiber orientation under this array was 24 ± 5° with respect to the horizontal. (Reprinted from Ref. 12 by permission of The American Society for Clinical Investigation, Inc.)

were parallel, with the highest gradients near the S2 mesh electrode. By introducing the S2 shock, it was possible to induce a leading circle activation pattern of circus reentry which led to VF in all animals. After the shock occurred, earliest activation appeared at the opposite side of the mapped region from the S2 electrode and at the edge of the directly excited regions, not in the region adjacent to the mesh S2 electrode where the shock field was the greatest. The "critical point" about which reentry was created was that point at which critical values of S2 field strength (approximately 5 V/cm) and refractoriness intersected. This was the area at which conduction propagated away from the directly excited border where potential gradients were weaker and blocked at the border where gradients were stronger. A circus reentrant pattern was formed by activation circling around this point. When the row of S1 electrodes was at the right and the S2 mesh electrode was at the top of the mapped region and when the S1 electrodes were at the left and the S2 mesh electrode was at the bottom of the mapped region, reentry proceeded in a clockwise manner, and a spatial shift of 180° in phase occurred. When the row of S1 electrodes was at the right and the S2 electrode was at the bottom and when the S1 electrodes were at the left and the S2 electrode was at the top of the mapped region, reentry proceeded in a counterclockwise manner but was also shifted spatially 180° in phase (Fig. 3). The location of the rotor could also be moved predictably by changing either the strength or the

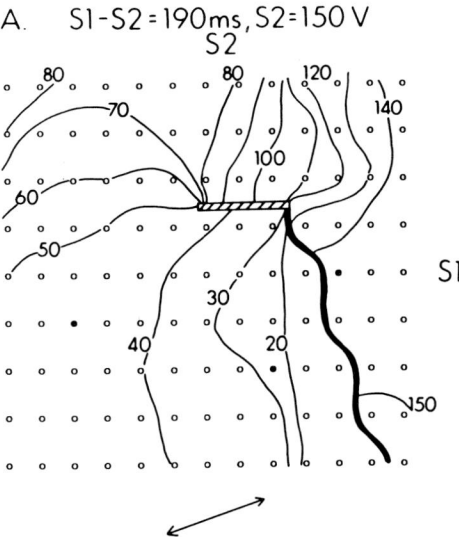

Figure 3 Effect of locations of S1 and S2 on direction of reentrant circuits. Activation times, shown in milliseconds, are measured from the start of the 3-ms S2 shock. Solid dots represent sites of inadequate recordings. The solid line represents the transition between successive activation maps and is called a "frame line." It is required because each static isochronal map can show only a single cycle of a continuous dynamic reentrant circuit. The hatched line represents a zone of conduction block and is called a "block line." Isochrones are at 10-ms intervals. The double-headed arrow for this figure represents the mean epicardial fiber orientation in the area of conduction block, in this case 21° with respect to the horizontal. (A) The first cycle of reentry following a 150-V S2 at an S1–S2 interval of 190 ms is shown with S2 at the top and S1 toward the septum. Earliest activation occurred distant from the S2 site, with activation wavefronts experiencing slow conduction near the S2 site and conducting in a clockwise manner around a line of block. The potential gradient was 5.4 V/cm, and the preshock interval was 172 ms (critical refractory period = 168 ms) at the critical point. In (B) and (C), earliest activation occurred distant from the S2 site with activation fronts forming a reentrant circuit by conducting around a line of block and through a region of slow conduction near the S2 site. In (B) (S2 of 150 V, S1–S2 of 197 ms), with S2 at the top and S1 at the side near the right ventricle, a counterclockwise reentrant circuit was formed. The potential gradient was 5.2 V/cm, and the preshock interval was 173 ms (critical refractory period = 171 ms) at the critical point. In (C) (S2 of 150 V, S1–S2 of 197 ms), with S2 at the bottom and S1 at the side near the right ventricle, a clockwise reentrant circuit was formed as in (A) (septal S1 with top S2). These two reentrant patterns differ in phase by approximately 180°. The potential gradient was 5.9 V/cm, and the preshock interval was 169 ms (critical refractory period = 170 ms) at the critical point. (Reprinted from Ref. 12 by permission of the American Society for Clinical Investigation, Inc.)

timing of the S2, which would change the location of the critical point. The study by Frazier and colleagues demonstrated that the initiation and location of reentry were functions of the interaction between the strength of the shock field and the degree of refractoriness and not just functions of the differences in refractoriness throughout the mapped region. Conduction block was caused by the interaction of a uniformly dispersed change in refractoriness and the shock field. This formed a critical point around which activation fronts rotated. Thus reentry was not caused by an activation front which conducted away in all directions from the S2 electrode and later blocked in a region where there was a large change in refractoriness, i.e., where recovery was nonuniformly dispersed.

The Process of Defibrillation

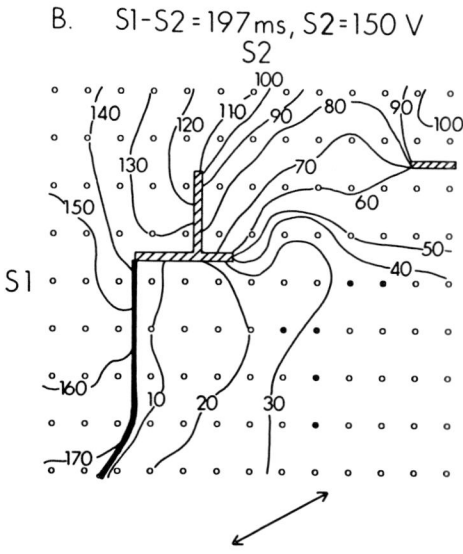

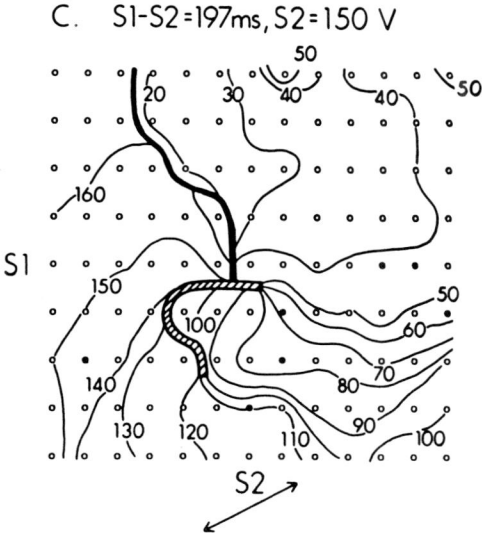

In this study and two others [13,14], a region that was excited directly by the S2 stimulus was present, and the location of the border of this directly excited region was dependent on both the strength of the S2 field and the stage of refractoriness of the cells. When the S2 potential gradient was weak and less than approximately 5 V/cm (as it was for 3-ms square monophasic waveforms), the border of the directly excited region was in cells that were only mildly refractory, and an activation front conducted away from this border through the tissue that was not directly excited by the S2 field. When the S2 potential gradient exceeded 5 V/cm, myocardium that was even more refractory was directly excited, so that a zone of temporary unidirectional block was created, and activation fronts did not conduct away from the border of the directly excited region. The electric field of the S2 stimulus probably prolonged refractoriness and resulted in block where the potential gradient was greater than 5 V/cm [15]. After S2 stimulation, activation could spread away from the border of the directly excited region where the potential gradient was less than 5 V/cm but not where it was greater than 5 V/cm. The locations of the S1 and S2 sites and the spatial relationship of the S2 isogradient field to the distribution of refractoriness determined whether reentry was leading circle or figure of eight. The type of reentrant pattern could be predicted from the different shapes and intersections of the isogradient and isorefractory lines [16,17]. Both monophasic and biphasic waveforms have been used to create leading-circle reentry following a shock. The gradient required to produce reentry differed with the type of waveform that was used [18].

II. MAINTENANCE OF VENTRICULAR FIBRILLATION

After VF is induced by the mechanisms just described or by some other mechanism, it is thought to be maintained by multiple, disorganized, wandering wavelets that follow constantly changing reentrant pathways. During the first minute of VF, it is likely that only a few wavelets are present. Wiggers [1] used cinematography to study VF and found that at the beginning of VF, large sections of myocardium activated together but in an uncoordinated and asynchronous manner relative to the rest of the heart. He described Stage I, the initial tachysystolic phenomena, which usually lasted less than a second in dogs, as a period in which two to eight peristaltic waves, which frequently appeared to arise from a single focus, swept rapidly across the ventricle. Stage II, the conclusive incoordination stage which usually lasted 15 to 40 s, had waves of contraction with distinctly different rhythms and sequences that passed over the ventricles. According to Wiggers, the stage of tremulous incoordination, Stage III, usually followed the coarse, convulsive stage and continued for 2 to 3 min. In Stage III, contraction waves appeared to spread very rapidly over short distances. Wiggers called the fourth stage the stage of progressive atonic incoordination. In Stage IV, the visible waves became coarser and slower and no longer maintained the even level of elevated intraventricular pressure that characterized Stages I–III. During this final stage, movement over the ventricular surface decreased in intensity until eventually only slight movements remained in a few regions.

When Garrey [19] dissected the heart into pieces of various sizes, he found that a critical mass of myocardium was necessary for VF to persist. In dogs, the critical mass is about one-fourth of the total ventricular mass. VF can only be sustained in larger hearts, e.g., in humans and dogs, and is frequently difficult to induce in smaller hearts, e.g., in frogs [1]. Although VF appears to be disorganized and asynchronous, frequency analysis in humans and dogs has resulted in a power spectrum of VF that has a well-defined peak and its higher harmonics [20]. The evidence that some degree of organization exists during VF has been recognized for decades and suggests that VF could be sufficiently organized to be mapped with closely spaced electrodes if the electrodes did not cause excessive damage to the tissue [11].

A. Multiple Wandering Wavelets

Moe [21] used the work of Garrey [19] and Mines [22] and a series of astute observations to revive the theory that reentry provides the basic mechanism for VF and to develop the well-known multiple wandering wavelet hypothesis. At the time Moe developed this theory, it was difficult to make simultaneous multichannel recordings from a large number of electrodes on the heart. With his colleagues, he tested his hypothesis by developing a mathematical computer model in which the heart was represented as an electrophysiologically inhomogeneous two-dimensional sheet of hexagonal cells [23]. Using this model, they were able to demonstrate activity that resembled fibrillation and consisted of multiple wandering wavelets which exhibited self-sustaining turbulence. These computer model studies strengthened the probability that the multiple wavelet hypothesis represented a mechanism for describing fibrillation in the heart.

Several groups have used multichannel recordings to study atrial fibrillation (AF) in the dog. Sano and Scher [24] induced AF by giving single electrical shocks and recorded an average of 20 bipolar electrograms at the onset of each instance of AF and during recovery. They concluded that ectopic impulse formation was the initiating mechanism but that reentry was probably the mechanism responsible for maintaining AF. Allessie et al. [25] conducted a series of in-vivo experiments using isolated Langendorff-perfused canine hearts and confirmed Moe's multiple wavelet theory as the basis for AF. They recorded 480 electrograms alternately from two solid egg-shaped multiple electrodes, one in the right atrium and the other in the left, and reconstructed excitation of the atria during stable AF. The right atrium was mapped during an episode of AF, and then the left atrium was mapped during a second episode which was initiated a couple of minutes later. They demonstrated that multiple wandering wavelets, which were due to intraatrial reentry of the leading circle type, provided the basis for the continuity of impulse conduction during AF [26]. They interpreted activation patterns in one atrium that appeared to be "foci" giving rise to new impulses as endocardial breakthrough sites of impulses coming from the other atrium. They also noted that it was possible that the presence of a normal or abnormal pacemaker might sometimes succeed in supporting the continuation of multiple wandering wavelets and that such a pacemaker might actually be necessary for the perpetuation of AF. They found that, shortly after the simultaneous extinction of all activation fronts had occurred by chance, the generation of an impulse either by the sinus node or by some abnormal pacemaker would almost certainly restart the arrhythmia. Thus it is possible that reentry and multiple rapidly firing ectopic foci may act together to maintain chronic AF [25].

B. Degree of Organization

Some evidence exists to suggest that VF is organized, at least during the 15 to 60-s period which follows the initial tachysystolic stage. Chen et al. [27] used 40 plunge needles, which were anchored 5 mm apart in the right ventricles of six dogs and contained three bipolar electrodes that had 1 mm between poles and 1 mm between recording sites, to provide transmural information after 20 s of VF. They observed coherent activation fronts with dimensions and path lengths of several centimeters. The cycle length averaged 96 ± 16 ms and was compatible with the frequency of activation of between 600 and 660 per minute that was observed by Wiggers [28] and described as Stage II VF. During Stage II, the activation fronts frequently collided or blocked when they approached tissue that remained refractory following a previous activation front. These findings were consistent with Moe's theory that fibrillation reflected a series of wandering wavelets of activation. Recent work using phase-plane plots and state-space diagrams of VF led Witkowski and Penkoske [29] to conclude that there is no evidence of recurring spatial patterns during VF mapping studies that used electrodes spaced 2 mm apart. However, Johnson et al. [30] mapped VF with 121 electrodes spaced 0.28 mm apart in pigs and found that organization increased during the first minute of VF, as evidenced by a sharper peak in the power spectra, by less conduction block, and by a high beat-to-beat repeatability of the activation sequences in some pigs. Recently, Damle et al. [31] used vector analysis to show that electrical activation was spatially (for electrodes spaced 2.5 mm apart) and temporally (from one beat to the next) organized at the onset of VF in both infarcted and noninfarcted canine hearts. They found that the degree of organization decreased during the first 5 s.

C. Frequency Characteristics

During VF, there is frequently a clear dominant frequency with a narrow bandwidth and a peak in the power spectrum around 9 to 12 Hz [20,32]. Carlisle et al. [33] used several different methods to induce VF in dogs (by ischemia, by reperfusion, or by electrical stimulation in the presence of ischemia) and fast Fourier transform analysis to determine frequency characteristics of the VF. They found that by 120 s after the onset of VF, the initial frequency of around 12 Hz, as measured from limb lead recordings, had fallen to 5 to 6 Hz. Endocardial recordings initially showed a dominant frequency similar to that recorded at the body surface, but after 3 min from onset there was still no significant drop in frequency. The reason for the decrease in frequency in the limb leads after 1 to 2 min of continued fibrillation is unknown, but the results are consistent with those presented by Worley et al. [34] In that study, direct bipolar recordings at five different levels throughout the left ventricular free wall showed that activation rates in the endocardium continued at a rapid rate for many minutes, even though activation rates in the myocardium and epicardium decreased markedly.

Since the success rate in the treatment of VF varies inversely with the duration of time between its onset and the initiation of cardiopulmonary resuscitation and transthoracic defibrillation, i.e., the downtime [35], the decrease in the peak frequency over time may be of clinical significance. The median frequency of the power spectrum during VF in pigs was used by Dzwonczyk et al. [36] to track the decrease in frequency with the increase in time. They developed an algorithm which could predict the total elapsed time since onset of VF with an average error of -0.86 min. This type of algorithm may eventually prove useful in the prehospital treatment of VF.

III. MECHANISMS OF DEFIBRILLATION

In order to determine the mechanisms responsible for defibrillation, it is necessary to determine the distribution of potential gradients and current densities that are generated through the heart by a shock of a particular strength that is given through a particular electrode set. These parameters can be estimated by means of computer modeling or direct experimentation. All types of computer modeling, including finite elements, finite differences, and integral equations [37–42], require estimates of the locations and sizes of the anatomical structures within the heart and thorax and estimates of the resistivities of these structures. Experimental measurements of potential gradients are invasive and require the placement of electrodes at known locations. These locations are either predetermined and have a fixed spacing or are determined after the study [43–46]. Potentials generated by the shock are recorded from these electrodes, and potential gradients are then calculated from the potential differences and the distances between electrodes. It is also possible to calculate current densities from the experimentally determined potential gradients if the resistivity of the tissue at each electrode site can be determined or estimated.

The myocardium can be considered to consist of two spaces, one extracellular and the other intracellular. Both of these spaces have a much lower resistivity than the cell membrane which separates them [47]. The potential gradient distributions that have been measured experimentally during the defibrillation shocks have been in the extracellular space, since the recording electrodes were located there [43–46]. The relationship between the distribution of the extracellular potential gradient and the potential difference across the cell membrane, i.e., the transmembrane potential, is the subject of much research, since it is thought that shocks defibrillate by changing the transmembrane potential [48]. Modeling [49] and experiments [50,51] with

The Process of Defibrillation

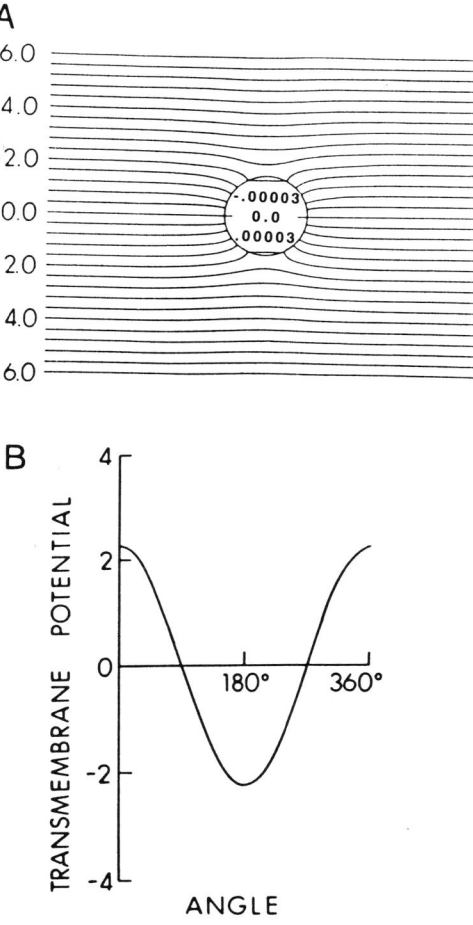

Figure 4 Single spheroidal cell in a uniform extracellular potential gradient field. (A) The cell is exposed to a uniform electrical field created by the cathode at the top and the anode at the bottom. Extracellular potentials are given in millivolts at the left, with isopotential lines spaced every 0.4 mV. As indicated by the isopotential lines spaced every 0.00003 mV, the potential within the cell changes much less than the extracellular potential. (B) The transmembrane potential in millivolts, which is equal to the difference between the intracellular and extracellular potentials in (A), is shown as a function of the location on the surface of the cell, as expressed by the polar angle, with 0° at the top of the cell and 180° at the bottom. The top half of the cell toward the cathode is depolarized, and the bottom half toward the anode is hyperpolarized. (Reprinted from Ref. 49 with permission of the Institute of Electrical and Electronics Engineers.)

isolated myocardial cells have both suggested that the end of the cell nearest the anode is hyperpolarized while the end of the cell nearest the cathode is depolarized, and the degree of hyperpolarization and depolarization is directly and linearly related to the extracellular potential gradient (Fig. 4). However, the relationship between the extracellular potential gradient and the transmembrane potential has not been established for a syncytium of coupled myofibers as occurs in the heart. Some models predict that within approximately a centimeter of an anodal electrode, all portions of all cells will be hyperpolarized; and that within the same distance from a cathodal electrode, all portions of all cells will be depolarized [52–55]. Another model predicts that cells will be hyperpolarized only a very short distance away from anodes and depolarized only a short distance away from cathodes, because the anisotropy in resistivity along and across fibers is different in the extracellular and intracellular spaces [56]. According to this model, all portions of cells more than a few millimeters away from the electrode along a line parallel to the long axis of the myofibers and passing through the electrode will be depolarized for anodes and hyperpolarized for cathodes. In the myocardium that is more than approximately one cm away from the defibrillation electrodes, i.e., most of the myocardium, one model predicts that there is no simple relationship between the extracellular potential gradient and the changes in transmembrane potential [57]. Neunlist and Tung [58] have recently shown experimentally that oppositely polarized regions coexisted within approximately 1 mm of the stimulating electrode when the electrode was used as either the anode or the cathode and the monophasic pulse was more than 15 times greater than that needed for the cathodal threshold of excitation. This is in contradiction to the models in which the amounts of hyperpolarization and depolarization are directly and linearly proportional to the extracellular potential gradient.

Experimental results from Frazier et al. [59] are consistent with a linear relationship between the extracellular potential gradient produced by a shock and the change in the transmembrane potential induced by the shock. They found that, for tissue located more than about 1 cm away from the stimulating electrodes, the extracellular potential gradient threshold for stimulation of fully recovered myocardium was relatively constant for a particular waveform. The extracellular potential gradient needed to stimulate an action potential in diastole in the intact heart is much less than that needed for an isolated myofiber. When the electric field is oriented parallel to the long axis of the myofibers, the intact canine heart requires about 0.6 V/cm for stimulation with a 3-ms truncated exponential waveform. About 1.8 V/cm is needed when the field is oriented perpendicular to the long axis [59]. When the electric field is parallel to the long axis of isolated frog ventricular myocytes, a potential gradient of approximately 1.5 V/cm is required for stimulation with a 3-ms rectangular waveform, while approximately 9 V/cm is needed when the field is perpendicular to the long axis [60,61]. One possible reason for the difference in stimulation requirements between isolated cells and intact myocardium is that myocardial cells are tightly coupled electrically, so that a bundle of myofibers responds to an extracellular electric field as a single unit, with the end of the unit closer to the anode hyperpolarized and the end closer to the cathode depolarized [54]. Since the ratio of the stimulation requirements along and across the isolated cells corresponds approximately to the ratio of the length to the width of the cells (100–120 μm/15–20 μm), the myofibril electrical unit has been estimated to be approximately 2000 μm long and 200 μm wide [54]. A width of 200 μm corresponds roughly to the distance between connective tissue septa that has been observed in the ventricles [62].

Models that predict a linear relationship between the extracellular potential gradient produced by a shock and the change in the transmembrane potential induced by the shock also predict that shock requirements for defibrillation should be almost completely independent of which electrode is the cathode and which is the anode. The results of experimental studies examining the effect of changing the polarity of the defibrillation electrodes are not clear cut. While all studies report a significant effect of polarity on defibrillation efficacy, the difference is either small or is inconsistent, with an anode on the left ventricle reported in some cases to be superior while in other cases a cathode on the left ventricle is reported to be superior [63–66].

The Process of Defibrillation

Relatively refractory myocardium requires a larger potential gradient field for stimulation of a new action potential than does fully recovered myocardium, whether the electric field is oriented along or across the long axis of the myocardial cells [67]. A stimulus that is less than about 5 V/cm (the exact value depends on the waveform and the orientation of the cells with respect to the electric field) causes an all-or-none response [67]. A new action potential will result only if the myocardium has recovered sufficiently, but will otherwise have almost no effect. An intermediate or graded response can be produced with a stimulus greater than 5 V/cm if the cells are too refractory to undergo a complete new action potential [15]. A graded response will prolong refractoriness and action potential duration, but not as much as would a new action potential. A propagating activation front usually does not occur after tissue has been stimulated to produce a graded response. This is probably because the neighboring tissue is refractory and a graded response has less stimulating ability than does a full action potential. The size and duration of the graded response vary directly with the size of the stimulus and the time since the last activation. Action potential prolongation can be induced almost immediately after phase zero of the previous activation if the stimulus is sufficiently strong [68].

Prolongation of refractoriness by the shock has been reported to be important for defibrillation [27,68–73]. It has also been suggested that prolongation of action potential duration by the shock is an important determinant of whether any activation fronts that are present just after the shock will block, reenter, and lead to refibrillation [73]. A particular potential gradient within a certain range of shock potential gradients will prolong refractoriness at almost the same time (Fig. 5), even though different cells are in different portions of their action potential during fibrillation. This means that the dispersion of refractoriness present just before the shock would be almost totally obliterated by the shock if all the ventricular myocardium were exposed to the same potential gradient within this certain range at the time the shock was given. Any activation fronts still present would be much less likely to block, reenter, and lead to the resumption of fibrillation, since all cells would recover at about the same time [73].

Unfortunately, signs of damage are seen at higher stimulus strengths. These include "hanging up" of the transmembrane potential near the plateau voltage for long periods [74], conduction block [75], and inhibition of normal automaticity [76–78]. These signs of myocardial damage occur at extracellular potential gradients of approximately 60 V/cm or more, while shocks of 200 V/cm lasting 5 ms have been shown to cause dielectric breakdown of the membranes of isolated chick embryo myocytes [79]. An extracellular potential gradient of 200 V/cm produces a voltage drop across the cell membrane of almost 1 V, which results in an extremely high potential gradient across the membrane because the cell membrane is so thin. This extremely high potential gradient causes the cell membrane to break down and form holes [79]. Indiscriminate flow of ions through the holes causes the membrane to depolarize and the potential to "hang up." Conduction is also blocked, and automaticity is inhibited. As the potential gradient of the shock is increased, the number and size of the holes in the membrane increase, as does the length of time before they close [79]. Cell death occurs when the potential gradient of the shock is more than 100–200 V/cm.

A. Critical Mass Hypothesis

Early work in defibrillation formed the basis for the hypothesis that electrical paralysis and conduction block lasting for several seconds after the shock and extending throughout the ventricles were the basic mechanisms at work in successful defibrillation [80]. This hypothesis has been shown to be incorrect by the results of several studies. First, successful shocks can defibrillate without creating such a strong potential gradient field (greater than 60 V/cm) through-

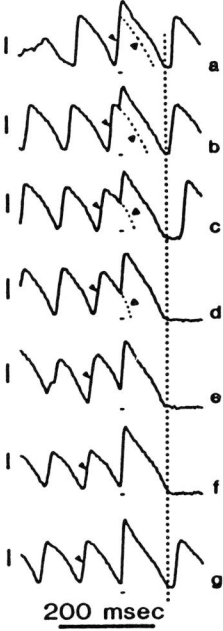
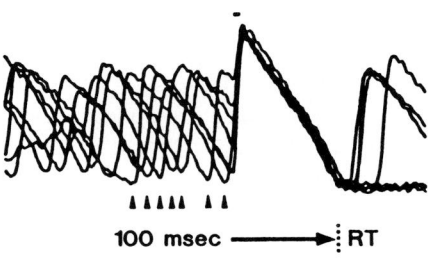

Figure 5 Optical recordings showing induction of a constant repolarization time by a shock during fibrillation. Seven different tracings are shown in the left panel. Shock time and durations are indicated by the horizontal black bar underlying each trace. Filled arrowheads indicate upstroke immediately preceding shock. Open arrowheads in traces a–d mark dashed curves showing likely time course of repolarization had the shock not been applied. Dashed curves were copied from the preceding action potential. Vertical dashed line indicates earliest repolarization time. Optical calibration bars on each trace show size of 1% fluorescence change. Shocks were 1.25 J. In the right panel, the optical recordings from the left are superimposed. The horizontal line at the top shows the time and duration of the shock. Beginnings of preshock upstrokes are indicated by filled arrowheads. A constant repolarization time (RT) of 100 ms occurred in all traces. Recordings also show a high degree of overlap from the peak of the shock response to repolarization and give the impression that the shock evokes a single response at all levels of the action potential. (Reprinted from Ref. 13 with permission from The American Heart Association.)

out the ventricles (Fig. 6). Second, one or two rapid activations frequently occur in the first 200-ms period which immediately follows a successful defibrillation shock [81–83]. The "critical mass" hypothesis of defibrillation developed from the last finding. The presence of activations almost immediately following the successful defibrillation shock led to the conclusion that it was not necessary to halt all fibrillatory activity in order to have defibrillation occur, but that it was sufficient to halt activation fronts within a critical mass (perhaps 75%) of the myocardium in the ventricles. In this theory, the assumption was made that, if all activation fronts are localized to a region smaller than the critical mass of myocardium, they are not capable of maintaining fibrillation and die out after one or two cycles [19,81,82].

The critical mass hypothesis of defibrillation has been supported by several recent observations from cardiac mapping. Activation fronts have been demonstrated to appear in almost all portions of the ventricles following shocks that are delivered through small defibrillation electrodes on the epicardium and are too weak to defibrillate [69]. This is consistent with the hypothesis that the shock field is too weak to halt fibrillation activation fronts throughout the

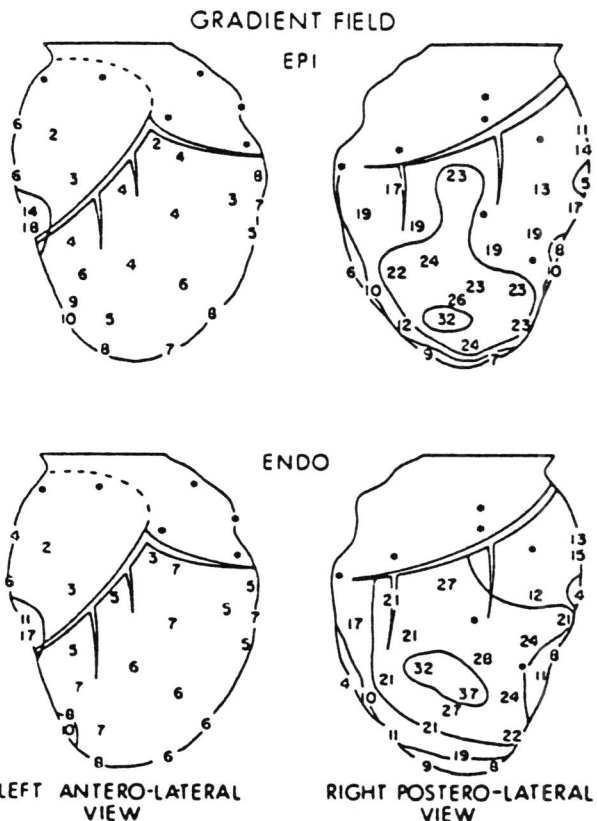

Figure 6 The potential gradient field created in a dog heart by a 500-V defibrillation shock from a catheter electrode in the right ventricular apex and a cutaneous patch electrode at the left lower thorax. The numbers are the potential gradients at each recording site in volts per centimeter. Asterisks represent the top row of electrodes on the atria and the right ventricular outflow tract, where potential gradients are not calculated because no recording sites are above them. Solid circles represent locations where potential gradients are not calculated, either because potentials at those locations are inadquate for interpretation or because the exact location of that electrode is not known. Isogradient lines are separated by 10 V/cm. (Reprinted from Ref. 3 with permission of The Institute of Electrical and Electronics Engineers.)

heart. As the shock strength is progressively increased, the region around the defibrillation electrodes in which the potential gradient exceeds approximately 6 V/cm (for a typical monophasic waveform) becomes larger. The fact that activation fronts no longer arise from this region is consistent with the interpretation that a gradient of more than 6 V/cm is needed to halt activation fronts during fibrillation. Only a small portion of the ventricles is exposed to a potential gradient of less than 6 V/cm when the shock strength is just slightly weaker than that needed to defibrillate, and activation fronts arise primarily from this region following the shock [45]. This is also consistent with the interpretation that the shock was too weak to halt the fibrillation activation fronts in this region and that the region was just slightly larger than the minimum mass of myocardium needed to sustain fibrillation. Another observation that is consistent with the critical mass hypothesis for defibrillation is that earliest activations following unsuccessful defibrillation attempts arise from the portion of the myocardium with the lowest potential gradients and occur at the time that this portion of myocardium would be expected to activate if the shock had not been given [44]. This is consistent with the hypothesis that the shock is so weak in this low-gradient region that it has no effect on the activation sequence in that area. Zhou et al. have recently shown that a low potential gradient in approximately 10% of the ventricular mass can cause defibrillation to fail in dogs [84].

Other studies have found that an unsuccessful shock that is slightly weaker than what is needed to defibrillate can alter the activation sequence in the ventricular regions exposed to the lowest potential gradients [27,84]. Although the first few activation sequences following such a failed defibrillation shock are sufficiently organized that they can be mapped with 128 electrodes spaced 1–2 cm apart throughout the ventricular free walls, more closely spaced electrodes are required to map the complex activation patterns that are present in fibrillation just before the shock. Two studies have recorded the epicardial spread of activation during VF both just before and just after a defibrillation shock. Chen et al. [27] used plunge needle electrodes spaced 5 mm apart to record the three-dimensional spread of activation, while Zhou et al. [84] used epicardial electrodes spaced 3.8 mm apart to record the epicardial spread of activation in dogs. Fibrillation activation fronts followed pathways that were typically several centimeters in length, could be tracked for up to 100 ms, and frequently exhibited some similarity from cycle to cycle during the first 15 s after the electrical induction of VF. It was possible, to a certain extent, to predict what the activation sequence would be for a few tens of milliseconds into the future due to this moderate amount of organization during fibrillation, as long as the sequence was not altered by another shock. Analysis of the studies of activation sequences that occurred following unsuccessful defibrillation attempts led to the development of a new hypothesis about the effect of shocks on activation wavefronts during successful defibrillation, i.e., the upper limit of vulnerability hypothesis for defibrillation.

B. Upper Limit of Vulnerability Hypothesis

The upper limit of vulnerability hypothesis for defibrillation states that a successful shock must halt existing activation fronts by directly exciting the myocardium or by prolonging refractoriness just in front of these activation fronts and must not give rise to new activation fronts at the border of the directly excited region. The same hypothesis predicts that the shock strength at the upper limit of vulnerability during regular rhythm should be approximately the same as the minimum shock strength needed to defibrillate, since the critical potential gradient that leads to the induction of fibrillation during the vulnerable period of regular rhythm is about the same as during defibrillation (about 5 V/cm for a typical monophasic waveform in both cases). This has been shown to be true in several animal studies (Fig. 7) [85–89]. In approximately half of the unsuccessful defibrillation attempts with shocks slightly weaker than that needed to defibrillate, activation spreads in all directions away from the site of earliest activation rather than primarily in one direction, as would be predicted by the upper limit of vulnerability hypothesis for defibrillation if activation is spreading away from the border of a region directly excited by the shock [27]. These focal patterns may represent activity that was triggered by the shock or small reentrant pathways that were missed because the electrode spacing was too great. The minimum spacing needed to map activation sequences during fibrillation has not been defined but may be only 1–2 mm [29,90]. Zhou et al. reported that postshock activation fronts after either monophasic or biphasic shocks that did not defibrillate exhibited either a focal origin or unidirectional conduction and were markedly different from those just before the shock [84]. If the upper limit of vulnerability hypothesis is correct, [11] the one or two rapid

The Process of Defibrillation

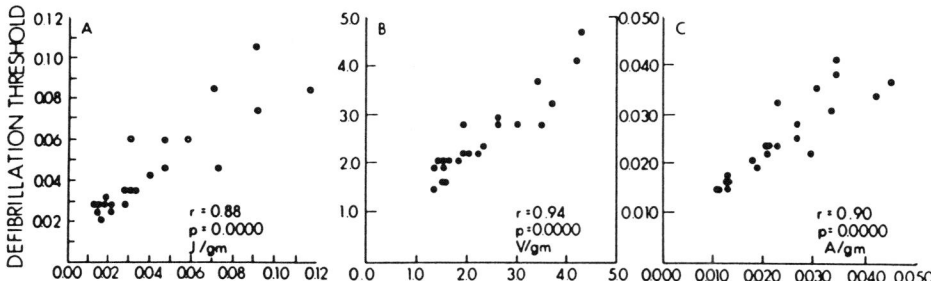

Figure 7 Relationship between defibrillation threshold and the upper limit of vulnerability for defibrillation electrodes with the right atrium as anode and the ventricular apex as cathode in 22 dogs. Results are expressed in units of energy (A), voltage (B), and current (C). All units are divided by the heart weight. (Reprinted from Ref. 87 with permission of The American Heart Association.)

activations sometimes observed following a successful defibrillation shock [81–83] may be equivalent to the one or two rapid responses that are frequently seen when a large premature stimulus is given in an attempt to induce fibrillation.

Probably as the result of slight changes in autonomic and metabolic state between stimulation trials in the same animal, it is sometimes possible for a premature stimulus of the same strength and timing to induce fibrillation and at other times to induce repetitive responses. This may also explain why a defibrillation shock of a given strength may sometimes succeed and other times fail in the same patient or animal [91]. There appears to be a range of shock strengths that may sometimes defibrillate, rather than a discrete defibrillation threshold value for shocks in which shocks greater or equal to this value always succeed and shocks less than this value always fail. Thus the probability of successful defibrillation increases as the shock strength increases [Fig. 8) [92]. Since the distribution of activation fronts and refractoriness at the time of a shock is different for every episode of fibrillation, a defibrillation shock of a

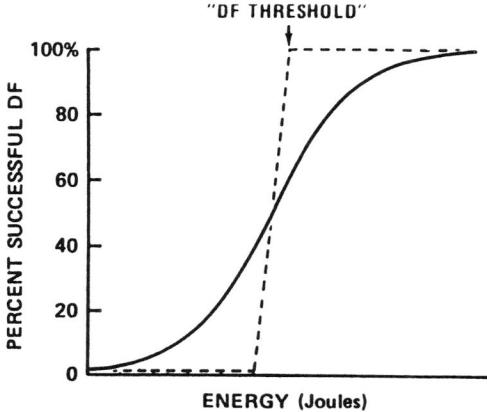

Figure 8 Comparison of the defibrillation threshold and defibrillation curve concepts. A defibrillation threshold implies a clear-cut distinction between effective and ineffective energies, while a curve implies a dose–response relationship with increasing energies associated with greater percentages of success. DF = defibrillation. (Reprinted from Ref. 92 with permission of the C. V. Mosby Company.)

particular strength may succeed during some defibrillation episodes but not others in the same patient.

C. Defibrillation Waveforms

In early attempts at defibrillation, large transformers were used with alternating current to generate shocks that were applied transthoracically [93–95]. Later, Lown et al. defibrillated by generating a damped sinusoidal waveform by capacitor discharge through a series inductor and the "resistor" formed by the paddles and thorax [96]. This group showed that direct-current shocks had fewer side effects in animals, e.g., postshock arrhythmias, myocardial injury, and deaths, than shocks from alternating current. Straight capacitor discharges without truncation were also investigated and were found to have high peak currents associated with myocardial depression [97,98]. Recent work has concentrated on the shape of the waveform that is generated by discharging capacitors, since the shape of the waveform directly influences the effectiveness of shocks given for internal defibrillation.

Several groups have found that monophasic truncated exponential waveforms are superior to straight capacitor discharges in implantable devices, since the refibrillatory effects of the low-voltage tail are avoided [97–100]. Wessale et al. [101] gave shocks through a bipolar catheter with electrodes in the apex of the right ventricle and superior vena cava of dogs and demonstrated that peak current dose (peak current divided by body weight) increased with decreasing pulse duration (20 ms to 2 ms) and increasing tilt (<5% to 80%), where tilt was defined as the difference between initial and final currents expressed as a percent of the initial current. Chapman et al. [102] showed that lower defibrillation energy requirements were associated with shorter pulse durations in monophasic truncated exponential waveforms with fixed pulse width and variable tilt when tested in dogs with a transvenous catheter in the right ventricle to subcutaneous patch system. The shortest (2.5-ms) and longest (20-ms) pulse width durations were associated with higher threshold voltages than were durations in the middle of the range. With their catheter-patch electrode system, Chapman's group found that pulse durations of 5 to 15 ms were associated with the best combination of low initial voltage (596–632 V), low energy (18–25 J), and low average current (5–7 A).

Sequential application of monophasic waveforms has also been investigated, but only small improvements were found for waveforms of the same magnitude, duration, and polarity that were separated in time [102]. Sweeney et al. [103] have reported that the optimum separation between two shocks is approximately 85% of the activation rate during fibrillation. Bourland et al. [104] tried to reduce defibrillation energy requirements by summing energy both temporally and spatially, with pulses separated in both time and space to achieve a more uniform field. Several groups have shown that sequential pulses given through separate lead systems result in lower defibrillation thresholds than is the case when single pulses are given simultaneously through each lead system [105–109]. The advantage of delivering sequential shocks disappears if the shocks are given more than 10 ms apart and is optimized if the separation time is between 0.2 and 1 ms [110].

The biphasic waveform, in which the waveform has two phases that are opposite in polarity, is another approach to dividing the shock into parts. Biphasic waveforms have been shown to defibrillate with lower voltage and energy than monophasic waveforms of the same duration [111–115]. Schuder et al. [112] found in calves that some symmetric biphasic waveforms could defibrillate at lower energies and currents than monophasic waveforms of similar durations. Biphasic waveforms with second phases having lower amplitudes than their first phases but equal durations were found to defibrillate at lower energies than symmetric biphasic waveforms [112,113]. Biphasics with second phases longer than the first require more energy and higher voltages for defibrillation [113,116]. The optimum separation between the phases is 5 ms or less [117]. Single-capacitor biphasic waveforms which have the leading-edge voltage of the second phase equal to the trailing-edge voltage of the first phase and are delivered from a 150-µf capacitor required less energy and lower leading-edge voltages to defibrillate than did monophasic or double-capacitor biphasic waveforms [118]. Human studies have confirmed that biphasics with a second phase shorter in duration and smaller in amplitude than the first phase are more effective than monophasic waveforms, and that a single-capacitor biphasic waveform is more effective than monophasics of the same or half the total duration [119,120]. These last findings have important implications for implantable defibrillators, since single-capacitor biphasic waveforms could result both in longer battery life by using less energy and in smaller devices by omitting the second capacitor.

Triphasic waveforms which have a third phase with the same polarity as the first phase have also been tested [121,122]. Dixon et al. [113] found no improvement for a triphasic waveform with phases 5 ms, 5 ms, and 2 ms in duration over a biphasic waveform that used the first two phases of the triphasic waveform. Chapman et al. [122] found that biphasic waveforms with 5-ms phases required significantly less energy (10.1 J) than either 10-ms monophasic waveforms (21.1 J) or 2.5–5–2.5 ms triphasic waveforms (14.3 J) when used for internal defibrillation in a nonthoracotomy system in dogs. Defibrillation thresholds for triphasic waveforms were significantly lower than those of monophasic waveforms. Triphasic waveforms have been shown to improve the safety factor, the ratio between the shock level that stimulates and the shock level that causes dysfunction, in cultured chick myocardial cells [121]. Jones et al. postulated that each of the three pulses has a different effect and that the first phase acts as a "conditioning prepulse," the second "excites" or "defibrillates," and the third "heals." Although further work needs to be done, it is possible that triphasic waveforms may cause less dysfunction at the suprathreshold shock strengths likely to be used in implantable defibrillators.

D. Electrode Systems

The finding that a minimum potential gradient is required for successful defibrillation has implications with regard to the placement of electrodes [123], since potential gradient distribution is uneven throughout the heart for most electrode configurations used for defibrillation. This has been shown by both computer modeling [37–39,41] and from experimental measurements [39,43–46]. This distribution is much more uneven when the electrodes are located on and in the heart than when they are located on the thorax. The ratio of the highest to the lowest potential gradients produced in the ventricles by a shock is approximately 20 to 1 when one or both defibrillation electrodes are located on or in the heart [39,43–46] and approximately 4 to 1 for transthoracic defibrillation [39]. The lowest potential gradient observed in the ventricles ranges from 3 to 9 V/cm for shocks that are just large enough to defibrillate [44,45,76,84]. The minimum potential gradient required for defibrillation is a function of the duration and shape of the shock waveform and probably follows a strength–duration relationship similar to that found for the total shock strength needed for defibrillation [101,102,124]. For a typical monophasic truncated exponential waveform, the minimum potential gradient for defibrillation is about 5 V/cm, while it is about 3 V/cm for a typical biphasic waveform [84]. Defibrillation configurations with electrodes on or in the heart produce gradients of 80 to 120 V/cm or more in the tissue adjacent to the electrodes in order to achieve this minimum gradient. Yabe et al. [75] gave shocks of 70 to 850 V through wire-mesh patches adjacent to an epicardial plaque containing 117 electrodes and found that gradients of 100 to 120 V/cm resulted in conduction

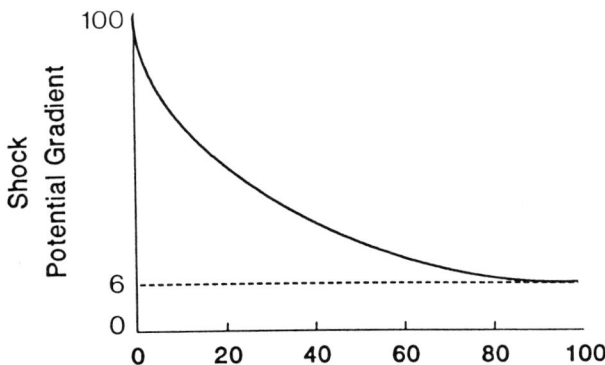

Figure 9 Idealized diagram of distribution of ventricular potential gradients, in volts per centimeter, generated by shocks from small epicardial defibrillation electrodes, demonstrating that most of the shock field is wasted. Every tick mark on the abscissa represents 20% of the ventricular volume. If the same minimum potential gradient is required throughout the ventricular myocardium for defibrillation (indicated by the dashed line), then that portion of the shock field above the dashed line is wasted. (Reprinted from Ref. 123 with permission of Futura Publishing Company, Inc.)

block that lasted from 2 to 10 s. Conduction block in an area for such an extended period of time would be likely to result in decreased wall motion after the shock.

The uneven distribution of potential gradients across the heart that results from most electrode configurations is wasteful. In order to increase the lowest gradients to the minimum level required for defibrillation, much of the shock strength is used to increase the potential gradient throughout the heart to values that are higher than than the minimum needed in most cardiac regions [Fig. 9]. Since the uneven distribution can also result in damage in high-gradient regions [75,79,125,126], the best defibrillation field is the one that can be created with the smallest shock voltage and energy and has low potential gradients that are close to the minimum required and are evenly distributed throughout the heart. Design requirements for configurations that would improve defibrillation with epicardial electrodes should include using electrodes with large surface areas that encompass most of the ventricular myocardium between the electrode outlines and have borders that are nearly equidistant at all points [123]. The electrodes should be located on the lateral surface of each ventricle so that current flows across the interventricular septum and should be placed to avoid the three major coronary arteries.

There is also some evidence that the superiority of biphasic over monophasic waveforms is dependent on the electrode system which is used. Bardy et al. [127] performed a prospective, randomized evaluation of defibrillation efficacy of monophasic and single-capacitor biphasic waveform pulses on 51 cardiac arrest survivors who were undergoing automatic defibrillator implantation. They tested a right ventricular patch–left ventricular epicardial patch system, a right ventricular catheter–chest patch nonthoracotomy system, and a coronary sinus catheter–right ventricular catheter nonthoracotomy system. Defibrillation with biphasic waveforms required lower energy for defibrillation than monophasic waveforms in the first two systems but was not significantly different for the third. In some individuals, monophasic waveforms were more efficient than biphasic waveforms, regardless of the lead system. Guse et al. [128] have shown in dogs that sequential biphasic shocks delivered through two different lead systems defibrillate with less energy and voltage than monophasic shocks delivered through the same lead systems. Saksena et al. [129] used a triple-electrode system that included catheters in the right ventricle and right atrium and a left thoracic patch to show that simultaneous biphasic shocks were more effective and reduced the energy requirements of bidirectional shocks when compared to either sequential or simultaneous monophasic shocks. Simultaneous biphasic shocks were successful at identical energy levels at which simultaneous monophasic shocks had failed to terminate polymorphic ventricular tachycardia or fibrillation in 9 of 11 patients. There was no patient in whom sequential monophasic shocks worked but simultaneous biphasic shocks did not.

As additional advances are made to lower defibrillation thresholds by refining the waveform shape and optimizing electrode placement, the success of implantable defibrillators will improve. Lowered defibrillation thresholds will enable manufacturers to produce smaller implantable defibrillators that can deliver more shocks over the lifetime of the battery. With further advances the nonthoracotomy approach will probably become the method of choice for the implantable cardioverter defibrillator in the large majority of patients [130].

ACKNOWLEDGMENTS

This work was supported in part by National Institutes of Health research grants HL-42760, HL-44066, HL-28429, and HL-33637, and by National Science Foundation Engineering Research Center grant CDR-86222011.

REFERENCES

1. Wiggers CJ. The mechanism and nature of ventricular defibrillation. Am Heart J 1940; 20:399-412.
2. Smith WM, Wharton JM, Blanchard SM, Wolf PD, Ideker RE. Direct cardiac mapping. In: Zipes DP and Jalife J, eds. Cardiac Electrophysiology, From Cell to Bedside. Philadelphia: Saunders, 1990:849-858.
3. Tang ASL, Wolf PD, Claydon FJ III, Smith WM, Pilkington TC, Ideker RE. Measurement of defibrillation shock potential distributions and activation sequences of the heart in three dimensions. Proc IEEE 1988; 76:1176-1186.
4. Mastrototaro JJ, Pilkington TC, Ideker RE, Massoud HZ. Thin-film multielectrode arrays for potential gradient measurements in the heart. In: Harris G, Walker C, eds. Proc. 10th Annual Conference of the IEEE Engineering in Medicine and Biology Society. New Orleans, LA: IEEE, 1988:90.
5. Cabo C, Wharton JM, Simpson EV, Ideker RE, Smith WM. Use of coherence in activation detection during ventricular fibrillation. In Kim Y, Spelman FA, eds. Proc. 11th Annual Conference of the IEEE Engineering in Medicine and Biology Society, Seattle, WA: IEEE, 1989:1733-1734.
6. Janse MJ, van Capelle FJL, Morsink H, et al. Flow of "injury" current and patterns of excitation during early ventricular arrhythmias in acute regional myocardial ischemia in isolated porcine and canine hearts: evidence for two different arrhythmogenic mechanisms. Circ. Res. 1980; 47:151-165.
7. Ideker RE, Klein GJ, Harrison L, et al. The transition to ventricular fibrillation induced by reperfusion following acute ischemia in the dog: a period of organized epicardial activation. Circulation 1981; 63:1371-1379.
8. Ideker RE, Bardy GH, Worley SJ, German LD, Smith WM. Patterns of activation during ventricular fibrillation. In Josephson ME, Wellens HJJ, eds. Tachycardias: Mechanisms, Diagnosis, Treatment, Philadelphia: Lea Febiger, 1984:519-536.
9. Pogwizd SM, Corr PB. Electrophysiologic mechanisms underlying arrhythmias due to reperfusion of ischemic myocardium. 1987; Circulation 76:404-426.
10. Pogwizd SM, Corr PB. Mechanisms underlying the development of ventricular fibrillation during early myocardial ischemia. 1990; Circ Res 66:672-695.
11. Moe GK, Harris AS, Wiggers CJ. Analysis of the initiation of fibrillation by electrographic studies. Am J Physiol 1941; 134:473-492.

12. Frazier DW, Wolf PD, Wharton JM, Tang ASL, Smith WM, and Ideker RE. Stimulus-induced critical point: mechanism for electrical initiation of reentry in normal canine myocardium. J Clin Invest 1989; 83:1039-1052.
13. Chen P-S, Wolf PD, Dixon EG, et al. Mechanism of ventricular vulnerability to single premature stimuli in open-chest dogs. Circ Res 1988; 62:1191-1209.
14. Shibata N, Chen P-S, Dixon EG, et al. Influence of shock strength and timing on induction of ventricular arrhythmias in dogs. Am J Physiol 1988; 255:H891-H901.
15. Kao CY, Hoffman BF. Graded and decremental response in heart muscle fibers. Am J Physiol 1958; 194:187-196.
16. Ideker RE, Frazier DW, et al. Experimental evidence for autowaves in the heart. In Jalife J, ed. Ann NY Acad Sci Vol 591, Mathematical Approaches to Cardiac Arrhythmias. New York: New York Academy of Sciences, 1990:208-218.
17. Winfree AT. When Time Breaks Down: The Three-Dimensional Dynamics of Electrochemical Waves and Cardiac Arrhythmias. Princeton, NJ: Princeton University Press, 1987.
18. Ideker RE, Alferness C, Hagler J, Wolf PD, and Smith WM. Rotor site correlates with defibrillation waveform efficacy (abstr). Circulation 1991; 84:II-499.
19. Garrey WE. The nature of fibrillatory contractions of the heart—its relation to tissue mass and form. Am J Physiol 1914; 33:397-414.
20. Herbschleb JN, Heethaar RM, Tweel L, Meijler RL. Frequency analysis of the ECG before and during ventricular fibrillation. In: Ripley KL, Ostrow HG, eds. Proc Computers in Cardiology. Washington, DC: IEEE Computer Society Press, 1980:365-368.
21. Moe GK. Cardiac Arrhythmias: introductory remarks to part III. Ann NY Acad Sci 1956; 64:540-542.
22. Mines GR. On circulating excitations in heart muscles and their possible relation to tachycardia and fibrillation. Trans Roy Soc Can 1914; 4:43-52.
23. Moe GK, Rheinboldt WC, Abildskov JA. A computer model of atrial fibrillation. Am Heart J 1964; 67:200-220.
24. Sano T, Scher AM. Multiple recording during electrically induced atrial fibrillation. Circ Res 1964; 14:117-125.
25. Allessie MA, Lammers WJEP, Bonke FIM, Hollen J. Experimental evaluation of Moe's multiple wavelet hypothesis of atrial fibrillation. In: Zipes DP, Jalife J, eds. Cardiac Electrophysiology and Arrhythmias. Orlando, FL: Grune & Stratton, 1985:265-275.
26. Allessie MA, Bonke FIM, Schopman FJG. Circus movement in rabbit atrial muscle as a mechanism of tachycardia. III. The "leading circle" concept: a new model of circus movement in cardiac tissue without the involvement of an anatomical obstacle. Circ Res 1977; 41:9-18.
27. Chen P-S, Wolf PD, Melnick SB, Danieley ND, Smith WM, Ideker RE. Comparison of activation during ventricular fibrillation and following unsuccessful defibrillation shocks in open chest dogs. Circ Res 1990; 66:1544-1560.
28. Wiggers CJ. Studies of ventricular fibrillation caused by electric shock: cinematographic and electrocardiographic observations of the natural process in the dog's heart: its inhibition by potassium and the revival of coordinated beats by calcium. Am Heart J 1930; 5:351-365.
29. Witkowski FX, Penkoske PA. Activation patterns during ventricular fibrillation. In Jalife J, ed. Mathematical Approaches to Cardiac Arrhythmias. New York: New York Academy of Sciences, 1990:219-231.
30. Johnson EE, Idriss SF, Cabo C, Melnick SB, Smith WM, Ideker RE. Evidence that organization increases during the first minute of ventricular fibrillation in pigs mapped with closely spaced electrodes (abstr). J Am Coll Cardiol 1992; 19:90A.
31. Damle RS, Kanaan NM, Robinson NS, Ge Y-Z, Goldberger JJ, Kadish AH. Spatial and temporal linking of epicardial activation directions during ventricular fibrillation in dogs: evidence for underlying organization. Circulation 1992; 86:1547-1558.
32. Carlisle EJF, Allen JD, Bailey A, et al. Fourier analysis of ventricular fibrillation and synchronization of DC countershocks in defibrillation. J Electrocardiol 1988; 21:337-343.

33. Carlisle EJF, Allen JD, Kernohan WG, Anderson J, Adgey AAJ. Fourier analysis of ventricular fibrillation of varied aetiology. Eur Heart J 1990; 11:173-181.
34. Worley SJ, Swain JL, Colavita PG, Smith WM, Ideker RE. Development of an endocardial-epicardial gradient of activation rate during electrically induced, sustained ventricular fibrillation in the dog. Am J Cardiol 1985; 55:813-820.
35. Yakaitis RW, Ewy A, Otto CW, Taren DL, Moon TE. Influence of time and therapy on ventricular defibrillation in dogs. Crit Care Med 1980; 8:157-163.
36. Dzwonczyk R, Brown CG, Werman HA. The median frequency of the ECG during ventricular fibrillation: its use in an algorithm for estimating the duration of cardiac arrest. IEEE Trans. Biomed. Eng. 1990; BME-37:640-646.
37. Rush S, Lepeschkin E, Gregoritsch A. Current distribution from defibrillation electrodes in a homogeneous torso model. J Electrocardiol 1969; 2:331-341.
28. Fahey JB, Kim Y, Ananthaswamy A. Optimal electrode configurations for external cardiac pacing and defibrillation: an inhomogeneous study. IEEE Trans Biomed Eng 1987; BME-34:743-748.
39. Claydon FJ III, Pilkington TC, Tang ASL, Morrow MN, Ideker RE. A volume conductor model of the thorax for the study of defibrillation fields. IEEE Trans Biomed Eng 1988; BME-35:981-992.
40. Kothiyal KP, Shankar B, Fogelson LJ, Thakor NV. Three-dimensional computer model of electric fields in internal defibrillation. Proc IEEE 1988; 76:720-730.
41. Ramirez IF, Eisenberg SR, Lehr JL, Schoen FJ. Effects of cardiac configuration, paddle placement and paddle size on defibrillation current distribution: a finite-element model. Med Biol Eng Comp 1989; 27:587-594.
42. Sepulveda NG, Wikswo JP Jr, Echt DS. Finite element analysis of cardiac defibrillation current distributions. IEEE Trans Biomed Eng 1990; BME-37:354-365.
43. Chen P-S, Wolf PD, Claydon FJ III, et al. The potential gradient field created by epicardial defibrillation electrodes in dogs. Circulation 1986; 74:626-636.
44. Witkowski FX, Penkoske PA, Plonsey R. Mechanism of cardiac defibrillation in open-chest dogs with unipolar DC-coupled simultaneous activation and shock potential recordings. Circulation 1990; 82:244-260.
45. Wharton JM, Wolf PD, Smith WM et al. Cardiac potential and potential gradient fields generated by single, combined, and sequential shocks during ventricular defibrillation. Circulation 1992; 85:1510-1523.
46. Tang ASL, Wolf PD, Afework Y, Smith WM, Ideker RE. Three-dimensional potential gradient fields generated by intracardiac catheter and cutaneous patch electrodes. Circulation 1992; 85:1857-1864.
47. Henriquez CS. Simulating the electrical behavior of cardiac tissue using the bidomain model. CRC Crit Rev Biomed Eng in press.
48. Jones JL, Jones RE, Balasky G. Improved cardiac cell excitation with symmetrical biphasic defibrillator waveforms. Am J Physiol 1987; 253:H1418-H1424.
49. Klee M, Plonsey R. Stimulation of spheroidal cells—the role of cell shape. IEEE Trans Biomed Eng 1976; BME-23:347-354.
50. Windisch H, Ahammer H, Schaffer P, Müller W, Koidl B. Optical monitoring of excitation patterns in single cardiomyocytes. In: Proc 12th Annual Conference of the IEEE Engineering in Medicine and Biology Society. New Orleans, LA: IEEE, 1990:1641.
51. Knisley S, Blitchington T, Hill B, et al. Transmembrane potential changes measured optically during field stimulation of ventricular cells (abstr). J Am Coll Cardiol 1992; 19:122A.
52. Plonsey R, Barr RC. Inclusion of junction elements in a linear cardiac model through secondary sources: application to defibrillation. Med Biol Eng Comp 1986; 24:137-144.
53. Krassowska W, Pilkington TC, Ideker RE. Periodic conductivity as a mechanism for cardiac stimulation and defibrillation. IEEE Trans Biomed Eng 1987; BME-34:555-560.
54. Krassowska W, Frazier DW, Pilkington TC, Ideker RE. Potential distribution in three-dimensional periodic myocardium. Part II. Application to extracellular stimulation. IEEE Trans Biomed Eng 1990; BME-37:267-284.

55. Plonsey R, Barr, RC, Witkowski FX. One-dimensional model of cardiac defibrillation. Med Biol Eng Comp 1991; 29:465-469.
56. Sepulveda NG, Barach JP, Wikswo JP Jr. A three dimensional finite element bidomain model for cardiac tissue. In Nagel JH, Smith WM, eds. Proc 13th Annual Conference of the IEEE Engineering in Medicine and Biology Society, Orlando, FL: IEEE, 1991:512-514.
57. Sepulveda NG, Wikswo JP Jr. Electric and magnetic fields from two-dimensional anisotropic bisyncytia. Biophys J 1987; 51:557-568.
58. Neunlist M, Tung L. Evidence of oppositely polarized regions in the myocardium around a stimulating point electrode (abstr). Circulation 1992; 86:I-560-I-560.
59. Frazier DW, Krassowska W, Chen P-S, et al. Extracellular field required for excitation in three-dimensional anisotropic canine myocardium. Circ Res 63:1988;147-164.
60. Tung L, Sliz N, Mulligan MR. Influence of electrical axis of stimulation on excitation of cardiac muscle cells. Circ Res 1991; 69:722-730.
61. Bardou AL, Chesnais J-M, Birkui PJ, et al. Directional variability of stimulation threshold measurements in isolated guinea pig cardiomyocytes: relationship with orthogonal sequential defibrillating pulses. PACE 1990; 13:1590-1595.
62. Sommer JR, Scherer B. Geometry of cell and bundle appositions in cardiac muscle: light microscopy. Am J Physiol 1985; 248:H792-H803.
63. Schuder JC, Stoeckle H, McDaniel WC, Dbeis M. Is the effectiveness of cardiac ventricular defibrillation dependent upon polarity? Med Instrum 1987; 21:262-265.
64. Bardy GH, Ivey TD, Allen MD, Johnson G, Greene HL. Evaluation of electrode polarity on defibrillation efficacy. Am J Cardiol 1989; 63:433-437.
65. Troup P, Wetherbee JN, Chapman PD, et al. Does electrode polarity affect defibrillation efficacy? (abstr). PACE 1990; 13:528.
66. O'Neill PG, Boahene KA, Lawrie GM, Harvill LF, Pacifico A. The automatic implantable cardioverter-defibrillator: effect of patch polarity on defibrillation threshold. J Am Coll Cardiol 1991; 17:707-711.
67. Knisley SB, Smith WM, Ideker RE. Effect of field stimulation on cellular repolarization in rabbit myocardium: implications for reentry induction. Circ Res 1992; 70:707-715.
68. Dillon SM. Optical recordings in the rabbit heart show that defibrillation strength shocks prolong the duration of depolarization and the refractory period. Circ Res 1991; 69:842-856.
69. Shibata N, Chen P-S, Dixon EG, et al. Epicardial activation following unsuccessful defibrillation shocks in dogs. Am J Physiol 1988; 255:H902-H909.
70. Ideker RE, Tang ASL, Frazier DW, Shibata N, Chen P-S, Wharton J. Ventricular defibrillation: basic concepts. In: El-Sherif N, Samet P, eds. Cardiac Pacing and Electrophysiology. Orlando: FL: Saunders 1991:713-726.
71. Ideker RE, Tang ASL, Frazier DW, et al. Basic mechanisms of ventricular defibrillation. In: Glass L, Hunter P, McColloch A, eds. Theory of the Heart. New York: Springer-Verlag, 1991:533-560.
72. Swartz JF, Jones JL, Jones RE, Fletcher R. Conditioning prepulse of biphasic defibrillator waveforms enhances refractoriness to fibrillation wavefronts. Circ Res 1991; 68:438-449.
73. Dillon SM. Synchronized repolarization after defibrillation shocks: a possible component of the defibrillation process demonstrated by optical recordings in rabbit heart. Circulation 1992; 85:1865-1878.
74. Moore EN, Spear JF. Electrophysiologic studies on the initiation, prevention, and termination of ventricular fibrillation. In: Zipes DP, Jalife J, eds. Cardiac Electrophysiology and Arrhythmias. Orlando, FL: Grune & Stratton, 1985:315-322.
75. Yabe S, Smith WM, Daubert JP, Wolf PD, Rollins DL, Ideker RE. Conduction disturbances caused by high current density electric field. Circ Res 1990; 66:1190-1203.
76. Lepeschkin E, Jones JL, Rush S, Jones RE. Local potential gradients as a unifying measure for thresholds of stimulation, standstill, tachyarrhythmia and fibrillation appearing after strong capacitor discharges. Adv Cardiol 1978; 21:268-278.

77. Jones JL, Lepeschkin E, Jones RE, Rush S. Response of cultured myocardial cells to countershock-type electric field stimulation. Am J Physiol 1978; 235:H214-H222.
78. Jones JL, Jones RE. Determination of safety factor for defibrillator waveforms in cultured heart cells. Am J Physiol 1982; 242:H662-H670.
79. Jones JL, Jones RE, Balasky, G. Microlesion formation in myocardial cells by high-intensity electric field stimulation. Am J Physiol 1987; 253:H480-H486.
80. Peleska B. Cardiac arrhythmias following condenser discharges and their dependence upon strength of current and phase of cardiac cycle. Circ Res 1963; 13:21-32.
81. Mower MM, Mirowski M, Spear JF, Moore EN. Patterns of ventricular activity during catheter defibrillation. Circulation 1974; 49:858-861.
82. Zipes DP, Fischer J, King RM, Nicoll A, Jolly WW. Termination of ventricular fibrillation in dogs by depolarizing a critical amount of myocardium. Am J Cardiol 1975; 36:37-44.
83. Chen P-S, Shibata N, Dixon EG, et al. Activation during ventricular defibrillation in open-chest dogs: evidence of complete cessation and regeneration of ventricular fibrillation after unsuccessful shocks. J Clin Invest 1986; 77:810-823.
84. Zhou X, Daubert JP, Wolf PD, Smith WM, Ideker RE. Epicardial mapping of ventricular defibrillation with monophasic and biphasic shocks in dogs. Circ Res 1993; 72:145-160.
85. Fabiato A, Coumel P, Gourgon R, Saumont R. Le seuil de réponse synchrone des fibres myocardiques. Application à la comparaison expérimentale de l'efficacité des différentes formes de chocs électriques de défibrillation. Arch Mal Coeur 1967; 60:527-544.
86. Lesigne C, Levy B, Saumont R, Birkui P, Bardou A, Rubin B. An energy-time analysis of ventricular fibrillation and defibrillation thresholds with internal electrodes. Med Biol Eng 1976; 14:617-622.
87. Chen P-S, Shibata N, Dixon EG, Martin RO, Ideker RE. Comparison of the defibrillation threshold and the upper limit of ventricular vulnerability. Circulation 1986; 73:1022-1028.
88. Wharton JM, Richard VJ, Murry CE, et al. Electrophysiologic effects in vivo of monophasic and biphasic stimuli in normal and infarcted dogs. PACE 1990; 13:1158-1172.
89. Chen P-S, Feld GK, Mower MM, Peters BB. Effects of pacing rate and timing of defibrillation shock on the relation between the defibrillation threshold and the upper limit of vulnerability in open chest dogs. J Am Coll Cardiol 1991; 18:1555-1563.
90. Bayly PV, Johnson EE, Idriss SF, Ideker RE, Smith WM. Minimum electrode spacing for mapping ventricular fibrillation using spatial sampling theory. Proc Comput Cardiol. In press.
91. Deale OC, Wesley RC Jr, Morgan D, Lerman BB. Nature of defibrillation: determinism versus probabilism. Am J Physiol 1990; 259:H1544-H1550.
92. Davy JM, Fain ES, Dorian P, Winkle RA. The relationship between successful defibrillation and delivered energy in open-chest dogs: reappraisal of the "defibrillation threshold" concept. Am Heart J 1987; 113:77-84.
93. Hooker DR, Kouwenhoven WB, Langworthy OR. The effect of alternating currents on the heart. Am J Physiol 1933; 103:444-454.
94. Beck CS, Pritchard WH, Feil HS. Ventricular fibrillation of long duration abolished by electric shock. JAMA 1947; 135:985-986.
95. Zoll PM, Linenthal AJ, Gibson W, Paul MH, Norman LR. Termination of ventricular fibrillation in man by externally applied electric countershock. N Engl J Med 1956; 254:727-732.
96. Lown B, Newman J, Amarasingham R, Berkovitz BV. Comparison of alternating current with direct current electroshock across the closed chest. Am J Cardiol 1962; 10:223-233.
97. Geddes LA, Tacker WA Jr. Engineering and physiological considerations of direct capacitor-discharge ventricular defibrillation. Med Biol Eng. 1971; 9:185-199.
98. Schuder JC, Stoeckle H, Keskar PY, Gold JH, Chier MT, West JA. Transthoracic ventricular defibrillation in the dog with unidirectional rectangular double pulse. Cardiovasc. Res. 1970; 4:497-501.
99. Schuder JC, Stoeckle H, Gold JH, West JA, Keskar PY. Experimental ventricular defibrillation with an automatic and completely implanted system. Trans Am Soc Artif Intern Organs 1970; 16:207-212.

100. Mirowski M, Mower MM, Reid PR, Watkins L, Langer A. The automatic implantable defibrillator. PACE 1982; 5:384-401.
101. Wessale JJL, Boulard JD, Tacker WA, Geddes LA. Bipolar catheter defibrillation in dogs using trapezoidal waveforms of various tilts. J Electrocardiol 1980; 13:359-366.
102. Chapman PD, Wetherbee JN, Vetter JW, Troup P, Souza J. Strength-duration curves of fixed pulse width variable tilt truncated exponential waveforms for nonthoracotomy internal defibrillation in dogs. PACE 1988; 11:1045-1050.
103. Sweeney RJ, Gill RM, Reid PR. Characterization of refractory period extension by transcardiac shock. Circulation 1991; 83:2057-2066.
104. Bourland JD, Tacker WA Jr, Wessale JL, Kallok MJ, Graf JE, Geddes ME. Sequential pulse defibrillation for implantable defibrillators. Med Instrum 1986; 20:138-142.
105. Jones DL, Klein GJ, Guiraudon GM, et al. Internal cardiac defibrillation in man: pronounced improvement with sequential pulse delivery to two different lead orientations. Circulation 1986; 73:484-491.
106. Jones DL, Klein GJ, Guiraudon GM, Sharma AD, Yee R, Kallok MJ. Prediction of defibrillation success from a single defibrillation threshold measurement with sequential pulses and two current pathways in humans. Circulation 1988; 78:1144-1149.
107. Bardou AL, Degonde J, Birkui PJ, Auger P, Chesnais J-M, Duriez M. Reduction of energy required for defibrillation by delivering shocks in orthogonal directions in the dog. PACE 1988; 11:1990-1995.
108. Jones DL, Klein GJ, Kallok MJ. Improved internal defibrillation with twin pulse sequential energy delivery to different lead orientations in pigs. Am J Cardiol 1985; 55:821-825.
109. Jones Dl, Klein GJ, Rattes MF, Sohla A, Sharma AD. Internal cardiac defibrillation: single and sequential pulses and a variety of lead orientations. PACE 1988; 11:583-591.
110. Jones DL, Sohla A, Bourland JD, Tacker WA Jr, Kallok MJ, Klein GJ. Internal ventricular defibrillation with sequential pulse countershock in pigs: comparison with single pulses and effects of pulse separation. PACE 1987; 10:497-502.
111. Gurvich NL, Markarychev VA. Defibrillation of the heart with biphasic electrical impulses. Kardiologiia 1967; 7:109-112.
112. Schuder JC, McDaniel WC, Stoeckle H. Defibrillation of 100-kg calves with asymmetrical, bidirectional, rectangular pulses. Cardiovasc. Res. 1984; 18:419-426.
113. Dixon EG, Tang ASL, Wolf PD, et al. Improved defibrillation thresholds with large contoured epicardial electrodes and biphasic waveforms. Circulation 1987; 76:1176-1184.
114. Chapman PD, Vetter JW, Souza JJ, Troup PJ, Wetherbee JN, Hoffmann RG. Comparative efficacy of monophasic and biphasic truncated exponential shocks for nonthoracotomy internal defibrillation in dogs. J Am Coll Cardiol 1988; 12:739-745.
115. Chapman PD, Vetter VJ, Souza JJ, Wetherbee JN, Troup PJ. Comparison of monophasic with single and dual capacitor biphasic waveforms for nonthoracotomy canine internal defibrillation. J Am Coll Cardiol 1989; 14:242-245.
116. Tang ASL, Yabe S, Wharton JM, Dolker M, Smith WM, Ideker RE. Ventricular defibrillation using biphasic waveforms: the importance of phasic duration. J Am Coll Cardiol 1989; 13:207-214.
117. Cooper RAS, Guse PA, Dixon-Tulloch EG, Smith WM, Ideker RE. The effect of phase separation on biphasic waveform defibrillation (abstr). PACE 1991; 14:667.
118. Kavanagh KM, Tang ASL, Rollins DL, Smith WM, Ideker RE. Comparison of the internal defibrillation thresholds for monophasic and double and single capacitor biphasic waveforms. J Am Coll Cardiol 1989; 14:1343-1349.
119. Bardy GH, Ivey TD, Allen MD, Johnson G, Mehra R, Greene L. A prospective randomized evaluation of biphasic versus monophasic waveform pulses on defibrillation efficacy in humans. J Am Coll Cardiol 1989; 14:728-733.
120. Winkle RA, Mead RH, Ruder MA, et al. Improved low energy defibrillation efficacy in man with the use of a biphasic truncated exponential waveform. Am Heart J 1989; 117:122-127.

121. Jones JL, Jones RE. Improved safety factors for triphasic defibrillator waveforms. Circ Res 1989; 64:1172-1177.
122. Chapman PD, Wetherbee JN, Vetter JW, Troup PJ. Comparison of monophasic, biphasic, and triphasic truncated pulses for non-thoracotomy internal defibrillation (abstr). J Am Coll Cardiol 1988; 11:57A.
123. Ideker RE, Wolf PD, Alferness CA, Krassowska W, Smith WM. Current concepts for selecting the location, size and shape of defibrillation electrodes. PACE 1991; 14:227-240.
124. Gold JH, Schuder JC, Stoeckle H. Contour graph for relating per cent success in achieving ventricular defibrillation to duration, current, and energy content of shock. Am Heart J 1979; 98:207-212.
125. Doherty PW, McLaughlin PR, Billingham M, Kernoff R, Goris ML, Harrison DC. Cardiac damage produced by direct current countershock applied to the heart. Am J Cardiol 1979; 43:225-232.
126. Lerman BB, Weiss JL, Bulkley BH, Becker LC, Weisfeldt ML. Myocardial injury and induction of arrhythmia by direct current shock delivered via endocardial catheters in dogs. Circulation 1984; 69:1006-1012.
127. Bardy GH, Troutman C, Johnson G, et al. Electrode system influence on biphasic waveform defibrillation efficacy in humans. Circulation 1991; 84:665-671.
128. Guse PA, Walcott GP, Rollins DL, Smith WM, Ideker RE. Defibrillation electrode configurations developed from cardiac mapping that combine biphasic shocks with sequential timing. Am Heart J 1992; 124:1491-1500.
129. Saksena S, An H, Mehra R, et al. Prospective comparison of biphasic and monophasic shocks for implantable cardioverter-defibrillators using endocardial leads. Am J Cardiol 1992; 70:304-310.
130. Akhtar M, Avitall B, Jazayeri M, et al. Role of implantable cardioverter defibrillator therapy in the management of high-risk patients. Circulation 1992; 85:I-131-I-139.

2

The Defibrillation Threshold: A Reliable Method for Rapid Determination of Defibrillation Efficacy

Douglas L. Jones

*University of Western Ontario and University Hospital
and John P. Robarts Research Institute
London, Ontario, Canada*

I. INTRODUCTION

In their pioneering studies on electrical stimulation for resuscitation, Prevost and Battelli [51] documented termination of ventricular fibrillation using alternating current (AC) or direct current (DC) electrical discharge from capacitors. They wrote in 1899: "... we have shown that the fibrillatory tremulations produced in the dog, in which they are definitely established, can under certain circumstances be arrested, the heart re-establishes its beats, if one submits the animal to passages of a current of high voltage (of 4800 volts, for example)" (quoted in Ref. 21). Documented clinical termination of fibrillation was subsequently described, following experiments with dogs, by Kouwenhoven and associates [28] in the 1930s, who initially used 60-Hz AC and subsequently DC shocks to defibrillate [39], and who gave us both direct heart defibrillation and closed-chest compression [21].

As the use of AC shocks fell from favor and DC shocks became the shock modality of choice, additional refinements led to the widespread availability of external defibrillators. A major impetus for further development was due to the constraints necessary for a totally implantable device. Two overriding factors came into play. First, as an ultimate clinical device, it became paramount to understand the factors which influence the likelihood of achieving successful defibrillation and long-term efficacy of implanted devices. Second, it was important to achieve successful defibrillation while optimizing reductions in electrical and physical components of the device. Implicit with both factors is the need to determine accurately the shock parameters for successful defibrillation.

The objective of this chapter is to provide an overview of a method for determining the efficacy of any electrode-device-waveform system to defibrillate a subject, with some variations in techniques. Other chapters in this book will deal in detail with factors which may alter efficacy due to changes in system components and/or subject. Although some of these will be alluded to briefly, they are *not* the focus of this chapter. This chapter deals specifically with the "assessment tool": the determination of a "defibrillation threshold" (DFT).

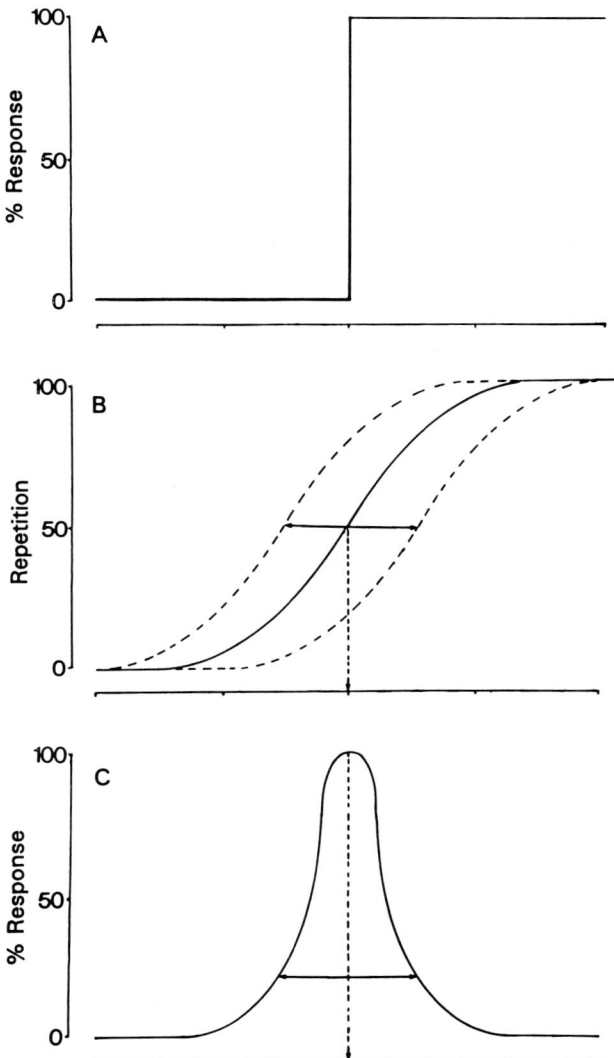

Figure 1 Generalized figures of biological responses related to a range of stimulation intensities. (A) The response with a virtual threshold. (B) The sigmoid response. Note that there is some variability around the midpoint in the curve. (C) The probability of finding the midpoint in the curve.

II. CONCEPTS

With any bioelectric stimulation device, it is essential to determine accurately the ability of that device to accomplish the task for which it was designed. If nature was truly constant, and infinitely small steps were used, theoretically it would be possible to define a limit, or threshold, below which no activation would occur and above which activation would occur 100% of the time (see Fig. 1A). In biological systems, such constancy is not possible. Instead, a balance point is the norm, at which activation occurs 50% of the time (Fig. 1B). In addition, even with all external variables constant, there remains the inherent problem of biovariability, both subject to subject and time-dependent, thus yielding a bell-shaped curve for finding the midpoint (Fig. 1C). For the investigator working with implantable defibrillators, variability is abundant, with some variables determinable, but most not, as they appear to vary either "randomly" or "chaoticly." Despite major design improvements and mathematical expertise in the last decade, our ability to understand the mechanisms of this variability has changed little since the classical experiments of Wiggers and colleagues over half a century ago [66]. Nevertheless, there have been several attempts to accurately assess defibrillation efficacy within a reasonable window of probability [10,11,20,23,25,30,31,40,44,52,58].

It is important to recognize that there is variation in the ability of any system to defibrillate at a particular instant in time (Fig. 1C). The spectrum of factors which may contribute to this variability are poorly understood. For example, the same setting on a defibrillator will fail on one attempt but be successful a few seconds later, with no obvious change in any measured variable.

There has been some suggestion that the mechanisms which alter efficacy due to the stochastic processes might be "random" or "chaotic" [24]. Although this has not been resolved, it seems implicitly clear that, as myocytes are not instantaneously depolarized and spontaneously repolarized, once a particular wave pattern of activation is established (at a given interval in time), in the next several milliseconds the pattern cannot be truly random since, to be truly random, all myocytes must have an equal chance of being reactivated. Clearly, those which are totally depolarized or are in the early phases of the activation will be in a refractory state and will not be reactivatable. Thus, for the subsequent several milliseconds, the movement of the wavefront(s) cannot be random. Therefore, although the tenant of randomness remains possible for the pattern in the first instant selected, a second selection within a short period of time thereafter cannot be random. Also, there may be some factors that influence defibrillation which are determinable.

III. INFLUENCE OF PATIENT SIZE ON DEFIBRILLATION

There is not widespread agreement on the energy needed for successful defibrillation, due to a number of factors including underlying cardiac disease, hypoxia, acidosis, electrode size and placement, as well as shock characteristics [40,63]. What is clear from a recent survey by Lehmann and associates [40] of current implantation practices is that despite wide variability, every center which implants automatic defibrillators ". . . assessed DFT regardless of the patients presenting arrhythmia . . . in every center the lowest tested energy that results in at least one successful defibrillation is taken as the 'DFT'. . ." [40].

Within a sample population there appears to be a Poisson distribution of defibrillation efficacy (Fig. 2), defined as the minimum energy which successfully defibrillated the patient [32,34]. The patients represented in Fig. 2 were normothermic, not on cardiopulmonary bypass, and undergoing surgery for correction of Wolff-Parkinson-White syndrome. Although the defibrillation energy requirements of the majority of the patients were within a narrow range, consistent with what has been reported anecdotally by several investigators, there are a small number of subjects skewing the curve at the upper end. The reason for these outliers is not known, although it is possible that body weight [62] or increased left ventricular mass [7,22] increases the energy requirement for defibrillation. In cross-species comparisons, Geddes and associates [23] found a correlation between defibrillation threshold and heart weight, the linear equation being $U = 161 \times 10^{-6} W^{1.83}$ (where U is the energy in joules and W is the body

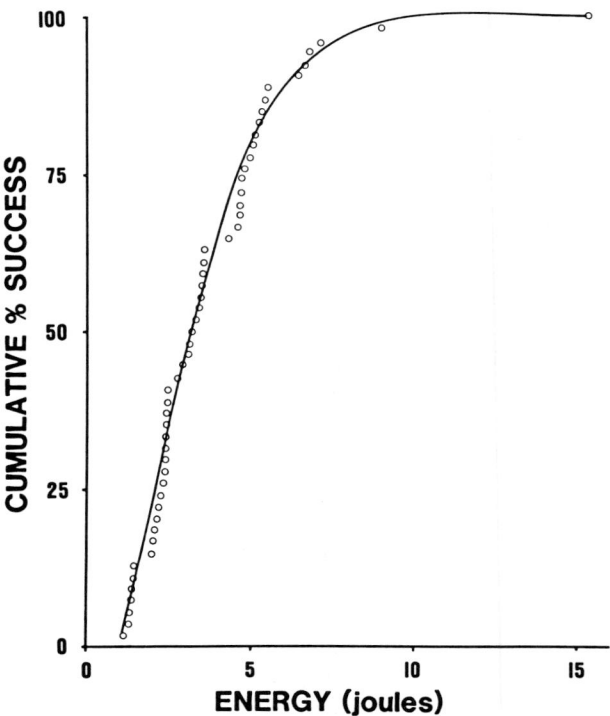

Figure 2 Cumulative defibrillation energies for 54 successive patients defibrillated in the operating room using a three-patch, sequential pulse defibrillation system. DFT was defined as the lowest energy which defibrillated the patient. The initial energy was set to deliver approximately 3–6 J. If the first shock was unsuccessful, subsequent shocks were delivered at approximately 1- 2 J increments until defibrillation was accomplished. If the first shock was successful, an additional ventricular fibrillation episode was permitted beginning at approximately 1 J, with similar increments until defibrillation was successful.

weight in kilograms). However, it is not always possible to know heart weight of the subject, although body weight can usually be determined.

A pediatric patient routinely requires less energy for transthoracic defibrillation than an adult. For transthoracic defibrillation or cardioversion in children, a dose of 2 J/kg has been recommended for children from pediatric to adolescent [27,61]. Although there is some thought that for the adult, left ventricular mass may negatively impact defibrillation, in single-species animal studies the correlations between defibrillation efficacy and body weight (Fig. 3A) or heart weight (Fig. 3B) are poor, with considerable scatter in the data, even when the same defibrillation system is used. An exception to this rule appears to be the relationship found in a model of heart failure in dogs [41], where there was a positive correlation between ventricular weight and defibrillation energy requirements. However, generally the data suggest that factors in addition to simple left ventricular mass also have major influences on defibrillation efficacy [32,34].

Given these constraints, the ultimate task of the investigator is to determine, with some degree of accuracy, the probability of a particular defibrillation system being capable of successfully extinguishing fibrillation, for a particular subject. Mathematical models and computer simulations have been helpful to examine some issues related to such a process, although in the final analysis, in-vivo studies on subjects in the setting of confirmed ventricular fibril-

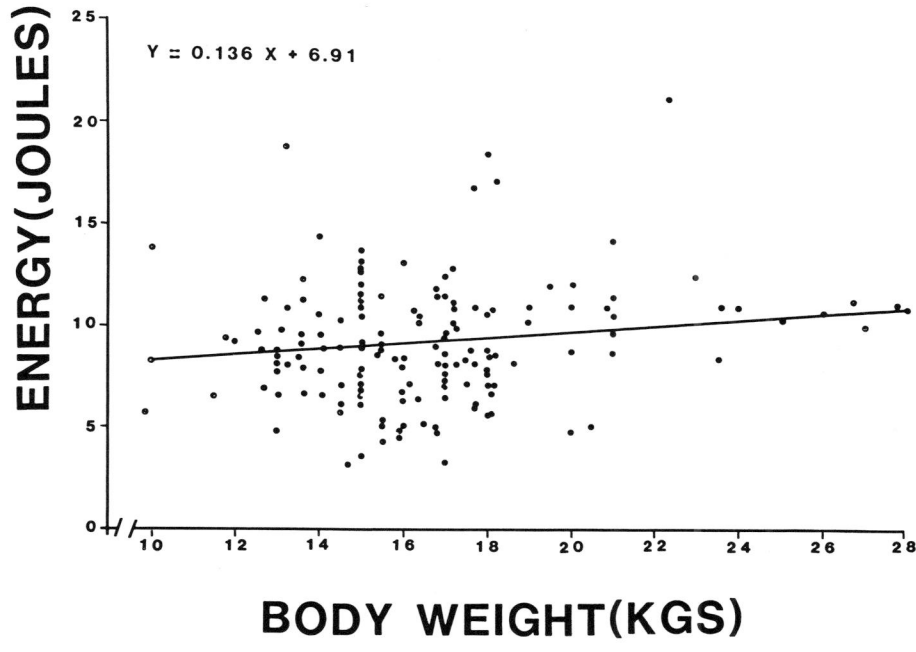

(A)

Figure 3 Relationships between the defibrillation thresholds of 163 successive pigs and body weight (A) and heart weight (B, $n = 96$). Defibrillation thresholds were determined using a Medtronic 6880 catheter and Medtronic TX-7 patch electrode. Correlation coefficients were not significant for either variable, as there was considerable scatter in the data.

lation must be assessed. In performing this assessment, the investigator needs to ensure that there is a reliable method for assessing defibrillation efficacy: optimizing the need to ensure accuracy by repeatedly inducing and terminating fibrillation, while keeping the number of fibrillation episodes to a minimum for subject safety [10,21,40,45,48,58].

IV. THE ASSESSMENT TOOL: DFT VERSUS DOSE–RESPONSE CURVE

To date there has not been a universally accepted "gold standard" for assessing defibrillation efficacy or a "safety margin" [40]. As has been alluded to above, due to several factors, the ability to defibrillate has variability, and there has been considerable controversy regarding the most appropriate diagnostic technique for assessing efficacy [11,25,31,44]. Early experiments [54,55] determined percent success with repeated fibrillation episodes with delivery of several replicates at multiple energy levels. A mathematical formula then derived a "best-fit" curve (dose–response curve), using one of several alternate formulas: logistic, exponential, or limited growth curves [11,15,25]. This process required in excess of 25–40 fibrillation episodes [11,26] and is not applicable to the clinical setting [40,67].

On the other hand, a calculation of defibrillation threshold usually requires fewer than five fibrillation episodes [45,52,53], and triplicate determinations can be routinely obtained with less than 10 episodes [21,30]. In a direct comparison of some of these methods for assessing defibrillation efficacy [31], three defibrillation threshold replicates using an up–down algorithm [52] were found to be equally reliable as the logistic model based on 36 fibrillation

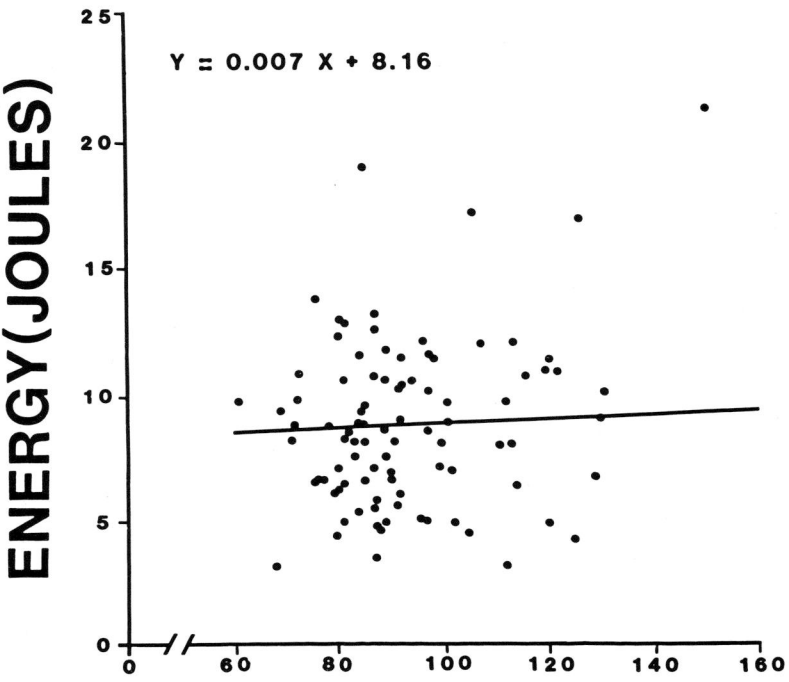

(B)

HEART WEIGHT (GMS)

episodes, and considerably more reliable than any of the other dose–response mathematical models [31]. Indeed, some of the mathematical formulas [17,25] were not capable of calculating dose–response data derived directly from 36 defibrillation attempts in two of the 20 pigs.

The "dose–response curve" (DRC) was estimated by regressing defibrillation success rates on energy doses using three mathematical models: (1) the logistic model and two reparameterizations of the model [11,15], (2) the exponential model [25], and (3) a standard exponential growth curve. With the logistic model, observed success rates were fitted to the following function:

$$Y_i = \frac{e^{B_0 + B_1 X_i}}{1 + e^{B_0 + B_1 X_i}} + E_i$$

For the Davy et al. [11] reparameterization, the success rates were fitted to the following function:

$$Y_i = \frac{A}{A + K}$$

For the Echt et al. [15] reparameterization, the success rates were fitted to the following function:

$$Y_i = \frac{e^x}{1 + e^x}$$

The Defibrillation Threshold

Table 1 Comparisons of the Coefficients of Variation as a Measure of Reliability of Various Mathematical Models

	DFT	Logit	Exponential	Davy	Echt	Growth
N	18	18	18	18	18	18
Median	0.092	0.076	0.313	1.135	0.367	0.810
Mean	0.103	0.101	0.535	1.072	1.252	1.579
S.D.	0.076	0.076	0.553	0.365	2.609	2.306
Range	0.022–0.274	0.032–0.288	0.050–2.200	0.120–1.56	0.169–11.085	0.610–10.19

Group differences were highly significant ($p < 0.00001$), based on Freidman's test [59], with and without the "growth" group. DFT: triplicate determinations for each animal. Logit: logistic regressions by SAS. Exponential: exponential curve cited in Gliner et al. [25]. Davy: reparameterization cited in Davy et al. [11]. Echt: reparameterization cited in Echt et al. [15].
Growth: growth curve based on $Y_i = e^{B_0 + B_1 X_i} - 1 + E_i$.
Source: From Ref. 31.

For the Gliner et al. [25] exponential model, the success rates were fitted to the following function:

$$Y_i = 1 - e^{-(B_0 + B_1 X_i)} + E_i$$

For the growth curve, the success rates were fitted to the following function:

$$Y_i = e^{B_0 + B_1 X_i} - 1 + E_i$$

where

e = 2.718, the base of natural logarithms (ln)
Y_i = percent success
X_i = delivered energy (also termed A by Davy et al. [11])
x = (ln 9[ED − ED$_{50}$])/(ED$_{90}$ − ED$_{50}$)
B_0 = intercept
B_1 = slope
E_i = an additive error term of discrepancies between real data and the model
ED$_{50}$ and ED$_{90}$ = energy associated with 50% and 90% defibrillation success respectively [17] (The ED$_{50}$ is also termed K by Davy et al. [11])

Models were fitted using nonlinear least squares [4,56], based on the natural logarithmic scale. The slope, B_1, is the change in percent success, Y_i, produced by a unit change in energy dose, X_i. The intercept B_0 is the percent success when energy does is 0. Table 1 compares the coefficients of variation as a measure of reliability of various mathematical models. Only data from the 18 animals for which all models would calculate values are included.

In addition, the DFT was found to reliably approximate the midpoint (ED$_{50}$) of the logit dose–response curve. Having some assurance of the reliability of this measurement tool, it is relevant to ask how it attains a measurement near the midpoint on the dose–response curve, and how it may be used to determine the energy necessary to achieve 80% or higher success for an individual subject. Mathematical models and computer simulations can again be helpful to answer such questions.

V. MATHEMATICAL MODELS AND COMPUTER SIMULATIONS

A simplified model [30] was developed using the concept of a linear relation between energy delivery from 0 to 20 J and percentage success (Fig. 4). The methodology described below was

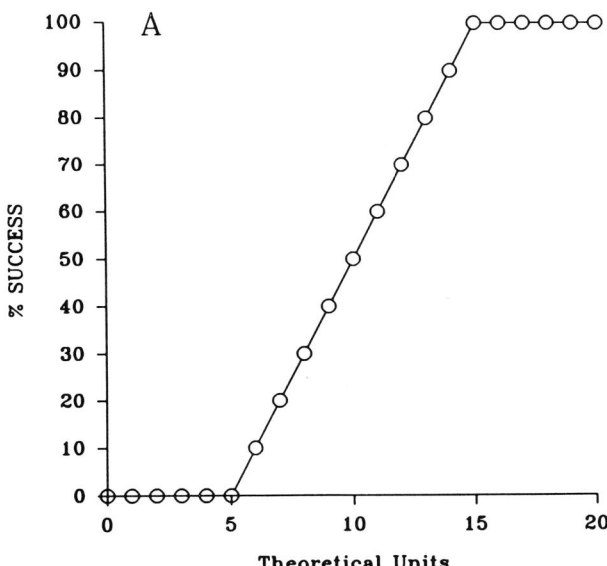

Figure 4 A linear model of defibrillation efficacy versus energy (A). In (B) is demonstrated the probability of obtaining a defibrillation threshold using the up–down algorithm and the criteria in the text and illustrated in Fig. 5.

used to determine defibrillation efficacy using an up–down algorithm [6,45,65] based on two assumptions. First, although the defibrillation range was constant, at the time of delivering a "test shock" the actual "energy necessary for defibrillation" was randomly located within the range. Thus the probability of "success" or "failure" was calculated from the curve. Second, multiple "ventricular fibrillation episodes" could be run without altering the basic characteristics of the relationship between defibrillation success and delivered energy. Using these assumptions, the methodology used with the model included the following. Increments or decrements of 1 J were applied, depending solely on the "success" or "failure" to defibrillate of the first test shock of a "ventricular fibrillation episode." If necessary, when the first shock was unsuccessful, a second test shock, at a 1-J increment above the first test shock, was allowed within a fibrillation episode. If both test shocks were unsuccessful, the episode was over (in the normal setting this would be equivalent to delivering a rescue shock). Defibrillation threshold (DFT) was established as the lowest test shock which was "successful," when the immediately lower test shock in the same, preceding, or following fibrillation episode was "unsuccessful" [52]. Calculating all the relationships, a bell-shaped curve of the probability of finding a DFT was obtained. In order to understand how this curve was constructed, consider, for example, the calculation of the probability of determining a DFT at the midpoint (ED_{50} = 10 J on the defibrillation energy scale).

For the immediately preceding episode (at one decrement), to establish a DFT (see Fig. 5A), both the first shock (at 9 J) and the second shock (at 10 J) of the preceding fibrillation episode had to be unsuccessful—if the second shock had been successful, the DFT would have been defined within that first episode, without a need of the second episode. Also, the first shock (at 10 J) of the second episode had to be successful. Now it is possible to assign prob-

The Defibrillation Threshold

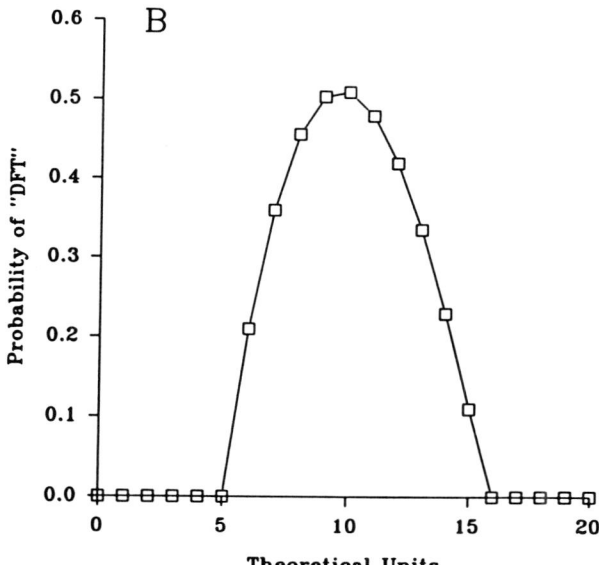

abilities (see Fig. 4A). The probability of the shock at 9 J being unsuccessful is 60% (0.6). The probability of the second shock (at 10 J) also being unsuccessful is 50% (0.5). The probability of the first shock of the second episode (at 10 J) being successful is also 50% (0.5). Thus the probability of the combination is the product of the probabilities (0.6 × 0.5 × 0.5 = 0.15). Second, calculate the probability of the DFT being determined in a single episode (see Fig. 5B). The probability of the immediately lower shock (at 9 J) being unsuccessful is 0.6. The probability of the second shock being successful is 0.5—but there are only 60% of the episodes remaining as they were unsuccessful at 9 J, so the probability is (0.6 × 0.5). Thus the probability is 0.6 × (0.6 × 0.5) = 0.18. Finally, calculate the probability that the DFT is established by the following shock (see Fig. 5C). In this case, the shock at 10 J (second episode) would have to be successful (probability 0.5). The following first shock (at 9 J, third episode) would have to be unsuccessful (probability 0.6). In addition, unless testing happened to begin at 10 J, the first episode would have had to be a success at 11 J (with a probability of 0.6). It could not have been a failure at 9 J, with a success in the same episode at 10 J, or this episode itself would have established a DFT at 10 J. Similarly, it could not have been a failure at 9 J and also at 10 J, or the success of episode 2 at 10 J would again have established a DFT. The only remaining possibility is that the first episode was a success at 11 J. Thus the probability of the subsequent episode establishing a DFT is the product: 0.6 × 0.5 × 0.6 = 0.18. The total probability of the three combined probabilities for establishing a DFT (at 10 J—from the previous, same or following episodes) is the sum of the three (0.15 + 0.18 + 0.18 = 0.51).

Using similar logic, the remainder of the probability curve can be determined. It is highly likely, therefore, that a DFT will be at or very near the midpoint (ED_{50}) of a defibrillation success curve, particularly if testing begins near the midpoint [44,45]. In the example provided, the highest probability of defining a "defibrillation threshold" was at the midpoint of the line, 51% at the midpoint, and very near that probability value at 1 J above and 1 J below that point. The existence of probabilities beside the midpoint and the presence of the bell-shaped curve

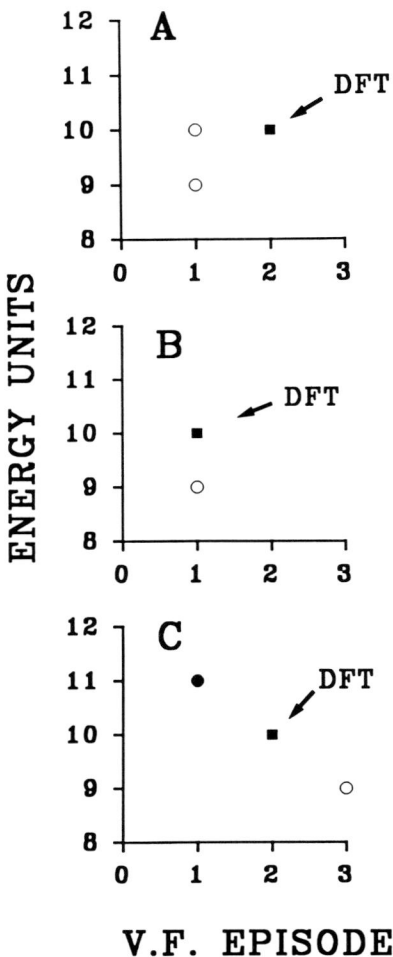

Figure 5 Schematic example of the three criteria for determining a defibrillation threshold. Open symbols represent unsuccessful shocks. Energy delivery follows those of the linear model. Closed symbols represent successful shocks. Squares and arrows indicate those values associated with the defibrillation threshold.

demonstrates that if the starting point approaches the outside values, it will still be possible to establish a DFT, although the value will be a poorer estimate of the true midpoint.

In the situation where only a single shock would be allowed before a "rescue shock," the shape of the curve would be identical. However, at each point on the curve the probability of determining a DFT would be lower. Thus there would be an increase in the number of episodes necessary to determine a DFT, and the scatter in the data would be increased, in turn widening the window of error.

To test some of these concepts, a series of experiments was performed using a computerized mathematical model. The mathematical model of defibrillation threshold determination used a logistic curve derived from defibrillation success data averaged from 20 pigs (Fig. 6). The logistic equation for the model was

$$Y_i = \frac{e^{B_0 + B_1 X_i}}{1 + e^{B_0 + B_1 X_i}} + E_i$$

The Defibrillation Threshold

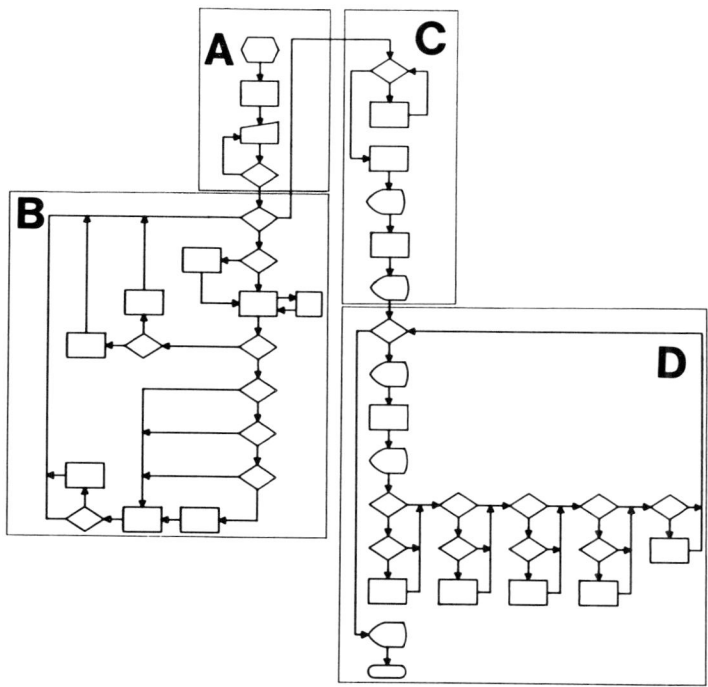

Figure 6 Mathematical model for computer simulation of multiple determinations of defibrillation threshold. The curve relating defibrillation success to energy is sigmoidal. Top is the overall logic tree. (A) The initiation of the simulation and establishment of starting energy. (B) Designated loop for 1000 replicates. (C) Short report of the overall mean and standard deviation. (D) Report of the results from each of the parameters. This final report is extended to provide the individual numbers and replicates.

A series of 1000 "fibrillation episodes" with 100 simulated subjects was run with the time of day and date used as random number seeds for each run, and for curve generation, values of $a = -3.8337$ and $b = 0.70144$.

Using this model, the midpoint (ED_{50}) was approximately 6 J. From the simulations of this model (Fig. 7), two findings were evident. First, confirming what had been proposed, the farther the starting point was from the midpoint, the more replicates were needed to be within the final average of all (usually over 400) calculated DFTs. Starting at 5, 6, or 7 J, the *first* DFT was consistently within the mean ±1 standard deviation (S.D.) of the mean (Fig. 7A), while starting with values well above or below this value progressively increased the number of replicates needed to approach the overall mean, although the final running average was always approximately 6 J. Second, acceptance of a wider window of error substantially reduced the number of replicates needed to reach criterion. With a starting position of 1 J, over 15 replicates were required to approach the group mean ±1 J (Fig. 7B), while with a window of ±3 J from the mean, criterion was reached within the first to second replicate for all but the starting position of 10 J, which required 5 replicates (Fig. 7D). This also demonstrated that starting well above the midpoint (ED_{50}), the *first* DFT would most likely be greater than the ED_{50}; and starting well below the ED_{50}, the *first* DFT would most likely be lower than the ED_{50}.

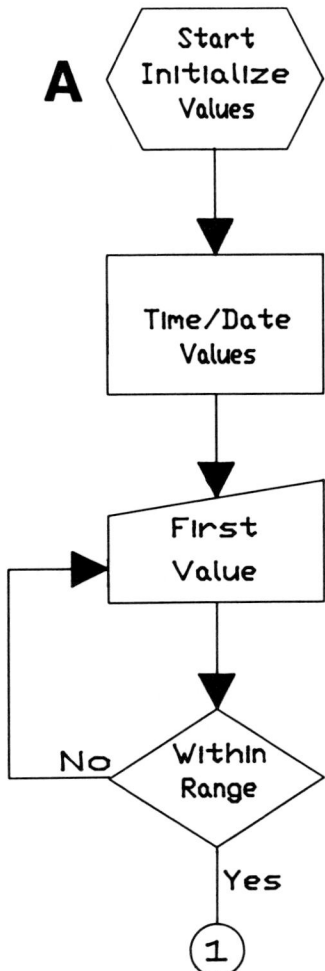

Figure 6 Continued

VI. IMPLICATIONS FROM THE MODELS

How can the investigator use this information for biological experiments and/or clinical testing? First, if there is a-priori indication of the average threshold for a subject, or group, when using a particular defibrillating system, that midpoint is the best initial test energy setting to reduce the number of fibrillation episodes [10,45,58], as in over 60% of the subjects the first determined threshold will be as reliable as multiple assessments [30]. This percentage will increase the wider the acceptable window of accuracy.

Second, although a single assessment has been used clinically [32,34], to improve accuracy, replication of the DFT determination is very helpful [21,30,31,58]. In animal and clinical studies, triplicate determinations have been routinely found to be as accurate as seven replications [21], and thresholds have been found to be stable over periods of 2.5 h, allowing multiple comparisons [1,5,53]. Also, animal and anecdotal human data [12,46] suggest that defibrillation efficacy does not change substantially with time [12,20,46], although disease progression or adjunct antiarrhythmic drug therapy may subsequently alter defibrillation efficacy [58,63].

The Defibrillation Threshold

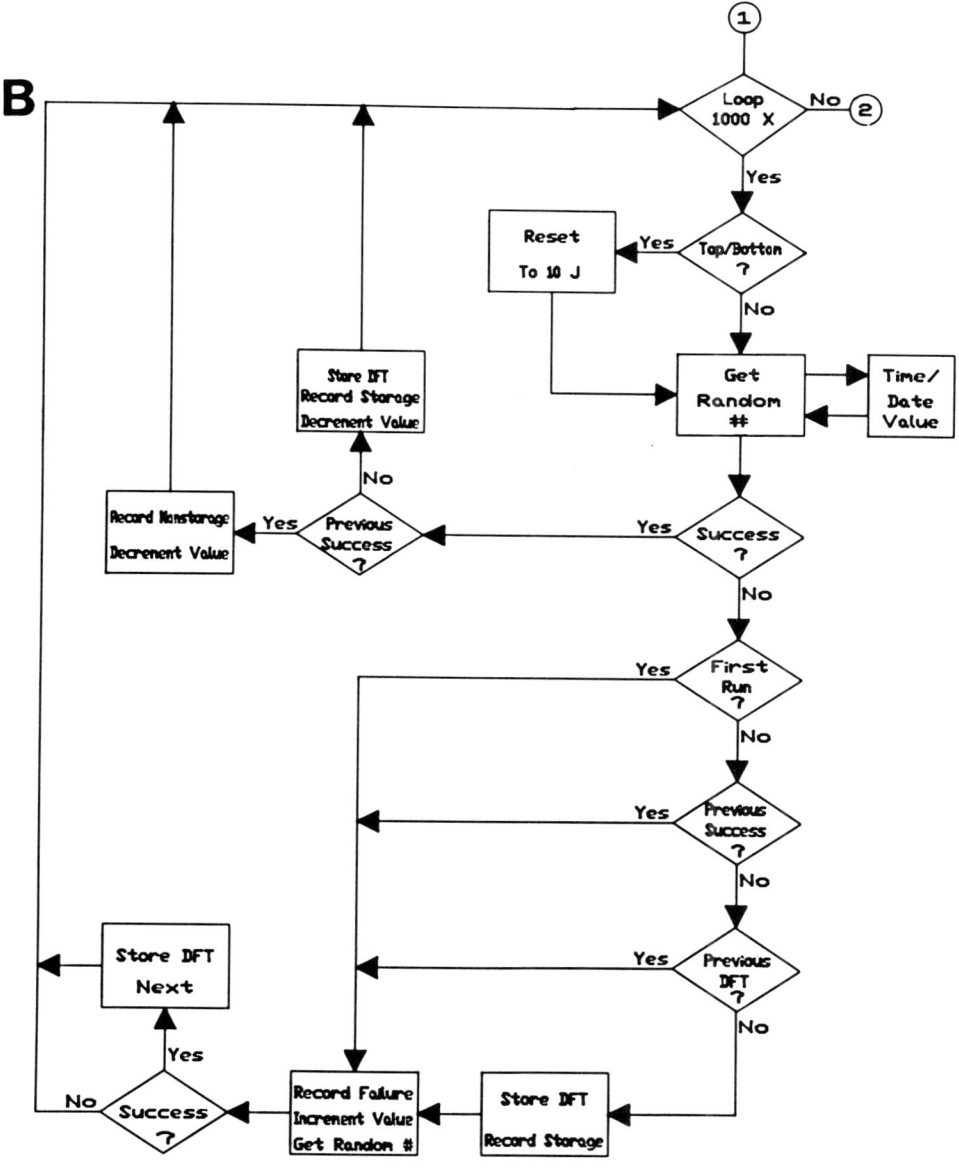

VII. PREDICATION OF EFFICACY FROM THRESHOLD DETERMINATIONS

The finding of an average coefficient of variation of approximately 10% for the defibrillation threshold determination provides a reasonable assurance of reliability of a measure. In addition, when starting near the midpoint, the approximately 90% reproducibility within ±1 J or ±15% of the mean, depending on electrode system, species tested, and mathematical algorithm, is found consistently [1,31,44]. However, it must be recognized that this will be influenced by the starting setting and energy steps [21,30,31,45].

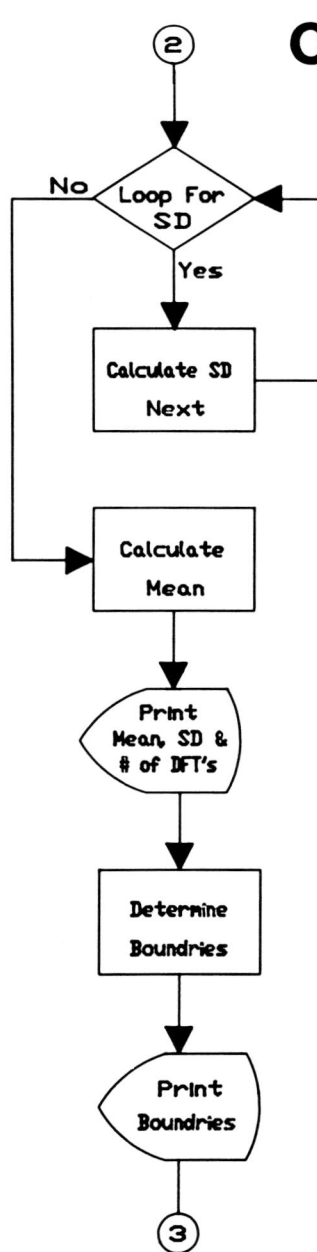

Figure 6 Continued

The question then arises: How much larger a shock does one need to deliver to achieve 90–95% success? Previous studies, even with single assessments of DFT [32,36,52], found better than 80% success when delivering energies of 1.5–2.6 × DFT [10,31,34,52,58] (Fig. 8). Using a particular defibrillating system, having titrated the specific energy requirements for a particular patient, there is a reasonable expectation of the ability to determine the safety margin for the patient with such ratios. If the starting point is well above the midpoint for a subject,

The Defibrillation Threshold

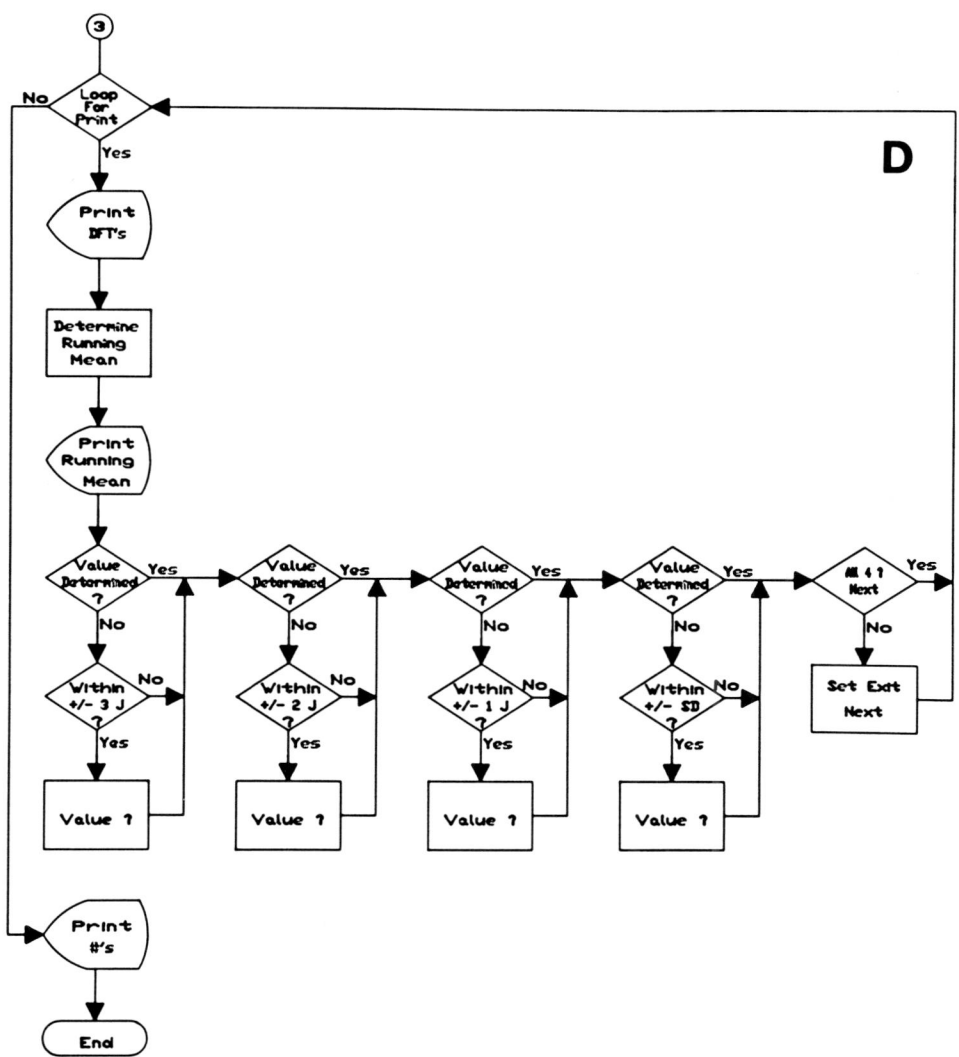

and defibrillation efficacy is determined using decrements, the estimated single DFT is likely to be high, and the safety margin ratio will be increased, although a lower ratio could be used. If the starting point is well below the midpoint, the estimated single DFT is likely to be low, the safety margin will be reduced, and a higher ratio should be used. However, relative error is reduced by using triplicate measurements [21,30,31]. "Thus the defibrillation threshold provides a reproducible estimate that should improve the accuracy of predicting defibrillation efficacy" [31].

VIII. ALTERNATIVE METHODS FOR ASSESSING DEFIBRILLATION

There are alternative methodologies used to determine defibrillating capabilities at the time of device implantation [40]. Does it really matter? Is there any improvement in long-term clinical

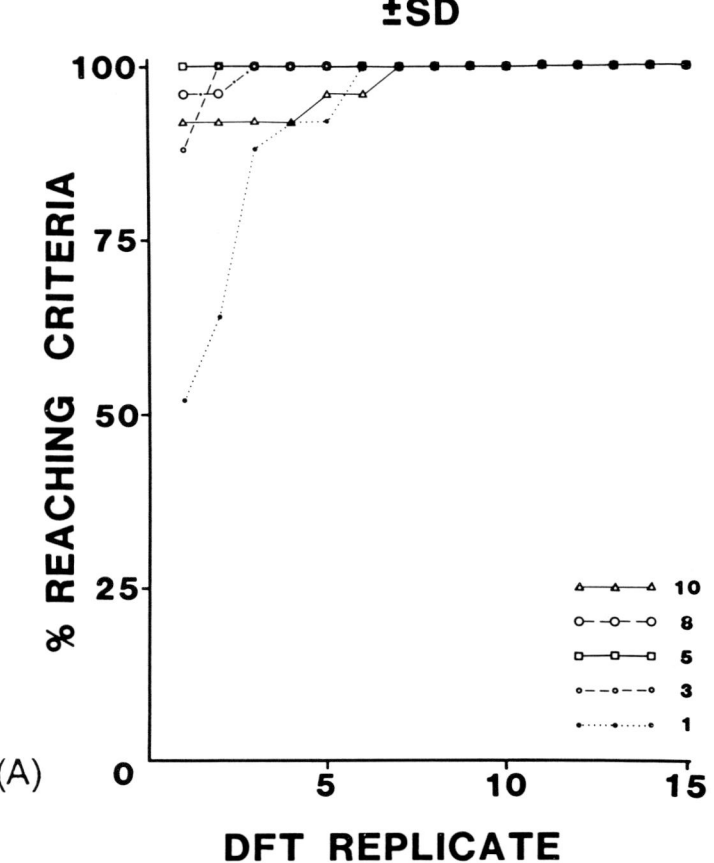

Figure 7 Representations of the DFT replicates meeting overall group criteria of: (A) within the range of the mean ± standard deviation (SD); (B) within the range of the mean ±1 J; (C) within the range of the mean ±2 J; and (D) within the range of the mean ±3 J.

outcome? Unfortunately, there is insufficient clinical data to answer these questions. However, it is important if the method selected does not allow device titration for subsequent changes in patient status. Here it may again be useful to look at some of the alternative computer and implantation methodologies.

Malkin et al. [43] used a Bayesian technique for estimating the 95% success and the absolute average difference was 8.7%, although this was highly dependent on ". . . significant prior knowledge [which] can be used to pick the test voltages . . ." [43]. In the previous section it was demonstrated that defibrillation thresholds differ depending on starting level and step size [21,30,31,44,45]. McDaniel and Schuder [44] argue that as few as 4 fibrillation episodes can be used to estimate the ED_{50} value with a standard deviation of 12% of the mean. In a revisitation of their model, McDaniel and Schuder have used the first reversal to initiate the four "up-down" steps [45], which more closely approximates the triplicate DFT technique [31], and provides the lowest total error [10]. However, in some clinical situations, the decision is simply to implant or not: "GO-NO GO."

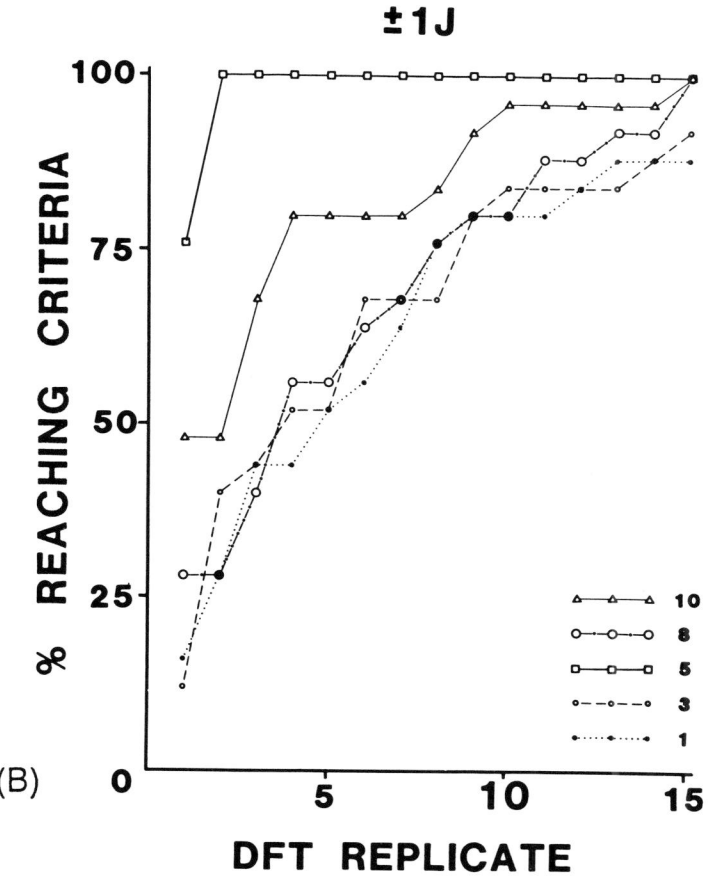

(B)

IX. ESTIMATED DEFIBRILLATION EFFICACY

A pragmatic method used at implant is to test a shock at a level approximately 10 J below the normal output of the device [40,58]. The number of successive defibrillations is then calculated with one or two repeat defibrillation shocks [40,58]. Thus the probability function determines an upper boundary only, using the "worst-case scenario." The principal behind this assessment relies on the concept that the relationship between the midpoint on the curve (ED_{50}) and the width of the curve is approximately equal to the ED_{50} value [58]. Therefore a width from 5% to 95% would be approximately three times the minimum "dose" (i.e., 5% = E_{min}). To provide some additional safety margin for the device, an additional 0.5 times the value is added. Thus, the total calculated safety margin would be 3.5 times the value of a single successful shock (E_{min}) [58]. Obviously, for a patient at implant, with a starting energy setting of 15 J, even with a single successful defibrillation, the calculated "safety margin" would be unacceptably high (3.5 × 15 = 52.5 J). However, this estimate can be reduced if a second or a third shock is employed. Two successes would require 2.5 × E_{min} (2.5 × 15 = 37.5 J), and three successes at 15 J would require 1.7 × E_{min} (1.7 × 15 = 25.5 J) [58]. This technique provides only the "go–no go."

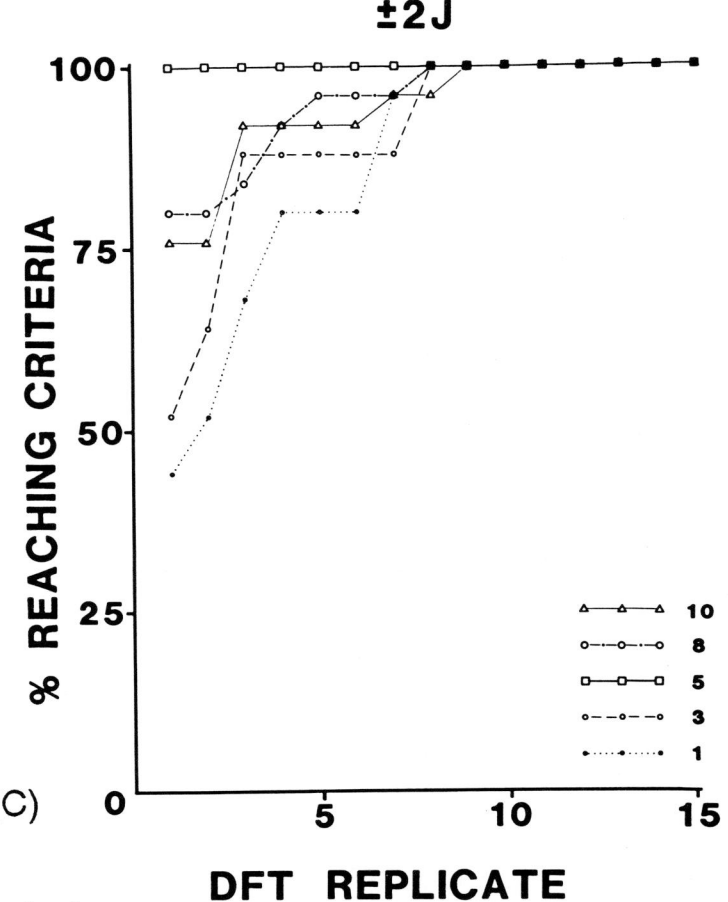

Figure 7 Continued

There are two additional limitations with this technique. The first is the lack of reliability in the measure. Even with three determinations, the variability is ⅓ for success versus failure. Thus, for patient safety, the "worst-case scenario" is accepted and implantation could be aborted inappropriately. The second disadvantage is that neither a curve nor a true DFT is established. Thus, further comparisons of interventions such as drugs, lead positions, or changes over time cannot be assessed [10,58].

A modification of this technique which partially overcomes this problem is to begin testing at 15–18 J (approximately 50% of the full device output), and to test successively lower values until a failure is recorded, then to retest the next higher level in a subsequent episode, similar to the "up–down" technique. Thus two successes at or below the midpoint of the device output is taken to provide reasonable assurance of "safety margin" for the patient, using a particular lead orientation [10,70].

X. UPPER LIMIT OF VULNERABILITY

These shock protocols are highly dependent on cooperation of all staff in the operating room, and are predicated on the clinical status of the patient undergoing repeated defibrillation test-

The Defibrillation Threshold

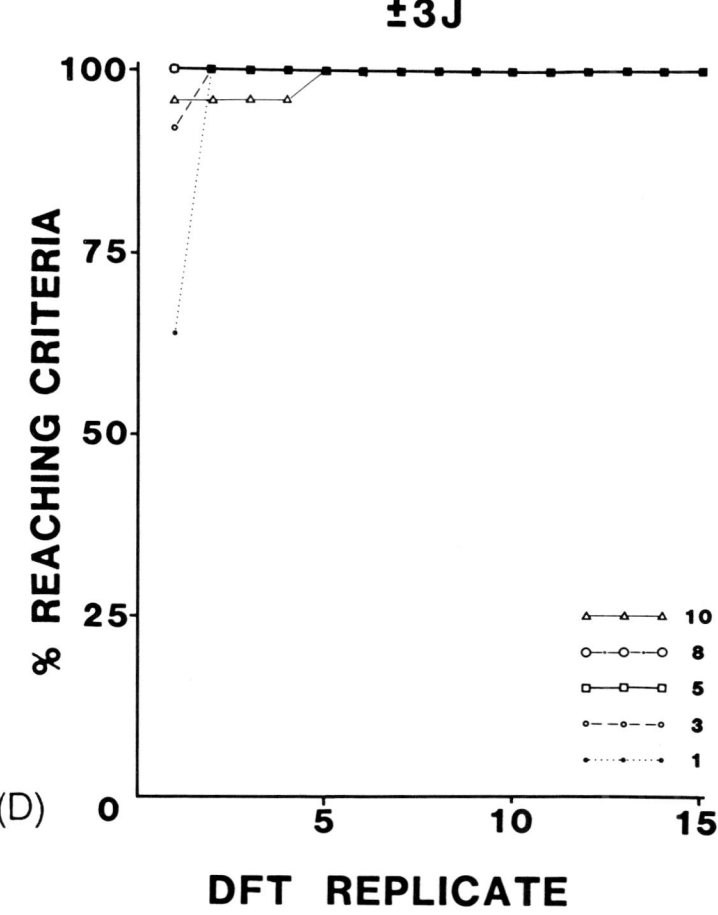

ing. Of particular interest is whether repeated defibrillation testing itself compromises patient safety. A novel methodology was recently proposed to reduce patient risk by reducing the number of fibrillation episodes using determination of the "upper limit of vulnerability" (ULV). An obvious concern with repeated fibrillation-defibrillation episodes is the prolongation of associated total ischemia time. Determination of a "defibrillation threshold" without inducing-fibrillation would alleviate some of this concern. Beginning with the findings from Ideker's laboratory using computerized mapping of voltage gradients during a defibrillation shock, Chen et al. [9] suggested that the phenomena described in the 1940s by Wiggers and associates might explain unsuccessful shocks. Their logic was that shock intensities which produced at least a minimum voltage gradient of approximately 6 V/cm exceeded the upper limit of vulnerability for refibrillation postshock. This concept was further developed to suggest that an alternative estimate of the energy necessary for defibrillation could be assessed without multiple inductions of fibrillation by determining the upper limit of vulnerability of shock strengths which will induce fibrillation during the vulnerable period (T wave) [8,9,13,37]. Using this technique, shocks initially at high intensity are delivered during the ventricular vulnerable period (paced or during sinus rhythm), with decreasing strength until a shock elicits fibrillation,

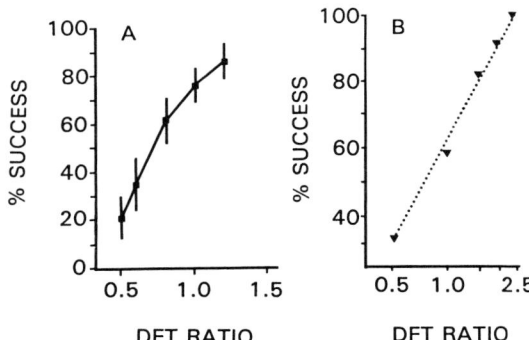

Figure 8 Defibrillation success curves for: (A) pigs [52], and (B) humans [34] when fixed ratios of the defibrillation threshold (DFT) were delivered after a single determination of the DFT.

which is rapidly terminated [8,9,13,37] to minimize fibrillation time. A significant correlation has been found between this ULV and the defibrillation threshold [8], although there are considerable discrepancies between the absolute DFTs and ULVs [8,9,13,37]. As pointed out by Singer and Lang [58], the ULV curve is also sigmoidal in shape and requires multiple estimates [58], and thus a simplified protocol needs to be established. In addition, repeated high-intensity shocks are required, and there are many reports of increased myocardial irritability and postshock arrhythmias with this technique [13], which are consistent with the concept that the degree of myocardial damage [48] and postshock arrhythmias are associated with shock intensity [29,48,63]. This begs the question: Is repeated fibrillation-defibrillation testing safe?

XI. DEFIBRILLATION TESTING: FRIEND OR FOE

The simple answer to this question is that it must be titrated to the individual patient. However, most investigators would agree that the assessment is unavoidable, but the potential for damage must be kept to a minimum, although there is not a consensus on that minimum level. There is clear evidence of damage due to transthoracic shocks and multiple direct cardiac shocks in animal studies [63], but little direct evidence in patients [18]. We [49], and others [16,47], have some anecdotal information indicating that the cardiac isoenzyme CPK is not significantly altered following normal defibrillation testing in humans. There is some data to indicate effects on cardiac function [38,58,60], but they are not detrimental beyond 10 min, and some of them might be due to shock-induced catecholamine release, or possibly in response to hypotension [63]. Singer and associates [57] presented data on the effects of defibrillation testing on patient EEG patterns. The results from 70 ventricular fibrillation episodes indicated that hypoperfusion with mean arterial pressures less than 30 mmHg elicited EEG alterations in five of five patients with less than six ventricular fibrillation episodes, but only one of five patients with greater than six ventricular fibrillation episodes. In addition, when hypoperfusion was prolonged beyond 20 sec, EEG changes persisted from several minutes up to an hour [57,58]. Although there was no neurological data provided on these patients, the authors comment that similar changes during coronary artery bypass surgery may be associated with confusion and perhaps even permanent neurological deficits [58]. Thus the authors recommend EEG monitoring during defibrillation testing [57].

On the other hand, Frame and associates [18] reported on a retrospective analysis of 84 patients having an average of 5.3 fibrillation episodes and up to 50 shocks during preimplantation of an automatic cardioverter-defibrillator. In this series, the authors did not have one patient demonstrate symptoms from cerebral hypoperfusion attributable to defibrillation testing [18]. Nevertheless, studies including EEG and neurological assessment with long-term follow-up are essential to establish clearly the effects of hypoperfusion during defibrillation testing.

XII. WAITING TIME BEFORE DELIVERING A TEST SHOCK

Even if there is limited problem with hypoperfusion during defibrillation testing, the questions remain: Does prolonged fibrillation alter defibrillation thresholds, and how long should one wait before delivering a defibrillation shock? The effects of fibrillation time are controversial, with suggestions that there is (1) a progressive increase [14,50], (2) a progressive decrease [1], or (3) no change over time [2,20,64] in the energy necessary to defibrillate. The reality is probably a combination of all three, depending on the time frame being considered. Several laboratories, including our own, have mapped the wavefronts at the onset of fibrillation. During the first several seconds there is a progressively more rapid tachycardiac rhythm, which eventually degenerates into multiple wavelets "chasing their tails in search of nonrefractory tissue." It is well known that true multiwavelet "fine" fibrillation requires several times more energy to defibrillate that ventricular tachycardia (and, by extension, probably ventricular flutter). This may explain why some defibrillation studies reported some successful very low defibrillation energy shocks, when the average time to shock delivery was only 4–7 s [14,48,68]. The question therefore is: When waiting, how long is long enough? This is undoubtably species, drug state, and wavefront activation time dependent. However, to get some handle on this problem, we reviewed over 400 fibrillation episodes in pigs, in which the shock was delivered at least 10 s after the onset of fibrillation. There were virtually no returns to sinus rhythm, from what was clearly fibrillation, after approximately 8 s had expired. However, the number of reversions was progressively increased below 8 s.

In the operating room, our experience has indicated that there is very little return from fibrillation after 20 s; however, this has not been explored systematically. When AC was used to induce fibrillation, there were some returns to sinus rhythm within 5 to 10 s after cessation of stimulation, and even one case with return to sinus rhythm after approximately 15 s (Fig. 9). Routinely, we now wait at least 20 s from the initiation of fibrillation by AC before beginning defibrillation testing. However, caution is warranted, as there is a limited time window for defibrillation testing before there are patient problems associated with prolonged defibrillation-induced ischemia time [20,57].

In a study on pigs [20], where defibrillation thresholds were determined in random order at 10, 20, 40, and 60 s after the onset of fibrillation, no difference in defibrillation thresholds was found. This is consistent with the findings of Murakawa et al. [48], who found significantly lower values at 5 s but no statistical differences between 10 and 20 s. However, they differ from those of Echt et al. [14], who found no difference between ED_{50} and ED_{90} values at 5 and 15 s but significant elevations at 30 s, and those of Platia et al. [50], who found progressive differences at 5, 15, and 25 s. However, caution is warranted with these results, as was indicated previously in this chapter: There may be a problem with the equation used by Echt and associates [14] in calculating the dose–response curve [31].

On the other hand, there are increases in electromechanical dissociation with protracted time before defibrillation [1,20,50], and the incidence of complete heart block even with shocks at 1.4 × DFT [20]. As a general rule of thumb, even in the early studies we did not allowed fibrillation to continue in any experiment beyond 90 s, and rarely does it go beyond 45 s from the onset of AC current. Babbs et al. [1] found that fibrillation bouts longer that 2 min became progressively easier to defibrillate, presumably due to the extracellular accumulation of potassium. However, Yakaitis et al. [69] found transthoracic defibrillation progressively more

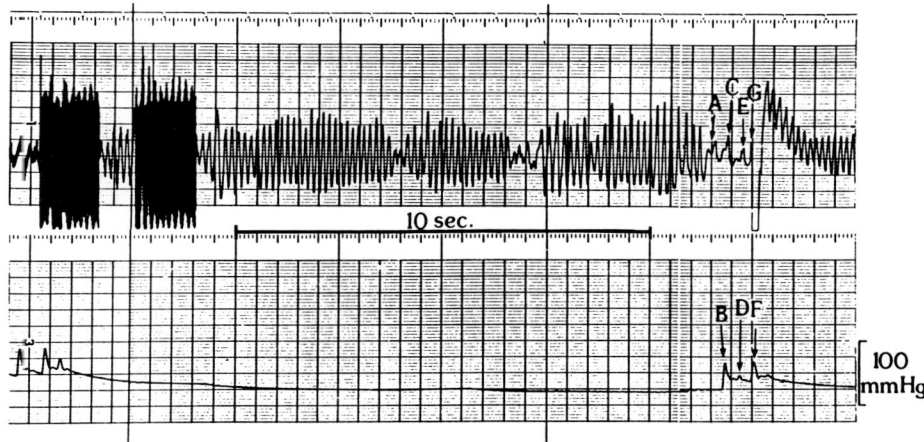

Figure 9 Example of return of contracture after presumed "ventricular fibrillation" induction. The tracings are continuous electrocardiographic (top) and blood pressure (bottom) recording from a patient in the operating room. Two brief trains of AC appeared to induce ventricular fibrillation with a precipitous fall in blood pressure. Eighteen seconds after the initiation of the first AC train, three spontaneous contractures (A, C, and E) clearly elicited return of blood pressure (B, D, and F, respectively). These were not noted in sufficient time to abort the delivery of a "defibrillation" shock (G), which promptly returned the heart to fibrillation.

difficult when tested at 1, 3, 5, and 9 min. At the present time there is no consensus on the effects of time, although with very early shocks it may be possible with lower-energy shocks to arrest tachyarrhythmias before they degenerate into true fibrillation.

XIII. SETTING THE LEVEL OF THE FIRST SHOCK THERAPY

Another controversial question facing the clinician at the time of implantation is: How high should the first shock therapy be programmed? Again, there is no consensus. However, if triplicate defibrillation thresholds have been determined and their mean is low, it seems reasonable to start with an initial shock below the maximum output of the device. The second or third shock may be programmed at device maximum. By not charging to the maximum of the device, the charge time and battery drain will be significantly reduced. In addition, if the first shock is at $1.5-2.0 \times$ DFT, greater than approximately 90% of the attempts should be successful on the first attempt; combined with the second or third shock, the maximum likelihood of success should be obtained. For the patient where only a "go–no go" has determined the eligibility for implantation, the first shock setting is more questionable. An initial setting at two-thirds of the maximum output of the device would be reasonable only if the criterion for accepting implantation was established with successes at or below 50% of the device output. This often is at 10 J below maximum device output for present devices [40].

There have been some suggestions of problems with delivering unsuccessful preshocks [3]. However, several laboratories have reported either no problem with initial low-energy shocks [20,64], or effects were attributable to the protracted time to deliver additional successful therapy [50]. Even with the present technology, within 60 s a third "rescue shock" at the full charge could be available if necessary. With the engineering developments to improve electrodes and allow faster charge times of even large capacitors, allowing multiple-phase shocks, plus the biological advances in improved electrode locations using these superior waveforms, as well as the potential of coupling a device-controlled drug delivery to improve defibrillation, there will be significantly enhanced patient safety margin in future-generation devices, as well as if low-energy shocks can be delivered early in the tachyarrhythmia stages to terminate the arrhythmia before it degenerates into true ventricular fibrillation.

XIV. SUMMARY

Ventricular fibrillation is a process with inherent variability, making the assessment of defibrillation efficacy difficult. In this chapter the theoretical basis of determining a "defibrillation threshold" using an up–down algorithm and triplicate replications was presented. In addition to computer-based mathematical models, data from animal and clinical experiments have demonstrated that such a defibrillation threshold is a reliable, reproducible, and rapid technique for estimating defibrillation efficacy. Regardless of method for assessing defibrillation efficacy, each model presumes a sigmoidal curve reaching and sustaining a maximum at 100% success. In addition, the presumption is that the curves do not have a parallel shift, but rather the slope changes with the midpoint (DFT or ED_{50}) [10,43,44,58]. Thus changes in patch configuration or waveform will change both the DFT and the steepness of the dose–response curve. As additional chapters in this book address the specifics of these differences directly, they were not elaborated in this chapter except to indicate the relationship between the DFT (ED_{50}) and the steepness of the dose–response curve. Although this relationship appears to be borne out in group data [10,11,25,31,54,58], it has not been rigorously tested experimentally. In addition, for some subjects, defibrillation success may not reach 100% or, having reached 100% success at a particular energy setting, at higher shock intensities, success may again decrease [55,63].

For the clinician at the time of implantation, there are additional considerations and constraints, such as the maximum allowable fibrillation time and number of shocks. Taking all these into consideration, a rational approach to titrating the defibrillation system to the specific needs of the individual patient can be achieved, even using an up–down, "go–no go" algorithm.

ACKNOWLEDGMENTS

This work would not have been completed without the contributions from collaborators, research fellows, students whose names are on the papers in the reference list (and therefore will not be listed separately here), and technicians, G. K. Wood, M. Densmore, D. McLellan, and E. Jarvis, as well as the surgical staff of OR #5, University Hospital, London. In addition, defibrillating electrodes and defibrillators were kindly provided through Dr. M. J. Kallok and more recently R. Mehra of Medtronic, Inc. Funding has been provided by the Medical Research Council of Canada, the Heart and Stroke Foundation of Ontario, and the Ontario Ministry of Health.

REFERENCES

1. Babbs CF, Whistler SJ, Yim GK. Temporal stability and precision of ventricular defibrillation threshold data. Am J Physiol (Heart Circ Physiol 4) 1978; 235: H553-H558.
2. Bardy GH, Ivey TD, Allen M, Johnson G. A prospective randomized evaluation of effects of ventricular fibrillation duration on defibrillation thresholds in humans. J Am Coll Cardiol 1989;13:1362-1366.

3. Bardy GH, Stewart RB, Ivey TD, et al. Potential risk of low energy cardioversion attempts by implantable defibrillators. J Am Coll Cardiol 1987; 9:168A.
4. Bates D, Watts D. Nonlinear Regression Analysis and Its Applications. New York: John Wiley, 1988.
5. Bourland JD, Tacker WA, Wessale JL, Kallok MJ, Graf JE, Geddes LA. Sequential pulse defibrillation for implantable defibrillators. Med Instrum 1986; 20:138-142.
6. Brownlee KA, Hodges JL, Rosenblatt M. The up-and-down method with small samples. J Am Statist Assoc 1953; 48:262-277.
7. Chapman PD, Sagar KB, Wetherbee JN, Troup PJ. Relationship of left ventricular mass to defibrillation threshold for the implantable defibrillator: a combined clinical and animal study. Am Heart J 1987; 114:274-278.
8. Chen P-S, Feld GK, Mower MM, Peters BB. The effects of pacing rate and timing of shocks on the relationship between defibrillation threshold and upper limit of vulnerability in open chest dogs. J Am Coll Cardiol 1991; 18:1555-1563.
9. Chen P-S, Shibata N, Dixon EG, Martin RO, Ideker RE. Comparison of the defibrillation threshold and the upper limit of ventricular vulnerability. Circulation 1986; 73: 1022-1028.
10. Church T, Martinson M, Kallok M, Watson W. A model to evaluate alternative methods of defibrillation threshold determination. PACE 1988; 11:2002-2007.
11. Davy J-M, Fain ES, Dorian P, Winkle RA. The relationship between successful defibrillation and delivered energy in open-chest dogs: reappraisal of the defibrillation threshold concept. Am Heart J 1987; 113:77-84.
12. Deeb GM, Griffith BP, Thompson ME, Langer A, Heilman MS, Hardesty RL. Lead systems for internal fibrillation. Circulation 1981; 64:242-245.
13. DeGroot PJ, Norenberg MS, Mehra R. Relationship between the upper limit of vulnerability and defibrillation threshold using a three-electrode system. PACE 1991; 14:689.
14. Echt DS, Barbey JT, Black JN. Influence of ventricular fibrillation duration on defibrillation energy in dogs using bidirectional pulse discharges. PACE 1988; 11:1315-1323.
15. Echt DS, Cato EL, Coxe DR. pH-dependent effects of lidocaine on defibrillation energy requirements in dogs. Circulation 1989; 80:1003-1009.
16. Ehsani AA, Ewy GA, Sobel BE. CPK isoenzyme elevations after electrical countershock. Am J Cardiol 1976; 37:12-18.
17. Ewy, GA, Horan WJ. Effectiveness of direct current defibrillation: role of paddle size II. Am Heart J 1977; 93:674-675.
18. Frame R, Brodman R, Furman S, et al. Clinical evaluation of safety of repetitive intraoperative defibrillation threshold testing. PACE 1992; 15:870-877.
19. Freund JE, Walpole RE. Point estimation: In: Mathematical Statistics, 3rd ed. Englewood Cliffs, NJ: Prentice Hall, 1980:310-325.
20. Fujimura O, Jones DL, Klein GJ. Effects of time to defibrillation and subthreshold preshocks on defibrillation success in pigs. PACE 1989; 12:358-365.
21. Fujimura O, Jones DL, Klein GJ. The defibrillation threshold: how many measurements are enough? Am Heart J 1989; 117:971-979.
22. Geddes LA. A short history of the electrical stimulation of excitable tissue including electrotherapeutic applications. The Physiologist 1984; 27 (suppl):S1-S47.
23. Geddes LA, Tacker WA, Rosborough JP, et al. The electrical dose for ventricular defibrillation with electrodes applied directly to the heart. J Thorac Cardiovasc Surg 1974; 68:593-602.
24. Glass L, Mackey MC. The Rhythms of Life. Princeton, NJ: Princeton University Press, 1988; XVIII:248.
25. Gliner BE, Murakawa Y, Thakor NV. The defibrillation success rate versus energy relationship. Part I—curve fitting and the most efficient defibrillation energy. PACE 1990; 13:326-338.
26. Gliner BE, Murakawa Y, Thakor NV. The defibrillation success rate versus energy relationship: Part II—estimation with the "Bootstrap." PACE 1990; 13:425-431.

27. Gutgesell HP, Tacker WA, Geddes LA, Davis JS, Lie JT, McNamara DG. Energy dose for ventricular defibrillation of children. Pediatrics 1976; 58:898-901.
28. Hooker DR, Kouwenhoven WB, Langworthy OR. The effect of alternating electrical currents on the heart. Am J Physiol 1933; 103:444-454.
29. Jones DL. Responses to a defibrillation shock: the good, the bad and the ugly. Am Heart J 1992; 124:834.
30. Jones DL, Fujimura O, Klein GJ. Minimum replications to estimate average threshold energy for defibrillation. Med Instrum 1988; 11:298-303.
31. Jones DL, Irish WD, Klein GJ. Defibrillation efficacy: comparison of defibrillation threshold versus dose–response curve determination. Circ Res 1991; 69:45-51.
32. Jones DL, Klein GJ, Guiraudon GM, et al. Internal cardiac defibrillation in man: pronounced improvement with sequential pulse delivery to two different lead orientations. Circulation 1986; 73:484-491.
33. Jones DL, Klein GJ, Guiraudon GM, et al. Sequential pulse defibrillation in man: comparison of thresholds in normal subjects and those with cardiac disease. Med Instrum 1987; 21:166-169.
34. Jones DL, Klein GJ, Guiraudon GM, Sharma AD, Yee R, Kallok MJ. Prediction of defibrillation success from a single defibrillation threshold measurement with sequential pulses and two current pathways in humans. Circulation 1988; 78:1144-1149.
35. Jones DL, Klein GJ, Kallok MJ. Improved defibrillation threshold with sequential pulse energy delivered to different lead orientations in pigs. Am J Cardiol 1985; 55:821-825.
36. Jones DL, Sohla A, Bourland JD, Tacker WA, Kallok MJ, Klein GJ. Internal ventricular defibrillation with sequential pulse counter shock in pigs: comparison with single pulses and effects of pulse separation. PACE 1987; 10:497-502.
37. Kavanagh KM, Harrison JH, Dixon EG, et al. Correlation of the probability of success curves for defibrillation and for the upper limit of vulnerability. PACE 1990; 13:536.
38. Kerber RE, Martens JB, Gascho JA, Marcus ML. Effects of direct-current countershocks on regional myocardial contractility and perfusion. Circulation 1981; 63:323-332.
39. Kowenhoven WB, Milnor WR. Treatment of ventricular fibrillation using a capacitor discharge. J Appl Physiol 1954; 7:253-257.
40. Lehmann MH, Steinman RT, Schuger CD, Jackson K. Defibrillation threshold testing and other practices related to AICD implantation: do all roads lead to Rome? PACE 1989; 12:1530-1537.
41. Lucy SD, Jones DL, Klein GJ. Defibrillation is increased over time in a dog model of congestive heart failure. Circulation 1990; 82:III-709.
42. Malkin RA, Pilkington TC. A new defibrillation efficacy estimator using upper limit of vulnerability testing. Am Heart J 1992; 124:832.
43. Malkin RA, Pilkington TC, Johnson EE, Ideker RE. Optimum estimation of the 95 percent effective defibrillation dose. Proc IEEE Eng Med Biol Soc 1991; 13:775-759.
44. McDaniel WC, Schuder JC. The cardiac ventricular defibrillation threshold: inherent limitations in its application and interpretation. Med Instrum 1987; 21:170-176.
45. McDaniel WC, Schuder JC. An up–down algorithm for estimation of the cardiac ventricular defibrillation threshold. Med Instrum 1988; 22:286-292.
46. Mead RH, Ruder M, Schmidt P, Gaudiane V, Winkle R. Improved defibrillation efficacy with chronically implanted defibrillation leads. Circulation 1986; 74:II-110.
47. Mower M, Mirowski M, Denniston RH, Staewen WS, Tabatznik B. The effects of intra-arterial and intra-ventricular countershock on the surrounding myocardium. Circulation 1971; 44:II-203.
48. Murakawa Y, Gliner BE, Thakor NV. Success rate versus defibrillation energy: temporal profile and the most efficient defibrillation threshold. Am Heart J 1989; 118:451-458.
49. Perkins DG, Klein GJ, Silver MD, Yee R, Jones DL. Cardioversion and defibrillation using a catheter electrode: myocardial damage assessed at autopsy. PACE 1987; 10:800-804.
50. Platia EV, Waclawski SH, Pluth TA, Brooks S, Mispireta L. Automatic implantable defibrillators (AICD): implications of delayed and subthreshold shocks. Circulation 1987; 76:IV-311.

51. Prevost JL, Battelli F. Some effects of electrical discharge on the hearts of mammals. Compt Rend Acad Sci 1899; 129:1267-1268.
52. Rattes MF, Jones DL, Sharma AD, Klein GJ. Defibrillation threshold: a simple and quantitative estimate of the ability to defibrillate. PACE 1987; 10:70-77.
53. Rattes MF, Jones DL, Sohla A, Sharma AD, Jarvis E, Klein GJ. Defibrillation with the sequential pulse technique: reproducibility with repeated shocks. Am Heart J 1986; 111:874-878.
54. Schuder JC, Gold JH, Stoeckle MD, Roberts SA, McDaniel WC, Moellinger DW. Defibrillation in the calf with bidirectional trapezoidal wave shocks applied via chronically implanted epicardial electrodes. Trans Am Soc Artif Inter Organ 1981; 37:467-470.
55. Schuder JC, Stoeckle MD, Dolan AM: Transthoracic ventricular defibrillation and square-wave stimuli, one-half cycle, one cycle, and multicycle waveforms. Circ Res 1964; 15:258-264.
56. Seber GAF. Nonlinear Regression. New York: John Wiley, 1989.
57. Singer I, Edmonds HL, van der Laken C, et al. Is defibrillation threshold testing safe? PACE 1991; 14:1899-1904.
58. Singer I, Lang D. Defibrillation threshold: clinical utility and therapeutic implications. PACE 1992; 15:932-949.
59. Sokal RR, Rohlf FJ. Biometry. San Francisco: Freeman, 1981:859.
60. Stoddard MF, Redd RR, Buckingham TA, McBride LR, Labovitz AJ. Effects of electrophysiologic testing of the automatic implantable cardioverter-defibrillator on left ventricular systolic function and diastolic filling. Am Heart J 1991; 122:714-719.
61. Suddaby EC, Riker SL. Defibrillation and cardioversion in children. Pediatr. Nurs. 1991; 17:477-481.
62. Tacker WA, Galioto G, Giuliani E, Geddes LA, McNamara DG. Energy dosage for human transchest defibrillation. N Engl J Med 1974; 290:214-215.
63. Tacker WA Jr, Geddes LA. Electrical Defibrillation. Boca Ratan, FL: CRC Press, 1979: 192.
64. Troup PJ, Chapman PD, Wetherbee JN, Duquette S, Vetter J. Do subthreshold shocks increase energy requirement for subsequent defibrillation attempts? Circulation 1987; 76:IV-311.
65. Wetherill GB, Levitt H. Sequential estimation of points on a psychometric function. Br J Math Stat Psychol 1965; 18:1-10.
66. Wiggers CJ. The physiological basis for cardiac resuscitation from ventricular fibrillation—method for serial defibrillation. Am Heart J 1940; 20:412-422.
67. Winkle RA, Stenson EB, Bach SM, Echt DS, Oyer P, Armstrong K. Cardioversion/defibrillation thresholds in man using truncated exponential waveform and an apical patch-SVC spring electrode configuration. Circulation 1984; 69:766-779.
68. Winkle RA, Mead RH, Ruder MA, et al. Improved energy defibrillation efficacy in man with the use of a biphasic truncated exponential waveform. Am Heart J 1989; 117:122-127.
69. Yakaitis RW, Ewy GA, Otto CW, Taren DL, Moor TE. The influence of time and therapy on ventricular defibrillation in dogs. Crit Care Med 1980; 8:157-163.
70. Yee R, Klein GJ, Sharma A, Guiraudon G, Jones DL, Norris C. The pacemaker/cardioverter-defibrillator: initial experience at the time of implant. New Trends in Arrhythmia 1988; IV(3):921-926.

3

Unipolar Defibrillation

Gust H. Bardy

University of Washington
Seattle, Washington

I. INTRODUCTION

Implantable cardioverter-defibrillators (ICDs) provide protection against sudden cardiac death (SCD) [1–10], a major cause of death in the United States. However, there have been some objections to the use of ICDs due to procedural morbidity and mortality [11–18], cost of thoracic surgery, and the prolonged inpatient hospitalization associated with epicardial implantation [19–22]. Present transvenous lead systems have helped reduce some of the morbidity, mortality, and cost associated with defibrillator implantation. But they are far from simple. In this chapter, a new unipolar, single-lead, single incision transvenous defibrillation system is described that is as efficient as epicardial lead systems, decreases surgical time and cost of defibrillator surgery, and potentially makes the use of ICDs a more practical preventive tool against SCD [23].

II. UNIPOLAR AND STANDARD NONTHORACOTOMY DEFIBRILLATION LEAD SYSTEMS: CLINICAL EXPERIENCE

The unipolar defibrillation lead system was tested in 40 consecutive patients. These cardiac arrest survivors had syncopal ventricular tachycardia (VT), ventricular fibrillation (VF), or both. Seventy-eight percent of these patients (31 of 40) were men. Ages ranged from 27 to 73 years, with a mean of 57 ± 13 years.

The unipolar defibrillation lead system consisted of a 10.5-F anodal 5-cm-long endocardial right ventricular (RV) defibrillation electrode (Medtronic model 6966) and a generator titanium shell electrode (Medtronic model 7219C). The cathodal shell electrode's surface area was 108 cm^2. The RV endocardial lead, which had standard bipolar pace and sense electrodes at the tip, was inserted into the left cephalic vein when possible; otherwise, the left subclavian vein was

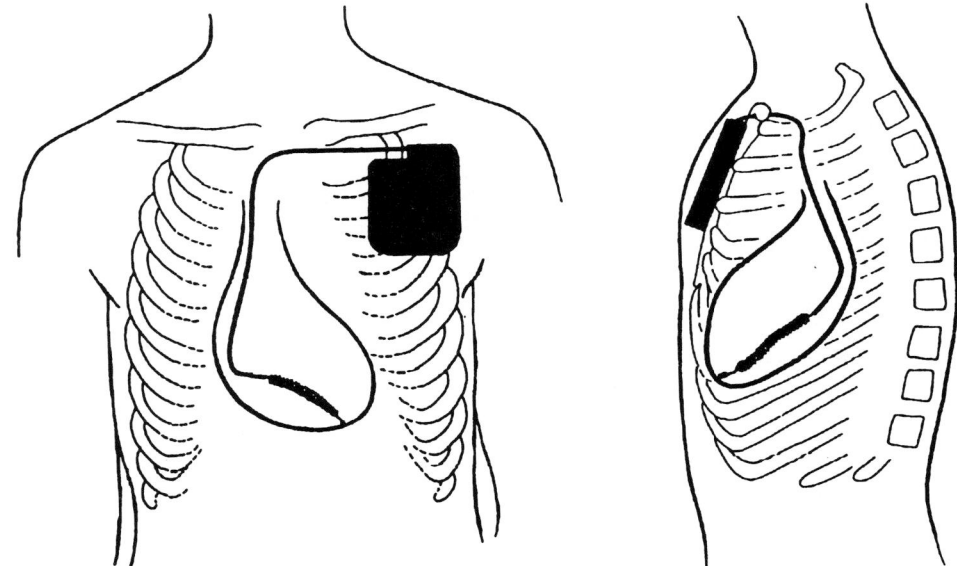

Figure 1 Unipolar transvenous defibrillation system showing a single tripolar lead inserted into the RV apex. (Reprinted with permission of the American Heart Association Bardy, et al., Circulation 1993; 88:543.)

used. The 7219C pulse generator shell was positioned on the pectoralis major muscle fascia (see Fig. 1).

The unipolar defibrillation system was compared to the best configuration found with a nonthoracotomy transvenous defibrillation lead system defined as the "standard" transvenous lead system and consisting of three defibrillation electrodes and a pulse generator (Medtronic model 7217B) [24]. The pulse generator was positioned in the abdomen, and its shell was not electrically active. Three leads were used. The two transvenous leads were the 110-cm, 10.5-F RV tripolar pace, sense, and defibrillation lead (Medtronic model 6966), and a 110-cm, 6.5-F catheter (Medtronic model 6963) that had a 5-cm-long coil electrode that could be positioned in either the superior vena cava or the coronary sinus. The third electrode was a 56-cm^2 subcutaneous chest patch electrode (Medtronic model 6921L). This electrode was positioned over the anterolateral left thorax.

III. DEFIBRILLATION THRESHOLD TESTING

The defibrillation threshold (DFT) was defined as the lowest pulse amplitude that could successfully terminate VF 10 s after its initiation [25,26]. Because of the limitations of repetitive VF induction and termination in humans, the DFT was measured only once for each defibrillation lead system examined.

A 65%-tilt asymmetric biphasic defibrillation pulse delivered between the RV endocardial electrode and the pulse-generator titanium shell electrode was used with the unipolar defibrillation lead system [27–29]. For the standard defibrillation lead system, a monophasic 65%-tilt dual-pathway pulse was delivered simultaneously or sequentially across the two pathways [10,24,30,31]. The first transvenous defibrillation test began with a 10-J stored energy pulse delivered 10 s after VF onset, including the time period during which alternating current was

Table 1 Comparative Defibrillation Data

	Unipolar	Standard
DFT stored energy	9.3 ± 6.0 J	11.3 ± 4.9 J
Leading-edge voltage	376 ± 119 V	424 ± 95 V
Leading-edge resistance	58 ± 7 Ω	62 ± 14 Ω
No. of VF inductions (to determine the best pulsing method and to measure DFT)	3.4 ± 0.8	7.4 ± 3.2
Time (lead insertion and DFT testing to meet implant criteria)	100 ± 28 min	183 ± 19 min

applied [28]. If the transvenous pulse was unsuccessful, a transthoracic rescue pulse was delivered immediately.

After a minimum rest period of 3 min between VF inductions, pulse output was increased or decreased, depending on transvenous shock failure or success. Between each VF induction and termination, care was taken to ensure that ECG ST-T segments, QRS duration, and arterial pressure had returned to baseline values before VF was reinitiated.

IV. UNIPOLAR DEFIBRILLATION TESTING RESULTS

Data on the unipolar defibrillation lead system compared favorably with the standard nonthoracotomy transvenous defibrillation lead system. As shown in Table 1, the unipolar defibrillation lead system outperformed even the best of the several standard defibrillation lead systems tested.

Thirty-seven of the 40 patients (93%) were defibrillated by less than 20 J using the unipolar defibrillation lead system, and 39 of 40 (98%) by less than 24 J (Fig. 2). With the stan-

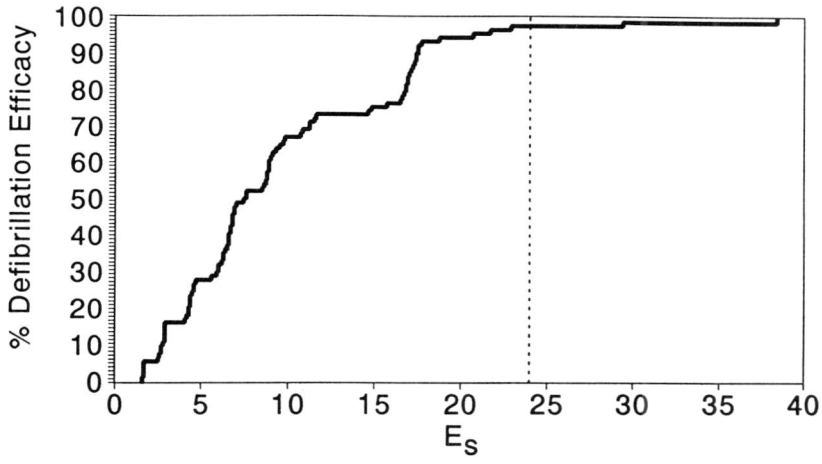

Figure 2 Defibrillation percent efficacy for the unipolar defibrillation system. (Reprinted with permission of the American Heart Association Bardy, et al., Circulation 1993; 88:543.)

dard defibrillation lead system, to achieve defibrillation efficacy comparable to that possible with the unipolar defibrillation lead system, an average of 4.0 ± 2.2 pulsing methods had to be tested to find a suitable nonthoracotomy transvenous defibrillation lead system that would satisfy the implant criterion.

V. DISCUSSION

The single-lead, single-incision unipolar defibrillation lead system is efficient and requires few VF inductions for confirmation of efficacy. The defibrillating efficiency is related to a number of factors. First, use of a 65% tilt biphasic waveform has been shown to be superior to monophasic waveform defibrillation, as demonstrated in earlier clinical studies [28,29]. Second, the vectors appear good. As shown in Fig. 1, current is directed from right to left and inferior to superior. Depending on the RV defibrillation coil location, the current also may be directed posterior to anterior. Third, electrode polarity may contribute to defibrillation success. Previous studies suggest that the electrode closest to the left ventricle should be anodal for optimal defibrillation [32,33]. Fourth, defibrillation is more efficient due to the use of a continuous-surface-area electrode (pulse generator's titanium casing), which decreases pulsing resistance and, in turn, increases current delivery.

There are several practical procedural advantages to the unipolar defibrillation lead system. First, only one standard infraclavicular incision is required. Currently, two or three incisions are needed to position the patches and pulse generator. Second, a standard lead length is used. Present transvenous lead systems are more than 100 cm long and require tunneling procedures under the thoracic skin to an abdominal pocket. With the unipolar defibrillation lead system, the pulse generator is small enough to be placed in an infraclavicular pocket, and therefore the lead length need only be the standard pacemaker length of 58 cm. This shortened lead is much easier to manipulate than long leads. Moreover, tunneling is no longer required. In addition, shorter leads are easier to replace should lead fractures occur.

A third advantage of the unipolar defibrillation lead system is that implantation may be possible using local anesthesia rather than general anesthesia. In the standard defibrillation lead system, general anesthesia is needed for two reason: (1) multiple incisions and tunneling of electrodes and (2) intubation to maintain ventilation during repetitive VF inductions. However, with the unipolar defibrillation lead system, only one incision is needed, and tunneling is avoided by the short lead length. Extensive testing is unnecessary due to the unipolar defibrillation lead system's reliable defibrillation at low DFTs.

With the possibility of defibrillators being implanted under local anesthesia, the procedure could be performed in the electrophysiology laboratory rather than in the operating room. Therefore, personnel requirements, time requirements, and costs should decrease. In addition, the procedure may be performed on an outpatient basis if there are no other indications for hospitalization. Finally, the simplified technology used in the unipolar defibrillation lead system will allow the physician to concentrate on SCD prevention.

VI. CONCLUSION

This study has demonstrated that the unipolar, single-lead, single-incision defibrillation lead system is effective in the treatment of VT and VF, while being more efficient and procedurally advantageous over standard transvenous defibrillation lead systems. The unipolar defibrillation lead system uses a simplified implant procedure, requires fewer VF inductions, and provides defibrillation at energy levels comparable or superior to other lead systems. This results in valuable cost and time savings to both the physician and patient, while increasing the quality of the implantable defibrillator's performance.

REFERENCES

1. Mirowski M, Reid PR, Mower MM, et al. Termination of malignant ventricular arrhythmias with an implanted automatic defibrillator in human beings. N Engl J Med 1980; 303:322-324.
2. Echt D, Armstrong K, Schmidt P, Oyers PE, Stinson EB, Winkle RA. Clinical experience, complications, and survival in 70 patients with the automatic implantable cardioverter defibrillator. Circulation 1985; 71:289-296.
3. Lehmann MH, Steinman RT, Schuger C, Jackson K. The automatic implantable cardioverter defibrillator as antiarrhythmic treatment modality of choice for survivors of cardiac arrest unrelated to acute myocardial infarction. Am J Cardiol 1988; 62:803-805.
4. Tchou PJ, Kadn N, Anderson J, Caceres JA, Jazayeri M, Akhtar M. Automatic implantable cardioverter defibrillators and survival of patients with left ventricular dysfunction and malignant ventricular arrhythmias. Ann Intern Med 1988; 109:529-534.
5. Winkle RA, Mead RH, Ruder MA, Gaudiani VA, Smith NA, Buch WS, Schmidt P, Shipman T. Long-term outcome with the automatic implantable cardioverter-defibrillator. J Am Coll Cardiol 1989; 13:1353-1361.
6. Manolis AS, Tan-DeGuzman W, Lee MA, et al. Clinical experience in seventy-seven patients with the automatic implantable cardioverter defibrillator. Am Heart J 1989; 118:445-450.
7. Fogoros RN, Elson JJ, Bonnet CA, Fiedler SB, Burkholder JA. Efficacy of the automatic implantable cardioverter-defibrillator in prolonging survival in patients with severe underlying cardiac disease. J Am Coll Cardiol 1990; 16:381-386.
8. Lehmann MH, Thomas A, Jackson K, et al. Long-term outcome with implantable cardioverter defibrillator (ICD) therapy in a multicenter investigator-edited database (abstr). Circulation 1990; 82(suppl III):III-166A.
9. Akhtar M, Avitall B, Jazayeri M, et al. Role of implantable cardioverter defibrillator therapy in the management of high-risk patients. Circulation 1992; 85(suppl I):I-131-I-139.
10. Bardy GH, Troutman C, Poole JE, et al. Clinical experience with a tiered therapy multiprogrammable antiarrhythmia device. Circulation 1992; 35:1689-1698.
11. Platia EV, Griffith LSC, Reid PR, et al. Complications with the automatic implantable cardioverter-defibrillator (abstr). J Am Coll Cardiol 1986; 7:200A.
12. Marchlinski FE, Flores BT, Buxton AE, et al. The automatic implantable cardioverter-defibrillator: efficacy, complications, and device failures. Ann Intern Med 1986; 104:481-488.
13. Kelley PA, Cannorn DS, Garan H, et al. The automatic implantable cardioverter-defibrillator: efficacy, complications and survival in patients with malignant ventricular arrhythmias. J Am Coll Cardiol 1988; 11:1278-1286.
14. Borbola J, Denes P, Ezri MD, Hauser RG, Sery C, Goldin MD. The automatic implantable cardioverter-defibrillator: clinical experience, complications, and follow-up in 25 patients. Arch Intern Med 1988; 142:70-76.
15. Gartman DM, Bardy GH, Allen MD, Misbach GA, Ivey TD. Short term morbidity and mortality of implantation of automatic implantable cardioverter-defibrillator. J Cardiovasc Thorac Surg 1990; 100:353-359.
16. Kim SG, Fisher JD, Furman S, et al. Exacerbation of ventricular arrhythmias during the postoperative period after implantation of an automatic defibrillator. J Am Coll Cardiol 1991; 18:1200-1206.
17. Gohn D, Edel T, Pollard C, et al. Determinants of operative mortality in implantable cardioverter defibrillators (abstr). J Am Coll Cardiol 1991; 17:86A.
18. O'Donoghue S, Platia EV, Waclawski S, Mispireta L. Transient electrical storm; prognostic significance of very numerous automatic defibrillator discharges (abstr.). J Am Coll Cardiol 1991; 17:352A.

19. Kuppermann M, Luce BR, McGovern B, Podrid PJ, Bigger JT Jr, Ruskin JN. An analysis of the cost-effectiveness of the implantable defibrillator. Circulation 1990; 31:91-100.
20. O'Donoghue S, Platia EV, Brooks-Robinson S, Mispireta L. Automatic implantable cardioverter-defibrillator: is early implantation cost-effective? J Am Coll Cardiol 1990; 16:1258-1263.
21. Larsen GC, Manolis AS, Sonnenberg AS, Beshansky JR, Estes NAM, Pauker SG. Cost effectiveness of the AICD: effect of improved battery life and comparison with amiodarone therapy. J Am Coll Cardiol 1992; 19:1323-1334.
22. Campbell RWF. Life at a price: the implantable defibrillator. Br Med J 1990; 64:171-173.
23. Bardy GH, Johnson G, Poole JE, et al. A simplified, single-lead unipolar transvenous cardioversion-defibrillation system. Circulation 1993; 88(2):1-5.
24. Bardy GH, Hofer B, Johnson G, et al. Implantable transvenous cardioverter-defibrillators. Circulation 1993; 87:1152-1168.
25. Bardy GH, Ivey TD, Allen MD, Johnson G. A prospective, randomized evaluation of ventricular fibrillation duration on defibrillation thresholds in humans. J Am Coll Cardiol 1989; 13:1362-1366.
26. Bardy GH, Ivey TD, Allen MD, Johnson G, Greene HL. Prospective comparison of sequential pulse and single pulse defibrillation using two different clinically available systems in man. J Am Coll Cardiol 1989; 14:165-171.
27. Bardy GH, Allen MD, Mehra R, Johnson G. An effective and adaptable transvenous defibrillation system for use in humans. J Am Coll Cardiol 1990; 16:887-895.
28. Bardy GH, Ivey TD, Allen MD, Johnson G, Mehra R, Greene HL. A prospective, randomized evaluation of biphasic vs monophasic waveform pulses on defibrillation efficacy in humans. J Am Coll Cardiol 1989; 14:728-733.
29. Bardy GH, Troutman C, Johnson G, et al. Electrode system influence on biphasic waveform defibrillation efficacy in humans. Circulation 1991; 84:665-671.
30. Yee R, Klein GJ, Leitch JW, et al. A permanent transvenous lead system for an implantable pacemaker cardioverter-defibrillator: nonthoracotomy approach to implantation. Circulation 1992; 85:196-204.
31. Fromer M, Schlapfer J, Fischer A, Kappenberger L. Experience with a new implantable pacer-cardioverter-defibrillator for the therapy of recurrent sustained ventricular tachyarrhythmias: a step toward a universal tachyarrhythmia control device. PACE 1991; 14:1288-1298.
32. Bardy GH, Ivey TD, Allen MD, Johnson G, Greene HL. Evaluation of electrode polarity on defibrillation efficacy. Am J Cardiol 1989; 63:433-437.
33. O'Neill PG, Boahene KA, Lawrie GM, Harvill LF, Pacifico A. Evaluation of electrode polarity on defibrillation efficacy. J Am Coll Cardiol 1991; 17:707-711.

4

Basic Concepts in Tachycardia Management by Pacing

James A. Roth and John D. Fisher

Montefiore Medical Center
Bronx, New York

I. BACKGROUND

It was first recognized three decades ago that ventricular tachycardia occurring in the setting of bradycardia could be prevented by pacing at physiologic rates [1–6]. The next decade saw the advent of initial efforts at the more complex problem of prevention, management, and termination of tachycardias occurring outside the setting of preexistent bradycardia. By the mid-1970s, implantable devices capable of manually activated or automated tachycardia termination became available, but their use for the management of ventricular tachycardia was limited by the unpredictable risk of acceleration to potentially lethal arrhythmias posed by antitachycardia pacing. By contrast, the implantable defibrillator was highly effective and safe. Initial attempts to unify the benefits of antitachycardia pacing with the safety of defibrillation combined a separate antitachycardia pacemaker with a first-generation implantable defibrillator and were complicated by the complex interactions between devices. The present decade has seen the introduction of devices capable of the tiered introduction of pacing and shock therapies dictated by tachycardia characteristics and the efficacy or lack thereof of pacing attempts. The availability of such devices greatly broadens the potential applicability of pacing methods for termination of ventricular tachycardia. At the same time, the addition of this new therapeutic dimension complicates further the decisions faced by physicians in selecting appropriate therapy. This chapter addresses the basic physiology and theory of antitachycardia pacing, the relative performance of the many available strategies, and how these factors relate to the use of these methods with concomitant defibrillator backup.

II. PREVENTION OF TACHYCARDIA

Clinical data regarding the use of pacing methods to prevent tachycardia are limited by the sporadic nature of sustained, clinically significant tachycardias and the absence of criteria to assess efficacy for chronic therapy. Although preventive methods have shown some merit in the acute stabilization of patients with very frequent or incessant ventricular tachycardia, little is known about the long-term efficacy of these techniques, and hence their clinical role in long-term management remains uncertain.

A. Rate Support and Overdrive Suppression

In those patients in whom tachycardia occurs only in the setting of clinical bradycardia, the use of backup rate support pacing at physiologic rates is well established [7,8]. Pacing is also clearly useful in the management of the idiopathic as well as drug-induced prolonged QT syndromes by prevention of bradycardia and pauses that commonly precede the onset of Torsades de Pointes [9–12]. However, for the majority of tachycardias that are not dependent on bradycardia for initiation, prevention has been more problematic. Pacing at moderately above physiologic rates (overdrive suppression) can be demonstrated to decrease significantly the frequency of spontaneous ventricular ectopy and nonsustained ventricular tachycardia (VT) on ambulatory recordings [13]. Several reports have shown some value of overdrive suppression in selected patients [2,4,6,14–21], however its use to prevent sustained tachycardia in the chronic setting has been limited by unpredictable long-term efficacy. As ventricular overdrive pacing implies the obligate loss of AV synchrony, there may be advantage to the use of atrial or dual-chamber pacing for this application [10,22,23].

B. Alteration of Repolarization and Refractoriness

The initiation of reentry relies on critical timing within the tachycardia substrate and attempts to disrupt this process have shown some promise in experimental preparations. Restivo et al. [24] have reported, in a canine model of late postinfarction VT, that precisely timed and positioned stimuli can alter repolarization patterns and prevent induction of VT. A related phenomenon may have been observed by Marchlinski et al [25], who were able to prevent the induction of VT in a limited number of coronary patients by high-current-strength stimulation close to the site of origin of tachycardia.

C. Subthreshold Stimulation, Summation, and Inhibition

A conditioning stimulus or train of stimuli delivered below diastolic threshold (subthreshold) or above diastolic threshold but within the myocardial effective refractory period does not elicit a propagated response. However, such stimuli may either facilitate or prevent capture or propagation of a subsequent stimulus. The former process has been called *summation* and appears to be favored by high output conditioning stimuli, and the latter is called *inhibition* and has been associated with low output subthreshold conditioning stimuli [26]. As no propagated response is generated, the effect is highly localized [27,28]. Shenasa et al. [29] performed subthreshold stimulation at the site of early activity in 15 patients undergoing catheter or surgical mapping of ventricular tachycardia. In eight of these patients subthreshold stimulation was capable of termination of tachycardia on at least one occasion. Others have made similar observations in isolated patients [30–32]. Both summation and inhibition could provide potential avenues for the prevention or modulation of tachycardia, either by inhibition or facilitation of propagation in areas critical to initiation and maintenance of tachycardia.

At present, simple rate support and overdrive suppression represent the most practical potential avenues for tachycardia prevention. However, the undesirable physiologic consequences of continuous rapid pacing, and the present absence of devices capable of both dual-chamber stimulation and tachycardia termination, gives overdrive pacing limited applicability in the chronic management of ventricular tachycardia.

III. HEMODYNAMIC STABILIZATION TECHNIQUES

With the onset of tachycardia, a variety of undesirable physiologic consequences rapidly ensue. Hypotension is frequently immediate and profound; coronary ischemia, hypoperfusion, and shock may rapidly follow. Several techniques can be used in selected patients to alter this process favorably until definitive therapy can be accomplished. Pacing of the atrium can be used during ongoing ventricular tachycardia to optimize the timing of atrial contraction. In slower ventricular tachycardias, pacing the atrium above the tachycardia rate may restore appropriate AV synchrony and, by virtue of overdrive of the ventricular mechanism, restore a normal sequence of ventricular activation [33]. Hamer et al. [34] performed ventricular-triggered atrial pacing (AVT pacing) during ventricular tachycardia in eight patients with left ventricular dysfunction. Mean arterial pressure rose significantly, by a mean of 19 mmHg, and cardiac index by a small but significant degree. Based on blood pressure criteria, the optimal time for atrial contraction was early in diastole which resulted from atrial pacing between 60% and 73% of the RR interval. Another palliative technique which has been occasionally useful is to synchronize ventricular activation by simultaneous pacing at more than one site, resulting in narrowing of the QRS complex. Another technique, ventricular paired pacing [33,35–37], may be used during ventricular or supraventricular tachycardia to improve effective systolic pressure without alteration in overall heart rate. This is accomplished by advancing electrical systole of alternate beats by ventricular pacing, resulting in a diminished mechanical systole on the paced cycle but a potentiated systole on the ensuing unpaced beat. These techniques have found their main use in the stabilization of the patient with refractory or incessant tachycardias until definitive therapy can be delivered. With the evolution of more sophisticated devices, techniques such as AVT pacing may find wider application in stabilizing hemodynamics while initial therapeutic pacing attempts are undertaken.

IV. MECHANISMS OF TACHYCARDIA INTERRUPTION [38–40]

A. Resetting

The physiologic basis of tachycardia termination by pacing is best understood by examination of the related phenomena of resetting and entrainment of ongoing tachycardia. A premature stimulus delivered during ongoing tachycardia is frequently followed by a less than compensatory pause. This phenomenon, referred to as resetting, is closely related to and usually precedes successful tachycardia termination by pacing. Almendral et al [41] have examined the characteristics of resetting in response to single, double, or multicapture bursts in 53 patients during well-tolerated induced tachycardia. Resetting could be demonstrated in 55%, 79%, and 85% of tachycardias with single, double, or multiple extrastimuli, respectively. Successfully reset tachycardias tended to be somewhat slower (369 ms versus 349 ms). The same investigators have also examined the pattern of resetting to successively more premature extrastimuli [42]. With the onset of resetting, the return cycle to QRS onset was shorter than the tachycardia cycle length in 41% and shorter in 76% when corrected for propagation time from the stimulation site to tachycardia substrate. This recovery cycle remained either flat or increased with successively earlier extrastimuli. Those tachycardias likely to be terminated by extrastimuli frequently display a rapid progressive increase in the recovery cycle length prior to tachycardia termination. This steep resetting curve likely reflects the conduction characteristics of the critical area of slowed conduction, which eventually fails to conduct at the point of tachycardia termination [43–45]. This observed resetting behavior is most consistent with a reentrant basis for most well-tolerated ventricular tachycardias. That the reset recovery cycle is shorter than

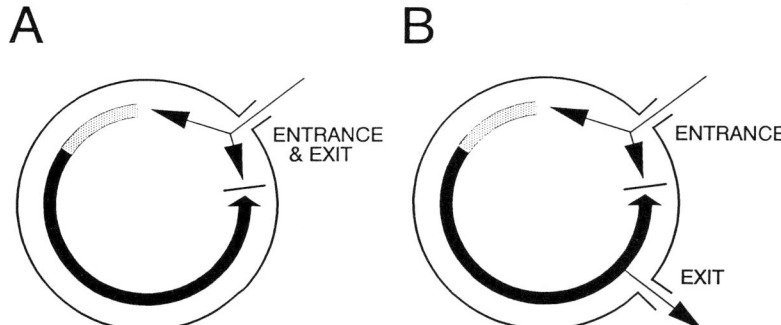

Figure 1 Single entrance and exit model (A) versus distinct entrance and exit model of reentrant ventricular tachycardia (B). In (A), a premature stimulus must traverse the entire circuit before reemerging as an advanced tachycardia beat. The resultant reset return cycle would be expected at greater than or equal to the tachycardia cycle length. In (B), a premature stimulus need traverse only a portion of the full tachycardia circuit, permitting the subsequent reset return cycle to occur at less than the tachycardia cycle length. Coronary VT most commonly conforms to the second model.

the unperturbed tachycardia cycle suggests that the paced beat traverses only a portion of the full circuit before emerging from the site of tachycardia origin as the advanced wavefront, and favors the concept of a anatomically distinct entrance and exit site to the tachycardia substrate (Fig. 1). The ability to reset most clinical tachycardias also implies the presence of a substantial excitable gap. Finally, the close association between a steep slope of resetting and ultimate termination suggests that successful pace termination relies on progressive failure followed by ultimate block in the area of slowed conduction by premature wavefronts.

B. Entrainment

Resetting is most easily observed during extrastimulus testing. However, during rapid ventricular pacing, resetting is frequently obscured by tachycardia termination [41]. Nonetheless, the closely allied phenomenon of transient entrainment or continuous resetting can be demonstrated (Fig. 2). In atrial flutter [46] and AV reentrant tachycardia [47], Waldo and co-workers have linked the characteristics of transient entrainment to the underlying reentrant mechanism of these tachycardias. The characteristic features of transient entrainment [47–49] include:

1. Constant fusion beats (or its electrogram equivalent) in the ECG during pacing except for the last captured beat, which is entrained but unfused. This is evidence of successive advancement or resetting of the tachycardia circuit with each paced cycle.
2. Constant but progressive fusion with increasing pacing rate.
3. Interruption of tachycardia associated with localized block for one beat followed by subsequent activation of that blocked site from a different direction. This is associated with a shift to a fully paced morphology on surface ECG.

These features appear to result from successive penetration and advancement without block (resetting) of the tachycardia circuit due to repeated premature excitation by the paced impulse. The fusion complex results from delayed emergence of the entrained tachycardia wavefront colliding with the ensuing paced wavefront. It is critical to recognize that because of the anatom-

Tachycardia Management by Pacing

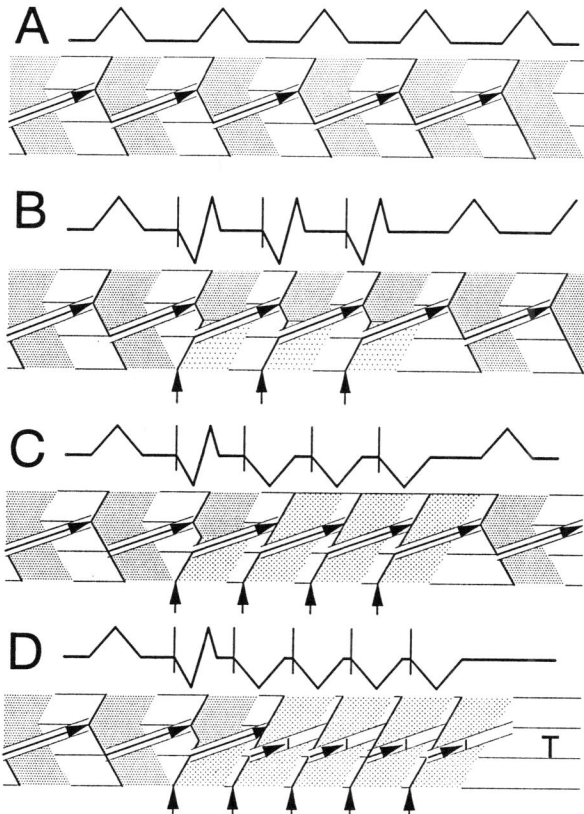

Figure 2 Entrainment of reentrant ventricular tachycardia by progressively faster bursts of ventricular pacing. Tachycardia is maintained by an anatomically or functionally isolated conduit of slowed conduction (diagonal long arrows) which bridges the diastolic interval and reexcites the ventricle from the tachycardia site or origin somewhere distant from the pacing site. The orthodromic emerging wavefront radiates from this site, generating the unperturbed tachycardia morphology (A). Pacing (vertical arrows) is applied into ongoing tachycardia at a site distant from the site of origin or exit site of the tachycardia circuit. With the introduction of pacing at moderate rates (B), the conduit of slowed conduction is engaged without tachycardia termination, resulting in a fused ventricular activation pattern. Pacing at faster rates (C) may be able to take over all ventricular activation, resulting in a shift to a fully paced morphology, but yet fail to induce block and hence terminate tachycardia. Pacing at still faster rates (D) induces block and termination (T) of the tachycardia. Stippled areas represent refractory myocardium left in the wake of the advancing depolarization wavefront.

ically distinct entry and exit of the area of slowed conduction, the paced wavefront is able to interact with the substrate via the entry without altering the initial ventricular activation induced by the orthodromic wavefront exiting from the site of origin of tachycardia. Increases in pacing rate typically result in a progressive shift toward the fully paced morphology. Block in the tachycardia circuit results in failure of entrainment, with consequent direct activation by the paced wavefront of sites near the tachycardia exit (the so-called site of origin during activation mapping studies). This forms the basis for the third criterion. The development of block for at least one cycle is an essential requisite for termination of reentrant tachycardia.

One or all of these criteria may be absent and yet entrainment may still be present. The ability to demonstrate transient entrainment on surface ECG depends on the site of stimulation being distant from the exit point of the reentrant circuit [50]. However, Almendral et al. [51], in a study of 16 coronary patients undergoing endocardial mapping, found that the physiology of entrainment was present in all, when recordings were made at the site of origin of tachycardia. In all cases where tachycardia was terminated by pacing, entrainment criterion 3 was satisfied. However, the development of block could be concealed if the pacing site was close to the site of origin or the refractory period of the circuit short. In this case initial activation of the site of origin was by the paced wavefront before emergence of the reentrant wavefront. It may be concluded that, in order to terminate reentrant tachycardia, pacing must:

1. Be able to penetrate the reentrant circuit. This may require multiple captures if the site of stimulation is far from the tachycardia substrate. Arrival at and interaction with the tachycardia substrate is frequently presaged by resetting and advancement of the ongoing tachycardia.
2. If termination is not immediate, entrainment or resetting of the circuit appears to occur, although its presence may be inapparent on the surface ECG.
3. Entrainment criterion 3, a failure of activation from the tachycardia wavefront followed by shift to a fully paced activation pattern, is a necessary but not sufficient requirement for termination.
4. Block must occur in the antegrade limb of the circuit. This may only be apparent following termination of pacing if entrainment criterion 3 has already been satisfied due to proximity of the pacing site to the site of origin of the tachycardia or relatively short refractory periods in the tachycardia circuit. Block in the antegrade limb is frequently preceded by progressive delay in the recovery cycle during pacing attempts which fail to terminate tachycardia.

V. MECHANISMS OF FAILURE OF ANTITACHYCARDIA PACING

Those tachycardias which fail to terminate during pacing attempts may do so for a variety of potential reasons. As suggested by observations during resetting, a single extrastimulus may fail to interact in any demonstrable way with the tachycardia substrate in nearly half of tachycardias. That this effect is rapidly overcome by addition of successive stimuli suggests that single-capture methods fail by inability to propagate to the tachycardia substrate due to intervening refractory myocardium. By contrast, burst pacing methods usually interact successfully with the tachycardia substrate, as evidenced by resetting or entrainment. Failure of these methods likely relates to multiple factors, including inability to induce block in the antegrade limb of the circuit due to short refractory periods, inability to achieve adequate pacing rates at the site of stimulation due to local refractoriness, successful termination followed by reinduction of the same tachycardia within the same burst, intercurrent hemodynamic deterioration of the patient before successful termination can be accomplished, or failure due to tachycardia acceleration by pacing. Tachycardia acceleration may occur secondary to exposure of a secondary shorter path through the same substrate, insertion of a second propagated wavefront in the same tachycardia circuit (so-called double wave reentry [52]), induction of a second distinct faster tachycardia by pacing, or the precipitation of heterogenous propagation and dispersion in refractoriness promoting development of polymorphic tachycardias or ventricular fibrillation. It is unfortunate that both tachycardia termination and acceleration are more likely to occur with more numerous and more tightly coupled extrastimuli.

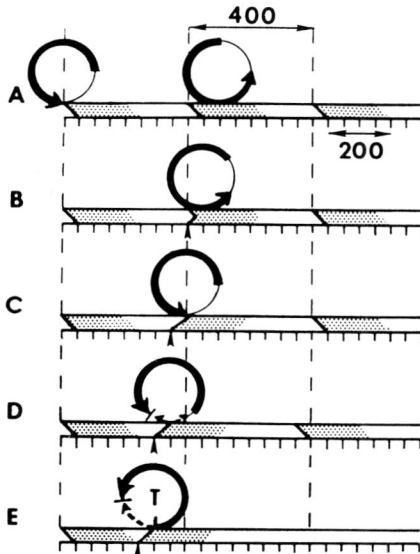

Figure 3 Tachycardia termination by a single extrastimulus. This diagram incorporates a simplified single entrance/exit model. Tachycardia circuit is represented by the circle, with the advancing wavefront and tail of refractory myocardium represented by the bold circular arrow. The pacing site is at the bottom (vertical arrows), and intervening myocardium is represented by the ladder diagram strip. A late coupled stimulus (B and C) fails to interact and does not reset the tachycardia. An earlier stimulus (D) interacts and resets the circuit without termination. An even earlier stimulus (E), often encroaching on local ventricular refractory period, interacts with and blocks the circuit, terminating tachycardia. Because of the competing sequences of activation and recovery, a single stimulus often fails, in faster tachycardias, to interact with the tachycardia substrate, making termination impossible. Reproduced with permission from Ref. 39.

VI. PACING STRATEGIES

A. Single-Capture Termination Methods

The least effective means of tachycardia termination, single-capture methods (Fig. 3) are also the least likely to result in acceleration. Asynchronous underdrive pacing at rates less than the tachycardia will terminate tachycardias of slow rate and wide termination zone by random scanning of the diastolic interval. This technique is inherently inefficient but is available as a magnet mode with most conventional pacemakers and has been incorporated into specialized "dual-demand" or "upside-down" pacers for automatic underdrive pacing on detection of tachycardia [53,54]. A scanning extrastimulus is more efficient and available in many specialized devices. In well-tolerated, relatively slow ventricular tachycardias, Fisher et al. [55] reported 139 or 290 (48%) episodes terminated with a single extrastimulus, with one (0.34%) episode of acceleration. With very rare exceptions, they observed that the termination zone began just outside the refractory period. Ultrarapid train stimulation at a rate of 100 Hz represents a very efficient means of achieving capture at this critical point just outside the ventricular refractory period. This method applies a train of stimuli at intervals much shorter than the ventricular refractory period, such that only one stimulus will result in capture. In the same study, Fisher et al. reported 67 of 120 (56%) episodes terminated by single-capture train stimulation, with one case (0.83%) of acceleration. The efficacy of a scanned extrastimulus and train stimulation were concordant in 94% of matched trials. Therefore both methods offered only approximately 50% efficacy but very low risk of acceleration in slow, well-tolerated tachycardias. Train stimulation was inherently more efficient, however, with a capture in the termination zone usually obtained on the first stimulation attempt. Single-capture methods are dependent on the fortuitous combination of slow tachycardia rate, relative proximity to the tachycardia substrate, and relatively short refractory period of the intervening myocardium, permitting a single capture to gain access to and block in the tachycardia circuit. As suggested in the earlier discussion, resetting may be observed in only 55% of well-tolerated tachycardias [41] with a single extrastimulus, suggesting that in the remainder, the extrastimulus fails even to interact with the tachycardia substrate, making termination impossible. Such conditions, although present in half of slow tachycardias, may not be present reliably. In one study, only one of 20 patients studied on multiple days had VT which was consistently terminable by a single extrastimulus during all induced episodes [56]. These factors make single-capture methods unreliable for long-term management of ventricular tachycardia. However, the low risk of acceleration gives single-capture methods a place in the first tier of therapy for slower, very well-tolerated tachycardias, where delay in therapy is unlikely to compromise hemodynamic stability. Careful placement of the stimulation electrode close to the tachycardia substrate may maximize the efficacy of this method.

B. Multiple-Capture Termination Methods

Additional captures result in an increase in efficacy but are accompanied by an increased risk of acceleration. Naccarelli et al. [57] compared single and double extrastimuli as well as multicapture bursts (Fig. 4) in 57 patients during 89 episodes of ventricular tachycardia. The overall efficacy of these techniques was 18%, 42%, and 61%, respectively, while acceleration occurred in 0%, 15%, and 18%, respectively. Therefore the addition of a second extrastimulus approximately doubled efficacy but was accompanied by an even more striking increase in risk of acceleration. By comparison, multicapture bursts were associated with a more than threefold improvement in efficacy but risk of acceleration comparable to that of double-capture termination. When only tachycardias with cycle length >350 ms were examined, the efficacy rose to 21%, 51%, and 76%, but risk of acceleration was not reduced. The benefit conferred by slow rate was the same whether spontaneous or drug-slowed. This beneficial effect of antiarrhythmic drugs has not been universally observed, and Roy et al. [58] reported that procainamide made termination more difficult in 26% of patients. However, the strong dependence of efficacy on tachycardia rate remains a universal observation [59,60]. Substantial evidence from studies of resetting and entrainment suggests that the early stimuli in the burst serve to progressively reverse the sequence of ventricular activation, permitting the latter stimuli actually to interact, advance, and induce block in the tachycardia circuit (Fig. 5). This phenomenon has been referred to as "peeling back of refractoriness" and is a major advantage of multicapture methods. As these early stimuli often fail to interact with the tachycardia substrate, Gardner et al. [61] examined the effect of an added one to two extrastimuli following a multicapture burst designed first to reverse ventricular activation and gain access to the substrate in 25 patients failing to respond to one to three extrastimuli and burst pacing alone. Utilizing a burst rate previously ineffective but which did not result in acceleration, this method had an efficacy of 84% without acceleration. Although acceleration was not noted in their series, others have reported acceleration with this technique as well [62]. The risk of acceleration during burst pacing in an individual patient may be difficult to predict based on initial experience in the electrophysiology laboratory. Fisher et al. [60] found that while 89% of *episodes* were terminated with pac-

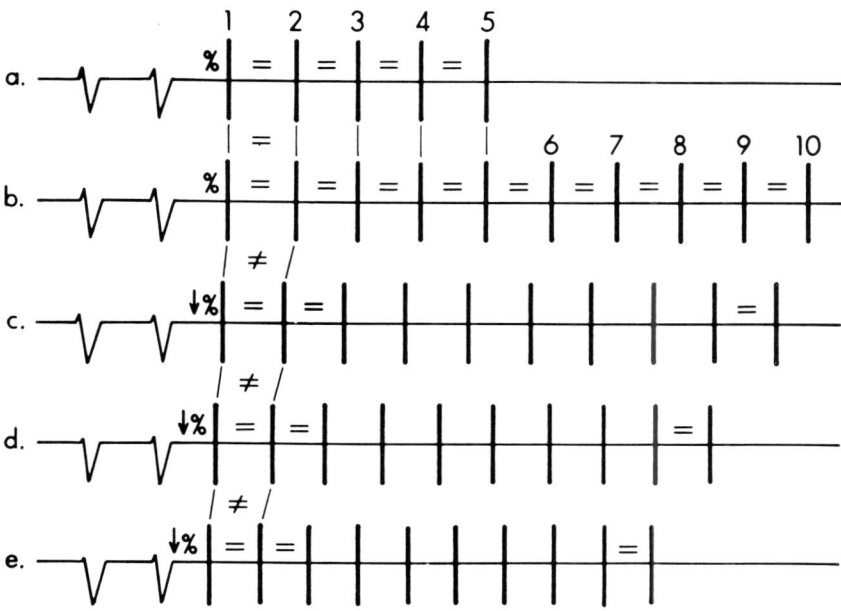

Figure 4 Synchronous rate-adaptive burst pacing. Stimuli are delivered at constant coupling intervals adapted at a percentage of the tachycardia cycle length. Therapy is titrated by addition of stimuli (b) or successive decrements in all coupling intervals (c–e). Reproduced with permission from Ref. 94.

ing, with only 4% resulting in acceleration, 43% of *patients* experienced acceleration on at least one occasion.

Autodecremental or ramp pacing (Fig. 6 and 7), in which the first stimulus is delivered at an adaptive percentage (typically 97%) of the tachycardia cycle length and each subsequent extrastimulus is delivered at successively shorter decrements of the first coupling interval (typically by approximately 3% or 10 ms), has been incorporated into several devices. Therapy is successively titrated by adding stimuli at the end of the sequence at successively shorter intervals. Relatively long initial coupling intervals and gradual decrements favor capture of all

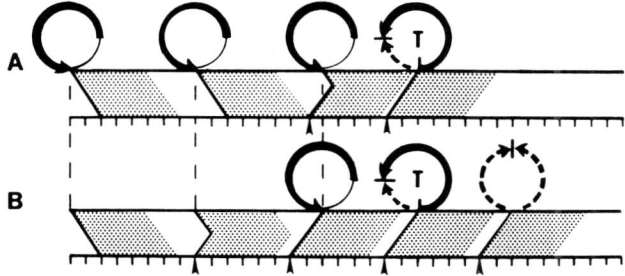

Figure 5 Peeling back of refractory periods by multiple stimuli. Conventions as in Fig. 3. Two (A) or multiple (B) stimuli are able to successively reverse the sequence of ventricular activation, permitting the latter stimuli to interact successfully with and induce block in the substrate and consequently terminate tachycardia. Reproduced with permission from Ref. 39.

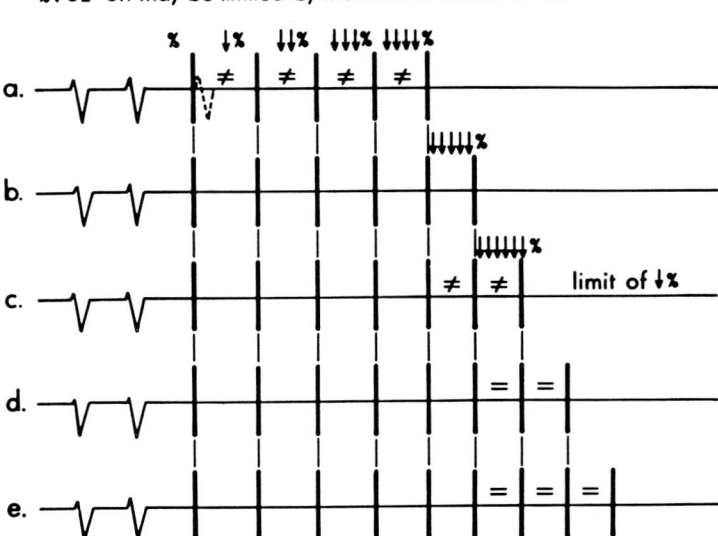

Figure 6 Autodecremental or ramp pacing. Intervals are decremented successively from a starting interval adapted to the tachycardia cycle length to a minimum programmed interval. Therapy is titrated by successive addition of stimuli at progressively shorter cycle lengths (a–c). Stimuli delivered beyond the minimum coupling interval are delivered at a constant rate (d, e). Reproduced with permission from Ref. 94.

stimuli, even with relatively rapid terminal pacing rates. Charos et al. [63] compared titrated autodecremental to a single conventional adaptive burst attempt during matched episodes of ventricular tachycardia with cycle length ≥280 ms. They found autodecremental effective in 71/77 (92%) of tachycardias with no acceleration and adaptive burst effective in 48/86 (56%) of episodes with 2% acceleration. Only a single fixed-rate burst attempt was made in this study, and therefore both efficacy and risk of acceleration may have been underestimated for fixed-rate bursts. Overall evaluation of autodecremental pacing in 204 tachycardias with cycle length ≥280 ms showed an aggregate efficacy of only 78% but continued very low 1% incidence of acceleration. Although each method has its strong proponents, both decremental and fixed-rate bursts have high and approximately equal efficacy and low risk of acceleration. In a recent comparison, Cook et al. [64] found 75% and 77% efficacy for decremental and fixed-rate burst pacing, respectively, with 3% and 2% risk of acceleration in 110 episodes treated randomly by either technique. Several subsequent randomized comparisons [65–68] have noted comparable efficacies but substantially higher risks of acceleration, ranging from 6% to 21%. However, no mode of pacing therapy has proved significantly superior with regard to either efficacy or risk of acceleration in these trials.

Numerous other multicapture sequences have been conceived, including shifting bursts [69], scanning bursts [69], scanning ramps, incremental-decremental (or centrifugal) scan [70], and so-called universal pacing [71]. However, none has proven clearly superior. Difference in efficacy and risk between these techniques may be subtle and only clarified by detailed analysis of the large number of episodes being logged in multicenter device trials.

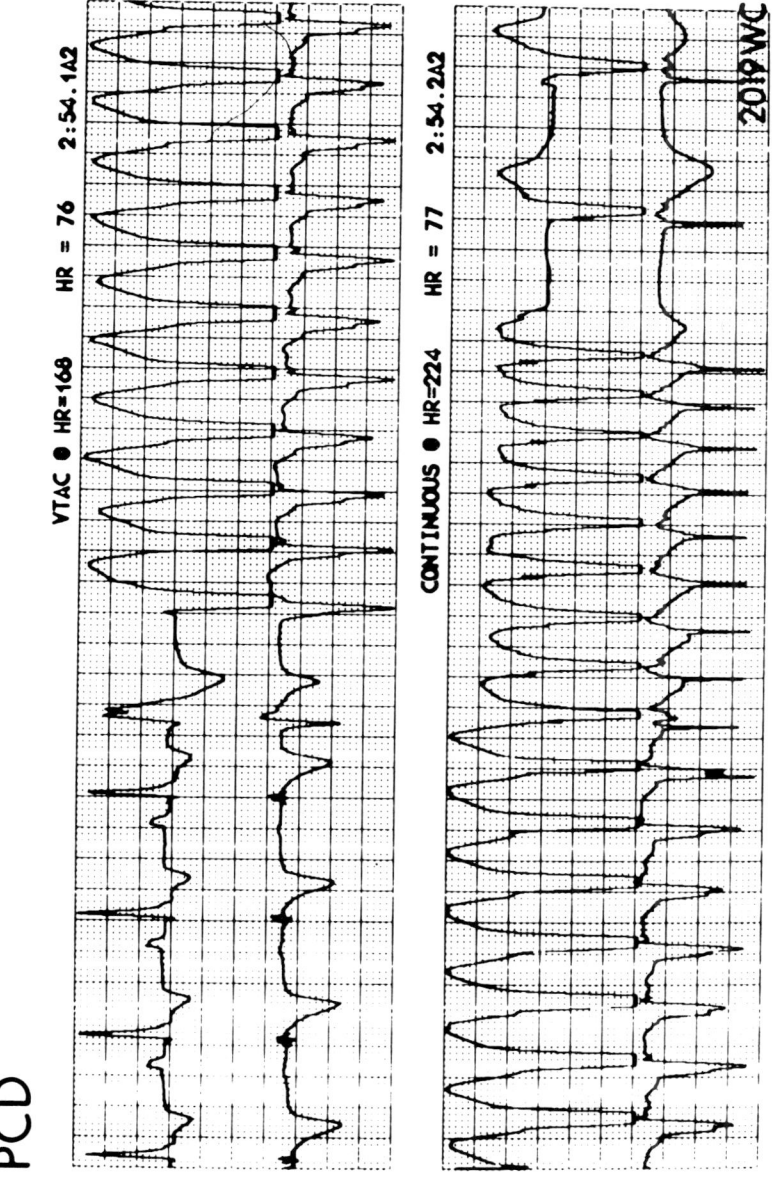

Figure 7 Ambulatory recording of a spontaneous ventricular tachycardia appropriately detected after 16 cycles and terminated with a single 10-stimulus ramp therapy by the Medtronic PCD model 7217B. VVI backup pacing follows successful termination. Reproduced with permission from Ref. 94.

C. Combined Use of Pacing and Low-Energy Cardioversion

Saksena and co-workers [72,73] have compared antitachycardia pacing using progressively decremented fixed-rate bursts with low- to moderate-energy transvenous cardioversion. In relatively slow tachycardias with mean cycle length 391 ms, both efficacy (cardioversion 83%, pacing 80%) and risk of acceleration (cardioversion 11%, pacing 6%) were comparable, but transient supraventricular arrhythmias were much more frequent following transvenous cardioversion, occurring in 23% of trials. In tachycardias with cycle length >270 ms, pacing terminated 77% of episodes. In those failing pacing, addition of transvenous cardioversion increased efficacy by only 8%, with a significant risk of acceleration [73]. Therefore, when compared to low-energy transvenous cardioversion, pacing had comparable efficacy and risk of acceleration. Once pacing failed, the gains added by low- to moderate-energy cardioversion are modest, with a significant risk of acceleration. Waspe et al., in a study of 13 patients, made similar observations [74]. Hammill [75] has recently presented a larger experience encompassing 71 patients during 488 episodes of VT induced as part of the multicenter Medtronic PCD investigation. Grouping all tachycardias with cycle length ≤300 ms, ramp pacing, burst pacing, and low- to moderate- energy cardioversion (0.2 to 5 J) had efficacies of 62%, 47%, and 63%, with acceleration in 12%, 17%, and 13%, respectively. Grouping all tachycardias >300 ms, efficacies were 63%, 60%, and 87%, with acceleration in 9%, 7%, and 4%, respectively.

D. Choice of Method

When rapid, poorly tolerated tachycardias are excluded, multicapture techniques have demonstrated efficacies in excess of 75% and variable risk of acceleration from 1% to as high as 35% [57–60,63,76] of episodes. Even when the risk of acceleration per episode is low, a given patient will frequently and unpredictably experience an episode of acceleration after multiple successful terminations. The extent to which variability among investigators reflects patient selection, differences in application/titration of pacing therapy, and actual differences among the pacing methods cannot be accurately assessed. It is likely that all are important factors. Successful termination is favored by slower tachycardia rate, either spontaneously or caused by concomitant antiarrhythmic therapy. Both efficacy and risk of acceleration are increased by greater number of stimuli and faster rates of stimulation. Rapid, hemodynamically unstable tachycardias are less likely to respond to pacing techniques of any type, although a fraction of even such tachycardias will respond to aggressive pacing. All pacing strategies consume time, and success is not assured. In more rapid tachycardias, where efficacy is lower and hemodynamic collapse more likely, careful consideration should be given to the potential risks of postponing high-output shock therapy (Fig. 8). The absolute threshold for pacing versus shock therapy remains unclear and will vary from patient to patient. In the ambulatory patient, tachycardias with cycle lengths shorter than 250 ms should be strongly considered for immediate shock therapy, while those longer than 350 ms will frequently respond to pacing methods with defibrillator backup. Between these limits, judgment will need to suffice until more sophisticated hemodynamic monitoring is incorporated into implantable devices. Because all methods pose a substantial risk of acceleration, pacing for termination of ventricular tachycardia should presently be applied only when either implanted or external rescue defibrillation is immediately available. For tachycardias with cycle length longer than 270 to 300 ms, pacing methods appear to have comparable efficacy and risk when compared to low- or moderate-energy transvenous cardioversion. However, current understanding is based on small numbers of patients and pre-

Tachycardia Management by Pacing

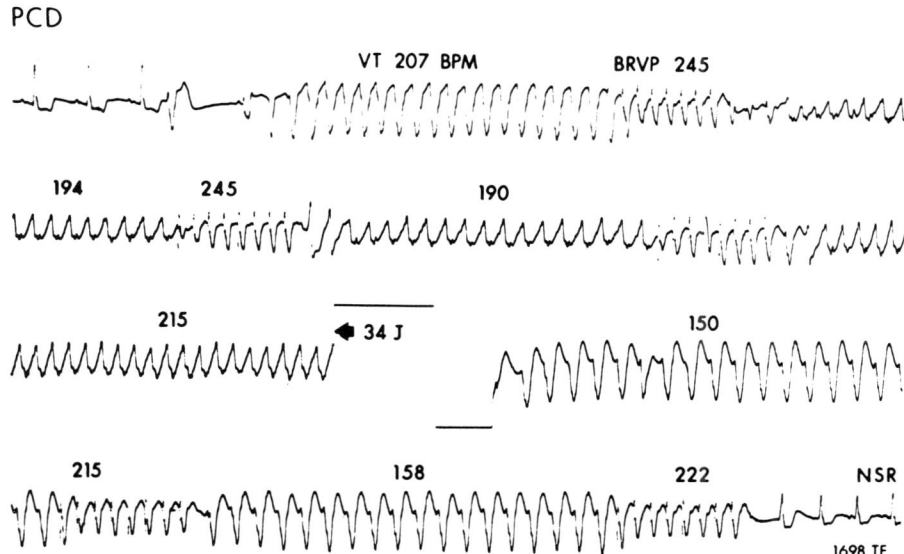

Figure 8 Complex interplay of antitachycardia pacing and cardioversion. A spontaneous VPC is followed by a pause terminated by a ventricular escape pace generated by the implanted pacer defibrillator. This is followed by ventricular tachycardia with a rate of 207, detected as VT and treated by an adaptive burst therapy. A change in morphology and acceleration of tachycardia ensues, and a second burst therapy is delivered without effect. A third treatment results in tachycardia acceleration to a rate of 215, now exceeding the fibrillation detection rate, resulting in delivery of a full-output internal countershock. This, however, fails to terminate tachycardia but results again in deceleration to a rate of 150, which is eventually terminated by further burst therapies. Backup pacing, burst pacing, and defibrillation therapies were all delivered automatically by an implanted Medtronic PCD model 7217B. Although tachycardia was eventually terminated, initial therapy was delayed by ineffective burst therapies. It is unknown whether the shock therapy delivered late in the tachycardia and only partially effective was compromised by the delay incurred by burst therapy. Reproduced with permission from Ref. 94.

liminary data. The relative merits of each technique in faster tachycardias, where both appear to pose substantial risks of acceleration, is still unclear.

VII. CLINICAL PERFORMANCE OF ANTITACHYCARDIA PACING

A. Pacing Without Defibrillator Backup

The reported clinical experience with implanted antitachycardia pacers in the absence of backup defibrillation encompasses more than 200 patients and is detailed in Table 1. The threshold for and criteria governing implantation of pacers for this indication vary widely between centers. In the absence of effective backup defibrillation, most devices have been utilized in an interactive or manually activated mode. In this capacity, patients with slow, well-tolerated recurrent tachycardia have been managed very effectively, with the majority of centers reporting good to excellent results. Most centers which have hazarded the implantation of automated antitachycardia devices for VT termination in the absence of defibrillator backup have required

Table 1 Ventricular Tachycardia Termination by Implanted Pacemakers

First author, year	No of patients	Pacer model	Pacer type	No. of preimplant tests	No. of postimplant tests	Drugs too?	Duration of follow-up (mo.)	Results Excellent	Results Good	Results Poor	Comments
Moss, 1974 [17]	1	Medt 5842	Manual via magnet	NS	NS	NS	6	1			No VT after pacer rate increased
Hartzler, 1979 [95]	2	Medt 5998	Manual RF	>30–100	>50–70	Yes	1–11	1			1 pt. VT at 4 wks—died
Ruskin, 1980 [96]	3	Medt 5998	Manual RF	>100	100 each	Yes	Mean 13.6	3			1 died, lung cancer
Greene, 1982 [97]	2	Cordis Orthocor	2PES	mult.	mult.	4, 9	2	0	0	0	Never used in 1 pt.
Luderitz, 1982 [98]	3	2 Magnet 1 Cordis Orthocor 234A	Manual, under Manual, burst	NS	NS	NS	Yes	NS	2	1	
Strasberg, 1982 [99]	2	Medt 5998	Manual RF	NS	NS	NS					1 pt. no recurrence 1 pt. 1 recurrence
den Dulk, 1984 [100]	6	Medt SPO500	Manual, variable modes	NS	NS	5	6–20	4	2		
Griffin, 1984 [101] (multicenter)	52	Intermedics Cybert	Auto, burst	NS	NS	NS	12	30			14 nontachy deaths, 4 sudden deaths
Reddy, 1984 [102]	1	PASAR 4151	Autoscanning PES	"Many"	"Several"	Yes	6	1			
Rothman, 1984 [103] (multicenter)	53	Cordis Orthocor	Manual burst, etc.	NS	NS	NS	1–41	45			3 sudden deaths, 3 doc. VT/VF deaths
Sowton, 1984 [70]	9	Siemens Elema Tachylog	Autoscanning PES or burst	NS	NS	3	6–14	5			
Spurrell, 1984 [69]	1	PASAR 4151	Auto, shifting	NS	NS	NS	NS	1			Unit explanted after pt. free of VT
Bertholet, 1985 [104]	3	Medt SPO500	Manual scanning or burst	"At least 100"	NS	Yes	17–30	3			

	Refs.	Pts.									
Herre, 1985 [105]	28		Medt 5998	Manual RF	NS	125 EP studies	18	1–25	97% success in 9 pts.			No spont. VT in 19 pts., 1 pt. sudden death
Higgins, 1985 [106]	1		PASAR 4151	Auto, scan burst or PES	NS	NS	No	16		1		
Peters, 1985 [107]	6		Medt 5998	Manual RF	NS	NS	Yes	3–36	1	5	2 accel. 3 refractory	
Tanabe, 1985 [108]	1		Medt Spect	Manual	NS	NS	NS					
Falkoff, 1986 [109]	2		Intermed Cybertach	Burst	Many	Many	2	7, 64	2	0	0	Pacer syndr. in 1
Saksena, 1986 [110]	11		Cordis Orthocor 234A	Manual burst	NS	NS	10	(0–28)	Not certain; see comments			4 for VT term; 7 mostly for PES
Fisher, 1987 [37]	20		Misc	Misc.	>100	>100	Yes	2–92	16	2	3	1 explant at 1 mo., 4 disarmed at 1 mo., 4 sudden, not pacer-related deaths
Fromer, 1987 [111]	1		Intermed Intertach	2PES scan	>25	NS	1	12	1	0	0	
Palakurthy, 1988 [112]	1		Telec PASAR 4171	Auto scan, 2PES	NS	NS	1	23	1	0	0	
Moller, 1989 [113]	2		Telec PASAR 4171	Bursts			2	26–27 = 26.5	2	0	0	
Occhetta, 1989 [114]	1		Cordis Orthocor	Bursts	10	>30	1	21	1	0	0	Finally failed AICD

Totals									Excellent to Good	Poor	Unstated
Number	24	212							135	8	69
Percent									64%	3.8%	32%

EP = electrophysiologic; NS = not stated; PES = programmed extrastimuli; RF = radiofrequency; spont = Spontaneous; tachy = tachycardia; VF = ventricular fibrillation; VT = ventricular tachycardia. Modified and expanded with permission from Ref. 115.

multiple successful terminations without acceleration, frequently exceeding 100 successful terminations [37]. Of necessity, this has represented a highly select group of patients who are not, in general, representative of the typical patient with VT.

B. Combined Use of Pacing and Defibrillation

Pacing techniques as sole therapy for recurrent ventricular tachycardia are presently rarely employed because of the potential catastrophic consequences of tachycardia acceleration. Table 2 summarizes the reported clinical experience to date with an automated antitachycardia pacemaker combined with an independent implantable defibrillator. Combining two distinct complex devices in the same patient poses special problems which will be addressed further. Table 3 encompasses the more recent clinical experience with integrated devices capable of antitachycardia pacing, cardioversion, and high-output defibrillation. The incidence of sudden death in these patients has been extremely low and the reported efficacy of antitachycardia pacing high, ranging from 50% to 92.4%. An important and consistent observation has been the relatively small number of episodes requiring shocks for termination. However, the apparent corollary that the number of tachycardias treated successfully by burst therapy is equivalent to the number of shocks prevented by these devices is not necessarily correct. The availability of pacing therapies may invite the programming of rate detection cutoffs slower than would have been used in shock-only devices. Some of the tachycardias terminated successfully by pacing might have been asymptomatic and self-terminating in a patient with a shock-only device. These early reports may also reflect some degree of selection or referral bias in favor of patients with frequent tachycardia that is amenable to pacing. Leitch and co-workers [77], reporting on their experience with the Medtronic PCD in 46 patients, classified 38 of 909 episodes of detected "VT" as likely sinus tachycardia. Another 257 episodes could not be classified, as they were clinically silent. The overlap in rate between clinical pace-terminable tachycardia and sinus rhythm, a problem compounded by antiarrhythmic therapy, is a potentially very important clinical problem and complicates the interpretation of the data derived from devices which do not provide detailed electrogram storage of episodes. Patients receiving a third-generation device appear to have 12- to 24-month survivals comparable to those reported with earlier shock-only devices [78,79]. A recent historical comparative study of all causes of mortality at 1 year following implantation of either a nonprogrammable (6605 patients), simple programmable (227 patients), or third-generation pacing ICD (291 patients) showed no significant difference in outcome [80].

C. Adverse Interactions Between Pacing and Defibrillation Systems

Several important adverse interactions have been noted when an independent pacemaker and defibrillator are implanted. These may conveniently be divided into effects of pacing on the defibrillation system and effects of defibrillation on the pacemaker system. Experience with these interactions is limited largely to interactions with the CPI AICD, which utilizes bipolar rate sensing governed by an automatic gain control designed to optimize sensing of low-amplitude signals during ventricular fibrillation. The independent pacemaker impulse may be sensed, and because of the short refractory period required for tachycardia detection, the propagated ventricular electrogram and even evoked T waves may be sensed independently, resulting in double or triple sensing and inappropriate initiation of shock therapy. Of more concern, if the pacing system fails to inhibit during ventricular fibrillation, due either to undersensing or noise mode reversion, the presence of pacer spikes may cause the AICD to automatically reduce sensing gain such that only the pacer artifact is detected and detection of tachycardia fails. This

Table 2 Ventricular Tachycardia Termination with Independent Defibrillator Backup

First author	Year publ.	No. of pts.	Pacer model	ICD model	Pacing mode	Percent req. drugs	Follow-up months range (mean)	No. of episodes Rx'd by pacing	Term	Failed/ Accel.	No. of episodes Rx'd by shock	Comments
Greve [116]	1988	11	Intermed Intertach	AICD	NS	NS	(12)	87	Approx. 50%	NS	43	2 died of CHF
Newman [117]	1989	11	Intermed Intertach	AICD	PES, Burst, Ramp	NS	3–35 (11.6)	>1998	NS	NS	2	2 died of CHF, ATP active in 8 pts.
Masterson [118]	1990	10	4 Cordis Orthocor 284A, 6 Intermed Intertach	AICD	PES, Burst, Ramp	100%	NS	1542	1373 (89%)	NS	179	
Bonnet [119]	1991	14	Cordis Orthocor 284A	AICD	Burst	10/14 (71%)	(25)	6029	NS	NS	103	No mortality
Luderitz [120]	1991	6	Siemens-Elema Tachylog	AICD	Burst	NS	1–47 (32.0)	1631	NS	NS	227	
Totals[a]		52						>11,287			554	

[a]Totals are estimates; multicenter reports may include patients already reported in other series. Abbreviations as in Table 1. Modified and expanded with permission from Ref. 94.

Table 3 Ventricular Tachycardia Termination with Integrated Defibrillator Backup

First author	Year publ.	No. of pts.	Pacer/ICD model	Pacing mode	Percent req. drugs	Follow-up months range (mean)	No. of episodes Rx'd by pacing	Term	Failed/accel.	No. of episodes Rx'd by shock	Comments
Fromer [121]	1991	4	Medtronic PCD 7216A, 7217B	Ramp	NS	12–19 (16.5)	16	70%	30%	19	
Leitch [77]	1991	46	Medtronic PCD 7216, 7217	Burst, Ramp	16/46 (35%)	1–13 (6.1)	909	840 (92.4%)	3.3%/4.3%	44	4 cardiopulmonary deaths, 1 sudden death
Saksena [122]	1991	16	Medtronic PCD 7216A	Burst, Ramp	8/16 (50%)	2–10 (6.0)	96	78 (81%)	19%	27	2 nonarrhythmic deaths
Singer [123]	1991	5	Telectron, Guardian ATP 4210	Burst	4/5 (80%)	6–8	226	NS	NS	127	
Block [124]	1991	21	Medtronic PCD	NS	NS	(5)	439	435 (99%)	3(.68%)/1(0.23%)	16	2 post-op pulmonary deaths, only 8/19 had ATP active
Ellenbogen [125] (multicenter)	1991	100	Telectron, Guardian ATP 4210	NS	NS	0–9 (2.3)	128	75 (59%)	22(17%)/31(24%)	9 VF (+31 ATP failures)	Inpatient follow-up only

Fromer [126] (European multicenter)	1992	102	Medtronic PCD	NS	NS	1–21 (9.4)	1,289	1,116 (86.5%)	173 (13.4%)	126 VT 286 VF (incl. ATP failures)	Survival 84% @ 18 mos. + 3.9% surg. mortality
Bardy [91]	1992	50	Medtronic PCD 7216A and 7217B	NS	9/50 (8%)	8–24 (15)	623	498 (80%)	125 (20%)	110 VT 144 VF (incl. ATP failures)	Survival 96% @ 24 mos.
Saksena [127] (PCD investigators, multicenter)	1992	751	Medtronic PCD 434 Epicard 317 Nonthor	NS	NS	0–22	10,320	9,446 (91.5%)	NS	874 VT 1410 VF (incl. ATP failures)	Survival 90.3% @ 12 mos. + 3.3% surg. mortality
Totals[a]		1095					14,046			3223	

[a]Totals are estimates; multicenter reports may include patients already reported in other series. Abbreviations as in Table 1. Modified and expanded with permission from Ref. 94.

interaction may have catastrophic consequences, resulting in failure to deliver shock therapy [81]. The likelihood of crosstalk occurring can be minimized by utilizing only bipolar pacing systems with pacing and AICD sensing leads positioned at a distance, and verifying the absence of crosstalk at the time of device implantation. When implantation of a pacemaker is undertaken in a patient with an independent ICD, induction of tachycardia and verification of appropriate detection and therapy is mandatory. Defibrillation therapy may also have important effects on pacemaker function. High-energy shocks may result in transient pacemaker undersensing, consequent asynchronous pacing [82], and possibly reinitiation of tachycardia. A transient rise in pacing threshold and noncapture has been observed following internal defibrillation, which may result in pacemaker noncapture [82–84]. However, this effect has not been universally observed [85]. Finally, shocks may cause pacemaker reprogramming or reversion to backup mode [82]. In a bipolar device which is also capable of unipolar pacing, the backup mode may utilize unipolar pacing, potentially resulting in unexpected crosstalk. In selecting a bipolar pacing system, it is therefore desirable to utilize a committed bipolar system which is incapable of reversion to unipolar pacing as a backup mode. Although reversion to unipolar backup mode is potentially catastrophic, Ching et al. [86] observed only two ICD shock-induced resets to unipolar mode during 846 shocks in 41 patients. At the time of implantation it is feasible to measure the size of the paced electrogram on the ICD sensing leads, and systematic mapping to find the optimal position for bipolar leads has been proposed [87]. Calkins et al. [82] reviewed the incidence of interactions in 30 patients undergoing combined implantation of a pacemaker and AICD defibrillation system. Transient sensing/pacing failure after shocks was noted in seven patients, double counting in one patient, AICD failure to sense VF due to pacer spike crosstalk in three patients (this occurred at usual outputs in unipolar devices but only at unusually high outputs in bipolar devices), and pacemaker reprogramming caused by AICD discharge in three patients. In two cases reprogramming consisted of reversion to backup mode; however, in one case the pacemaker program turned the device off entirely. Others have also reported adverse interactions of potential clinical import [88].

The use of an independent pacemaker capable of antitachycardia pacing poses additional concerns. This combination has been used to render pacing therapy before shock therapy. The limitations of this configuration are several. If the tachycardia rate exceeds the AICD detect rate, the time available for burst therapy is brief, typically 4–8 s before the AICD begins a charge cycle and committed shock. This may leave little room for titration of therapy, with time for usually only one to two attempts at pace termination [89]. If the pacemaker tachycardia detection rate is set slower than the AICD detect rate, then multiple attempts may be undertaken. However, if pacing fails, the pacemaker must intentionally accelerate tachycardia to initiate shock therapy or leave the tachycardia untreated. In summary, the potentially adverse interactions between independent pacing and defibrillation systems may result in both inappropriate therapy as well as failure or delay in delivery of appropriate therapy. Most such interactions have been observed during in-hospital evaluation and not in ambulatory settings. It is unknown whether these effects result in increased jeopardy to patients with combined independent systems, but the possibility cannot be dismissed. Although many of these interactions are effectively eliminated in the new generation of integrated pacing defibrillators, new forms of interaction have already been noted [90].

D. Antiarrhythmic Medication in Combination with Antitachycardia Pacing

In the 9807-patient CPI AICD database [78], 55.1% of patients required concomitant antiarrhythmic therapy. By contrast, in the two largest series of third-generation devices reporting this data, Leitch et al. [77] required concomitant medication in 16/46 (35%) and Bardy et al. [91] in only 9/50 (8%) of patients. Therefore the use of antiarrhythmic medication has declined along with the availability of the more robust capabilities of the most recent generation of devices. Other factors, including patient selection and a growing recognition of the potential adverse effects of antiarrhythmic agents, may also be important factors in this evolution. As noted above, antiarrhythmic medication often, but not consistently, improves the success of antitachycardia pacing. Although many episodes of tachycardia treated by antitachycardia pacing are asymptomatic, patients who develop frequent transient symptoms prior to effective pacing therapy may require antiarrhythmic medication to alleviate symptoms. Differentiation of more rapid monomorphic tachycardias from VF may also be facilitated by the use of drugs which slow the rate of tachycardia. However, the same drugs may render slower tachycardias too slow to be reliably distinguished from sinus rhythm. Paul et al. [92] looked at the relationship between maximum sinus rate with exercise or during ambulatory recording and rate of sustained tachycardia in 108 patients. In the absence of medication, only 11% had sinus rates exceeding the rate of VT. However, on antiarrhythmic medication, 35% receiving Class 1A, 33% on amiodarone, 41% on Class 1C, and 63% on combination therapy had VT rates slower than maximum physiologic sinus rates. Of note, beta blockade had a favorable effect on maximum sinus rate with no effect on VT rate. Several presently investigational third-generation devices provide some electrogram storage capability, and future morphology recognition schemes may simplify management. Exercise testing and ambulatory recording are essential to screen for this potential problem. Because of the known adverse effects of antiarrhythmic medications, including proarrhythmia, myocardial depression, and increase in defibrillation threshold, as well as the difficulty of predicting which medications are likely to prevent shocks in patients who fail serial drug testing [93], caution should be exercised in the initiation of concomitant antiarrhythmic medication in patients whose symptoms do not mandate such therapy. Whether concomitant beta blockade might exert favorable effects in this setting by prevention of inappropriate therapy for sinus tachycardia or SVT, or through its other complex actions, is currently unknown.

VIII. SUMMARY

Pacing methods provide both an important probe into the underlying mechanism of tachycardia as well as an elegant, efficient, and painless means of its termination. The addition of these capabilities requires little or no sacrifice in terms of device size or longevity when compared to simple shock-only devices. Preventive methods currently have a limited role in the management of tachycardias occurring in the absence of bradycardia. Methods currently exist to improve hemodynamic toleration during ongoing tachycardia and may find a place with the development of more advanced, dual-chamber systems. Observations during resetting and entrainment suggest a reentrant substrate with distinct entry and exit sites and an excitable gap in the vast majority of clinical monomorphic ventricular tachycardias. The success or failure of pacing methods depends on multiple factors, including the characteristics of the tachycardia substrate, local refractoriness at the stimulation site, location of stimulation, availability of other potential tachycardia mechanisms, and hemodynamic stability of the patient. Despite these competing factors, the large majority of well-tolerated tachycardias are amenable to pace termination. Early clinical experience with integrated pacing-cardioversion-defibrillation systems suggests very high efficacy in termination of events detected as ventricular tachycardia. If these early results are borne out, then it is likely that the clinical indications for implantation of defibrillation systems will be greatly expanded to include not only those patients at high risk of sudden death but also those for whom rescue from acceleration due to antitachycardia pacing is the primary indication for implantation.

REFERENCES

1. Escher DJ. The treatment of tachyarrhythmias by artificial cardiac pacing. Am Heart J 1969; 78:829-832.
2. Lew HT, March HW. Control of recurrent ventricular fibrillation by transvenous pacing in the absence of heart block. Am Heart J 1967; 73:794-797.
3. Zipes DP, Festoff B, Schaal SF, Cox C, Sealy WC, Wallace AG. Treatment of ventricular arrhythmia by permanent atrial pacemaker and cardiac sympathectomy. Ann Intern Med 1968; 68:591-597.
4. DeFrancis NA, Giordano RP. Permanent epicardial atrial pacing in the treatment of refractory ventricular tachycardia. Am J Cardiol 1968; 22:742-745.
5. DeSanctis RW, Kastor JA. Rapid intracardiac pacing for treatment of recurrent ventricular tachyarrhythmias in the absence of heart block. Am Heart J 1968; 76:168-172.
6. Friedberg CK, Lyon LJ, Donoso E. Suppression of refractory recurrent ventricular tachycardia by transvenous rapid cardiac pacing and antiarrhythmic drugs. Report of seven cases. Am Heart J 1970; 79:44-50.
7. Jensen G, Sigurd B, Sandoe E. Adams-Stokes seizures due to ventricular tachydysrhythmias in patients with heart block: prevalence and problems of management. Chest 1975; 67:43-48.
8. Steinbrecher UP, Fitchett DH. Torsade de pointes. A cause of syncope with atrioventricular block. Arch Intern Med 1980; 140:1223-1226.
9. Moss AJ, Liu JE, Gottlieb S, Locati EH, Schwartz PJ, Robinson JL. Efficacy of permanent pacing in the management of high-risk patients with long QT syndrome. Circulation 1991; 84:1524-1529.
10. Wilmer CI, Stein B, Morris DC. Atrioventricular pacemaker placement in Romano-Ward syndrome and recurrent torsades de pointes. Am J Cardiol 1987; 59:171-172.
11. Keren A, Tzivoni D, Golhman JM, Corcos P, Benhorin J, Stern S. Ventricular pacing in atypical ventricular tachycardia. J Electrocardiol 1981; 14:201–205.
12. Smith WM, Gallagher JJ. "Les torsades de pointes": an unusual ventricular arrhythmia. Ann Intern Med 1980; 93:578-584.
13. Fisher JD, Teichman SL, Ferrick A, Kim SG, Waspe LE, Martinez MR. Antiarrhythmic effects of VVI pacing at physiologic rates: a crossover controlled evaluation. PACE 1987; 10:822-830.
14. Till JA, Rowland E. Atrial pacing as an adjunct to the management of post-surgical His bundle tachycardia. Br Heart J 1991; 66:225-229.
15. Hsu I, Lumia FJ, Siegel FA, Halberstam MJ, Rios JC. Pacemaker overdrive causing recurrence of rate-dependent ventricular tachycardia. Chest 1974; 65:558-560.
16. Johnson RA, Hutter AM Jr, DeSanctis RW, Yurchak PM, Leinbach RC, Harthorne JW. Chronic overdrive pacing in the control of refractory ventricular arrhythmias. Ann Intern Med 1974; 80:380-383.
17. Moss AJ, Rivers RJ Jr. Termination and inhibition of recurrent tachycardias by implanted pervenous pacemakers. Circulation 1974; 50:942-947.
18. Lichstein E, Chadda K, Fenig S. Atrial pacing in the treatment of refractory ventricular tachycardia associated with hypokalemia. Am J Cardiol 1972; 30:550-553.
19. Beller BM, Kotler MN, Collens R. The use of ventricular pacing for suppression of ectopic ventricular activity. Am J Cardiol 1970; 25:467-473.
20. Cohen LS, Buccino RA, Morrow AG, Braunwald E. Recurrent ventricular tachycardia and fibrillation treated with a combination of beta-adrenergic blockade and electrical pacing. Ann Intern Med 1967; 66:945-949.
21. McCallister BD, McGoon DC, Connolly DC. Paroxysmal ventricular tachycardia and fibrillation without complete heart block. Report of a case treated with a permanent internal cardiac pacemaker. Am J Cardiol 1966; 18:898-903.

22. Hill PE, Neill WA, Denes P. Adverse response to ventricular pacing but favorable response to atrial pacing in polymorphous ventricular tachycardia. Am Heart J 1988; 116:1355-1357.
23. Adornato E, Pennisi V, Pangallo A, et al. La stimolazione DDD R nella prevenzione della tachicardia ventricolare sostenuta indotta dall'esercizio. Cardiostimolazione 1990; 8:118-122.
24. Restivo M, Gough WB, el Sherif N. Reentrant ventricular rhythms in the late myocardial infarction period: prevention of reentry by dual stimulation during basic rhythm. Circulation 1988; 77:429-444.
25. Marchlinski FE, Buxton AE, Miller JM, Josephson ME. Prevention of ventricular tachycardia induction during right ventricular programmed stimulation by high current strength pacing at the site of origin. Circulation 1987; 76:332-342.
26. Swerdlow CD, Liem LB, Franz MR. Summation and inhibition by ultrarapid train pacing in the human ventricle. Circulation 1987; 76:1101-1109.
27. Prystowski EN, Zipes DP. Inhibition in the human heart. Circulation 1983; 68:707-713.
28. Stevenson WG, Wiener I, Weiss J, Klitzner T. Limitations of bipolar and unipolar conditioning stimuli for inhibition in the human heart. Am Heart J 1987; 114:303-310.
29. Shenasa M, Cardinal R, Kus T, Savard P, Fromer M, Page P. Termination of sustained ventricular tachycardia by ultrarapid subthreshold stimulation in humans. Circulation 1988; 78:1135-1143.
30. Ruffy R, Friday KJ, Southworth WF. Termination of ventricular tachycardia by single extrastimulation during the ventricular effective refractory period. Circulation 1983; 67:457-459.
31. Garan H, Ruskin JN. Reproducible termination of ventricular tachycardia by a single extrastimulus within the reentry circuit during the ventricular effective refractory period. Am Heart J 1988; 116:546-550.
32. Podczeck A, Borggrefe M, Martinez-Rubio A. Termination of re-entrant ventricular tachycardia by a subthreshold stimulus applied to the zone of slowed conduction. Eur Heart J 1988; 9:1146-1150.
33. Fisher JD, Kim SG, Mercando AD. Electrical devices for treatment of arrhythmias. Am J Cardiol 1988; 61:45A-57A.
34. Hamer AW, Zaher CA, Rubin SA, Peter T, Mandel WJ. Hemodynamic benefits of synchronized 1:1 atrial pacing during sustained ventricular tachycardia with severely depressed ventricular function in coronary heart disease. Am J Cardiol 1985; 55:990-994.
35. Waldo AL, Krongrad E, Kupersmith J, Levine OR, Bowman FO Jr, Hoffman BF. Ventricular paired pacing to control rapid ventricular heart rate following open heart surgery. Observations on ectopic automaticity Report of a case in a four-month-old patient. Circulation 1976; 53:176-181.
36. Fisher JD, Kim SG, Furman S, Matos JA. Role of implantable pacemakers in control of recurrent ventricular tachycardia. Am J Cardiol 1982; 49:194-206.
37. Fisher JD, Johnston DR, Furman S, Mercando AD, Kim SG. Long-term efficacy of antitachycardia pacing for supraventricular and ventricular tachycardias. Am J Cardiol 1987; 60:1311-1316.
38. Fisher JD. Pacing for tachycardias. Med Times 1980; 108:87-9, 93-4, 9.
39. Fisher JD, Kim SG, Waspe LE, Matos JA. Mechanisms for the success and failure of pacing for termination of ventricular tachycardia: clinical and hypothetical considerations. PACE 1983; 6:1094-1105.
40. Fisher JD, Kim SG, Matos JA, Waspe LE. Pacing for ventricular tachycardia. PACE 1984; 7:1278-1290.
41. Almendral JM, Rosenthal ME, Stamato NJ, et al. Analysis of the resetting phenomenon in sustained uniform ventricular tachycardia: incidence and relation to termination. J Am Coll Cardiol 1986; 8:294-300.
42. Almendral JM, Stamato NJ, Rosenthal ME, Marchlinski FE, Miller JM, Josephson ME. Resetting response patterns during sustained ventricular tachycardia: relationship to the excitable gap. Circulation 1986; 74:722-730.
43. Kay GN, Epstein AE, Plumb VJ. Resetting of ventricular tachycardia by single extrastimuli: relation to slow conduction within the reentrant circuit. Circulation 1990; 81:1507-1519.
44. el Sherif N, Gough WB, Restivo M. Reentrant ventricular arrhythmias in the late myocardial infarction period: 14. Mechanisms of resetting, entrainment, acceleration, or termination of reentrant tachycardia by programmed electrical stimulation. PACE 1987; 10:341-371.

45. Hailing F, Frame LH. Why a steep slope of the resetting response curve predicts termination of reentry by premature stimuli (abstr). Circulation 1991; 84(suppl 2):497.
46. Waldo AL, Maclean WA, Karp RB, Kouchoukos NT, James TN. Entrainment and interruption of atrial flutter with atrial pacing: studies in man following open heart surgery. Circulation 1977; 56:737–745.
47. Waldo AL, Plumb VJ, Arciniegas JG, et al. Transient entrainment and interruption of the atrioventricular bypass pathway type of paroxysmal atrial tachycardia. A model for understanding and identifying reentrant arrhythmias. Circulation 1983; 67:73-83.
48. Brugada P, Wellens HJ. Entrainment as an electrophysiologic phenomenon. J Am Coll Cardiol 1984; 3:451-454.
49. Waldo AL, Henthorn RW, Plumb VJ, Maclean WA. Demonstration of the mechanism of transient entrainment and interruption of ventricular tachycardia with rapid atrial pacing. J Am Coll Cardiol 1984; 3:422-430.
50. Mann DE, Lawrie GM, Luck JC, Griffin JC, Magro SA, Wyndham CR. Importance of pacing site in entrainment of ventricular tachycardia. J Am Coll Cardiol 1985; 5:781-787.
51. Almendral JM, Gottlieb CD, Rosenthal ME, et al. Entrainment of ventricular tachycardia: explanation for surface electrocardiographic phenomena by analysis of electrograms recorded within the tachycardia circuit. Circulation 1988; 77:569-580.
52. Brugada J, Boersma L, Kirchhof C, et al. Double-wave reentry as a mechanism of acceleration of ventricular tachycardia. Circulation 1990; 81:1633-1643.
53. Curry PV, Rowland E, Krikler DM. Dual-demand pacing for refractory atrioventricular re-entry tachycardia. PACE 1979; 2:137-151.
54. Fisher JD, Furman S. Automatic termination of tachycardia by an implanted "upside down" demand pacemaker (abstr). Clin Res 1978; 26:231a.
55. Fisher JD, Ostrow E, Kim SG, Matos JA. Ultrarapid single-capture train stimulation for termination of ventricular tachycardia. Am J Cardiol 1983; 51:1334-1338.
56. Fisher JD, Kim SG, Matos JA, Ostrow E. Comparative effectiveness of pacing techniques for termination of well-tolerated sustained ventricular tachycardia. PACE 1983; 6:915-922.
57. Naccarelli GV, Zipes DP, Rahilly GT, Heger JJ, Prystowsky EN. Influence of tachycardia cycle length and antiarrhythmic drugs on pacing termination and acceleration of ventricular tachycardia. Am Heart J 1983; 105:1-5.
58. Roy D, Waxman HL, Buxton AE, et al. Termination of ventricular tachycardia: role of tachycardia cycle length. Am J Cardiol 1982; 50:1346-1350.
59. Keren G, Miura DS, Somberg JC. Pacing termination of ventricular tachycardia: influence of antiarrhythmic-slowed ectopic rate. Am Heart J 1984; 107:638-643.
60. Fisher JD, Mehra R, Furman S. Termination of ventricular tachycardia with bursts of rapid ventricular pacing. Am J Cardiol 1978; 41:94-102.
61. Gardner MJ, Waxman HL, Buxton AE, Cain ME, Josephson ME. Termination of ventricular tachycardia. Evaluation of a new pacing method. Am J Cardiol 1982; 50:1338-1345.
62. Jentzer JH, Hoffmann RM. Acceleration of ventricular tachycardia by rapid overdrive pacing combined with extrastimuli. PACE 1984; 7:922-924.
63. Charos GS, Haffajee CI, Gold RL, Bishop RL, Berkovits BV, Alpert JS. A theoretically and practically more effective method for interruption of ventricular tachycardia: self-adapting autodecremental overdrive pacing. Circulation 1986; 73:309-315.
64. Cook JR, Kirchhoffer JB, Fitzgerald TF, Lajzer DA. Comparison of decremental and burst overdrive pacing as treatment for ventricular tachycardia associated with coronary artery disease. Am J Cardiol 1992; 70:311-315.
65. Gillis AM, Leitch JW, Wyse DG, et al. Randomized comparative trial of modes of ventricular tachycardia pace termination (abstr). PACE 1992; 15:505.
66. Newman D, Dorian P, Hardy J. A randomized prospective comparison of ventricular antitachycardia pacing modalities (abstr). PACE 1992; 15:506.
67. Klein H, Hofmann R, Troster J, Trappe HJ, Kielblock B. Efficacy of various antitachycardia pacing modes with ICD therapy (abstr). PACE 1992; 15:506.

68. Calkins H, el Atassi R, Kalbfleisch S, Langberg J, Morady F. Comparison of fixed burst versus decremental burst pacing for termination of ventricular tachycardia. PACE 1993; 16:26-32.
69. Spurrell RA, Nathan AW, Camm AJ. Clinical experience with implantable scanning tachycardia reversion pacemakers. PACE 1984; 7:1296-1300.
70. Sowton E. Clinical results with the Tachylog antitachycardia pacemaker. PACE 1984; 7:1313-1317.
71. den Dulk K, Kersschot IE, Brugada P, Wellens HJ. Is there a universal antitachycardia pacing mode. Am J Cardiol 1986; 57:950-955.
72. Saksena S, Chandran P, Shah Y, Boccadamo R, Pantopoulos D, Rothbart ST. Comparative efficacy of transvenous cardioversion and pacing in patients with sustained ventricular tachycardia: a prospective, randomized, crossover study. Circulation 1985; 72:153-160.
73. Calvo RA, Saksena S, Pantopoulos D. Sequential transvenous pacing and shock therapy for termination of sustained ventricular tachycardia. Am Heart J 1988; 115:569-575.
74. Waspe LE, Kim SG, Matos JA, Fisher JD. Role of a catheter lead system for transvenous countershock and pacing during electrophysiologic tests: an assessment of the usefulness of catheter shocks for terminating ventricular tachyarrhythmias. Am J Cardiol 1983; 52:477-484.
75. Hammill S, Stanton M, Packer D. The effect of therapy type (autodecremental, burst, cardioversion) on subsequent ventricular tachycardia cycle length in patients with an implantable antitachycardia pacing-cardioversion-defibrillation device (abstr). PACE 1991; 14:623.
76. Mason JW, Winkle RA. Electrode-catheter arrhythmia induction in the selection and assessment of antiarrhythmic drug therapy for recurrent ventricular tachycardia. Circulation 1978; 58:971-985.
77. Leitch JW, Gillis AM, Wyse DG, et al. Reduction in defibrillator shocks with an implantable device combining antitachycardia pacing and shock therapy. J Am Coll Cardiol 1991; 18:145-151.
78. Nisam S, Mower M, Moser S. ICD clinical update: first decade, initial 10,000 patients. PACE 1991; 14:255-262.
79. Winkle RA, Mead RH, Ruder MA, et al. Long-term outcome with the automatic implantable cardioverter-defibrillator. J Am Coll Cardiol 1989; 13:1353-1361.
80. Nisam S, Mower MM, Thomas A, Hauser R. Patient survival comparison in the three generations of automatic implantable cardioverter defibrillators: review of 12 years, 25,000 patients. PACE 1993; 16:174-178.
81. Kim SG, Furman S, Waspe LE, Brodman R, Fisher JD. Unipolar pacer artifacts induced failure of an automatic implantable cardioverter/defibrillator to detect ventricular fibrillation. Am J Cardiol 1986; 57:880-881.
82. Calkins H, Brinker J, Veltri EP, Guarnieri T, Levine JH. Clinical interactions between pacemakers and automatic implantable cardioverter-defibrillators. J Am Coll Cardiol 1990; 16:666-673.
83. Slepian M, Levine JH, Watkins L Jr, Brinker J, Guarnieri T. Automatic implantable cardioverter defibrillator/permanent pacemaker interaction: loss of pacemaker capture following AICD discharge. PACE 1987; 10:1194-1197.
84. Guarnieri T, DaTorre SD, Bondke H, Brinker J, Myers S, Levine JH. Increased pacing threshold after an automatic defibrillator shock in dogs: effects of class I and class II antiarrhythmic drugs. PACE 1988; 11:1324-1330.
85. Khastgir T, Lattuca J, Aarons D, et al. Ventricular pacing threshold and time to capture postdefibrillation in patients undergoing implantable cardioverter-defibrillator implantation. PACE 1991; 14:768-772.
86. Ching E, Carlblom D, Wilkoff BL, Castle LW. Risk of pacemaker damage induced by implantable defibrillator shocks (abstr). PACE 1991; 14:629.
87. Epstein AE, Kay GN, Plumb VJ, Shepard RB, Kirklin JK. Combined automatic implantable cardioverter-defibrillator and pacemaker systems: implantation techniques and follow-up. J Am Coll Cardiol 1989; 13:121-131.
88. Ahern TS, Nydegger C, McCormick DJ, et al. Device interaction—antitachycardia pacemakers and defibrillators for sustained ventricular tachycardia. PACE 1991; 14:302-307.
89. Luderitz B, Gerckens U, Manz M. Automatic implantable cardioverter/defibrillator (AICD) and antitachycardia pacemaker (Tachylog): combined use in ventricular tachyarrhythmias. PACE 1986; 9:1356-1360.

90. Callans DJ, Hook BG, Marchlinski FE. Paced beats following single nonsensed complexes in a "codependent" cardioverter defibrillator and bradycardia pacing system: potential for ventricular tachycardia induction. PACE 1991; 14:1281-1287.
91. Bardy GH, Troutman C, Poole JE, et al. Clinical experience with a tiered-therapy, multiprogrammable antiarrhythmia device. Circulation 1992; 85:1689-1698.
92. Paul V, Bashir Y, Anderson M, Ward DE, Camm AJ. Antitachycardia pacing and antiarrhythnmics combined: a recipe for misdiagnosis? (abstr). PACE 1991; 14:722.
93. Kou WH, Kirsh MM, Bolling SF, et al. Effect of antiarrhythmic drug therapy on the incidence of shocks in patients who receive an implantable cardioverter defibrillator after a single episode of sustained ventricular tachycardia/fibrillation. PACE 1991; 14:1586-1592.
94. Roth JA, Fisher JD. Antitachycardia pacing: ATP-ICD Interaction. In: Naccarelli GV, Veltri E, eds. Implantable Cardioverters/Defibrillators. Cambridge: Blackwell, In press.
95. Hartzler GO. Treatment of recurrent ventricular tachycardia by patient-activated radiofrequency ventricular stimulation. Mayo Clin Proc 1979; 54:75-82.
96. Ruskin JN, Garan H, Poulin F, Harthorne JW. Permanent radiofrequency ventricular pacing for management of drug-resistant ventricular tachycardia. Am J Cardiol 1980; 46:317-321.
97. Greene HL, Gross BW, Preston TA, et al. Termination of ventricular tachycardia by programmed extrastimuli from an externally-activated permanent pacemaker. PACE 1982; 5:434-439.
98. Luderitz B, DAlnoncourt CN, Steinbeck G, Beyer J. Therapeutic pacing in tachyarrhythmias by implanted pacemakers. PACE 1982; 5:366-371.
99. Strasberg B, Fetter J, Palileo E, Levitsky S, Rosen KM. Postoperative electrophysiological studies with a modified radiofrequency system. Technical aspects and clinical usefulness. PACE 1982; 5:688-693.
100. den Dulk K, Bertholet M, Brugada P, et al. Clinical experience with implantable devices for control of tachyarrhythmias. PACE 1984; 7:548-556.
101. Griffin JC, Sweeney M. The management of paroxysmal tachycardias using the Cybertach-60. PACE 1984; 7:1291-1295.
102. Reddy CP, Todd EP, Kuo CS, DeMaria AN. Treatment of ventricular tachycardia using an automatic scanning extrastimulus pacemaker. J Am Coll Cardiol 1984; 3:225-230.
103. Rothman MT, Keefe JM. Clinical results with Omni-Orthocor, an implantable antitachycardia pacing system. PACE 1984; 7;1306-1312.
104. Bertholet M, Demoulin JC, Waleffe A, Kulbertus H. Programmable extrastimulus pacing for long-term management of supraventricular and ventricular tachycardias: clinical experience in 16 patients. Am Heart J 1985; 110:582-589.
105. Herre JM, Griffin JC, Nielsen AP, et al. Permanent triggered antitachycardia pacemakers in the management of recurrent sustained ventricular tachycardia. J Am Coll Cardiol 1985; 6:206-214.
106. Higgins JR, Swartz JF, Dehmer GJ, Beddingfield GW. Automatic scanning extrastimulus pacemaker to treat ventricular tachycardia. PACE 1985; 8:101-109.
107. Peters RW, Scheinman MM, Morady F, Jacobson L. Long-term management of recurrent paroxysmal tachycardia by cardiac burst pacing. PACE 1985; 8:35-44.
108. Tanabe A, Ikeda H, Fujiyama M, et al. Termination of ventricular tachycardia by an implantable atrial pacemaker and external pacemaker activator. PACE 1985; 8:532-538.
109. Falkoff MD, Barold SS, Goodfriend MA, Ong LS, Heinle RA. Long-term management of ventricular tachycardia by implantable automatic burst tachycardia-terminating pacemakers. PACE 1986; 9:885-895.
110. Saksena S, Pantopoulos D, Parsonnet V, Rothbart ST, Hussain SM, Gielchinsky I. Usefulness of an implantable antitachycardia pacemaker system for supraventricular or ventricular tachycardia. Am J Cardiol 1986; 58:70-74.
111. Fromer M, Shensa M, Kus T, Page P. Management of a patient with recurrent sustained ventricular tachycardia with a new software-based antitachycardia pacemaker. J Electrophysiol 1987; 1:133-139.

112. Palakurthy PR, Slater D. Automatic implantable scanning burst pacemakers for recurrent tachyarrhythmias. PACE 1988; 11:185-192.
113. Moller M, Simonsen E, Ing PA, Oxhj H. Long-term follow-up of patients treated with automatic scanning antitachycardia pacemaker. PACE 1989; 12:425-430.
114. Occhetta E, Bolognese L, Magnani A, Francalacci G, Rognoni G, Rossi P. Clinical experience with Orthocor II antitachycardia pacing system for recurrent tachyarrhythmia termination. J Electrophysiol 1989; 3:289-300.
115. Fisher JD, Johnston DR, Kim SG, Furman S, Mercando AM. Implantable pacers for tachycardia termination: stimulation techniques and long-term efficacy. PACE 1986; 9:1325-1333.
116. Greve H, Koch T, Gulker H, Heuer H. Termination of malignant ventricular tachycardias by use of an automatical defibrillator (AICD) in combination with an antitachycardial pacemaker. PACE 1988; 11:2040-2044.
117. Newman DM, Lee MA, Herre JM, Langberg JJ, Scheinman MM, Griffin JC. Permanent antitachycardia pacemaker therapy for ventricular tachycardia. PACE 1989; 12:1387-1395.
118. Szabo TS, Klein GJ, Guiraudon GM, Yee R, Sharma AD. Localization of accessory pathways in the Wolff-Parkinson-White syndrome. PACE 1989; 12:1691-1705.
119. Bonnet CA, Fogoros RN, Elson JJ, Fiedler SB, Burkholder JA. Long-term efficacy of an antitachycardia pacemaker and implantable defibrillator combination. PACE 1991; 14:814-822.
120. Luderitz B. The impact of antitachycardia pacing with defibrillation. PACE 1991; 14:312-316.
121. Fromer M, Schlapfer J, Fischer A, Kappenberger L. Experience with a new implantable pacer-cardioverter-defibrillator for the therapy of recurrent sustained ventricular tachyarrhythmias: a step toward a universal ventricular tachyarrhythmia control device. PACE 1991; 14:1288-1298.
122. Saksena S, Mehta D, Krol RB, et al. Experience with a third-generation implantable cardioverter-defibrillator. Am J Cardiol 1991; 67:1375-1384.
123. Singer I, Austin E, Nash W, Gilbo J, Kupersmith J. The initial clinical experience with an implantable cardioverter defibrillator/antitachycardia pacemaker. PACE 1991; 14:1119-1128.
124. Block M, Borggrefe M, Hammel D, et al. Pacer-cardioverter-defibrillator (PCD): utilization, efficacy and complications of antitachycardia pacing (abstr). J Am Coll Cardiol 1991; 17:54A.
125. Ellenbogen K, Welch W, Luceri R, et al. Clinical evaluation of the Guardian ATP 4210 implantable pacemaker/defibrillator: worldwide experience (abstr). PACE 1991; 14:623.
126. Fromer M, Brachmann J, Block M, et al. Efficacy of automatic multimodal device therapy for ventricular tachyarrhythmias as delivered by a new implantable pacing cardioverter-defibrillator. Results of a European multicenter study of 102 implants. Circulation 1992; 86:363-374.
127. Saksena S, Lehmann M, Mitchell LB, Sakun V. Device use and clinical results with a third-generation cardioverter-defibrillator using endocardial or epicardial leads (abstr). Circulation 1992; 86:I-60.

5

Low-Energy Cardioversion

Connor J. Haugh, Antonis S. Manolis, and N. A. Mark Estes III

*Tufts University School of Medicine
and New England Medical Center
Boston, Massachusetts*

The advent of low-energy internal cardioversion can be traced to the transcatheter defibrillation demonstrated by Mirowski et al. in 1973 [1]. Subsequently, investigators modified this technique to deliver lower-energy, synchronized shocks for the termination of ventricular tachycardia in an attempt to decrease myocardial damage and increase patient tolerance. Early internal cardioverters employed a temporary endocardial lead connected to an external power source and were used in controlled settings such as the electrophysiology lab or cardiac care unit for patients requiring frequent cardioversion [2–4]. The first implantable cardioverter was reported in 1984 [5], but it did not remain long in clinical investigational use [6] because of the risk of tachycardia acceleration and degeneration into ventricular fibrillation. Backup defibrillation capacity was required. Since that time refinements in lead and device technology have led to the current state-of-the-art ventricular tachycardia (VT) control device, which offers the option to deliver low-energy cardioversion and antitachycardia pacing in the setting of backup high-energy defibrillation capacity [7–9].

Low-energy cardioversion (LEC) shocks are commonly defined as shocks with energies up to 2–5 J [2,10]. Shocks with energies of 5–15 J are considered as intermediate-energy shocks, and those with energies >15 J are considered high-energy shocks [11].

I. ADVANTAGES OF LOW-ENERGY CARDIOVERSION

The addition of low-energy cardioversion into the device-therapy hierarchy creates a variety of potential advantages. Low-energy cardioversion is delivered promptly, with less patient discomfort and less battery drain than high-energy countershock. These advantages are not always realized, however; if the low-energy cardioversion is unsuccessful, definitive therapy with high-energy cardioversion is delivered with more delay, discomfort, and battery drain. The clinical utility of low-energy cardioversion is frequently limited by conversion failure, tachycardia accelerations, induction of supraventricular tachycardia, bradyarrhythmias, and patient

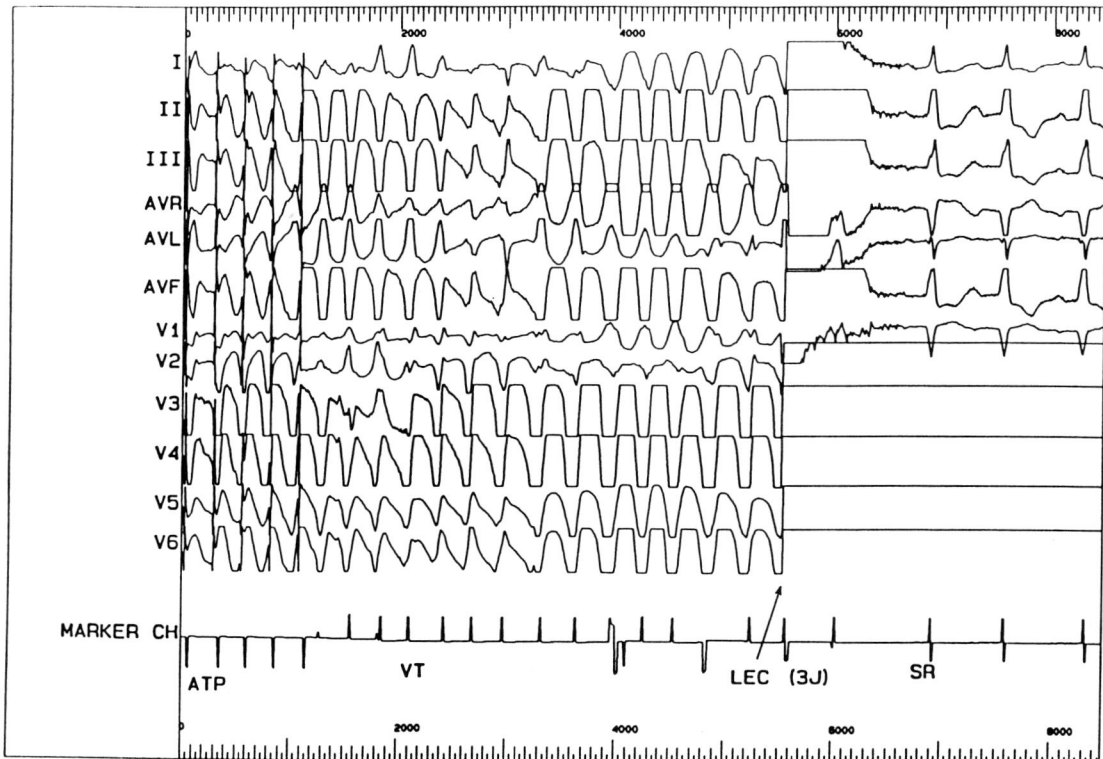

Figure 1 Antitachycardia pacing (ATP) in this patient failed to terminate sustained ventricular tachycardia (VT) and was followed by a 3-J low-energy cardioversion (LEC) shock, which successfully converted the arrhythmia into sinus rhythm (SR). MARKER CH = marker channel.

intolerance. Consequently, low-energy cardioversion should be employed only when it is likely to be effective, preferably after this has been initially demonstrated reliable by appropriate testing (Figs. 1–3).

A. Time to Delivery of Therapy/Battery Drain

When compared to high-energy defibrillation, low-energy cardioversion can be delivered more rapidly (Figs. 1 and 2) and affords less battery drain. Typical charge time for a 1-J countershock is less than half a second, compared to approximately 6.5 s for a 30-J charge. Postulating a detection time of 2.5 s, a delay of 2.5 s, and a synchronization time of 1.5 s, two low-energy cardioversion attempts could be delivered in the time required to deliver one 30-J shock.

This reduction in time to therapy may make it more effective through two mechanisms. The early cycles of ventricular tachycardia may be less stable than after it has become sustained, and hence tachycardia may be more amenable to conversion at its onset [12]. The second is a statistical phenomenon. If an energy's likelihood of converting tachycardia to sinus rhythm is represented as a probability function, one high-energy shock should have a success probability of 0.96 to be equivalent to two low-energy shocks with a success probability of 0.8. It should be noted that low-energy cardioversion is not delivered any faster than antitachycardia pacing, so that neither advantage is a valid consideration for that comparison.

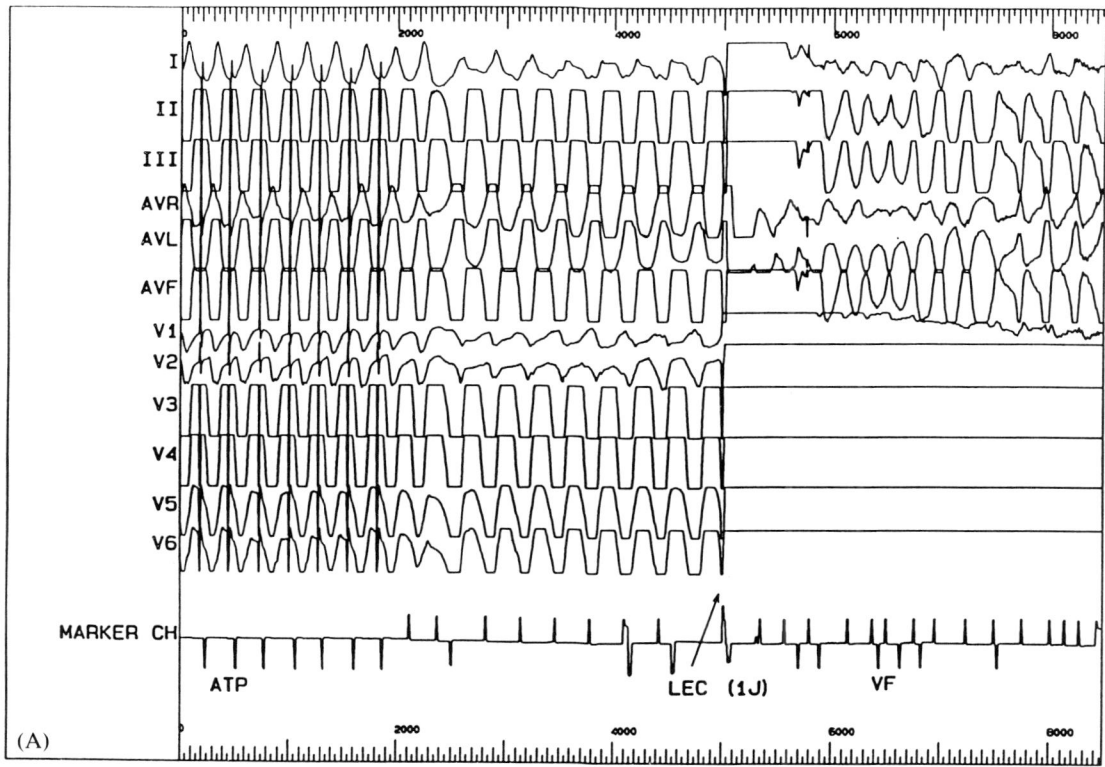

Figure 2 Delivery of a 1-J low-energy cardioversion (LEC) shock after failed antitachycardia pacing (ATP) for the patient in Fig. 1 could not terminate the ventricular tachycardia, which degenerated into ventricular fibrillation (VF) (A), requiring high-energy (34 J) shock for conversion (B).

B. Patient Tolerance

Patients' tolerance of low-energy cardioversion varies with delivered energy. Energies less than 0.5 J were typically described as "minimally uncomfortable" and generally well tolerated [2,4,9], although in one series 44% of patients described shocks of 0.03 to 0.5 J as "intolerable" [13]. Shocks of 0.5 to 1.0 J were less well received; patients frequently sought sedation or anesthesia prior to device testing at these energy levels [2,13]. Discharges of greater than 2.0 J were almost uniformly described as "severely painful" [2,13,14]. Patients' subjective comparison between these energies and high-energy (greater than 25-J) shocks were not studied. Although precise comparisons are not available, lead configuration (endocardial, epicardial patch, subcutaneous patch, etc.) did not seem to influence perception of shock.

II. EFFICACY OF LEC

Low-energy cardioversion must terminate the ventricular tachycardia if the advantages described above are to be obtained. The ability of internal, low-energy, synchronized, direct current shocks to terminate stable, monomorphic ventricular tachycardia is well documented [6]. Low-energy cardioversion terminates ventricular tachycardia by depolarizing regions or critical

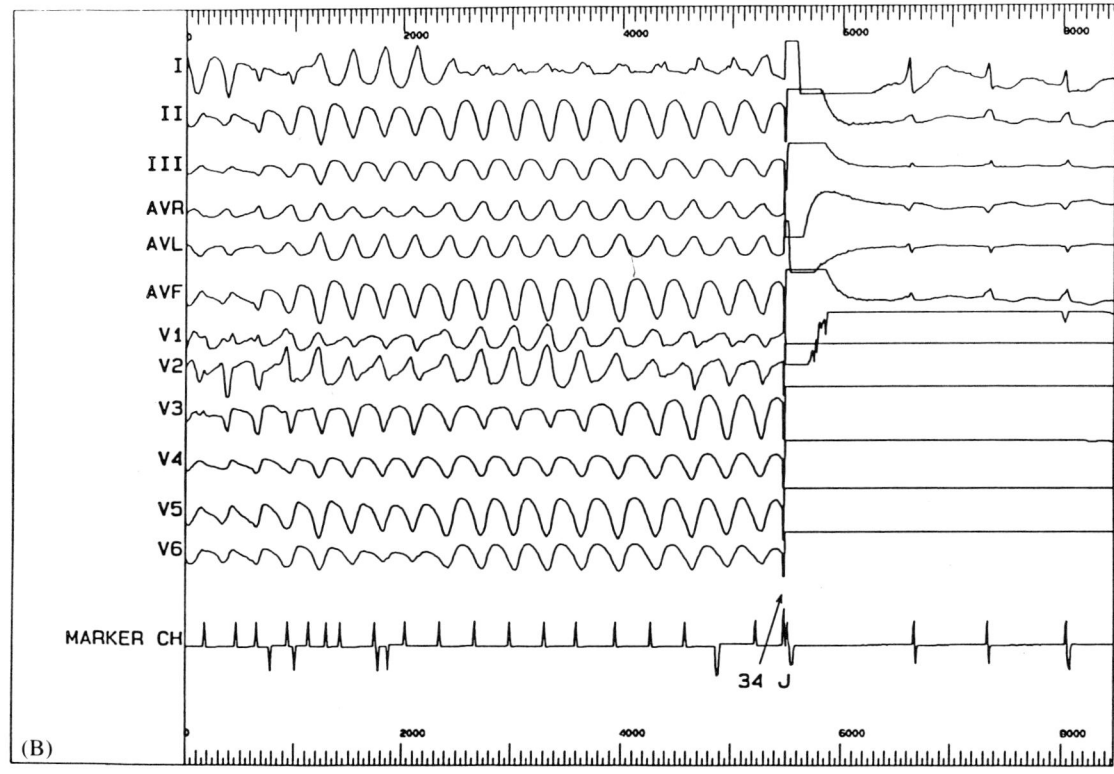

Figure 2 Continued

components of the ventricular tachycardia circuit, creating areas of conduction block, which either promptly terminate the circulating wavefront (type I cardioversion), or induce circuit instability causing delayed tachycardia termination (type II cardioversion) [15]. If the LEC shock fails, the success of subsequent higher-energy therapy may or may not be adversely affected [16,17]. The efficacy of a 1-J shock in terminating stable ventricular tachycardia is reported as varying between 28% and 77% [18,19]. Different electrode and waveform configurations and current pathways may influence cardioversion energy requirements and success. The data support a correlation between cardioversion success and tachycardia cycle length [2,12,13,17,20]. One study suggests that the likelihood of low-energy cardioversion terminating ventricular tachycardia correlates with shock energy and inversely with the duration of the sinus rhythm QRS and duration of ventricular tachycardia [12]. These correlations have both theoretical bases and important clinical implications.

A. Lead/Waveform Configuration

A variety of cathode/anode configurations are available for the delivery of low-energy cardioversion. The most frequently employed include combinations of electrodes placed at the right ventricular apex, superior vena cava, coronary sinus, and pericardial and subcutaneous patches. The configuration selected may depend on many factors: implanter experience, lead/device availability, the patient's anatomy, history of previous surgery, planned concomitant surgery, and results on intraoperative testing.

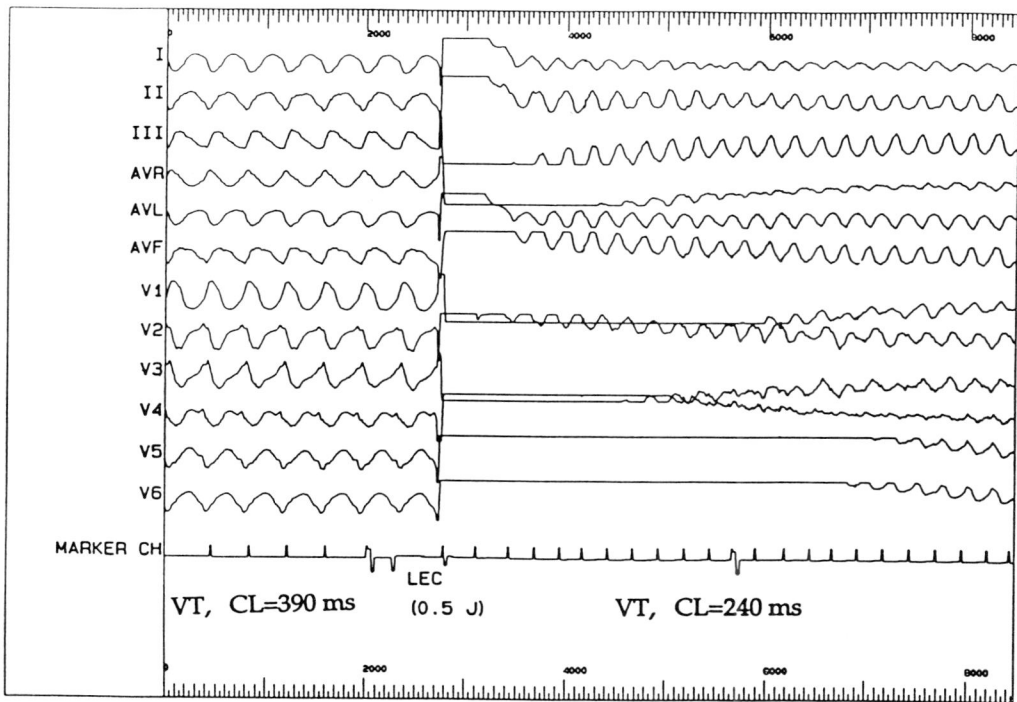

Figure 3 Testing of a 0.5-J low-energy cardioversion shock in this patient demonstrated failure to terminate sustained monomorphic ventricular tachycardia (VT). Rather, the VT accelerated to a much faster one, from 154 bpm (cycle length CL = 390 ms) to 250 bpm (CL = 240 ms).

Animal data demonstrate that the combination of right ventricular apex and pericardial "cone" patch reduced cardioversion energy requirements 25- to 250-fold when compared to right ventricular apex/coronary sinus or right ventricular apex/superior vena cava combinations [20]. This improved efficiency probably reflects less energy waste through "short circuiting" by the low-resistance intraventricular blood pool. The patches' larger surface area and consequent smaller impedance may have contributed as well. Human data demonstrate that the combination of right ventricular apex/subcutaneous patch was neither more efficient nor more effective than a right ventricular apex/superior vena cava system [21]. In a triple-electrode, bidirectional system (right ventricular apex cathode, right atrial anode, thoracic patch anode), simultaneous biphasic shocks improved efficacy and reduced cardioversion energy requirements, but energies tested were in the middle- (5–15 J) rather than low-energy range [22]. In general, studies have shown that bidirectional and/or biphasic shocks [22,23] are more efficacious for defibrillation, but similar systematic studies have not been performed with these current pathways and waveforms for LEC.

B. Tachycardia Cycle Length

Many investigators found a direct correlation between tachycardia cycle length and likelihood of cardioversion [2,12,13,17,20,24]. In a canine model, Jackman et al. showed that shock energies of 1 J or less terminated 83% of ventricular tachycardia with a cycle length of 200 ms or greater, but only 20% of those with a cycle length less than 200 ms [20]. A study in humans showed a 94.7% efficacy when the tachycardia rate was less than 180 beats/min as opposed to an 83% efficacy for rates over 180 beats/min. [17]. These results are supported by several investigators' findings of significant differences between the tachycardia cycle lengths of successful versus unsuccessful cardioversion attempts [2,12,13].

The tachycardia cycle-length dependence of cardioversion success can be explained as a consequence of the reentrant mechanism of ventricular tachycardia. As the cycle length of a monomorphic ventricular tachycardia decreases, the size of the excitable gap would also be expected to decrease. If the tachycardia cycle length approached the refractory period of the ventricular tissue, the leading edge of the depolarization wavefront would begin to impinge on relatively refractory tissue. Consequently, little or no excitable tissue would remain for the cardioversion pulse to capture, resulting in ineffective or no conduction block. Without the creation of conduction block, the tachycardia would continue, and the cardioversion attempt would be ineffective.

C. Shock Energy

Although intuitively appealing, the hypothesis that higher cardioversion energies are more likely to be successful is less well supported. One study, using sequences of cardioversion attempts ranging from 0.03 J to 10 J, demonstrated that higher-energy sequences were more likely than lower-energy ones to terminate ventricular tachycardia [12]. In contrast, Winkle et al. found that increasing cardioversion energy from 1 J to 25 J did not significantly improve the likelihood of converting stable, monomorphic ventricular tachycardia [18]. Intermediate-energy (5–15 J) shocks increase the risk of VT acceleration [11]. The flat dose-response curve of the Winkle et al. study might be explained by the energies studied; for stable monomorphic ventricular tachycardia, the likelihood of cardioversion may have been energy dependent for energies less than 1 J (the-less-than-1-J range).

It is precisely in this less-than-1-J range that basic investigation suggests variation in cardioversion waveform propagation. Electrophysiological mapping during very low-energy cardioversion (0.03 J) demonstrated immediate local depolarization of the right ventricle followed by depolarization of left ventricular sites by intraventricular propagation rather than by instantaneous shock-induced depolarization. Higher-energy shocks (0.5 J) depolarized left ventricular sites instantaneously. Examples of intraventricular propagation resetting tachycardia and instantaneous depolarization terminating tachycardia have been demonstrated, suggesting a mechanism for the energy dependence of cardioversion success [15].

D. Other Correlations

One study found that successful cardioversion also correlated inversely with duration of sinus QRS and time to initial cardioversion [12]. A longer sinus QRS would suggest the presence of intraventricular conduction delay, which in turn could hamper the propagation of low-energy cardioversion impulses. It could also mean delayed sensing and increased chance of a shock not being delivered within the QRS complex and thus increased likelihood of inducing acceleration or degeneration [20,24]. Furthermore, delay in cardioversion could reduce efficacy through two potential mechanisms. For patients with coronary artery disease, ventricular tachycardia could reduce perfusion and thereby increase ischemia, creating more conduction blocks and potential tachycardia circuits. It is also suggested that the reentrant circuit of some ventricular tachycardias may be initially unstable, and hence more amenable to disruption by cardioversion. It should be noted that a different study found no correlation between efficacy and time

Table 1 Comparative Trials of LEC Versus ATP[a]

Author/Year	Pts	Episodes	ATP Success	ATP Accel.	LEC Success	LEC Accel.
Waspe et al. [2], 1983[b]	13	25	100%	0%	84%	14%
Bardy et al. [10], 1993[c]	24	96	63%	17%	75%	21%
Saksena et al. [13], 1985[d]	15	62	80%	6%	83%	11%

[a]Accel. = acceleration; ATP = antitachycardia pacing; LEC = low-energy cardioversion; pts = (number of) patients.
[b]LEC energy = 0.01–5 J; induction of atrial arrhythmias: 0% versus 15% (ATP versus LEC).
[c]LEC energy = 0.2–2 J.
[d]LEC energy = 0.5–2.7 J; induction of atrial arrhythmias: 3% versus 23% (ATP versus LEC).

to cardioversion, a fact which may be explained by their generally later use of cardioversion and their population's better left ventricular function [2].

III. DISADVANTAGES AND LIMITATIONS
A. Ventricular Tachycardia Acceleration

The addition of low-energy cardioversion to the therapy tier is not without potential disadvantages. Any unsuccessful therapy attempt would be deleterious simply by prolonging the arrhythmia, but low-energy cardioversion attempts pose other risks as well. Foremost among these is the risk of acceleration, with the cardioversion attempt producing a faster ventricular tachycardia or ventricular fibrillation (Figs. 2 and 3).

Acceleration of ventricular tachycardia by low-energy cardioversion is not uncommon (Table 1). Precise comparisons between studies are difficult, but the reported risk of acceleration varies between 7.5% and 23% [2,10,13,14,17,18]. The risk of acceleration appears to vary with tachycardia cycle length, but this relationship may simply be an extension of the cycle-length/success correlation. In a canine model, Jackman et al. found that the risk of acceleration and repetitive ventricular responses was increased by delivery of the cardioversion energy during the last quarter of the surface QRS [20]. No data relating accelerations to lead position or current path are available. Prospective randomized studies suggest that low-energy cardioversion and antitachycardia pacing cause ventricular tachycardia acceleration with similar frequency [10,13] (Table 1).

The mechanism by which low-energy cardioversion induces VT acceleration is not clearly defined. Very rapid ventricular tachycardias may have one QRS's repolarization extending into the following QRS; a shock synchronized to one QRS could be delivered into the vulnerable period of the previous complex [20]. Mapping during cardioversion acceleration demonstrated alteration of slow-region conduction with development of new areas of conduction block. This circuit, newly created by the cardioversion attempt, can result in acceleration of ventricular tachycardia [15].

B. Supraventricular Tachyarrhythmias

Low-energy cardioversion, unlike antitachycardia pacing [25], is also associated with the induction of supraventricular tachycardia, primarily atrial fibrillation or atrial flutter. The reported incidence in humans is as high as 23% of delivered shocks [13]. Most episodes are transient, but they may be sustained, particularly in patients with the atrial substrate to support fibrillation or flutter. Even nonsustained episodes can be problematic; if the device is unable to discriminate between supraventricular and ventricular tachycardia, the therapy algorithm would continue, resulting in inappropriate shocks.

Ventricular tachycardia frequently causes AV disociation. Energy delivery synchronized to ventricular electrical systole may be delivered during the vulnerable period of atrial recovery. Data comparing the incidence of atrial fibrillation/flutter induction of different lead systems and current paths are not available in humans, but minimization of atrial involvement in the current path would intuitively minimize atrial arrhythmia induction. Animal studies demonstrated an energy dependence of atrial arrhythmia induction; shocks greater than 0.5 J were more likely than lower-energy shocks to induce atrial arrhythmias, suggesting that higher-energy shocks, with their instantaneous rather than propagated depolarization of distant tissue, are more likely to involve the atrium [15,20].

IV. COMPARISON WITH ANTITACHYCARDIA PACING

Both low-energy cardioversion and antitachycardia pacing are frequently programmable options for the early tiers of the therapy hierarchy; their relative utility merits consideration. Antitachycardia pacing has the advantage of being universally painless; low-energy cardioversion is variably tolerated, as discussed earlier. Two randomized prospective trials addressed the relative clinical efficacy of low-energy cardioversion and antitachycardia pacing for termination of ventricular tachycardia [10,13]. These trials showed that the likelihood of antitachycardia pacing and low-energy cardioversion to terminate stable, monomorphic ventricular tachycardia were similar (Table 1). Bardy et al. [10] demonstrated conversion to sinus rhythm in 75% and 63% with low-energy cardioversion and ramp antitachycardia pacing, respectively; using a more aggressive protocol, Saksena et al. [13] demonstrated conversion to sinus rhythm in 83% with cardioversion and 80% with burst pacing. The successful therapy concordance of 78% demonstrated by Saksena et al. was strikingly higher than that of the 33% shown by Bardy et al., a difference that may be explained by differences in therapy protocols. Saksena et al. did show that low-energy cardioversion was more likely than antitachycardia pacing to cause acceleration, atrial fibrillation, or supraventricular tachycardia, a difference not evident in the trial by Bardy et al.

V. GUIDELINES FOR THE USE OF LEC

Several guidelines for the use of low-energy cardioversion are evident. Low-energy cardioversion should be used only with backup defibrillation capacity. The success rate of low-energy shocks for the termination of very fast ventricular tachycardia or ventricular fibrillation is very low, and accelerations are frequent for this application. As the duration of ventricular fibrillation may affect defibrillation efficacy [21], recent data also show that low-energy shocks for ventricular fibrillation may prejudice later attempts at defibrillation; consequently, low-energy shocks should not be programmed into therapy zones for fast ventricular tachycardia that may include ventricular fibrillation [16]. However, according to other data there is no correlation between nonconversions and accelerations by LEC, while no patient failed to be reverted by the second 30-J rescue shock [17].

Several studies show antitachycardia pacing and low-energy cardioversion to have similar efficacy; antitachycardia pacing is clearly better tolerated. Consequently, antitachycardia pacing should typically precede low-energy cardioversion attempts when both therapeutic modalities are available. The concordance between the success of these two modalities remains unclear [10,13]. A very high concordance would suggest little utility for low-energy cardioversion if antitachycardia pacing is available, a lower concordance would suggest it to be more useful. It appears that some patients may respond better to one than to the other form of therapy.

The use of low-energy cardioversion after failed antitachycardia pacing (Fig. 1) is supported by two clinical series. A report of European experience of tiered therapy for 1204 and a U.S. report of 623 episodes of ventricular tachycardia both demonstrated an initial 60% success rate of low-energy cardioversion after failed antitachycardia pacing, saving a total of more than 100 high-energy shocks [9,27]. Repeated attempts at low-energy cardioversion, however, were futile; the success rate dropped to 40% for second cardioversion shocks in the European study. This substantial clinical experience supports the secondary role of low-energy cardioversion for control of ventricular tachycardia. Caution must still be exercised not to commit too much time to low-energy cardioversion attempts. Following LEC, high-energy shocks should be programmed to be delivered (Fig. 2B), rather than intermediate-energy (5–15 J) shocks, which have been associated with unacceptably high risk of accelerating the tachycardia or inducing ventricular fibrillation [11].

In summary, low-energy cardioversion represents a useful modality for the treatment of monomorphic ventricular tachycardia in the setting of defibrillation capacity. Slower ventricular tachycardia is more effectively terminated; lower-energy shocks are better tolerated. Whenever possible, patients should have cardioversion thresholds demonstrated at programming (Figs. 1–3), and data logging should be checked frequently to minimize episodes of acceleration. Use of the proper hierarchy with tiered therapy devices contributes to better patient tolerance and increase in battery longevity, with need for fewer high-energy shocks without compromising patient safety [7–10,13,17,25–28].

REFERENCES

1. Mirowski M, Mower MM, Gott VL, Brawley RK. Feasibility and effectiveness of low-energy catheter defibrillation in man. Circulation 1973; XLVII:79-85.
2. Waspe LE, Kim SG, Matos JA, Fisher JD. Role of a catheter lead system for transvenous countershock and pacing during electrophysiologic tests: an assessment of the usefulness of catheter shocks for terminating tachyarrhythmias. Am J Cardiol 1983; 52:477-484.
3. Yee R, Zipes DP, Gulamhusein S, Kallok MJ, Klein GJ. Low energy countershock using an intravascular catheter in an acute cardiac care setting. Am J Cardiol 1982; 50:1124-1129.
4. Bucknall CA, Lewis S, Vincent R, Jackson G, Jewitt DE, Chamberlain DA. Transvenous cardioversion for the management of recurrent ventricular arrhythmias. Br Heart J 1987; 58:245-250.
5. Zipes DP, Heger JJ, Miles WM, et al. Early experience with an implantable cardioverter. N Engl J Med 1984; 311:485-490.
6. Miles WM, Prystowsky EN, Heger JJ, Zipes DP. The implantable transvenous cardioverter: long-term efficacy and reproducible induction of ventricular tachycardia. Circulation 1986; 74:518-524.
7. Fromer M, Schlapfer J, Fischer A, Kappenberger L. Experience with a new implantable pacer-cardioverter-defibrillator for the therapy of recurrent sustained ventricular tachyarrhythmias: a step toward a universal tachyarrhythmia control device. PACE 1991; 14:1288-1298.
8. Saksena S, Mehta D, Krol RB, et al. Experience with a third generation implantable cardioverter defibrillator. Am J Cardiol 1991; 67:1375-1384.
9. Bardy GH, Troutman C, Poole JE, et al. Clinical experience with a tiered therapy multiprogrammable antiarrhythmia device. Circulation 1992; 85:1689-1698.

10. Bardy GH, Poole JE, Kudenchuk PJ, Dolack GL, Kelso D, Mitchell R. A prospective randomized repeat-crossover comparison of antitachycardia pacing with low-energy cardioversion. Circulation 1993; 87(6):1889-1896.
11. Lindsay BD, Saksena S, Rothbart ST, Wasty N, Pantopoulos D. Prospective evaluation of a sequential pacing and high-energy bidirectional shock algorithm for transvenous cardioversion in patients with ventricular tachycardia. Circulation 1987; 76:601-609.
12. Ciccone JM, Saksena S, Shah Y, Pantopoulos D. A prospective randomized study of the clinical efficacy and safety of transvenous cardioversion for termination of ventricular tachycardia. Circulation 1985; 71:571-578.
13. Saksena S, Chjandran P, Shah Y, Boccadomo R, Pantopoulos D. Comparative efficacy of transvenous cardioversion and pacing in sustained ventricular tachycardia: a prospective, randomized crossover study. Circulation 1985; 52:377-384.
14. Calvo RA, Saksena S, Pantopoulos D. Sequential transvenous pacing and shock therapy for termination of sustained ventricular tachycardia. Am Heart J 1988; 115(3):569-575.
15. Saksena S, Pantopoulos D, Hussain SM, Gielchinsky I. Mechanisms of ventricular tachycardia termination and acceleration during transvenous cardioversion as determined by cardiac mapping in man. Am Heart J 1987; 113:1495-1506.
16. Bardy GH, Stewart RB, Ivey TD, et al. Potential risk of low energy cardioversion attempts by implantable defibrillators (abstr). J Am Coll Cardiol 1987; 9:168A.
17. McVeigh K, Mower MM, Nisam S, Voshage L. Clinical efficacy of low energy cardioversion in automatic implantable cardioverter defibrillator patients. PACE 1991; 14(II):1846-1849.
18. Winkle RA, Stinson EB, Bach SM, Echt DS, Oyer P, Armstrong K. Measurement of cardioversion defibrillation thresholds in man by a truncated exponential waveform and an apical patch-superior vena caval spring electrode configuration. Circulation 1984; 69:766-771.
19. Gottlieb C, Powers M, Kay H, et al. Efficacy and safety of the implantable defibrillator's programmable functions. PACE 1990; 13:518.
20. Jackman WM, Zipes DP. Low-energy synchronous cardioversion of ventricular tachycardia using a catheter electrode in a canine model of subacute myocardial infarction. Circulation 1982; 66:187-195.
21. Saksena S, An H. Clinical efficacy of dual electrode systems for endocardial cardioversion of ventricular tachycardia: a prospective randomized crossover trial. Am Heart J 1990; 119:15-22.
22. Saksena S, An H, Mehra R, et al. Prospective comparison of biphasic and monophasic shocks for implantable cardioverter defibrillators using endocardial leads. Am J Cardiol 1992; 70:304-310.
23. Saksena S, Luceri R, Krol RB, et al. Endocardial pacing, cardioversion and defibrillation using a braided endocardial lead system. Am J Cardiol 1993; 71:834-841.
24. Perelman MS, Rowland E, Krikler DM. Assessment of a prototype implantable cardioverter for ventricular tachycardia: relation between synchronisation of sensing and origin of the tachycardia. Br Heart J 1984; 52:385-391.
25. Wietholt D, Block M, Isbruch F, et al. Clinical experience with antitachycardia pacing and improved detection algorithms in a new implantable cardioverter defibrillator. J Am Coll Cardiol 1993; 21:885-894.
26. Winkle RA, Mead RH, Ruder MA, Smith NA, Buch WS, Gaudiani VA. Effect of duration of ventricular fibrillation on defibrillation efficacy in humans. Circulation 1990; 81:1477-1481.
27. Fromer M, Brachmann J, Block M, et al. Efficacy of automatic multimodal device therapy for ventricular tachyarrhythmias as delivered by a new implantable pacing cardioverter-defibrillator. Results of an European multicenter study of 102 implants. Circulation 1992; 86:363-374.
28. Leitch JW, Gillis AM, Wyse DG, et al. Reduction in defibrillator shocks with an implantable device combining antitachycardia pacing and shock therapy. J Am Coll Cardiol 1991; 18:145-151.

6

Stored Ventricular Electrogram Analysis in the Management of Patients with Implantable Cardioverter-Defibrillators

Bruce G. Hook
Catholic Medical Center
Manchester, New Hampshire

Henry H. Hsia
Temple University School of Medicine
Philadelphia, Pennsylvania

David J. Callans and Francis E. Marchlinski
Philadelphia Heart Institute
Presbyterian Medical Center
Philadelphia, Pennsylvania

Raman L. Mitra
Rush-Presbyterian Medical Center
Chicago, Illinois

The implantable cardioverter-defibrillator (ICD) has been shown to be highly efficacious in the treatment of patients with sustained ventricular tachyarrhythmias (VTs) [1–7]. Since the introduction of the original ICD in 1980 [1], considerable advances have occurred, including the introduction of nonthoracotomy implant techniques for energy-delivering lead placement, availability of antitachycardia pacing, low- and high-energy cardioversion, noninvasive programmed stimulation, and a fully integrated bradycardia pacemaker [8]. One of the most exciting developments has been the availability in some third-generation ICDs of ventricular electrogram storage capabilities. Information obtained by analysis of stored electrograms provides accurate insight into the electrical events preceding ICD responses. This chapter focuses on our experience with stored ventricular electrogram analysis in the Cadence (Ventritex, Sunnyvale, CA) ICD. This device stores electrograms obtained using local bipolar recordings from the rate-sensing electrodes of the ICD. Other manufacturers (Cardiac Pacemakers, Inc.) are evaluating the use of wide bipolar electrogram recordings from energy-delivering or shocking leads. Preliminary reports [8a] suggest that these recordings may also be helpful in providing an accurate recording of electrical events that lead to ICD therapy.

I. THE USE OF SYMPTOMS PRECEDING ICD RESPONSES AS AN INDEX OF THE APPROPRIATENESS OF ICD INTERVENTION

Since the initial reports on outcome in patients who received the ICD [1–7], it has been apparent that many patients do not experience symptoms of hemodynamic compromise prior to shock therapy. Those patients receiving shocks preceded by severe presyncope or syncope, with prompt resolution of symptoms following the shock, were assumed to have received an appropriate shock for a ventricular tachyarrhythmia. Several reports [9–11] subsequently used the presence of such symptoms prior to ICD shocks to estimate the benefit of the ICD in prolonging survival. However, it has been estimated that up to 52% of patients receiving the ICD will receive shocks without any preceding symptoms [12], thereby making classification of the events preceding such shocks difficult. Recent studies [13–15], limited to devices capable of delivering shock therapy only, have documented the electrocardiographic rhythm prior to ICD shock. Maloney et al. [15] reported 121 episodes of ICD shock recorded on a Holter monitor. Of 68 episodes of sustained uniform VT which lead to shock therapy, 32 (47%) were not preceded by any symptoms. Marchlinski et al. [13] documented the electrocardiographic rhythm in 35 patients who received ICD shocks in the absence of significant symptoms, noting appropriate intervention for sustained VT in 9 (26%) patients. The absence of significant symptoms occurred in one patient even in association with a VT cycle length of 260 ms and an arrhythmia duration of 16 s prior to device discharge. Clearly, classifying only those device discharges preceded by symptoms as appropriate will lead to an underreporting of the incidence of ICD responses for ventricular tachyarrhythmias.

II. VENTRICULAR ELECTROGRAM STORAGE IN THE CADENCE ICD

The limitations in using symptoms as the sole means of determining the appropriateness of ICD discharge lead to the incorporation of ventricular electrogram storage capability in some of the newer, third-generation ICDs. The Ventritex Cadence ICD stores ventricular electrograms corresponding to 1–7 tachycardia events of 16–64 s each (one 64-s event, three 32-s events, or seven 16-s events, depending on programmed values), with the date and time of the event. The stored electrograms may be transferred to a chart recorder for hard-copy display. Bipolar electrograms are filtered by the device using a bandpass centered at 20 Hz. We routinely program storage of the ventricular electrograms to be triggered by return of the heart rate to less than the minimum programmed cutoff rate that satisfies tachycardia detection (Fig. 1). Storage can also be programmed to be triggered by a device response, such as antitachycardia pacing or a shock. By using return of the heart rate to less than the minimum programmed cutoff rate that triggers tachycardia detection to initiate electrogram storage, tachycardias terminating spontaneously will also be stored (see below). With the device programmed in this fashion, termination of the tachycardia is always the final portion of any stored event. However, if the total duration of tachycardia from onset to termination is greater than the programmed storage time for an individual event, the onset of the tachycardia will not be available for review. Furthermore, if the number of spontaneous tachycardia episodes exceeds the programmed number of stored electrogram events, only the most recent tachycardia episodes will be available for review. In addition to permitting display of electrograms corresponding to a tachycardia, it is possible to record real-time electrograms at the time the device is interrogated, thereby allowing comparison of electrogram morphology between that recorded during a tachycardia and that recorded during the baseline rhythm [16].

III. CRITERIA FOR ARRHYTHMIA DIAGNOSIS USING STORED ELECTROGRAM ANALYSIS (TABLE 1)

A. Ventricular Tachycardia

Activation of the ventricles during VT typically results in a change in the ventricular electrogram morphology during the tachycardia relative to that recorded during the baseline rhythm [17] (Figs. 1 and 2). While automated analysis of electrogram morphology is capable of

Stored Ventricular Electrogram Analysis

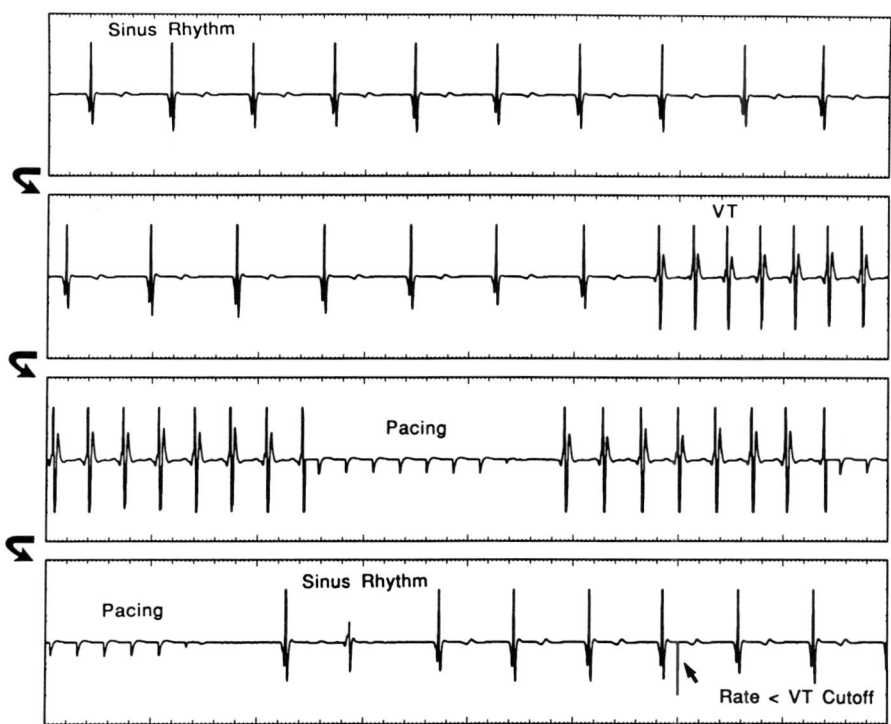

Figure 1 Continuous recording (25 mm/s) of stored electrograms from an episode characterized as uniform VT. The initial rhythm is regular, with a cycle length of 800 ms, and is presumably sinus. At the end of the second panel there is the abrupt onset of a tachycardia with a cycle length of approximately 360 ms. Coincident with the onset of the tachycardia is a distinct change in the morphology of the electrogram consistent with VT. Two bursts of antitachycardia pacing are delivered, with successful termination of VT following the second burst (fourth panel).

Table 1 Criteria for Arrhythmia Diagnosis Using Stored Ventricular Electrograms

	Heart Rate (bpm)	R–R Interval Variability >60ms	Morphology
Sinus tachycardia	<200	No	Same as NSR
Atrial fibrillation	Variable	Yes	Same as NSR
Atrial flutter	140–160	No	Same as NSR
Monomorphic VT	Variable	No	Ventricular
Polymorphic VT/VF	Usually >250	Variable	Polymorphic

VT = Ventricular tachycardia
VF = Ventricular fibrillation
NSR = Normal sinus rhythm

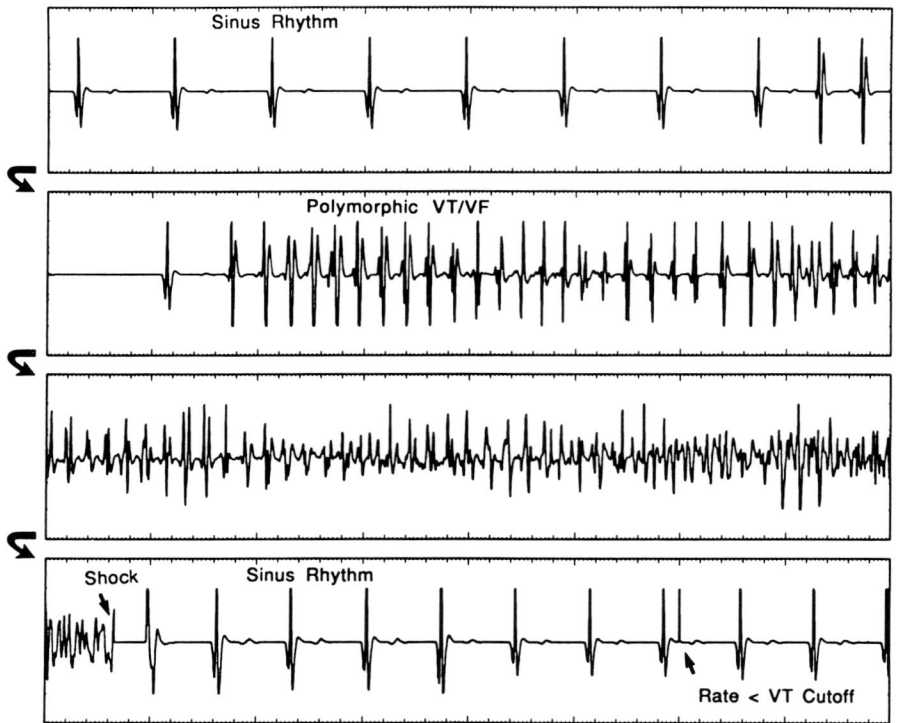

Figure 2 Continuous recording (25 mm/s) of stored electrograms from an episode characterized as polymorphic VT/VF. The initial rhythm is regular and presumably sinus. Two premature beats with a different morphology (end of the first panel) are associated with the onset of a very rapid tachycardia (second and third panels). During the tachycardia, the electrogram morphology and rate are both variable, consistent with polymorphic VT or VF. A single shock (fourth panel) successfully restores sinus rhythm.

discriminating ventricular from supraventricular rhythms [18], these techniques are not currently available in any ICD. Thus, we rely on visual analysis of the stored electrograms in establishing an arrhythmia diagnosis. Differences in electrogram morphology are considered present if there is any alteration in the number or polarity of individual electrogram components during the tachycardia relative to the baseline rhythm. Ventricular electrograms of uniform morphology at very rapid rates (>250 beats/min) or of continuously changing configuration at any rate are always designated as VT (uniform or polymorphic, respectively). Previous work from our laboratory [17] has demonstrated that VT induced at intraoperative and postoperative testing fullfil these criteria in over 90% of cases. Supraventricular tachycardias are not associated with an electrogram morphology change. An important limitation of this technique is that development of rate-dependent bundle branch block during supraventricular tachycardia may alter the electrogram morphology relative to sinus rhythm, particularly when the recording electrodes are located ipsilateral to the side of the bundle branch block [19]. Information related to the status of AV conduction, the history of preimplant supraventricular tachycardias, and the morphology of electrograms during all induced ventricular tachycardias make this important exception of lesser clinical importance.

B. Atrial Fibrillation

The presence of variability in R–R intervals of more than 60 ms for three or more of 10 consecutive intervals with no change in the electrogram morphology relative to the baseline rhythm is used to classify a rhythm as atrial fibrillation (Figs. 3 and 4). Of note, while there may be less R–R interval variability during atrial fibrillation associated with very rapid ventricular rates, the ability to record ventricular electrograms for up to 30 s prior to device response in the majority of episodes permits inspection of a large number of intervals for analysis of R–R variability.

C. Supraventricular Tachycardia

A tachycardia without the R–R interval variability described for atrial fibrillation and with no change in the electrogram morphology relative to the baseline rhythm is classified as supraventricular tachycardia. While the type of supraventricular tachycardia cannot be established using ventricular electrograms alone, a history of atrial tachycardia, atrial flutter, atrioventricular

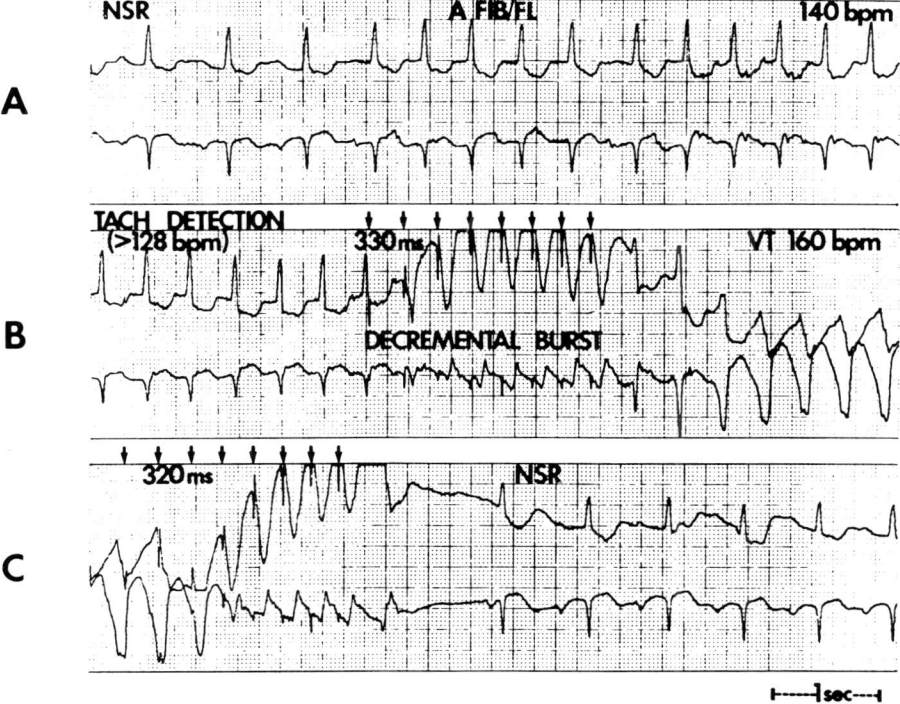

Figure 3 Continuous recording of two surface electrocardiographic leads from an episode of atrial fibrillation/flutter (AFIB/FL) leading to device therapy. The onset of AFIB/FL at 140 beats/min (A) was greater than the programmed cutoff rate for tachycardia detection (128 beats/min, B), leading to a decremental burst of antitachycardia pacing. This in turn induced ventricular tachycardia at 160 beats/min. A second burst of antitachycardia pacing successfully terminated ventricular tachycardia (C). (Reprinted with permission from Ref. 31.)

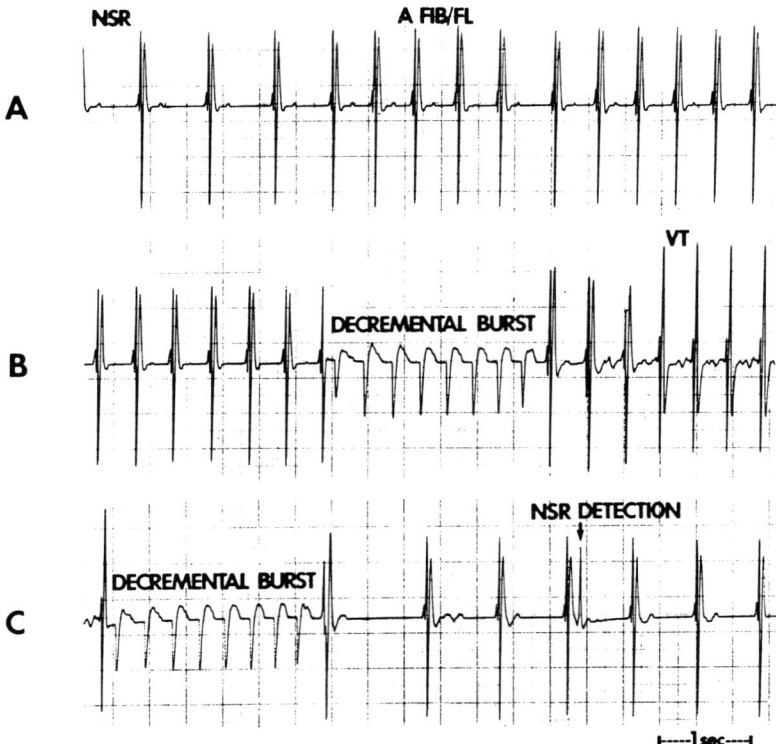

Figure 4 Continuous recording of stored electrograms corresponding to the episode shown in Fig. 3. Note that, with the onset of atrial fibrillation/flutter (A), the local electrogram remains identical to that recorded during sinus rhythm. Following induction of ventricular tachycardia by a decremental burst of antitachycardia pacing (B), the electrogram demonstrates a definite change in morphology relative to sinus rhythm. Termination of ventricular tachycardia (C) is associated with a return of the sinus rhythm electrogram. (Reprinted with permission from Ref. 31.)

nodal reentry tachycardia, or activities consistent with sinus tachycardia prior to device response are helpful in establishing a probable diagnosis.

D. Rate-Sensing Lead Disruption

High-frequency, high-amplitude signals recorded from the sensing leads consistent with an intermittent make–break phenomenon are useful in establishing a diagnosis of rate-sensing lead disruption (Fig. 5). The diagnosis is confirmed by an abnormal lead impedance recorded during real-time measurements and by reproducing the electrical artifact on a real-time electrogram recording channel with manipulation of the ICD generator/lead system at the bedside or during the intraoperative repair.

E. Indeterminate

Tachycardias with the same electrogram morphology as that during the baseline rhythm, but which terminate abruptly with antitachycardia pacing or shock, can be difficult to classify.

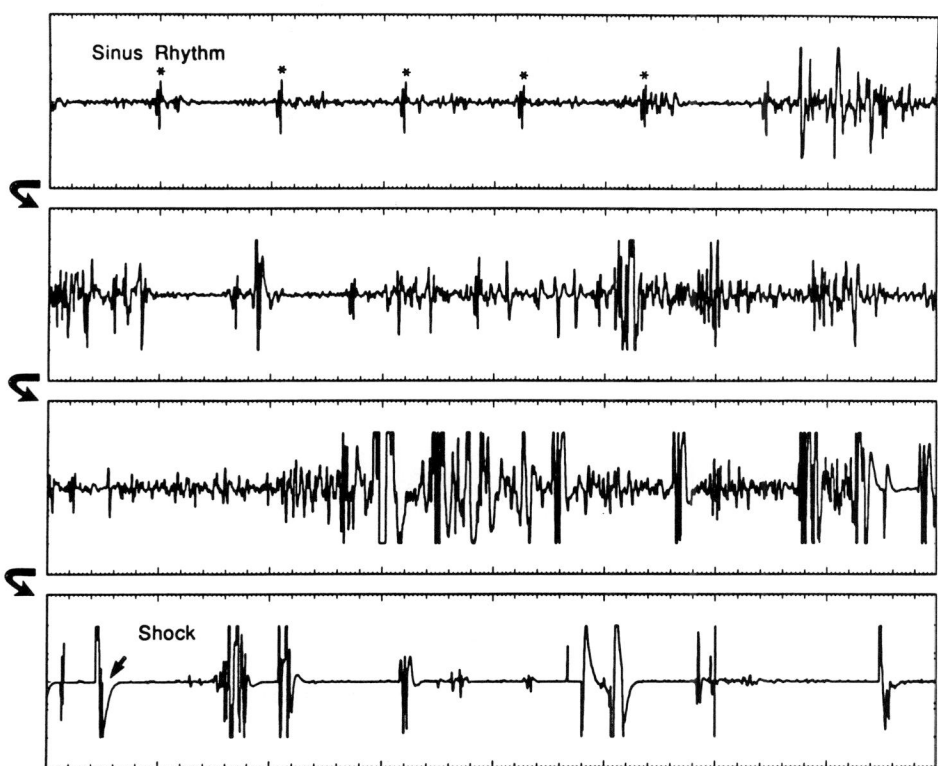

Figure 5 Continuous recording (25 mm/s) of stored electrograms from an episode characterized as electrical artifact. The most prominent feature of this example is the high-frequency, high-amplitude signals present throughout the recording, consistent with disruption of the rate-sensing lead system. The underlying rhythm is probably sinus, as regular electrograms are visible in the first panel (asterisks). These electrograms are subsequently obscured by the electrical artifact. These high-frequency signals were sensed by the device, and a shock was delivered (fourth panel).

While atrial fibrillation or atrial tachycardia occasionally terminate with delivery of a shock, termination of such rhythms with antitachycardia pacing is uncommon. In such instances when electrogram analysis suggests a supraventricular arrhythmia, but termination is consistent with an arrhythmia of ventricular origin, ventricular electrograms corresponding to all VTs induced during electrophysiological testing are reviewed to determine if any VT demonstrates the same morphology as sinus rhythm. Using this technique, a probable arrhythmia diagnosis can then be established. In our experience with stored electrogram analysis, indeterminate rhythms account for only about 3% of all stored events [20].

IV. VALUE OF STORED VENTRICULAR ELECTROGRAMS IN ASYMPTOMATIC ICD THERAPY

We recently reported the incidence of asymptomatic ICD therapy in 48 patients who received the Cadence for treatment of sustained ventricular tachyarrhythmias [20]. During a mean follow-up of 15 ± 8 months, 29 (60%) of the 48 patients experienced at least one episode of antitachycardia pacing or shock which was preceded by no or only minimal symptoms. Twenty-five of the 29 patients received at least one shock from the device which was not preceded by significant symptoms. Nine patients experienced device responses for VT only; 10 patients for non-VT rhythms only; 8 patients for both VT and non-VT rhythms; 2 patients for VT, non-VT, and indeterminate rhythms; and one patient for VT and an indeterminate rhythm. There were 74 episodes of VT, 24 episodes of non-VT rhythms, and 3 episodes classified as indeterminate rhythms. Of the 74 VT episodes, 45 were treated successfully with antitachycardia pacing and 28 with shock therapy. Of those episodes requiring shock therapy, 19 were delivered as initial therapy (11 patients) for rapid VT and 9 after antitachycardia pacing had failed to terminate the arrhythmia (4 patients). Non-VT rhythms included 13 episodes of atrial fibrillation, 6 episodes of supraventricular tachycardia, 4 episodes of rate-sensing lead disruption, and one episode of T-wave oversensing.

Based on the diagnostic information provided by stored electrogram analysis, changes in tachycardia detection criteria and/or antiarrhythmic regimens were implemented in an effort to reduce the frequency of device responses for non-VT rhythms and to improve the efficacy of antitachycardia pacing for termination of VT. During 11 ± 7 months of additional follow-up, there were only 3 recurrent device responses for non-VT rhythms (atrial fibrillation in 3 patients). Of the 4 patients in whom antitachycardia pacing failed to terminate VT, 3 patients required no further shocks for termination of 13 episodes of VT with antitachycardia pacing after device reprogramming. Thus, diagnostic information provided by analysis of stored electrograms permits changes in tachycardia detection criteria and/or antiarrhythmic regimens, which can reduce the need for shock therapy for VT and also markedly limit device responses for non-VT rhythms.

V. VALUE OF STORED ELECTROGRAMS IN STUDYING THE INITIATION OF VT

Since our current understanding of the events precipitating VT initiation is limited, the ability to record and subsequently analyze the initiation of VT in a large number of patients could lead to a better understanding of these events and hopefully offer new therapies designed to prevent spontaneous arrhythmia development. Using the criteria for rhythm classification described in the preceding sections, we have reported preliminary information on the electrical events preceding the onset of uniform VT [21]. We divided the events preceding VT into three categories. Although most VT episodes were preceded by a regular supraventricular rhythm at a rate <110 beats/min, up to 40% of VT episodes were preceded by a supraventricular tachycardia (usually atrial fibrillation) or ICD therapy directed at the patient's supraventricular tachycardia. We also noted that abrupt changes in heart rate frequently preceded VT, with over 25% of VT episodes preceded by short–long–short coupling intervals. Long–short intervals were defined as an increase of ≥100 ms followed by a decrease of ≥100 ms in the R–R intervals when compared to the preceding stable supraventricular rhythm. These preliminary observations have potential therapeutic implications for decreasing the frequency of spontaneous episodes of VT. Aggressive treatment designed to prevent or slow the ventricular response to rapid atrial fibrillation may be of value in selected patients. In addition, pacing techniques which prevent abrupt and marked cycle length changes may be capable of preventing VT in patients susceptible to long–short initiation sequences. Whether these interventions can reduce the frequency of spontaneous VT requires further study.

VI. IMPORTANCE OF ABORTIVE SHOCK CAPABILITY AND STORED ELECTROGRAMS

A significant limitation of first- and second-generation ICDs was that they were committed to deliver shock therapy once tachycardia detection criteria were satisfied, thereby resulting in shocks for nonsustained VT or other self-limited tachycardias. Most third-generation ICDs circumvent this problem either by sensing continuously during capacitor charging or by taking a "second look" prior to capacitor discharge. The Cadence stores the electrograms corresponding to such aborted events, and these can be retrieved and analyzed in a manner similar to that used for the electrical events triggering antitachycardia pacing or shock. To determine the utility of the stored electrograms obtained at the time of the aborted shock, we analyzed the stored electrograms obtained from 49 patients during a mean follow-up period of 10 ± 7 months [22]. Of 406 events satisfying tachycardia detection criteria, there were 55 aborted episodes registered in 18 of the 49 patients, including 32 events in 15 patients for which electrograms were stored and available for analysis using the previously described criteria for rhythm classification. Electrical events leading to aborted capacitor discharge included rate-sensing lead disruption ($n = 13$) in 6 patients, nonsustained uniform morphology VT ($n = 10$) in 5 patients, atrial fibrillation ($n = 5$) in 2 patients, supraventricular tachycardia ($n = 2$) in 2 patients, and polymorphic VT ($n = 2$) in 1 patient. Rate-sensing lead disruption was caused almost exclusively by fracture of a "Y" adapter used to connect the two epicardial leads to the generator header. This problem has been obviated by the use of endocardial rate-sensing leads with the Cadence ICD and by the development by the manufacturer of a generator header which accepts epicardial leads directly, without requiring an adaptor. The ability to store the events leading to an aborted shock in patients with a disrupted rate-sensing lead adaptor revealed a potentially life-threatening problem which would not otherwise have been detected. The ability to abort the discharge upon spontaneous tachycardia termination or with intermittent make–break phenomenon associated with the lead disruption prevented unnecessary shock delivery (Fig. 6). Clearly, analysis of stored electrograms can reveal important information about the integrity of the rate-sensing lead system and has also documented the value of abortive shock capability in reducing shocks for nonsustained tachycardias.

VII. VALUE OF ELECTROGRAM RECORDINGS IN THE DIAGNOSIS OF LOGICAL SENSING ERRORS

The ability to review real-time and stored electrogram sequences provides a significant advantage in the recognition of sensing errors. By combining bradycardia pacing, antitachycardia pacing, and cardioversion-defibrillation capabilities into a single device, the potential for adverse interactions between physically and logically separate cardioverter-defibrillators and bradycardia pacemakers [23–26] is markedly reduced. However, this creates the potential for unique types of sensing errors. Typically both brady and tachy sensing are governed by a codependent decision algorithm, and are often performed using a single lead system. The sensing requirements for a codependent device are much more demanding than those developed for bradycardia pacemakers. Rapid detection of ventricular fibrillation requires accurate sensing of R-wave amplitudes that may suddenly change over an order of magnitude. This is usually accomplished by employing an automatic variable-gain amplification system (or a variable-sensing threshold system), which allows rapid adjustment to detect signals as small as 0.2 mV [27]. This obviously countermands the concept of a fixed, programmable sensing threshold

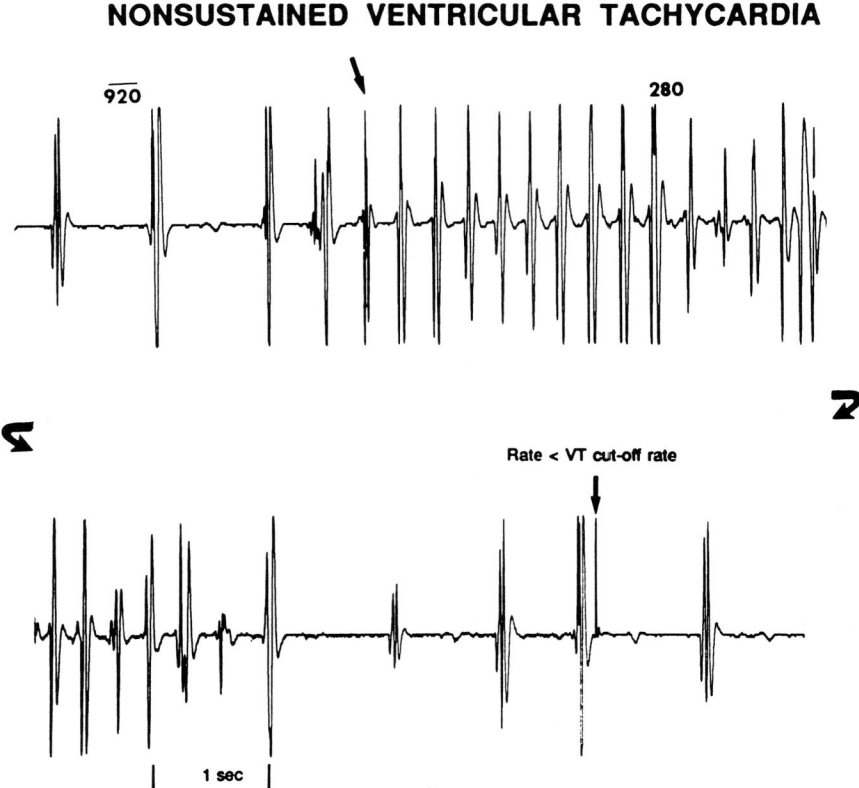

Figure 6 Continuous recording (25 mm/s) of stored electrograms from an aborted shock for nonsustained VT. As in Figs. 1 and 2, the onset of tachycardia is associated with a change in the electrogram morphology, suggesting VT as the diagnosis. In contrast to those examples, the tachycardia terminates spontaneously (second panel), and thus no therapy is delivered. (Reprinted with permission from Ref. 22.)

typically used in bradycardia pacing, where signal characteristics (R-wave amplitude and slew rate) are much more constant. Despite the distinct advantage this offers in the detection of low-amplitude signals associated with ventricular fibrillation, codependent sensing algorithms cannot avoid the inherent conflicts that exist between brady- and tachy-sensing paradigms. For example, when confronted with the sudden absence of sensed R waves, two potentially life-threatening conditions with mutually exclusive treatment strategies must be distinguished: complete heart block requiring bradycardia pacing versus ventricular fibrillation requiring amplifier gain adjustments for proper detection.

We have recently published two reports [28,29] concerning the potential for logical sensing errors in third-generation ICDs. We used the term ''logical sensing error'' to describe errors in interpreting sensed events caused by the contradictions presented by combining brady- and tachy-sensing paradigms into a single algorithm. In a series of 61 patients with third-generation devices (Cadence and PCD, Medtronic), we found that logical sensing errors that resulted in symptoms, device inefficacy, or delivery of inappropriate therapy occurred in 12 patients (19.7%). A total of five different categories of logical sensing errors were observed. The two

A. Transient Sensing Failure During Sinus Rhythm Caused by Spontaneous Variation in Signal Amplitude (Fig. 7).

The sense amplifier adjusts to the characteristics of the predominant R wave during spontaneous rhythm. Single atrial or ventricular premature beats do not change the gain setting, but do cause a transient alteration in the sinus cycle length. We have shown that abrupt changes in heart rate can cause considerable variations in the sinus rhythm R-wave amplitude [30]. The electrogram of the sinus beat that follows the pause induced by a premature beat can be sufficiently smaller than the preceding sinus beats, which can result in transient sensing failure. In the absence of a sensed R wave, a bradypacing stimulus is delivered at the programmed pacing interval, producing a long–short sequence that can result in device-mediated tachycardia initiation in susceptible patients.

B. Inappropriate Inhibition of Bradycardia Pacing due to T-Wave Oversensing (Fig. 8)

When the lead system is used for pacing, sensing functions are temporarily suspended (blanking). In 100% paced rhythms, the largest signal available for sensing is the T wave and the local afterdepolarization at the lead–tissue interface. The sense amplifier increases the gain to detect these low-amplitude events, magnifying the amplitude and duration of repolarization signals in a way that is not predictable from assessment of the surface QT interval. This magnification can result in T-wave oversensing, which inhibits the delivery of the next pacing stimulus, potentially leading to significant bradycardia in pacing-dependent patients.

In all cases, information from real-time electrograms during implantation and predischarge testing or stored electrogram sequences from spontaneous events was essential in the accurate diagnosis of sensing errors. After error recognition, device reprogramming was successful in preventing further errors in 9 of 10 patients over an average follow-up of 10 months.

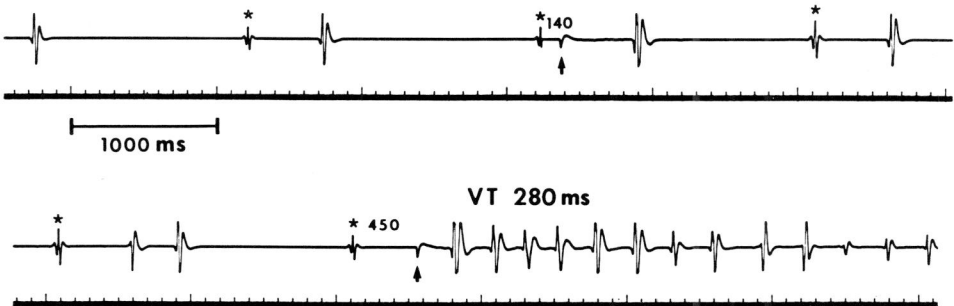

Figure 7 Continuous recording of stored electrograms from an episode of VT initiated by inappropriate bradycardia pacing by the device. The underlying rhythm is sinus (asterisks), with ventricular bigeminy. The larger amplitude of the ventricular complexes causes the automatic gain amplifier to reduce its sensitivity, resulting in intermittent failure to sense the sinus complexes. The device detects a prolonged asystolic interval and delivers bradycardia pacing stimuli (arrows). The coupling interval of the first stimulus (top panel) is too short to achieve ventricular capture; however, the second stimulus (bottom panel) falls later in diastole and initiates VT. (Reprinted with permission from Ref. 28.)

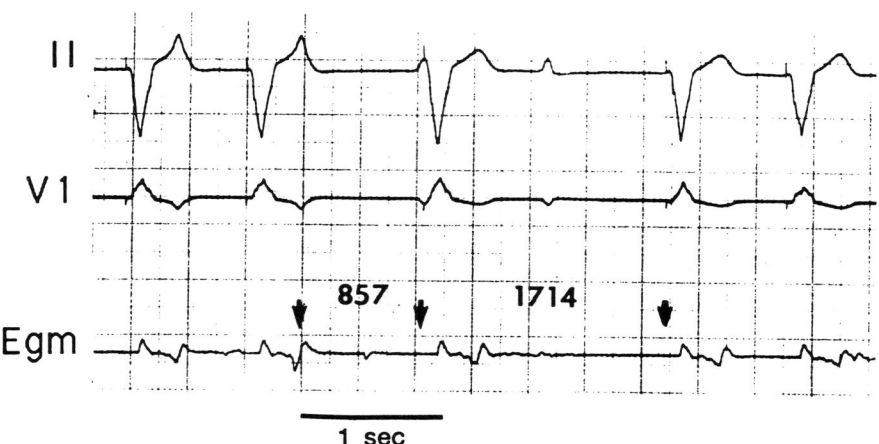

Figure 8 Real-time surface ECG and intracardiac electrograms from an episode of bradycardia pacemaker oversensing. Complete heart block is present with ventricular demand pacing set at a rate of 70 beats/min (857 ms). Following the second paced complex there is a local afterdepolarization (first arrow) of sufficient amplitude to reset the counter. This results in the third complex being delivered at an interval longer than the programmed pacing value (second arrow). Following the third paced complex, an afterdepolarization is again sensed; however, the amplitude is slightly less than that of the preceding beat. Although this afterdepolarization is sensed, the smaller amplitude signal triggers a unique software design feature that results in complete pacing inhibition for one cycle. Thus, the fourth stimulus is delivered at twice the programmed pacing interval (third arrow). (Reprinted with permission from Ref. 29.)

In summary, logical sensing errors are an important cause of symptomatic bradyarrhythmias and inappropriate therapy delivery in patients with combination bradycardia pacing and antitachycardia therapy devices. The diagnosis of sensing errors is usually impossible from surface electrocardiographic data alone, and requires monitoring of real-time and/or stored electrogram sequences. Accurate diagnosis of logical sensing errors can lead to specific reprogramming steps that can prevent further errors, even though the inherent conflicts between brady and tachy sensing paradigms cannot be resolved.

VIII. SUMMARY AND FUTURE DIRECTIONS

The ability of third-generation devices to store the electrogram sequences preceding device therapy represents a major advance in diagnostic technology. We have demonstrated that this information may be useful in several scenarios, including evaluation of asymptomatic device responses, documenting the value of abortive shock capability, studying the events immediately preceding initiation of VT, and diagnosing sensing errors. In many instances, this information has permitted device reprogramming to improve the sensitivity and specificity of device responses.

While this diagnostic information represents an important advance in ICD therapy, several additional developments can be expected. The capacity for electrogram storage will increase in future devices, thereby permitting review of all spontaneous episodes, and allowing more detailed analysis of the events preceding spontaneous VT. Diagnostic information will be transmitted via telephone linkage, allowing immediate access by the electrophysiologist. Automated electrogram analysis may be used as a criteria for arrhythmia classification by the device prior to intervention. Techniques such as template matching, gradient pattern detection, fast Fourier transformation, and the use of an atrial recording lead may improve the specificity of tachycardia detection criteria and increase the diagnostic capabilities related to ICD signal analysis, storage, and retrieval.

ACKNOWLEDGMENTS

This work was supported in part by grants from the American Heart Association, Southeastern Pennsylvania Chapter, and grant #HL07346-13 from the National Institutes of Health, Bethesda, Maryland.

REFERENCES

1. Mirowski M, Reid PR, Mower MM, et al. Termination of malignant ventricular arrhythmias with an implanted automatic defibrillator in human beings. N Engl J Med 1980; 303:322-324.
2. Echt DS, Armstrong K, Schmidt P, Oyer PE, Stinson EB, Winkle RA. Clinical experience, complications, and survival in 70 patients with the automatic implantable cardioverter/defibrillator. Circulation 1985; 71:289-296.
3. Marchlinski FE, Flores BT, Buxton AE, et al. The automatic implantable cardioverter-defibrillator: efficacy, complications, and device failures. Ann Intern Med 1986; 104:481-488.
4. Fogoros RN, Fiedler SB, Elson JJ. The automatic implantable cardioverter-defibrillator in drug-refractory ventricular tachy-arrhythmias. Ann Intern Med 1987; 107:635-641.
5. Gabry MD, Brofman R, Johnston D, et al. Automatic implantable cardioverter defibrillator: patient survival, battery longevity and shock delivery analysis. J Am Coll Cardiol 1987; 8:1349-1356.
6. Kelly PA, Cannom DS, Garan H, et al. The automatic implantable cardioverter-defibrillator: efficacy, complications and survival in patients with malignant ventricular arrhythmias. J Am Coll Cardiol 1988; 11:1278-1286.
7. Tchou PJ, Kadri N, Anderson J, Caceres JA, Jazayeri M Akhtar M. Automatic implantable cardioverter defibrillators and survival of patients with left ventricular dysfunction and malignant ventricular arrhythmias. Ann Intern Med 1988; 109:529-534.
8. Klein LS, Miles WM, Zipes DP. Antitachycardia devices: realities and promises. J Am Coll Cardiol 1991; 18:1349-1362.
8a. Block M, Isbruch F, Clerc G, Dees H, Breithardt G. ECGs of defibrillation electrodes yield more information than ECGs of sensing electrodes (abstr). Eur JCPE 1992; 2(2):122A.
9. Myerburg RJ, Luceri RM, Thurer R, et al. Time to first shock and clinical outcome in patients receiving an automatic implantable cardioverter-defibrillator. J Am Coll Cardiol 1989; 14:508-514.
10. Fogoros RN, Elson JJ, Bonnet CA, Fiedler SB, Burkholder JA. Efficacy of the automatic implantable cardioverter-defibrillator in prolonging survival in patients with severe underlying cardiac disease. J Am Coll Cardiol 1990; 16:381-386.
11. Levine JH, Mellits ED, Baumgardner RA, et al. Predictors of first discharge and subsequent survival in patients with automatic implantable cardioverter-defibrillators. Circulation 1991; 84:558-566.
12. Fogoros RN, Elson JJ, Bonnet CA. Actuarial incidence and pattern of occurrence of shocks following implantation of the automatic implantable cardioverter defibrillator. PACE 1989; 12:1465-1473.
13. Marchlinski FE, Buxton AE, Flores BF. The automatic implantable cardioverter defibrillator: Follow-up and complications. In: El-Sherif N, Samet P, eds. Cardiac Pacing and Electrophysiology. Orlando, FL: Grune & Stratton, 1990:743-758.

14. Steinberg JS, Sugalski JS. Cardiac rhythm precipitating automatic implantable cardioverter-defibrillator discharge in outpatients as detected from transtelephonic electrocardiographic recordings. Am J Cardiol 1991; 67:95-97.
15. Maloney J, Masterson M, Khoury D, et al. Clinical performance of the implantable cardioverter defibrillator: electrocardiographic documentation of 101 spontaneous discharges. PACE 1991; 14(II):280-285.
16. Hook BG, Marchlinski FE. Value of ventricular electrogram recordings in the diagnosis of arrhythmias precipitating electrical device shock therapy. J Am Coll Cardiol 1991; 17:985-990.
17. Callans DJ, Hook BG, Marchlinski FE. Use of bipolar recordings from patch-patch and rate sensing leads to distinguish ventricular tachycardia from supraventricular rhythms in patients with implantable cardioverter defibrillators. PACE 1991; 14(II):1917-1922.
18. Pannizzo F, Mercando AD, Fisher JD, Furman S. Automatic methods for detection of tachyarrhythmias by antitachycardia devices. J Am Coll Cardiol 1988; 11:308-316.
19. Sarter BH, Hook BG, Callans DJ, Marchlinski FE. Effect of bundle branch block on local electrogram morphology: potential cause of arrhythmia misdiagnosis. PACE 1992; 15(4), part II:562.
20. Hook BG, Callans DJ, Kleiman RB, Flores BF, Marchlinski FE. Implantable cardioverter defibrillator therapy in the absence of significant symptoms: rhythm diagnosis and management aided by stored electrogram analysis. Circulation 1993; 87:1897–1906.
21. Marchlinski FE, Hook BG, Cadence Phase I Investigators. Electrical events initiating ventricular tachycardia requiring device therapy. Circulation 1990; 82(suppl II)(4):547.
22. Hurwitz JL, Hook BG, Flores BT, Marchlinski FE. Importance of abortive shock capability with electrogram storage in cardioverter-defibrillator devices. J Am Coll Cardiol 1993; 21:895–900.
23. Calkins H, Brinkler J, Ventri EP, et al. Clinical interactions between pacemakers and automatic implantable cardioverter-defibrillators. J Am Coll Cardiol 1990; 16:666-673.
24. Kim SG, Furman S, Waspe LE, et al. Unipolar pacer artifacts induced failure of an automatic implantable cardioverter/defibrillator to detect ventricular fibrillation. Am J Cardiol 1986; 57:880-881.
25. Cohen AI, Wish MH, Fletcher RD, et al. The use and interaction of permanent pacemakers and the automatic implantable cardioverter defibrillator. PACE 1988; 11:704-711.
26. Epstein AE, Kay GN, Plump VJ, et al. Combined automatic implantable cardioverter-defibrillator and pacemaker systems: implantation techniques and follow-up. J Am Coll Cardiol 1989; 13:121-131.
27. Troup PJ. Implantable cardioverters and defibrillators. Curr Probl Cardiol 1989; 12:675-815.
28. Callans DJ, Hook BG, Marchlinski FE. Paced beats following single nonsensed complexes in a "codependent" cardioverter defibrillator and bradycardia pacing system: potential for ventricular tachycardia induction. PACE 1991; 14:1281-1287.
29. Callans DJ, Hook BG, Kleiman RB, Mitra RL, Flores BT, Marchlinski FE. Unique sensing errors in third generation implantable cardioverter-defibrillators. J Am Coll Cardiol 1993; 22:1135-1140.
30. Callans DJ, Hook BG, Marchlinski FE. Effect of rate and coupling interval on endocardial R wave amplitude variability in permanent ventricular sensing lead systems. J Am Coll Cardiol 1993; 22:746-750.
31. Johnson NJ, Marchlinski FE. J Am Coll Cardiol 1991; 18(5):1418-1425.

7
Engineering Considerations in the Design of ICD Systems

Eliot L. Ostrow and Stephen J. Whistler

*Intermedics, Inc., A Company of Sulzermedica
Angleton, Texas*

I. INTRODUCTION

Implantable cardioverter-defibrillators (ICDs) are often likened to cardiac pacemakers in terms of their design demands, and, indeed, they do share much in common: the need for high-reliability, low-power components; the ability to sense cardiac activity, and, when appropriate, to deliver energy to the heart; the ability to deal with external sources of electromagnetic interference, radiation, and high energy; and the need to manage the interactions among the various functional subsections of the circuitry. Yet the nature of the disease which ICD technology is designed to treat, and of the therapy it is meant to deliver, present many unique challenges to the teams of engineers charged with the development of ICD systems.

The simplified block diagram shown in Fig. 1 illustrates the major components of a typical "fourth-generation" ICD system: the *microprocessor*, which orchestrates the interplay between the various subsections of the system; the *memory section*, containing both *read-only memory (ROM)* and *random-access memory (RAM)*, utilized by the microprocessor to store program instructions that determine the functional characteristics of the ICD, the programming information that tailors those characteristics to the needs of the individual patient, and the diagnostic information that allows the physician to assess device function and patient–device interactions over time; the *power source* (i.e., batteries); the *pacing and high-voltage output sections*, which take the modest 3 to 10 V provided by the batteries and convert them into device discharges that may range from less than 1 V (for pacing) to 750 V or more (for defibrillation); the *sense amplifier*, which must adjust to endocardial signals during sinus rhythm, tachycardia, and fibrillation that may vary widely without significant undersensing or oversensing; the *communications section*, which allows the ICD to exchange information with the programmer or other external devices; and, finally, the *isolation circuit*, which protects the ICD from the damage that could be caused if a defibrillation shock (generated by the ICD itself or an external defibrillator) were to be coupled into the device via the electrodes.

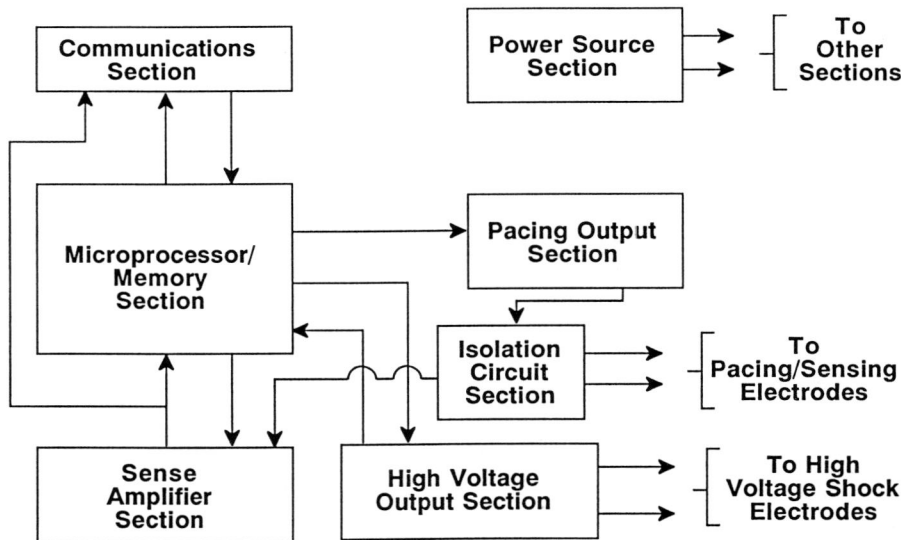

Figure 1 Simplified block diagram of major component sections in a typical "third-generation" ICD.

Other chapters in this volume deal, in specific terms, with many of the components of an implantable cardioverter-defibrillator: power sources; capacitors used in the high-voltage output circuit; communications circuits for providing programming information to, and receiving telemetry data from, the implanted system; sensing and detection circuits and algorithms; and the logic circuitry that orchestrates the activities of the various subsystems within the ICD. In this chapter we seek to provide insight into the general considerations that must be taken into account in the overall design of such systems.

II. FUNCTIONAL CHARACTERISTICS

A. The Microprocessor

Most, if not all, of the latest-generation of ICDs employ microprocessor technology, rather than discrete logic circuits, in their control sections. Microprocessors are unparalleled in terms of their size, their energy efficiency, and, equally important, their flexibility. Given the size and power consumption constraints inherent in the design of implantable devices such as these, the extensive programming and data storage capabilities of the fourth-generation ICDs and beyond would not be possible without them.

ICD design teams must decide early in the development process whether they will use a commercially available "off-the-shelf" microprocessor, or will design and procure a custom component. A suitable commercial microprocessor holds great allure. The ready availability of the processor, as compared to its custom counterpart, would dramatically reduce product development time, allowing the manufacturer to bring the product to market sooner. This, in turn, would increase the product's life cycle, and would confer a significant competitive advantage upon the manufacturer. The need for fewer in-house engineering resources, the already-available software development tools, and the existing pool of available programmers experienced in developing software for the commercial processor are all distinct advantages that

Engineering Considerations

translate into reduced development costs. However, the higher current drains and operating voltage requirements associated with most, if not all, of today's commercial microprocessors make this a choice of compromise for implantable systems, where longevity is a major design consideration. Because of this, many device manufacturers have developed custom microprocessors, which deal more effectively with these specific design constraints (although usually at the expense of faster operating speeds). The shortcomings of commercially available microprocessors are, however, rapidly diminishing; the demand for small, portable, computationally powerful, battery-powered consumer products, such as laptop computers, is driving the development of low-power commercial microprocessors that may ultimately prove suitable for ICD applications.

B. Memory

Closely associated with the microprocessor is the device's memory, or data storage, section. In fact, the relationship between the two may be thought of as symbiotic: The microprocessor could not function without the associated ROM (its fixed set of instructions) and RAM (its alterable memory), while memory is useless without a means of organizing and accessing it.

Although today's devices may have in the area of 5–10 kilobytes of ROM and 300–20,000 bytes of RAM (versus 1–2 kilobytes of ROM and 64 bytes of RAM just a few years ago), the demand for additional memory will undoubtedly continue to increase as more sophisticated devices emerge, incorporating more complex rhythm detection and discrimination algorithms, dual-chamber rate-responsive pacing, and increased diagnostic data storage.

Diagnostic data storage features provide an excellent illustration of the ever-increasing need for memory. Physicians have expressed an ardent desire for information that will allow them to reconstruct clinical events (delivery of shocks, acceleration of arrhythmias, prolonged arrhythmic episodes, etc.) and to better assess the appropriateness of device behavior [1–4]. This information may take any or all of several forms: cumulative event counters; detailed descriptions of significant events; storage of part or all of a clinical episode interval by interval; and/or recordings of intracardiac electrograms (IEGMs).

These diagnostics require varying amounts of memory. For example, the RAM necessary to store 1 min of annotated IEGM data (with adequate resolution to be clinically useful) would allow for an hour or more of stored interval data. Because device memory is not limitless, trade-offs will always be necessary. However, as the amount of memory increases, these trade-offs become less significant.

As is the case with microprocessor technology development, the rapidly expanding interest in commercial uses of low-power memory storage for products such as laptop computers, and the enormity of those markets, will drive the development of new, energy-efficient memory technologies, such as dynamic RAM (DRAM), in a way that the implantable device manufacturers never could.

C. Pacing and High-Voltage Output Sections

The circuitry for delivering pacing pulses is very similar to that found in a standard bradycardia pulse generator. Voltage multipliers incorporate a series of capacitors, some or all of which are selectively charged and discharged to provide outputs that are multiples or fractions of the supply (power source) voltage. The only additional consideration in ICD pacing output circuit design is to ensure that the output capacitor can charge quickly enough, even as the power source approaches end-of-service voltages, to deliver the bursts of closely spaced pacing pulses typically used for arrhythmia induction or termination, without a significant dropoff in pulse voltage from the first pulse in the burst to the last. This means that the design team must pay particular attention to minimizing sources of energy loss within the device output circuitry.

The more significant engineering challenge is to charge up the high-voltage capacitors to a point where they can deliver a defibrillation-sized shock of up to 800 V using a power source two orders of magnitude lower in voltage, and to generate it quickly enough to be of optimal clinical utility. This is typically accomplished by using a transformer-coupled flyback oscillator circuit, similar in concept to that used in a television set to generate the large voltages needed to power the picture tube from the 110-V power supply. In such a system, the oscillator generates large voltages, which are then stepped up and delivered to an output capacitor. This process is rapidly repeated until the capacitor is charged to the desired level. To implement circuitry that can accomplish this task, and to do so in a fashion that meets the size and efficiency requirements for an implantable device, is another formidable challenge for the design team.

D. Isolation/Protection Circuits

Implantable bradycardia pulse generators have, for years, incorporated circuitry to protect their components from damage caused by external cardioversion or defibrillation. This protection typically consists of the incorporation of zener diodes [5], which, when voltage levels begin to exceed a prescribed maximum, lower their impedance to increase current flow through the devices while clamping the voltage.

An implantable cardioverter-defibrillator must deal not only with the occasional exposure to external sources of high voltage (e.g., external defibrillation), but also with potentially frequent self-generated cardioversion/defibrillation shocks. Moreover, the close proximity of the pacing/sensing electrodes to the shock electrodes could provide a ready pathway from the high-voltage shock delivery site back to the low-power circuitry of the ICD. This results in a higher probability of exceeding the power rating of the zener diodes, in which case protection would no longer be afforded to the circuitry. Thus, this method of protection, by itself, may not be sufficient for such devices.

To protect the zener diodes, an ICD could incorporate circuitry that would monitor current flow independently, and increase the series impedance in this current path before the power rating of the zener diodes is exceeded [6]. This would provide additional protection against both device-generated shocks and external high-energy sources. In addition, the device could proactively open switches to "break" circuit pathways leading to sensitive inputs when it delivers a shock.

Regardless of the method or methods chosen (some of those described above are not in widespread use today), the means for protecting sensitive circuit inputs merits careful consideration in the overall design of an implantable cardioverter-defibrillator.

III. IMPLEMENTATION CONSIDERATIONS

Once the functional subsections of an ICD are defined, they must be combined into a cohesive unit within which each can perform its function in conjunction with, and with minimal interference from, the others, all the while striving to minimize size, weight, and cost while maximizing longevity, reliability, manufacturability, and testability.

A. Power Considerations

Probably the single most significant challenge facing ICD circuit designers is the integration of components with vastly different power requirements into the same circuit, often in close proximity on the same assembly. The sensing and logic control circuits, which ICDs share with traditional pacemakers, consume energy in the microjoule range. The pacing output circuit, also common to both types of devices, develops and delivers outputs in the 1- to 10-V range (microjoules of energy), and will have peak demands from the power source in the milliampere range. By comparison, the converter circuits for defibrillation outputs, which develop and deliver outputs of up to 750 V (approximately 30–40 J), can impose peak current drain demands of several amperes on the power source [7]. These factors have implications in the selection of a power source, in the design of the circuitry, and in the relative positioning of components in an assembly (i.e., circuit layout).

Some of the conflicts inherent in combining high- and low-power circuits could be mitigated by using two separate power sources. For examples, a lithium iodide cell, the standard for bradycardia pacemakers, could be employed to run the low-power circuitry, while a cell with a high-rate, low-internal-impedance chemistry, such as lithium-silver vanadium oxide, could be used for the high-output circuitry. Such an arrangement would alleviate concerns regarding maintenance of an adequate supply voltage to the logic circuitry during peak current demands from the defibrillation circuits, and would allow the choice of the optimum power source for each need. However, additional cells add size and weight to the ICD, while practical demands require that size and weight be reduced. Moreover, the engineering considerations involved in the interconnection of, and interaction between, circuits that operate at different voltages are not trivial. For those reasons, most ICD designs employ only one battery chemistry, and the supply circuit complexity is increased slightly to deal with the differing circuit demands previously mentioned.

When a single power source is used, the logic circuitry must be provided with a voltage supply that remains within a range that ensures consistent operation under widely varying battery loads. If the supply voltage were to become inadequate, even briefly, the possibility exists that the logic circuitry could lose control of the high-voltage circuit. One approach to resolving this concern would be to design the circuit to operate down to levels below the minimum supply voltage that might be expected under worst-case conditions, i.e., charging to deliver a maximum output when the power supply is at its end-of-service voltage. A second alternative might be to design circuitry that would independently monitor the voltage being delivered to the logic control circuitry, and prioritize the distribution of power to ensure adequate voltage to this control circuitry, even if that were to require the temporary suspension of charging of the high-voltage circuits [8].

While the precise method of power distribution and prioritization may vary from manufacturer to manufacturer, and from device to device, this issue is one to which the design team pays particular attention.

B. Integration

Serious consideration must be given to the processes and technologies that will be used to implement the many functions demanded in a completed assembly. The first consideration is the level of circuit integration that is practical. Integration is the process of combining components, or entire functional subsections, into a single circuit. Such an *integrated circuit* (IC) might, for example, incorporate the microprocessor, the memory section, and the necessary input/output (I/O) interface circuitry (sense amplifiers, pulse generator circuits, etc.) onto a single "chip." The use of integrated circuits can greatly improve overall reliability, permit further optimization of circuit current consumption (with associated improvements in device longevity), and reduce the physical size and complexity of the device by reducing the total number of discrete components included in the design. In addition, the cost of components and of device manufacturing/assembly may also be greatly reduced, provided circuit integration is not carried out to an extreme point where it starts to affect IC manufacturability/yield. Due to the wide disparity in the technologies needed to realize low-power/low-voltage circuitry and high-power/high-voltage circuitry in the same device, and an inability to integrate certain circuit components (high-value capacitors, adjustable resistors, etc.), circuit integration has its practical limits, and provides only one means of achieving size reduction without compromise.

C. Hybridization

Although early ICDs were designed using primarily discrete components and printed circuit board assemblies, today virtually all of these devices utilize some form of hybrid circuit technology. Circuit hybridization reduces size, weight, and current consumption while improving overall device reliability, but to a lesser extent than does integration. However, it does offer advantages over integration in the timeliness with which design changes can be realized (which is especially important in the later stages of product development).

High-density hybrid circuits combine discrete components and integrated circuits (ICs) on a single substrate. These substrates are typically of a multilayered ceramic composition. The integrated circuits and discrete components are mounted on these substrates and connected to one another via metal pathways, known as traces, that run along and between the layers of the ceramic substrate. When only low-voltage/low-current circuitry is involved (as is typical for standard pacemaker applications), these traces can be very narrow and densely packed, thus reducing circuit size dramatically. However, when high-voltage/high-current circuitry is incorporated, the traces must conduct much higher currents, which greatly increases the possibility of interference between traces due to capacitive or inductive coupling. For this reason, the hybrid circuit designers must always be cognizant of the potential for unwanted interactions, and must space potentially vulnerable traces at greater distances from one another or provide appropriate shielding between them. Today's hybrid CAD (computer-aided design) packages provide a vehicle for the design engineer to specify these critical circuit interactions in advance of the layout process. With this information, the layout computer can provide immediate insight into layout areas that may be problematic in the final assembly. This greatly enhances the probability that these design issues will be addressed early in the design phase.

The hybrid designer must also consider the placement of discrete components in relation to one another, and to the integrated circuits. Some of the high-power conversion circuits, which provide the energy necessary for defibrillation, may generate considerable electrical "noise," or interference, which may interfere with the proper functioning of other parts of the circuitry. If the device is to have the ability, during charging, to sense, to communicate bidirectionally with external support equipment (such as programmers), to read and store intracardiac electrograms, and to internally monitor and record certain circuit functions, careful attention must be paid to component layout on the hybrid circuit, and advanced electrical shielding techniques may need to be employed.

D. Size/Shape/Weight

Until recently, the use of epicardial/extrapericardial patch electrodes made the abdominal region the preferred site for implantation of ICDs; thus, relatively minor variations in the size, shape, weight, and volume were not of great significance. However, transvenous lead systems, now widely available in Europe and in the United States, are proving to be mechanically reliable and clinically efficacious, with defibrillation thresholds somewhat higher than with patch systems, but still within the acceptable range. Studies have demonstrated that the transvenous approach reduces surgical mortality and morbidity, postoperative patient discomfort, the risk of infection, length of hospital stay, and overall hospitalization costs, making it the approach of choice in the overwhelming majority of cases. This development has, in turn, led to the demand for ICDs that can be implanted pectorally, in much the same fashion as bradycardia pacemakers are. Thus, size and shape once again become critical factors, and device manufacturers are being subjected to the same pressures they faced years ago with pacemakers.

From a design standpoint, the size and shape of ICDs are currently constrained by practical considerations. For example, a large portion (up to two-thirds [9]) of the volume of current ICDs is consumed by the batteries and the high-voltage capacitors. Existing battery technologies already permit the designer some flexibility in specifying desirable mechanical properties to optimize the overall shape of the completed device. However, the currently available aluminum electrolytic capacitors, in addition to being relatively large, have traditionally been available only in a cylindrical shape, which is suboptimal in terms in their effect on overall device size and shape. Thus, the most critical factor influencing the transition to a smaller, lighter, more "physiologically" shaped device suitable for pectoral implantation will be the availability of smaller, lighter, higher-energy-density capacitors that can be appropriately form-factored. This may result from the evolution of existing capacitor technologies and/or the development of new technologies.

Other factors that may allow ICDs to become smaller include improvements in lead systems and enhancements to our basic understanding of cardiac physiology, both of which may contribute to an overall reduction in defibrillation thresholds. When low DFTs are consistently achievable, the maximum shock output capacity of the ICD can be reduced, resulting in concomitant reduction in the size of batteries and capacitors.

Technological advances in many areas will allow manufacturers to produce devices with physical characteristics suitable for pectoral implantation in the near future, and ongoing developments will result in continued improvements that will, in many ways, parallel the developments seen in pacemakers over the last 30 years.

IV. OTHER DESIGN CONSIDERATIONS

A. Protection Against Memory Errors and Component Failures

With the incorporation of microprocessors into ICDs, the appropriate function of the device depends on the integrity of the processor and of the instructions stored in memory for use by the processor. Any disruption or corruption of these instructions could result in inappropriate device behavior. Such software corruption could result from the coupling of high currents into the device, such as might arise from the use of electrocautery or external defibrillation; incomplete or incorrect communication of programming information from the programmer to the implanted ICD; a software "bug" that manifests itself only when a particular combination of values or sequence of events occurs; a transient drop in battery voltage below that which is required to maintain microprocessor function, as might occur if an attempt is made to deliver a high-output shock when the power source has been depleted beyond its recommended level; or a component failure.

The preferable way to deal with this potential problem is, of course, to prevent it from occurring in the first place. In some cases, this is possible. For example, programming routines typically contain safeguards that do not allow a programming sequence to be implemented if communication of the programming sequence is interrupted, or if the programming information is incorrectly received by the ICD. (This topic is covered in depth in another chapter.) Extensive testing of the device and programmer software is done as part of the premarket qualification of the device, in an attempt to minimize the likelihood of a significant bug being found in the clinical setting.

If corruption of the instructions does occur, or if the microprocessor fails, the device should recognize that fact, and shift into a safe mode of operation. Many techniques exist for having the software check itself on a cycle-to-cycle or periodic basis. Several ICD systems employ backup or "shutdown" modes similar to those used in pacemakers, which contain unalterable instructions that are invoked in the event that the backup circuit is triggered, and which typically cause the device to revert to a safe set of bradycardia pacing parameters. However, there is no universally appropriate set of tachyarrhythmia detection and therapy parameters. Thus, the most common form of reversion to backup mode in today's ICDs involves disabling all antitachyarrhythmic functions. It is therefore highly desirable that the device be designed in such a way that reversion to a backup mode of operation would occur only when the memory is actually corrupted, and when failure to revert to backup would put the patient at greater risk. Future technological advances might allow device software to incorporate self-diagnostic functions that would be able to ascertain the nature of the problem and, where appropriate, correct the software anomaly and return the device to normal operation.

B. Protection From Noncardiac Interference

Inappropriate sensing of extracardiac signals, whether physiological in nature (e.g., myopotentials) or from external sources (e.g., electromagnetic interference, or EMI), has long been a concern of bradycardia pacemaker designers [10]. While the metal "can" used to encapsulate the circuitry provides a great deal of shielding, the leads serve as antennae by which extracardiac signals can be brought into the sensing circuit inputs. A combination of bandpass filtering (typically using filter capacitors to shunt high-frequency noise away from the sense amplifier inputs), sensitivity programmability, and various time-domain noise detection and noise reversion schemes, has worked reasonably well, although myopotential sensing still remains a significant problem in unipolar devices [11].

ICD design teams have additional factors to consider as well. For example, many ICDs incorporate some form of automatic gain control (AGC) sensing circuitry, to ensure that sinus, tachycardia, and fibrillation electrograms are sensed appropriately. Since the AGC is designed to increase its sensitivity when low-amplitude fibrillation electrograms may be present, this increased sensitivity may also make it more likely that the ICD will sense EMI signals that would be below the sensing threshold for a typical bradycardia pacemaker. Elaborate algorithms incorporated into the AGC routines attempt, as much as possible, to minimize these problems, since oversensing could cause the EMI to be incorrectly identified as a tachyarrhythmia, with the resultant inappropriate delivery of a therapy which could initiate a real episode of tachycardia or fibrillation. Unipolar sensing, as traditionally employed in bradycardia pacemakers (i.e., sensing between a cathode in or on the heart and the device itself acting as the anode), has a demonstrated susceptibility to far-field sensing of inappropriate intracardiac and extracardiac signals, and is therefore generally considered unacceptable for use in antitachyarrhythmia devices. Bipolar sensing, whether between a traditional pacing/sensing electrode pair (epicardial or endocardial) or between a single pacing/sensing electrode and a high-voltage shock electrode in close proximity, is standard in all ICD systems available today.

When bradycardia pacemakers encounter continuous interference which can be identified as such, they are typically designed to revert to an asynchronous noise reversion mode (e.g.,

VOO or DOO) to prevent inappropriate device inhibition, which could result in a period of asystole for the pacemaker-dependent patient. For an ICD patient who is not pacemaker dependent, asynchronous pacing could result in competition between the intrinsic rhythm and the pacing function, which could, in turn, result in the initiation of a tachyarrhythmia. To avoid this, it is possible to design an ICD such that its noise reversion mode is programmable, so that pacemaker-dependent patients can receive asynchronous pacing, while nondependent patients can have pacing inhibited as long as the noise is present.

C. Ionizing Radiation

CMOS (complementary metal oxide semiconductor) circuitry, which is used in virtually all implantable bradycardia pacemakers and ICDs, has many advantages, among them low power consumption and high reliability. However, CMOS circuitry is susceptible to damage when exposed to ionizing radiation [12]. Accounts of the amount of exposure required to cause damage vary widely, but the effect of exposure is cumulative. Moreover, because the ionizing radiation attacks the physical structure of the circuit directly, it is impossible to predict the mode of failure due to exposure; all of the tens of thousands of transistors in the circuit are under bombardment.

No effective, acceptable way of shielding CMOS circuitry in an ICD from ionizing radiation has been developed, and device labeling usually contraindictates the use of therapeutic levels of radiation administered at or near the device implant site. However, considerable interest exists, particularly within the space program and the military, in developing "radiation-proof" circuitry. Due to this interest, it is possible that improvements to, or alternatives for, CMOS circuitry will be developed in the future, which will minimize this potential problem even further.

V. CONCLUSION

Although the technology for pacemakers and implantable defibrillators has been in use for many years, the merging of these technologies into today's state-of-the-art implantable ICDs, which incorporate bradycardia pacing, antitachycardia pacing, cardioversion, and defibrillation capabilities, has been, and continues to be, a daunting engineering undertaking. Nonetheless, a period of rapid evolution of ICD technology can be expected, bringing dramatic decreases in size, and equally dramatic increases in therapeutic and diagnostic capabilities, to patients once doomed to die a sudden arrhythmic death.

REFERENCES

1. Tullo NG, Saksena S, Krol RB. Technological improvements in future implantable defibrillators. Cardiology 1990 (May); 107-111.
2. Coumel P. Historical milestones of implanted defibrillation. PACE 1992; 15:598-603.
3. Veltri EP, Mower MM, Mirowski M. The automatic implantable cardioverter-defibrillator: clinical experience. In: El-Sherif N, Samet P, eds. Cardiac Pacing and Electrophysiology. 3d ed. Philadelphia: W.B. Saunders, 1991:737-758.
4. Troup P. Early development of defibrillation devices. IEEE Eng Med Biol 1990 (June); 19-24.
5. Barold SS, Falkoff MD, Ong LS, Heinle RA. Interference in cardiac pacemakers: exogenous factors. In: El Sherif N, Samet P, eds. Cardiac Pacing and Electrophysiology. 3d ed. Philadelphia: W.B. Saunders, 1991:608-633.
6. Protection apparatus for patient-implantable device. U.S. Patent 4,745,923, May 24, 1988.
7. Troup P. Implantable cardioverters and defibrillators. Curr Probl Cardiol 1989; 12:675-843.

8. Power priority system. U.S. Patent 4,599,523, July 8, 1986.
9. Troup P. Implantable cardioverters and defibrillators. Curr Probl Cardiol 1989; 12:675-843.
10. Gross JN, Platt S, Ritacco R, Andrews C, Furman S. The clinical relevance of electromyopotential oversensing in current unipolar devices. PACE 1992; 15:2023-2027.
11. Barold SS, Falkoff MD, Ong LS, Heinle RA. Interference in cardiac pacemakers: exogenous factors. In: El Sherif N, Samet P, eds. Cardiac Pacing and Electrophysiology. 3d ed. Philadelphia: W.B. Saunders, 1991:608-633.
12. Rodriguez F, Filimonov A, Henning A, Coughlin C, Greenberg M. Radiation-induced effects in multiprogrammable pacemakers and implantable defibrillators. PACE 1991; 14:2143-2153.

8
Energy Storage and Delivery

Esther S. Takeuchi and William D. K. Clark

Wilson Greatbatch Ltd.
Clarence, New York

I. INTRODUCTION

For implantable defibrillators, unique challenges arise for the electrical energy system, as one needs a capability for high power density over a long period but also wants it in a package that is as small as possible. A successful defibrillation requires a voltage of several hundred volts, with the energy delivered in a millisecond time frame. The electrical system must be capable of delivering a few hundred such pulses at any time during a design life of several years. The following list of items gives a more detailed synopsis of the requirements and operating environment for the energy system.

Develop a voltage of 700–800 V
Deliver 35–40 J in a 10- to 20-ms pulse
Deliver >300 pulses
5-year usable life
Duty cycle of 10–90 days
Operate in an isothermal (37°C) environment

In order to satisfy the above requirements, all implantable device designers have used a battery/capacitor combination to provide the energy/power needs for the device. The capacitor provides the high-voltage pulse to the heart; the battery serves as the energy storage reservoir and charges the capacitor. Suitable interfacing electronics in the form of a DC/DC converter must exist between the battery and capacitor. The converter consists of three functional subunits. An inverter converts the nominal 6-V DC battery output to AC, and a transformer boosts this low-AC voltage to 700–800 V. A rectifier converts this boosted AC signal to DC, which is the output that is used to charge the capacitor. At present, the capacitor technology is generally a commercially available photoflash product, whereas the battery technology is a custom-designed article. The following sections present the information related to both these technologies.

II. BATTERIES AND BATTERY TECHNOLOGY

A. Introduction to Battery Technology

A battery converts chemical energy to electrical energy. This is accomplished by having two materials with different electrode potentials present in the battery. One material serves as the anode, readily gives up electrons, and is thus oxidized. The other material acts as the cathode, accepts electrons, and is reduced. External to the battery, the transfer of electrons from the anode to the cathode occurs through the circuit the battery is powering. Inside the battery, transfer of ions between the anode and cathode is made possible by the electrolyte, which provides high ionic conductivity but little or no electronic conductivity. Figure 1 shows a schematic displaying the electrochemical function of a battery.

Some standard terminology is used in describing battery characteristics. The open-circuit voltage (OCV) of a cell describes the difference in electrode potential between the anode and the cathode. The closed-circuit voltage (CCV) is the cell voltage during application of a load. Capacity in ampere-hours (Ah) is a measure of the amount of charge a battery can deliver. For example, the drain of 1 A for 1 h is 1 Ah of battery capacity. The total energy of a battery is described in watt-hours (Wh), obtained by multiplication of the battery capacity (Ah) by the voltage (V). Battery energy can be related to the size or weight of the battery to provide energy

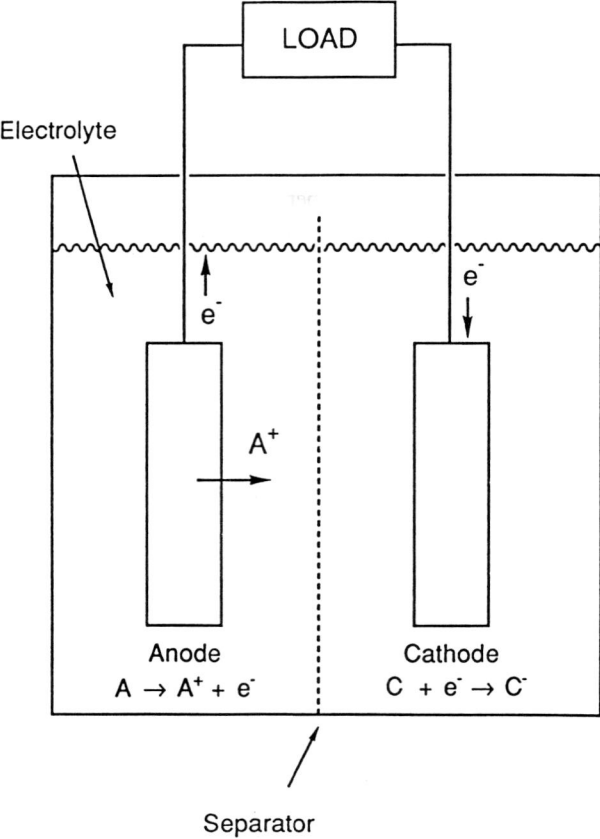

Figure 1 Schematic depiction of electrochemical cell showing the presence of electrolyte, the anode reaction, and the cathode reaction.

density. The units of gravimetric energy density are typically watt-hours/kilogram (Wh/kg), and the units of volumetric energy density are watt-hours/liter (Wh/L).

Two major classes of batteries exist. Those discharged a single time, providing only one use, are called primary batteries. Secondary batteries can be recharged and used several times. Since at this time all batteries used in cardioverter defibrillators are primary, nonrechargeable types, the discussion in this chapter will focus on this class of battery. In addition, the use of the words "cell" and "battery" have come to be used interchangeably to indicate power source and will be used in that manner.

B. Batteries for the Cardioverter-Defibrillator

1. Battery Requirements

The battery for the cardioverter-defibrillator must meet a stringent set of requirements. It must be able to deliver high pulse currents when fibrillation is sensed to charge capacitors which defibrillate the heart. The cells must provide low background current for extended periods of time to power the device. The cells must provide state-of-charge indication, in order to allow assessment of the remaining life of the cell and device. Low self-discharge is necessary to provide reasonable shelf life for the device and provide extended service during low-current operation. Safety and reliability must be consistent with implantable device requirements. In addition, it is important that the cells are as small as possible to allow the design of small patient-acceptable devices.

2. Battery Chemistry

The first type of cell used to power implantable cardiac defibrillators was based on the lithium/vanadium oxide couple [1]. Lithium (Li) as an anode material provides high cell voltage and light weight. Lithium metal has an atomic number of 3, an atomic weight of 6.9, and a density of 0.53 g/cm^3. It reacts readily with water and must be handled in a dry environment. A lithium anode delivers the electrons necessary for current flow and is converted to lithium ions during cell discharge. The vanadium oxide cathode material accepts electrons and is reduced during discharge. Vanadium oxide is an orange-yellow powder with a formula of V_2O_5. During battery discharge the oxidation state of the vanadium atoms in the material are reduced from a state of V(V) to V(IV) and then later to V(III). The reactions taking place in the lithium/vanadium oxide cell are shown in Eqs. (1)–(3) [2].

Anode: $$Li \rightarrow Li^+ + e^- \tag{1}$$

Cathode: $$e^- + V_2O_5 \rightarrow V_2O_5^- \tag{2}$$

Cell: $$Li + V_2O_5 \rightarrow Li\,V_2O_5 \tag{3}$$

Lithium/vanadium oxide cells used to power cardiac defibrillators contained an organic electrolyte consisting of a mixed lithium salt dissolved in methyl formate solvent [1]. Cells based on this chemistry were implanted until 1989.

Subsequent generations of cells used to power cardiac defibrillators are based on the lithium/silver vanadium oxide chemistry, and practically all cells being implanted today are based on this chemistry [3,4]. Silver vanadium oxide (SVO) has two characteristics which allow it to provide higher volumetric energy density in a battery than vanadium oxide: It is more conductive and more dense. The increased conductivity allows SVO cathodes with minimal conductive additive to discharge, while vanadium oxide demands larger amounts of carbon or graphite as inert additives. The increased density of SVO provides higher weight per volume of cathode material. Both of these characteristics, acting in concert, provide higher-energy-density cells. Since it is the SVO chemistry that is in such widespread use, the discussion in this chapter will focus on this chemistry. The anode is lithium metal and functions as described above. The cathodes consist of silver vanadium oxide prepared by the thermal treatment of vanadium oxide and a silver salt, typically silver nitrate. SVO has the dark color and electronic conductivity characteristic of metal oxide bronzes [5]. The optimum formula for the material used in lithium batteries is $Ag_2V_4O_{11}$ [6]. Discharge of the SVO cathode in a lithium cell progresses by the reduction of V(V) to V(IV), reduction of Ag(I) to Ag(0), and then reduction of V(IV) to V(III) [7]. The reactions are summarized in Eqs. (4)–(6). A total of 7 equivalents of lithium can be incorporated into one mole of SVO cathode. The cells utilize a mixed organic solvent with a dissolved lithium salt as electrolyte.

Anode: $\qquad 7Li \rightarrow 7Li + 7e^-$ (4)

Cathode: $\qquad 7e^- + Ag_2V_4O_{11} \rightarrow Ag_2V_4O_{11}^{-7}$ (5)

Cell: $\qquad 7Li + Ag_2V_4O_{11} \rightarrow Li_7Ag_2V_4O_{11}$ (6)

3. Cell Construction and Configuration

Cells for the defibrillator application must deliver current pulses of up to 2.0 A. In order to do this, the cells are constructed with high electrode surface areas [8]. The large surface areas allow delivery of high current pulses with acceptable voltage drop during the pulse. Typically, cells contain a strip anode fabricated from lithium foil pressed onto a nickel current collector. Cathodes are fabricated by compressing a mixture of SVO, binder, and conductive additives onto metal current collectors. The anode and the cathodes are encased in polypropylene membranes, which allow electrolyte and ion flow but prevent mechanical contact of the anode and cathode. Assembly of the cell stack is accomplished by folding the anode strip into an accordion-like structure and placing a cathode between each fold of the anode. The cell stack is inserted into a 304-L stainless steel case, where the anode is welded to the case to provide a case-negative design. The cell is then equipped with a header that contains a small hole for vacuum filling with electrolyte and a corrosion-resistant glass-to-metal feedthrough. The cathode tabs are welded to the pin of the feedthrough, and the header is welded to the case. After filling with electrolyte and welding a small plug to cover the fill hole, the cells provide a hermetic package. The hermeticity and appropriate choice of materials provide long-term stability for the cell and its components. At the time of this writing, eight different cell configurations of varying sizes and shapes are in production.

A typical configuration of the Li/SVO cell is designated as the model 8830. The cell has a rectangular configuration with dimensions of 42.9 × 26.9 × 8.9 mm. The stoichiometric capacity is 2.2 Ah, and the nominal weight of the cell is 28 g. Information for this cell type will be used in the examples for consistency.

4. Cell Discharge Performance

Lithium/silver vanadium oxide cells have an open-circuit voltage at beginning of life of 3.2 V. The voltage decreases with discharge, showing a second major plateau at 2.6 V. This gradual decrease in voltage aids in the determination of the cell state of charge. A typical discharge curve obtained by discharge over 6 months under a 5-kΩ load is shown in Fig. 2. This curve shows the voltage plateaus at 3.2 and 2.6 V, and a delivered capacity of about 2.0 Ah to 2.0 V.

Under field-use conditions, the cells would be expected to deliver background current of 10 to 20 µA for extended periods of time and intermittently to deliver pulses to charge capacitors. Testing methods have been developed to reflect field use. Charging of the capacitors is imitated by having the cell deliver four 10-s, 2.0-A pulses in a pulse train. Figure 3 shows the voltage response of a cell during one pulse train where four 10-s pulses with 15 s of rest between pulses are applied. Note the rapid voltage drop upon application of the pulse and more gradual

Energy Storage and Delivery

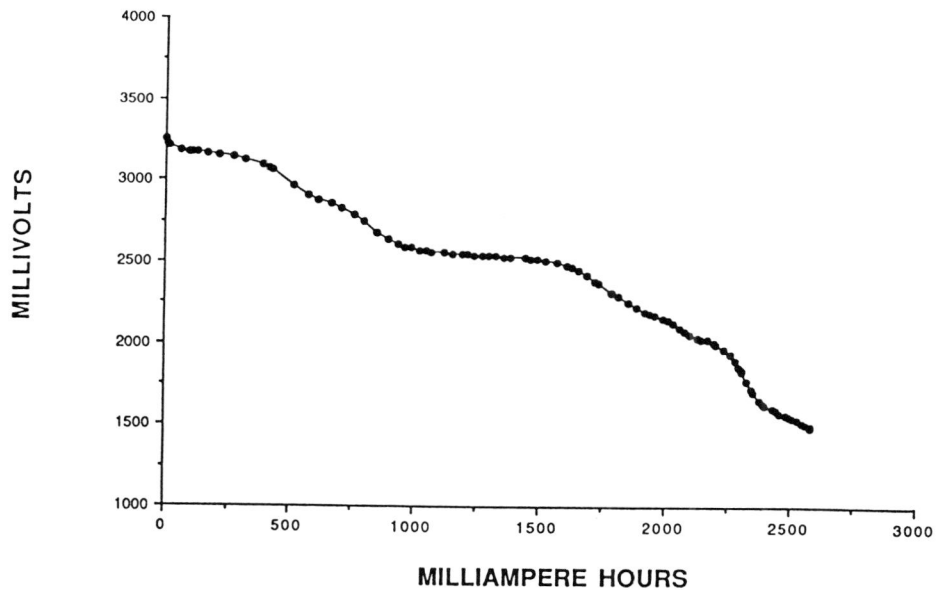

Figure 2 Discharge of a lithium/silver vanadium oxide defibrillator battery under a 5-kΩ load at 37°C.

voltage decay during continued pulse application. When the current is stopped there is a rapid period of recovery, followed by a more gradual recovery to stable OCV. If more than four pulses are applied in sequence, the cell voltage under pulse continues to decrease. The relationship of pulse voltage and number of pulses is a complicated one that depends on the depth of discharge.

Accelerated discharge under a pulse scheme can be accomplished by applying one pulse train every 30 min. Figure 4 shows the discharge of a model 8830 cell under such a scheme. The data plotted represent the cell voltage measured before the first pulse, at the minimum of the first pulse, and at the minimum of the fourth pulse of the train. Note that the open-circuit voltage as well as the loaded voltage decrease with discharge. Under accelerated testing, the resistance of the cell decreases to a minimum at about 50% depth of discharge and then increases again as the cell approaches end of life. This type of test requires about 3 days to complete.

Cell testing is also done under schemes where the discharge requires one or several years for completion. Figure 5 shows the discharge of a cell under a background load of 17.4 kΩ and the application of one pulse train every 2 months. The background voltage before pulse is indicated, as well as the pulse minima under the first and fourth pulses. The time on test was greater than one year. Schemes for three- and five-year testing involve application of pulse trains every 4 and 6 months, respectively, with lighter background loads.

Assessment of the state of charge of a cell is an important determination. Various approaches have been used. The open-circuit voltage of the silver vanadium oxide cells decreases with depth of discharge, but the voltage is also dependent on the time since the last pulse. Further, the open-circuit voltage provides no indication of the internal resistance of a cell. It is often the voltage under pulse that determines end of life, which is determined by the internal resistance of a cell. Another approach that has been used for the state of charge determination is the assessment of capacitor charge time. The charge time increases as the cell voltage decreases. If there are increases in cell internal resistance, the charge time will also increase.

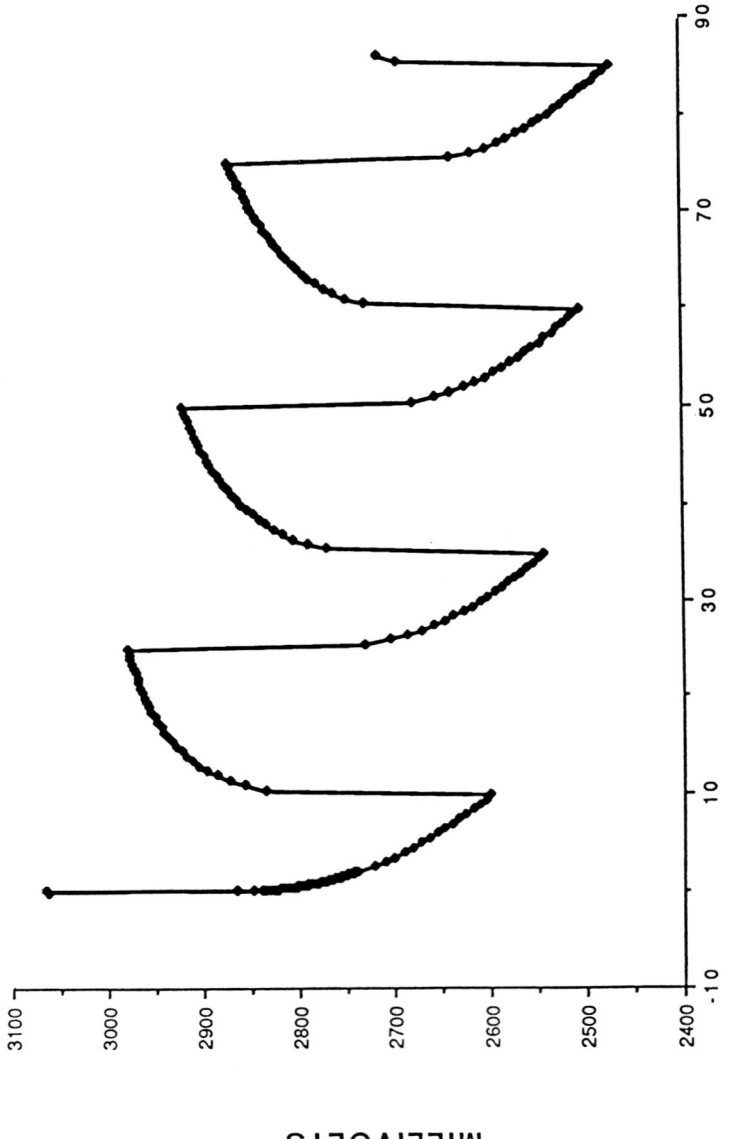

Figure 3 Voltage response of a lithium/silver vanadium oxide cell during a pulse train. Current was delivered by the cell in four 10-s pulses beginning at 0 s. Each pulse was followed by a 15-s rest.

Energy Storage and Delivery

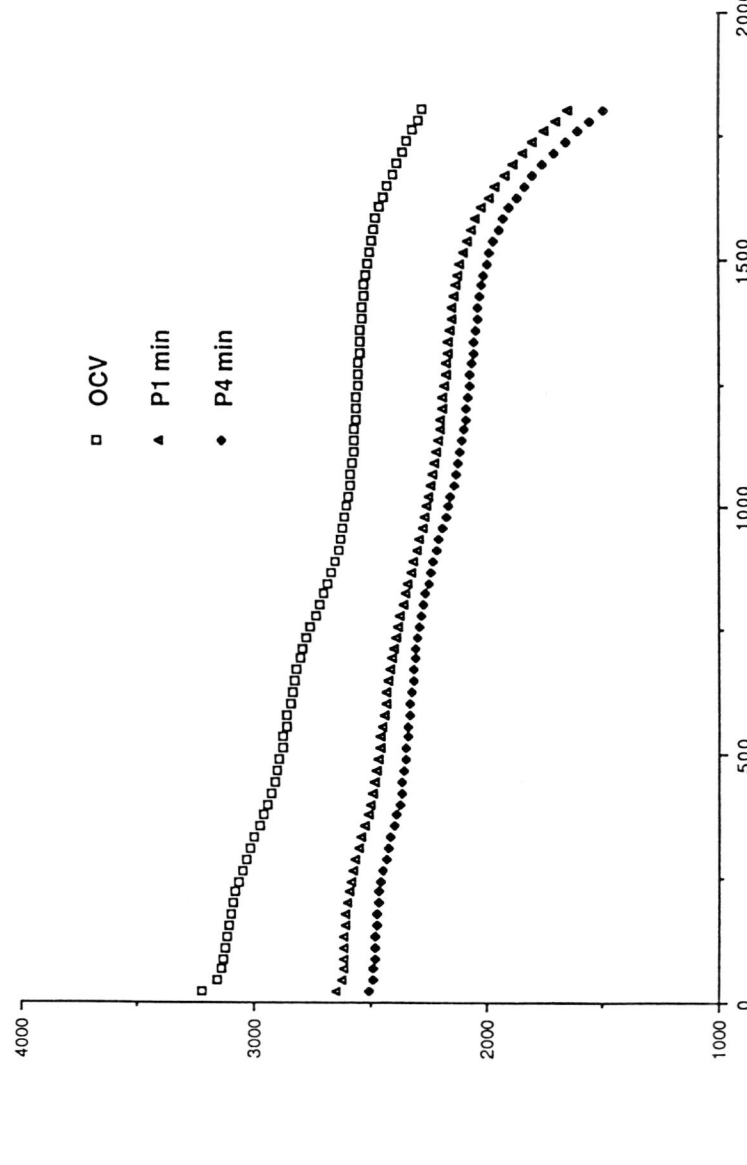

Figure 4 Discharge of a lithium/silver vanadium oxide battery under an accelerated pulse test at 37°C. Four 10-s, 2-A pulses were applied every 30 min.

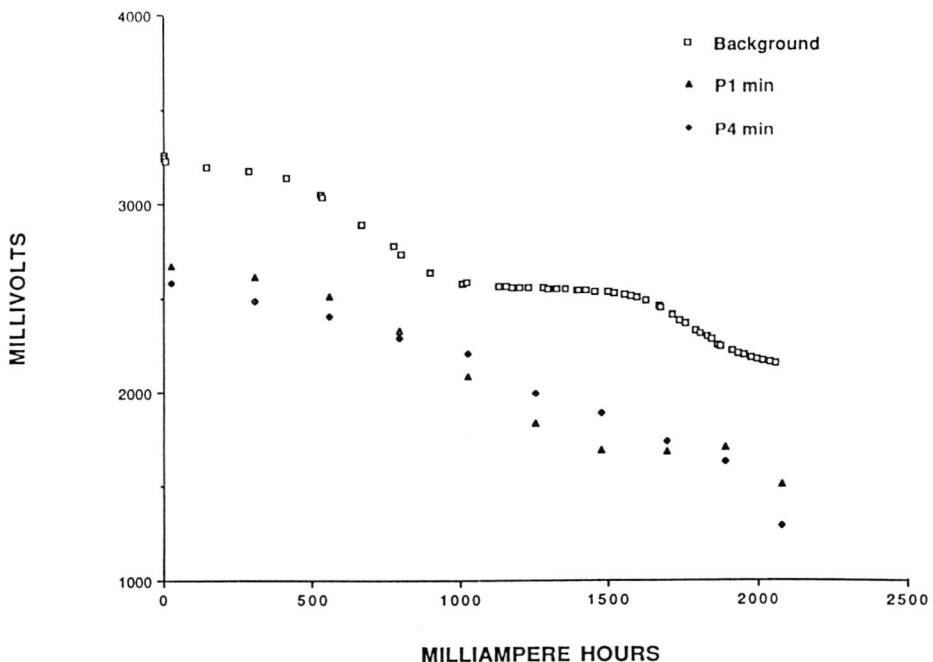

Figure 5 Discharge of a lithium/silver vanadium oxide battery under a 1.5-year pulse test at 37°C. The cell was discharged under a 17.4-kΩ background load, and four 10-s, 2-A pulses were applied every 2 months.

Charge time will be longer if voltage delay is present, but should decrease in subsequent pulses as the voltage delay decreases. Voltage delay is a drop in voltage at the leading edge of the first pulse that generally lasts less than 2 or 3 seconds. Thus, charge time is more effective for the determination of state of charge than open-circuit voltage alone.

5. Battery Qualification and Electrical Testing

  a. Battery Qualification Testing. Along with characterizing the performance of cells under normal discharge conditions, it is important to characterize cells under normal and abnormal environmental conditions. The testing determines the response of cells to environmental conditions that might be experienced during transportation, handling, storage, assembly, or final use. This type of testing is done in the design stage of a new cell model to determine limits on certain design criteria as well as on each new cell model before that cell can be designated as implantable grade. The results of the tests are summarized in a cell qualification document.

  The environmental tests that are run on cells are summarized below. The tests are done on cells that are fresh, half depleted, and fully depleted. Characterization after the testing includes visual and dimensional examination as well as X-radiography. For a cell model such as the 8830 as described above, none of the test conditions results in the rupture or leakage of a battery. The application of a short circuit does result in depletion of cell capacity and an increase in temperature of about 100°C.

Thermal cycling from 70°C to −40°C with 1-min transition time
High-pressure testing at 90 and 120 psi
Low-pressure testing in vacuum equivalent to 4,500, 12,030, and 15,000 m

Low- and high-temperature exposure
Short circuit at room temperature and at 37°C
Forced overdischarge at the $C/10$ rate, where C is the cell capacity
Forced discharge of a depleted cell by a fresh cell
Shock testing with a $1000g$ force
Vibration testing at frequencies ranging from 5 to 5000 Hz

Cells are also subjected to tests that are abusive in nature. These tests include: dent and puncture by a sharp metal rod; a crush test, where the cells are crushed to generate an internal short; recharge at a current of $C/10$; and high-rate, forced overdischarge at a current of 1.6 A. These tests are used to characterize and demonstrate the behavior of a cell under extreme conditions. There are no pass/fail criteria associated with the tests. The information gained can be used to define proper handling of the cells to maintain safety.

b. Electrical Test Sampling Plan. All cells manufactured are subjected to an electrical test protocol prior to being released for shipment. The electrical information from the predischarge, which removes 1–3% of the cell capacity, is examined to determine acceptability. In addition, cells are sampled from the production stream and placed on accelerated pulse test, where one pulse train is applied every 30 min. This sampling and testing of cells is an ongoing procedure and ensures the acceptability and consistency of the cells being manufactured.

Further performance data on batteries are obtained by selecting cells from the production line in random fashion and placing them on tests called "life tests." These tests consist of either low-level background loads such as 100 kΩ applied for the life of the cell, or low-level loads with one four-pulse train applied once per month. Figure 6 shows life test data for model 8830 cells. The background cell voltage under 100-kΩ load is shown along with the pulse minima under the first pulse and fourth pulse of a pulse train. Such application rate-discharge data provide information about the consistency of the product and the expected behavior in field use.

6. The Future

Currently, only primary batteries are used for cardioverter defibrillators, but secondary batteries may be considered at some point. It is likely that secondary batteries would serve as the source of the high current needed to charge capacitors, but less likely that they would provide the low-level maintenance current needed to power the other functions of the device. Secondary cells generally do not maintain voltage or state of charge as well as primary cells do. Thus, more detailed evaluation would be needed to assess whether the frequency of patient intervention to charge the cells would be acceptable. Further, secondary batteries generally have about half the energy density of a primary cell, or less. The impact secondary cells would have on device size would need to be evaluated considering the inherent loss in cell energy density compared to primary cells and the additional device features that would be needed to charge the cells.

Nuclear batteries have been considered and used in the past in implantable devices [9]. The cells can likely deliver only the low-level current needs of the device. The high currents needed for capacitor charging would still require an additional power source. The eventual application of nuclear power sources in cardioverter-defibrillators will be limited by the same forces that limited application in other areas. The regulatory requirements of implementing a nuclear power source may make the option unfavorable.

C. Conclusions

Chemically based power sources have been developed to power the cardioverter-defibrillator. Those in most widespread use today are lithium/silver vanadium oxide cells. The cell voltage

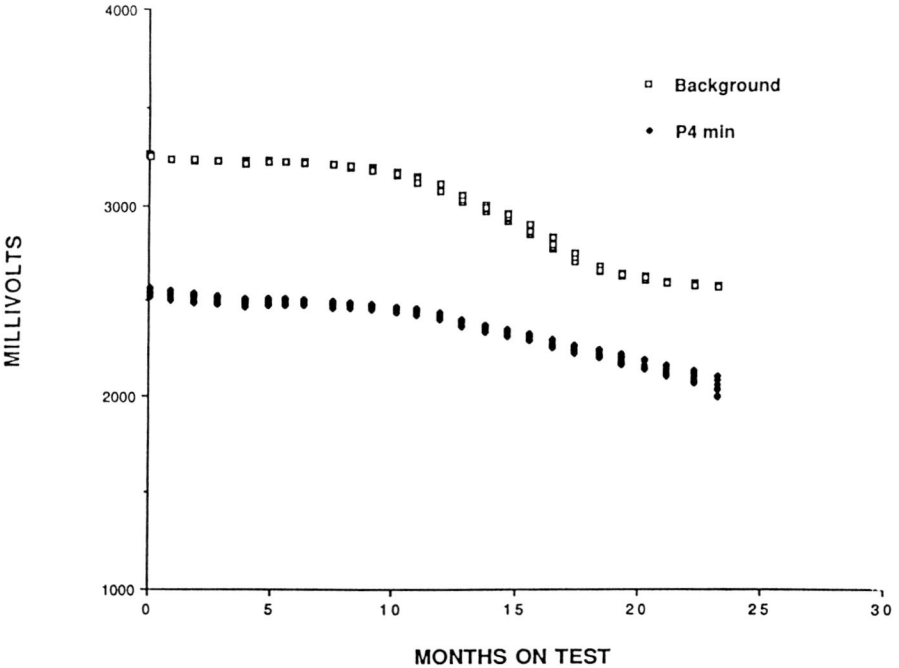

Figure 6 Discharge of a group of model 8830 cells on life test where a 100-kΩ background load was applied to the cells and a pulse train was applied once per month. A pulse train consists of four 10-s, 2.0-A pulses.

is initially 3.2 V and decays as the cells are discharged. In order to meet the high current requirements of the defibrillator, the cells are assembled with high electrode surface areas. Extensive electrical, environmental, and abuse testing has been conducted on lithium/silver vanadium oxide cells to demonstrate their suitability for use with the cardiac defibrillator.

III. CAPACITORS AND CAPACITOR TECHNOLOGY

A. Introduction to Capacitor Technology

Whereas the energy for batteries is stored in the form of chemical energy, in the case of the capacitors it is stored in the form of static charge. As a result, a capacitor does not need to have a conversion take place from one form of energy to another in order to generate an electrical output. The basic construction of a capacitor involves two metal electrodes separated from each other by an insulating, dielectric material. The static charges are accumulated at the electrode/dielectric interfaces. A potential difference of hundreds to thousands of volts can be developed across the dielectric, depending on the nature of the material and the construction of the device. The governing equation relating the dimensional and material properties and the capability to store charge is

$$C = k \cdot e \frac{A}{d} \tag{7}$$

where C is the capacitance, e is the permittivity constant, k is the dielectric constant for the material, A is the cross-sectional area, and d is the thickness of the dielectric material. The energy that can be stored in the capacitor can be calculated from the following relationship:

$$U = C \cdot \frac{V^2}{2} \tag{8}$$

where U is the energy and V is the voltage. However, the capacitor can only withstand the application of a certain voltage before dielectric breakdown occurs. This field strength, E, is related to the applied voltage and the thickness as follows:

$$E = \frac{V}{d} \tag{9}$$

The interaction of these parameters results in practical limitations for the energy densities and thus the size of the capacitor that can be used.

B. Capacitors for Cardioverter Defibrillators

1. Capacitor Requirements

The following list of items gives a more detailed synopsis of the requirements and operating environment for the capacitor(s).

Voltage of 700–800 V, capacitance of 100–150 μF
Deliver 35–40 J in a 10- to 20-ms pulse
A possible volume form factor is 20–22 mm diameter, 65–75 mm long
5-year usable life
Nominal leakage current of 0.1–1 mA
Energy density >1.5 J/cm^3
Duty cycle of 10–90 days
Capacitor sits in the uncharged state
Operates in an isothermal (37°C) environment

2. Capacitor Types

The common energy-storage capacitors that rely on storage in the form of static charge can exist in three material forms, differentiated primarily on the basis of the nature of the material and its dielectric layer: electrochemically formed metal oxides, ceramics, and plastic thin films. At present, electrolytic photoflash capacitors which exhibit an energy density of about 1.7 J/cm^3 are used in implantable defibrillators under the above parameters. The following descriptions of each of the respective technologies will give an indication of the potential for each to meet the requirements for the implantable defibrillator application and possible approaches that could lead to reducing the size of the capacitive storage element.

a. Electrolytic Capacitors. Aluminum electrolytic capacitors have traditionally been the capacitors most commonly used for energy storage. Their ability to store energy relies not so much on the dielectric constant of the aluminum oxide that serves as the insulating charge separator or its high-voltage stress levels, but on the fact that large surface areas of material can be formed by the use of special etching techniques for the aluminum foil that have been developed over the years. At present, up to 80% of the foil can be etched away in the form of columnar wells in the foil. The foil is then treated electrochemically to grow a thin aluminum oxide surface on the foil surface. The high surface area of the resultant structure allows the storage of a large amount of charge and its rapid dissipation in the external circuit due to the low impedance of the structure. However, the high percentage of material that has been etched to create the high surface area, as well as the ability to do this primarily with aluminum only, limits what can be done in the way of further improvements. A representation of these structures is shown in Fig. 7. The total thickness of the elements is of the order of a few thousandths of an inch. The contact for a lower-surface-area, second aluminum electrode is made through the use of an electrolyte that can flow into the pores of the foil to achieve contact with this high surface area. The two aluminum electrodes are separated by the use of a thin, porous insulating medium and wound into a jellyroll construction. The wound element is inserted into a cylindrical can, which is then filled with the electrolyte. Common electrolytes use various salts in a glycol-like solvent, while the separating medium can be made from special paper for this application.

Table 1 lists energy densities for a number of capacitors, illustrating the relatively wide range of values for a technology that has been manufactured for several decades. The one model manufactured by the Rubycon Corporation has the highest value for energy density. The voltage ratings and dimensional parameters were taken from the manufacturers' catalogs. The other parameters are calculated values. As one can see from the values for the voltages in the table, one needs two capacitors of this type in series in order to achieve the voltages needed for defibrillation.

Concerns have been voiced with the electrolytic capacitor technology over the need to re-form the capacitors periodically. The re-forming process involves the application of the rated voltage for a period of a few minutes in order to repair any imperfections or damage that has occurred in the oxide film on the aluminum foil anode as a result of the capacitor aging over several weeks or months. The re-forming process results in the flow of current that subsides as the full insulating characteristics of the oxide layer are restored. Frequent re-forming would thus represent a parasitic load for the battery and thus could shorten operational life for the device. The newer electrolytic capacitors cited in Table 1, especially the Rubycon product, require minimal re-forming, so this issue is no longer a significant technical concern.

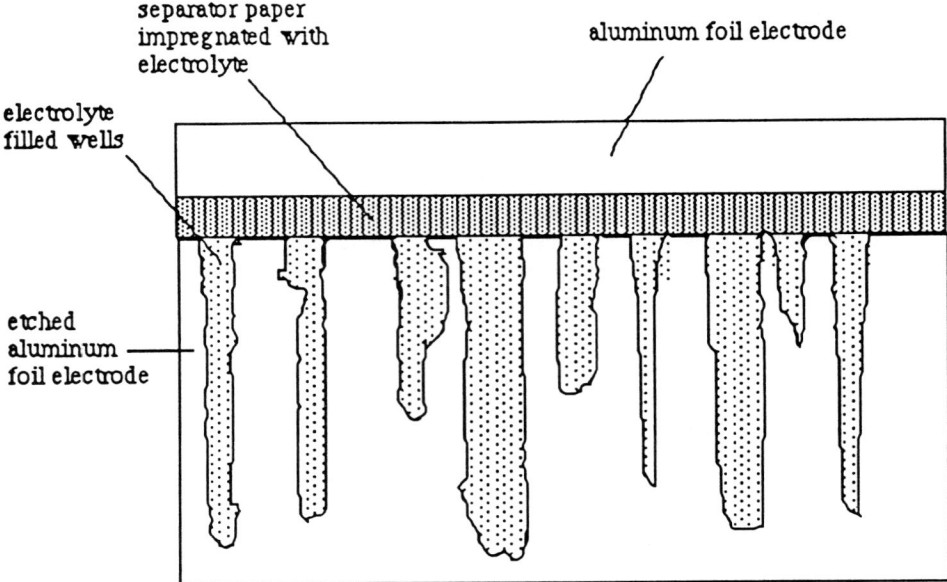

Figure 7 Cross section of structural elements of an electrolytic capacitor.

Table 1 Energetics of Electrolytic Capacitors

Capacitor manufacturer model	Voltage (V)	Capacity (μF)	Energy (J)	Charge (C)	Energy density (J/cm³)	Length (mm)	Diameter (mm)
Nichicon							
VX-2V/151	350	150	9.19	0.0525	0.53	35	25
VX-2F/331	315	330	16.37	0.10395	0.56	60	25
Sprague							
TVA1622	350	150	9.19	0.0525	0.21	66.78	28.575
TVA1628	350	300	18.38	0.105	0.25	92.08	31.75
Rubycon							
FKX	360	300	19.44	0.108	1.72	47	17.5
FXT	330	300	16.34	0.099	1.24	33	22.5
FW	330	200	10.89	0.066	1.00	40.5	18.5
SF	450	300	30.38	0.135	0.85	49	30.5
RTE Aerovox							
AGA	350	150	9.19	0.0525	0.30	61	25.4

b. Plastic Film Capacitors. This class of capacitors relies mainly on the availability of very thin films (1–10 μm) of polymeric materials which can be metallized and rolled into compact bundles of high energy density. The polymer materials, while having lower dielectric constants than the metal oxides, can withstand much greater voltage stress levels (a few hundred volts per micrometer) and thus allow for the construction of high-voltage capacitors. Typical polymers used for this type of construction include polypropylene, Mylar, and other materials falling into the realm of engineered plastics. The basic structural element is shown in Fig. 8.

Energy densities higher than those observed for the electrolytic capacitors have been reported, with recent work [10] citing values >4 J/cm³. However, these values are for capacitors at voltages in the range of a few hundred kilovolts, and thus the energy density is achieved by the leveraging of the energy density from the squared-term dependence on the voltage. Charging the capacitors to only the 800-V value reduces the realized energy density to values below that for aluminum electrolytic capacitors. Improvements in the form of higher dielectric constants and voltage stress levels for the plastics, as well as the ability to make thinner films, are needed to give the desired energy densities in the 1000-V range.

c. Ceramic Capacitors. Ceramic materials hold the promise for having the highest energy density of the three material classes, because the values for the dielectric constants can be up to 1000 times larger [11]. However, the dielectric constants exhibit strong variations for both temperature and applied voltage [11]. Energy density values for commercially available mul-

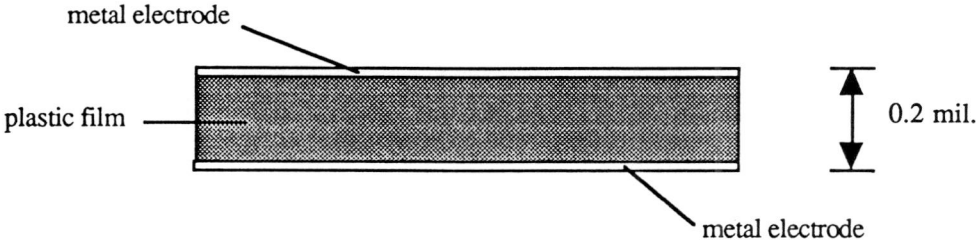

Figure 8 Cross section of structural elements of a plastic film capacitor.

tilayer constructions are only 0.1 J/cm^3 [12]. Therefore, a focused program to develop improved materials is needed in order to increase the energy density for this class of capacitors beyond the values for the electrolytic capacitors. Titanates are the general class of ceramic material used for this type of capacitor, and barium titanate has been used extensively. Ceramic capacitors are constructed in a multilayer structure, where thin tapes of ceramic powder and binder are painted with metal contacts, cut into the desired shape, and stacked to heights of a few hundred elements. The unit is then fired at high temperature to fuse the ceramic powders. A depiction of a few elements of a multilayer structure is shown in Fig. 9.

d. Electrochemical Capacitors. Energy storage "capacitors" exist that can nominally exceed the above energy density of storage of the conventional capacitors. The so-called pseudocapacitors [13], ultracapacitors [14], or electrochemical capacitors [15] (which are basically a form of high-power rechargeable battery, as there is a significant coulombic character to their charge storage) exhibit energy densities in the 10's of J/cm^3 range [14]. The "double-layer capacitors" [16] are nominally electrochemical in nature, but rely on the static charge formed at an electrode/electrolyte interface that exists in all systems of this type. Both types present formidable manufacturing challenges, as a few hundred unit voltage cells must be connected in series to achieve the voltages for defibrillation, and thus are seen only as a longer-term replacement for the above capacitor technologies.

3. Capacitor Discharge/Charge Performance

Because all capacitors are dissipating static electric charge, the same physics governs the discharge of the devices, and the form of the discharge is an exponential decay of the voltage. The pulse for the defibrillator application generally takes the form of a truncated exponential decay of 10–30 ms width as shown in Fig. 10. The charging curve has an analogous rising exponential voltage increase, but the charging times are generally of the order of 5–15 s.

4. Capacitor Electrical and Qualification Testing

Each manufacturer of defibrillator devices subjects the lots of capacitors to performance and environmental tests appropriate for the environment in which they will be used. Each manufacturer has its own protocols, the details of which are not generally available.

C. Conclusions

The electrolytic capacitors provide an adequate pulse power source for the defibrillator application. However, the nearer- and longer-term successes in attempts to improve energy density

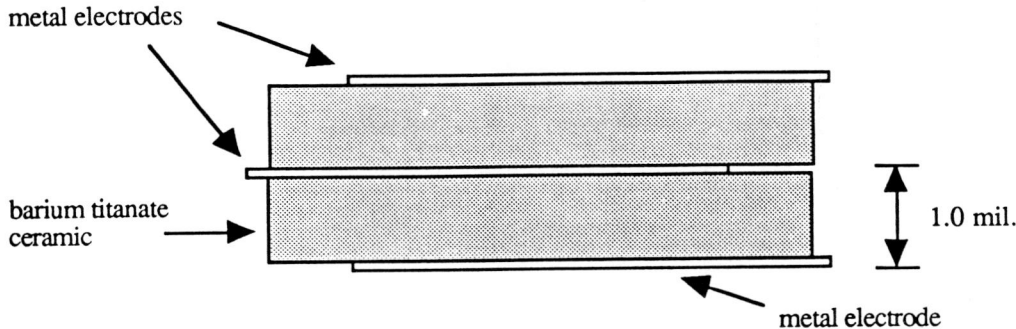

Figure 9 Cross section of structural elements of a ceramic capacitor.

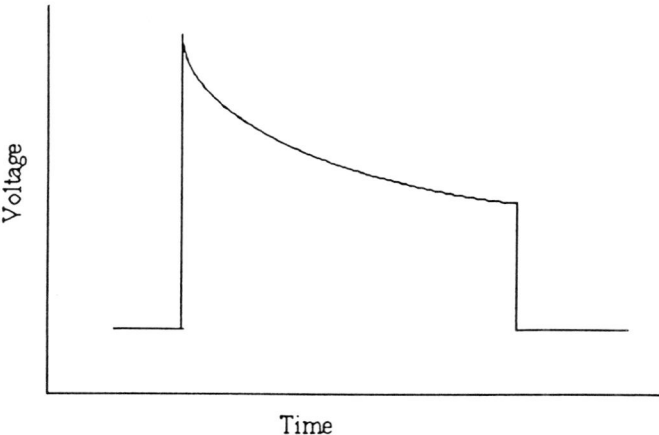

Figure 10 Waveform for the defibrillator pulse.

for capacitors that have to function in the 800-V range would appear to be with the plastic film or ceramic material devices. The "electrochemical"-based systems present formidable assembly problems to achieve the necessary voltages.

REFERENCES

1. Horning RJ, Viswanathan S. High rate lithium cell for medical application. Proc. 29th Power Sources Conference, Electrochemical Society, Pennington, NJ, 1980:64.
2. Walk CR. In: Gabano JP, ed. Lithium Batteries. New York: Academic Press, 1983:265.
3. Liang CC, Bolster ME, Murphy RM. U.S. Patents 4,310,609 and 4,391,729, 1982.
4. Holmes CF, Visbisky M. Long-term testing of defibrillator batteries. PACE 1991; 14:341.
5. Hagenmuller P. In: Bailer JC, Emeleus HJ, Nyholm R, Trotman-Dickenson AF, eds. Comprehensive Inorganic Chemistry. New York: Pergamon Press, 1973:541.
6. Takeuchi ES, Piliero P. Lithium/silver vanadium oxide batteries with various ratios of silver to vanadium. J Power Sources 1987; 21:133.
7. Takeuchi ES, Thiebolt WC. The reduction of silver vanadium oxide in lithium/silver vanadium oxide cells. J Electrochem Soc 1988; 135:2691.
8. Takeuchi E. Design evolution of defibrillator batteries. Proc. Sixth Annual Battery Conference on Applications and Advances, California State University, Long Beach, 1991.
9. Purdy DL. In: Owens BB, ed. Batteries for Implantable Biomedical Devices. New York: Plenum Press, 1986:285.
10. Ennis JB, Haskell DK, Sevigny JA. Proc. 34th International Power Sources Symposium, June 25-28, 1990:392–394.
11. Sarjeant WJ. IEEE Trans Electrical Insulation 1990; 25(5):861-922.
12. Catalogue of Olean Advanced Products, (a division of AVX Corporation), Olean, NY.
13. Conway BE. Proc. 34th International Power Sources Symposium, June 25-28, 1990:319-327.
14. Tong RR, Mason GE, Lee HL, Bullard GL. Proc. 34th International Power Sources Symposium, June 13-16, 1988:600-606.
15. Sarangapani S, Lessner P, Forchione J, Griffith A, LaConti AB, Proc. 25th IECEC Meeting, Aug 12-17, 1990; 3:137-142.
16. Rose, FM. Proc. 34th International Power Sources Symposium, June 13-16, 1988:572-592.

9

The Effects of External Interference on ICDs and PMs

Walter H. Olson

Medtronic, Inc.
Minneapolis, Minnesota

I. INTRODUCTION

Prior to the mid-1970s, when pacemaker circuits became hermetically sealed in titanium cans and there were few interference rejection circuits, the pacemaker electromagnetic interference (EMI) literature was rich with interactions due to household appliances such as microwave ovens and radiofrequency transmitting systems. Today's pacemakers (PMs) and implantable cardioverter-defibrillators (ICDs) are immune to most common sources of electromagnetic energy in homes and workplaces. Important exceptions include primarily specific diagnostic and therapeutic medical equipment and very-high-energy sources that are encountered by a few patients with specific occupations. The clinical consequences of EMI oversensing for ICDs may be inappropriate shocks, whereas for PMs inhibition of pacing in pacemaker-dependent patients may cause syncope. Exposure to intense energy such as radiation, shock waves, heating, pressure, and mechanical trauma can permanently damage or alter the function of ICDs and PMs.

Many factors combine to make generalizations about the effects of external interference on PMs and ICDs difficult. The spatial proximity and orientation of the patient with an implanted device to the source of energy that causes interference is probably the single most important factor. Electric and magnetic fields usually decrease inversely with the square of the distance from the source. Many energy sources restrict emission of energy to a particular direction, and the invisible nature of most electromagnetic radiation makes it difficult for patients to appreciate hazards that may exist.

The frequency of technical service telephone calls that Medtronic, Inc., receives with questions on electromagnetic compatibility for PMs ranges from 80 to 140 per month and represents about 5% of the total calls received. About half of these calls pertain to medical or dental equipment, 10% concern transmitters, 8% deal with arc welding, 6% relate to consumer products, 3% for electric power, and 3% are industrial sources. The remaining 17% are miscellaneous or not categorized. For the medical and dental equipment calls, electrosurgery and ionizing radiation each account for 25%, while 16% concern magnetic resonance imaging, 10% transcutaneous nerve stimulators, 7% ultrasound, 4% defibrillation, 3% diathermy, and 3% ablation, leaving about 10% miscellaneous or not categorized. Toll-free technical consultation is readily available from all PM and ICD manufacturers.

This chapter on the effects of external interference on ICDs and PMs was written based on a review of the literature by the author and may be incomplete or inaccurate. This review contains opinions of the author which may differ from the legal positions of Medtronic, Inc. Of course, the author also disclaims responsibility for the consequences of statements herein, although he hopes you are still interested in reading what follows.

II. TYPES OF INTERFERENCE, TIMING, AND SPATIAL FACTORS

Many types of energy are used in homes, public places, workplaces, and medical facilities. Some forms of energy can adversely affect the operation of implanted electronic devices and very rarely even alter or damage these devices (Fig. 1). A broad description of the energy types and the possible mechanisms of interactions with implanted electronic devices will be discussed here with examples.

A. Radiated Electromagnetic Fields

Radiated electromagnetic fields have both an electric field measured in volts/meter (Fig. 1A) and an orthogonal magnetic field measured in amperes/meter (Fig. 1C). These sources can be broadly divided into low-frequency sources from 0.1 Hz to 10 kHz, with examples such as electric power and audio entertainment equipment; and high-frequency sources from 10 kHz to 12 GHz, with examples being radar transmitters, radio and television transmitters, microwave ovens, and antitheft systems. There have been very few confirmed effects from these sources and even fewer clinically significant incidents. The most likely adverse effects for radiated electromagnetic fields are induction of voltage into loops of noncoaxial sensing leads, which causes oversensing that inhibits or causes reversion pacing by PMs, and erroneous detections and shocks for ICDs. Extremely intense electromagnetic fields could theoretically induce current in lead wires that could stimulate or possibly fibrillate the heart. Unused or abandoned leads should be capped to avoid inadvertent conductive pathways to the heart that have much lower fibrillation thresholds [1]. Electromagnetic fields could mimic radiofrequency telemetry and alter implanted device operating parameters; however, this is extremely unlikely due to the access codes required to establish a telemetry link, parity checks of transmitted messages, and the requirement for simultaneous magnetic reed switch closure by at least a 10-gauss steady magnetic field.

B. Directly Conducted Galvanic Currents

Directly conducting galvanic currents flowing through the body are measured in amperes/meter^2 and require two physical contacts at different locations on the body (Fig. 1B). A wide range of frequencies may affect implanted devices, although the power frequencies of 50 Hz (Europe), 60 Hz (United States), and 400 Hz (aircraft) predominate. These currents may cause oversensing, although it is unclear whether such currents would be above or below the threshold of perception, which is about 1 mA/cm^2 for moist skin and depends largely on skin resistance for constant voltage sources. The author is aware of only one anecdotal case of an ICD patient receiving an inappropriate shock while using a radial-arm wood-cutting saw outside in wet weather. A likely source for these currents is by physical contact with improperly grounded electrical equipment. Other sources of conducted electric current that may cause malfunctions or damage include external defibrillators and electrosurgery. Electrostatic discharge at high voltage but low current may cause electrical resetting of memory to reset values during handling and implantation, but resetting has not been reported for devices fully implanted under the skin.

C. DC Magnetic Fields

DC magnetic fields from permanent magnets and electromagnets are measured in units of telsa (T), which equals 10,000 gauss. Most PMs and ICDs contain a magnetic reed switch that is closed by approximately a 10-gauss magnetic field. Continuous application of at least a 10-gauss magnetic field for at least 30 s to most AICDs manufactured by Cardiac Pacemakers, Inc., results in deactivation of the ICD. While this feature is useful in emergency situations, it has lead to many case reports of inadvertent deactivation of AICDs by speaker magnets, bingo wands, and other devices with large permanent magnets [2-6]. For many ICDs, a strong magnet placed over the device temporarily suspends automatic detection and therapies. The very intense magnetic fields in magnetic resonance imaging (MRI) have reportedly exerted forces on implanted metallic devices including PMs and ICDs [7]. Large magnetic fields may interfere with the transformers used to charge the ICD capacitors. It is very unlikely that high magnetic fields will be present during the brief and rare charging period of ICDs.

D. Ionizing Radiation Dose

The ionizing radiation dose is the amount of energy absorbed per unit mass of material, with units of joule per kilogram or gray (Gy). The rad (rd) is an obsolete unit which is 0.01 Gy. Radiation found in the environment and medical imaging equipment probably have no effect on implanted electronic devices. Therapeutic radiation used in oncology can damage the oxide layers of CMOS semiconductor circuits in ICDs and PMs, and these effects are cumulative.

E. Acoustic Radiation

Acoustic radiation from lithotripsy machines is used to disintegrate kidney and gallbladder stones. About 1500 discharges from a 20-kV spark gap generate pressure shock waves that are typically 45 MPa at the 12-mm-diameter focal area. If pressure waves of this magnitude are applied directly to a PM or ICD, the electronic circuits could be damaged (Fig. 1D).

F. Thermal Heating

Thermal heating of the electronics by electrical diathermy, focused therapeutic ultrasound, or other means could damage the circuits, battery, or capacitors of ICDs or PMs. Such heat would quickly conduct to the fluid around the implanted device if the exposure to the heat source is brief.

G. External Pressure

External pressure applied to the whole body in hyperbaric chambers or during SCUBA diving could exert large forces on the "can" of the ICD or PM. This force could push on the sides of the can enough to possibly cause short circuits or to mechanically damage components or internal connections.

H. Mechanical Trauma and Twiddling

Mechanical trauma and twiddling of implanted lead wires has caused dislodgements and lead fractures.

I. Temporal Factors

The frequency of electromagnetic interference affects both the efficiency of coupling the energy to the device and the nature of the effect created. The interference may be modulated in amplitude and/or frequency, and it may occur in bursts or single large pulses. The duration of exposure is particularly important for ICDs, because they all use some method to determine whether the tachyarrhythmia is sustained, either by counting the number of beats at high rates or the time of beating at high rate. Therefore the duration of the interference will determine whether inappropriate detection occurs. Also, the timing of the interference with respect to cardiac events and bradycardia pacing pulses can affect the type and severity of interference.

J. Geometric Factors

The distance from the source of interference to the patient with an implanted device and leads is extremely important, as is the orientation of the implanted device electrodes with respect to the direction of the radiated or conducted interference. Little effect will occur if the electrodes

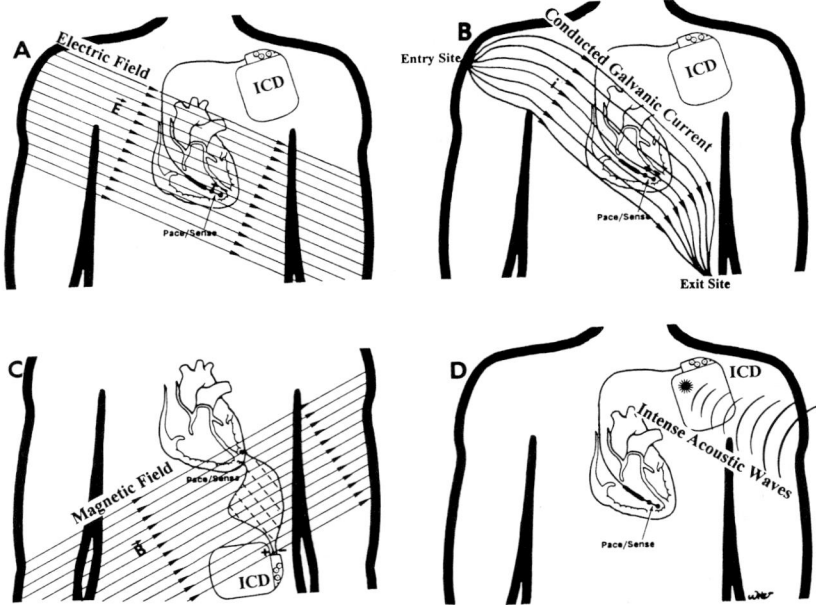

Figure 1 Schematic diagrams for types of ICD interference. Panel A: A strong time varying electric field (E) when passing through the heart could induce an interference voltage (+ −) at the sensing electrodes in the right ventricular apex. The electric field lines are actually curved due to the nonuniform conductivity of body tissues. Panel B: AC conducted glavanic current (i) that enters and exits the conductive human body at two sites could induce an interference voltage at the sensing electrodes in the right ventricular apex. Panel C: A strong time varying magnetic field (B) can induce an interference voltage in the lead wires that depends on the area between the wires (dashed area) that is perpendicular to the magnetic field. The induced interference voltage appears at the input terminals of the ICD (+ −). For coaxial leads, the area is extremely small so the induced interference voltage would be nil. The magnetic field lines would actually be curved due to the nonuniform permeability of the medium. Panel D: Intense focused acoustic waves from lithotripsy that fall on ICD internal components could cause damage. Most of the acoustic waves would be reflected by the metal case of the ICD.

are perpendicular to the direction of the electric field, whereas the effect will be maximal if the field and the device with its lead are parallel. For conducted interference, both the entry and exit points for the electric current, the types of intervening tissues, and the location of the device and lead within the path of current flow all affect the amount of interference that occurs. The type of coupling media between the source of interference and the various parts of the human body can be critical. For example, acoustic energy does not conduct well through air, so some liquid medium between the source and the human body will greatly affect possible acoustic interference.

III. DIFFERENCES BETWEEN IMPLANTABLE CARDIOVERTER-DEFIBRILLATORS AND PACEMAKERS

ICDs designed to terminate tachyarrhythmias have much technology in common with PMs, but there are important differences. Antitachycardia pacing, cardioversion, and defibrillation therapies are typically needed less frequently than bradycardia pacing therapy. The consequences of oversensing can be inappropriate shocks from ICDs, compared to inhibition of pacemakers or reversion pacing. The result of undersensing ventricular fibrillation by ICDs is usually death, compared to asynchronous bradycardia pacing by pacemakers.

ICDs use only bipolar sensing; however, the sense amplifiers are almost 10 times more sensitive—as high as 0.15 mV. ICDs may use standard bipolar sensing between two epicardial screw-in electrodes with recommended spacing of 1 cm. If the two epicardial electrodes are implanted more than 1 cm apart, the opportunity for sensing interference increases. For transvenous endocardial leads the sensing is either standard bipolar between tip and ring electrodes, similar to bipolar bradycardia leads, or integrated bipolar between the tip electrode and the right ventricular coil electrode, that is also used for shock delivery. The larger length and surface area of the right ventricular coil electrode compared to a sense ring increases the opportunity for interference to be sensed.

The large-surface-area epicardial and subcutaneous patch electrodes and the large transvenous coil electrodes can be thought of as antennas for coupling interference to the circuits of the ICD. Furthermore, the abdominal implant sites require long lead lengths, which must be tunneled under the skin. The projected area of any loops in noncoaxial electrode systems represents an opportunity for electromagnetic fields to induce voltage on the sensing lead conductors. The larger size of the ICD cans and their location in the abdomen rather than the pectoral region probably increases susceptibility to many forms of interference. Transvenous leads with coaxial conductors and ICDs small enough for pectoral implantation have little susceptability to interference.

IV. INTERFERENCE FROM OTHER MEDICAL DEVICES AND INSTRUMENTS

A. External Cardiac Defibrillation

External transthoracic defibrillation using paddles or disposable defibrillation electrodes can apply several thousand volts and tens of amperes of current to implanted PMs, ICDs, and their leads [8]. To protect the pacing output circuits and the sense amplifiers in PMs, back-to-back zener diodes are placed to shunt the current and limit the voltage at the terminals of the device. While these diodes prevent permanent damage to the internal circuitry, defibrillation-shock transient voltages may cause PMs and ICDs to "reset." The reset operation is a protection mechanism designed into PMs and ICDs to sense conditions that may jeopardize the integrity of memory parameters that affect device operation. If battery voltage dips below some critical value, even for a very short time, or if very high voltage appears within circuits, or if special timers in microprocessors are triggered, then the contents of volatile memory are abandoned and default values are retrieved from read-only memories and device operation is restarted. Some ICDs reset with defibrillation detection and therapy "on," and others reset with them "off."

External paddles or disposable defibrillation electrodes should not be placed directly over the implanted PM or ICD. For ICDs with epicardial patch electrodes, external defibrillation should aim to pass current through the heart perpendicular to a line between the epicardial patch electrodes to maximize the flow of current through the myocardium [9,10]. Following any defibrillation or electroconvulsive transcranial shock therapy, PMs and ICDs should be tested for proper function and interrogated.

B. Electrosurgery

Radiofrequency (RF) currents are used in many surgical procedures to cut and coagulate tissue. Sinusoidal and modulated RF from 100 kHz to 5 MHz, with power levels from 10 to 500 W, is usually delivered in a unipolar mode between an active probe and a large-surface-area disposable dispersive electrode. For desiccation and coagulation the RF energy is pulsed at 20 kHz, and for cutting the RF energy is continuous.

The critical factor for electrosurgical interference is the geometric coupling of this RF energy to the PM or ICD and its lead system. The electric current density close to the active probe is very high, and it decreases as the current spreads out as it flows to the large dispersive electrode. Chauvin et al. [11] demonstrated that electrosurgical electrodes positioned close to either the can or the lead tip electrode produce maximal interference. The effect was a function of the distance between the leads and was negligible when applied to the path followed by the lead. All forms of interference, including inhibition and oversensing, resetting of all memory and parameters, or permanent damage have been observed for ICDs and PMs. If the active probe gets very close to or touches the leads or can, then permanent damage to internal circuits may occur. The amplitude of the electric current is critical, and the duration of damaging exposure may be very short. Although newer ICD and PM designs are more resistant to electrosurgery, these effects cannot be eliminated.

If electrosurgery must be used for ICD and PM patients, position both the active and the dispersive electrode as far from the leads and can as possible, and never within 15 cm of the leads or can. Use minimal electrosurgical current, and all manufacturers recommend deactivating the ICD to avoid undesired shocks. Wilson et al. [12] implanted CPI AICDs epicardially in canines and applied electrosurgery to the edge of the thoracotomy incision with 112 W in cut mode and 255 W in coagulation mode. No oversensing, charging, or damage was observed. In three patients with AICDs activated, electrosurgery with 30–40 W performed on abdominal and peripheral organs did not affect the AICDs. Improper grounding or disconnected cables did result in electrosurgical oversensing.

Note that the term "electrocautery" means electrical heating of a metal instrument tip without passage of electric current through the patient. However, "electrocautery" is often used synonymously with "electrosurgery."

C. Radiofrequency Catheter Ablation

Many cardiac arrhythmias are being cured with RF catheter ablation, which permanently damages a small arrhythmogenic intracardiac tissue segment. Chin et al. [13] studied the effects of catheter ablation on implanted cardiac pacemakers in 12 canines with an ablation electrode positioned 1 cm from the tip of the pacing lead. During the ablation with 15 W applied for 30 s, the pacemakers inhibited even in asynchronous mode, paced at abnormally high rates, and reverted to reset parameters. None of the pacemakers was permanently damaged. Careful monitoring, backup external pacing during ablation, and complete pacing system analysis after the ablation are recommended.

D. Magnetic Resonance Imaging (MRI)

The very large static and gradient magnetic fields (1.5–4 T) from newer MRI scanners close the reed switch of pacemakers within several meters of the scanner, resulting in asynchronous pacing or suspension of ICD detection. The physical force exerted on a pacemaker case was judged as large enough to result in pacemaker movement within the pocket unless prohibited by fibrotic tissue encapsulation [14]. These forces are increased for ICDs because of the large ferrous transformer material. In-vitro and in-vivo animal studies [15] have shown that application of 64-MHz radiofrequency power, required to produce MRI scans, results in rapid pacing at pulsing periods between 200 ms and 1000 ms that can stimulate the heart at that period and may induce ventricular fibrillation. This rapid pacing requires an intact lead that is connected to a pacemaker. The mechanism for rapid pacing by the pulsed radiofrequency field apparently uses the lead to couple energy to the pacemaker defibrillation protection diodes or the output circuits. Inhibition of both the atrial and ventricular outputs of dual-chamber pacemakers by MRI has been reported [16]. In the abstract literature, several cases of successful MRI on patients with pacemakers without adverse effects on pacemaker operation have been reported [17–20]. However, there was one patient whose pacemaker was disabled by the MRI magnetic field, resulting in cardiac arrest, successful CPR, but severe brain damage [21]. One in-vitro study of the effects of MRI on ICDs showed that voltage amplitude and frequency sufficient to produce ventricular fibrillation appear on the leads alone and when connected to ICDs [22]. The very strong MRI magnetic field may prevent detection and could cause damage to the ICD if charging occurs while in the magnetic field. The use of MRI for patients with PMs or ICDs is generally contraindicated.

E. Lithotripsy

Extracorporeal shock-wave lithotripsy is a noninvasive method for dissolution of renal or uretheral calculi. Electromechanical shock waves are created by 18- to 30-kV electrical discharges between spark plug electrodes. The explosive shock wave is focused by an ellipisoid reflector to a focal point that is about 2 cm in diameter. To avoid cardiac arrhythmias, each of the typically 1500 shock waves is synchronized to the R wave on the electrocardiograph. The pressure of the shock wave may mechanically damage PM or ICD components, or the electromagnetic field from the discharge may cause electromagnetic interference. During in-vitro studies two single-chamber, rate-responsive pacemakers placed at focal point F2 had the piezoelectric crystal shattered, while two identical pacemakers placed 5 cm away were not damaged [23]. A survey of 131 pacemaker patients treated with lithotripsy found only four complications: one reset to default parameters, one irregular heart rhythm if more than 22 kV was used, one intermittent asynchronous operation, and one 10-beats/min pacing-rate increase with several extrasystoles [24]. Only two of these pacemakers were in the abdominal position, and both were considered to be outside the lithotripsy field. Most ICDs, because of their size, must be implanted in the abdomen. In one case report, preceded by a strap-on test in another patient, a right renal calculus was treated successfully with lithotripsy without damage to the AICD that was implanted an unknown distance away on the left side [25]. The ICD was deactivated for the duration of the procedure to avoid inappropriate shocks. PMs should be programmed to fixed-rate VVI with the lowest usable sensitivity. ICD and PM patients apparently can receive lithotripsy treatment safely if the device and the target are at least 18 cm apart. The effects of lithotripsy on leads are unknown [26].

F. Ionizing Radiation

CMOS semiconductor circuits used in implantable devices can be permanently damaged by very-high-energy radiation, including X-rays, gamma rays, electrons, protons, neutrons, and cosmic particles used primarily in oncology therapy, including cobolt radiators, linear accelerators, and betatrons. The effects of this intense radiation on thin oxide layers on the integrated circuits (ICs) are cumulative, can alter the transistor parameters, or create undesired electrical shorts that may result in premature battery depletion. The effects on device operation are extremely unpredictable, and PM rate runaway has been reported [27]. A report on 23 PMs and 4 nonprogrammable, rate-only ICDs [28] showed PM failure for doses as low as 14 Gy. Although none of the ICDs failed at less than 50 Gy, the charge times increased catastrophically for less than 50 shocks delivered compared to no failures after more than 79 shocks delivered for a control group of 6 patients with implanted ICDs. In a policy statement for oncologists, Mellenberg [29] recommended 2 Gy as a dosage limit for PMs to be achieved by altering the treatment plan (Fig. 2), requiring PM repositioning or PM replacement after completion of the treatment plan.

G. Medical Diathermy

Short-wave diathermy (27 MHz) is usually preferred to microwave diathermy (2450 MHz), because it penetrates deeper to heat tissue for treatment of musculoskeletal pain, primarily in

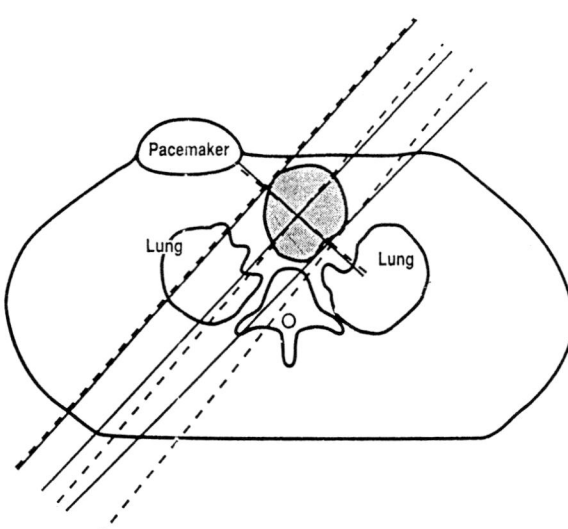

Figure 2 Transverse section of a patient showing how an oblique field of radiation treatment for a tumor (shaded area) can minimize exposure of the pacemaker to the radiation that can damage the electronic circuits (Ref. 29).

the shoulder, spine, back, and knee. The field intensity is highest close to the applicator, so exposure of a PM or ICD depends on their relative positioning. PM inhibition and ICD oversensing and inappropriate shocks are the primary risks. If an applicator is placed directly over an ICD, then thermal heating is possible, although conduction of the heat to adjacent tissue occurs rapidly [30,31].

H. TENS and Other Stimulators

Transcutaneous electrical nerve stimulators (TENS) and implantable spinal-cord stimulators for relief of chronic pain produce trains of pulses that can be inappropriately sensed by PMs or ICDs. This stimulation is usually bipolar, and adequate separation of the two electrode systems is the most important factor. The short duration of the stimulus pulses contain frequencies that are heavily filtered by the sense amplifiers. PM inhibition from oversensing of these stimulus pulses have been reported, but usually only a few beats on Holter monitors [32–38]. Although reports of interaction of these stimulators with ICDs was not found, the concern is that the bursts of stimuli that are sometimes used in these stimulators could be sensed as ventricular fibrillation by an ICD and result in an inappropriate shock.

I. Hyperbaric Chambers

Hyperbaric oxygen treatment is used for skin trauma and gas poisoning. The high static pressure could cause mechanical deformation of the cans of PMs and ICDs and damage the internal circuits. Four PM models (Medtronic Elite, Synergyst II, Legend, and Legend II) were tested for up to 4 h at a pressure equivalent to 165 f of seawater (FSW) with no adverse effects [39]. Informal testing of the Medtronic PCD has shown it can withstand 200 FSW for 15 min or 100 FSW for 2 h.

J. Miscellaneous Equipment

Many other possible interactions of medical devices with PMs have been investigated without significant clinical consequences. Examples include various dental equipment [40–43], electroconvulsive shock therapy [44,45], EEG [46], fetal monitoring [47], intraaortic balloon counterpulsation [48], and cardiomyoplasty (unpublished animal tests).

V. ENVIRONMENTAL INTERFERENCE IN HOMES AND PUBLIC PLACES

Normal operation of household appliances and electrical devices found in most workplaces do not affect modern PMs or ICDs. This includes microwave ovens, cellular telephones, operation of automobiles, small internal-combustion engines, computer terminals, televisions, and audio equipment. Patients with bipolar sensing leads are much less likely to be affected by electromagnetic interference than patients with unipolar PMs.

Radiated electromagnetic energy with frequencies from 10 kHz to 3000 MHz is widely used for communications and radar. The peak electric field strengths in public areas close to the transmitter source are less than 200 V/m rms, except for ham radio, which can be 325 V/m rms, and microwave radar, which is estimated to be as high as 1400 V/m rms. Several abstracts describe testing with some pacemaker inhibition, but clinically significant case reports could not be found for PMs or ICDs.

A. Power Frequency (50–60 Hz) Electromagnetic Energy

The effects of power-line-frequency electric fields up to 20 kV/m in 35 patients with 16 different PMs were studied [49]. The Medtronic and some Vitatron PMs had normal sensing and pacing, while PMs from other manufacturers exhibited varying degrees of inhibition and reversion to fixed-rate pacing. Another study of directly injected 50-Hz currents in the range of 0–600 μA were applied directly to 18 patients [50]. Reversion to fixed-rate pacing which indicates oversensing, occurred for currents in the range of 29–250 μA, and was dependent on the pacemaker model, location of the injecting electrodes, posture, and respiration. Fifteen patients with 12 different PMs were tested at a high-voltage substation in the vicinity of 110- and 400-kV/m power lines [51]. Several PMs oversensed in moderate (1.2–2.7 kV/m) and strong (7–8 kV/m) electric fields in unipolar mode, whereas only one bipolar PM inhibited at high sensitivity (0.5–1.0 mV) for the strongest field. Thus the programmed sensitivity and the lead configuration were important factors that affected inhibition. In one anecdotal ICD case, a patient received a shock while operating a large orbital electric sander that was pressed against his abdomen directly over the AICD [52]. The presumed mechanism in this case was electromagnetic induction into the sensing system from electromagnetic fields generated by the electric motor, which was very close to the ICD and its leads.

B. Security Systems

No effects were observed while monitoring over 100 patients in airport security metal detectors [53]. Electronic article surveillance systems for retail merchandise use either low-frequency magnetic fields of about 16 Hz to 60 kHz or radiofrequency electromagnetic fields with 2–10 MHz, broadband RF, or microwave frequencies. During in-vitro and in-vivo testing of these antitheft devices, only the low-frequency magnetic field devices caused inhibition of the PMs [54]. No changes to programmed parameters of the PMs were observed.

C. Aviation Environments

Electromagnetic radiation in aircraft from radio communication transmitters, radar, and the 400-Hz power system might cause PM inhibition or ICD oversensing, detection, and inappropriate shocks. Although in-vitro testing within aircraft has shown inhibition, similar results for PMs implanted in patients have not been found [55], and a search could not identify clinical case reports. Medical helicopters may have higher levels of electromagnetic interference, and operation of telemetry to pace terminate arrhythmias may represent additional risks [56].

D. SCUBA Diving

The external pressure testing described above for hyperbaric chambers is applicable to SCUBA diving. For modern pacemakers, deformation of the titanium can began to occur at 132 FSW, so restricting SCUBA divers to 100 FSW is recommended. Rate responsive pacing began to diminish for pressures greater than 60 FSW.

E. Stun Guns

Devices designed to produce large electrostatic voltage pulses up to 100 kV at 5 to 20 pulses/s are being used for personal security. These stun guns were tested in animals with implanted pacemakers and found to induce ventricular fibrillation [57]. Apparently, the lead and pacemaker provide a means for inducing voltage that is applied directly to heart muscle. No clinical cases of this hazard have been reported.

VI. INTERFERENCE IN SPECIFIC OCCUPATIONS AND ACTIVITIES

Specific work environments have long been recognized as being capable of inhibiting or resetting PMs. Electric arc welding up to 225 A did not inhibit or affect bipolar pacemakers (Pacesetter: Synchrony II, Solus, Phoenix, Phoenix II, and Sensolog III) when used by patients or while standing within 2–3 m of the equipment [58]. The welding cables were not coiled, and the welding site and the power generator were kept away from the PMs. Larger arc welding machines with currents exceeding 1000 A did inhibit PMs during an in-vitro test within 1 or 2 m of the machines or the weld site. In this same study, interference was observed for a 200-A gas tungsten arc welding machine that also used a superimposed 25-kHz square wave. High voltage, up to 4000 V, in a neon sign burn-in room caused interference, as did the magnetic field from several types of industrial degaussing coils. Other sources of large voltages, currents, or magnetic fields include but are not limited to resistance welding, electric steel furnaces, dielectric heaters, induction heaters, electric power generators, large transformers, railroad locomotives, and radar transmitters.

VII. STANDARDS FOR ICD AND PM INTERFERENCE TESTING

Test methods for measuring susceptibility of PMs to electromagnetic interference date back to an August 1975 Pacemaker Standard developed by the Association for the Advancement of Medical Instrumentation under contract from the U.S. Food and Drug Administration [59]. Section 4.1.8 specifies radiated electromagnetic interference at 450 MHz with 100% modulation using rectangular pulses 200 V/m peak pulse amplitude at 125% of the PM basic rate. The 450-MHz frequency is a "compromise frequency that represents good body penetration." The 200-V/m electric field strength was recommended by the U.S. Air Force as "representing a reasonable choice based upon maximum expected electromagnetic environments" and is consistent with the established exposure limit of 10 mW/cm^2. The PM is tested with a straight lead in a test cell at least 20 cm × 40 cm × 80 cm to "represent the human chest cavity" filled with saline having 375 Ω-cm resistivity. The worst-case orientation of the electric field is parallel to the device and lead. For conducted galvanic currents, the power-line frequencies of 50 Hz (Europe), 60 Hz (United States), and 400 Hz (aircraft) are used, and the amplitude of 100 mV root mean square (rms), injected directly to appear directly at the pulse generator terminals, is "based on human threshold of perception" assuming a 2-mA threshold, a total body impedance of 1000 Ω, and 2 V applied at the skin. Clearly, these testing conditions are somewhat arbitrary and attempt to represent a reasonable and practical worse-case scenario. They have also stood the test of time for the pacemaker industry, for physicians, and for patients.

A modern European Standard for "Safety of Implantable Cardiac Pacemakers," CENELEC EN 50 061 [60], did not include Section 6.3 on electromagnetic compatibility. A "final draft" of this Section 6.3 has specific requirements for maximum induced currents applied to the heart, avoiding damage to the PM, oversensing that would change PM timing, and static magnetic fields that would not alter device function when removed. To prevent electromagnetic induction of currents through the lead into the heart that may cause fibrillation or tissue damage near the electrodes, the current should be limited to 50 μA (rms) from 20 Hz to 1 kHz. Larger currents are allowed at higher frequencies. Test voltages of 1 V continuous sinusoidal peak-to-peak amplitude and 20 Hz to 500 kHz frequency must be applied without causing malfunction or damage of the PM. With the PM programmed to its highest sensitivity, a 2-mV peak-to-peak modulated common-mode test voltage from 20Hz to 1 kHz should not cause oversensing. PMs should not be affected by static magnetic fields with flux densities less than 1 mT, and lasting effects should not occur upon removal of magnetic fields up to 10 mT.

A draft European Standard for ICDs and the functions of active implantable medical devices intended to treat tachycardia, prEN 45502-#, Ver. 4.00 [61] is under review. Protection from electromagnetic nonionizing radiation are similar to EN 50061 for pacemakers except unipolar sensing from epicardial or endocardial electrodes is not applicable to ICDs. When one high voltage lead is used as the pace/sense indifferent electrode, the ICD is tested in the same way as a unipolar pacemaker. New common mode and differential tests for malfunction due to voltages induced on the high voltage leads were added. Testing to avoid confusion between sensed beats and commonly encountered electromagnetic fields has not been specified.

REFERENCES

1. Olson WH. Electrical Safety. In: Webster JG, ed. Medical Instrumentation: Application and Design. 2d ed. Boston: Houghton Mifflin, 1992.
2. Schmitt C, Brachmann J, Waldecker B, Navarete L, Beyer T, Pfeifer A, Kubler, W. Implantable cardioverter defibrillator: possible hazards of electromagnetic interference. PACE 1991; 14(6): 982-984.
3. Ferrick KJ, Johnston RN, Kim SG, Roth J, Brodman R, Zimmerman J, Fisher JD. Inadvertent AICD inactivation while playing bingo. Am Heart J 1991; 121(1 pt 1):206-207.
4. Bonnet CA, Elson JJ, Fogoros RN. Accidental deactivation of the automatic implantable cardioverter defibrillator. Am Heart J 1990; 120(3):696-697.
5. Vlay SC, Olson LC, Burger L. Automatic internal cardioverter defibrillator lockout. Am Heart J 1990; 120(3):677-698.
6. Karson TH, Grace K, Denes P. Stereo speaker silences automatic implantable cardioverter-defibrillator. N Engl J Med 1989; 320(24):1628-1629.
7. Bach SM., Shapland JE. Engineering aspects of implantable defibrillators. In: Saksena S, Goldschlager N, eds. Electrical Therapy for Cardiac Arrhythmias: Pacing, Antitachycardia Devices, Catheter Ablation. 1990, Philadelphia: Saunders, 1990:376-377.
8. Levine PA. Effect of cardioversion and defibrillation on implanted cardiac pacemakers. In: Barold SS, ed. Modern Cardiac Pacing. Mount Kisco, NY: Futura, 1985.
9. Walls JT, Schuder JC, Curtis JJ, Stephenson HE, McDaniel WC, Flaker GC. Adverse effects of permanent cardiac internal defibrillator patches on external defibrillation. Am J Cardiol 1989; 64:1144-1147.
10. Pinski SL, Arnold AZ, Mick M, Maloney JD, Trohman RG. Safety of external cardioversion/defibrillation in patients with internal defibrillation patches and no device. PACE 1991; 14(1):7-12.
11. Chauvin M, Crenner F, Brechenmacher C. Interaction between permanent cardiac pacing and electrocautery: the significance of electrode position. PACE 1992; 15(11 pt 2):2028-2033.
12. Wilson JH, Lattner S, Jacob R, Stewart R. Electrocautery does not interfere with the function of the automatic implantable cardioverter defibrillator. Ann Thorac Surg 1991; 51(2):225-226.
13. Chin MC, Rosenqvist M, Lee MA, Griffin JC, Langberg JJ. The effect of radiofrequency catheter ablation on permanent pacemakers: an experimental study. PACE 1990; 13(1):23-29.
14. Pavlicek W, Geisinger M, Castle L, et al. The effects of nuclear magnetic resonance on patients with cardiac pacemakers. Radiology 1983; 147:149-153.
15. Hayes DL, Holmes DR, Gray JE. Effect of 1.5 Telsa nuclear magnetic resonance imaging scanner on implanted permanent pacemakers. J Am Coll Cardiol 1987; 10(4):782-786.
16. Erlebacher JA, Cahill PT, Pannizzo F, Knowles JR. Effect of magnetic resonance imaging on DDD pacemakers. Am J Cardiol 1986; 57(6):437-440.
17. Hardage M, Winsor D. Pacemakers in the magnetic resonance imaging environment. Asian Pacific Symposium on Cardiac Pacing and Electrophysiology, 3d., Melbourne, Australia: Organizing Committee, 1985.

18. Iberer F, Justich E, Stenzl W, et al. Behavior of the Activitrax pacemaker during in-vitro nuclear magnetic resonance investigation. PACE 1987; 10(5):1215.
19. Iberer F, Justich E, Stenzl W, Tscheliessnigg KH, Kapeller J, Machler H. Experimental and clinical experience with the magnetic resonance imaging of pacemaker patients. PACE 1989; 12(7 pt II):1183.
20. Alagona P, Toole JC, Maniscalco BS, Glover MU, Abernathy GT, Prida XE. Nuclear magnetic resonance imaging in a patient with a DDD pacemaker. PACE 1989; 12(4 pt I):619.
21. Avery JK. Not my responsibility. J Tenn Med Assoc 1988; 81(8):523.
22. Stanton MS, Stahl W, Gray JE. Interaction between magnetic resonance imaging and implantable defibrillators. J Am Coll Cardiol 1992; 19(3):243A.
23. Cooper D, Wilkoff B, Masterson M, et al. Effects of extracorporeal shock wave lithotripsy on cardiac pacemakers and its safety in patients with implanted cardiac pacemakers. PACE 1988; 11(11 pt I):1601-1616.
24. Drach GW, Weber C, Donovan JM. Treatment of pacemaker patients with extracorporeal shock wave lithotripsy: experience from 2 continents. J Urol 1990; 143:895-896.
25. Long AL, Venditti FJ. Lithotripsy in a patient with an automatic implantable cardioverter defibrillator. Anesthesiology 1991;74:937-938.
26. Anon. Use of shock wave lithotripsy on pacemaker patients. Medtronic Cardiovascular Technical Note 1986; 86:1-2.
27. Lee RW, Huang SK, Mechling E, Bazgan I. Runaway atrioventricular sequential pacemaker after radiation therapy. Am J Med 1986; 81(5):883-886.
28. Rodriguez F, Filimonov A, Henning A, Coughlin C, Greenberg M. Radiation-induced effects in multiprogrammable pacemakers and implantable defibrillators. PACE 1991; 14(12):2143-2153.
29. Mellenberg DE. A policy for radiotherapy in patients with implantable pacemakers. Med Dosimetry 1991; 16:221-223.
30. Agarwal A, Redding VJ. Interference effect of two commonly used (Megatherm and Megapulse) physiotherapy diathermy (27 MHz) on VVI pacemakers; do recommendations need reviewing? Indian Heart J 1988; 40(5 abstr):374.
31. Martin CJ. An evaluation of radiofrequency exposure from therapeutic diathermy equipment in the light of current recommendations. Clin Phys Physiol Meas 1990; 11(1):53–63.
32. Chen D, Philip M, Philip PA, Monga TN. Cardiac pacemaker inhibition by transcutaneous electrical nerve stimulation. Arch Phys Med Rehabil 1990; 71:27-30.
33. Rasmussen MJ, Hayes DL, Vliestra RE. Can transcutaneous electrical nerve stimulation be safely used in patients with permanent cardiac pacemakers? Mayo Clin Proc 1988; 63:443-445.
34. LaBan MM, Petty D, Hauser AM, Taylor RS. Peripheral nerve conduction stimulation: its effect on cardiac pacemakers. Arch Phys Med Rehabil 1988; 69:358-362.
35. Shade SK. Use of transcutaneous electrical nerve stimulation of a patient with a cardiac pacemaker. Physical Therapy 1985; 65(2):206-208.
36. Cazzin R, Pinato G, Rota P, Piccolo E. Management of dual chamber cardiac pacemaker in patients with spinal cord stimulators. Report of three observed cases and review of the literature. Cardiostimolazione 1991; 9:56-61.
37. Andersen C, Oxhoj H, Arnsbo P. Management of spinal cord stimulators in patients with cardiac pacemakers. PACE 1990; 13(5):574-577.
38. Anon. Pacemaker patients who use transcutaneous electrical nerve stimulators. Medtronic Cardiovascular Technical Note 1982:82-4.
39. Eichers P. Hyperbaric chamber and pressure vessel tests. Medtronic Design Assurance Rep PE92-292, 1992.
40. Luker J. The pacemaker patient in the dental surgery. J Dentistry 1982; 10(4):326-332.
41. Simon AB, Linde B, Bonnette GH, Schlentz RJ. The individual with a pacemaker in the dental environment. JADA 1975; 91:1224-1229.
42. Rahn R, Beckmann D, Kreuzer J, Zegelman M. Influence of dental appliances to the body activity directed pacemaker. Herz-schrittmacher 1988; 8:30-34.

43. Agarval A, Hewson J, Redding V. Ultrasound dental scalers and demand pacing. PACE 1988; 11(6):853.
44. Alexopoulos GS, Frances RJ. ECT and cardiac patients with pacemakers. Am J Psychiatry 1980; 137(9):1111-1112.
45. Abiuso P, Dunkelman R, Proper M. Electroconvulsive therapy in patients with pacemakers. JAMA 1978; 240(22):2459-2460.
46. Clark S, Goldberg M, Gorman R, Gerwer A. Interference of automated electroencephalographic processing by an endocardial pacemaker. J Clin Monit 1989; 5(1):22-25.
47. Goodlin RC, Cheatham JP. Electronic fetal monitor paced by maternal implanted pacemaker. Am J Obstet Gynecol 1985; 153(5):570-571.
48. Robicsek F, Morency RP. Failure of intraaortic balloon counterpulsation caused by pacing or other electrical artifacts: a new method of correction. J Cardiac Surg 1987; 2:407-410.
49. Butrous GS, Male JC, Webber RS, et al. The effect of power frequency high intensity electric fields on implanted cardiac pacemakers. PACE 1983; 6(6):1282-1292.
50. Kaye GC, Butrous GS, Allen A, Meldrum SJ, Male JC, Camm AJ. The effect of 50 Hz external electrical interference on implanted cardiac pacemakers. PACE 1988; 11(7): 999-1008.
51. Toivonen L, Valjus J, Hongisto M, Metso R. The influence of elevated 50 Hz electric and magnetic fields on implanted cardiac pacemakers: the role of the lead configuration and programming of the sensitivity. PACE 1991; 14(12):2114-2122.
52. Herre JM. Personal communication, Feb 28, 1993.
53. Cooperman Y, Zarfati D, Laniado S. The effect of metal detector gates on implanted permanent pacemakers. PACE 1988; 11(10):1386-1387.
54. Dodinot B, Godenir JP, Costa AB. Electronic article surveillance: a possible danger for pacemaker patients. PACE 1993; 16(1 pt I):46-53.
55. Toff WD, Edhag OK, Camm AJ. Cardiac pacing and aviation. Eur Heart J 1992; 13(suppl H):162-175.
56. Sumchai A, Sternbach G., Eliastam M, Liem LB. Pacing hazards in helicopter aeromedical transport. Am J Emerg Med 1988; 6:236-240.
57. Roy OZ, Podgorski AS. Tests on a shocking device—the stun gun. Med Biol Eng Comp 1989; 27:445-448.
58. Marco D, Eisinger G, Hayes DL. Testing of work environments for electromagnetic interference. PACE 1992; 15(11 pt II):2016-2022.
59. Anon. Pacemaker Standard: labeling requirements, performance requirements, and terminology for implantable artificial cardiac pacemakers. Assoc Adv Med Instr. 1975; Section 4.1.8, 53-56, 94-96.
60. Anon. Safety of implantable cardiac pacemakers, protection against electrical-magnetic interferences, Final draft EN 50-061, Section 6.3, 1991.
61. Anon. Draft European Standard for Active Implantable Medical Devices, particular requirements for implantable cardioverter defibrillators and the functions of active implantable medical devices intended to treat tachycardia. prEN 45502 Ver. 4.000 93-11-19.

10

Data Storage

Richard Lu

Telectronics Pacing Systems
Englewood, Colorado

I. INTRODUCTION

In a little over a decade, the implantable cardioverter-defibrillator (ICD) has evolved from a "simple" device to a sophisticated life saver. The initial ICD was a nonprogrammable, shock-only device. With advances in technology and clinical experience gained from early ICDs, the functions as well as the complexity of modern ICDs have increased manyfold. As a minimum, the following features can be found in current-generation ICDs: more than one tachycardia detection criterion; tiered therapy which combines bradycardia support pacing with various antitachycardia pacing modes, low-energy cardioversion, and defibrillation; and some sort of data logging capability. The data storage of modern ICDs has become increasingly important, since the amount of required data increases proportionally with the increase of ICD functions. Efficient handling of a large amount of data has become possible with the incorporation of a microprocessor and memory into the ICD.

Different types of data are stored in the memory of an ICD, including program instructions, programmable parameters, and other temporary data. Throughout this chapter, the storage of data in memory in general is termed "data storage," whereas "data logging" is a subset of data storage and refers to the recording of data associated with arrhythmia sensing, detection, and therapy delivery for patient management. Among the stored data, data which might be of interest to users include: administrative data (model number, serial number, date of implant, defibrillation lead type, pacing lead type, etc); tachyarrhythmia detection parameters (tachycardia detection interval, ventricular fibrillation detection interval, onset detection enable, etc); bradycardia therapy parameters (escape interval, pacing amplitude, pulse width, etc); antitachycardia pacing (ATP) parameters (ATP therapy enabled, number of ATP trains, number of ATP paces, etc); shock therapy parameters (number of shocks in a series, first shock energy, second shock energy, etc); noninvasive induction parameters (induction mode, number of paces, etc); other measurement parameters and data logging; etc.

Among the data stored in a modern ICD, the data logging facility has become increasingly important in the management of the device. The importance of such a data logging facility has been well recognized [1,2]. It has been stated that "The [early ICD] devices did not make any permanent record of the arrhythmia at the time of shocks. This necessitated frequent monitoring with transtelephonic devices, 24-hour ambulatory ECGs, and expensive hospitalizations to determine the cause of shocks. Shocks had to be classified as appropriate or inappropriate based on arbitrary clinical criteria. There was no way to evaluate the integrity of sensing and shocking leads" [3]. The problems and costs associated with such arbitrary decisions can easily be markedly reduced with the incorporation of an internal data logging facility in the ICDs. Such a facility was only wishful thinking a few years ago. As stated in a 1985 publication, a ". . . major problem with the [ICD] device has been the inability to easily determine the cause for the majority of pulse discharges received by the patient. . . . Until the [ICD] device incorporates a memory feature, the arrhythmias initiating each discharge cannot be tabulated" [4]. In recent years, the usefulness of a data logging facility in an ICD has been well established [5–9].

II. HOW ARE DATA STORED?

A. Microprocessor System

A microprocessor is an electronics device which accepts data from peripheral input circuits, such as telemetric circuits and sensing amplifiers. It then processes and manipulates the input data, outputting new data (therapy sequencing, shock energy, pacing amplitude, etc) to peripheral output circuits. A microprocessor system consists of a microprocessor, or central processing unit (CPU), memory, peripheral input/output circuits, and a clock (see Fig. 1). The heart of the system is the CPU, whose electronic architecture enables it to respond to instructions and data stored in memory in accordance with predetermined conditions or rules. Peripheral input circuits, such as telemetric circuits and sense amplifiers, provide inputs from the outside world. On the other hand, peripheral output circuits, such as pacing circuits and high-energy delivery systems, provide outputs to the outside world. Since a microprocessor uses clocked logic, a clock is needed to allow synchronous operations.

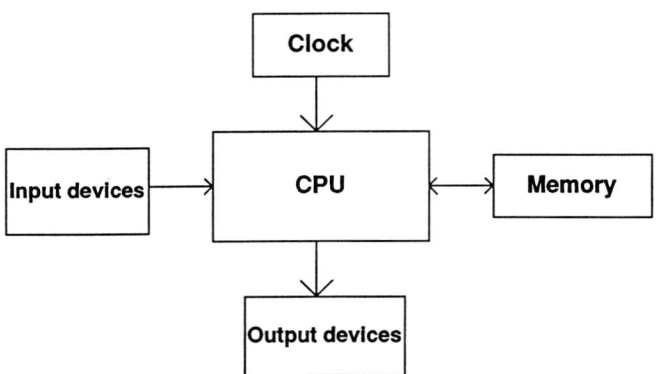

Figure 1 A microprocessor system consists of a central processing unit (CPU), memory, peripheral input devices, peripheral output devices, and a clock.

B. Binary Number System

In a binary number system, each digit is called one *bit* and has a value of either 1 or 0. For example, if a person tosses a coin and announces the outcome (either heads or tails), then each outcome is a "bit" of information. In this example, a 1 might represent heads while a 0 would represent tails. Eight bits are called a *byte*. Large amounts of memory are expressed in terms of "kilo" (abbreviated K) and "mega" (abbreviated M) bits or bytes. A "kilo" in the binary system is 1024, and a "mega" is 1024 × 1024 = 1,048,576. For example, 8K bytes of memory refers to 8192 bytes, or 65,536 bits of memory.

In a binary number, the weighing of each digit is 2^n, where n is the digit (bit) number. The rightmost digit is bit 0. For example, the binary number 01011001 is the decimal number 89 ($2^7 \times 0 + 2^6 \times 1 + 2^5 \times 0 + 2^4 \times 1 + 2^3 \times 1 + 2^2 \times 0 + 2^1 \times 0 + 2^0 \times 1$). If only positive numbers are required, a binary number of N bits can represent decimal numbers in the range of 0 to $2^N - 1$. Thus, an 8-bit binary number can represent 0 to 225 in decimal. Negative numbers can also be represented in a similar fashion. The only change is that the leftmost (or most significant) bit has a weighting of -2^{N-1} instead of 2^{N-1}. Hence, an N-bit binary number can represent decimal numbers from -2^{N-1} to $2^{N-1} - 1$. An example is given in Fig. 2.

It is also necessary to represent characters, as well as numbers, in a microprocessor system. Several standard methods have been developed. ASCII representation is the most common method and requires 7 bits for each character. An example is shown in Fig. 3.

C. Memory

Digital logic is used in microprocessor systems. Each component of a digital circuit can be either a HI or a LO state, corresponding to the measured voltage. A HI state in a digital circuit corresponds to the value 1 in the binary number system; similarly, a LO state is 0 in binary. For the example shown in Fig. 4, a HI state or 1 is established at the output when the switch is closed and electrical current passes through the load. Hence a voltage (V_{cc}) is established across the load. On the other hand, when the switch is open, no current passes through the load. Hence no voltage can be measured across the output, and the output is LO or 0.

Each component of a digital circuit can hold 1 bit of information. For a memory of 8K bytes (8 bits form 1 byte), $8 \times 1024 \times 8 = 65,536$ digital components are needed. Many of these digital components and their associated microelectronic networks can be fabricated into a memory chip using integrated circuit technology. In an integrated circuit memory, each of these components is called a *memory cell*. The requirement of low power consumption makes the integrated circuit technology called *complementary metal oxide semiconductor* (CMOS) the logical choice for an implantable memory.

Unlike human memory, which can be retrieved by seeing familiar things, memory cells in a microprocessor system must be accessed by specific addresses or locations. Since the specific location of a bit in a byte is known, every memory cell can be accessed by knowing the address of a byte in an 8-bit memory. Similarly, for a 16-bit or a 32-bit memory, each memory cell can be addressed if the address of the 16-bit unit or 32-bit unit of memory is known. In order to provide access to every single memory cell, the memory cells must be organized in a structured way.

In a memory chip, memory cells are organized in a matrix structure. The matrix is not necessarily square: Any configuration may be used. One possible arrangement is a matrix of 16 rows and 64 columns, with each row consisting of 8 bytes. A particular byte can be addressed by enabling the correct combination of row-select and column-select lines. To

Decimal number	Binary representation
-128	10000000
-127	10000001
-126	10000010
-125	10000011
-124	10000100
-123	10000101
-122	10000110
-121	10000111
⋮	⋮
-4	11111100
-3	11111101
-2	11111110
-1	11111111
0	00000000
1	00000001
2	00000010
3	00000011
⋮	⋮
120	01111000
121	01111001
122	01111010
123	01111011
124	01111100
125	01111101
126	01111110
127	01111111

Figure 2 Two's complement representations of 8-bit binary numbers from -128 to 127 in decimal range. Negative numbers can be identified by a 1 in the leftmost (most significant) bit, while the most significant bit is 0 for positive numbers.

illustrate, 128×8 memory cells can be organized as shown in Fig. 5. There are 16 row-select lines and 8 column-select lines. When row X_3 and column Y_0 are HI, the byte $X_3 - Y_0$ will be addressed for reading or writing.

There are two types of commonly used integrated circuit memory: Read-only memory (ROM), and random-access memory (RAM). The major difference between these two types of memories is that RAM can be both read from and written to by the microprocessor, while ROM can only be read from by the microprocessor. A ROM is a network that stores a fixed program. Writing is not possible after a ROM is fabricated. Fabrication consists of forming microelectronic circuits at each cell location. Before a ROM is fabricated as a matrix of fixed logical 1's and 0's which cannot be changed thereafter, the customer supplies the manufacturer with programming instructions. Reading of a ROM by the microprocessor is nondestructive, and the memory is nonvolatile. In contrast, a RAM is volatile. A volatile memory is one in which the data are lost when power is removed. However, both ROM and RAM are accessed in the same way by the microprocessor, by specific locations which can be used to link data together in a microprocessor system. For example, at power-up, the microprocessor reads data at

Data Storage

Character	ASCII representation
.	.
.	.
.	.
A	1000001
B	1000010
C	1000011
D	1000100
E	1000101
F	1000110
G	1000111
H	1001000
I	1001001
J	1001010
K	1001011
L	1001100
M	1001101
N	1001110
O	1001111
P	1010000
Q	1010001
R	1010010
S	1010011
T	1010100
U	1010101
V	1010110
W	1010111
X	1011000
Y	1011001
Z	1011010
.	.
.	.
.	.

Figure 3 ASCII representations of characters in 7-bit binary notation.

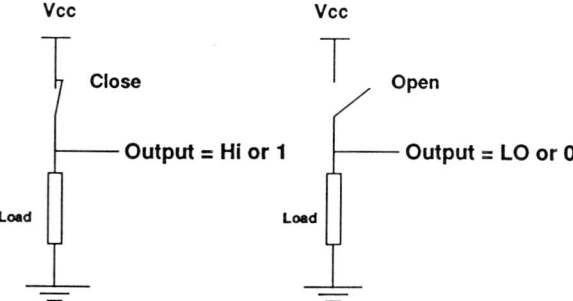

Figure 4 Logic states. V_{cc} is the supply voltage. Left panel: HI or 1 state is established at the output when the switch is closed and current passes through the load. Right panel: LO or 0 state is established at the output when the switch is open and no current passes through the load.

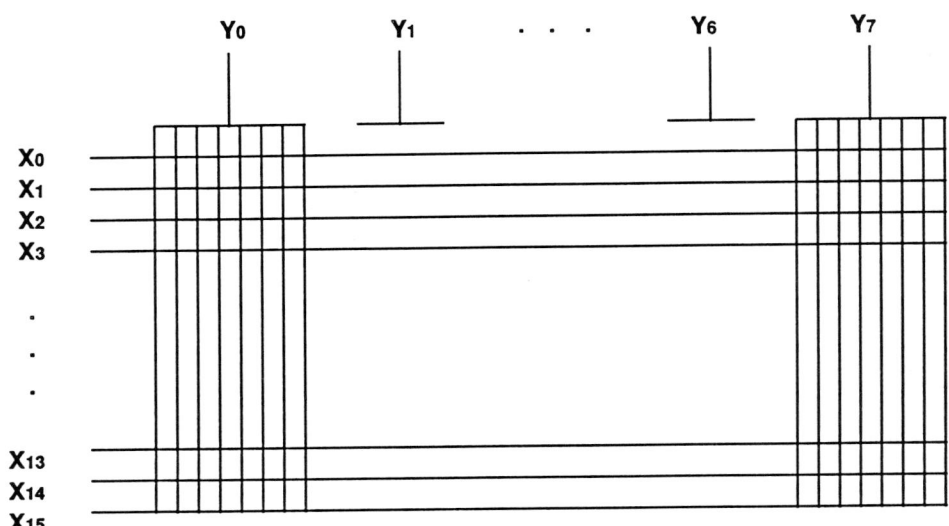

Figure 5 A memory organization of 128 × 8 memory cells. Each byte of memory can be addressed by enabling the correct combination of row-select and column-select lines.

predetermined addresses, which may contain the starting address of the operating program. The microprocessor then follows instructions of the operating program. Required data (e.g., a constant) may be stored within the operating program, or addresses of required data (e.g., the value of a programmed parameter) may be given, so that the data can be obtained by the microprocessor to execute the programmed instructions. Both RAM and ROM are usually used in a microprocessor system. However, the size of each type of memory required may vary with different applications.

Operating programs or instructions which a microprocessor follows to make a decision are usually stored in ROM before the device leaves the manufacturing factory. To accommodate the flexibility of software changes, RAM may also be used to store operating programs in some applications. An example of a hypothetical program in pseudo-code which may be stored in an ICD in binary representation is shown in Fig. 6. Temporary data stored in RAM can be written to and read from by a microprocessor, and includes values of programmable parameters (e.g., ventricular fibrillation detection interval, escape interval shown in Fig. 6), data logging counters (e.g., number of tachyarrhythmia detections, number of noise detection), and detailed episodic logs (e.g., R–R intervals).

Two types of errors may occur in memory devices: hard and soft errors. A hard error is a physical failure of the memory device (e.g., an internal short). A soft error is a random occurrence of a memory location change from a high level to a low level and vice versa. In an ICD, the former may be avoided by better design and better quality control before the device leaves the manufacturing facility. The latter may be more a concern for an implanted ICD. Soft errors may be caused by the following environmental conditions: cosmic rays, alpha-particle radiation, extreme temperature, abnormal pressure, vibrations, electromagnetic interference, power supply fluctuations, or power surges. Some of these conditions may be difficult to control, while others may be avoided by better system design, e.g., better power regulation to prevent power supply fluctuations, or a better defibrillation protection circuit to prevent power surges during high-energy shocks. Simple error detection-correlation methods, such as range

If (8/10 R-R intervals < Fibrillation detection interval)

    then start shock therapy

else if (8/10 R-R intervals < tachycardia confirmation interval) and

    (8/10 R-R intervals > minimum cycle length for ATP)

    then start ATP therapy

else if (R-R interval > standby interval)

    then start bradycardia therapy

else stay in monitoring state

Figure 6 A hypothetical program in pseudo-code which may be stored in an ICD.

checking, can be applied for programmable parameters: During a test, the value of a parameter must fall within a valid range, otherwise, nominal values are programmed. To detect soft errors in operating programs, error detection methods, such as check-sum checking or parity checking, must be used. Check-sum checking is a simple error detection method which performs an arithmetic sum of all data in memory within the range of tested addresses and compares the result with the predetermined check sum stored at one or more memory locations in a predetermined format. If the newly calculated check sum and the stored check sum do not match, one or more errors must have occurred. Parity checking normally requires each memory byte to be extended with an extra parity bit. This is called horizontal parity checking. The parity bit can be determined in one of two ways: (1) even parity, where each byte (including the parity bit) contains an even number of 1-bits; or (2) odd parity, where each byte (including the parity bit) contains an odd number of 1-bits. In order to detect as well as to correct errors, more sophisticated algorithms and memory requirements will be needed. For example, horizontal parity checking may be combined with vertical parity checking to achieve single-error detection and correction. Vertical parity checking requires a parity bit for each column of bits (a column consists of several bytes). Obviously, the better the error detection-correction scheme, the more memory and power consumption are needed. Therefore, a trade-off between costs (memory and power) and data reliability must be reached.

III. HOW ARE STORED DATA PRESENTED TO USERS?

After a device is implanted, it can only communicate with the outside world via a telemetric link. Hence, data in the RAM are read by the microprocessor, the microprocessor transfers the data to the peripheral devices, which then communicate with the clinical programmer via its telemetric link. To program a parameter, the reverse process is carried out to transfer a value from the clinical programmer to the implant device's RAM memory. For example, the first 2 bits of the byte at address AA00 is assigned to store the sensing configuration, and the next 2 bits are for the pacing configuration, while the last 4 bits are for the sensitivity. After the data

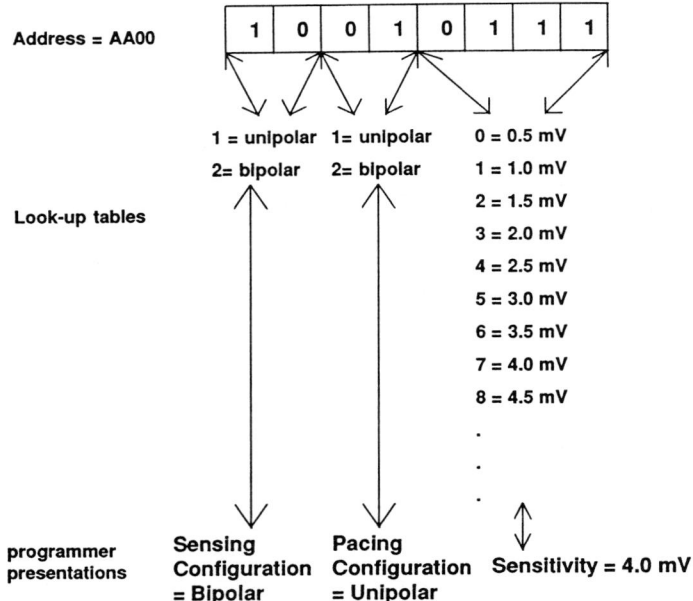

Figure 7 Mapping of memory data to user presentations and vice versa. The first two bits at address AA00 are assigned to store the sensing configuration, the next two bits are for the pacing configuration, while the last four bits are for the sensitivity. Look-up tables are used to convert the data obtained from address AA00 to user presentations displayed on a programmer.

at address AA00 are retrieved by the programmer, the data will be matched with look-up tables to convert the binary data to user-understandable values, as shown in Fig. 7. A clinical programmer with a telemetric wand is shown in Fig. 8.

IV. DATA LOGGING OF EVENTS

With the increased complexity of modern ICDs, internal data logging has become an important facility which improves the ease of ICD management. Data logging in an ICD can be grouped into three types: long-term cumulative data, detailed episodic data ("episode log") including sense history data, and intracardiac electrograms. Refer to Section VI for the data logging facilities which are available in various ICDs.

A. Long-Term Log

A long-term cumulative data log consists of event counters which register the occurrences of events cumulatively since the time the counters were cleared using a clinical programmer. Examples of these events are number of shocks delivered to the patient, number of defibrillator activations, number of tachyarrhythmia detections, number of noise detections, etc. The quantity and range of available event counters vary in different devices. There are only three in the Guardian 4202/4203 and the Ventak 1550. There are as many as 17 counters in the Guardian ATP 4210. An example programmer printout is shown in Fig. 9.

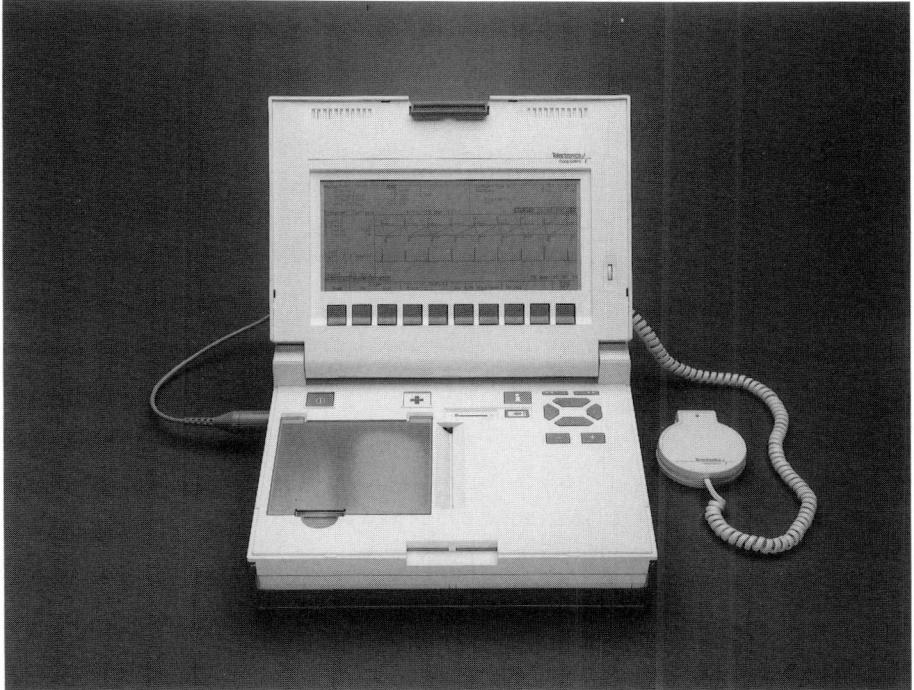

Figure 8 A clinical programmer with a telemetric wand with which the ICD communicates for data transmission.

B. Detailed Record of Tachyarrhythmia Episodes

Detailed "episode logs" record information about each episode, such as date and time of a tachyarrhythmia detection, average tachycardia cycle length and criteria for detection, type of each therapy delivered, details of each therapy, and defibrillation electrode impedance. An example can be seen in Fig. 10. The amount of data in each "episode log" and the number of episodes logged differs among various ICDs, and depends on the programmed parameters and the patient response to the delivered therapy. A sense history of each tachyarrhythmia episode, which lists sensed intervals prior to detection, during tachyarrhythmia confirmations, and after reversion, may also be stored in the devices. The numbers of stored intervals vary depending on the device.

C. Intracardiac Electrogram

As part of the "episode logs," segments ("snapshots") of intracardiac electrograms can also be stored in more sophisticated ICD devices, such as the Cadence V-100 and the Guardian ATP 4210. Data logging of intracardiac electrograms requires the largest amounts of memory. The number of episodes and the length of each episode of stored intracardiac electrograms vary in different devices. An example is shown in Fig. 11.

```
Tachy Episodes from 13:34 08 Jan 92 to 14:22 13 Jan 92

Total Detections                3        Total Shocks                 31
 Tachy       Detections         2         Reversions by Shock 1        0
 Onset       Detections         0         Reversions by Shock 2        0
 VF          Detections         1         Reversions by Shock 3        0
                                          Reversions by Shock 4+       0
Noise         Detections        0
                                         Last Shock at 13:27 08 Jan 92
Spontaneous  Reversions         2         Nominal Energy            Max J
Delayed      Reversions         0         Delivered Energy         37.2 J
Other        Reversions         0          Impedance                 44 ohms

ATP          Reversions         1
 Accelerations > 50 ms          0        Percent Pacing               0 %
 Accelerations to VF            0        Life Remaining            > 40 %
 Max ATP Attempts Used          0        Equiv BOL Max Charges     19.1
```

Figure 9 A programmer printout of event counters.

Data Storage

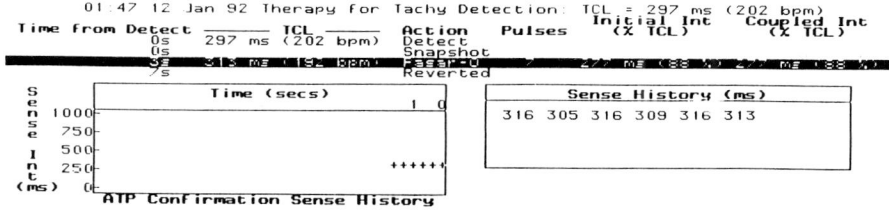

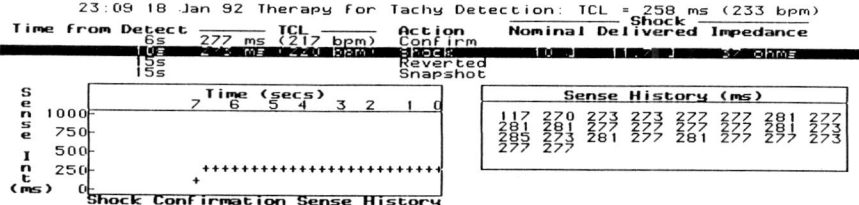

Figure 10 Programmer printouts of detailed "episode logs" with sense histories. Top panel: An ATP train of 7 pulses was delivered. Bottom panel: A shock of 11.7 J, 37 Ω, was delivered.

V. UTILITIES OF DATA LOGGING

There are at least three major utilities of the data logging facility in an ICD: (1) clinical utility, (2) engineering utility, and (3) research utility.

A. Clinical Utility

One of the major disadvantage of early ICDs was that the appropriateness of delivered therapies could not be assessed easily [3]. In a modern ICD, the sequence of events, and the response of the device to each rhythm classification, including each form of subsequent therapy, can be reconstructed from the stored data. Hence, the correctness of each response of the device can be determined. For example, the stored tachycardia cycle lengths were used to assess the accuracy of rhythm classification of ICDs by Wang et al. [6] and Mehta et al. [10]. The clinical applications of stored intracardiac electrograms were demonstrated by Hurwitz et al. [8]. The benefits of easy acquisition and retrieval of various stored data (long-term counters, detailed records of tachyarrhythmia episodes, and stored intracardiac electrograms) were also demonstrated by Luceri et al. [5].

With increasing device complexity, logged data have become very important in guiding patient-specific programming of the modern ICD [7,9]. From the event counters, the frequency of each therapy application can be obtained. The effectiveness of each therapy and changes in therapy requirements can also be determined. Hence, reprogramming of the ICD to tailor it to an individual's need at a certain time can be performed in an optimal way, or a change in pharmacological application can also be decided. For example, a patient's follow-up data may show that the frequency of tachycardia detected by the fibrillation detector has decreased while the frequency of tachycardia detected by the tachycardia detector increases. This may indicate that the tachycardia rate has been slower during the current follow-up period than during the previous period, possibly due to the effectiveness of a certain antiarrhythmic drug. Hence, the prescription of medication can be carefully controlled. In addition, antitachycardia therapy

Figure 11 A printout of logged intracardiac electrograms and main timing events postdetection.

may be reprogrammed to allow for antitachycardia pacing therapy before the delivery of shock therapy. Another example is that, if the spontaneous reversion counter is high, the tachycardia detection criteria may be reprogrammed (e.g., from 8/10 intervals less than detection interval to 16/20 intervals less than detection interval), so that nonsustained ventricular tachyarrhythmias or supraventricular tachyarrhythmias will be less likely to initiate unnecessary charging of capacitors.

Detailed "episode log" data provide information about therapy sequencing as well as the decision making of the device. This information not only provides occurrences of events in a timely order for diagnostic purposes, it also provides the users a view of the logical reasoning of the device. Since the interactions between therapies and functions in the ICD have become very complex, providing a record of the device's decision making helps increase users' confidence in the device. Furthermore, the detailed data provide confirmation and correlation to reassure the physician of trends shown from the event counters. For example, if antitachycardia pacing therapy is more successful during a recent period than the previous follow-up period, the long-term counters should indicate this. However, the episode logs would provide a confirmation of successful terminations of tachycardia by antitachycardia pacing therapy. The pacing train which terminates a certain episode of a tachycardia can be identified exactly. The integrity of defibrillation leads can also be determined from the defibrillation impedance of each shock.

The logged intracardiac electrograms and sensed markers provide information for out-of-hospital sensing assessment following onsets of tachyarrhythmias. This is important because in-hospital real-time assessment during implantation and follow-up visits provide information only in an artificial setting. The sensing performance can further be confirmed with the additional information of R–R intervals from the sense history prior to the detection, confirmation of a tachycardia, and after the reversion of a tachycardia. The sense history also provides information to verify the satisfaction of detection or confirmation criteria.

The combination of event counters, "episode logs," and intracardiac electrograms as well as sense histories has proved to be a useful tool in making clinical decisions. For example, when the noise-detection counter shows a high number of occurrences, this could be attributable to real noise interference, intermittent lead connection problems, or other causes. Without other information, the real cause of these detections can be difficult to determine. If the following data were also observed: the spontaneous reversion counter is high, the R–R intervals in the sense history of the last episode vary significantly, with some short intervals which fall inside the noise detection window (e.g., between 70 and 100 ms), and logged intracardiac electrograms show irregularity of interference (different from regular line frequency), then it is very likely that the noise detections are due to sensing lead connection problems.

B. Engineering Utility

During the development and validation of the ICD, the data logging facility can be a reliable debugging tool to determine whether the device is functioning according to specification, since the device logic and sequencing can be recorded accurately in the memory. The data logging facility has been shown to be a very useful tool for device validation on the bench with prerecorded signals [11]. Since the characteristics of input signals are known, the outputs can be expected. Logged data then can be used to determine whether the decisions of the device agree with expectation. Besides the benefits of making the validation job easier, information gathered in the data log can also provide concrete evidence of correct functioning of the device for regulatory purposes.

From time to time, engineers in the office are faced with bits and pieces of information received from the field with the suspicion that a device is functioning abnormally. With the availability of logged data, the explanation for a certain behavior can be determined more easily and in a timely fashion, since the "states" of the defibrillator machine can be logged and the performance can be traced. Without the data logging facility, the task of piecing the information together itself is already a difficult job. Problem solving may even be impossible.

C. Research Utility

With the availability of data logging in the ICD, many clinical questions can now be answered. Since data obtained from ICD patients are most appropriate as test signals for algorithm fine-tuning or for the development of future ICD algorithms, many efforts have been made by ICD researchers to record data from ICD patients. In some cases, data gathering by other means can be difficult or impossible. For example, data necessary to study whether prophylactic pacing can prevent the onsets of tachyarrhythmias can only be obtained in an interactive clinical pacing–data gathering setting. Another example is the investigation of morphological changes in the intracardiac electrograms before the onset of an arrhythmia. Other issues, such as "rate stability," sudden deaths, efficacy of drugs, and progression of diseases, may also be addressed by monitoring premature ventricular contractions, couplets, R-on-T, etc. Such kinds of questions can potentially be answered by using the data logging facility. Therefore, the data logging facility can be a very powerful scientific tool to investigate new therapies and detection algorithms.

Furthermore, reports of ICD therapy and survival have focused mainly on symptomatic shocks. With the availability of stored data, databases of stored events may be constructed. This might provide another method for determining the likely rhythm for which therapy was delivered, and a better way for estimating the mechanisms of onset and terminations of arrhythmias. Hence, studies such as those regarding projected survival without an ICD may be predicted more accurately. For example, a hypothetical survival curve was constructed by using stored data of defibrillation shocks in ICDs by Fromer et al. [12].

VI. DEVICE COMPARISON—DATA LOGGING

At the time of this writing, advanced ICDs are available from at least six manufacturers. The data logging facilities of various devices are compared in Fig. 12. The first column lists the names of manufacturers. The second column lists model names of different ICDs. The last three columns show data logging facilities of different devices in three groups: long-term counters, "episode logs," and intracardiac electrograms. All ICDs have at least a few counters. Most devices have some forms of "episode logs." Only the Guardian ATP 4210 (Telectronics Pacing Systems, Englewood, CO) and the Cadence-V-100 (Ventritex, Sunnyvale, CA) have intracardiac electrogram logs. The Guardian ATP 4210 logs short simultaneous "snapshots" of intracardiac electrograms and main timing events for each logged episode, while the Cadence V-100 logs longer segments of intracardiac electrograms with three variable lengths depending on the number of logged events.

VII. FUTURE DEVELOPMENT

Advanced data logging facilities in ICDs will likely require the storage of more data. In order to store more data, larger memory will be needed. It is important to note that a larger memory

Data Storage

Company	Model	Counter	Episode Log	Intracardiac electrograms
CPI	Ventak AICD series	3	none	none
CPI	Ventak PRx	3	128 episodes with minimal data, and last 16 shock episodes with 16 sense intervals prior to therapy and 16 intervals prior to episode end	none
Intermedics	Res Q	14	last episode timing data only	none
Medtronic	PCD	15	last episode, sensed intervals only	none
Siemens	Siecure	several	48 episodes, 16 episodes for each of the three rate classes. Rate and 64 intervals prior to detection and 64 intervals post reversion	none
Telectronics	Guardian 4202/4203	3	none	none
Telectronics	Guardian ATP 4210	17	average 25 episodes including sense history. Maximum 5 episodes of full length therapies.	intracardiac electrogram and main timing event snapshots of each logged episode
Ventritex	Cadence V-100	3	11 episodes	1 event/64 secs or 3 events/32 secs each or 7 events/16 secs each

Figure 12 A comparison of available data logs in different ICDs.

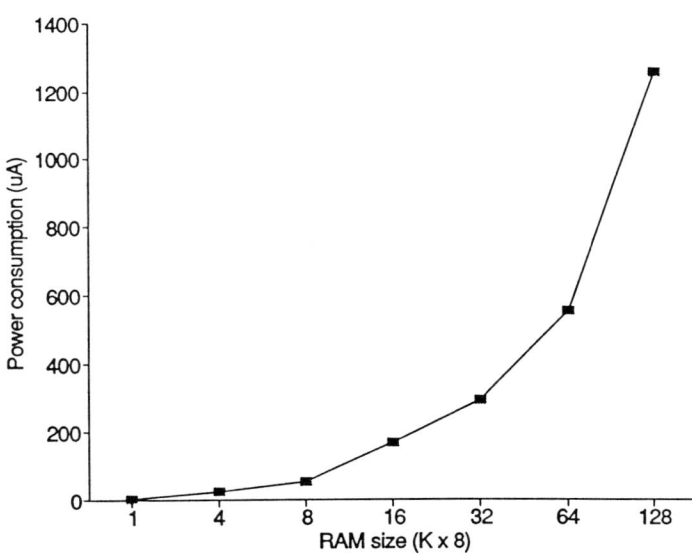

Figure 13 A comparison of operating power consumption of different RAM sizes.

may necessitate higher power consumption (see Fig. 13 for a comparison of operating currents which are consumed when the memory is accessed), and larger package size. In addition, other factors limiting RAM size in ICDs are microprocessor speed, telemetry speed, and programmer speed, since these are the crucial components required to transmit and retrieve data from memory. Due to power consumption, size, and other constrains in implantable devices, there is generally a lag between technology used in implantable pulse generators and available technology. Even though other high-memory-capacity technologies, such as the magnetic bubble memory, and larger memory capacity in a single-chip CMOS RAM, are available on the market, only 8K × 8 RAM with approximately 3K for data logging is used in the Guardian ATP 4210, and 64K × 8 RAM with approximately 24K for data logging in the Guardian ATP 4211 (Telectronics Pacing Systems, Englewood, CO), due to the stringent limitations of implantable devices. Although the operating current shown in Fig. 13 increases with increasing memory size, the operating current is consumed only when memory is accessed. Therefore, the operating current is relevant only when data are read from or stored to the data storage facility. Another type of power consumption is the standby current. The standby current for a new 128K × 8 RAM can be approximately $\frac{1}{5}\mu$A. Thus, with some minor technology improvements, a memory size of 128K × 8 for data logging in an ICD may be realized in the next few years. Despite these limitations, the improvements in data storage capabilities as described in the following paragraphs can be expected in the near future.

Data logs in present-generation ICDs are read by using a programmer, and are usually cleared at the end of a follow-up visit. Information obtained from the data logs may be printed on paper for record keeping. However, paper recordings can be lost, damaged, or even not printed. This problem can be solved by transferring the logged data automatically to a storage medium, such as a hard disk or floppy disk file of the programmer, every time the device is read, regardless of whether the user requires the logged data to be displayed on the programmer or not. The data can then be transferred to a storage medium on another computer, where the data can be incorporated into an individual patient database. Besides the database keeping a permanent record of each patient's therapy history, it can also be used with a software expert system to determine optimal parameter settings, which can in turn be used as a guide for reprogramming the device. As the ICD has become increasingly complex, the programming of the device can be a challenge and a time-consuming task for some users. This improvement can potentially lead to the realization of automatic analysis of data to aid reprogramming of the ICD by the physician. Furthermore, other automatic algorithms may be used to analyze patient databases to aid the physician in classification of rhythms and to provide interpretations of stored data. For example, variable ventricular R–R intervals suggest that a detected episode is likely to be associated with atrial fibrillation, or frequent noise detections with variable lead impedances may be due to lead problems, or warnings of increased defibrillation thresholds due to certain interventions (e.g., a change of medications) may be given.

It has been learned from the current-generation ICDs that a Holter function can be essential in some cases. For example, the availability of data obtained from Holter monitoring proved to be very useful, as reported by Birgersdotter-Green et al. [13]. Without Holter data, the cause of death of this particular patient could not have been determined. However, data storage of intracardiac electrograms requires vast amounts of memory. For example, at a sampling rate of 250 Hz (sampling period = 4 ms), 900,000 samples will be needed for 1 h of recording. If 8 bits are used for each sample, then 900K bytes of memory are needed. At the present time, a sampling rate of up to 500 Hz may be realized in an implantable device. To reduce memory allocation, only shorter passages of signals triggered by certain events, such as repeated ectopic beats, potential onsets of arrhythmias, morphological changes, a detected arrhythmia within a certain rate zone, or the delivery of a certain therapy, etc. could be recorded. In addition, other memory management techniques, such as data compression [14–17], could be used. These memory management techniques have not been used to date because their added complexities do not fully warrant their uses. The major costs associated with these data compression techniques are memory allocations for algorithm storage, power consumption, and the compromise of the microprocessor speed, as well as other costs associated with external devices, such as telemetric link and programmer speed limitations, etc. Therefore, technology improvements as well as algorithmic simplifications for data compression and reconstruction will be required before these techniques can be used in implantable devices. Longer segments of intracardiac recordings not only provide better diagnostic information, they can also be used to re-create the response of different devices to identical signals for comparison and learning purposes on the bench. The latter helps to further understanding of device interactions and decision making. Potentially, in addition to the sensed signal in the ventricle (usually bipolar), the following signals can also be recorded: unipolar signals, surface electrograms, atrial signals, and event markers from both chambers. Unipolar signals may be established using a subcutaneous patch or the defibrillator can to provide better electrogram timing information [18]. Surface electrograms may be recorded using subcutaneously implanted leads in order to provide additional morphological data. Atrial signals may be obtained when dual-chamber ICDs become available, and may improve the specificity of tachyarrhythmia detection [19].

Transtelephonic interrogation and transmission of stored data from ICDs have been proved to be feasible and useful for patient management [20–22]. A system of an ICD with transtelephonic transmission capability can reduce the number of unscheduled clinic visits. Early diagnoses can be made following unexpected deliveries of shocks. The benefits are more significant when patients reside far away from the implanting center. Such a system may be offered more widely to patients with ICDs in the near future, so that stored data can managed more efficiently. Since the telemetric link provides bidirectional communications between an implantable device and the outside world, stored data not only can be read from the device but new data can also be written to the device. Therefore, it is possible to reprogram an implanted device with new operating programs and new parameters (stored in RAM), if regulatory approval is obtained. In addition, reprogramming of implanted devices via transtelephonic links may also be realized. The major drawbacks of such a system are costs associated with the rigorous error detection and recovery scheme required to ensure data integrity, and the length of time required for data transmission.

Memory for data logging in an implantable device is required only for temporary storage, until the data are read. Thus, if the stored data can be read more often and stored in an external device, then the requirement of a larger memory may become less important. In one scenario, advanced telemetric links which span several meters would allow automatic transtelephonic transmission of data to a physician's office without limiting patients' activities in their own homes. The data would then be processed for review by the physician. The physician might also set patient-specific alarms depending on the urgent nature of the diagnosis. This might open up the possibility of automatic follow-ups of ICDs at the patients' own homes.

ACKNOWLEDGMENT

The author wishes to express appreciation to Bruce Steinhaus, Tibor Nappholz, and Saul Greenhut for reviewing this chapter.

REFERENCES

1. Chapman PD, Troup P. The automatic implantable cardioverter-defibrillator: evaluating suspected inappropriate shocks. J Am Coll Cardiol 1986; 7:1075.
2. Baker G, Hunt L. Experience of data logging in an implantable defibrillator. PACE 1989; 12:1255.
3. Winkle RA, State-of-the-art of the AICD. PACE 1991; 14:961-966.
4. Echt DS, Armstrong K, Schmidt P, et al. Clinical experience, complications, and survival in 70 patients with the automatic implantable cardioverter/defibrillator. Circulation 1985; 71:289-296.
5. Luceri RM, Puchferran RL, Brownstein SL, et al. Improved patient surveillance and data acquisition with a third generation implantable cardioverter defibrillator. PACE 1991; 14:1870-1874.
6. Wang PJ, Mandalakas N, Clyne C, et al. Accuracy of rhythm classification using a data log system in implantable cardioverter defibrillators. PACE 1991; 14:1911-1916.
7. Ellenbogen K, Luceri R, Dorian P. et al. Clinical evaluation of implantable cardioverter defibrillator (ICD) function: importance of data logging to assess device efficacy. Circulation 1991; 84:II-426.
8. Hurwitz JL, Hook BG, Callans DJ, et al. Importance of abortive shock capability with electrogram storage in cardioverter-defibrillator devices. Circulation 1991; 84:II-427.
9. Sowton E. Advances in diagnostics for implantable ICD systems. PACE 1990; 13:1211.
10. Mehta D, Saksena S, Krol RB, et al. Diagnostic use of significant symptoms underestimates appropriate ventricular tachyarrhythmia reversions by programmable pacemaker defibrillators. PACE 1992; 15:531.
11. Lu RMT, Matthews R, Leer T, et al. Data logging and noninvasive facilities for electrophysiological studies by an arrhythmia control system. Proc IEEE/EMBS Annual Conference 1990; 12:646-648.
12. Fromer M, Brachmann J, Block M. et al. Efficacy of automatic multimodal device therapy for ventricular tachyarrhythmias as delivered by a new implantable pacing cardioverter-defibrillator. Results of a European multicenter study of 102 implants. Circulation 1992: 86(2):363-374.
13. Birgersdotter-Green U, Rosenquist M, Lindemans F, et al. Holter documented sudden death in a patient with an implanted defibrillator. PACE 1992; 15:1008-1014.
14. Jalaleddine S, Hutchens C, Strattan R, et al. ECG data compression techniques—a unified approach. IEEE Trans Biomed Eng 1990; 37:329-343.
15. Bohs LN, Barr RC. Prototype for real-time adaptive sampling using the fan algorithm. Med Biol Eng Comput 1988; 26:574-583.

16. Moody GB, Mark RG, Goldberger AL. Evaluation of the "trim" ECG data compressor. Comput Cardiol 1989; 167-170.
17. Tai SC. Slope—a real time ECG data compressor. Med Biol Eng Comput 1991; 29:175-179.
18. Kroll M, Remole S, Asso A, et al. Pulse correlation for arrhythmia discrimination in the implantable defibrillator. Eur J CPE 1992; 2:A113.
19. Chiang C, Jenkins J, DiCarlo L. Realtime automatic detection of complex cardiac arrhythmias using rate augmented by intraatrial and intraventricular electrogram analysis. PACE 1992; 15:529.
20. Steinberg JS, Sugalski JS, Harotonik K, et al. Cardiac rhythm precipitating automatic implantable cardioverter defibrillator discharge in outpatients: observations from transtelephonic recordings. Circulation 1989; 80:II-530.
21. Fetter J, Stanton M, Trusty J, et al. Transtelephonic interrogation and transmission of stored data from an implantable cardioverter defibrillator. PACE 1992; 15:505.
22. Anderson MH, Paul VE, Jones S, et al. Transtelephonic interrogation of the implantable cardioverter defibrillator. PACE 1992; 15:1144-1150.

11

Historical Development of the AICD

Morton M. Mower

Cardiac Pacemakers, Inc.
St. Paul, Minnesota

Robert G. Hauser

Minneapolis Heart Institute
Minneapolis, Minnesota

The automatic implantable cardioverter-defibrillator (AICD) has now become a fairly well-accepted treatment for many patients with serious ventricular arrhythmias [1], although some controversy may still remain as to its true benefit in some cases [2]. The progression of this therapy from initial concept and design through early clinical application and to its present status was a long, difficult, and often fascinating journey. Both of the above authors played significant roles, at somewhat different but overlapping times, in the application of this new and novel therapeutic modality.

The original concept of the AICD is rightly attributed to Dr. Michel Mirowski (Fig. 1) [3]. In the mid-1960s, he had served as chief of cardiology at a government hospital in Israel. He was deeply touched by the sudden arrhythmic death of his chief of medicine. As a result of this experience, he left his position there in 1969, and came to Sinai Hospital of Baltimore (Fig. 2) in order to work on the concept of an implantable automatic defibrillator [4], which seemed far-fetched to some [5,6] when he first proposed it. He was joined in the endeavor by the first author (MMM) [7].

One of the most striking aspects of the initial design and fabrication of the circuits was the rapidity with which the initial work progressed. Within 3 months, a battery-operated device was ready for testing in the animal laboratory. The shocks were given between a subcutaneous electrode and an intravascular catheter (Fig. 3). In some cases, both electrodes were contained on a single transvenous lead (Figs. 4 and 5). Because defibrillation efficacy was heavily dependent on the stability and exact positioning of the distal end of the catheter, an extensive array of potential electrode possibilities was investigated (Fig. 6). Patch electrodes in the form of a cup fitting directly over the cardiac apex (and later a flexible patch serving the same purpose) were also developed (Fig. 7). Most episodes were able to be automatically reverted with single shocks, but the devices could recycle if necessary. They automatically returned themselves to a standby mode following each episode. The initial parameter that was monitored by the circuitry and served to signal the onset of the malignant arrhythmia was the pressure in the right

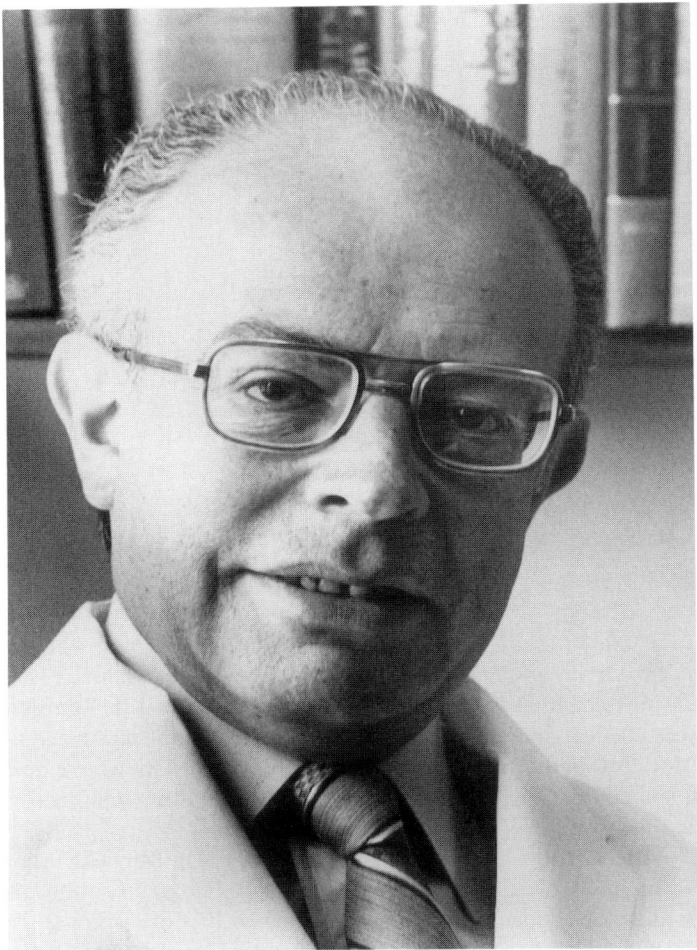

Figure 1 Photograph of Dr. Michel Mirowski taken in the late 1980s. At the time, he was professor of medicine at The Johns Hopkins University School of Medicine and director of the Coronary Care Unit at Sinai Hospital of Baltimore.

ventricle (Fig. 8). While this worked very well initially, an electrocardiographic method using probability density function (Fig. 9) was selected for the early chronically implanted devices [8], because suitable chronically implanted long-term pressure transducers were not readily available.

In the mid-1970s, a series of 25 long-term chronic animal implants was performed. As part of this effort, a battery-powered, implantable, 60-cycle current generator was built so that the animals could be fibrillated at will. Also, a fuse was developed for the output circuit that would indicate the occurrence of any discharge in the interim. Several movies were made of automatic defibrillation sequences in these awake animals (Fig. 10). Over the space of 60 implant months and 97 episodes of automatic resuscitation, there were only four failures, all due to lead damage, most of them caused by surgical technique [9].

In this same time frame, there were two clinical investigations of interest which were carried out. The first concerned establishing the required energy levels needed in humans. For this

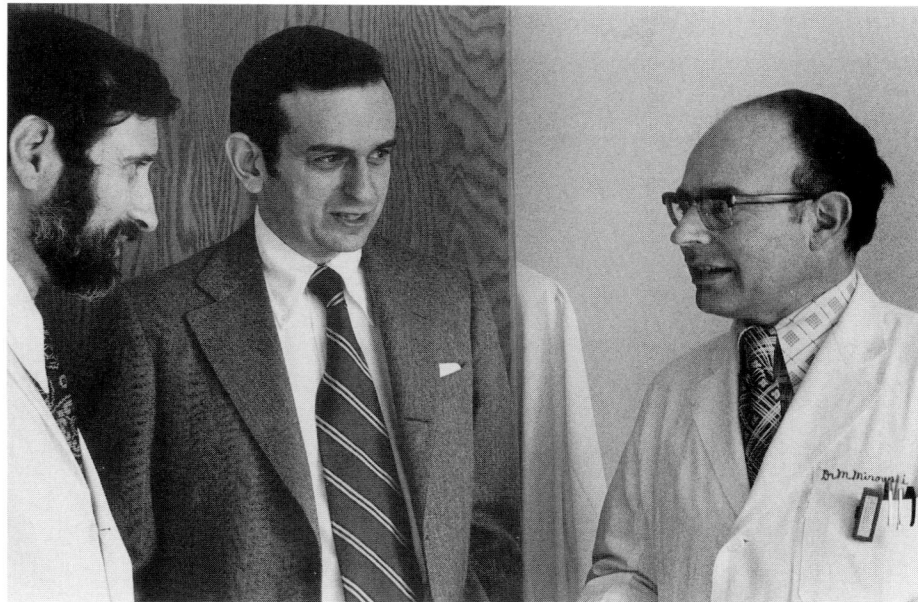

Figure 2 Photograph of Dr. Mirowski (at the right) taken in the mid-1970s, just after the initial animal laboratory work on the AICD had been done. The first author (MMM) is shown on the left, along with Dr. Arthur Moss, who was visiting them at Sinai Hospital of Baltimore at the time. There had been considerable controversy in the medical literature at the time over this early work, and Dr. Moss had written in support of the right of investigators to engage freely in even such high-risk research without having clearly defined and universally accepted eventual outcomes.

purpose, patients undergoing coronary artery bypass grafting under aortic cross-clamping were selected. Such patients often develop ventricular fibrillation after the clamps are removed and rewarming occurs, and need to be defibrillated anyway. Instead of delivering the defibrillation pulses conventionally through paddles, electrodes simulating intravascular location of catheter electrodes were incorporated into the cannulae used in the aorto-pulmonary bypass apparatus (Fig. 11). We found that intravascular defibrillation could be easily accomplished with energies of 15 J and below [10].

A second study was performed to determine the subjective effects of delivery of defibrillatory shocks to awake patients. This was performed in the setting of reverting atrial fibrillation in patients for whom it was determined that progression to external cardioversion under anesthesia would be done anyway if the attempt at transvenous cardioversion were unsuccessful (Fig. 12).

Concurrently, the device was subjected to stringent environmental testing, including resistance to electromagnetic interference, pressure, mechanical shock, temperature, etc., by outside industrial laboratories, and the design was extensively reviewed by the Applied Physics Laboratory of The Johns Hopkins University [11].

In late 1979, as the device was just finishing this entire range of preclinical testing and qualifications, project planning for an FDA clinical trial was in full swing. It was obvious that this phase of the research might involve too much patient risk for a small community hospital to assume, so The Johns Hopkins Hospital was chosen as the initial implanting center.

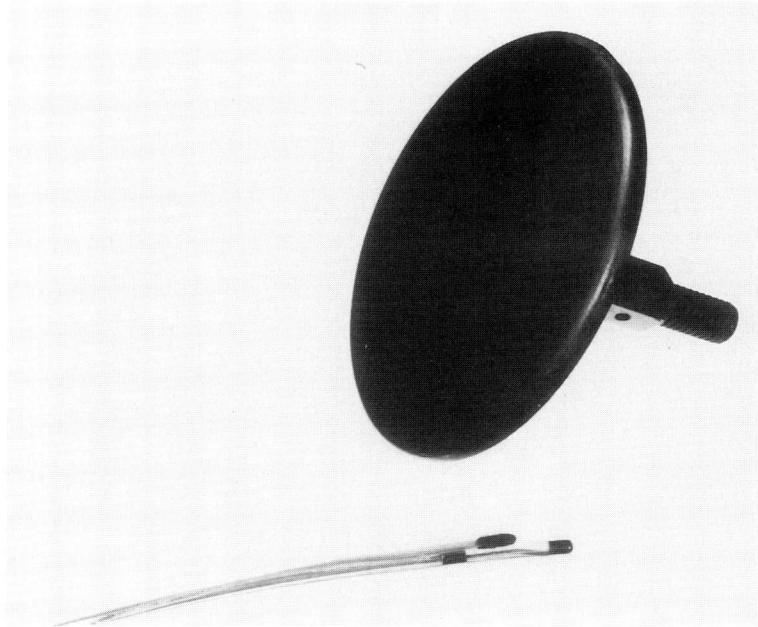

Figure 3 Photograph of intravascular electrode catheter (note the solid-state pressure transducer affixed with medical adhesive near the catheter tip) and subcutaneous plate electrode (derived from a discarded external defibrillator paddle) used in the initial animal laboratory experiments.

The first patient (Fig. 13) had a history of previous myocardial infarction and recurrent episodes of drug-resistant ventricular fibrillation requiring resuscitation. After the implantation on February 4, 1980, it was thought absolutely essential to prove that the patient's arrhythmias could be reverted by the implanted device. She was induced with alternating current [12] and the device was allowed to rescue her automatically. This kind of testing has remained routine ever since.

A number of the initial patients in the series had spontaneous episodes of arrhythmia while still being monitored in the hospital. Also, following hospitalization, many instances of automatic termination of malignant arrhythmias were reported. Typically, the scenario was a discrete episode of palpitations and weakness, followed by dizziness or frank collapse, and then by a diffuse muscular contraction caused by the internal discharge, followed by prompt recovery and a feeling of well-being. Often, the underlying arrhythmias were documented electrocardiographically during the subsequent hospitalization.

After the first three implantations, a paper describing these initial results was readily accepted for publication [13]. Following this, we quickly became aware that it was not uncommon for ventricular fibrillation to be preceded by a period of ventricular tachycardia. Accordingly a synchronizing circuit was added to the design, and the device was made able to perform cardioversion in addition to being able to defibrillate [14].

The data were analyzed following the first 52 patient implantations through September 1982, and the 1-year sudden death mortality of 8.5%, and the mortality from all causes of 22.9% were considered striking improvements on the natural history of the disease. An esti-

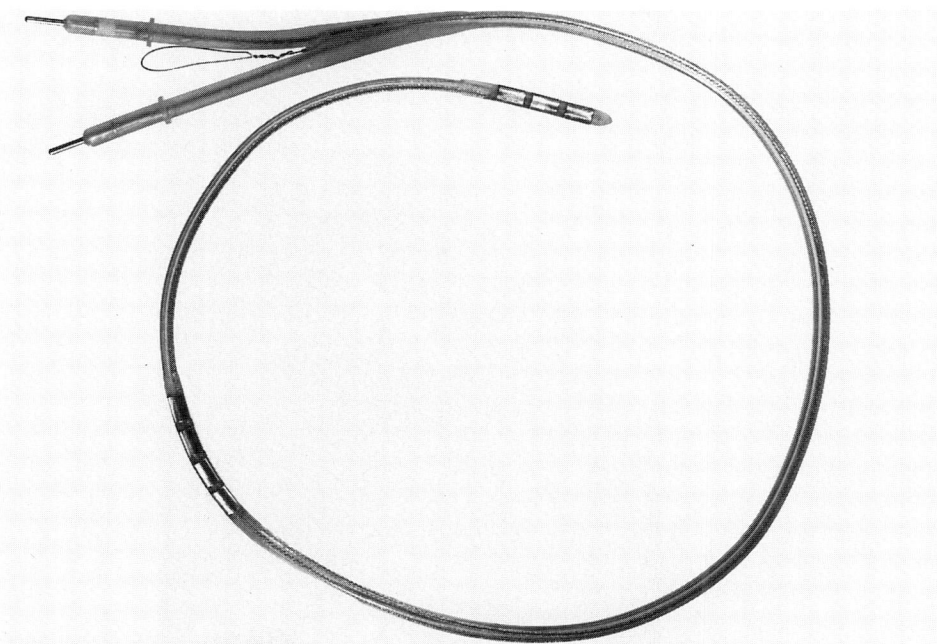

Figure 4 Photograph of one of the original intravascular defibrillating catheters. Each of the two electrodes in the pair consisted of physically separated (for flexibility) metallic rings, each set being connected together electrically.

mated sudden death rate, based on initial defibrillator discharges assumed to be life-saving, indicated a figure as high as 48% would have occurred if the defibrillator had not been implanted [15].

In the early 1980s, the second author (RGH) was assistant director and then co-director of the Cardiology Section at the Rush-Presbyterian–St. Lukes Medical Center in Chicago. This facility was among the first dozen centers to become part of the clinical trial, and he gained considerable familiarity with the device at that time.

In 1985, FDA approval for marketing the AICD was obtained. CPI assumed responsibility for the further application of this therapy, and began developing an integrated-circuit version of the original device. Successive improvements in actuarial curves were noted with the improvements in hardware [16], and the number of implantees grew rapidly. Advanced programmable models, the VENTAK P and the closely related VENTAK 1550, were then developed. The initial data regarding these devices, collated toward the end of their FDA clinical trials, showed that survivals were uniformly high. Since market release, some differences in favor of the advanced devices have even emerged.

A substantial body of data has now been collected with regard to the clinical results that can be obtained with AICD therapy; however, to understand why randomized clinical trials were not done immediately, it is necessary to recall the climate into which this therapeutic modality was initially brought forward. The implantable defibrillator concept was developed during an era in which it was firmly believed that, primary prevention aside, drugs were going to be the answer to sudden cardiac death. The problem was simply to develop the proper drug,

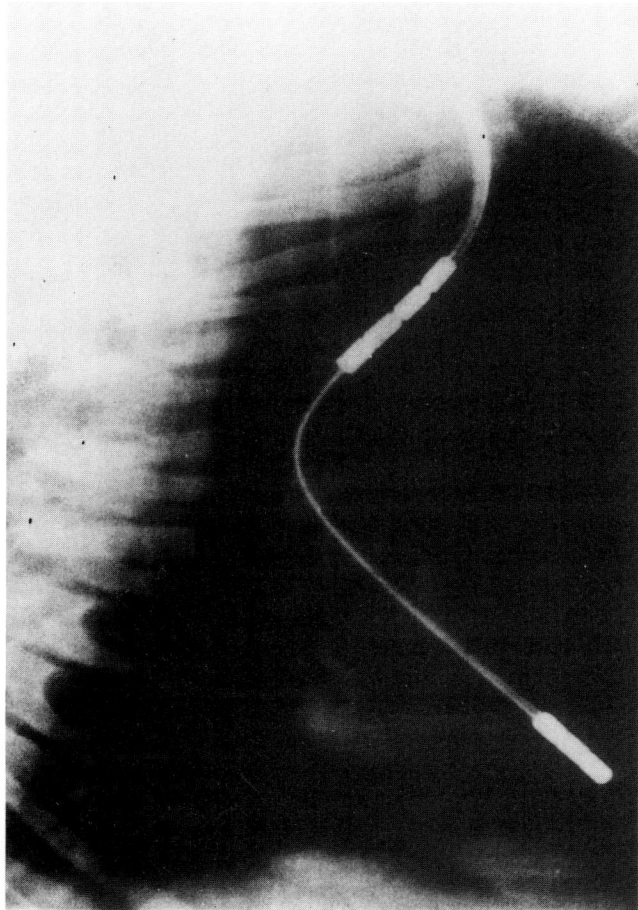

Figure 5 Photograph of lateral chest X-ray of experimental animal in which an early single intravascular defibrillating catheter was implanted. The distal electrode is wedged into the right ventricular apex of the heart, and the proximal one lies in the superior vena cava at about its juncture with the right atrium. This arrangement was very satisfactory for internal defibrillation, although it was also very dependent on the stability of the position of the distal electrode.

if indeed it did not already exist, and to identify those individuals who would need it. It is not unfair to recall that device therapy was considered a waste of time and money, serving only to divert attention from any of the really important work which investigators should have been doing. Given the virtual universal lack of support for the concept, and the high recurrence rates known to occur in patients resuscitated from episodes of cardiac arrest, the initial implantees had to be chosen from the very worst of the worst. They were in fact required to have undergone not one but two cardiac arrests, one of which had to have been a breakthrough on what was presumably effective therapy. Thus there was little enthusiasm on the part of potential investigators to randomize this type of patient.

Worldwide, since the beginning of the clinical uses of all the devices, cumulative survival rates have continued to be quite high. The present patient group consists of over 25,000 patients, with average ejection fraction of 33%. The statistics for CPI are compiled quarterly and

Historical Development of the AICD

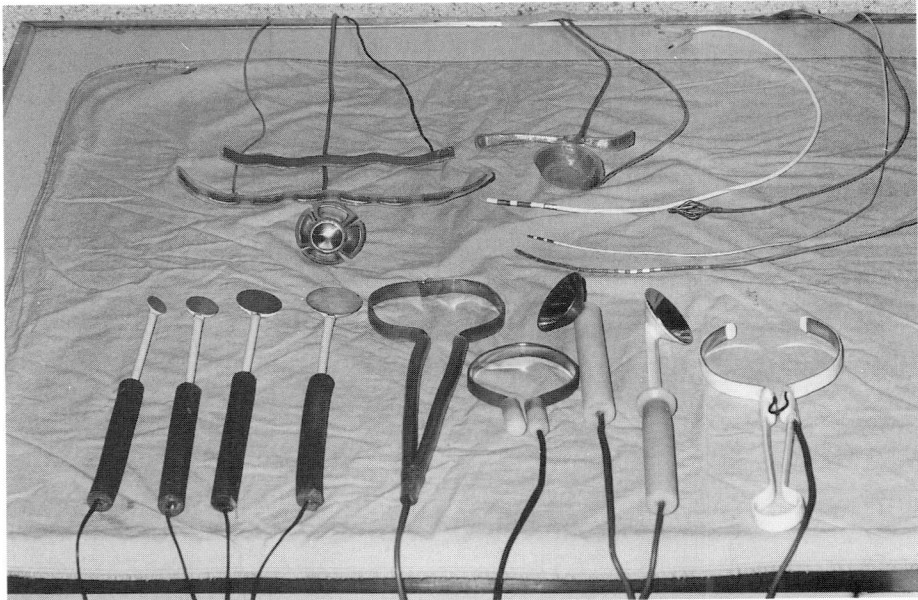

Figure 6 Display on a surgical table of the variety of defibrillating electrode configurations utilized in the initial animal laboratory investigations.

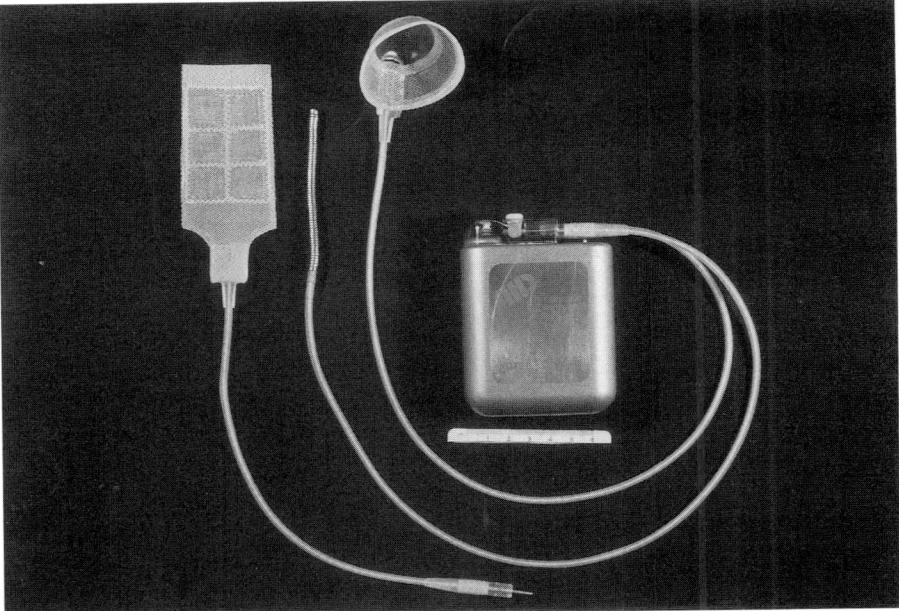

Figure 7 Early implantable-grade defibrillator with original apical cup electrode (and superior vena cava electrode as the second one) and the subsequent flexible patch electrode later developed. This latter was easier to apply surgically, and conformed to whatever radius of curvature was present on the ventricular surface.

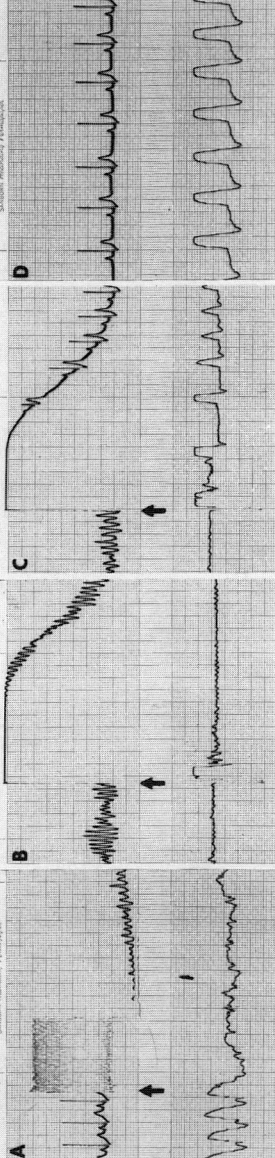

Figure 8 Simultaneous ECG (above) and right ventricular pressure (below) curves in an episode of fibrillation-automatic defibrillation: (A) induction of ventricular fibrillation with alternating current; (B) unsuccessful defibrillating shock; (C) automatic recycling and successful second shock; (D) normal curves approximately 15 s later.

Historical Development of the AICD

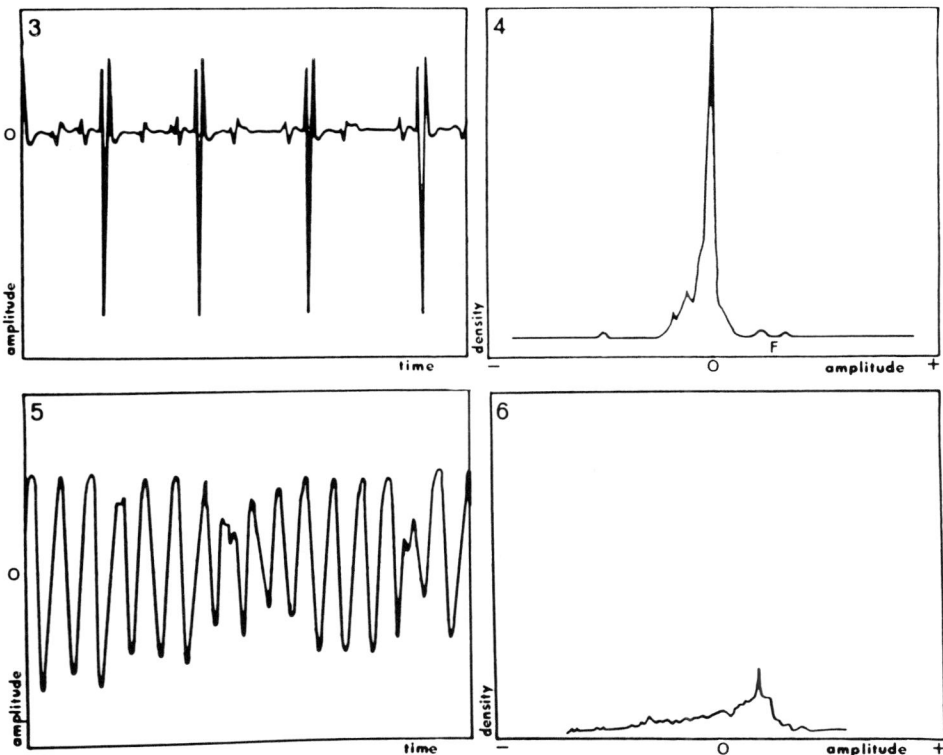

Figure 9 Oscilloscope tracings illustrating functioning of probability density function circuitry in normal versus malignant rhythms. Upper panels show differentiated sinus rhythm (left) and its probability density function (right), with its large peak at the zero line. This indicates that the ECG signal spends a relatively large amount of time near the baseline. Lower panels show differentiated ventricular fibrillation signal (left) and its corresponding probability density function (right). The absence of the large peak near the zero line indicates that the original signal spends relatively little time at or near the baseline, and is a reliable indicator of the presence of this malignant arrhythmia.

show freedom from sudden death at 99.1% at 1 year, and total survival through 5 years in excess of 84%. Thus, despite the relatively short time the AICD has been clinically available, it is a major treatment modality, and one for which the indications for use are still evolving in a very dynamic manner.

In the natural course of evolution of this modality, both authors were asked to join CPI, the company further developing the AICD, as full-time employees. The second author (RGH) became vice president of medical sciences and services in 1987, and was named president and CEO in 1988. The first author (MMM) had been a consultant to CPI since 1985 and then joined the company as vice president of medical sciences and services in 1989.

During the phases of development conducted at CPI, the device naturally became more versatile. The new features included: (1) improved defibrillation waveforms, (2) development of permanent transvenous lead systems not requiring thoracotomy for implantation, (3) availability of antitachycardia pacing, (4) programmability of energy outputs for cardioversion and defibrillation, (5) incorporation of bradycardia pacing, and (6) extensive telemetric capabili-

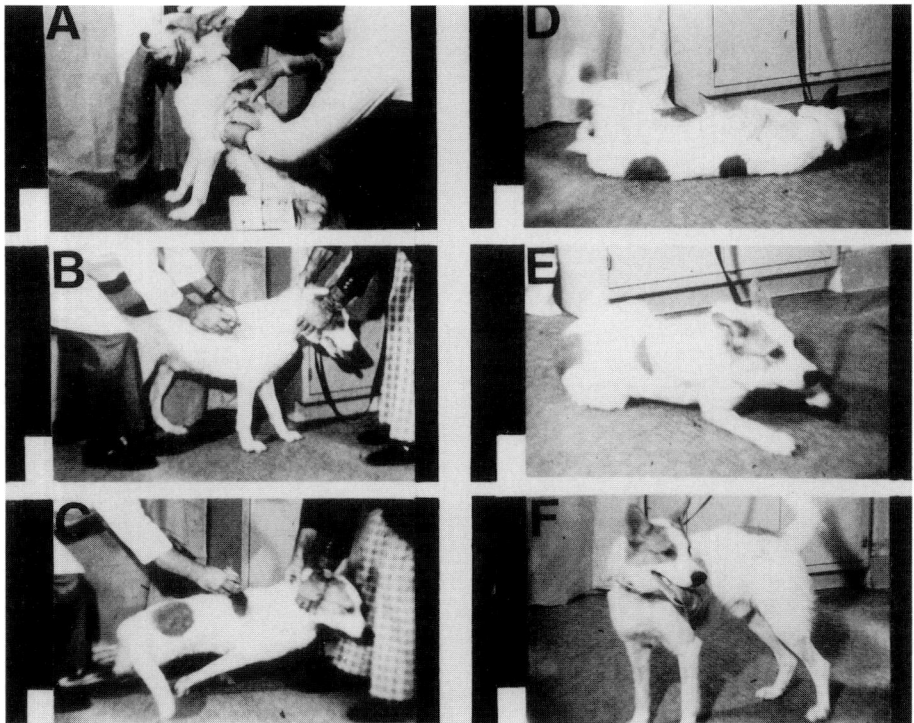

Figure 10 One of a series of 25 chronic implant animals from the mid-1970s: (A) testing of charge time of the defibrillator; (B) induction of ventricular fibrillation with an implanted alternating current generator; (C) resultant syncope; (D) instant of shock; (E) immediately after shock; (F) 15 s later.

ties. Other refinements can still be anticipated in the future, with improvements in sensing, arrhythmia differentiation, and classification, further reduction in device size, and improvements in transvenous defibrillation leads.

Along with the improvements in device design and increased device programmability, the applications of AICD therapy have also been evolving. These changes in indications come about by consensus within the medical profession, FDA approvals, and Medicare reimbursement decisions. One of the most important recent advances was the dropping of inducibility as a requirement for device reimbursement. Organized professional societies have played an important role in shaping opinions in both private and public sectors on behalf of improvements such as these. For example, the American College of Cardiology decided that "we must conclude that the level of risk in the noninducible patient is sufficiently high to justify the cost and morbidity of the AICD. Since defibrillation is a 'final common pathway' therapy, it is effective for either ventricular tachycardia or fibrillation and does not require inducibility" [17].

The results of scientific studies are one of the very important drivers for change from previously accepted indications. This is true both with respect to research directly involving devices and to that involving the alternative forms of therapy. The use of electrophysiological testing to guide drug therapy in cardiac-arrest victims is proving disappointing. In one recent study of 241 out-of-hospital ventricular fibrillation survivors studied by electrophysiological testing, 42% were noninducible, ventricular fibrillation was induced in 16%, and sustained

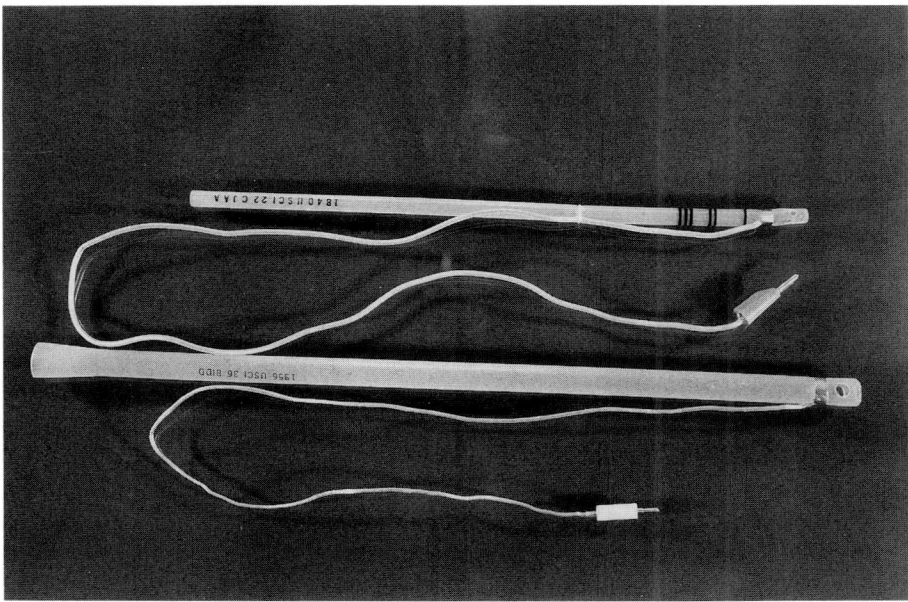

Figure 11 Electrodes simulating intravascular location incorporated into cardiopulmonary bypass canulae for the purpose of determining defibrillation threshold requirements in patients undergoing coronary artery bypass surgery.

ventricular tachycardia was induced in 27%. Recurrences of sudden cardiac death ranged as high as 28% in the various groups, and those with drug-induced suppression of baseline-induced arrhythmia did not do any better than the nonsupressible ones. Randomized drug trials such as CASCADE have indicated 17% 1-year and 35% 3-year incidences of recurrent cardiac arrest with amiodarone [18]. The results of CAST are well known, and even the moricizine arm of CAST has shown excess mortality in the treated population. In the case of implantable defibrillators, however, evidence from multiple large series indicates sudden cardiac death rates of under 2% and 5% at 1 and 3 years, respectively [19]. As more data become available, physicians will undoubtedly become more willing to abandon ineffective treatments. This in itself will result in a larger pool of patients being available for device therapy.

Another important trend is that there appears to be a growing application of device therapy to the slower and more organized ventricular tachycardia class of arrhythmias [20]. Data from the CPI medical records database for market-released devices show that the proportion of patients receiving units for sustained monomorphic tachycardia, rather than the more traditional indications of the two rhythms which are associated with cardiac arrests, i.e., true ventricular fibrillation, and those rhythms of a more polymorphic nature not exactly fitting that criteria, has been increasing over the past 5 years. The trends are even more marked with regard to the devices used within clinical studies, which are still under FDA aegis and which can probably be thought of as being on the cutting edge of thinking with regard to AICD applications (Fig. 14).

Evidence of still more forward thinking is also at hand. A widespread feeling is developing that it may be possible to identify patients at high risk of sudden death, prior to an overt serious arrhythmic event, and to protect them by early, so-called prophylactic, device implantation

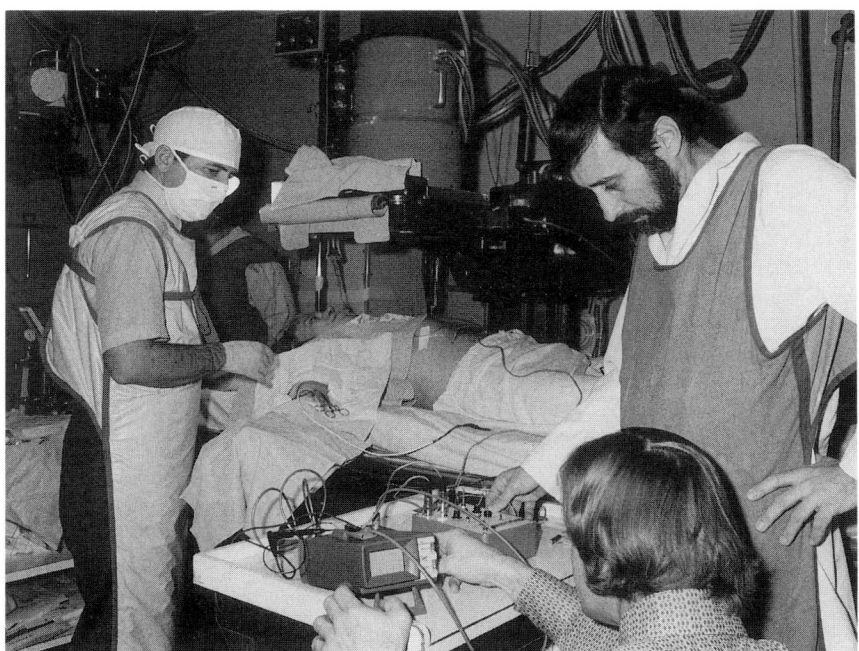

Figure 12 Catheterization laboratory experiments in intravascular reversion of atrial fibrillation done in patients lightly sedated, primarily to determine the subjective responses of awake subjects to internal defibrillatory shocks. The first author is shown at the right of the photograph (circa 1973).

[21]. It has been recognized that such a radical change in indications needs to have solid scientific backing, and a number of large-scale, multicenter, cooperative studies of devices for prophylactic use, some with National Institutes of Health co-funding, have been launched [22]. These studies include CABG Patch, MADIT, and MUSTT. In general, the results of these studies will not be available for several more years, but if they are positive, they may be expected to dramatically affect the accepted indications for implantation at that time.

Another area of possible use developing for the AICD involves the concept of using the device as a temporizing strategy for congestive heart failure patients who will ultimately receive heart transplantation—in essence, a bridge to transplantation for those patients. Many are at high risk of dying suddenly prior to the availability of a suitable donor heart. Scientific studies involving this possible indication are now being developed and are expected to be launched shortly.

In retrospect, therefore, despite the relatively short time that AICD therapy has been available, we have seen major, and very impressive, shifts in how it is being used. Moreover, the indications for this therapy are still progressing in a very dynamic manner. The AICD concept has thus evolved from a nonprogrammable committed device capable only of treating ventricular fibrillation and rapid ventricular tachycardia to a programmable, noncommitted device incorporating antitachycardia and bradycardia pacing with extensive data logging capabilities, and has extended device treatment into an effective therapeutic modality that has revolutionized treatment of patients with malignant ventricular dysrhythmias. Viewed initially as a treatment

Historical Development of the AICD

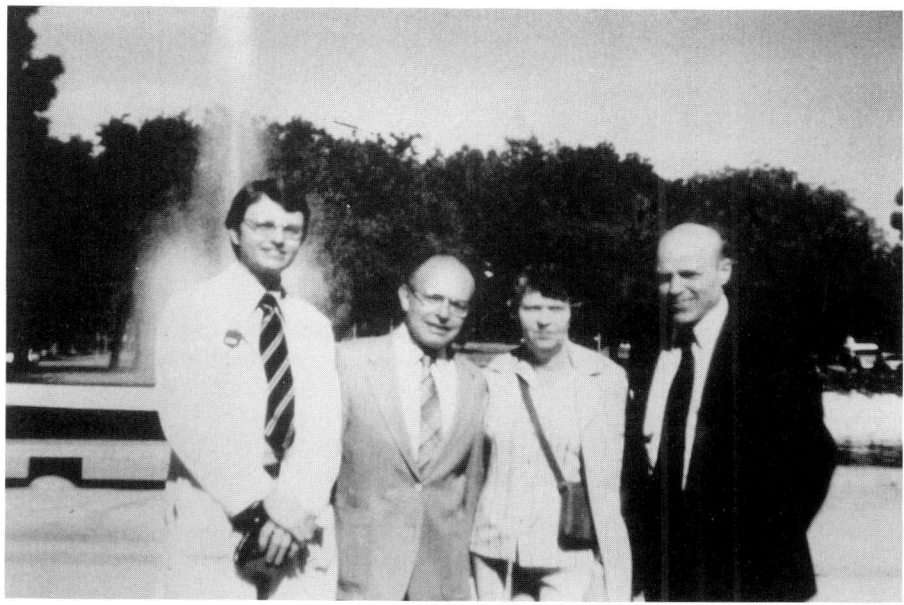

Figure 13 The original patient (third from left), shown with her personal cardiologist, Dr. Roger Winkle (left), Dr. Mirowski (second from left), and Dr. M. S. Heilman (right), who was president of Medrad/Intec Systems, the company which brought the implantable defibrillator through the FDA clinical trials.

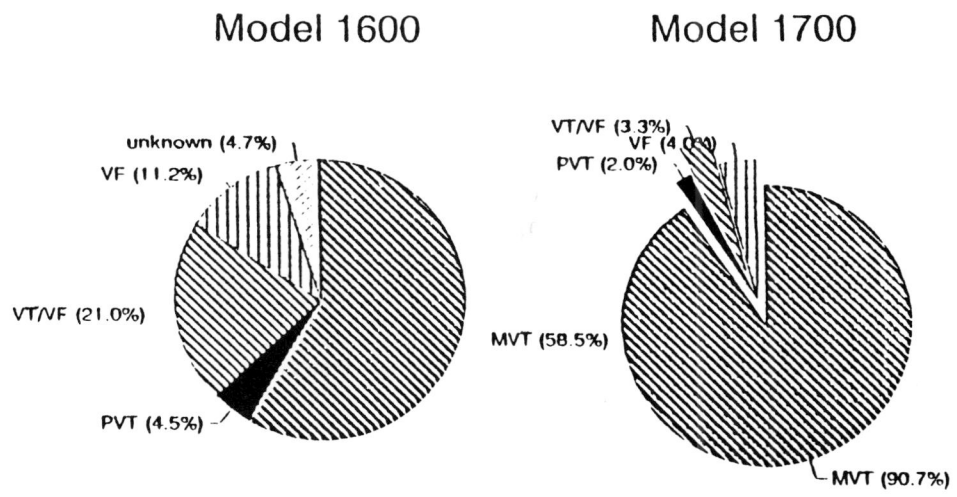

Figure 14 Piecharts depicting presenting arrhythmia of patients in two recent FDA clinical trials. The model 1600 is the VENTAK P, now market-released, and the Model 1700 is the VENTAK PRx device, which is still investigational. Note the much higher proportion of patients with monomorphic ventricular tachycardia in the latter case. PVT = polymorphic ventricular tachycardia, VT = ventricular tachycardia, VF = ventricular fibrillation, and MVT = monomorphic ventricular tachycardia.

of last resort, this therapeutic approach for therapy of ventricular fibrillation and ventricular tachycardia is now advocated by some as the "gold standard" against which other therapies should be compared.

REFERENCES

1. Nisam S, Mower M, Moser S. ICD clinical update: first decade, initial 10,000 patients. PACE 1991; 14:255–262.
2. Lehmann MH, Saksena S. Implantable cardioverter defibrillators in cardiovascular practice: report of the policy conference of NASPE. PACE 1991; 14:969–979.
3. Moss AJ. Implanted standby defibrillators. Circulation 1973; 47:1135.
4. Mirowski M, Mower MM, Staewen WS, Tabatznik B, Mendeloff AI. Standby automatic defibrillator: an approach to prevention of sudden coronary death. Arch Int Med 1970; 29:158–161.
5. Lown, B, Axelrod P. Implanted standby defibrillators. Circulation 1972; 46:637–639.
6. Harken DW. Implanted standby defibrillators. JAAMI 1971; 5:310.
7. Mower MM. Building the AICD with Michel Mirowski. PACE 1991; 14:928–934.
8. Langer A, Heilman MS, Mower MM, Mirowski M. A novel ventricular fibrillation detector for implantable defibrillator. Circulation 1975; 52:II-205.
9. Mirowski M, Mower MM, Langer A, Heilman MS, Schreibman J. A chronically implanted system for fibrillation-defibrillation in active conscious dogs: experimental model for treatment of sudden death from ventricular fibrillation. Circulation 1978; 58:90–94.
10. Mirowski M, Mower MM, Gott V, Brawley RK. Feasibility and effectiveness of low-energy cardioversion in man. Circulation 1973; 47:79–85.
11. Mirowski M, Mower MM, Bhagavan BS, Langer A, Fischell RE, Heilman MS. Chronic animal and bench testing of the implantable automatic defibrillator. Proc VIth World Symposium on Cardiac Pacing, Montreal, Canada, Oct 2–5, 1979. Meere C, ed. Pacesymp chap 27-2.
12. Mower MM, Reid PR, Watkins L Jr, Mirowski M. Use of alternating current during diagnostic electrophysiologic studies. Circulation 1983; 67:69–72.
13. Mirowski M, Reid PR, Mower MM, et al. Termination of malignant ventricular arrhythmias in man with an implanted automatic defibrillator. N Engl J Med 1980; 303:322–324.
14. Reid PR, Mirowski M, Mower MM, Griffith LSC, Platia E, Watkins L. Treatment of ventricular tachycardias with an R-wave synchronized automatic implantable defibrillator. Circulation 1982; 66:II-216.
15. Mirowski M, Reid PR, Watkins L, Weisfeldt ML, Mower MM. Clinical treatment of life-threatening ventricular tachyarrhythmias with the automatic implantable defibrillator. Am Heart J 1981; 102:265–270.
16. Reid PR, Mower MM, Griffith LSC, et al. Comparative effects of the first and second generation implantable defibrillators. Abstracts 3rd European Symposium on cardiac pacing. PACE 1985; 8:A–58.
17. American College of Cardiology Board of Trustees statement, Oct 22, 1989.
18. Greene L, Bardy G, CASCADE Investigators. Cardiac arrest in Seattle: conventional versus amiodarone drug evaluation (The CASCADE Study). Am J Cardiol 1991; 67:578–584.
19. Winkle R, Mead H, Ruder M, et al. Ten year experience with implantable defibrillators. Circulation 1991; 84:II-426.
20. Mower MM, Nisam S. AICD indications (patient selection): past, present, and future. PACE 1988; 11:2064–2070.
21. Nisam S, Thomas A, Mower M, Hauser R. Identifying patients for automatic implantable cardioverter-defibrillator therapy: status of prospective studies. Am Heart J 1991; 122:607–612.
22. Nisam S, Thomas A, Mower M. Prospective studies to identify high risk patients for prophylactic AICD therapy. In: L'Elettrostimolazione Cardiaca Tra Clinica E Technologia. Edizioni-Luigi Pozzi, 1990: 91–102.

12

Indications for the Implantable Cardioverter-Defibrillator

Arun Gadhoke and N. A. Mark Estes III

*Tufts University School of Medicine
and New England Medical Center
Boston, Massachusetts*

David S. Cannom

*Hospital of the Good Samaritan
and UCLA School of Medicine
Los Angeles, California*

I. INTRODUCTION

The implantable cardioverter-defibrillator (ICD) emerged from the 1980s as the "gold-standard therapy" [1] for sudden-cardiac-death (SCD) survivors, with guidelines for use [2] which had undergone considerable evolution. Initially the device was restricted to patients who had survived two episodes of cardiac arrest. As the impact of the ICD on reduction in sudden death [3–12] in those with malignant ventricular arrhythmias refractory to pharmacologic therapy [13–19] was defined, the appropriate use of the device has been reevaluated and indications expanded. The treatment strategies to prevent a recurrence of ventricular tachycardia (VT), fibrillation (VF), and SCD in those not responding to conventional drugs [13–20] have included investigational antiarrhythmic agents, mapping guided surgery, catheter ablation techniques, and the ICD. Of these the ICD has become the dominant strategy. Currently, new technologic developments coupled with physician enthusiasm for the device leave the potential for expansion of indications for the device beyond what may be warranted on the basis of appropriately designed clinical trials [1].

II. BACKGROUND

Sudden cardiac death presently accounts for approximately one-half of all cardiovascular mortality in this country, and sustained ventricular tachycardia and fibrillation represent the most common mechanism [2]. In the United States, approximately 350,000 to 450,000 individuals suffer an episode of out-of-hospital cardiac arrest every year, with less than 25% surviving the first episode. Several prior reports have demonstrated that if sudden-death survivors are untreated, the recurrence rate is extremely high, with an annual sudden-death mortality of 30% [17,21]. Empiric drug therapy without serial drug testing carries a 1-year sudden-death rate of 20–30% [12–14,17,21]. With drug treatment guided by programmed ventricular stimulation, between 5%–10% of patients who have no inducible arrhythmias on drug therapy will have arrhythmia recurrence or sudden death in 18–24 months of follow-up [16,18–20]. Patients with an ejection fraction greater than 30% have a lower chance of recurrence (5% at 2 years) when compared to patients with ejection fraction of less than 30% (15% at 2 years) [16]. Patients in whom ventricular tachycardia cannot be suppressed by programmed stimulation, who are discharged on an ineffective drug regimen, have a sudden-cardiac-death mortality of approximately 20% per year [15].

Antiarrhythmic therapy guided by noninvasive approaches such as ambulatory monitoring has been shown to result in subsequent sudden-cardiac-death rate of 5–12% in the first year [22,23], with 20–40% dying by the fourth year. These data likely underestimate the arrhythmia recurrence and sudden cardiac death, because they are derived from patient populations that largely included sustained ventricular tachycardia patients who had not had a cardiac arrest [24]. This subgroup of patients represents a lower-risk group for sudden death compared to those with ventricular tachycardia with hemodynamic collapse or prior ventricular fibrillation. Other limitations of antiarrhythmic drug therapy guided by noninvasive approaches include the fact that one-third of patients with prior out-of-hospital cardiac arrest lack adequate PVC frequency to be used as a therapeutic endpoint for guiding drug therapy. In the 40% of patients in whom spontaneous arrhythmias cannot be satisfactorily suppressed, alternate therapeutic modalities are needed, since the arrhythmia recurrence and SCD is extremely high [22,23].

Amiodarone has been reported to reduce sudden cardiac death to approximately 6–10% per year, although there is a high risk of toxicity [25]. It remains an option in sustained ventricular tachycardia patients or sudden-death survivors who are otherwise pharmacologically refractory and refuse or are poor candidates for the ICD. Mapping guided subendocardial resection remains an option in appropriately selected patients with sustained ventricular tachycardia [26]. Recent operative mortality with this approach has been less than 5%, with long-term freedom from arrhythmia recurrence in over 90% of patients [27].

The automatic implantable cardioverter-defibrillator was introduced in the early 1980s as "last-resort therapy" for patients who had survived two episodes of cardiac arrest. The indications for devices from 1980 to 1982 included documentation of VT or VF at the time the patient was unconscious, recurrent VT/VF while on antiarrhythmic medication, and electrophysiological (EP) study during which VT or VF was induced and the patient lost consciousness [28]. Other restrictions included the need for emotional maturity and geographic stability for long-term follow-up, as well as a life expectancy of at least 6 months. With multiple investigators reporting the annual sudden-cardiac-death rate as low as 1–2%, the device became accepted by many electrophysiologists as the antiarrhythmic treatment modality of choice for most sudden-cardiac-death survivors [24]. In 1985, the Food and Drug Administration (FDA) approved the use of the implantable cardioverter-defibrillator for patients who were at high risk of sudden cardiac death [28]. In this group were those patients who had survived at least one episode of cardiac arrest in the absence of an acute myocardial infarction. Also included were those who, in the absence of such previous arrest, had experienced recurrent ventricular tachyarrhythmias and were inducible into sustained hypotensive ventricular tachycardia and/or fibrillation despite conventional antiarrhythmic drug therapy [28]. It was required that all patients undergo a complete cardiovascular evaluation, including electrophysiological testing, prior to implantation. In January 1986, the Health Care Financing Administration (HCFA) reworked guidelines for reimbursement for Medicare and Medicaid beneficiaries requiring the ICD [28]. Patients were required to have an electrophysiology study and have a ventricular arrhythmia unresponsive to medical or surgical therapy or be an unsuitable candidate for surgical therapy. Coverage for reimbursement purposes was provided if the device was used as therapy of last resort. The guidelines stressed that if a ventricular arrhythmia could not be induced, then payment for the device would not be provided. It was not until July 1991, after multiple appeals by physicians to HFCA, that the requirements for inducibility was eliminated [29]. Both the North American Society of Pacing and Electrophysiology (NASPE) and the American College of Cardiology (ACC) ratified the 1985 FDA guidelines, reserving the ICD for only the highest-risk patients [2,30]. Generally, reimbursement was provided when implantation of the ICD met these originally proposed guidelines [2,30].

III. NASPE GUIDELINES FOR ICD IMPLANTATIONS

Guidelines for the use of the ICD were published in 1991 by the North American Society of Pacing and Electrophysiology [2]. Three classes of indications were proposed for implantable cardioverter-defibrillator use, which included patients in whom there is a consensus that ICD therapy is warranted (Class I). Class II indications were those in which the ICD is a therapeutic option but consensus does not exist. Those clinical situations in which the ICD is generally not justified are considered Class III. The Class I, II, and III NAPSE indications for ICD implantation are as follows.

Class I
1. One or more episodes of sustained VT/VF in a patient in whom EP testing and/or spontaneous ventricular arrhythmias cannot be used to accurately predict efficacy of other therapies.
2. Recurrent episodes of spontaneous sustained VT/VF in a patient despite antiarrhythmic drug treatment guided by either electrophysiologic testing or noninvasive methods.
3. Spontaneous sustained VT/VF in a patient in whom antiarrhythmic treatment is limited by intolerance or noncompliance.
4. Persistent inducibility of clinically relevant sustained VT/VF at EP study on the best available drug treatment or despite surgical/catheter ablation in a patient with spontaneous sustained VT/VF.

Class II
1. Syncope of undetermined etiology in a patient with clinically relevant sustained VT/VF induced at EP study in whom antiarrhythmic drug treatment is limited by inefficacy, intolerance, or noncompliance.

Class III
1. Sustained VT/VF mediated by acute ischemia/infarction or toxic/metabolic etiology amenable to corrections or reversibility.
2. Recurrent syncope of undetermined etiology in a patient without inducible sustained VT.
3. Incessant VT/VF.
4. VF secondary to atrial fibrillation in the WPW syndrome and in the patient whose bypass tract is amenable to surgical or catheter ablation.
5. Surgical, medical, or psychiatric contraindications.

Although the NASPE guidelines do not qualify the induced arrhythmia based on hemodynamic stability, the ACC guidelines call for the induced ventricular tachycardia to be hemodynamicallly significant [2,30]. By the FDA, NASPE, and ACC guidelines, there is no clear definition of a drug response [2,28,30]. Some investigators have contended that significant slowing of ventricular tachycardia by more than 100 ms or hemodynamic tolerance of ventricular tachycardia on antiarrhythmic drugs during EP testing indicates a good long-term prognosis [15]. There no uniform approach currently to such patients, with many laboratories accepting this endpoint and giving the patient a trial on antiarrhythmic drugs, and other laboratories going on to implant an ICD in such a patient. Similarly, the number of drug trials evaluated during EP testing remains unspecified. There is a very clear trend toward fewer drug trials based on a low response rate, and a continued risk in drug responders of sudden cardiac death that exceeds that of those treated with the ICD. Some laboratories currently will acutely test intravenous procainamide and, if the patient remains persistently inducible, they will consider the patient pharmacologically refractory. The precise role of isoproterenol infusion in attempting to provoke arrhythmias in patients who otherwise respond to an antiarrhythmic agent remains to be defined. Similarly, no guidelines address the issue of the role of amiodarone in patients who do not respond to alternate antiarrhythmic drugs. Although EP-guided pharmacological therapy has a good predictive value, it is not as good in patients who do not have coronary artery disease. The recurrence rate of ventricular tachycardia in patients with cardiomyopathy, or other forms of noncoronary heart disease, is greater than in those with coronary artery disease [13,14].

Similarly, none of the indications currently make specific recommendations regarding the patient's ejection fraction and how it should be factored into the decision to place an ICD. The subgroup of patients with prior cardiac arrest or sustained VT with ejection fractions less than 35% have a response rate to antiarrhythmic drugs which is approximately 20% [14–21]. Furthermore, the recurrence rate in this patient patient group is as high as 15% at 2 years in those in whom electrophysiological testing predicts effective therapy [16]. To that extent, many clinicians have become skeptical of the use of EP testing in this patient population, and tend to have a lower threshold for ICD implantation.

IV. ICD USE IN PATIENTS WITH NO INDUCIBLE ARRHYTHMIAS

It is accepted that the prognostic significance of noninducibility in survivors of cardiac arrest is uncertain but by no means benign. The reported incidence of recurrent VT/VF or SCD for these patients ranges from 8% to 50%, with over half of them dying at the time of recurrence [13,14,17–19,29,31–35]. In the majority of series, the recurrence rate of life-threatening ventricular arrhythmias in patients in whom arrhythmias cannot be induced remains clinically significant [31–35]. Most physicians currently feel that this would logically obligate therapy. Although it was initially controversial, there is a growing consensus regarding the appropriateness of use of the implantable cardioverter-defibrillator in patients without an inducible arrhythmia [29].

Noninducibility has been reported in between 0 and 40% of patients with prior sudden cardiac death [13,14, 17–19,29–35]. Inducibility at electrophysiology studies is dependent on a number of factors, including the underlying structural heart disease and the protocol used for programmed ventricular stimulation. Initially, Medicare would not reimburse for implantation in survivors of cardiac arrest without an inducible tachycardia or fibrillation. Guidelines for coverage were revised such that after July 1991, the implantation of an automatic defibrillator is a covered service for patients who have had a documented episode of life-threatening ventricular tachyarrhythmia or cardiac arrest not associated with a myocardial infarction [29]. This revised guideline effectively eliminates the need for inducibility for reimbursement.

The NAPSE guidelines have indicated that implantation of an ICD is treatment of choice for patients resuscitated from VT/VF with no inducible ventricular arrhythmias [2,29]. Caveats regarding patient selection include that the patient's life expectancy is greater than 6 months and that adequate psychological resources are present. Additionally, the cardiac arrest or hypotensive VT should not be associated with a myocardial infarction, correctable ischemic event, or other reversible cause. Similarly, the American College of Cardiology [29,30] indicated that the ICD was reasonable in certain patients in whom VT/VF is not inducible during EP studies. Included in the category are patients who have one or more documented episodes of hemodynamically significant VT/VF and in whom EPS and Holter monitoring cannot be used to accurately predict the efficacy of therapy, and that mapping-directed therapies such as surgery or ablation are not appropriate. Recurrent syncope of undetermined cause was not regarded as a significant indication for the ICD [29]. Similarly, the National Institutes of Health, concluded that implantation of the ICD should no longer be considered a treatment of last resort and was appropriate in noninducible patients if there was existence of a documented episode of symptomatic VT or VF or SCD unrelated to an acute myocardial infarction [29]. The presence of poorly controlled myocardial ischemia at the time of the arrhythmic event or ischemia that was not medically or surgically correctable was also felt to be an indication for ICD therapy in noninducible patients. Adequacy of the patient's psychological resources and a life expectancy of at least 6 months were caveats for defibrillator use in this patient population.

V. CONTRAINDICATIONS TO ICD IMPLANT

Patients with terminal illnesses or with a life expectancy of less than 6 to 12 months are not considered as candidates for ICD implant [2,29,30]. Included in this population would be those with malignancy, congestive heart failure, unstable medically refractory coronary artery disease not amenable to surgical therapy or angioplasty, or other medical or surgical consideration which would likely preclude survival for 6 months. Previous psychiatric problems that would interfere with meticulous care and follow-up necessary for the ICD patient are contraindications to such therapy. Patients with a history of continued intravenous drug abuse are at high risk for device infection. Patients who have ventricular tachycardia or other arrhythmias in the setting of correctable causes such as ischemia, metabolic or toxic abnormalities should not be considered candidates for the ICD [2,29,30]. Finally, patients who have frequent arrhythmias which might trigger shock therapy, such as sustained ventricular tachycardia not responsive to pharmacological or antitachycardia therapy are not ICD candidates. Such arrhythmias would frequently trigger device shock therapy.

VI. FUTURE INDICATIONS FOR ICD IMPLANTATIONS

It is clear that the indications for ICDs continue to evolve. There is currently a consensus among cardiac electrophysiologists that patients should receive a device if they suffered out-of-hospital cardiac arrest with ventricular tachycardia or ventricular fibrillation or have hemodynamically compromising ventricular tachycardia without a reversible cause if they are pharmacologically refractory or arrhythmias cannot be induced to guide drug therapy [24]. Since it is widely recognized that the yield declines sharply with each successive antiarrhythmic drug trial, there is a definite trend toward undertaking fewer antiarrhythmic trials [6,18,19–21]. Some electrophysiologists believe that the ICD is the treatment of choice for patients presenting with ventricular fibrillation, independent of the results of drug testing [24]. Nonetheless, electrophysiological evaluation provides important information regarding concomitant conduction system disease and supraventricular arrhythmias. Additionally, information regarding the rate and ability to terminate ventricular tachycardia with low-energy cardioversion or pacing techniques are critical for appropriate decisions regarding tiered therapy available in third-generation devices.

A number of multicenter clinical trials are in progress, which examine prospectively the role of ICD therapy in high-risk, "pre-event" patients [36–38]. The CABG Patch Trial is randomizing patients undergoing coronary bypass surgery who have a left ventricular ejection fraction below 36% and an abnormal signal-averaged EKG to receive an ICD or no device at the time of CABG [36,37]. The primary endpoint of the study is all-cause mortality or nonfatal, sustained ventricular arrhythmias that require drug treatment or cardioversion for termination.

The Multicenter Automatic Defibrillator Implantation Trial (MADIT) is another trial evaluating the prophylactic use of ICDs [38]. Postinfarction patients with ejection fractions less than 36%, nonsustained ventricular tachycardia, and inducible sustained VT which is not suppressed with procainamide will be enrolled in this trial. Conventional therapy may include drug therapy guided by further electrophysiological testing and/or amiodarone. The final endpoint of this study will be death of all causes. The Multicenter Unsustained Tachycardia Trial (MUSTT) will enroll patients with coronary artery disease, ejection fraction less than 41%, a late potential on the signal-averaged EKG, and nonsustained ventricular tachycardia [36,37]. Those patients with inducible sustained ventricular tachycardia will be randomized either to no therapy or EP-guided therapy. Those found to be pharmacologically refractory in the EP-guided therapy limb will receive an ICD. The results of these and other trials will clarify the role of the ICD in high-risk patients who have not yet had lethal ventricular arrhythmias.

It has become increasingly evident that many patients with congestive heart failure awaiting heart transplantation die suddenly [39–41]. It is estimated that of the total cardiac deaths in this patient population, approximately one-half are arrhythmic and might be preventable with an ICD [39]. The strategy of prophylactically implanting the ICD into patients awaiting heart transplant has been proposed in a study in which the defibrillator is used as a bridge to transplant (DEFIBRILAT study) [41].

At the same time that trials are being initiated to clarify the role of the ICD in patients who have not yet had a cardiac arrest, the National Heart, Blood, and Lung Institute (NHLBI) has recognized the need for a prospective evaluation of the ICD in survivors of cardiac arrest compared to alternate pharmacological therapy [42]. Prior studies reporting on the benefit of the ICD have used historical control subjects, projected sudden death rates based on number of appropriate shocks, concurrent, unmatched nonrandomized groups receiving and not receiving the ICD, or concurrent matched controlled subjects [3–12]. Such comparisons have significant limitations. The best method of evaluating the benefits of the ICD is with a randomized, controlled comparison of a treatment group with a control group that is not treated, treated with placebo, or actively treated with another method [42]. Additionally, there is a growing consensus that the most appropriate primary endpoint for such a study is total mortality rather than sudden death [42]. The Hamburg Cardiac Arrest Study has recently published interim data on 139 patients randomized to receive either ICD, amiodarone, propafenone, or metoprolol [43]. After a mean follow-up of 11 months, the ICD reduced the sudden death rate to 0%, compared with 9% in those receiving amiodarone and 11% each for the metoprolol and propafenone groups. However, overall mortality was not different between the ICD and drug therapy group (14% ICD, 14% metoprolol, 15% amiodarone, and 20% propafenone). As future results from this trial, CABG Patch, MUSTT, MADIT, the randomized controlled study of antiarrhythmic drugs versus implantable defibrillators (AVID) [44,45], and other trials become available, it is evident that the indications for the ICD will continue to evolve.

REFERENCES

1. Cannom DS. Implantable cardioverter defibrillator: the promise and perils of an evolving technology. PACE 1992; 15:1-4.
2. Lehmann M, Saksena S. NASPE Policy Conference Committee. Implantable cardioverter defibrillator in cardiovascular practice: report of the policy of the North American Society of Pacing and Electrophysiology. PACE 1991; 969-978.
3. Newman D, Suave NJ, Herre J, et al. Survival after implantation of the cardioverter defibrillator. Am J Cardiol 1992; 69:899-903.
4. Manolis AS, Tan-DeGuzman W, Lee MA, et al. Clinical experience in 77 patients with the automatic implantable cardioverter defibrillator. Am Heart J 1989; 118:445-450.
5. Marchlinski FE, Flores BT, Buxton AE, et al. The automatic implantable cardioverter defibrillator: efficacy, complications, and device failure. Ann Intern Med 1986; 104:481-488.
6. Winkle RA, Mead RH, Gandiani VA, et al. Long term outcome with automatic implantable cardioverter defibrillator. J Am Coll Cardiol 1989; 13:1353-1361.
7. Manolis AS, Rastegar H, Estes NAM III. Automatic implantable cardioverter defibrillator: Current status. JAMA 1989; 262(10):1362-1368.
8. Hombach V, Kochs M, Weismuller P, et al. Clinical dilemmas in patient selection for ICD treatment. In: Luderitz B, Saksena S, eds. Interventional Electrophysiology. Mt. Kisco, NY: Futura, 1991: 415-424.
9. Tchou PJ, Kadry N, Anderson J, et al. Automatic implantable cardioverter defibrillation and survival of patients with LV dysfunction and malignant ventricular arrhythmias. Ann Intern Med 1988; 109:529-534.
10. Kelley PA, Cannom DS, Garan H, et al. The automatic implantable cardioverter defibrillator: efficacy, complications and survival in patients with malignant ventricular arrhythmias. J Am Coll Cardiol 1988; 11:1278-1286.
11. Edel T, Maloney JD, Moore SL. Analysis of death in patients with an implantable cardioverter defibrillator. PACE 1992; 15:60-70.
12. Fisher JD, Brodman RF, Kim SG. VT/VF 60/60 protection. PACE 1990; 13:218-222.
13. Swerdlow CD, Winkle RA, Mason JW. Determinants of survival in patients with ventricular tachyarrhythmias. N Engl J Med 1983; 24:1436-1442.
14. Roy D, Waxman HL, Kienzle MG, et al. Clinical characteristics and long term follow-up in 119 survivors of cardiac arrest: relation to inducibility at electrophysiologic testing. Am J Cardiol 1983; 52:969-974.
15. Waller TJ, Kay HR, Speilman SR, et al. Reduction in sudden death and total mortality by antiarrhythmic therapy evaluated by electrophysiologic drug testing: criteria of efficacy in patients with sustained ventricular tachyarrhythmias. J Am Coll Cardiol 1987; 10:83-89.
16. Wilbur DJ, Garan H, Finklestein D, et al. Out-of-hospital cardiac arrest: use of electrophysiological testing in the prediction of long term outcome. N Engl J Med 1983; 318:19-24.
17. Baum RS, Alvarez H, Cobb LA. Survival after resuscitation from out-of-hospital cardiac arrest. Circulation 1974; 50:1231-1235.
18. Horowitz LN, Josephson ME, Farshidi A, et al. Recurrent sustained ventricular tachycardia: role of electrophysiological study in selection of antiarrhythmic regimen. Circulation 1978; 58:986-94.
19. Mason JW, Winkle RA. Accuracy of the ventricular tachycardia induction study for predicting long term efficacy and inefficacy of antiarrhythmic drugs. N Engl J Med 1980; 303:1073-1080.
20. Ruskin JN, Schoenfield MH, Garan H. Role of EP techniques in the selection of antiarrhythmic drug regimen for ventricular tachycardia. Am J Cardiol 1983; 52:41-15.
21. Myerburg RJ, Kessler KM, Estes D, et al. Long-term survival after prehospital cardiac arrest: analysis of outcome during an 8 year study. Circulation 1984; 70:538-546.
22. Mason JW. A comparison of electrophysiologic testing with Holter monitoring to predict antiarrhythmic-drug efficacy for ventricular tachyarrhythmias. N Engl J Med 1993; 329: 445–451.

23. Hession MJ, Lampert S, Podrid PJ, Lown B. Ethmozine (Moricizine HCL) therapy for complex ventricular arrhythmias. Am J Cardiol 1987; 60:59F-66F.
24. Lehmann MH, Steinman RT, Schuger CD, Jackson K. The automatic implantable cardioverter defibrillator as antiarrhythmic treatment modality of choice for survivors of cardiac arrest unrelated to acute myocardial infarction. Am J Cardiol 1988; 62:803-805.
25. Manolis AS, Urichio F, Estes NAM III. Prognostic value of early electrophysiologic studies for ventricular tachycardia recurrence in patients treated with amiodarone. J Am Coll Cardiol 1989; 63:1052-1057.
26. Manolis AS, Rastegar H, Payne D, Cleveland R, Estes NAM III. Surgical therapy for drug refractory ventricular tachycardia: results with mapping guided subendocardial resection. J Am Coll Cardiol 1989; 14:199-208.
27. Foote C, Wang PJ, Clyne C, et al. The role of left ventricular reconstruction in preserving cardiac function in patients undergoing endocardial resection (abstr.) PACE 1992; 533.
28. Healthcare Finance Administration (HCFA)-Section 35-85, Implantation of Automatic Defibrillator, Jan 1986, and Interim Payment Procedures for Defibrillator Implant, Mar 1986.
29. Handlesman H. Implantation of the automatic implantable cardioverter defibrillator: noninducibilty of ventricular tachyarrhythmias as a patient selection criteria. AHCPR 91-0041, Health Technology Assessment Rep 1990; 10:1-7.
30. Dreifus LS, Fisch C, Griffin J, et al. Guidelines for implantation of cardiac pacemakers and antiarrhythmic devices. July 1991. A report of the American College of Cardiology/American Heart Association Task Force on Assessment of Diagnostic and Therapeutic Cardiovascular Procedures. Committee on Pacemaker Implantation. J Am Coll Cardiol 1991; 18:1–13.
31. Sager PT, Ranjiv, Choudhary LC. Long term prognosis of patients with out-of-hospital cardiac arrest but no inducible ventricular tachyarrhythmias. Am Heart J 1990; 120:1334-1342.
32. Elder M, Suave MJ, Schnieman MM. Electrophysiological testing and follow-up of patients with aborted sudden death. Circulation 1974; 49:790-798.
33. Wellens JHH, Brugada P, Stevenson WG. Programmed electrical stimulation of the heart in patients with life threatening ventricular arrhythmias: what is the significance of induced arrhythmias and what is the correct stimulation protocol? Circulation 1985; 72:1-17.
34. Friedman RA, Swerdlow CD, Soderholm-Difatte V, et al. Prognostic significance of arrhythmia inducibility or noninducibility at initial electrophysiologic study in survivors of cardiac arrest. Am J Cardiol 1988; 61:578-82.
35. Eldar M, Suaveman J, Schneiman MM. Electrophysiological testing and follow-up of patient with aborted sudden deaths. J Am Coll Cardiol 1987; 10:291-298.
36. Bigger JT Jr. Future studies with the implantable cardioverter defibrillator. PACE 1991; 14:883-889.
37. Bigger JT Jr. Prophylactic use of implantable cardioverter defibrillators: medical, technical and economic considerations. PACE 1991; 14:376.
38. MADIT Executive Committee. Multi-center automatic defibrillator implantation trial (MADIT): design and clinical protocol. PACE 1991; 14:920-927.
39. Stevenson LW, Milton MA, Tillisch IH, et al. Decreasing survival benefit from cardiac transplantation for outpatients as the waiting list lengthens. J Am Coll Cardiol 1991; 18:919-25.
40. Bolling SF, Deeb GM, Morady F, et al. Automatic internal cardioverter defibrillator: a bridge to heart transplantation. J Heart Lung Transplant 1991; 10:562-566.
41. Lehmann M, for the DEFBRILAT Study Group. Actuarial risk of sudden death while awaiting cardiac transplantation in patients with atherosclerotic heart disease. Am J Cardiol 1991; 68:545-546.
42. Epstein AE. AVID Necessity, PACE 1993; 1773–1775.
43. Kuck KH, Siehels J, Schneider M, Hamburg GM. Cardiac arrest study group (abstr.). Rev Eur Tech Biomed 1990; 12:110.

13

Survival of Patients with Implantable Cardioverter-Defibrillators

Richard N. Fogoros

*Medical College of Pennsylvania
and Allegheny General Hospital
Pittsburgh, Pennsylvania*

I. INTRODUCTION

Over 25,000 patients have received the implantable cardioverter-defibrillator (ICD) in the first dozen years of its clinical use. During that time, the ICD has come to be regarded as one of the most important tools available for preventing sudden cardiac death. Nonetheless, each year an additional 1 million individuals in the United States develop conditions which place them at high risk for sudden death, and 400,000 actually die suddenly. Implanting the ICD in an average of slightly over 2000 patients per year, then, has not made a measurable impact on the overall problem of sudden cardiac death. If the ICD is ever to make such an impact, its usage will have to be vastly increased.

In fact, the impetus to expand the usage of the ICD is becoming very strong. Given the expense of this new technology, a major increase in the usage of ICDs would have an important impact on the cost of health care, and therefore, should be preceded by firm data justifying that increase. Now is the time, while the use of the ICD is still relatively limited, to take a sober look at the data accumulated to date on the efficacy of this device. The purpose of this chapter is to review the available data on the efficacy of the ICD in prolonging the survival of its recipients. An attempt will be made to assess the benefits of therapy with the ICD as it has been used so far, and to examine the extent to which the available data support the expansion of therapy with the ICD to new groups of patients.

II. EFFICACY OF THE ICD IN PREVENTING SUDDEN DEATH

Early studies on the efficacy of the ICD are notable for their assumption that successfully preventing sudden cardiac death is a worthwhile end in itself. This assumption stems directly from Mirowski's original stimulus for the development of the ICD [1], namely, the sudden, premature demise from ventricular tachyarrhythmias of an admired and productive colleague.

Preventing unnecessary sudden death was the vision that drove Mirowski and his colleagues to design, build, and test the ICD despite (to say the least) the lack of encouragement from the general medical community. The notion that prevention of sudden cardiac death was a sufficient goal for documenting efficacy of the ICD was the major theme of early investigations with this device, and remains an arguably legitimate point of view in the eyes of many investigators.

The earliest published results with the ICD in human subjects documented beyond a reasonable doubt that the ICD could indeed efficiently and reliably abort fatal ventricular tachyarrhythmias. The first important report on clinical results with the ICD was published by Mirowski et al. [2] in 1983. Mirowski's study included the first 52 patients to receive the ICD at Johns Hopkins and Stanford Universities (the original implanting centers). In this series, the ICD was implanted only in patients who had survived at least *two* episodes of arrhythmic cardiac arrest, and whose arrhythmias had proven refractory to pharmacological therapy. After implantation, the ICDs in this series successfully converted all 82 documented episodes of spontaneous malignant ventricular tachyarrhythmias, and 81 of 99 episodes of induced ventricular tachyarrhythmias. During a mean follow-up period of 14 months, 62 episodes of symptomatic recurrent arrhythmias in 17 patients were automatically terminated by the ICD. The 1-year actuarial incidence of sudden death was 8.5%, and of overall death was 22%. The estimated mortality had the ICD not been implanted (based on the incidence of successful resuscitations by the ICD) was 48% at 1 year, and the estimated reduction in mortality was 52% at 1 year. Given the primitive nature of the ICD used in this study, and the fact that the patient population was probably "sicker" than in later series (the requirement for surviving two cardiac arrests was dropped after this first series of patients), these results were quite impressive.

Subsequent reports from other implanting centers confirmed a very low incidence of sudden death in recipients of the ICD. Borbola et al. [3] reported an overall 1-year survival rate of 86%, and a sudden-death survival rate of 100% in 25 patients who received the ICD. Kelly et al. [4] reported only one sudden death among 91 patients who received the ICD, and an overall 1-year survival rate of 95%. In 77 recipients of the ICD, Manolis et al. [5] described sudden-death survival rates of 100% at 1 and 2 years, and 92% at 3 years, while overall actuarial survival in this series was 94% at 1 and 2 years, and 75% at 3 years. Veltri et al. [6] reported the 2-year actuarial sudden-death survival rate to be 96% in 163 recipients of the ICD. Data from the author's center [7] for 70 survivors of sudden death who received the ICD showed the actuarial sudden-death survival rate to be 99% at 1 year and 97% at 5 years, and the overall survival rate to be 96% at 1 year and 79% at 5 years. Winkle et al. [8], in the largest published single-center series, reported the actuarial sudden-death survival rate among 270 recipients of the ICD to be 99% at 1 year and 96% at 5 years, and overall survival to be 92% at 1 year and 74% at 5 years. Data from the registry maintained by Cardiac Pacemakers, Inc. (the company that manufactured the first ICD to be approved by the FDA) showed that the first 3610 recipients of the ICD had a sudden-death survival rate of 98% at 1 year, and 94% at 5 years; and an overall survival of 90% at 1 year and 70% at 5 years [9].

To further assess the efficacy of the ICD in preventing sudden death, a report from our center compared the actuarial incidence of sudden death in similar patients who did and who did not receive the ICD [10]. All 50 patients in our study had presented with ventricular tachyarrhythmias which produced loss of consciousness, and all had inducible ventricular tachyarrhythmias which could not be suppressed with antiarrhythmic drugs. Twenty-one patients received the ICD, and 29 patients (who had either refused the ICD or who presented at a time when the ICD was not available) did not receive the device. The 29 patients treated without the

ICD received empiric therapy with amiodarone. Among the 21 patients who received the ICD, there were no sudden deaths, although 13 patients had apparent recurrences of their arrhythmias which were treated successfully by their ICDs. Among the 29 who did not receive the ICD, the actuarial incidence of sudden death was 31% at 1 and 2 years (incidence of sudden death in patients with an ICD versus in patients without an ICD, $p < 0.003$).

In an editorial published in late 1988, Lehmann et al. [11] compared the reports on the efficacy of the ICD in preventing sudden death in high-risk patients to reports on the efficacy of other commonly used therapies. In general, the long-term incidence of sudden death with the ICD was less than 10%, while the long-term incidence of sudden death with other therapies was most often between 20 and 70%. Lehmann's analysis of the available information led him to suggest that the ICD, instead of being considered a treatment of last resort, should be considered the "gold standard" in the prevention of sudden cardiac death in high-risk patients.

Thus, by the late 1980s, it was well established that the ICD was extraordinarily successful in doing exactly what it was designed to do, that is, preventing sudden cardiac death in patients who were at high risk for this event. The Food and Drug Administration agreed that the ICD was effective, and approved the device in 1985. Several medical device companies were sufficiently moved by these early results to make major commitments toward developing their own ICD technology.

III. CHALLENGING THE EFFICACY OF THE ICD

While early studies with the ICD had shown convincingly what they were designed to show, there was nonetheless a significant shortcoming, namely, the lack of a randomized, controlled study with the ICD. The failure to perform randomized studies was not an oversight— it simply was not feasible to perform a randomized study at the time of the first clinical trials with the ICD. Given the negative atmosphere at the time toward the very concept of implantable defibrillators, the early investigators felt extraordinary pressure to demonstrate as expeditiously as possible whether the implantable defibrillator could indeed automatically detect and terminate ventricular fibrillation. Further, several issues regarding the optimal use of the implantable defibrillator were not worked out at the time of the initial clinical investigations. These issues included patient selection, arrhythmia detection algorithms, lead design, lead positioning, surgical approaches, and intraoperative testing. All these issues were, in fact, addressed and altered during the first clinical trials. Thus, at the time that the ICD was first coming into clinical use, it was simply not possible to organize a meaningful randomized study.

As noted, the ability of the ICD to prevent sudden death was, in fact, quickly documented. And, once documented, the effective prevention of sudden death immediately rendered a randomized study with the ICD (in the type of high-risk patient who received the device in those early years) extremely difficult. Thus, the original decision not to do a randomized study proved to be difficult to reverse. As long as the efficacy of the ICD was measured in terms of its ability to prevent sudden death, however, the failure to conduct a randomized study was not considered a major problem.

In the late 1980s, some influential physicians began to take issue with the published data on the efficacy of the ICD [12,13]. These physicians accept the fact that the ICD reliably prevents sudden cardiac death, but they ask, in effect, "While the ICD is effective at preventing sudden cardiac death, what is the benefit (and what is the cost) of preventing sudden death with the ICD?" Essentially, they have challenged the original assumption that the benefit of preventing sudden death was self-evident.

IV. THE EFFECT OF THE ICD ON OVERALL SURVIVAL

The question of whether the ICD has prolonged the overall survival of its recipients is an important one. This question is vital in deciding whether therapy with the ICD has been, after all, worthwhile.

Since there are no randomized studies published using the ICD in patients at high risk for sudden death, every published study is, almost by definition, flawed. Some critics of the ICD have used this fact to suggest that the most appropriate course would be to avoid using the ICD until randomized studies are completed. However, if physicians were to stop using all therapies whose efficacy has not been rigidly proven, then medical practitioners would be impotent indeed. Further, in the case of the ICD, available data (despite the fact that there are no statistically perfect studies), present compelling evidence that the ICD has, in fact, prolonged the survival of its recipients.

In reviewing the literature on the efficacy of the ICD, there are at least six lines of evidence suggesting that the ICD has prolonged the overall survival of its recipients.

First, among survivors of cardiac arrest, the selective use of the ICD in drug nonresponders (those patients who have inducible ventricular tachycardia which is not suppressible during serial drug testing) has resulted in an actuarial incidence of sudden death and of overall death which is the same as for "low-risk" survivors of cardiac arrest (that is, patients whose arrhythmias were noninducible during baseline electrophysiological testing or whose inducible arrhythmias were suppressed during serial drug testing) [7]. This outcome in the nonresponders occurred despite the fact that their actuarial risk of recurrent arrhythmic events was significantly higher than for the lower-risk groups. The most reasonable explanation for this finding is that the selected use of the ICD in the nonresponders eliminated the "excess" mortality that otherwise would have occurred as a result of these recurrent arrhythmias.

Second, among recipients of the ICD, the overall survival of those patients who have received appropriate shocks has been the same as the overall survival of patients who have never received appropriate shocks. In our series, actuarial survival in both groups was greater than 90% at 30 months after implantation, even though the patients who received shocks tended to receive their first shocks during the first 6–12 months after implantation, and they also had a significantly lower mean left ventricular ejection fraction than patients who did not receive shocks [14]. Since patients whose arrhythmias recurred had the same overall survival as patients whose arrhythmias did not recur, the only reasonable conclusion is that the ICD removed the excess mortality that would have occurred among the patients who had recurrent arrhythmias.

Third, several studies have used the actuarial incidence of appropriate shocks after implantation of the ICD to estimate the predicted incidence of death had the ICD not been implanted. Tchou et al. [15], analyzed results of therapy in 70 consecutive patients who received the ICD for sustained ventricular tachyarrhythmias which could not be controlled with medication. Twenty-five recipients of the ICD had left ventricular ejection fractions less than 0.3. During follow-up, only one of the 25 had sudden death. The 2-year overall survival of these patients with severe underlying heart disease was 87%, compared to a projected survival without the ICD (based on the incidence of appropriate shocks) of 57% ($p = 0.025$). Patients treated with the ICD whose left ventricular ejection fractions were greater than 0.3 had an overall 2-year survival of 100%, compared to a projected survival of 60% ($p < 0.0015$).

Our group performed a similar analysis in 119 consecutive patients who received the ICD [16]. Forty of these patients had left ventricular ejection fractions less than 0.3. The 3-year overall survival rate for these 40 patients was 67%, compared to a projected survival without the ICD of 6% ($p \leq 0.001$). The 79 patients treated with the ICD whose left ventricular ejection fractions were ≥ 0.3 had a 3-year survival of 96%, compared to a projected survival without the ICD of 46% ($p < 0.001$). These studies strongly indicate that the ICD significantly prolonged the survival of its recipients, whether they had severe or only moderate underlying cardiac disease.

The major criticism of studies estimating projected survival based on appropriate shocks (aside from the fact that they are not prospective, randomized studies) is that it is impossible to tell whether an ICD shock has prevented sudden death. While this is strictly true, we have presented evidence that the commonly used definition of "appropriate shock" (a shock preceded by syncope or presyncope) actually underestimates the true incidence of appropriate shocks [17]. Further, among cardiac-arrest survivors, our data indicate that a recurrent arrhythmic event in a patient unprotected by the ICD has nearly an 80% chance of causing death [7,10]. Singer has presented evidence that even if only 20% of ICD shocks were actually life-saving, the actuarial survival with an ICD would still be significantly higher than the projected survival without the ICD [18].

Fourth, we have performed an actuarial estimate of the prolongation of survival conferred by the ICD in 89 patients who received appropriate shocks, using the date of the first appropriate shock as the date of entry into the actuarial analysis [14]. Survival was 94% at 1 year, 75% at 3 years, and 53% at 5 years after the first appropriate ICD discharge. Since there was no control group in this study, the reader is left to decide if this magnitude of survival is worthwhile. However, since it is likely that without the ICD the majority of these patients would have died on "day zero" of the actuarial analysis, it seems reasonable to conclude that the ICD was beneficial in these patients.

Fifth, several authors [14,19,20] have calculated the prolongation of survival conferred by the ICD by considering only those patients who have received appropriate shocks and then subsequently died. In our series [14], 17 patients have died after being rescued by their ICDs. Their mean survival after the first appropriate shock was 22 months. Others have reported similar results [19,20]. Since the majority of ICD-recipients who have received appropriate shocks remain alive, these estimates should be seen as "worst-case" estimates.

Sixth, Newman et al. [21] have recently published a case control study in which the actuarial survival of 60 consecutive recipients of the ICD was compared to the survival of 120 matched control patients treated with drug therapy. Overall survival in the patients treated with ICDs was significantly better than for the patients treated with drugs.

Thus, there are several careful analyses in the literature which, while they all suffer the flaw of not being randomized prospective trials, offer much evidence (some would say compelling evidence) that the ICD as it was applied in the 1980s significantly prolonged the survival of its recipients. Based on this evidence, it is appropriate to continue using the ICD in patients presenting with symptomatic sustained ventricular tachyarrhythmias which cannot be suppressed by antiarrhythmic drugs. In fact, in the author's opinion, evidence of the ICD's efficacy is at least as strong as for most of the commonly used therapies in medicine, and thus one is obligated to at least strongly consider using the ICD in such high-risk patients.

The author's opinion notwithstanding, two recent editorials discuss the need for randomized prospective trials to examine the use of the ICD in survivors of cardiac arrest [13,22], and the NHLBI has concurred. At least two randomized trials with the ICD in cardiac-arrest survivors are underway [13]. In the Canadian Implantable Defibrillator Study (CIDS), patients with symptomatic ventricular tachyarrhythmias are being randomized to therapy with the ICD or with amiodarone. The Cardiac Arrest Study of Hamburg (CASH) involves randomizing survivors of cardiac arrest to therapy with the ICD, metoprolol, amiodarone, or propafenone. In this latter study, survival with propafenone has already proven to be significantly worse than with the ICD, and the propafenone arm of the study has been terminated (personal communication).

Well-designed randomized trials are correctly regarded as the best way to evaluate the usefulness of a medical therapy. However, one needs only to consider the confusion brought about by the maze of conflicting results from studies assessing thrombolytic therapy in acute myocardial infarctions to recognize that, in order for a randomized trial to be useful, the right question has to be asked.

In the case of the ICD, asking the right question is vitally important. The question that is being asked seems to be "Does the ICD prolong overall survival?" Since the ability of the ICD to reliably prevent sudden death from ventricular arrhythmias is accepted by virtually everybody, this question really becomes "Does the prevention of sudden death prolong overall survival?" The answer to this question seems self-evident: In some patients the prevention of sudden death will lead to prolonged survival, and in other patients it will not. Thus, the "efficacy" of the ICD in prolonging overall survival depends almost entirely on how it is used.

If you give a carpenter a hammer and direct him to build a mansion, you may get a mansion, or you may get a shed. If you get a shed, however, it is not the hammer's fault. It is important to recognize that the ICD is merely a tool, a tool that is very effective in doing what it was designed to do. It is our use of the tool, and not the tool itself, which is useful or not useful.

Thus, asking "Does the ICD prolong overall survival?" is the wrong question. A study which merely examines the outcome of the way in which we happen to be using the ICD, even if it is a randomized prospective study, may give us the "wrong" answer. Such a study risks declaring as not useful a tool which unquestionably has enormous potential for good.

Instead, studies should be designed which will help us to use this clinical tool in the most beneficial way. Which patients are the most likely to experience prolonged survival with the ICD? Which underlying illnesses, and what degree of underlying illness, limits the long-term benefit of the ICD? Is there an age after which the prevention of sudden death with the ICD ceases to prolong overall survival? The answers to these and similar questions will help us to use this clinical tool in the most useful, cost-effective way. Since it is not clear that current or planned randomized trials with the ICD will help to answer these questions, the results of those trials will have to be interpreted with caution.

V. WHY AVAILABLE DATA MAY NOT SUPPORT EXPANDED USAGE OF THE ICD

As noted at the beginning of this chapter, the impetus to increase the usage of the ICD is becoming very strong. This impetus comes from the perceived efficacy of the ICD, the perceived inefficacy of antiarrhythmic drug therapy, the steadily increasing availability of electrophysiological facilities, and the whole-hearted commitment of the biomedical industry to ICD technology. For all of these reasons, we are now poised at a time when the use of the ICD stands to be greatly expanded. If this expansion approaches the levels being discussed by manufacturers of ICDs, the cost in health-care dollars would be astronomical. Implanting ICDs in every individual who enters a "high-risk" category might cost, in hardware alone, as much as $20–30 billion per year.

Expenditures anywhere near this level would need to be predicated on firm data supporting the efficacy of the ICD. While, as noted in the above discussion, the data support the use of the ICD of the 1980s as it was employed in the 1980s, data justifying the widely expanded usage

Survival of Patients with ICDs

of new generations of ICDs in new categories of patients are lacking. There are several reasons why the data cited in this chapter cannot be used to justify widespread expansion of the usage of the ICD. Among those reasons are that new groups of patients will be receiving ICDs, new devices will be used, and new centers will be implanting ICDs.

A. New Patients

Until recently, the use of the ICD has been limited to patients who have survived at least one episode of a spontaneous, sustained, life-threatening ventricular tachyarrhythmia. The vast majority of recipients of the ICD have had inducible sustained ventricular tachyarrhythmias which have not been suppressible by serial drug testing. For these patients, as described above, available survival data with the ICD is sufficiently convincing to justify the usage of the device, despite the lack of a randomized, controlled trial.

The same would not be the case with the use of the ICD in lower-risk patients (such as patients with underlying heart disease and asymptomatic ventricular ectopy and/or positive signal-averaged ECGs). Because the risk of sudden death in these patients is substantially lower than for survivors of sustained lethal arrhythmias, and because any perioperative mortality will be proportionally more important in lower-risk patients than in high-risk patients, a nonrandomized study almost certainly will not be sufficient to document efficacy of the ICD in such patients. The expansion of the use of ICDs to lower-risk groups, then, while tempting, must await the results of randomized clinical trials.

Conversely, new technology (such as nonthoracotomy lead systems) will tempt clinicians to apply ICD therapy to patients who might have been considered "too sick" for the implantation of the ICD in the past. As noted above, the ICD may not offer significant benefit to critically ill patients, even if implantation of the devices prevents sudden death. Well-designed clinical studies will be required before expanding the use of the ICD in this direction, also.

B. New Devices

The advent of nonthoracotomy lead systems will change the outcome of patients treated with ICDs. Presumably (and early data tends to bear this out), perioperative mortality will be improved if the ICD can be implanted without requiring a thoracotomy. However, the long-term integrity of these new lead systems remains to be proven, and long-term survival with these new lead systems will need to be assessed carefully.

The new, third-generation ICD generators which are in development may yield long-term results which are different than with earlier generations. This is particularly important to note since, now that the era of therapy with the ICD is about to truly begin, these new devices (and not the ICDs with which all the available survival data have been collected), are the ones which will be used. The new "tiered-therapy" devices offer much more flexibility than earlier generations of ICDs, including bradycardia pacing, antitachycardia pacing, and low-energy cardioversion. This new flexibility will no doubt help many patients. The new ICDs can be set up into literally scores of configurations, having been designed with the idea that one can tailor these devices very specifically and very precisely for the individual patient.

The price paid for this flexibility is a new complexity, and the presence of potential problems which appear to be generic to this type of device. The complexity of these new ICDs is far greater than for earlier devices, which were either nonprogrammable or minimally programmable. This complexity requires much sophistication on the part of the electrophysiologist, who must have a clear understanding of both the device itself and the individual patient's arrhythmias in order to assure that the device will be set up to function safely and effectively.

One of the generic risks in using tiered-therapy devices is that, by offering so many therapeutic options, these devices by their very nature tempt one to delay high-energy shocks in order to try "milder" therapies first. Allowing a patient to remain in a ventricular tachyarrhythmia for a prolonged period of time while attempting to pace-terminate the arrhythmia may reduce the efficacy of a high-energy shock when it is finally delivered.

Thus, it is by no means clear that the survival data collected with earlier generations of ICDs will apply to these new devices. Studies using these new devices will need to be conducted. Unfortunately, such studies will be relatively difficult to design, since the new ICDs can be programmed to behave in so many different ways.

C. New Centers

It should also be kept in mind that most of the data related to survival of patients with ICDs has been collected by centers specializing in the management of patients with malignant rhythm disturbances, and by physicians who have had an abiding interest in ICD technology. For many of the investigators whose results have been described in this chapter, for instance, the selection of patients for the ICD, the implantation of the ICD, and the follow-up of patients with ICDs have formed a major aspect of their careers.

A marked expansion in the use of ICDs will almost certainly mean that therapy with the ICD will be directed by physicians who have had relatively minimal training in electrophysiology. That this may lead to suboptimal results is obvious, considering the complex nature of the arrhythmias being treated and the complexity of the newer ICDs themselves. Manufacturers of ICDs stand ready to help new centers establish ICD programs. Given the competitive nature of the market, however, it is clear that industry is unable (even if it were willing) to attempt to screen new programs for competence in the management of arrhythmias. It may be that the survival statistics which are reported in the literature will be out of reach for many new implanting centers.

For the safety of patients, and for the integrity of the electrophysiology community, it is important that survival statistics be tracked by (or for) each implanting center. Each center must continuously assess its success with the ICD, and must assure that certain minimum standards are maintained. A confidential national database registry for therapy with ICDs is one means by which a center can compare its results to the nationwide experience. One such database is under development by the American College of Cardiology, and may prove to be an important tool in assuring the safe delivery of therapy with ICDs.

VI. SUMMARY

The evidence that therapy with the ICD effectively prevents sudden death from cardiac tachyarrhythmias was well established from the earliest reports on the clinical usage of this device. While no randomized controlled study exists using the ICD in patients at very high risk for sudden death, several studies using historical controls, nonrandomized contemporary control groups, and recipients of the ICD as their own controls (by approximating the projected mortality rate had the ICD not been present), document to the satisfaction of most observers that the ICD has significantly prolonged the overall survival of appropriately selected patients. For this reason, and because other therapies have been perceived as yielding disappointing results, there is a major impetus to greatly expand the use of the ICD.

It is likely that the ICD can benefit many more patients than have received the device so far. However, it is important to recognize that the survival statistics reported in this chapter apply only to "traditional" high-risk patients (i.e., those who have had spontaneous, symptomatic, sustained ventricular tachyarrhythmias unresponsive to drug therapy), who have received a "traditional" ICD (a minimally programmable device which delivers shock therapy only). ICDs which are now being marketed are fundamentally different in design from these earlier devices, and patients who will be receiving them are likely to be in lower-risk groups than previous recipients of the ICD. Before vastly expanding the use of ICDs, careful, randomized studies are needed to establish both the safety and efficacy of these new devices in new groups of patients.

REFERENCES

1. Kastor JA. Michel Mirowski and the automatic implantable defibrillator. Am J Cardiology 1989; 63:977-982.
2. Mirowski M, Reid PR, Winkle RA, et al. Mortality in patients with implanted automatic defibrillators. Ann Intern Med 1983; 98:585-588.
3. Borbola J, Denes P, Ezri MD, Hauser RG, Serry C, Goldin MD. The automatic implantable cardioverter-defibrillator: clinical experience, complications, and follow-up in 25 patients. Arch Intern Med 1988; 148:70-76.
4. Kelly PA, Cannom DS, Garan H, et al. The automatic implantable cardioverter-defibrillator: efficacy, complications and survival in patients with malignant ventricular arrhythmias. J Am Coll Cardiol 1988; 11:1278-1286.
5. Manolis AS, Tan-DeGuzman W, Lee MA, et al. Clinical experience in seventy-seven patients with the automatic implantable cardioverter defibrillator. Am Heart J 1989; 118:445-450.
6. Veltri EP, Mower MM, Mirowski M, et al. Follow-up of patients with ventricular tachyarrhythmia treated with the automatic implantable cardioverter defibrillator: programmed electrical stimulation results do not predict clinical outcome. J Electrophysiol 1989; 467-476.
7. Fogoros RN, Elson JJ, Bonnet CA, Fiedler SB, Chenarides JG. Long-term outcome of survivors of cardiac arrest whose therapy is guided by electrophysiologic teting. J Am Coll Cardiol 1992; 19:780-788.
8. Winkle RA, Mead RH, Ruder MA, et al. Long-term outcome with the automatic implantable cardioverter-defibrillator. J Am Coll Cardiol 1989; 13:1353-1361.
9. Thomas AC, Moser SA, Smutka ML, Wilson PA. Implantable defibrillation: eight years clinical experience. PACE 1988; 11:2053-2058.
10. Fogoros RN, Fiedler SB, Elson JJ. The automatic implantable cardioverter-defibrillator in drug-refractory ventricular tachyarrhythmias. Ann Intern Med 1987; 107:635-641.
11. Lehmann MH, Steinman RT, Schuger CD, Jackson K. The automatic implantable cardioverter defibrillator as antiarrhythmic treatment modality of choice for survivors of cardiac arrest unrelated to acute myocardial infarction. Am J Cardiol 1988; 62:803-805.
12. Furman S. AICD benefit. PACE 1989; 12:399-400.
13. Connolly SJ, Yusuf S. Evaluation of the implantable cardioverter defibrillator in survivors of cardiac arrest: the need for randomized trials. Am J Cardiol 1992; 69:959-962.
14. Fogoros RN, Elson JJ, Bonnet CA. Survival of patients who have received appropriate shocks from their implantable defibrillators. PACE 1991; 14:1842-1845.
15. Tchou PJ, Kadri N, Anderson J, Caceres JA, Jazayeri M, Akhtar M. Automatic implantable cardioverter defibrillators and survival of patients with left ventricular dysfunction and malignant ventricular arrhythmias. Ann Intern Med 1988; 109:529-534.
16. Fogoros RN, Elson JJ, Bonnet CA, Fiedler SB, Burkholder JA. Efficacy of the automatic implantable cardioverter defibrillator in prolonging survival in patients with severe underlying cardiac disease. J Am Coll Cardiol 1990; 16:381-386.
17. Fogoros RN, Elson JJ, Bonnet CA. Actuarial incidence and pattern of occurrence of shocks following implantation of the automatic implantable cardioverter defibrillator. PACE 1989; 1465-1473.

18. Interview of I. Singer. In: The validity of AICD survival statistics: an analysis. CPI AICD Advances 1991; 2nd quarter:6-9.
19. Myerburg RJ, Luceri RM, Thurer R, et al. Time to first shock and clinical outcome in patients receiving an automatic implantable cardioverter defibrillator. J Am Coll Cardiol 1989; 14:508-514.
20. Mercando AD, Furman S, Johnston D, et al. Survival of patients with the automatic implantable cardioverter defibrillator. PACE 1988; 11:2059-2063.
21. Newman D, Sauve MJ, Herre J, et al. Survival after implantation of the cardioverter defibrillator. Am J Cardiol 1992; 69:899-903.
22. Saksena S, Camm AJ. Implantable defibrillators for prevention of sudden death. Technology at a medical and economic crossroad. Circulation 1992; 85:2316-2321.

14

Implantable Cardioverter-Defibrillators in Children and Adolescents

Michael J. Silka
Jack Kron

Oregon Health Sciences University
Portland, Oregon

Paul C. Gillette

Medical University of South Carolina
Charleston, South Carolina

I. INTRODUCTION

The use of implantable cardioverter-defibrillators (ICDs) in young patients raises a number of unique issues in the use of these devices. The purpose of this chapter is to discuss these issues and their potential solutions, based on a collaborative analysis involving both pediatric and adult cardiologists/electrophysiologists. The differences and similarities between the child or adolescent and the adult who are survivors of, or at risk for, sudden cardiac death (SCD) provides the basis for much of this analysis. For the purposes of this chapter, the terms "child, adolescent, and young" will refer to patients between 1 and 19 years of age.

II. SUDDEN CARDIAC DEATH IN THE YOUNG

Sudden death is an uncommon event in young patients, with an estimated frequency of 1–13 events per 100,000 patient years [1–3]. Given the infrequency of sudden death due to cardiovascular disease in young patients, few studies have provided a systematic analysis of this problem [4–6]. Consequently, there is limited data on which to reference specific recommendations. However, with the evolution of rapid-response emergency medical systems and improvements in resuscitative techniques [7], an increasing number of young SCD survivors are being identified [5]. Simultaneously, advances in technology which have been incorporated into second- and third-generation devices, along with expanded clinical indications approved for use of ICDs, have increased the number of young patients who are potential candidates for such therapy [8–10]. Thus, there is currently a need to define the role of ICD therapy in young patients at risk for, or resuscitated from SCD, with recognition that such recommendations will continue to evolve.

Certain fundamental aspects of SCD in young patients require differentiation from SCD in adults. Asystole is the most common documented arrhythmia associated with SCD in young patients (77%), in contrast to ventricular fibrillation (9%) [11]. Second, based on historical analysis, approximately 7% of young patients resuscitated from cardiac arrest survive to hospital discharge, compared to 20% of adult patients [11]. However, one similarity is that victims of SCD resuscitated from ventricular fibrillation, regardless of age, are more likely to survive than victims found in asystole or electromechanical dissociation [12].

Young patients with *cardiovascular disease* are much more likely to experience ventricular tachycardia or fibrillation as immediate causes of sudden death, in contrast to young patients whose cardiac arrest is *not* associated with a cardiac etiology [13]. The focus of this chapter, on the use of ICDs in young patients, will consider primarily the first subset of patients. However, a basic limitation which remains is that a significantly lower percentage of young patients, both with and without previously recognized cardiovascular disease, will be successfully resuscitated from SCD than adult counterparts. The ability to prospectively identify young patients at "high risk" for SCD may allow one of the greatest benefits in the use of ICDs.

In the following sections, the recognized substrates of cardiovascular disease associated with SCD in young patients will be discussed, along with rationale for the use of the ICD or alternative therapies, followed by a discussion of anatomical and electrophysiological considerations in the use of ICDs in young patients.

III. CARDIOVASCULAR DISEASES AND SUDDEN CARDIAC DEATH

SCD in children or adolescents is associated with three principal forms of cardiovascular disease: (1) congenital heart disease; (2) cardiomyopathies; and (3) primary electrical diseases [5]. The arrhythmic mechanisms of SCD, and thus indications for ICD implantation, appear to vary among the differing substrates of cardiovascular disease (Table 1). Therefore, SCD and the use of ICDs will be discussed independently for each type of cardiovascular disease.

Table 1 Sudden Cardiac Death in the Young—Relative Risk Profile

	SCD risk (per year)	Electrophysiologic mechanism of SCD	Associated risk factors
Congenital heart disease			
Tetralogy of Fallot	0.1–1.5%	VT → VF AV block (??)	RV / LV dysfunction
Aortic stenosis	0.3–1.0%	ischemia → VF	LV hypertrophy/fibrosis
Transposition of the great arteries	0.2–2.0%	Atrial flutter 1:1 conduction VT → VF (?) Bradycardia → asystole (??)	RV dysfunction
Cardiomyopathies			
Idiopathic dilated	0.4–1.5%	Bradycardia → asystole Electromechanical dissociation VT → VF(?)	Congestive heart failure Sustained VT
Hypertrophic	3.0–6.0%	VT → VF SVT → VF (??)	Familial SCD Inducible VT
Primary electrical diseases			
Idiopathic V F	1.0–11.0%	Polymorphic VT → VF	Syncope
Long QT syndromes	4.0–6.0%	Torsade de pointes → VF	Syncope AV block

A. Sudden Cardiac Death and Congenital Heart Disease

The initial studies of SCD in the young were retrospective analyses of patients with congenital heart disease, who had experienced sudden, unexplained death [14,15]. Three basic differences between SCD in pediatric patients with congenital heart disease and adult patients with ischemic heart disease were defined: First, bradyarrhythmias were more prevalent as terminal events in young patients than adults [13]; second, atrial tachyarrhythmias, specifically atrial flutter, were correlated with sudden death in the young [16]; and third, coronary artery disease or anomalies could not be implicated as the etiology of SCD in the majority of young patients [14].

Definition of the relative risks of SCD associated with congenital heart defects continues to evolve. During the past decade, improvements in myocardial preservation and advances in cardiovascular surgical techniques have reduced the prevalence of two factors associated with SCD in patients with congenital heart disease: myocardial dysfunction and advanced pulmonary obstructive vascular disease [14,15]. Thus, evaluation of the relationship between congenital heart disease and risk of SCD must be viewed as a function of patient era [17]. In the current era, three specific congenital heart lesions are most commonly associated with SCD: tetralogy of Fallot, aortic stenosis, and transposition of the great arteries.

1. Tetralogy of Fallot

Sudden death has been estimated to occur in 0.1–1.5% of patients per year following surgical repair of tetralogy of Fallot [18,19]. Two mechanisms of SCD have been proposed in these patients: (1) progressive conduction system disease, with the development of late complete atrioventricular (AV) block [20], and (2) malignant postoperative ventricular tachyarrhythmias [21]. Conduction disturbances, specifically right bundle branch block (94%) and left anterior hemiblock (9%), are common following surgical repair of tetralogy of Fallot [22]. However, progression to complete AV block has rarely been documented during childhood or adolescence.

Ventricular arrhythmias are commonly detected (10–50%) during ambulatory monitoring in patients following repair of tetralogy of Fallot, and appear to be correlated with late sudden death [18,21]. Sustained ventricular arrhythmias are frequently inducible in these patients during programmed ventricular stimulation [23]; however, the specificity of this response remains uncertain. In a study of over 300 patients with prior repair of tetralogy of Fallot, inducibility of ventricular tachycardia was not predictive of SCD [24].

Although prospective methods have not been established to identify patients at risk for SCD following repair of tetralogy of Fallot, current medical evidence suggests that ventricular tachyarrhythmias are the probable immediate cause of SCD [21]. A number of studies have also cited ventricular dysfunction as an important risk factor for SCD in these patients [18,19,24]. Reported effective treatments for ventricular tachycardia in these patients include map-guided cryosurgery [25], pulmonary valve replacement in patients with severe right ventricular enlargement [26], and either Holter or electrophysiological guided pharmacologic therapy [21,27]. ICD therapy for patients with previous repair of tetralogy of Fallot would appear to be primarily indicated for SCD survivors with no inducible, or drug-refractory, inducible, sustained ventricular tachyarrhythmias.

2. Aortic Stenosis

Sudden death has been estimated to occur in 0.3–1% of children with aortic stenosis per annum [28]. There is minimal data regarding the prevalence of either ambulatory or inducible ventricular arrhythmias in these patients. SCD is hypothesized to be related to decreased cardiac output during exertion, followed by hypotension and coronary insufficiency, culminating in myocardial ischemia and ventricular arrhythmias [29]. Thus, primary evaluation of SCD in a young patient with aortic stenosis is directed toward left ventricular outflow tract obstruction. However, in the patient with a severely hypertrophied, and potentially fibrotic left ventricle, the potential for malignant ventricular arrhythmias may persist following reduction in the transaortic gradient. Persistent inducibility of ventricular arrhythmias following surgical relief of outflow tract obstruction in a SCD survivor with aortic stenosis would constitute a rational indication for ICD implantation.

Two other lesions, also with potential for an ischemic basis of SCD in young patients, are (1) anomalous origin of the left coronary artery, either from the pulmonary artery or the right sinus of Valsalva [5,30]; and (2) acquired, progressive coronary insufficiency as a sequelae of Kawasaki's disease [31]. Coronary arteriography is indicated in young SCD survivors to exclude congenital coronary abnormalities, which are amenable to surgical reimplantation or revascularization. However, prior myocardial infarction associated with these lesions may establish an anatomic basis for reentrant ventricular arrhythmias (Fig. 1). Our experience in the evaluation of these patients suggest electrophysiological responses similar to adults with sustained ventricular tachycardia postinfarction [32].

3. Transposition of the Great Arteries

Sudden death has been reported in 2–8% of patients with transposition of the great arteries who have undergone a Mustard procedure for physiological correction of their defect [17,33,34]. A variety of atrial and ventricular arrhythmias have been implicated as the causes of SCD in these patients. There appears to be a strong correlation between atrial flutter and sudden death in these patients [16]. Second, recent concern has focused on sustained ventricular tachyarrhythmias, particularly in association with progressive right ventricular dysfunction [35]. And third, bradyarrhythmias, which may be a primary cause of SCD, or predispose to the subsequent development of tachyarrhythmias, are recognized to occur in 60–80% of these patients [36,37].

Determination of the mechanism of SCD in a patient with transposition of the great arteries requires consideration of the patient's basal rhythm, as well as atrial and ventricular tachyarrhythmias. In patients with atrial flutter and documented 1:1 AV conduction, AAI-antitachycardia pacing may represent an effective prophylaxis for recurrent life-threatening arrhythmias, if atrial flutter has been documented as the precursor of SCD [38]. For other patients, ventricular arrhythmias require definitive therapy, such as an ICD, while in other patients, the cause of SCD may not be clearly defined, in which case an ICD may also be indicated. In the initial report of ICD use in patients with congenital heart disease, transposition of the great arteries was the most commonly cited form of congenital heart disease [39].

With the extended use of the Fontan type of repair for a variety of complex congenital heart defects, an increased number of patients may be at risk for severe hemodynamic compromise and SCD associated with either atrial or ventricular tachyarrhythmias [40]. This concern is substantiated by the recent observation of the abrupt transition of a primary atrial tachycardia to ventricular fibrillation in a young patient with a prior atrial baffle procedure (Fig. 2) [41]. In contrast to patients with tetralogy of Fallot and, perhaps, aortic stenosis, a corrective surgical procedure is not an option in patients with transposition of the great arteries or single ventricle complex. In these patients, a primary application of the ICD may be to serve as a ''bridge'' to orthotopic heart transplantation [42]. As of this time, however, there is limited experience to support this proposal.

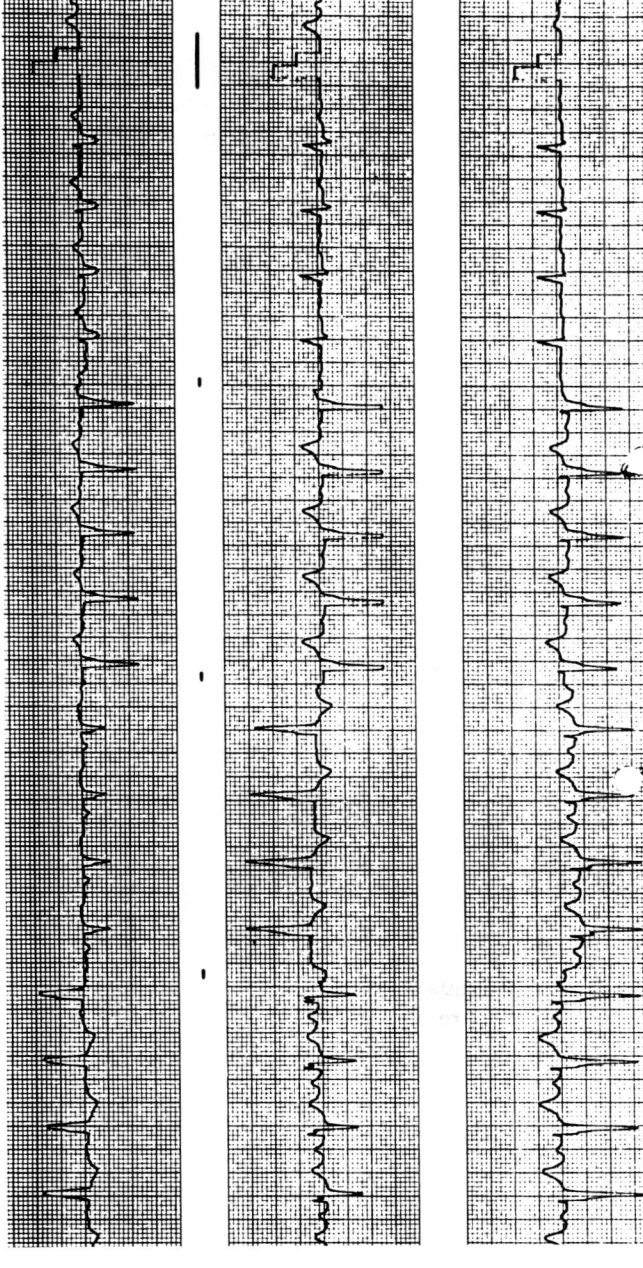

Figure 1 Electrocardiogram from a 13-year-old who was resuscitated from ventricular fibrillation, demonstrating a prior anterolateral myocardial infarction. Postresuscitation, coronary arteriography demonstrated anomalous origin of the left coronary artery from the left pulmonary artery. A left internal mammary artery graft to the left anterior descending was performed. No arrhythmias were inducible postoperatively, and none have been observed during ambulatory monitoring.

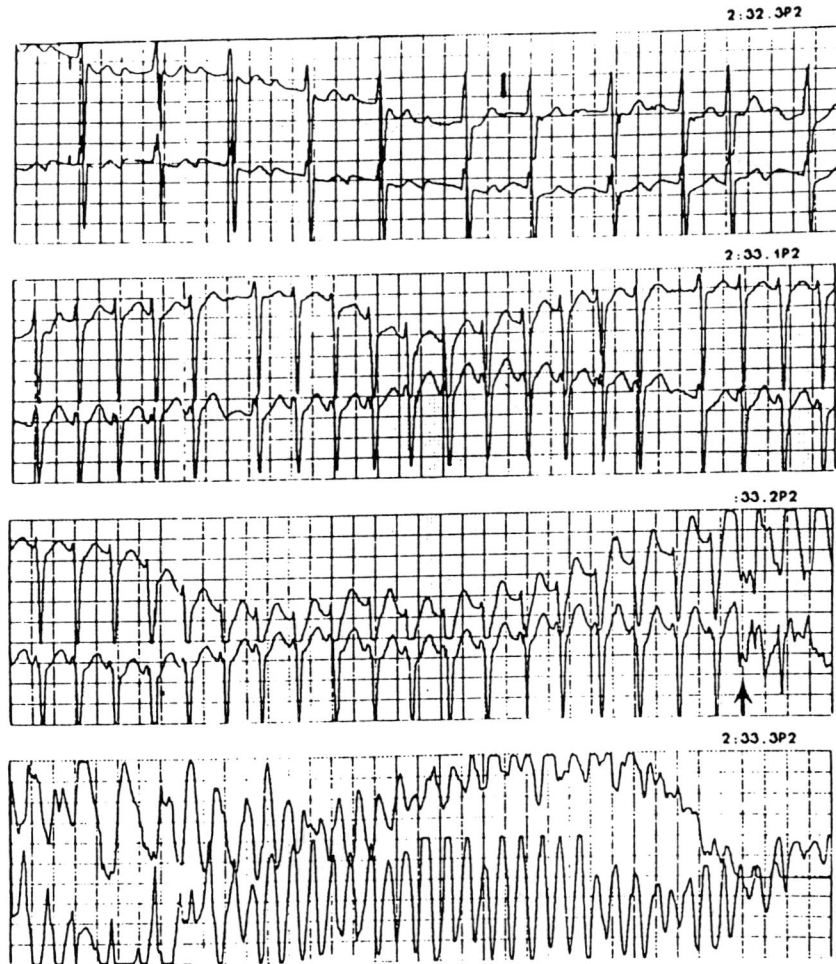

Figure 2 Ambulatory electrocardiographic recording in a 14-year-old with prior repair of anomalous pulmonary venous return. Supraventricular tachycardia, with 2:1 AV conduction, is initiated in the top panel. AV conduction changes to 1:1 in the second panel, with an abrupt change to ventricular fibrillation (arrow) in the third panel. Discharge of the ICD restored sinus rhythm 15 s after the onset of ventricular fibrillation. (From Ref. 40, with permission.)

B. Sudden Cardiac Death and Cardiomyopathies

1. Idiopathic Dilated Cardiomyopathies

Sudden death has reported in 4–15% of young patients with dilated cardiomyopathies, with a particularly poor prognosis in patients older than 2 years of age at time of diagnosis, and in those with persistent clinical congestive heart failure [43–45]. The precise role of ventricular arrhythmias in the genesis of SCD in patients with chronic congestive heart failure, and thus potential benefit of ICD therapy, remains controversial [46,47]. In a study of ambulatory ECG recordings preceding SCD in patients with dilated cardiomyopathy, either asystole, profound bradycardia or electromechanical dissociation were identified as the primary causes of SCD in patients *without* prior myocardial infarction [48]. Chen et al. have reported similar observations of bradyarrhythmic sudden death in children with dilated cardiomyopathy, while Friedman et al. have reported that neither atrial or nonsustained ventricular arrhythmias were independently predictive of sudden death [44,45].

Elucidation of the role of ventricular arrhythmias in SCD has been confounded by the lack of specificity of responses to programmed ventricular stimulation in patients with dilated cardiomyopathies [49]. It has been suggested that ventricular function is the primary determinant of long-term prognosis in these patients, and that nonsustained ventricular arrhythmias are a secondary manifestation of advanced cardiac dysfunction [47]. In contrast, symptomatic (syncopal) or sustained ventricular tachyarrhythmias do appear of critical prognostic importance [50]. In two studies of ICDs in young patients with dilated cardiomyopathies [51,52], inducibility of sustained ventricular arrhythmias was correlated with recurrent syncope or SCD.

In the initial study of the use of ICDs in young patients, dilated cardiomyopathies constituted the most frequent form of underling cardiovascular disease [52]. Given the negative inotrophic and proarrhythmic properties of antiarrhythmic drugs, sustained ventricular arrhythmias associated with dilated cardiomyopathies in young patients would appear to represent a rational substrate for ICD therapy, particularly second- and third-generation devices incorporating backup antibradycardia pacing capabilities [48].

Similar to patients with complex congenital heart defects, one consideration for ICD therapy in patients with dilated cardiomyopathies and symptomatic ventricular arrhythmias may be use as a "bridge" to orthotopic heart transplantation [42]. It is estimated that 25% of adults with severe congestive heart failure die suddenly while awaiting transplantation [53]. Although comparable data in children are not available, the period for donor procurement is two to four times longer for young patients than for their adult counterparts [54]. With the evolution of nonthoracotomy and transvenous ICD systems, this approach may acquire increased acceptance.

One specific subset of dilated cardiomyopathy which has been associated with SCD in young patients is arrhythmogenic right ventricular dysplasia (ARVD) (Fig. 3) [55]. Although the prevalence and natural history of ARVD have not been defined, familial clustering of cases of SCD has been reported [55]. The relative importance of the hemodynamic consequences of this disease versus the significance of ventricular tachycardia as related to SCD in ARVD remain controversial. In the initial report of ICD (automatic implantable defibrillator) use in humans in 1980, the second patient to receive a device was a 16-year-old boy with probable ARVD [56]. Use of ICDs in other patients with ARVD has subsequently been reported, although alternative forms of treatment, such a such disarticulation of the right ventricle or catheter fulguration of the sites of tachycardia, have also been advocated.

2. Hypertrophic Cardiomyopathy

Hypertrophic cardiomyopathy is one cardiovascular disease which has been consistently cited in studies of SCD in young patients [1–4]. SCD is a major problem in these young patients, with an estimated annual event rate of 3–6%, compared to a 2–3% annual SCD event rate in adults [57]. In a collaborative study of children and adolescents with hypertrophic cardiomyopathy, preexcitation and a positive family history were correlated with SCD [58]. Of note, the severity of left ventricular hypertrophy has not been demonstrated to be a predictive correlate of SCD in young patients [59].

Ventricular arrhythmias have been documented to be one mechanism of SCD in adults with hypertrophic cardiomyopathy [60,61]. Although a causal relationship is less certain in young patients, McKenna et al. have reported improved survival with the empiric use of amiodarone

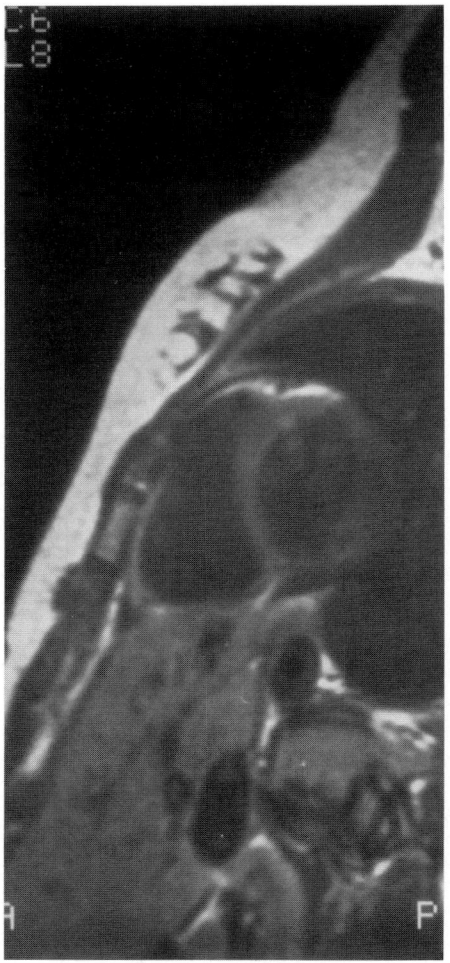

Figure 3 (A) T2 weighted, LAO projection magnetic resonance image of the right and left ventricles in a patient with arrhythmogenic right ventricular dysplasia who had documented polymorphic ventricular tachycardia and syncope during strenuous exercise. The right ventricle can be seen to be enlarged in this diastolic frame when compared to the left ventricle. (B) Lateral projection of diastolic frame of a right ventricular angiogram in same patient, showing scalloping of the diaphragmatic surface of the right ventricle and a lumpy, foamy appearance of the anterior surface of the right ventricle. (C) PA diastolic frame of the same patient as in (A) and (B), showing a scalloped appearance of the right ventricular anterior septum and enlarged total right ventricular volume.

in young patients with hypertrophic cardiomyopathies and documented tachyarrhythmias, syncope, or a positive family history of SCD [62].

The mechanisms of SCD may be age-related in young patients with hypertrophic cardiomyopathy, who are at the age when the risk of SCD is perceived to be the greatest [57,62]. Evaluation for supraventricular tachycardias, in particular those involving accessory AV connections, as well as ventricular tachycardias, is mandated. Electrophysiological testing may be

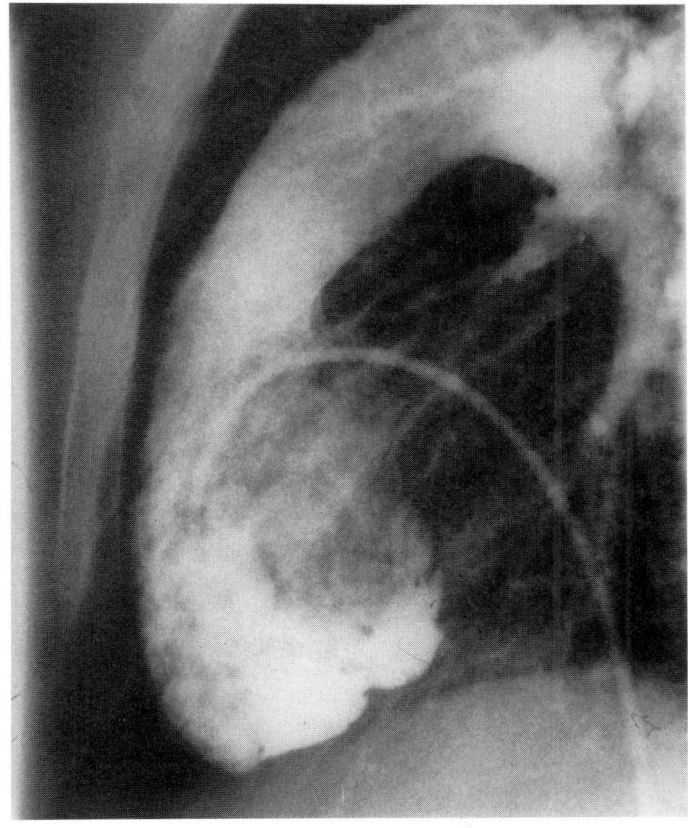

(B)

of prognostic value, as inducible, sustained ventricular arrhythmias appear to be associated with cardiac arrest or prior syncope [63]. Recently, the results of programmed ventricular stimulation have been reported in 30 patients with hypertrophic cardiomyopathy who were survivors of SCD: Sustained ventricular arrhythmias were inducible in 21, of whom 17 received an ICD. During follow-up there were 4 sudden deaths and ICD discharge in 4 other patients [63].

Studies of the long-term outcome of patients with hypertrophic cardiomyopathy successfully resuscitated from SCD suggest that approximately 40% will experience another event [64]; however, criteria to risk stratify these patients remain elusive. Successful utilization of ICDs in young patients with hypertrophic cardiomyopathy with either syncope or aborted SCD have been reported in three series to date [39,51,52].

C. Sudden Death and Primary Electrical Diseases

Primary electrical diseases, either idiopathic ventricular fibrillation or long QT syndromes, were the cardiovascular diagnoses in 45% of young patients to receive ICDs in the initial analysis of these devices [52]. While two other primary electrical diseases, the Wolff-Parkinson-White syndrome and complete atrioventricular block, may also result in SCD in young patients [6], ICD therapy will not be considered as an appropriate therapy in these patients.

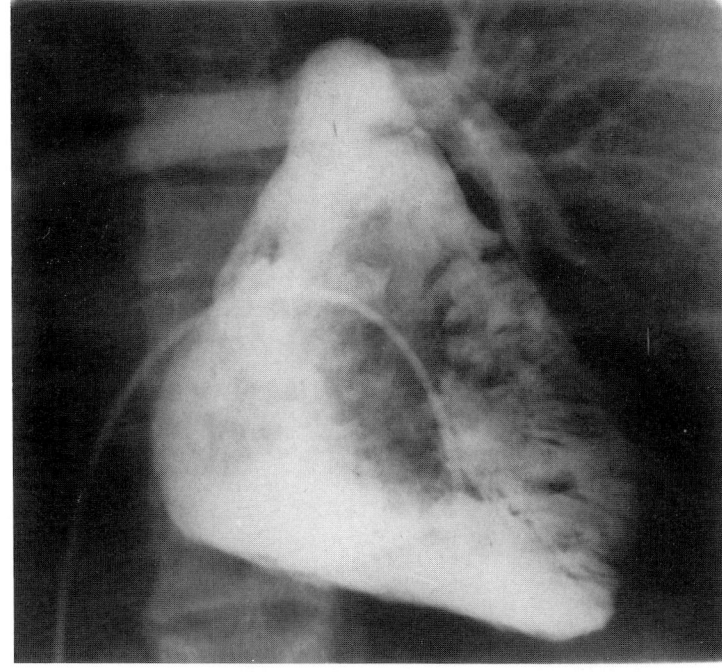

(C)

Figure 3 continued

1. Idiopathic Ventricular Fibrillation

It is estimated that in 8% of *young* patients referred for evaluation after resuscitation from ventricular fibrillation, an etiology cannot be defined, in spite of extensive evaluation [65]. In these patients the term "idiopathic ventricular fibrillation" has been applied [66]. Idiopathic ventricular fibrillation appears to be a clinical entity involving primarily adolescents and young adults. Awareness of this diagnosis is critical, as the annual recurrence risk of SCD has been estimated to be as high as 11% [66]. Although limited data are available to characterize these patients, recurrences of polymorphic, nonsustained ventricular tachycardia appear to be the primary clinical marker [67] (Fig. 4). In approximately 25%, syncope in association with palpitations has also been reported [66].

A distinction must be made between idiopathic ventricular fibrillation and idiopathic monomorphic ventricular tachycardia of childhood, which generally has a favorable prognosis [68]. The primary clinical entities which deserve consideration in a young patient with unexplained SCD are the long QT syndromes, myocarditis, myocardial bridging, coronary spasm, or ARVD. Although the definitive exclusion of many of these entities may be debated, the guarded prognosis for the young patient with unexplained (or idiopathic) ventricular fibrillation mandates caution and an exhaustive evaluation.

Electrophysiological testing in these patients has resulted primarily in induction of polymorphic ventricular tachycardia or ventricular fibrillation [69]. Electropharmacological testing has indicated potential suppression of inducibility with class IA drugs (primarily quinidine), although long-term efficacy has not been reported [67]. Given the guarded prognosis (based on limited data), and the questionable significance of polymorphic ventricular tachycardia or ven-

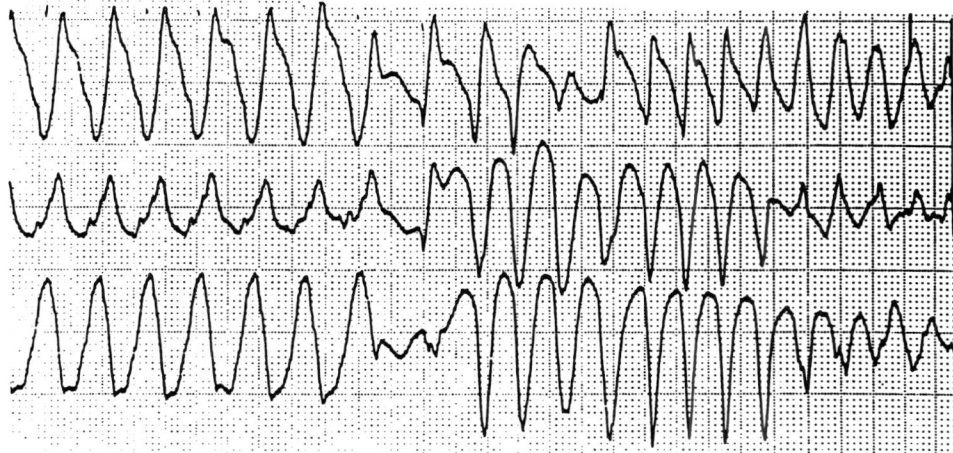

Figure 4 Electrocardiographic monitoring demonstrating polymorphic, nonsustained, ventricular tachycardia in a 16-year-old with recurrent syncope but no identifiable cardiovascular disease. Ventricular fibrillation was inducible during programmed stimulation.

tricular fibrillation as responses to programmed ventricular stimulation [70], use of ICD therapy would appear to be a rational approach to such patients. Limited clinical data thus far reported appear to validate this conclusion [66,71].

2. Prolonged QT Syndromes

The prolonged QT syndromes represent a spectrum of electrophysiological disorders, characterized by electrocardiographic corrected QT (QTc) interval >0.45 s, repolarization abnormalities, and a propensity for the development of recurrent polymorphic ventricular tachycardia, termed "torsade de pointes" [72]. The prolonged QT interval syndromes may represent a more malignant form of disease in younger patients, with an estimated annual risk of SCD of 4–6%, compared to 1–2% in adults [73].

Consideration of a spectrum of prolonged QT syndromes is required in young patients, some of whom have bradycardia-mediated ventricular tachyarrhythmias, at times associated with rate-dependent atrioventricular block [74]. In these patients, pacemaker implantation for chronotrophic support appears to be an effective form of prophylaxis in the prevention of recurrent syncope and polymorphic ventricular tachycardia [75]. Conversely, other forms of the prolonged QT syndrome appear to be due to autonomic imbalance, with various degrees of efficacy reported for treatment with beta-blockade or left cervicothoracic sympathectomy [76,77].

In approximately 5% of patients with the prolonged QT syndromes, the aforementioned forms of therapy will not provide an effective form of prophylaxis against recurrent syncope, ventricular arrhythmias, or SCD [78]. Hence, an estimated 70 patients with long QT syndromes have received an ICD to date [79,80]. Given the limited value of programmed ventricular stimulation in patients with the long QT syndrome [81], increased utilization of ICD therapy, in conjunction with beta-blockade, as a primary mode of therapy for the long QT syndromes is probable.

IV. CONSIDERATIONS IN THE USE OF ICDS IN YOUNG PATIENTS

Following the decision to implant an ICD in a young patient, considerations of anatomy, electrophysiology, patient size and body habitus must be made. These factors must be made evaluated individually, tailored to specific parameters of each patient. The following analysis of these factors is based on our experience in the use of these devices in young patients.

A. Anatomy

Approximately 20–25% of young patients evaluated for ICD implantation will have some form of congenital heart disease [52]. In these patients, two types of anatomic abnormalities associated with congenital heart disease must be considered prior to ICD implantation: anomalies of systemic and pulmonary venous return, and variations of coronary artery anatomy.

Due to relatively small patient size, or extensive adhesions due to prior cardiac surgery, a superior vena cava-right atrial spring to apical patch configuration of the defibrillation electrodes may be preferable [82]. A precise evaluation of systemic venous return is warranted in young patients, due to the potential for persistence of the left superior vena cava to coronary sinus, or stenosis of the right atrial/superior vena caval junction as a consequence of prior atrial surgery.

Persistence of the left superior vena cava to the coronary sinus is usually associated with absence (involution) of the left brachiocephalic vein [83]. Thus, the spring must be inserted via the right internal jugular or right subclavian vein to achieve conventional location at the superior vena cava-right atrial junction (Fig. 5). Persistence of the left superior vena cava also may result in relative hypoplasia of the right superior vena cava, with an increased risk of caval obstruction and subsequent thrombosis. Considerations for thromboembolic risk must be made in any patient with potential for an intracardiac right-to-left shunt [84].

Abnormalities of coronary artery distribution associated with certain congenital heart defects may require angiographic definition prior to the placement of epicardial patches, to allow a surgical approach to avoid positioning the patch electrodes directly over the main coronary arteries. Figure 6 demonstrates the ICD patch configuration in a young patient with ventricular inversion.

One general consideration is the surgical approach to ICD placement in the young patient. This will be predicated on a number of factors, including prior surgery, anatomical abnormalities, and concommitant surgical procedures. In general, an anterolateral thoracotomy has been our preferred approach for a two-patch system, unless the patient is undergoing concommitant cardiac surgery. For patients with the long QT syndrome, defibrillator patch placement may be combined with performance of a left cervicothoracic sympathectomy via a left thoracotomy (Fig. 7). These surgical considerations may be superseded by the further development of nonthoracotomy and transvenous ICD systems in the near future [85,86].

The potential for problems related to placement of defibrillator patches on the growing heart have not been defined. Given small patient size and limitations of epicardial surface area, utilization of two 10-cm^2 patches is frequently required. Studies to provide prospective serial evaluation of ventricular function and long-term stability of defibrillation thresholds are required in young patients [87]. However the significance of these concerns remains conjectural, and may be superseded by further development of nonthoracotomy and transvenous patch configurations (Fig. 8).

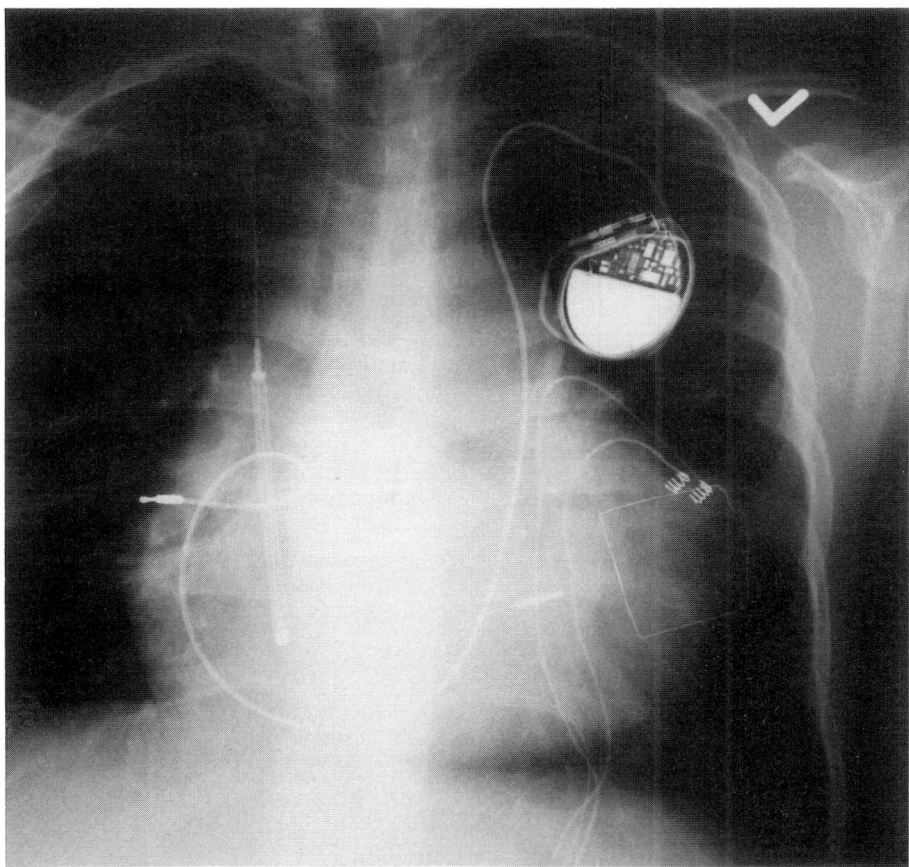

Figure 5 Tandem implantation of a transvenous atrial pacemaker and a spring-coil ICD in a young patient with persistence of the left superior vena cava in association with congenital heart disease. The spring was inserted via the right internal jugular vein and advanced to the high right atrium. A 10-cm^2 apical patch and two epicardial ventricular rate-sensing electrodes are present. The bipolar atrial pacing lead was inserted via the left subclavian vein and advanced through the left superior vena cava to the coronary sinus with lead fixation at the high right atrial free wall.

B. Electrophysiology

The capability of ICDs to detect and terminate sustained ventricular tachyarrhythmias in adults has been clearly documented [88]. However, as noted earlier, there is less certainty regarding the role of ventricular tachyarrhythmias in the genesis of SCD in young patients, in whom both bradyarrhythmias and atrial tachyarrhythmias have been implicated as etiologies of SCD.

1. ICD Tachycardia Detection

The use of rate criteria to differentiate sinus or supraventricular (SVT) from ventricular tachycardia (VT) in a young patient is a difficult problem. As the rates of sinus tachycardia may exceed 200 beats/min in young patients, differentiation of sinus from pathological tachycardias by rate criteria alone remains problematic [89]. Programmable ICD functions (tachycardia

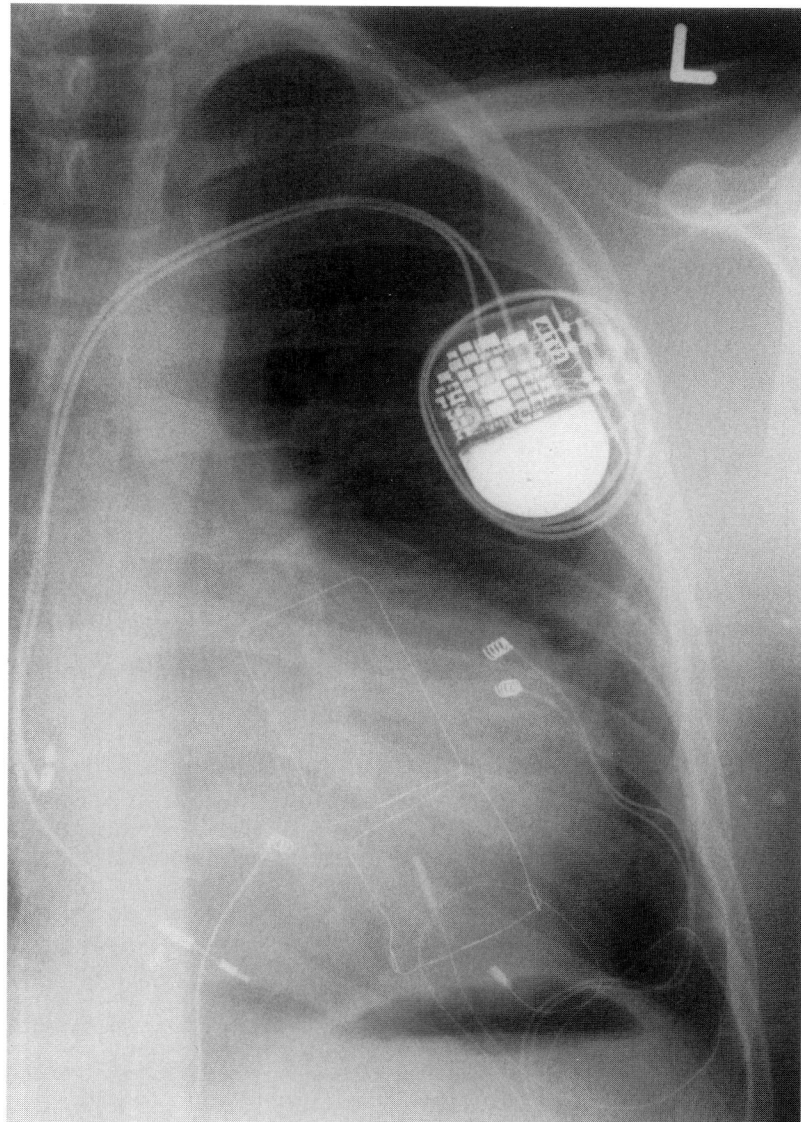

Figure 6 Chest roentgenogram (posteroanterior) demonstrating epicardial ICD patch, rate-sensing, and transvenous pacemaker lead configurations in an 18-year-old with ventricular inversion, atrioventricular block, and recurrent syncopal ventricular tachycardia. The endocardial bipolar ventricular pacing lead is at the apex of the morphologic left ventricle. The ICD patches and rate-sensing electrodes are positioned to the right of the left anterior descending coronary artery, over the systemic (morphologic) right ventricle.

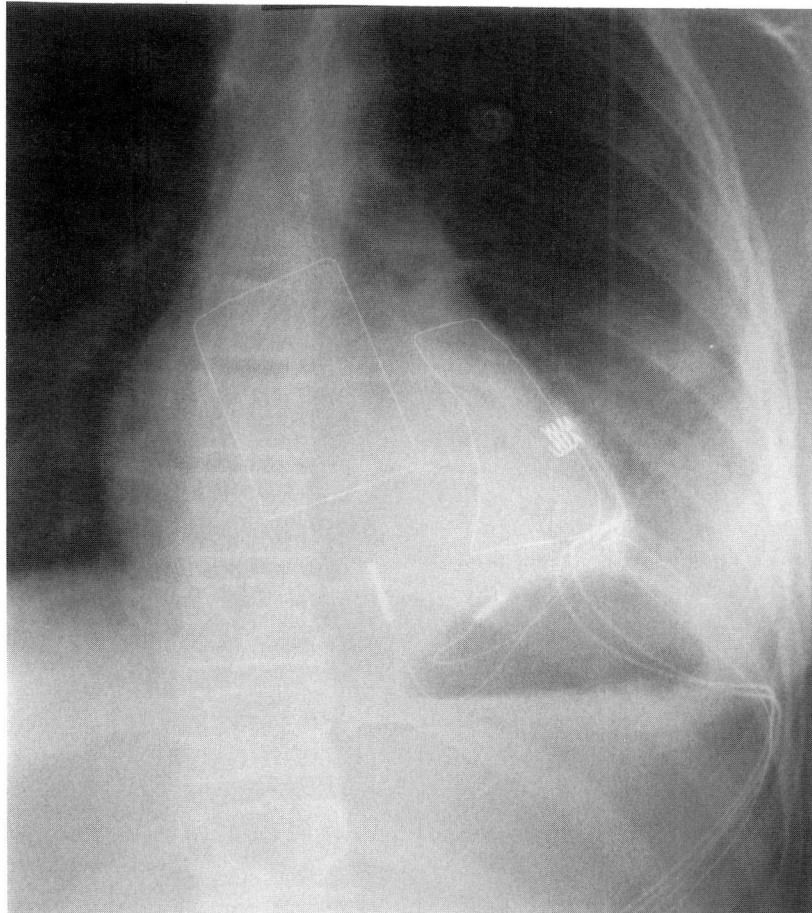

Figure 7 Chest roentgenogram of the ICD patch configuration placed via a left thoractomy in a patient resuscitated from ventricular fibrillation associated with the long QT syndrome. A left cervicothoracic sympathectomy was concomitantly performed via extension of the left thoracotomy at the time of ICD implantation.

detection interval) may allow this differentiation, provided the cycle length of sinus tachycardia is distinctly longer than that of the pathological tachycardia; otherwise, concomitant use of beta-blockade, or perhaps low-dose amiodarone, may be required [82].

Differentiation between SVT and VT presents even greater complexities, as the two frequently cannot be differentiated by rate criteria [90]. Future-generation devices may address this problem, by incorporating both atrial and ventricular sensing leads as a means of differentiating VT from SVT, in patients with VA dissociation during VT or less than 1:1 AV conduction during SVT [91]. Conversely, morphological analysis of the ventricular electrogram, based on template-matching methods, may allow the differentiation of SVT from VT, without the requirement for an additional pair of atrial sensing electrodes [92].

Due to extremely rapid rates, ventricular fibrillation has been reliably differentiated from other tachycardias by electrogram rate (or probability density function) methods. One

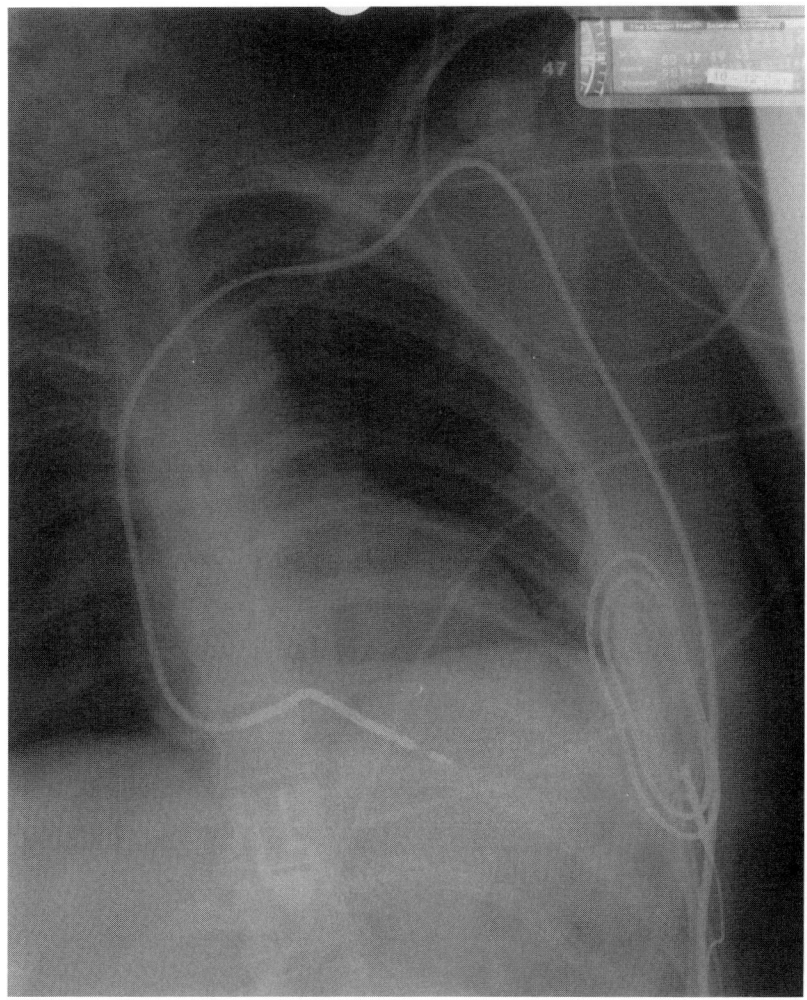

Figure 8 Chest roentgenogram (posteroanterior view) of a 12-year-old survivor of ventricular fibrillation associated with the long QT syndrome. The transvenous electrode catheter, positioned at the apex of the right ventricle, is capable of sensing and pacing, and functions as the common cathode during ICD discharge. An epicostal patch electrode (anode) has been positioned at the left midaxillary line at the fourth intercostal space.

theoretical concern in young patients, due to their relatively thin-walled ventricles, is the adequacy and consistency of local ventricular electrogram amplitudes during VF to allow consistent electrogram detection [93]. Thus far, this has not been reported as a clinical problem.

A final sensing consideration are the episodes of polymorphic, nonsustained VT associated with the long QT syndrome or its variants. The average sense time for rate-only devices is between 6 intervals and 10 s. The use of ICDs with the capability of ''second-look'' electrogram rate analysis following capacitor charging, or programmable extension of the duration of

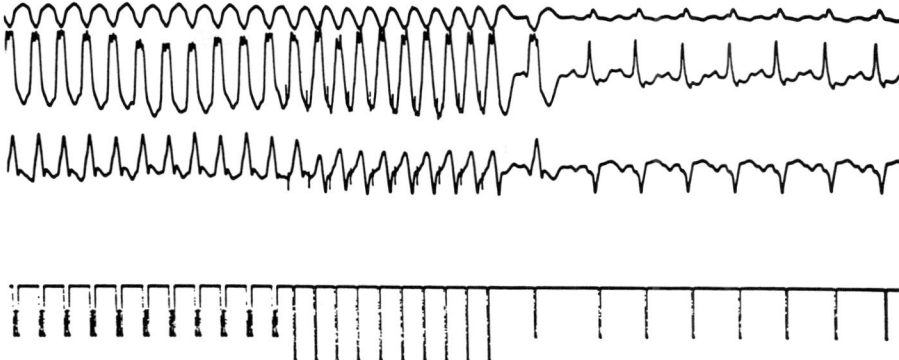

Figure 9 Overdrive pace termination of sustained monomorphic ventricular tachycardia (VT) by an ICD in a 15-year-old who had an anterolateral myocardial infarction associated with Kawasaki disease. Three electrocardiographic leads and a fourth marker channel are presented. The first 11 beats are sensed VT, cycle length 380 ms, followed by 10 paced beats at cycle length 300 ms. Sinus rhythm is restored following the termination of overdrive pacing. Bundle branch aberrancy is present in the first beat of sinus rhythm.

tachycardia to satisfy detection criteria prior to patient shock, may prove valuable in these patients. This may prevent a number of "spurious" ICD discharges, which may be painful for the patient and potentially arrhythmogenic [94,95].

2. ICD Therapies

Given the relative prevalence of bradyarrhythmias as etiologies of SCD in young patients, many patients who received first-generation devices also required implantation of a separate pacemaker system. This resulted in a number of problems related to ICD–pacemaker interactions, along with additional complexities of patient care and follow-up [96]. The incorporation of backup VVI pacing in second-generation ICDs has resolved some of these complexities and concerns regarding primary or postshock bradyarrhythmias as mechanisms of SCD [48,97]. The use of devices incorporating backup pacing capabilities appear warranted in young patients who require ICD therapy.

Similar to epicardial pacing leads, threshold problems have been a problem with pacing and sensing in ICD systems incorporating epicardial lead systems. Given the need for extended longevity of the ICD lead systems in younger patients, the placement of a third (extra) epicardial lead, at time of initial implant, may prevent the need for later reoperation due to lead sensing/capture failure.

As discussed earlier, the long-term stability of defibrillation thresholds (DFTs) in young patients, with growing hearts, has not been studied. Due to the potential for an increase in DFTs with time, the goal of a first-shock rescue, at a DFT of 5 J or less, should be the target at the time of initial ICD implant in a young patient.

The develoment of ICDs capable of tiered therapies, i.e., overdrive pacing, cardioversion, and defibrillation, may expand the indications for, and utilization of, these devices in young patients [98]. This may apply particularly to young patients with recurrent sustained VT (Fig. 9). Overdrive pace termination of VT may provide the only therapy required; however, backup defibrillator capability is mandated, due to the potential for acceleration and degeneration of VT into VF [99].

One proposed, but not approved, indication for implantation of an ICD is recurrent atrial flutter with a rapid ventricular response. Although this is a relatively common problem and has been demonstrated to be a cause of SCD in the young, we are unaware of any device implantations specifically for this indication. However, we have observed the termination of atrial flutter in one young patient with a superior vena cava spring-apical patch electrode configuration on several occasions (Fig. 2). Additionally, placement of one defibrillator patch on the right atrium, in patients with unacceptable defibrillation thresholds with a patch over the infero-basal right ventricle, has been reported [100]. With this configuration, device discharge in response to a detected ventricular cycle length satisfying tachycardia detection criteria would in theory also terminate reentrant atrial tachyarrhythmias. However, there are many concerns regarding the use of ICDs for atrial arrhythmias. One is that a patient likely would not lose consciousness prior to discharge, resulting in painful shocks. Continued advances in device technology will be required to resolve this problem. With the current configuration of ICDs, patients with atrial flutter and a 1:1 ventricular response would satisfy "ventricular" tachycardia detection criteria.

V. FUTURE CONSIDERATIONS

Sudden cardiac death in the young patient represents a final common mode of expression for a number of heterogeneous substrates of cardiovascular diseases and associated arrhythmias. Given the diversity of disease processes and arrhythmias, the use of ICDs in young patients requires devices capable of a number of complex arrhythmia termination algorithms. The development of second-generation ICDs with both software-based programmable sensing and backup VVI pacing functions, and third-generation devices capable of tiered therapies, clearly represent improvements over earlier devices. Furthermore, the clinical trials of completely transvenous systems suggests the potential for even greater application of these devices.

As the vast majority of these devices are implanted in adults, there appears to be minimal impetus for industry to develop alternative capacitor systems, which would allow further reduction in generator size [101]. The use of biphasic, sequential shocks may reduce the absolute energy requirements for defibrillation, although this remains investigational [102].

The greatest benefit, and potentially the primary application of ICD therapy in young patients, will be the prophylactic prevention of SCD [103]. The identification of young patients who have not yet experienced a life-threatening arrhythmia, but also have a clinical profile suggesting that this is likely, is one of the primary contemporary challenges of pediatric electrophysiology. However, the prophylactic use of ICDs in high-risk young patients will likely be confounded by economic as well as medical and technical considerations [104,105].

REFERENCES

1. Molander N. Sudden natural death in later childhood and adolescence. Arch Dis Child 1982; 57:572-576.
2. Neuspiel DR, Kuller LH. Sudden and unexpected death in childhood and adolescence. JAMA 1985; 254:1321-1325.
3. Driscoll DJ, Edwards JE. Sudden unexpected death in children and adolescents. J Am Coll Cardiol 1985; 5:118B-121B.
4. Benson DW, Benditt DG, Anderson RW, et al. Cardiac arrest in young, ostensibly healthy patients: clinical, hemodynamic, and electrophysiologic findings. Am J Cardiol 1983; 52:65-69.
5. Silka MJ, Kron J, Walance CG, Cutler JE, McAnulty JH. Assessment and follow-up of pediatric survivors of sudden cardiac death. Circulation 1990; 82:341-349.

6. Denfeld SW, Garson A. Sudden death in children and young adults. Ped Clin N Am 1990; 37:215-231.
7. Eisenberg MS, Cummins RO, Damon S, Larsen MP, Hearne TR. Survival rates from out-of-hospital cardiac arrest: recommendations for uniform definitions and data to report. Ann Emerg Med 1990; 19:1249-1259.
8. Dreifus LS, Fisch C, Griffin JC, Gillette PC, Mason JW, Parsonnet V. Guidelines for implantation of cardiac pacemakers and antitachycardia Devices. Circulation 1991; 84:455-464.
9. Lehmann MH, Snksena S. Implantable cardioverter defibrillators in cardiovascular practice: reports of the policy Conference of the North American Society of Pacing and Electrophysiology. PACE 969–979.
10. Winkle R. State-of-the-art of the AICD. PACE 1991; 14:961-966.
11. Eisenberg M, Bergner L, Hallstrom A. Epidemiology of cardiac arrest and resuscitation in children. Ann Emerg Med 1983; 12:672-674.
12. Valenzuela TD, Spiate DW, Meislin HW, Clark LL, Wright AL, Ewy GA: Case and survival definitions in out-of-hospital cardiac arrest. JAMA 1992; 267:272-274.
13. Walsh CK, Krongrad E. Terminal cardiac electrical activity in pediatric patients. Am J Cardiol 1983; 51:557-561.
14. Lambert EC, Menon VA, Wagner HR, Vlad P. Sudden unexpected death from cardiovascular disease in children. Am J Cardiol 1974; 34:89-96.
15. Garson A, McNamara DG. Sudden death in a pediatric cardiology population, 1958–1983: relation to prior arrhythmias. J Am Coll Cardiol 1985; 5:134B-137B.
16. Garson A, Bink-Boelkens M, Hesslein PS, et al. Atrial flutter in the young: a collaborative study of 380 cases. J Am Coll Cardiol 1985; 6:871-878.
17. Morris CD, Menashe VD. 25 year mortality after surgical repair of congenital heart defect in childhood. JAMA 1991; 266:3447-3452.
18. Kavey REW, Blackman MA, Sondheimer HM. Incidence and severity of chronic ventricular dysrhythmias after repair of tetralogy of Fallot. Am Heart J 1982; 103:342-350.
19. Garson A, Nihill MR, McNamara DG, Cooley DA. Status of the adult and adolescent after repair of tetralogy of Fallot. Circulation 1979; 59:1232-1240.
20. Wolff GS, Rowland TW, Ellison TC. Surgically induced right bundle block with left anterior hemiblock. Circulation 1972; 46:587-594.
21. Garson A, Randall DC, Gillette PC, et al. Prevention of sudden death after repair of tetralogy of Fallot: treatment of ventricular arrhythmias. J Am Coll Cardiol 1985; 6:221-227.
22. Gillette PC, Yoeman MA, Mullins CE, et al. Sudden death after repair of tetralogy of Fallot: electrocardiographic and electrophysiologic abnormalities. Circulation 1977; 56:566-571.
23. Garson A, Porter CJ, Gillette PC, McNamara DG. Induction of ventricular tachycardia during electrophysiologic study after repair of tetralogy of Fallot. J Am Coll Cardiol 1983; 1:1493-1502.
24. Chandar JS, Wolff GS, Garson A, et al. Ventricular arhythmias in postoperative tetralogy of Fallot. Am J Cardiol 1990; 65:655-661.
25. Harken AH, Horowitz LN, Josephson ME. Surgical correction of recurrent sustained ventricular tachycardia following complete repair of tetralogy of Fallot. J Thor Cardiovasc Surg 1980; 80:779-781.
26. Zahka KG, Horneffer PJ, Rowe SA. Long-term valvular function after total repair of tetralogy of Fallot. Circulation 1988; 78(suppl I):14-19.
27. Deal BJ, Scagliotti D, Miller SM, Gallastegui JL, Hariman RJ, Levitsky S. Electrophysiologic drug testing in symptomatic ventricular arrhythmias after repair of tetralogy of Fallot. Am J Cardiol 1987; 59:1380-1385.
28. Campbell M. Natural history of congenital arotic stenosis. Br Heart J 1968; 30:514-526.
29. Richards AM, Nicholls MG, Ikram H, Hamilton EJ, Richards RD. Syncope in aortic valvular stenosis. Lancet 1984; II:1113-1117.
30. Cheitlin MI, DeCastro CM, McAllister HA. Sudden death as a complication of anomalous left coronary artery origin from the anterior sinus of Valsalva. Circulation 1974; 50:780-787.

31. Nakano H, Saito A, Ueda K. Nojima K. Clinical characteristics of myocardial infarction following Kawasaki disease: report of 11 cases. J Pediatr 1986; 108:198-203.
32. Silka MJ, Kron J, Cutler JE, McAnulty JH. Analysis of programmed stimulation methods in the evaluation of ventricular arrhythmias in patients 20 years old and younger. Am J Cardiol 1990; 66:826-830.
33. Scott LP, Saallouke MG, Shapiro SR, et al. Sudden unexpected death following Mustard's procedure for transposition of the great arteries. Circulation 1976; 54 (Suppl II):89 (ABS)
34. Flinn CJ, Wolff GS, Dick II, M, et al. Cardiac rhythm after the Mustard operation for complete reposition of the great arteries. N Engl J Med 1984; 310:1635-1638.
35. Gewellig M, Cullen S, Mertens B, Lesaffre, Deanfield J. Risk factors for arrhythmia and death after Mustard operation for simple transposition of the great arteries after atrial switch. Circulation 1991(suppl III):187-192.
36. Silka MJ, Manwill J, Kron J, McAnulty JH. Bradycardia-mediated tachyarrhythmias in congenital heart defects and responses to pacing at physiologic rates. Am J Cardiol 1990 65:488-493.
37. Hayes CJ, Gersony WM. Arrhythmias after the Mustard operaton for transposition of the great arteries: a long-term study. J Am Coll Cardiol 1986; 7:133-137.
38. Gillette PC, Wampler DG, Shannon C, et al. Use of cardiac pacing after the Mustard operation for transposition of the great arteries. J Am Coll Cardiol 1986; 7:138-141.
39. Kral MA, Spotnitz HM, Hordof A, Bigger JT, Steinberg JS, Livelli FD. Automatic implantable cardioverter defibrillator implantation from malignant ventricular arrhythmias associated with congenital heart disease. Am J Cardiol 1989; 63:118-119.
40. Silka MJ, Kron J, McAnulty J. Supraventricular tachyarrhythmias, congenital heart disease, and sudden cardiac death. Ped Cardiol 1992; 13:116-118.
41. Bolling SF, Deeb M, Morady F, et al. Automatic internal cardioverter-defibrillator: a bridge to heart transplantation. J Heart Lung Transplant 1991; 10:562-566.
42. Weber HS, Hellenbrand WE, Kleinman CS, Perlmutter RA, Rosenfeld LE. Predictors of rhythm disturbances and subsequent morbidity after the Fontan operation. Am J Cardiol 1989; 64:762-767.
43. Griffin ML, Hernandez A, Martin TC, et al. Dilated cardiomyopathy in infants and children. J Am Coll Cardiol 1988; 11:139-144.
44. Chen S-C, Nouri S, Balfour I, Jureidni S, Appleton RS. Clincal profile of congestive cardiomyopathy in children. J Am Coll Cardiol 1990; 15:189-193.
45. Friedman RA, Moak JP, Garson A. Clinical course of idiopathic dilated cardiomyopathy in children. J Am Coll Cardiol 1991; 18:152-156.
46. Gersony WM. The child with dilated cardiomyopathy: prognostic considerations and management decisions. J Am Coll Cardiol 1991; 18:157-158.
47. Packer M. Lack of relation between ventricular arrhythmias and sudden death in patients with chronic heart failure. Circulation 1992; 85(suppl I):50-56.
48. Luu ML, Stevenson WG, Stevenson LW, Baron K, Walden J. Diverse mechanisms of unexpected cardiac arrest in advanced heart failure. Circulation 1989; 80:1675-1680.
49. Poll DS, Marchlinski FE, Buxton AE, Josephson ME. Usefulness of programmed stimulation in idiopathic dilated cardiomyopathy. Am J Cardiol 1986; 58:992-997.
50. de Luna AB, Coumel P, Leclercp JF. Ambulatory sudden cardiac death: mechanisms of production of fatal arrhythmias on the basis of data from 157 cases. Am Heart J 1989; 117:151-159.
51. Kaminer SJ, Pickhoff AS, Dunnigan A, Sterba R, Wolff GS. Cardiomyopathy and the use of implanted cardio-defibrillators in children. PACE 1990; 13:593-597.
52. Kron J, Oliver RP, Norsted S, Silka MJ. The automatic implantable cardioverter defibrillator in young patients. J Am Coll Cardiol 1990; 16:896-902.
53. Stevenson WG, Stevenson LW, Weiss J, Tillisch JH. Inducible ventricular arrhythmias and sudden death during vasodilator therapy of severe congestive heart failure. Am Heart J 1986; 116: 1447-1454.
54. Evans RW. Can society afford pediatric heart transplantations? J Heart Lung Transplant 1991; 10:867-871.

55. Theine G, Nava A, Corrado D, Rossi L, Pennelli N. Right ventricular cardiomyopathy and sudden death in young people. N Engl J Med 1988; 318:129-133.
56. Mirowski M, Reid PR, Mower MM, et al. Termination of malignant ventricular arrhythmias with an implanted automatic defibrillator in humans. N Engl J Med 1980; 303:322-324.
57. Maron BJ, Fananapazir L. Sudden cardiac death in hypertrophic cardiomyopathy. Circulation 1992; 85(suppl I):57-63.
58. Hordof A, Kuehl K, Vetter V. Risk factors for sudden death in patients with hypertrophic obstructive cardiomyopathy (abstr). Circulation 1988; 78:595.
59. Romeo F, Cianfrocca C, Pelliccia F, Collorida V, Cristofani R, Reale A. Long-term prognosis in children with hypertrophic cardiomyopathy: an analysis of 37 patients aged < 14 years at diagnosis. Clin Cardiol 1990; 13:101-107.
60. Nicod P, Polikar R, Peterson KL. Hypertrophic cardiomyopathy and sudden death. N Engl J Med 1988; 318:1255-1257.
61. Gillgan DM, Missouris CG, Boyd MJ, Oakley CM. Sudden death due to ventricular tachycardia during amiodarone therapy in familial hypertrophic cardiomyopathy. Am J Cardiol 1991; 68:971-973.
62. McKenna WJ, Franklin RCG, Nihoyannopoulos P, et al. Arrhythmia and prognosis in infants, children and adolescents with hypertrophic cardiomyopathy. J Am Coll Cardiol 1988; 11:147-153.
63. Fananapazir L, Epstein SE. Hemodynamic and electrophysiologic evaluation of patients with hypertrophic cardiomyopathy surviving cardiac arrest. Am J Cardiol 1991; 67:280-287.
64. Cecchi F, Maron BJ, Epstein SE. Long-term outcome of patients with hypertrophic cardiomyopathy successfully resuscitated from cardiac arrest. Am J Coll Cardiol 1989; 13:1283-1288.
65. Topaz O, Perin E, Cox M, Mallon SM, Castellanos A, Myerburg RJ. Young adult survivors of sudden cardiac arrest; analysis of invasive evaluation of 22 subjects. Am Heart J 1989; 118:281-287.
66. Viskin S, Belhassen B. Idiopathic ventricular fibrillation. Am Heart J 1990; 120:662-671.
67. Lemery R, Brugada P, Bella PD, Duginier T, Wellens HJJ. Ventricular fibrillation in six adults without overt heart disease. J Am Coll Cardiol 1989; 13:911-916.
68. Deal BJ, Miller SM, Scagliotti, Prechel D, Gallastegui JL, Hariman RJ. Ventricular tachycardia in a young population without overt heart disease. Circulation 1986; 73:1111-1118.
69. Belhassen B, Shapira I, Shosani D, Paredes A, Miller H, Laniado S. idiopathic ventricular fibrillation: inducibility and beneficial effects of class I antiarrhythmic agents. Circulation 1987; 75:809-816.
70. Wellens HJJ, Brugada P, Stevenson WG. Programmed electrical stimulation of the heart in patients with life-threatening ventricular arrhythmias: what is the signficance of induced arrhythmias and what is the correct stimulation protocol? Circulation 1985; 72:1-7.
71. Wellens HJJ, Lemery R, Smeets JL, et al. Sudden arrhythmic death without overt heart disease. Circulation 1992; 85 (suppl I):92-97.
72. Schwartz PJ, Periti M, Malliani A. The long QT syndrome. Am Heart J 1975; 89:378-390.
73. Weintraub RG, Gow RM, Wilkinson JL. The congenital long QT syndromes in childhood. J. Am Coll Cardiol 1990; 16:674-680.
74. VanHare GF, Franz MR, Roge C, Scheinman MM. Persistent functional atrioventricular block in two patients with prolonged QT intervals: elucidation of the mechanism of block. PACE 1990; 13:608-618.
75. Eldar M, Griffin JC, Abbott JA, et al. Permanent cardiac pacing in patients with the long QT syndrome. J Am Coll Cardiol 1987; 10:600-607.
76. Schwartz PJ: Idiopathic long QT syndrome: progress and questions. Am Heart J 1985; 109:399-411.
77. Schwartz PJ, Locati E, Moss AJ, Crampton RS, Trazzi R, Ruberti U. Left cardiac sympathetic denervation in the therapy of congenital long QT syndrome. Circulation 1991; 84:503-511.
78. Moss AJ, Robinson J. Clinical features of the idiopathic long QT syndrome. Circulation. 1992; 85 (suppl I):140-144.

79. Platia EV, Griffith LSC, Watkins L, Mirowski M, Mower MM, Reid PR. Managment of the prolonged QT syndrome and recurrent ventricular fibrillation with an implantable automatic cardioverter-defibrillator. Clin Cardiol 1985; 62:1319-1321.
80. Denes P. The role of the autonomic nervous system in ventricular arrhythmias. AICD Advances 1991; 3:8-9.
81. Bhandari AK, Shapiro WA, Morady F, Shen EN, Mason J, Scheinman MM. Electrophysiologic testing in patients with the long QT syndrome. Circulation 1985; 71:63-71.
82. Winkle RA, Stinson EB, Rcht DS, Mead RH, Schmidt P. Practical aspects of automatic cardioverter/defibrillator implantation. Am Heart J 1984; 108:1335-1346.
83. Dosios T, Gorgogiannis D, Sakorafas G, Karamptsas K. Persistent left superior vena cava: a problem in the transvenous pacing of the heart. PACE 1991; 14:389-391.
84. Silka MJ, Rice MJ. Paradoxic embolism due to altered hemodynamic sequencing following transvenous pacing. PACE 1990; 14:499-503.
85. McCowan R, Maloney J, Wilkoff B, et al. Automatic implantable cardioverter-defibrillator implantation without thoracotomy using an endocardial and submuscular patch system. J Am Coll Cardiol 1991; 17:415.
86. Bardy GH, Allen MD, Mehra R, et al. An effective and adaptable transvenous defibrillation system using the coronary sinus in man. J Am Coll Cardiol 1990; 16:887-895.
87. Troup P, Chapman PD, Olinger GN, et al. The implanted defibrillator: relation of the defibrillating lead configuration and clinical variables to defibrillation threshold. J Am Coll Cardiol 1985; 6:1315-1321.
88. Troup P. Programmed stimulation guided-therapy compared with implantable cardioverter-defibrillator therapy in the treatment of ventricular tachyarrhythmias. PACE 1991; 14:267-272.
89. Brown JP, Gillette PC, Goh TH, Arzbaecher RC. Discrimination of tachycardia by rate of onset. IEEE Proc 1986; 98-101.
90. Fisher JD, Goldstein M, Ostrow E, et al. Maximal rate of tachycardia development: sinus tachycardia with sudden exercise versus spontaneous ventricular tachycardia. PACE 1983; 6:221-228.
91. Schuger CD, Jackson K. Steinman RT, Lehmann MH. Atrial sensing to augment ventricular detection by the automatic implantable cardioverter-defibrillator: a utility study. PACE 1988; II; 1456-1464.
92. Langberg J, Gibb W, Auslander D, et al. Identification of ventricular tachycardia with use of the morphology of the ventricular electrogram. Circulation 1988; 77:1363-1369.
93. Bardy G, Ivey TD, Stewart R, Graham EL, Greene HL. Failure of the automatic implantable defibrillator to detect ventricular fibrillation. Am J Cardiol 1986; 85:1107-1108.
94. Saksena S, Stout R, Poliseno M, et al. Tachycardia detection and treatment with a third generation implantable cardioverter-defibrillator: an international experience (abstr). J Am Coll Cardiol 1992; 19:286.
95. Cohen TJ, Chein WW, Lurie KG, et al. Implantable cardioverter defibrillator proarrhythmia: case report and review of the literature. PACE 1991; 14:1326-1328.
96. Calkins H, Brinkler J, Veltri EP, et al. Clinical interactions between pacemakers and automatic implantable cardioverter defibrillators. J Am Coll Cardiol 1990; 16:666-673.
97. Khastgir T, Aarons D, Veltri E. Sudden bradyarrhythmic death in patients with implantable cardioverter-defibrillator: report of 2 cases. PACE 1991; 14:395-397.
98. Akhtar M, Avitall B, Jazayeri M, et al. Role of implantable cardioverter defibrillator therapy in the management of high-risk patients. Circulation 1992; 85 (suppl I):131-139.
99. Fisher JD, Mehra R, Furman S. Termination of ventricular tachycardia with rapid bursts ofl ventricular pacing. Am J Cardiol 1978; 41:94-102.
100. Lawrie GM, Wright-Harris J, Lin HT, Wyndham CRC. High defibrillation threshold with the AICD: management with right atrial patch electrode (abstr). Am J Coll Cardiol 1988; 11:209.
101. Troup P. Implantable cardioverter defibrillators. Curr Probl Cardiol 1989; 675-815.
102. Jones DL, Klein GJ. Guiraudon GM, et al. Sequential pulse defibrillation in humans: orthogonal sequential pulse defibrillation with epicardial electrodes. J Am Coll Cardiol 1988; 11:590-596.

103. Garson A. Jr. Electrophysiology and arrhythmias in young patients: considerations for antiarrhythmic drug regulation. J Cardiovasc Electophysiol 1991; 2:450-455.
104. Nisam S, Thomas A, Mower M, Hauser R. Identifying patients for prophylactic implantable cardioverter defibrillator therapy: status of prospective studies. Am Heart J 1991; 122:607-612.
105. Bigger JT Jr. Prophylactic use of implantable cardioverter defibrillators: medical, technical, economic considerations. PACE 1991; 14:376-380.

15

Strategies for Management of Malignant Ventricular Arrhythmias: Role of Pharmacotherapy, Surgery, Ablation, and the Implantable Cardioverter-Defibrillator

N. A. Mark Estes III

*Tufts University School of Medicine
and New England Medical Center
Boston, Massachusetts*

Multiple pharmacological and nonpharmacological therapeutic options currently are available for the treatment of patients who have survived previous episodes of malignant clinical arrhythmias such as sustained ventricular tachycardia (VT) or ventricular fibrillation (VF) [1–217]. Without therapy, such patients remain at high risk for recurrence of these ventricular arrhythmias and sudden death. With the development of numerous antiarrhythmic agents for the treatment of ventricular arrhythmias over the past decade, the pharmacological therapy available for treatment of these ventricular arrhythmias has expanded considerably (Table 1). These 12 antiarrhythmic agents currently used in the United States represent more than a doubling of those available a decade ago. During this same time, multiple studies have evaluated the role of using spontaneous or induced arrhythmias as endpoints for guiding drug therapy [14–60,213–215]. Although retrospective analyses of antiarrhythmic drug therapy guided by electrophysiological testing and Holter monitoring had strongly suggested a better overall predictive accuracy of the former technique, one recent prospective comparative trial assessing electrophysiological study versus electrocardiographic monitoring (ESVEM) for selection of antiarrhythmic drug therapy has shown no difference in the ability of the techniques to prevent arrhythmia recurrence and sudden death [34,46,213–215]. Retrospective analyses of series of patients in whom amiodarone has been used to prevent recurrence of malignant ventricular arrhythmias have demonstrated that the drug is extremely effective in suppressing spontaneous ventricular arrhythmias and may prolong survival [61–76]. A prospective trial of the drug versus conventional antiarrhythmic agents in survivors of out-of-hospital ventricular fibrillation determined that survival free of the endpoints of cardiac death, VT recurrence, or implantable cardioverter-defibrillator (ICD) shocks was improved with amiodarone [76]. A Canadian trial randomizing sudden-death survivors to amiodarone or an ICD is currently being performed, and a German study randomizing cardiac-arrest survivors to propafenone, metoprolol, amiodarone, or the ICD has begun [77]. Additional trials are currently underway enrolling patients at high risk for sudden cardiac death, who have not yet had sustained ventricular tachycardia or ventricular fibrillation, into studies evaluating the role of prophylactic ICD use [78–80]. The results of these studies will

Table 1 Pharmacological Therapy for Ventricular Arrhythmias: Approved Antiarrhythmic Agents

Class IA
    Quinidine, procainamide, disopyramide
Class IB
    Lidocaine, mexiletine, tocainide
Class IC
    Flecainide, propafenone
Class I
    Moricizine
Class III
    Bretylium, amiodarone, sotalol

provide useful information on the benefit of pharmacological and nonpharmacological management strategies to prevent sudden death in high-risk "pre-event" patients [8]. Guidelines for the use of the ICD have been established as appropriate therapy for sustained ventricular tachycardia and sudden-death survivors who have ventricular tachycardia presistently inducible by programmed ventricular stimulation despite pharmacological therapy or for those who have no inducible ventricular arrhythmias at the baseline drug-free study [81–85]. With refinement of patient selection, mapping, and surgical techniques, the operative mortality and efficacy of mapping-guided surgery for treating ventricular arrhythmias have improved [86–124]. Ablative techniques, with direct current and radiofrequency energy and percoronary techniques, are currently being investigated as potentially curative approaches in highly selected patients with sustained monomorphic VT [125–143]. Although antitachycardia pacemakers have been shown to have limited utility in long-term sudden-death prevention in the absence of backup defibrillation capability, the experience gained with arrhythmia detection and termination algorithms has been applied to current third-generation, tiered-therapy ICDs [144–160].

The ICD has emerged as the accepted primary therapeutic option for patients at continuing high risk for fatal arrhythmias [6,206]. It has evolved from a short-lived, nonprogrammable, committed device capable only of recognition of VF to a multiprogrammable, noncommitted, therapeutic option for VT and VF [206]. Initially regarded as "last resort" therapy, the ICD is considered by many to be the option of choice [6,206] for high-risk ventricular arrhythmia patients. The low sudden-death rates in patients with the ICD, when compared to nonrandomized cohorts as controls, has increasingly made this the dominant strategy for pharmacologically unresponsive malignant ventricular arrhythmias [161–194]. Although there is consensus that the ICD can prevent sudden death, the magnitude of benefit has not been demonstrated conclusively by appropriately designed, randomized prospective trials with concurrent controls [216,217]. Additional legitimate concerns have been raised regarding the impact of the device on total mortality. The Antiarrhythmics Versus Implantable Defibrillators (AVID) trial currently underway randomizing patients to ICD or pharmacological therapy with either sotalol or amiodarone will provide vital information on the relative benefits of device and drug therapy [77,188,205,216,217].

For patients with previous episodes of sustained VT or VF, pharmacological therapy directed by programmed ventricular stimulation has been the accepted initial approach to management, with surgical, ablative, or device therapy reserved for patients who do not respond to antiarrhythmic agents. A minority of patients with previous episodes of sustained ventricular tachycardia or fibrillation respond to drug therapy guided by EP endpoints [14–60,216,217]. Drug therapy is palliative, dependent on patient compliance, and frequently accompanied by side effects. There is growing skepticism about the ability of drugs to reduce arrhythmia recurrence and sudden death in patients with markedly reduced ejection fractions [29]. Based on these considerations and the considerable refinement in the last several years in mapping-guided surgery, ablative techniques, and ICD therapy, nonpharmacological approaches have emerged as accepted and, in many patients, primary treatment options. This chapter reviews the pharmacological and nonpharmacological strategies for management of malignant ventricular arrhythmias.

I. PHARMACOLOGICAL THERAPY

The evaluation of patients with previous lethal or malignant arrhythmias such as sustained VT or VF includes as an initial step the characterization of the underlying anatomical and electrophysiological substrate. Evaluation and treatment of congestive heart failure, ischemia, metabolic disorders, or drug toxicities is a critical initial step. This is followed by tests such as echocardiogram, gated blood pool scan, cardiac perfusion imaging, Holter monitoring, and signal-averaged electrocardiogram. Cardiac catheterization with characterization of the hemodynamics, coronary arteriography, and left ventriculography is a requisite for any patient with malignant ventricular arrhythmias. The therapeutic challenge faced by the clinician in the setting of malignant ventricular arrhythmias involves not only choosing arrhythmia therapy that maximizes the risk/benefit ratio but in detecting and effectively treating ischemia and congestive heart failure, which are frequently progressive and can account for significant cardiac mortality.

In the patient with previous out-of-hospital cardiac arrest from sustained ventricular tachycardia or ventricular fibrillation, studies have indicated that in the absence of antiarrhythmic therapy guided by invasive or noninvasive techniques, survival is poor, with only 30% of patients living 3 years past the index cardiac arrest [195–199]. Antiarrhythmic therapy given empirically without invasive or noninvasive assessment of efficacy is associated with a 1-year sudden death rate of 20–30% and a 5-year total mortality of over 70–80% [194–198]. Empiric antiarrhythmic therapy without use of suppression of spontaneous or induced arrhythmia endpoints has no proven benefit is reduction in the risk of sudden death [199].

Currently, Holter monitoring or electrophysiological studies (EPS) are the two options available for assessing the efficacy of antiarrhythmic therapy in patients with recurrent sustained ventricular tachycardia or ventricular fibrillation. Ambulatory electrocardiographic monitoring and stress testing have been used based on the premise that ventricular ectopic activity serves as a marker for sustained arrhythmias or fibrillation, and that reduction or elimination of spontaneous ectopy prevents recurrences of these lethal arrhythmias [12,13,34,35–38,40–48,51–55]. The PVC hypothesis was developed based on the observations that the presence of complex or frequent spontaneous ventricular premature beats or nonsustained VT identifies patients at higher risk for future sustained arrhythmias or cardiac arrest [41]. The PVC hypothesis held that suppression of these ventricular arrhythmias with antiarrhythmic therapy prevented future arrhythmic events. Grayboys et al. reported on 122 sustained VT or VF survivors followed for an average of 32 months, in whom assessment of drug efficacy was made with a rigorous noninvasive protocol which included Holter monitoring and exercise testing [43]. The criteria for a response to an antiarrhythmic agent included a 50% reduction in VPBs, 90% reduction in couplets, and 100% reduction in ventricular tachycardia [43]. With 6 sudden deaths in patients who responded to therapy and 17 in the 25 patients who did not, the positive predictive value of response to therapy was 68% and the negative predictive value was 73% by this approach [43,44].

Although therapy guided by ambulatory monitoring and stress testing has the advantage of being noninvasive and readily available to many physicians, the technique has clear limitations. Up to 30% of patients with prior sustained VT or VF have insufficient frequency of ventricular premature contractions, couplets, and runs of ventricular tachycardia to be used as a therapeutic endpoint on the baseline ambulatory monitor [34–38,40–48]. In such patients, alternative methods of directing antiarrhythmic therapy, such as programmed stimulation with use of the induced arrhythmia as endpoint, must be used.

Recently, the PVC hypothesis has been demonstrated to be invalid for patients at risk for arrhythmic mortality with PVCs or asymptomatic nonsustained ventricular tachycardia within the first 2 years of a myocardial infarction [45]. The Cardiac Arrhythmia Suppression Trial demonstrated a 2.5-fold increase in mortality in patients treated with encainide and flecainide compared to placebo, despite suppression of spontaneous arrhythmias. Additionally, the continuation of the CAST Trial with moricizine (CAST II) failed to show any beneficial effect despite suppression of spontaneous arrhythmias [200]. Hine et al. recently analyzed 10 additional studies assessing the benefits and risks of antiarrhythmic therapy in a total of 4122 patients who were randomized to antiarrhythmic therapy post-MI, including mexiletine, tocainide, flecainide, encainide, apridine, dilantin, and moricizine [58]. Meta-analysis of these studies suggested that despite PVC suppression, these agents probably shorten post-MI survival [58]. Additional data undermining the PVC hypothesis comes from Furberg, who reviewed short- and long-term postinfarction trials of class IA agents and found no support for an overall survival advantage with antiarrhythmic drug therapy [59]. With 1642 patients on active therapy with class IA drugs and 1563 on placebo, there were 122 deaths in the treatment group and 112 deaths in the placebo group ($p = 0.78$) [59]. Although these analyses have been conducted in patients who are at high risk for, but have not yet had, sustained ventricular tachycardia or ventricular fibrillation, they raise serious questions regarding suppression of spontaneous arrhythmias in any patient population as the endpoint for guiding antiarrhythmic drug therapy.

The invasive approach is based on the premise that patients with previous spontaneous malignant arrhythmias who had a sustained arrhythmia induced in the drug-free state which becomes noninducible on antiarrhythmic agents would be at low risk for arrhythmia recurrence. Multiple investigators have reported the results of an invasive approach in assessing drug efficacy for malignant ventricular arrhythmias (Table 2) [12,13,15–40,46–50]. Recurrence of ventricular tachycardia or sudden cardiac death in individuals in whom antiarrhythmic agents are determined to prevent arrhythmia induction in the EP lab is rare, with 80–100% of such patients remaining free of subsequent arrhythmic events [12,13,15–40,46–50]. However, a drug regimen that prevents VT induction can be identified in only a minority of patients [12,13,15–40,46–50]. When patients are discharged on a drug regimen that failed to prevent arrhythmia induction, the annual mortality from sudden death is over 20% [177]. The persistent induction of ventricular tachycardia during drug therapy is highly predictive of spontaneous arrhythmia recurrence [36,177]. During programmed stimulation, sustained ventricular arrhythmias are reproducibly induced in over 90% of coronary artery disease patients who have had spontaneous sustained VT and in greater than 75% of patients with ventricular fibrillation [12,13,15–40,46–50,81–85]. Long-term administration of antiarrhythmic agents predicted to be effective by programmed ventricular stimulation have been shown to be associated with prevention of sudden cardiac death in over 80% at up to 3 years of follow-up [12,13,15–40, 46–50]. Although the risk for life-threatening arrhythmia recurrence with pharmacological

Management of Malignant Arrhythmias

Table 2 Results with Pharmacologic Therapy Guided by Programmed Electrical Stimulation

Author	Year	Ref.	Number of pts. evaluated	Mean F/U period	Percent response	Responders			Nonresponders		
						Recurrence (%)	SCD (%)	Recurrence and/or SCD (%)	Recurrence (%)	SCD (%)	Recurrence and/or SCD (%)
Mason	1978	15	33	8	—	—	7	7	—	67	67
Ruskin	1980	17	31	15	—	—	0	0	—	50	50
Benditt	1983	18	34	18	60	0	6	6	6	33	—
Morady	1983	20	45	18	26	22	11	33	—	12	18
Roy	1983	19	119	20	33	—	15	17	—	21	—
Swerdlow	1983	23	239	15	59	—	12	—	—	32	—
Platia	1984	35	44	18	—	0	6	6	46	43	89
Kim	1986	38	52	19	40	—	—	40	—	—	35
Poll	1986	22	47	18	25	0	17	17	22	28	50
Skale	1986	21	58	22	34	0	0	0	15	22	37
Eldar	1987	39	108	26	23	18	11	29	14	10	24
Mitchell	1987	48	57	28	54	14	4	18	—	—	—
Rae	1987	49	38	21	44	44	0	0	21	14	36
Waller	1987	50	258	21	40	7	3	10	46	24	70
Freedman	1988	81	150	16	—	—	—	—	—	—	—
Kehoe	1988	25	38	27	73	0	0	0	100	75	100
Liem	1988	26	64	29	43	0	0	0	17	50	67
Milner	1988	28	19	17	69	11	44	56	50	0	50
Wilber	1988	29	166	21	70	—	12	12	—	33	33
Bonnett	1988	32	174	—	44	—	—	18	—	—	—
Mitchell	1990	37	57	60	44	—	—	27	—	—	—

—indicates data not presented by authors.
Source: Modified from Ref. 5.

therapy guided by programmed electrical stimulation is less than 5% at 24 months in patients presenting with out-of-hospital cardiac arrest with an ejection fraction of over 30%, the recurrence rate is considerably higher (15%) in patients with ejection fractions of less than 30% [29]. Similarly, electrophysiological testing to guide pharmacological therapy after nonfatal cardiac arrest in patients with a dilated cardiomyopathy without coronary disease has a lesser sensitivity and poorer predictive value than in patients with coronary artery disease [12,22,26,28].

One study has suggested that the persistent induction of VT with pharmacological therapy during programmed ventricular stimulation in selected patients does not necessarily preclude a good outcome, if there is suppression of spontaneous arrhythmias [38]. Partial responses to drugs such as slowing of the tachycardia by at least 100 ms to tolerable rates can offer protection against sudden death [50]. This study suggests that the use of alternative endpoints besides noninducibility, such as slowing of VT, may provide some benefit in reducing the risk of sudden death [50].

Although electrophysiological testing requires placement of intravascular catheters, the risks of the technique are minimal [14], and are related to placement of the catheter in the vascular system rather than to arrhythmia induction or termination. Its greatest utility is in patients with coronary artery disease with a lesser sensitivity and predictive accuracy in patients with cardiomyopathy [12,13,22,26,28,49]. An advantage of the electrophysiological approach is that in the absence of total suppression of the induced arrhythmia, induction and termination characteristics of the arrhythmias can be used to guide nonpharmacological approaches such as antitachycardia pacing. Lack of inducibility at the baseline EP evaluation or failure of drugs to suppress the induced arrhythmia are considered requisites for ICD implantation [161–194]. In the patient with coronary artery disease, a single morphology of sustained monomorphic ventricular tachycardia, and discrete left ventricular wall motion abnormality, mapping-guided surgical resection would have a high probability of cure [86–112]. By contrast, in the patient with noncoronary heart disease or multiple different morphologies of tachycardia, particularly if originating from regions of the myocardium that are anatomically distinct, the probability of mapping-guided subendocardial resection being curative is lower [93]. In such patients, therapy with an implantable cardioverter-defibrillator may be associated with a lower operative risk. If the tachycardia was reproducibly pace-terminable, a tiered-therapy device with antitachycardia pacing or low-energy cardioversion may be a reasonable option [201–202]. Finally, in the patient with a hemodynamically stable monomorphic ventricular tachycardia who fails drug therapy, catheter mapping of the region of origin of the tachycardia may allow for catheter ablation or ablation with precoronary techniques [125–143]. In patients undergoing cardiac electrosurgery or ablative techniques, if the ventricular arrhythmia is persistently inducible, addition of antiarrhythmic drugs may subsequently prevent arrhythmia induction despite failure prior to the ablation attempt. If this approach fails, an ICD can be considered.

Comparative studies between invasive and noninvasive approaches for assessing efficacy of antiarrhythmic therapy in patients with prior episodes of sustained VT, VF, or lethal arrhythmias have been performed [21,34,36–38,40,46,48]. It has been determined in retrospective, nonrandomized studies that patients who are treated with an effective regimen by programmed electrical stimulation criteria have better outcomes than those treated with a regimen effective by Holter criteria. However, due to the nonrandomized nature of these trials, retrospective studies comparing Holter and EP-guided pharmacological for prevention of sudden death suggest, but do not conclusively prove, that EP-guided therapy is superior in guiding pharmacological therapy. In one prospective, randomized study comparing the two techniques, therapy directed by invasive criteria was found to have a better predictive value than that guided by noninvasive criteria [37,48]. However, the small number of patients qualifing for the study, based on sufficient ambient ventricular arrhythmias and inducibility, and frequent use of amiodarone, make interpretation of this study difficult [37,48].

Based on this trial and prior retrospective analyses, the evidence had strongly suggested that EPS was preferrable to Holter monitoring for guiding drug therapy [36]. However, a recently conducted Electrophysiology Study Versus Electrocardiographic Monitoring (ESVEM) trial did not find any difference in the predictive accuracy of the two techniques [36,46,213–215]. This was the first prospective, large, randomized study to compare the accuracy of selecting drug therapy by ambulatory electrocardiography or electrophysiological study in patients eligible for both [34,46,213–215]. The patients randomized to ESVEM were selected from a larger group of 2103 patients with sustained VT, aborted sudden death, or unmonitored syncope. For entry into the study, patients were required to have greater than 10 PVCs per hour during a 48-h Holter monitor and reproducibly inducible VT on EPS, using a protocol employing a maximum of three extrastimuli and up to two pacing sites in the right ventricle. Between October 1, 1985, and February 5, 1991, 2103 patients were screened for enrollment based on documented sustained VT, aborted sudden death, or unmonitored syncope with inducible VT. Exclusion criteria were identified in 569 patients. A myocardial infarction was present within 3 weeks in 223 patients, concomitant medical illness or probably cardiac surgical intervention within 2 months in 316 patients, and arrhythmia-related problems such as ventricular preexcitation, presence of an ICD, or prior responsiveness to one of the study drugs in 72 patients. Of the 1534 eligible subjects, 1048 were not randomized. Holter monitoring or EPS criteria or both were not met in 519 patients. Enrollment was refused in 498 patients, and 31 others died or were not randomized for other reasons.

The remaining 486 patients were randomized to undergo serial drug testing by either electrophysiological study ($N = 242$) or ambulatory monitoring ($N = 244$). Up to six drugs were used in a random order until one was predicted to be effective [34,46,213–215]. The initial drugs selected included imipramine, mexiletine, procainamide, quinidine, and sotalol. Propafenone and pirmenol were added later, and impirimine was removed, as its efficacy and tolerance were substantially below those of the other drugs. Sotalol, propafenone, and pirmenol were withheld from patients with severe congestive heart failure, and mexiletine, pirmenol, and propafenone were not given to patients with second- or third-degree AV block in the absence of a pacemaker [34,46].

In the Holter monitoring limb, drug efficacy was defined as greater than 70% decrease in PVCs, greater than 80% decrease in couplets, and greater than 90% decrease in runs of 3 to 15 beats and a complete absence of runs greater than 15 beats [34,46]. Patients were required to have no VT during exercise stress testing in the Holter limb. EPS efficacy was defined as the suppression of previously inducible VT of greater than 15 beats using an equivalently aggressive stimulation protocol as that used originally to induce the target arrhythmia. Exercise stress testing was done on discharge but was not used to determine drug efficacy. If ventricular tachycardia developed on exercise testing in patients in whom EP had predictive efficacy, this was considered a drug failure and the patient was terminated from the study [34,46,213–215].

Of the randomized patients, sustained ventricular tachycardia was the presenting arrhythmia in 74%, aborted sudden death in 21%, and unmonitored syncope in 5%. Potentially effective drugs were found by Holter monitoring more efficiently than by EP testing. Overall, an effective drug was identified for 77% of patients assessed by the noninvasive method, compared to 45% of those in the EPS group, for a total of 296 patients discharged on predicted effective therapy. Of the 1281 drug trials, 24% resulted in the selection of a potentially effective drug. This included 15% of EP-guided drug trials and 38% of those guided by Holter mon-

Table 3 Electrophysiology Study Versus Electrocardiographic Monitoring (ESVEM) Results: Arrhythmia Recurrences Among Patients Receiving Drugs Predicted to Be Effective

	No. (%) of patients		
	All patients (N = 296)	Holter monitoring (N = 188)	Electrophysiologic study (N = 108)
Arrhythmic death	34 (11)	18 (10)	16 (15)
Cardiac arrest	16 (5)	11 (6)	5 (5)
Sustained VT	78 (26)	52 (27)	26 (24)
Syncope	8 (3)	6 (3)	2 (2)
Unsustained VT	11 (4)	6 (3)	5 (5)
Torsade de pointes VT	3 (1)	1 (1)	2 (2)
Total recurrences	150 (51)	94 (50)	56 (52)

itoring. The duration of hospital stay was approximately twice as long using the EP compared to Holter monitor endpoints.

Arrhythmia recurrence was defined as sudden death, ventricular tachycardia greater than or equal to 15 beats (with or without symptoms), or unmonitored syncope which the investigator felt was due to a tachyarrhythmia. Overall arrhythmia recurrence is shown in Table 3 for the 296 patients in whom drug efficacy was predicted. There were no significant differences in the predictive accuracy between the two methods, despite a trend at 1½ years of follow-up with greater accuracy of EP testing. The sudden-death, cardiac, and all-cause mortality were not statistically significantly different for the two methods.

Independent predictors of arrhythmia recurrences included previous antiarrhythmic therapy, age greater than 60 years, greater than 30 PVCs per hour, and treatment with drugs other than sotalol [34,46,213–215]. Independent predictors of all-cause mortality or severity of heart failure and treatment with drugs other than sotalol. The arrhythmia recurrence rate was 21% at 1 year for sotalol, compared to 44% for the other study drugs. This proved to be highly statistically significant, and persisted in even patients with poor left ventricular function. Although it did not reach statistical significance, there was a trend toward lower all-cause mortality with sotalol ($p = 0.69$).

Without a placebo arm in the ESVEM Trial, it is impossible to assess the true benefits or risks of antiarrhythmic agents guided by either Holter monitoring or EP testing [34,46,213–215]. It should be kept in mind that the comparison of the 1-year mortality of 7–8% in patients treated with encainide or flecainide in the CAST Trial might have been interpreted as a benefit of the drugs compared to historical controls had a placebo group not been included in the trial [45]. The endpoint of assessing drug efficacy in the EP lab in the ESVEM included use of the programmed stimulation protocol to the point that induced arrhythmia at the baseline study. Recent data suggest that using the baseline induction endpoint overestimates the number of patients responding by EP testing and leads to incorrect predictions of long-term drug efficacy [203]. These findings have important implications in interpreting recurrence rates in clinical trials assessing the accuracy of EP predictors. Furthermore, without a control group, the possibility that both techniques identified drug responders who have a better prognosis than nonresponders, even without therapy, cannot be excluded. One of the striking features of the trial was the very small percentage of patients who qualified for entry based on spontaneous and inducible arrhythmias. This has obvious implications for the utility of both techniques for assessing drug efficacy.

II. AMIODARONE

Multiple prior retrospective studies of amiodarone use in patients with malignant ventricular arrhythmias have suggested but not conclusively proven that this drug may reduce the rate of sudden cardiac death [61–76]. In previous series of patients treated with the class III drug, sudden-death rates have ranged from 2% to 10%, with a weighted averaged of 8% annually [61–76,177]. Several investigators have evaluated the predictive value of invasive and noninvasive techniques in patients taking amiodarone [61–76]. There is a consensus that noninducibility by programmed electrical stimulation predicts a low probability of future major arrhythmic events [61–76]. However, persistent inducibility, particularly of a ventricular tachycardia that is more difficult to induce and hemodynamically tolerated, does not preclude a good clinical outcome [59,61–76]. Ambulatory monitoring appears to have a high negative predictive value in patients taking amiodarone. In the multiple reported series, it is rare for clinical recurrences if the Holter monitor is free of ventricular tachycardia and has a significant reduction of ventricular premature contractions [50,61–76]. In the patient in whom amiodarone fails to prevent spontaneous arrhythmias on Holter monitoring, the incidence of arrhythmia recurrence is high. Currently, several prospective trials are being conducted to assess the efficacy of amiodarone [77,188]. The Canadian Implantable Defibrillator Study (CIDS) is randomizing patients with prior sustained VT or VF to empiric amiodarone versus ICD therapy [77]. The Hamburg Cardiac Arrest Study is randomizing sudden-death survivors to receive either non-pharmacological therapy with the ICD or pharmacological therapy with amiodarone, propafenone, or metoprolol. [77,188]. In the United States a multicenter NIH sponsored trial randomizing patients at very high risk for sudden death to ICD therapy or amiodarone or sotalol, the AVID trial, [205,216,217] is in its initial stages.

The results of the Cardiac Arrest in Seattle—Conventional versus Amiodarone Drug Evaluation [CASCADE) Trial recently have suggested a benefit to amiodarone compared to conventional therapy [76]. A total of 228 patients with out-of-hospital VF arrest were randomized to amiodarone or conventional drug therapy guided by EP testing and/or Holter monitoring. In this study, 113 received amiodarone and 115 patients received conventional therapy. The endpoints included cardiac death, recurrence of ventricular tachycardia, or ICD shocks [76,76a]. In a mean follow-up of 33 ± 23 months, 90%, 81%, and 62% of patients were free of an endpoint in the amiodarone group at 1, 2, and 3 years respectively. By contrast in the conventional treatment group, 76%, 68%, and 45% were free of an endpoint at 1, 2, and 3 years, respectively. The investigators concluded that survival free of an endpoint is better with amiodarone than conventional therapy [76,76a].

The role of low-dose amiodarone on mortality in cardiac patients with prior myocardial infarctions, congestive heart failure, or ventricular arrhythmias, who are at risk but have not yet had sustained ventricular tachycardia or ventricular fibrillation, was recently reviewed [204]. A total of 1283 patients have been enrolled in seven prospective preventative trials. In the patients randomized to amiodarone therapy there have been 110 deaths, compared to 153 in the placebo group, for an odds ratio of 0.66. The prophylactic use of low-dose amiodarone has been associated with a 34% reduction in total mortality in high-risk cardiac patients ($p < 0.02$). Although there are limitations inherent in pooling the results of a heterogenous patient population in these different trials, if these results are confirmed by current or future trials, amiodarone may be regarded as having the potential to favorably affect the management of ventricular arrhythmias resulting in deaths in high-risk patients who have not yet had sustained VT or VF [204].

Studies have been conducted retrospectively that have matched patients who have been treated with amiodarone with similar patients who have received implantable cardioverter-defibrillator therapy after out-of-hospital ventricular fibrillation or sustained ventricular tachycardia [178,185,187]. A total of 29 patients with sustained ventricular tachycardia or fibrillation were treated with amiodarone alone during a temporary lack of availability of ICDs [187]. They were compared with a group of 21 patients who were matched for age, sex, left ventricular ejection fraction, and rate of induced sustained ventricular tachycardia. The amiodarone group had a 24-month actual risk of sudden death of 31%, compared to 0% for those treated with the ICD [187]. It should be noted, however, that nonsudden death was more frequent in the patients receiving amiodarone alone (14% versus 5%), raising the possibility of an imbalance in the baseline of risk factors that were not measured or documented in the two groups [178].

In another retrospective case control study from one center, 60 patients who received the ICD were compared to 120 control patients matched for clinical variables such as duration of amiodarone use, age, left ventricular ejection fraction, type of heart disease, and type of presenting arrhythmia [185]. In 19 months of follow-up for the ICD group and 24 months for the control group, patients treated with an ICD had a lower sudden death rate than those treated with amiodarone [185]. Sudden deaths were reduced by 50% with the ICD (10% versus 5%, $p < 0.01$), and 3-year actuarial mortality was reduced by 31% (51% versus 35%, $p < 0.01$). These authors also reported an apparent reduction in nonsudden deaths by the ICD (39 versus 17%) [178,185]. Because neither of these trials was randomized, it is possible that there are inherent biases in patient selection or an adverse effect of amiodarone on total survival. No results of mortality trials comparing the ICD to amiodarone have been reported. To that extent the results of prospective randomized trials of amiodarone will help clarify the relative benefits and risks of its use compared to alterative drugs or the ICD [77,188,205,216,217].

III. MANAGEMENT OF PATIENTS WITH NO INDUCIBLE ARRHYTHMIAS AT BASELINE, ELECTROPHYSIOLOGICAL EVALUATION

In patients resuscitated from out-of-hospital sudden cardiac death, up to 30% will have no inducible arrhythmia at the time of initial drug-free electrophysiological evaluation [15–33, 81–85]. Inducibility of ventricular arrhythmias is dependent on many factors, including the protocol for programmed stimulation, the definition of noninducibility, the nature of the underlying structural heart disease, the presenting ventricular arrhythmia, left ventricular function, and any acute reversible causes such as metabolic disturbances or ischemia at the time of the clinical arrhythmia [31]. Although previously the management of patients with no inducible ventricular arrhythmia was controversial, a growing consensus has developed that the benefits of therapy with an implantable cardioverter-defibrillator outweigh the relatively low risks particularly with the extremely low risk of nonthoracotomy defibrillator implantation [85]. Recently follow-up on a series of 196 consecutive patients resuscitated from sudden cardiac death in whom no ventricular arrhythmias could be induced at the initial study were reported [84]. The ICD was used in one-half of the patients (98 patients) in a nonrandom manner. There were

Table 4 Arrhythmia Recurrence and Sudden Cardiac Death in Patients with No Inducible Tachyarrhythmia at Baseline Electrophysiologic Evaluation[a]

Author	Year	Ref.	Pts	Months F/U	Arrhythmia recurrence (%)	Sudden death (%)	Recurrence/ SCD (%)
Ruskin	1982	17	14	15	0	0	0
Benditt	1983	18	4	25	50	50	50
Roy	1983	19	47	20	—	32	—
Morady	1984	20	19	26	5	5	5
Skale	1985	21	14	22	—	13	—
Poll	1986	22	23	18	0	39	39
Swerdlow	1986	23	59	26	10	12	22
Eldar	1987	39	33	27	15	9	24
Freedman	1988	24	38	16	8	5	13
Kron	1988	27	25	21	—	5	—
Kehoe	1988	25	16	38	0	0	0
Liem	1988	26	21	29	—	—	—
Milner	1988	28	6	17	17	33	50
Wilber	1988	29	35	21	—	—	17
Zheutin	1988	30	43	32	5	2	7
Bonnett	1990	32	66	36	—	—	22
Sager	1990	33	26	16	4	38	42

[a]NI = noninducible; — = not reported by author.
Source: Modified from Ref. 5.

no differences in outcome predictors except a younger age in the ICD group. The overall 2-year sudden-death rate was lower for the ICD patients, with 3% dying compared to 11% of those not treated with an ICD ($p = 0.02$) [84]. The results of studies evaluating arrhythmia occurrence in sudden cardiac death in patients with no inducible tachyarrhythmia at baseline electrophysiologic evaluation are summarized in Table 4 [17–30,32,33,84].

From these series, several observations merit emphasis. In many patients the initial spontaneous ventricular arrhythmia occured while the patient was taking an antiarrhythmic agent [29]. In such patients it is frequently the case that no arrhythmia can be induced at the baseline electrophysiological evaluation, but with reinstitution of the antiarrhythmic agent, the arrhythmia becomes inducible [29]. Another potential trigger for life-threatening ventricular arrhythmias is acute ischemia [82–85]. It has been reported that selected patients with no inducible ventricular arrhythmias who have well-preserved left ventricular function can do well after coronary artery bypass surgery without antiarrhythmic agents or implantable cardioverter-defibrillators [29,39,121]. Patients who have suffered from out-of-hospital ventricular fibrillation more frequently are noninducible at the baseline drug-free study than those with sustained monomorphic ventricular tachycardia [29,121]. The outcome of patients with noninducibility of any ventricular arrhythmia at the baseline study, particularly when there is poor ventricular function, is sufficiently unfavorable to warrant implantable cardioverter-defibrillator implantation. Guidelines for implantation of the device, as discussed in Chapter 12, have now been extended to include those with prior sustained VT or VF without inducible arrhythmias [29,85]. This holds particularly true in patients with dilated cardiomyopathy, in whom the sensitivity of EP testing is less than in patients with coronary artery disease [12,22,26,28].

IV. SURGICAL THERAPY FOR VENTRICULAR ARRHYTHMIAS

Although coronary artery bypass grafting is frequently indicated as therapy for patients with critical coronary artery lesions, ischemia, and prior episodes of sustained ventricular tachycardia or ventricular fibrillation, it uncommonly impacts on inducibility of sustained monomorphic ventricular tachycardia [86,121]. Coronary artery bypass surgery improves symptoms, decreases the frequency of myocardial infarction, and decreases total mortality and sudden cardiac death in patients with left main or three-vessel coronary artery disease [207]. Additionally, it is appreciated that revascularization can impact favorably on outcome in patients with prior episodes of out-of-hospital cardiac arrest [23,25,86,121,122]. In our series of 56 patients studied preoperatively and postoperatively, one-third of patients with preoperatively induced arrhythmias showed a favorable effect on arrhythmia induction with bypass grafting [121]. Revascularization is reasonable therapy in patients with significant coronary artery disease, ischemia, well-preserved left ventricular function, and no inducible ventricular arrhythmias [121]. The response may also be favorable in patients with inducible VF, but sustained monomorphic ventricular tachycardia in patients with coronary artery disease less commonly responds to revascularization alone [121,122]. Accordingly, placement of an ICD or mapping-guided subendocardial resection in appropriate candidates is commonly performed at the time of coronary bypass surgery [114,121,122].

The initial attempts at blind aneurysm resection as the therapy for patients with ventricular tachycardia were unsuccessful [124]. Surgical techniques evolved with an isolation procedure called the encircling endocardial ventriculotomy [108], with which an endocardial incision was made around the myocardial scar. The intent was to electrically isolate this part of the myocardium from the remainder of the heart [107,108]. Although it was moderately successful in prevention of recurrent ventricular tachycardia, it frequently resulted in severe left ventricular dysfunction [1,107,108]. With refinement of techniques of mapping, it was determined that the region of tachycardia origin could be identified and was commonly at the margin of normal and scar tissue [94,97,115,116]. In patients with monomorphic ventricular tachycardia, preoperative endocardial catheter and pace mapping localizes the region of origin of the tachycardia. In the operating room, ventricular tachycardia is again initiated, and mapping is repeated from the endocardial and epicardial surface. The most valuable information comes from endocardial activation sequence mapping during the tachycardia, looking for the earliest site of origin relative to the onset of the QRS complex [94,97,115,116]. The inability to induce and adequately map a tachycardia intraoperatively, which can occur in up to 40% of patients, precludes identification of the earliest site of subendocardial activation and mandates reliance on the preoperative endocardial catheter map or a nondirected surgical procedure [86,93,95]. The extended endocardial resection technique was developed as a surgical technique to eliminate all subendocardial scar [104–107] without mapping. The most commonly used mapping-guided surgical technique is the subendocardial resection (94,97,115,116). This surgical technique has been supplemented with cryoablation [93,102], and laser ablation [103]. More recently, the technique of "sequential resection" was developed [91], with which the heart is maintained on normothermic cardiopulmonary bypass and cycles of induction mapping and resection are performed.

When programmed ventricular stimulation is repeated, over 80% of such patients are free of inducible ventricular tachycardia [87–93, 208]. The overall operative mortality and percentage of patients free of an inducible or spontaneous sustained ventricular tachycardia are represented in Table 5. It should be considered that this represents the experience of the decade starting with the late 1970s. It has been noted that the presence of a myocardial infarction

Table 5 Surgical Therapy for Ventricular Tachycardia

Author	Year	Ref.	Pts.	Operative mortality (%)	Noninducible post-op (%)
Garan	1986	86	45	9	78
Krafcek	1986	89	39	10	79
Swerdlow	1986	87	105	16	61
McGiffen	1987	88	123	19	33
Ostermeyer	1987	90	93	10	54
Colloborative Registry	1987	210	655	12	74
Haines	1988	91	92	6	87
Hargrove	1989	92	269	15	68
Manolis	1989	93	30	10	70
Foote	1992	208	18	0	88
Cox	1989	209	65	14	98

within 2 months, inability to map the tachycardia completely intraoperatively, disparate sites of origin of ventricular tachycardia, absence of a discrete left ventricular aneurysm, multiple ventricular tachycardia configurations, posterior wall site of ventricular tachycardia, and limited size of endocardial patch or resection all predict postsurgical arrhythmia induction or clinical recurrence [93]. Based on these observations, patient selection has improved, and operative mortality is currently approximately 5%. In appropriately selected patients, such as those with one morphology of sustained monomorphic ventricular tachycardia and a discrete anterior or anteroapical aneurysm, operative success as defined by prevention of induction or spontaneous ventricular tachycardia should be 90% [1]. Some centers have advocated implantation of a full defibrillator system at this time of subendocardial resection [112,113]. It had been our policy to place "prophylactic" patches in selected patients who, based on clinical and electrophysiological factors, are at high risk for arrhythmia induction postoperatively [114]. In such patients, if a ventricular tachycardia is present and pharmacologically unresponsive postoperatively, the defibrillator could be placed with local anesthesia. Currently prophylactic patches are not placed with the development of nonthoracotomy transvenous lead systems.

V. ABLATION TECHNIQUES

For patients with sustained monomorphic VT tolerated with sufficient hemodynamic stability to allow catheter mapping, catheter ablation may be an option [125–132,136–143]. The principal of this investigational procedure involves localizing the site of origin of tachycardia and then delivering a direct-current shock or radiofrequency energy to modify the anatomic substrate. Identification of a site of origin of VT requires a hemodynamically tolerated tachycardia to allow mapping. Patients with ventricular fibrillation, hemodynamically unstable tachycardia, or multiple sites of origin of ventricular tachycardia are poor candidates for this technique. Definition of success with this technique has not been uniform. However, in two series [128,137] summarizing the experience with the direct-current technique, only 25% of patients remain free of recurrent ventricular tachycardia. This technique has considerable risks, including strokes, myocardial infarction or rupture, and worsening of arrhythmias, with fatal complications reported [128,137]. Although radiofrequency ablation has been extremely successful in managing patients with supraventricular arrhythmias from dual AV nodal pathways or bypass tracts, the reported experience for ventricular tachycardia has been limited to relatively small series of patients without long-term follow-up. It may be curative in patients with sustained monomorphic ventricular tachycardia, with highest efficacy rates reported in those with right ventricular outflow tract tachycardias. However, the experience in the more common setting of coronary artery disease is limited, and radiofrequency ablation should be performed only in individuals with back-up ICDs.

Newer percoronary techniques of arrhythmia ablation with intracoronary ethanol [133–136] have been proposed. To date, patients in whom this procedure has been tried have been highly selected based on stability of their tachycardia and suitability of their coronary anatomy. In one prospective, randomized trial, efficacy was achieved in one-third of patients [135].

VI. ANTITACHYCARDIA PACEMAKERS

Devices with the capability of recognizing and pace-terminating sustained monomorphic ventricular tachycardia currently play a minor role in the management of patients with lethal arrhythmias [144–160]. The risk of lack of efficacy or arrhythmia acceleration have made this mode of therapy unacceptable without the backup of an implantable cardioverter-defibrillator [144–160]. In the past, candidates for antitachycardia pacemakers for ventricular tachycardia have undergone careful electrophysiological evaluation to assess for reliable detection and arrhythmia termination. Those patients who had arrhythmia-related syncope or tachycardia acceleration would be excluded. Although in highly selected patients the 5-year mortality has been reported to be comparable to that of other modalities [145], there remains a significant risk of sudden cardiac death. Antitachycardia pacing is currently being used only in tiered-therapy implantable devices which include cardioversion and defibrillation capability in the event of failure of the antitachycardia algorithm to terminate the tachycardia or ventricular fibrillation.

VII. IMPLANTABLE CARDIOVERTER-DEFIBRILLATOR THERAPY

ICD therapy has evolved from over a decade of development through the first clinical implant in 1980 to a widely used modality for treatment of sustained VT or VF [161–193,201,202]. The initial devices were able only to recognize ventricular fibrillation and deliver a high-energy shock to more sophisticated programmable devices [10]. Currently, all clinically available devices also recognize ventricular tachycardia. Many devices in clinical use or in development have tiered therapy, with antitachycardia pacing, cardioversion, defibrillation, and bradycardia pacing [210,202], as well as memory to store electrograms or data regarding detected arrhythmias. The clinical results with respect to operative mortality, sudden-death rate, and total cardiac mortality are represented in Table 6. It should be noted that there is a consistent sudden-death rate reported at less than 2% per year, and in the largest independent series it has been reported at 1% per year [175]. The benefit of the ICD persists for sudden-death reduction in patients with low ejection fraction [181]. Although there is impressive reduction in sudden cardiac death compared to historical controls, there remains a considerable total cardiac mortality.

Controlled trials comparing the ICD to alternative forms of therapy have not yet been completed, and to that extent it is not possible to make final conclusions with respect to comparative efficacy [178]. Although some investigators have proposed that implantable cardioverter-defibrillators be considered the "antiarrhythmic treatment modality of choice" for sudden-cardiac-death survivors, appropriate prospective studies are only now being performed to

Table 6 Results with the Implantable Cardioverter Defibrillator

Author	Year	Ref.	Pts.	Operative Mortality	F/U (months)	SCD (%)	Cardiac Mortality (%)	Total Mortality (%)
Mirowski	1983	161	52	0	14	7.7	15	23
Echt	1985	162	70	1.4	9	1.4	4.1	7.1
Luceri	1986	163	21	0	19	4.8	4.8	9.5
Marchinski	1986	164	26	3.8	13	0	11.5	27
Gabry	1987	165	22	0	20	9	13.6	22.7
Reid	1987	166	129	3.8	17	7.2	22.2	24.8
Fogoros	1987	187	65	—	25	1.5	9.2	10.8
Barbola	1988	167	25	8.0	20	4.3	8.0	25
Kelly	1988	169	94	3.1	17	1.1	5.5	8.2
Olinger	1988	170	77	0	27	2.6	5.1	9.0
Tchou	1989	171	70	1.4	18	1.0	1.0	7.1
Hargrove	1989	172	77	3	14	1.3	—	—
Manolis	1989	173	77	2.6	15	2.6	6.5	7.8
Myerburg	1989	174	60	2.0	25	1.7	18.3	21.7
Winkle	1989	175	270	1.5	25	2.6	9.2	14.8
Edel	1992	176	171	4.0	17	4.0	9.0	15
Newman	1992	185	60	3.3	36	5	12	22
Bardy	1992	201	50	0	15	0	0	4
Fromer	1992	212	102	3.9	9.4	1	3.5	4.6

determine the benefit of this therapy relative to drugs [6,213–215]. It is possible that patient selection, the influence of concomitant surgery, pharmacological therapy, or close follow-up may have influenced the results of these nonrandomized trials [178]. Currently, the device is reserved for patients who have had episodes of sustained ventricular tachycardia or ventricular fibrillation who are either noninducible at the initial drug-free study or are refractory to pharmacological therapy [85]. With improved detection algorithms, flexible adaptive antitachycardia pacing, backup cardioversion-defibrillation, data and electrogram storage, and reduced size, the ICD may become the dominant strategy for managing patients with prior life-threatening ventricular arrhythmias. As nonthoracotomy lead systems allow for increased ease of implantation, cost effectiveness of the defibrillator relative to other therapy is evaluated, and benefit is evaluated in lower-risk patient populations, it is also feasible that the device indications may be extended to prophylactic use in "pre-event" patients [8,77–80].

The data with regard to the reduction in sudden cardiac death with the ICD in survivors of cardiac arrest come largely from restrospective follow-up studies without any comparison or control groups [162–177]. However, there is inherent bias in patient selection and therapy, such as concomitant CABG surgery, and bias due to differences in time from cardiac arrest to entering the study, which makes this line of evidence weaker than that obtained from prospective studies [178,216]. The claims for reduction in sudden death based on comparison of actual sudden-death survival with projected sudden-death rates based on the number of appropriate shocks has definite limitations. With third-generation devices it is evident that not all arrhythmias which trigger shocks would have been fatal. In one recent series, over 70% of episodes of ventricular tachycardia which would have triggered a committed ICD were self-terminating [202]. There are also biases inherent in matching patients who have received ICDs with similar patients who received amiodarone treatment without ICD treatment [185,187]. Because none of these studies was randomized, it is possible that factors not examined or recognized by the authors could differentially have effected the comparisons [178]. The only data available from a prospective randomized trial of the ICD versus amiodarone [188] has shown no difference in overall mortality in preliminary analysis. This ongoing trial is currently randomizing patients who have had cardiac arrest and inducible VT or VF to ICD treatment or one of three drugs, each with different electrophysiological properties, including propafenone, metoprolol, and amiodarone. An interim analysis of 139 patients with a mean follow-up of 11 months has shown that the ICD reduced the rate of sudden death to zero compared with 9% receiving amiodarone and 11% each with metroprolol and propafenone. However, overall mortality was not different between the ICD and drug therapy groups (14% ICD, 14% metroprolol, 15% amiodarone, and 20% propafenone) [178,188].

In 1990 the Canadian Implantable Defibrillator Study (CIDS) began randomizing patients with malignant ventricular arrhythmias to amiodarone or ICD treatment as first-line therapy to test the hypothesis that the initial decision to use an ICD instead of amiodarone reduces the risk of an arrhythmic death [77]. The primary endpoint for this study is arrhythmic death. With plans to enroll 400 patients over 4 years, following them for an average of 3 years, the study is designed to have an 80% power to detect a 58% difference in 3-year arrhythmic mortality between the groups [77]. The CIDS and Hamburg study will be helpful in determining the relative merits of ICD and pharmacological therapy in patients with malignant ventricular arrhythmias. A multicenter trial to assess whether the use of the implantable cardioverter defibrillator will result in improved total mortality compared with pharmacological therapy in patients who have been resuscitated from sudden cardiac death due to ventricular fibrillation or are otherwise at very high risk of mortality from ventricular tachycardia (AVID trial) is currently enrolling patients [205,216,217]. The study will determine whether a treatment strategy based on initial placement of an ICD or one based on antiarrhythmic drug therapy results in longer survival. Patients considered candidates for both the ICD and antiarrhythmic drug therapy will be randomized to ICD placement versus sotalol or amiodarone and followed until death or the end of study. The primary endpoint of this study will be total mortality. Secondary endpoints will be quality of life, costs, mode of death, surgical morbidity, and ICD and lead failure. The patients assigned to drug therapy will be randomly allocated to empiric amiodarone or sotalol therapy guided by EP testing and/or Holter monitoring, as determined to be appropriate by the enrolling center [205,216,217]. Those patients assigned to but unable to have EP or Holter-guided therapy (less than 20 PVCs per hour and noninducible VT/VF) and patients with contraindications for sotalol will receive empiric amiodarone therapy [205,216,217]. The trial will be conducted with an intention to treat analysis. This trial, as well as the Hamburg and CIDS, should help to provide information regarding the impact of the ICD relative to pharmacological therapy on sudden death, total mortality, and other endpoints [77,188,205]. At the same time, some investigators feel that a potentially greater opportunity for ICD therapy exists when it is used as prophylaxis in patients at high risk for lethal sustained arrhythmias [77]. Device application in asymptomatic high-risk patients is now being evolved as a therapeutic strategy to reduce the risk of sudden cardiac death [211].

The Coronary Artery Bypass Graft Patch Trial (CABG Patch Trial) is a trial designed to test the hypothesis that use of an ICD in patients at high risk for sudden death undergoing planned bypass surgery will decrease the mortality [77]. The patient population eligible for this trial are those undergoing coronary bypass grafting with left ventricular ejection fraction less than 36% and a positive signal-averaged ECG. Those patients who have already had sustained ventricular arrhythmias are excluded from the study [77]. Intraoperatively, patients will be randomized to receive an implantable defibrillator or conventional treatment. The primary endpoint of the study is all-cause mortality or nonfatal sustained ventricular arrhythmias that require intravenous drug treatment or cardioversion for treatment. The pilot study, including five clinical centers, demonstrated the feasibility of this trial, and the full-scale trial is currently enrolling patients.

The Multicenter Automatic Defibrillation Trial (MADIT) is evaluating the prophylactic use of ICD in those patients at high risk for sudden cardiac death [77,80]. The trial's primary objective is to determine if the survival of the high-risk patients can be improved with the ICD. Patients who have had prior transmural myocardial infarctions, unsustained ventricular tachycardia, left ventricular ejection fraction of less than 36%, and inducible sustained VT or VF that is not suppressed with intravenous procainamide will be included in the trial [77,80]. Patients will be randomized to ICD treatment or conventional therapy. The primary endpoint of the trial will be death from all causes with the intention to treat analysis [77,80].

The Multicenter Unsustained Tachycardia Trial (MUSTT) began enrollment of patients who have had a prior myocardial infarction and a left ventricular ejection fraction less than or equal to 40% and asymptomatic or minimally symptomatic nonsustained VT in 1991. All patients will undergo programmed ventricular stimulation with the endpoint of induction of sustained monomorphic VT. Of those induced, one-half will be randomized to receive antiarrhythmic drug therapy in an effort to eliminate VT inducibility or achieve hemodynamically stable VT. If neither is achieved, patients will receive an ICD. The other one-half of patients will be randomized to no treatment. Other planned trials to examine potential new indications for ICD therapy include the Defibrillator Implant as a Bridge to Later Transplant (DEFIBRILAT Trial), Postmyocardial Infarction Trial (FIRST-AID), and European Dilated Cardiomyopathy Trial [211].

VIII. CONCLUSIONS

It is evident from the above discussion that, in patients with previous sustained ventricular tachycardia or fibrillation, and in patients at high risk for these arrhythmias, management strategies continue to emerge based on the evolving knowledge of the risks and benefits of the available therapies. At the present time the optimal approach must be individualized in each patient. If a patient has no inducible arrhythmia at the initial drug-free study, or if spontaneous or induced arrhythmias are not suppressed with a limited number of drug trials, nonpharmacological options should be considered. Mapping-guided subendocardial resection would be reasonable in a patient with a discrete aneurysm and preserved function of the nonaneurysmal portion of the ventricle. ICD therapy would provide optimal sudden-death protection in those who have no inducible arrhythmia at baseline or who are still inducible on drugs. The role of amiodarone in prevention of sudden death and arrhythmia recurrence will be clarified by current trials involving its safety and efficacy. Although it is widely accepted that the ICD can almost eliminate sudden-death recurrences, the extent of its benefit in improving total mortality compared to amiodarone or other pharmacological therapy remains to be accurately determined in currently ongoing trials.

REFERENCES

1. DiMarco JP. Nonpharmacologic therapy of ventricular arrhythmias. 1990; 13:1527–1533.
2. Marchlinski F. Treatment of sustained arrhythmias: which therapy to use. Ann Intern Med 198; 522–524.
3. Fisher JD, Kim SG, Roth JA, et al. Ventricular tachycardia/fibrillation: therapeutic alternatives. PACE 1991; 14:370–375.

4. Estes NAM III, Garan H, McGovern B, Ruskin JN. Class I antiarrhythmic agents, classification, electrophysiologic considerations, and clinical effects. In: Reister HJ, Horowitz LN, eds. Mechanisms and Treatment of Cardiac Arrhythmias: Relevance of Basic Studies to Clinical Management. Baltimore: Urban and Schwartzenberg, 1985:183–201.
5. Troup PJ. Programmed stimulation-guided therapy compared with implantable cardioverter defibrillator device therapy in the treatment of ventricular tachyarrhythmias. PACE 1991; 14:267–272.
6. Lehmann M, Steinman RT, Schuger CP, Jackson K. The automatic implantable cardioverter defibrillator as antiarrhythmic treatment modality of choice for survivors of cardiac arrest unrelated to acute myocardial infarction. Am J Cardiol 1988; 62:803–805.
7. Kim SG. Management of survivors of cardiac arrest: is electrophysiologic testing obsolete in the era of implantable defibrillators? J Am Coll Cardiol 1990; 16:756–62.
8. Cannom DS. Implantable cardioverter defibrillator: the promise and perils of an evolving technology. PACE 1992; 15:1–4.
9. Bigger JT. Prophylactic use of implantable cardioverter defibrillators: medical, technical, economic considerations. PACE 1991; 14:376–80.
10. DiMarco JP, Haines DE. Sudden cardiac death. Curr Probl Cardiol 1990; 18–232.
11. Fisher JD, Brodman RF, Kim SG, et al. VT/VF: 60/60 protection. PACE 1990; 13:218–222.
12. Cameron J, Isner J, Salem D, Estes NAM. Cardiac electrophysiologic testing: a review of the technique and its role in the selection of antiarrhythmic drug regimens for supraventricular and ventricular arrhythmias. Pharmacotherapy 1985; 5:95–107.
13. Rabinowitz, AJ, Maloney JD. Survivors of sudden cardiac death: a rational approach to evaluation and therapy of patients surviving ventricular fibrillation. Cleve Clin J Med 1992; 52:166–172.
14. Horowitz LN, Kay HR, Kutalek SP, et al. Risks and complications of clinical cardiac electrophysiologic studies: a propsective analysis of 1000 consecutive patients. J Am Coll Cardiol 1987; 9:1261–1268.
15. Mason JW, Winkle RA. Electrode-catheter arrhythmia induction in the selection and assessment of antiarrhythmic drug therapy for recurrent ventricular tachycardia. Circulation 1978; 58:971–985.
16. Wellens HJJ, Brugada P, Stevenson WG. Programmed electricle stimulation: its role in the management of ventricular arrhythmias in coronary heart disease. Prog Cardiovas Disc 1986; 29:165–180.
17. Ruskin JN, DiMarco JP, Garan H. Out-of-hospital cardiac arrest: electrophysiologic observations and selection of long-term antiarrhythmic therapy. N Engl J Med 1980; 303:607–613.
18. Benditt DG, Benson, DW, Klein GJ, et al. Prevention of recurrent sudden cardiac arrest: role of provocative electropharmacologic testing. J Am Coll Cardiol 1983; 2:418–425.
19. Roy D, Waxman HL, Kienzle MG, Buxton AE, Marchlinski FE, Josephson ME. Clinical characteristics and long-term follow-up in 119 survivors of cardiac arrest: relation to inducibility at electrophysiologic testing. Am J Cardiol 1983; 52:969–974.
20. Morady F, Scheinman MM, Hess DS, et al. Electrophysiologic testing in the management of out-of-hospital cardiac arrest. Am J Cardiol 1983; 54:85–89.
21. Skale BT, Miles WM, Heger JJ, Zipes DP, Prystowsky EN. Survivors of cardiac arrest: prevention of recurrence by drug therapy as predicted by electrophysiologic testing or electrocardiographic monitoring. Am J Cardiol 1986; 57:113–119.
22. Poll DS, Marchlinski FE, Buxton AE, Josephson ME. Usefulness of programmed stimulation in idiopathic dilated cardiomyopathy. Am J Cardiol 1986; 58:922–997.
23. Swerdlow CD, Winkle RA, Mason JW. Determinants of survival in patients with ventricular tachyarrhythmias. N Engl J Med 1983; 24:1436–1442.
24. Freedman RA, Swerdlow CD, Soderholm-Difatte V, et al. Prognostic significance of arrhythmic inducibility or noninducibility at initial electrophysiologic study in survivors of cardiac arrest. Am J Cardiol 1988; 61:578–582.
25. Kehoe R, Tommaso C, Zheutline T, et al. Factors determining programmed stimulation responses and long-term arrhythmic outcome in survivors of ventricular fibrillation with ischemic heart disease. Am Heart J 1988; 116:355–363.

26. Liem LB, Swerdlow CD. Value of electropharmacologic testing in idiopathic dilated cardiomyopathy and ventricular tachyarrhythmias. Am J Cardiol 1988; 62:611–616.
27. Kron J, Kudenchuk K, Murphy FS, et al. Ventricular fibrillation survivors in whom tachyarrhythmia cannot be induced: outcome related to therapy. PACE 1987; 10:1291–1300.
28. Milner PG, Dimarco JP, Lerman BB. Electrophysiologic evaluation of sustained ventricular tachyarrhythmias in idiopathic dilated cardiomyopathy. PACE 1988; 11:562–568.
29. Wilber DJ, Garan H, Finkelstein D, et al. Out-of-hospital cardiac arrest. Use of electrophysiologic testing in the prediction of long-term outcome. N Engl J Med. 1989; 318:19–24.
30. Zeutlin TA, Steinman RT, Mattioni TA, et al. Long-term arrhythmic outcome in survivors of ventricular fibrillation with absence of inducible ventricular tachycardia. Am J Cardiol 1988; 62:1213–1217.
31. Estes NAM III, Garan H, McGovern B, Ruskin JN. Influence of drive cycle length during programmed stimulation on induction of ventricular arrhythmias: analysis of 403 patients. Am J Cardiol 1986; 578:108–112.
32. Bonnet CA, Elson JJ, Fogoros RN. Prognostic significance of noninducibility during baseline electrophysiologic study vs. noninducibility during serial drug testing in cardiac arrest survivors. J Am Coll Cardiol 1990; 15:124A.
33. Sager PT, Ranjiv L, Choudhary LC. Long-term prognosis of patients with out-of-hospital cardiac arrest but no inducible ventricular tachyarrhythmias. Am Heart J 1990; 120:1334–1342.
34. ESVEM Investigators. Determinants of predicted efficacy of antiarrhythmic drugs in the electrophysiologic study versus electrocardiographic monitoring trial. Circulation 1993; 87:232–329.
35. Platia EV, Raid PR. Comparison of programmed electrical stimulation and ambulatory electrocardiographic (Holter) monitoring in the management of ventricular tachycardia and ventricular fibrillation. J Am Coll Cardiol 1984; 4:493–500.
36. Gottlieb C, Josephson ME. The preference for programmed stimulation guided therapy for sustained ventricular arrhythmias. In: Brugada P. Wellens HJJ, eds. Cardiac Arrhythmias: Where to Go from Here? Mt. Kisco, NY: Futura, 1987:421–434.
37. Mitchell LB, Duff HJ, Gillis AM, Manyari DE, Wyse DG. Long-term follow-up of the randomized comparison of noninvasive and invasive approaches to drug therapy for ventricular tachyarrhythmia (abstr). Circulation 1991; 84:II-126.
38. Kim SG, Seiden SW, Felder SD, et al. Is programmed stimulation of value in predicting the long-term success of antiarrhythmic therapy for ventricular tachycardias? N Engl J Med 1986; 315:356–362.
39. Eldar M, Sauve MJ, Scheinman MM. Electrophysiologic testing and follow-up of patients with aborted sudden death. J Am Coll Cardiol 1987; 10:291–298.
40. Kim SG. Value and limitations of programmed stimulation and ambulatory monitoring in the management of ventricular tachycardia. Am J Cardiol 1988; 62:71–121.
41. Lown B. Management of patients at high risk for sudden death. Am Heart J 1982; 103:689–697.
43. Graboys TB, Lown B, Podrid PJ, et al. Long-term survival of patients with malignant arrhythmia treated with antiarrhythmic drugs. Am J Cardiol 1982; 50:437–443.
44. Lampert S, Lown B, Graboys TB, et al. Determinants of survival in patients with malignant ventricular arrhythmia associated with coronary artery disease ease. Am J Cardiol 1988; 61:791–797.
45. The Cardiac Arrhythmia Suppression Trial (CAST) Investigators. Effect of encainide and flecainide on mortality in a randomized trial of arrhythmia suppression after myocardial infarction. N Engl J Med 1989; 321:406–412.
46. The ESVEM Investigators. The ESVEM Trial. Electrophysiologic study versus electrocardiographic monitoring for selection of antiarrhythmic therapy of ventricular tachyarrhythmias. Circulation 1989; 79:1354–1360.
48. Mitchell LB, Duff HJ, Manyari DE, et al. A randomized clinical trial of the noninvasive and invasive approaches to drug therapy of ventricular tachycardia. N Engl J Med 1987; 317:1681–1687.

49. Rae AP, Spielman SR, Kutalek SP, et al. Electrophysiologic assessment of antiarrhythmic drug efficacy for ventricular tachyarrhythmias associated with dilated cardiomyopathy. Am J Cardiol 1987; 59:291–295.
50. Waller TJ, Kay HR, Spielman SR, et al. Reduction in sudden death and total mortality by antiarrhythmic therapy evaluated by electrophysiologic drug testing: criteria of efficacy in patients with sustained ventricular tachyarrhythmia. J Am Coll Cardiol 1987; 10:83–89.
51. Pratt CM, Slymen DJ, Wierman AM, et al. Analysis of the spontaneous variability of ventricular arrhythmias: consecutive ambulatory electrocardiographic recordings of ventricular tachycardia. Am J Cardiol 1985; 56:67–72.
52. Vlay SC, Kallman CH, Reid PR. Prognostic assessment of survivors of ventricular tachycardia and ventricular fibrillation with ambulatory monitoring. Am J Cardiol 1984; 54:87–90.
53. Pratt CM, Thornton BC, Margo SA, Wyndham C. Spontaneous arrhythmia detected on ambulatory electrocardiographic recording lacks precision in predicting inducibility of ventricular tachycardia drug electrophysiologic study. J Am Coll Cardiol 1987; 10:97–104.
54. Morganroth J, Michelson EL, Horowitz LN, Josephson ME, Pearlman AS, Dunkman WB. Limitations of routine long-term electrocardiographic monitoring to assess ventricular ectopic frequency. Circultation 1978; 58:408–414.
55. Brugada P, Lemery R, Talajie M, Della Bells P, Wellens Hein JJ. Treatment of patients with ventricular tachycardia or ventricular fibrillation: first lessons from the "Parallel Study." In: Brugada P, Wellens HJJ, eds. Cardiac Arrhythmias: Where to Go from Here? Mount Kisco, NY: Futura, 1987:457–470.
56. Chua W, Roth H, Summers C, Zheutlin TA, Kehoe RF. Programmed stimulation versus ambulatory monitoring for malignant ventricular arrhythmias (abstr). Circulation 1983; 67(suppl III):III–55.
57. Poole JE, Mathisen TL, Kudenchuk PJ, et al. Long-term outcome in patients who survive out of hospital ventricular fibrillation and undergo electrophysiologic studies: evaluation by electrophysiologic subgroups. J Am Coll Cardiol 1990; 16:657–65.
58. Hine LK, Laird PM, Hewitt P, Chalmers TL. Meta-analysis of empirical long-term antiarrhythmic therapy for myocardial infarction. JAMA 1989; 262:3037–3044.
59. Furberg CD. Effect of antiarrhythmic drugs on mortality after myocardial infarction. Am J Cardiol 1983; 52:32C.
60. Steinbeck G, Andersen D, Bach P, et al. A comparison of electrophysiologically guided antiarrhythmic drug therapy with beta-blocker therapy in patients with symptomatic sustained ventricular tachyarrythmias. N Engl J Med 1992; 372:987–992.
61. Manolis AS, Urrichio F, Estes NAM. Prognostic value of early electrophysiologic studies for ventricular tachycardia recurrence in patients with coronary artery disease treated with amiodarone. Am J Cardiol 1989; 63:1052–1057.
62. Kim SG, Felder SD, Figura I, Johnston DR, Wapse LE, Fisher JD. Value of Holter monitoring in predicting long-term efficacy and inefficacy of amiodarone used alone and in combination with class IA antiarrhythmic agents in patients with ventricular tachycardia. J Am Coll Cardiol 1987; 9:169–174.
63. Veltri EP, Griffith LSC, Platia EV, Guarnieri T, Reid PR. The use of ambulatory monitoring in the prognostic evaluation of patients with sustained ventricular tachycardia treated with amiodarone. Circulation 1986; 74:1054–1060.
64. McGovern B, Garan H, Malacoff RF, et al. Long-term clinical outcome of ventricular tachycardia or fibrillation treated with amiodarone. Am J Cardiol 1984; 53:1558–63.
65. Naccarelli GV, Fincberg NS, Zipes DP, Higger JJ, Duncan G, Prystowsky EN. Amiodarone: risk factors for recurrence of symptomatic ventricular tachycardia indentified at electrophysiologic study. J Am Coll Cardiol 1985; 6:814–821.
66. Nademanee K, Hendrickson J, Kannan R, Singh BN. Antiarrhythmic efficacy and electrophysiologic actions of amiodarone in patients with life-threatening ventricular arrhythmias: potent suppression of spontaneously occuring tachyarrhythmias versus inconsistent abolition of induced ventricular tachycardia. Am Heart J 1982; 103:905–909.

67. Kim Sg, Felder SD, Figura I, Johnston DR, Waspe LE, Risher JD. Value of Holter monitoring in predicting long-term efficacy and inefficacy of amiodarone used alone and in combination with class IA antiarrhythmic agents in patients with ventricular tachycardia. J Am Coll Cardiol 1987; 9:169–174.
68. Stamato NJ, Marchlinski FE. Role of Holter monitoring in the management of patients with ventricular tachycardia treated with amiodarone. Clin Prog Electrophysiol Pacing 1986; 4:395–401.
69. Sokoloff NM, Spielman SR, Greenspan AM, et al. Utility of ambulatory electrocardiographic monitoring for predicting recurrence of sustained ventricular tachyarrhythmias in patients receiving amiodarone. J Am Coll Cardiol 1986; 7:938–941.
70. Marchlinski FE, Buxton AE, Flores BT, Doherty JU, Waxman HL, Josephson ME. Value of Holter monitoring in identifying risk for sustained ventricular arrhythmia recurrence on amiodarone. Am J Cardiol 1985; 55:709–712.
71. Veltri EP, Reid RP, Platia EV, Griffith LSC. Amiodarone in the treatment of life-threatening ventricular tachycardia: role of Holter monitoring in predicting long-term clinical efficacy. J Am Coll Cardiol 1985; 6:806–813.
72. Kadish AH, Buxton AE, Waxman HL, Flores B, Josephson ME, Marchlinski PE. Usefulness of electrophysiologic study to determine the clinical tolerance of arrhythmia recurrences during amiodarone therapy. J Am Coll Cardiol 1987; 10:790–796.
73. Herre JM, Suave MJ, Malone P, et al. Long-term results of amiodarone in patients with recurrent sustained ventricular tachycardia or ventricular fibrillation. J Am Coll Cardiol 1989; 13:442–449.
74. Morady F, Sauve MJ, Malone P, et al. Long-term efficacy and toxicity of high-dose amiodarone therapy for ventricular tachycardia or ventricular fibrillation. Am J Cardiol 1983; 52:975–979.
75. Fogoros RN, Fiedler SB, Elson JJ. Empiric amiodarone versus "ineffective" drug therapy in patients with refractory ventricular arrhythmias. PACE 1988; 11:1009–1017.
76. Greene HL, Poole JE, Fellows CL, Broudy DR, Kudenchuk PJ, Dolack GL, Bardy G, Maynard C, Hallstrom AP, Graham-Renfroe E, Powell JL, Main CC, Busch M, Sanders JB, Herity DL, CASCADE Investigators. Cardiac arrest in Seattle-Conventional versus amiodarone drug evaluation (CASCADE): Mortality Results. Circulation 1992; 86:2610.
77. Bigger JT. Future studies with the implantable cardioverter defibrillator. PACE 1991; 14:883–889.
78. CABG Patch Investigators. Results of the Pilot Study. Progress in Cardiovascular Disease. Drug in Cardiovas D 1993; 36:97–114.
79. Moss AJ. MUSTT and MADITT Trials. Examined the role of antiarrhythmic therapy in nonsustained VT patients. AICD Advances 1990: 5–7.
80. MADIT Executive Committee: Multicenter Automatic Defibrillator Implantation Trial (MADIT): design and clinical protocol. PACE 1992; 14:920(part II).
81. Freedman RA, Swerdlow CD, Soderholm-Difatte V, Mason JW. Clinical predictors of arrhythmia inducibility in survivors of cardiac arrest: importance of gender and prior myocardial infarction. J Am Coll Cardiol 1988; 12:973–978.
82. Kron J, Kudenchuck PJ, Murphy ES, et al. Ventricular fibrillation survivors in whom tachyarrhythmia cannot be induced: outcome related to selected therapy. PACE 1987; 10:1291–1300.
83. Freedman RA, Swerdlow CD, Soderholm-Difatte V, Mason JW. Prognostic significance of arrhythmia inducibility or noninducibility at initial electrophysiologic study in survivors of cardiac arrest. Am J Cardiol 1988; 61:578–582.
84. Candall BG, Morris CD, Culter JE, et al. The implantable defibrillator in non-inducible sudden death survival (abstr). Circulation 1991; 84:II–609.
85. Handelsman H. Implantation of the automatic implantable cardioverter defibrillator: noninducibility of ventricular tachyarrhythmias as a patient selection criteria. AHCPR 91-0041 Health Technology Assessment Report 1990; 10:1–7.
86. Garan H, Nguyen K, McGovern B, et al. Perioperative and long-term results after electrophysiologically directed ventricular surgery for recurrent ventricular tachycardia. J Am Coll Cardiol 1986; 8:201–209.

87. Swerdlow CD, Mason JW, Stinson EB, et al. Results of operations for ventricular tachycardia in 105 patients. J Thorac Cardiovasc Surg 1986; 92:105–113.
88. McGiffin DC, Kirklin JK, Plumb VJ, et al. Relief of life-threatening ventricular tachycardia and survival after direct operations. Circulation 1987; 76(suppl 5):93–103.
89. Krafchek J, Lawrie GM, Roberts R, et al. Surgical ablation of ventricular tachycardia; improved results with a map-directed regional approach. Circulation 1986; 73:1239–1247.
90. Ostermeyer J, Borggrefe M, Breithardt G, et al. Direct operations for the management of life-threatening ischemic ventricular tachycaardia. J Thorac Cardiovasc Surg 1987; 94:848–865.
91. Haines DE, Lerman BB, Kron IL, et al. Surgical ablation of ventricular tachycardia with sequential map-guided subendocardial resection: electrophysiologic assessment and long-term follow-up. Circulation 1988; 77:131–141.
92. Hargrove WE, Josephson ME, Marchlinski FE, et al. Surgical decisions in the management of sudden cardiac death and malignant ventricular arrhythmias. J Thorac Cardiovasc Surg 1989; 97:923–928.
93. Manolis AS, Rastegar H, Payne D, Cleveland R, Estes NAM III. Drug refractory ventricular tachycardia: results with mapping guided subendocardial resection. J Am Coll Cardiol 1989; 14:199–200.
94. Harken AH, Josephson ME, Horowitz LN. Surgical endocardial resection for the treatment of malignant ventricular tachycardia. Circulation 1979; 190:456–60.
95. Witting JH, Boineau JP. Surgical treatment of ventricular arrhythmias using epicardial, transmural, and endocardial mapping. Ann Thorac Surg 1975; 20:117–26.
96. Cuiraudon GM, Klein GJ, Sharma AD, Yee R. Use of old and new anatomic, electrophysiologic, and technical knowledge of direct operative approaches ot tachycardia: predictors of surgical success. Circulation 1984; 70:624–631.
97. Miller JM, Kienzle MG, Harken AH, Josephson ME. Subendocardial resection for ventricular tachycardia: predictors of surgical success. Circulation 1984; 70:624–631.
98. Miller JM, Gottlieb CD, Marchlinski FE, Hargrove WC, Josephson ME. Does ventricular tachycardia mapping influence the success of antiarrhythmic surgery? (abstr). J Am Coll Cardiol 1988; 11:112A.
99. Mason JW, Stinson EB, Winkle RA, et al. Surgery for ventricular tachycardia: efficacy of left ventricular aneurysm resection compared with operation guided by electrical activation mapping. Am J Cardiol 1982; 49:221–240.
100. Gallagher JJ, Kasell JH, Cox JL, Smith WM, Ideker RE, Smith WM. Techniques of intraoperative electrophysiologic mapping. Am J Cardiol 1982; 49:221–240.
101. Gallagher JJ, Selle JG, Stevenson RH, et al. Surgical treatment of arrhythmias. Am J Cardiol 1988; 61:27A–44A.
102. Caceres J, Werner P, Jazayeri M, Akhtar M, Tchou P. Efficacy of cryosurgery alone for refractory monomorphic sustained ventricular tachycardia due to inferior wall infarction. J Am Coll Cardiol 1988; 11:1254–1259.
103. Selle JG, Svenson RH, Sealy WC, et al. Successful clinical laser ablation of ventricular tachycardia: a promising new therapeutic method. Ann Thorac Surg 1986; 42:380–384.
104. Harken AH, Horowitz LN, Josephson ME. Comparison of standard aneurysmectomy with directed endocardial resection for the treatment of recurrent sustained ventricular tachycardia. J Thorac Cardiovasc Surg 1980; 80:527–534.
105. Mason JW, Stinson EB, Winkle RA, Oyer PE, Griffin JC, Ross DL. Relative efficacy of blind left ventricular aneurysm resection for the treatment of recurent ventricular tachycardia. Am J Coll Cardiol 1986; 8:201–209.
106. Kron IL, Lerman BB, DiMarco JP. Extended subendocardial resection: a surgical approach to ventricular tachyarrhythmias that cannot be mapped intraoperatively. J Thorac Cardiovasc Surg 1985; 90:586–591.
107. Landymore RW, Kinley CE, Gardner M. Encircling endocardial resection with complete removal of endocardial scar without intraoperative mapping for the ablation of drug-resistant ventricular tachycardia. J Thorac Cardiovasc Surg 1985; 89:18–24.

108. Guiraudon G, Fontaine G, Frank R, Escande G, Etievent P, Cabrol C. Encircling endocardial ventriculotomy: a new surgical treatment for life-threatening ventricular tachycardias resistant to medical treatment following myocardial infarction. Ann Thorac Surg 1978; 26:438–444.
109. Sami M, Chaitman BR, Bourassa MG, Charpin D, Chabot M. Long-term follow-up of aneurysmectomy for recurrent ventricular tachycardia or fibrillation. Am Heart J 1978; 96:303–308.
110. DiMarco JP, Lerman BB, Kron IL, Sellers TD. Sustained ventricular tachyarrhythmias within 2 months of acute myocardial infarction: results of medical and surgical therapy in patients resuscitated from the initial episode. J Am Coll Cardiol 1985; 6:759–768.
111. Miller JM, Josephson ME. Malignant ventricular arrhythmias early after myocardial infarction: brighter prospects. J Am Coll Cardiol 1985; 6:769–771.
112. Watkins L, Platia EV, Mower MM, Griffith LSC, Mirowski M, Reid PR. The treatment of malignant ventricular arrhythmias with combined endocardial resection and implantation of the automatic defibrillator: preliminary report. Ann Thorac Surg 1984; 37:60–66.
113. Platia EV, Griffith LSC, Watkins L, et al. Treatment of malignant ventricular arrhythmias with endocardial resection and implantation of the automatic cardioverter-defibrillator. N Engl J Med 1986; 314:213–216.
114. Manolis As, Rastegar H, Estes NAM. Prophylactic automatic implantable cardioverter-defibrillator patches in patients at high risk for post-operative ventricular tachyarrhythmias. J Am Coll Cardiol 1989; 13:1367–1373.
115. Josephson ME, Harken AH, Horowitz LN. Endocardial excision—a new surgical technique for the treatment of recurrent ventricular tachycardia. Circulation 1979; 60:1430–1439.
116. Horowitz LN, Harken AH, Kastor JA, et al. Ventricular resection guided by epicardial and endocardial mapping for treatment of recurrent ventricular tachycardia. N Engl J Med 1980; 302:589–593.
117. Moran KM, Kehoe R, Leob JM, et al. Extended endocardial resection for the treatment of ventricular tachycardia and fibrillation. Ann Thorac Surg 1982; 34:538–551.
118. Mittleman RS, Wang PJ, Rastegar H, Estes NAM III. Surgical therapy for drug refractory ventricular tachycardia: results with mapping guided approach. Choices in Cardiol 1989; 5:198–202.
119. Passamani E, Davis KB, Gillespie MJ, et al. A randomized trial of coronary artery bypass surgery. Survival of patients with a low ejection fraction. N Engl J Med 1985; 312:1665–1671.
120. Garan H, Ruskin JN, DiMarco JP, et al. Electrophysiologic studies before and after myocardial revascularization in patients with life-threatening ventricular arrhythmias. Am J Cardiol 1983; 51:519–524.
121. Manolis AS, Rastegar H, Estes NAM III. Effects of coronary artery bypass grafting on ventricular arrhythmias: results with electrophysiologic testing and long-term follow-up. PACE 1993; 16:984–999.
122. Kelly P, Ruskin J, Vlachakes GJ, Buckley MJ, Freeman CS, Garan H. Surgical coronary revascularization in survivors of pre-hospital arrest: its effect on inducible arrhythmias and long-term survival. J Am Coll Cardiol 1990; 15:267–273.
123. Tresch DD, Wetherbee JN, Siegel R, et al. Long-term follow-up of survivors of pre-hospital sudden cardiac death treated with coronary bypass surgery. Am Heart J 1985; 110:1139–1145.
124. Couch OA. Cardiac aneurysm with ventricular tachycardia and subsequent excision of aneurysm. Circulation 1959; 20:251–253.
125. Fontaine G, Tonet JL, Frank R, et al. La fulguration endocavitaire: une nouvelle methode de traitement des troubles du rhythme? Ann Cardiol Angeiol (Paris) 1984; 33:543–561.
126. Morady F. A perspective on the role of catheter ablation in the management of tachyarrhmnias. PACE 1988; 11:98–102.
127. Hartzler GO. Electrode catheter ablation of refractory focal ventricular tachycardia. J Am Coll Cardiol 1983; 2:1107–1113.
128. Evans, GT, Scheinman MM, Zipes DP, et al. The percutaneous cardiac mapping and ablation registry: final summary of results. PACE 1988; 11:1621–1626.
129. Scheinman MM, Evans GT. Catheter ablation of cardiac arrhythmias: a summary report of the percutaneous cardiac mapping and ablation registry. In: Brugada P, Wellens HJJ, eds. Cardiac Arrhythmias: Where to Go from Here? Mount Kisco, NY: Futura, 1987:529–538.

130. Fitzgerald DM, Friday KJ, Wah JA, et al. Electrogram patterns predicting successful catheter ablation of ventricular tachycardia. Circulation 1988; 77:806–814.
131. Stevenson WG, Weiss J, Weinder I, et al. Localization of slow conduction in a ventricular tachycardia circuit: implications for catheter ablation. Am Heart J 1987; 114:1253–1258.
132. Scheinman MM, Evans GT Jr. Catheter electrical ablation of cardiac arrhythmias. A summary report of the percutaneous cardiac mapping and ablation registry. In: Brugada P. Wellens HJJ, eds. Cardiac Arrhythmias: Where to Go from Here? Mount Kisco, NY: Futura, 1987: 529–538.
133. Chilson DA, Peigh PS, Mahomed Y, et al. Chemical ablation of ventricular tachycardia in the dog. Am Heart J 1986; 111:1113–1118.
134. Brugada P, de Swart H, Smeets JL, et al. Transcoronary chemical ablation of ventricular tachycardia. Circulation 1989; 79:475–482.
135. Plumb V, Epstein AE, Kay NW. A prospective trial of intracoronary ETOH ablation for recurrent sustained ventricular tachycardia. Circulation 1989.
136. Oeff M, Langberg JJ, Chin M, Finkbeiner WE, Scheinman MM. Ablation of ventricular tachycardia using multiple sequential transcatheter application of radiofrequency energy. PACE 1992; 15:1167–1176.
137. Davis MJ, Murdock C. Radiofrequency catheter ablation of refractory ventricular tachycardia. PACE 1988; 11:725–729.
138. Belhassden B, Miller HI, Geller E, et al. Transcatheter electrical shock ablation of ventricular tachycardia. J Am Coll Cardiol 1986; 7:1347–1355.
139. Morady F, Scheinman MM, Di CLJ, et al. Catheter ablation of ventricular tachycardia with intracardiac shocks: results in 33 patients. Circulation 1987; 75:1037–1049.
140. Garan H, Kuchard D, Freeman C, et al. Early assessment of the effect of map-guided transcatheter intracardiac electric shock on sustained ventricular tachycardia secondary to coronary artery disease.
141. Evans GT, Scheinman MM, Zipes DP, et al. The percutaneous cardiac mapping and ablation registry: summary of results. PACE 1987; 10:1395–1399.
142. Oeff M, Langberg JJ, Franklin JO, et al. Effects of multipolar electrode radiofrequency energy delivery on ventricular endocardium. Am Heart J 1990; 119:599–607.
143. Klein LS, Shih HT, Hackett FK, Zipes DP, Miles MV. Radiofrequency catheter ablation of ventricular tachycardia in patients without structural heart disease. Circulation 1992; 85:1666–1674.
144. Morady F, Harvey M, Kalbfleisch SJ, el-Atassi R, Calkins H, Langberg JJ. Radiofrequency catheter ablation of ventricular tachycardia in patients with coronary artery disease. Circulation 1993; 87(2):363–72
145. Wilber DJ, Baerman J, Olshansky B, Kall J, Kopp D, Adenosine-sensitive ventricular tachycardia. Clinical characteristics and response to catheter ablation. Circulation 1993; 87(1):126–34.
146. DeLacey WA, Nath S, Haines DE, Barber MJ, DiMarco JP. Adenosine and verapamil-sensitive ventricular tachycardia originating from the left ventricle: radiofrequency catheter ablation. PACE 1992; 15(12):2240–4.
147. Chinushi M, Aizawa Y, Kuwano H, Hosono H, Kitazawa H, Kusano Y, Naitho N, Tamura M, Shibata A. Successful radiofrequency current catheter ablation of sustained ventricular tachycardia. PACE 1992; 15(10 Pt 1):1460–6.
148. Tanabe A, Ikeda H, Fujiyama M, et al. Termination of ventricular tachycardia by an implantable atrial pacemaker and external pacemaker activator. PACE 1985; 8:532–538.
149. Bertholet M, Demoulin JC, Waleffe A, Kulbertus H. Programmable extrastimulus pacing for long-term management of supraventricular and ventricular tachycardias: clinical experience in 16 patients. Am Heart J 1985; 110:582–589.
150. den Dulk K, Bertholet M, Brugada P, et al. Clinical experience with implantable devices for control of tachyarrhythmias. PACE 1984; 548–556.
151. Luderitz B, d'Alnoncourt CN, Steinbeck G, Beyer J. Therapeutic pacing in tachyarrhythmias by implanted pacemakers. PACE 1982; 5:366–371.

152. Saksena S, Pantopoulos D, Parsonnet V, Rothbart ST, Hussian SM, Gielchinsky I. Usefulness of an implantable antitachycardia pacemaker system for supraventricular or ventricular tachycardia. Am J Cardiol 1986; 58:70–74.
153. Griffin JC, Sweeney M. The management of paroxysmal tachycardias using the Cybertach-60. PACE 1987; 7:1291–1295.
154. Rothman MT, Keefe JM. Clinical results with Omni-Orthocor implantable antitachycardia pacing system. PACE 1987; 7:1306–1312.
155. Reddy CP, Todd EP, Kuo SC, DeMaria AN. Treatment of ventricular tachycardia using an automatic scanning extrastimulus pacemaker. J Am Coll Cardiol 1984; 3:225–230.
156. Hartzler GO. Treatment of recurrent ventricular tachycardias by patient-activated radiofrequency ventricular stimulation. Mayo Clin Proc 1979; 54:75–82.
157. Ruskin JN, Garan H, Poulin F, Harthorne JW. Permanent radiofrequency ventricular pacing for management of drug-resistant ventricular tachycardia. Am J Cardiol 1980; 46:317–321.
158. Herre JM, Griffin JC, Nielsen AP, et al. Permanent triggered antitachycardia pacemakers in the management of recurrent sustained ventricular tachycardia. JAM Coll Cardiol 1985; 6:206–212.
159. Strasberg B, Fetter J, Palileo E, Levitsky S, Rosen KM. Postoperative electrophysiological studies with a modified radiofrequency system. Technical aspects and clinical usefulness. PACE 1982; 688–693.
160. Higgins JR, Swartz JF, Dehmer GH, Beddingfield GW. Automatic scanning extrastimulus pacemakers to treat ventricular tachycardia. PACE 1989; 8:101–109.
161. Mirowski M, Reid PR, Winkle RA, et al. Mortality in patients with implantable automatic defibrillator. Ann Intern Med 1983; 98:585–588.
162. Echt DS, Armstrong K, Schmidt P, Oyer PE, Stevenson EB, Winkle RA. Clinical experience, complications, and survival in 70 patients with the automatic implantable cardioverter defibrillator. Circulation 1985; 71:289–296.
163. Luceri RM, Thurer RJ, Palateanos GM, Fernandez PR, EL-Shalakway A, Castellanos A. The automatic implantable cardioverter defibrillator: results, observations, and comments. PACE 1986; 9:1343–1348.
164. Marchlinski FE, Flores BT, Buxton AE, et al. The automatic implantable cardioverter-defibrillator: efficacy, complications, and device failures. Ann Intern Med 1986; 104:481–488.
165. Gabry MD, Brodman R, Johnston D, et al. Automatic implantable cardioverter-defibrillator: Patient survival, battery longevity, and shock delivery analysis. J Am Coll Cardiol 1987; 9:1349–1356.
166. Reid PR, Griffith LSC, Platia EV, et al. The automatic implantable cardioverter-defibrillator: five year clinical results. In: Breithardt G, Borggrefe M., eds. Nonpharmacologic Treatment of Tachyarrhythmias. Mount Kisco, NY: Futura, 1987:477–486.
167. Barbola J, Denes P, Ezri MD, et al. The automatic implantable cardioverter-defibrillator: clinical experience, complications, and follow-up in 25 patients. Arch Intern Med 1988; 148:70–76.
168. Troup PJ, Chapman PD, Olinger GN, Kleinman LH. The implanted defibrillator: relation of defibrillator lead configuration and clinical variable to defibrillator threshold. J Am Coll Cardiol 1985; 6:1315–1321.
169. Kelly PA, Cannom DS, Gara H, et al. The automatic implantable cardioverter-defibrillator: efficacy, complications and survival in patients with malignant ventricular arrhythmias. J Am Coll Cardiol 1988; 11:1278–1286.
170. Olinger GN, Chapman PD, Troup PJ, Almassi GH. Stratified application of the automatic implantable cardioverter defibrillator. J Thorac Cardiovasc Surg 1988; 96:141–149.
171. Tchou P, Kadri N, Anderson J, Caceres J, Jazayeri M, Akhtar M. Automatic implantable cardioverter defibrillators and survival of patients with left ventricular dysfunction and malignant ventricular arrhythmias. Ann Intern Med 1988; 109:529–534.
172. Hargrove WC, Miller JM. Risk stratification and management of patients with recurrent ventricular tachycardia and other malignant ventricular arrhythmias. Circulation 1989; 79(suppl 1):178–181.

173. Manolis AS, Tan-DeGuzman W, Lee, et al. Clinical experience in seventy-seven patients with the automatic implantable cardioverter defibrillator. Am Heart J 1989; 118:445–449.
174. Myerburg RJ, Luceri RM, Thurer R, et al. Time to first shock and clinical outcomes in patients receiving an automatic implantable cardioverter-defibrillator. J Am Coll Cardiol 1989; 14:508–514.
175. Winkle RA, Mead RH, Ruder MA, et al. Long-term outcome with the automatic implantable cardioverter-defibrillator. J Am Coll Cardiol 1989; 13:1353–1361.
176. Edel B, Maloney JD, Moore SL, et al. Analysis of deaths in patients with an implantable cardioverter defibrillator. PACE 1992; 15:60–70.
177. Larsen GC, Manolis AS, Sonnenberg FA, Beshansky JR, Estes NAM III, Pauker SG. Cost-effectivenss of the automatic implantable cardioverter defibrillator: effects of improved battery life and comparison with amiodarone. J Am Coll Cardiol 1992; 19:1–12.
178. Connolly SJ, Yusef S. Evaluation of the implantable cardioverter defibrillator in survivors of cardiac arrest: the need for randomized trials. Am J Cardiol 1992; 69:959–962.
179. Furman S, Kim S. The present status of implantable cardioverter defibrillator therapy. J Cardiovasc Electrophysiol 1992; 3:602–624.
180. Maloney J, Materson M, Khoury D, et al. Clinical performance of the implantable cardioverter defibrillator: electrocardiographic documentation of 101 spontaneous discharges. PACE 1991; 14:280–285.
181. Tchou PJ, Kadri N, Anderson J, Caceres JA, Jazayeri M, Akhtar M. Automatic implantable cardioverter defibrillators and survival in patients with left ventricular dysfunction and malignant ventricular arrhythmias. Ann Intern Med 1988; 109:529–534.
182. Manolis AS, Rastegar H, Wang PJ, Estes NAM III. Implantation of the automatic defibrillator system in elderly and younger patients: comparative results. J Am Coll Cardiol 1993; 21; 212A.
183. Winkle RA. Nonpharmacologic therapy for tachycardia: the role of implanted devices. PACE 1989; 11:109.
184. Guarnieri T, Levin JH, Griffith LSC, Veltri EP. When "sudden cardiac death" is not so sudden: lessons learned from the automatic implantable defibrillator. Am Heart J 1988; 115:205–207.
185. Newman D, Sauve MJ, Herre J, et al. Survival after implantation of the cardioverter defibrillator. Am J Cardiol 1992; 69:899–903.
186. Sowton E, Sulke N. Clinical experience with the Siemens Pacesetter Siecure. J Cardiovasc Electrophysiol 1992; 3:515–522.
187. Fogoros RN, Fiedler SB, Eslon JJ. The automatic implantable cardioverter-defibrillator in drug refractory ventricular tachyarrhythmias. Ann Intern Med 1987; 106:635–641.
188. Kuck KH, Siebels J, Schneider M, Guger M. Hamburg Cardiac Arrest Study group (abstr). Rev Eur Tech Biomed 1990; 12:110.
189. Mosteller RRD, Lehmann MH, Thomas AC, Jackson K, participating investigators. Operative mortality with implantation of the automatic cardioverter defibrillatorr. Am J Cardiol 1991; 68:1340–1345.
190. Pinski SL, Sgarbossa EB, Maloney JD, Trohman RG. Survival in patients declining implantable cardioverter defibrillator. Am J Cardiol 1991; 68:800–801.
191. Levine JH, Mellits ED, Baumgardner RA, et al. Predictors of first discharge and subsequent survival in patients with automatic implantable cardioverter defibrillators. Circulation 1991; 84:558–566.
192. Marchena E, Chakko S, Fernandez P, et al. Usefulness of the automatic implantable cardioverter defibrillator in improving survival of patients with severely depressed left ventricular function associated with coronary artery disease. Am J Cardiol 1991; 67:812–816.
193. Myerburg RJ, Luceri RM, Thurer R, et al. Time to first shock and clinical outcome in patient receiving an automatic implantable cardioverter defibrillator.
194. Yusuf S, Teo KK. Approaches to prevention of sudden death: the need for fundamental re-evaluation. J Cardiovasc Electrophysiol 1991 (suppl 2):S233–S239.

195. Liberthson RR, Nagel EL, Hirschman JC, et al. Prehospital ventricular defibrillation. Prognosis and follow-up course. N Engl J Med 1974; 291:317–321.
196. Cobb LA, Werner JA, Trobaugh GB. Sudden cardiac death. I. A decade's experience with out-of-hospital resuscitation. Mod Concepts Cardiovasc Dis 1980; 49:31–36.
197. Myerburg RJ, Kessler KM, Estes D, et al. Long-term survival after prehospital cardiac arrest: analysis of outcome during an 8 year study. Circulation 1984; 70:538-546.
198. Baum RS, Alvarez H, Cobb LA. Survival after resuscitation from out-of-hospital ventricular fibrillation. Circulation 1974; 50:1231–1235.
199. Moosvi AR, Goldstein S, Medendorp SVB, et al. Effect of empiric antiarrhythmic therapy in resuscitated out-of-hospital cardiac arrest victims with coronary artery disease. Am J Cardiol 1990; 1192–1197.
200. The Cardiac Arrhythmia Suppression Trail II. Effect of the antiarrhythmic agent moricizine on survival after myocardial infarction. N Engl J Med 1992; 327:227–233.
201. Bardy G, Troutman C, Poolr J, et al. Clinical experience with a tiered-therapy multiprogrammable antiarrhythmic device. Circulation 1992; 85:1689–1694.
202. Thomas A, Moser S, Smutka ML, Wilson PA. Implantable defibrillation: eight years clinical experience PACE 1988; 11:1278–86.
203. Packer D, et al. Predicting drug efficacy in patients with sustained ventricular tachycardia: implications of differences in programmed stimulation endpoints. Circulation 1992; 86:534.
204. Teo K, Yusuf S, Furberg C. Overview of randomized trials of low dose amiodarone on mortality in cardiac patients. Circulation 1992; 86:534.
205. Hallstrom A, Greene L, McBride R. A controlled trial of implanted cardiac defibrillators versus antiarrhythmic therapy. ICD Clinical Trial Center. Univ. of Washington, Nov 23, 1992.
206. Myerburg RJ, Castellanos A. Evolution, evaluation, and efficacy of implantable cardioverter defibrillator technology. Circulation 1992; 86:691–693.
207. Holmes DR, Davis KB, Mock MR, et al. Participants in the Coronary Artery Surgery Study. The effect of medical and surgical treatment on subsequent sudden cardiac death in patients with coronary artery disease: a report from the Coronary Artery Surgery Study. Circulation 1986; 73:1254–1263.
208. Foote C, Wang PJ, Clyne C, et al. The role of left ventricular reconstruction in preserving cardiac function in patients undergoing endocardial resection. PACE 1991; 15:533.
209. Cox JL. Patient selection criteria and results of surgery for refractory ischemic ventricular tachycardia. Circulation 1989; 79(suppl I):1–163–I–77.
210. Borggrefe M, Podczeck A, Ostermeyer J, et al. Long-term results of electrophysiologically guided antitachycardia surgery in ventricular tachyarrhythmias: a collaborative report on 665 patients. In: G. Briethardt, Borggrete M, DP Zipes, eds. Nonpharmacological Therapy of Tachyarrhythmias. Mt. Kisco, NY: Futura, 1987:109–132.
211. Saksena S, Camm J. Implantable defibrillators for prevention of sudden death—technology at medical and economic crossroads. Circulation 1992; 85:2316–2322.
212. Fromer M, Brachman J, Block M, et al. Efficacy of automatic multimodal device therapy for ventricular tachyarrhythmias as delivered by a new implantable pacing cardioverter-defibrillator. Results of a European Multicenter Study of 102 implants. Circulation 1991; 86:363–374.
213. Mason JW. A comparison of electrophysiologic testing with Holter monitoring to predict antiarrhythmic drug efficacy for ventricular tachyarrhythmias. N Engl J Med 1993; 329:445–451.
214. Mason JW. A comparison of seven antiarrhythmic drugs in patients with ventricular tachyarrhythmias. N Engl J Med 1993; 329:452–458.
215. The ESVEM Investigators: Determinants of predicted efficacy of antiarrhythmic drugs in the Electrophysiologic Study Versus Electrocardiographic Monitoring Trial 1993; 97:323–329.
216. Epstein, AE. AVID Necessity. PACE 1993;16:1773–1775.
217. Greene, HL. Antiarrhythmic drugs versus implantable defibrillators: The need for a randomized controlled study. Am Heart J 1994 (in press).

16

Preoperative Evaluation for Cardioverter-Defibrillator Implant

Joseph Zebede and Antonis S. Manolis

*Tufts University School of Medicine
and New England Medical Center
Boston, Massachusetts*

The preoperative evaluation of a patient who presents with a life-threatening ventricular tachyarrhythmia and finally becomes a candidate for a cardioverter-defibrillator (ICD) implant must address several separate issues, which will constitute the topic of this chapter. At first, prompt measures are taken to stabilize the patient's rhythm. After initial resuscitative interventions and conversion of the arrhythmia, either medically or electrically, reversible causes of the arrhythmia should be sought, such as electrolyte and metabolic abnormalities, ischemia, or drug toxicity, and a myocardial infarction should be ruled out. Subsequently and once the medical condition of the patient is stabilized, noninvasive and invasive tests are performed to define the underlying anatomical cardiac substrate and to determine the electrophysiological (EP) characteristics of the patient's arrhythmia. Evaluation via EP studies will further determine such patient's candidacy for nonpharmacological therapy including an ICD implant. Comprehensive preoperative evaluation will also define the risk of ICD therapy for a particular patient. Furthermore, an assessment should be made regarding the type of concomitant surgery an individual patient might require, the surgical access to be used, and the type of ICD device the patient should receive. To accomplish all these preoperative goals, a rational, stepwise approach to the evaluation of the ICD candidate will be outlined in this chapter (Fig. 1).

The obvious requirement for ICD implantation is presenting clinically with a life-threatening ventricular tachyarrhythmia and being at risk for arrhythmia recurrence or sudden death [1–6] (see Chapter 12). On the other hand, contraindications to ICD implantation in a patient with such an arrhythmia also need to be recognized. When the life expectancy of the patient is severely compromised, it would not be appropriate to recommend this procedure, which has its own inherent morbidity and mortality. Patients on life-support systems or those with severe congestive heart failure or angina pectoris, in whom no further therapy is possible, would not qualify for ICD implantation.

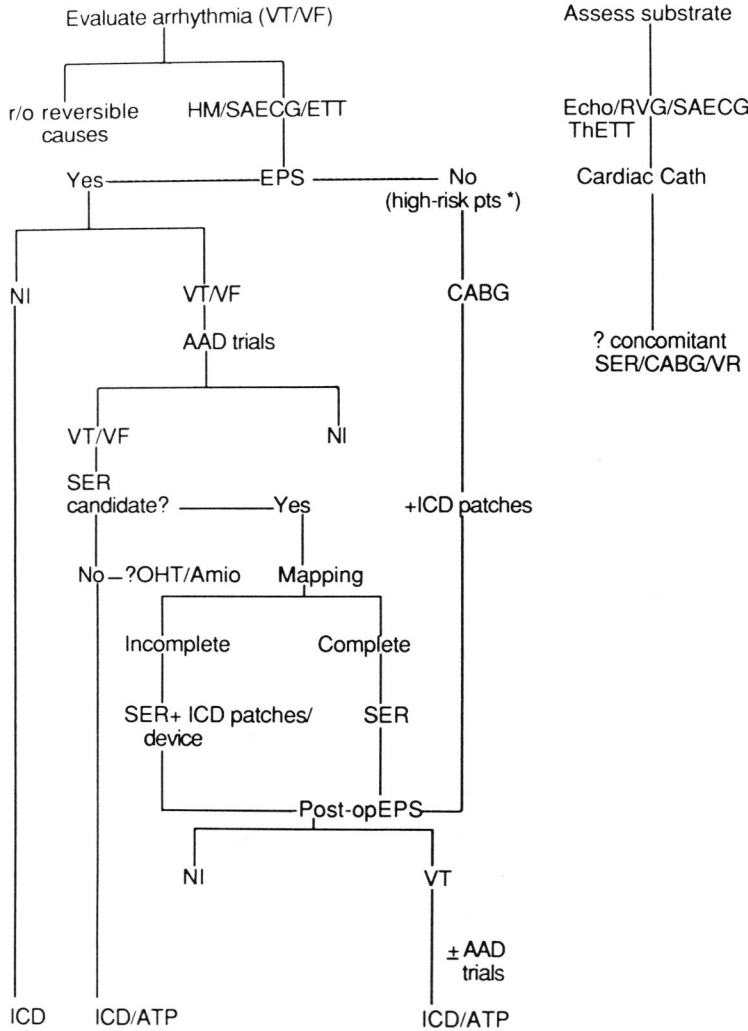

Figure 1 The flow chart indicates important steps in the preoperative evaluation of a patient who may be a candidate for an automatic implantable cardioverter defibrillator (ICD). AAD = antiarrhythmic drugs; Amio = amiodarone; ATP = antitachycardia pacing (device); CAD = coronary artery disease; CABG = coronary artery bypass grafting surgery; Cath = catheterization; Echo = echocardiogram; EPS = electrophysiology studies; ETT = exercise tolerance testing; HM = Holter monitor; NI = noninducible; OHT = orthotopic heart transplant; r/o = rule out; RVG = radionuclide ventriculogram; SAECG = signal-averaged electrocardiogram; SER = subendocardial resection; ThETT = thallium stress test; VF = ventricular fibrillation; VR = valve replacement; VT = ventricular tachycardia.

I. MEDICAL STATUS OF THE PATIENT

During the preoperative assessment of a patient being evaluated for ICD implantation, conditions which can be improved should be addressed prior to surgery. Most important, the functional status of the patient, including ambulation, nutrition, and recovery from a recent procedure such as cardiac catheterization should be optimized. Attention should also be given to addressing issues of anxiety and/or misconceptions involving both the surgical procedure and the device.

Reversible metabolic abnormalities should be normalized. Electrolyte imbalances, calcium and magnesium deficiencies, and significant anemia should be corrected. Aspirin therapy should be discontinued preoperatively, especially in patients undergoing concomitant coronary artery bypass surgery, in order to minimize bleeding complications [7–10].

Infection is generally a contraindication to any surgical procedure. This is especially true for ICD implantation. Patients should be screened for the presence of common infections by chest X-ray and urinalysis, in addition to routine hematological parameters. Treatment of the infection must be complete, and negative repeat culture results must be documented prior to surgery. Skin integrity should be optimized, as well as treatment for folliculitis and minor skin infections in the areas of proposed surgical incisions. Evaluation by a dentist or oral surgeon should be obtained if there is evidence of dental or periodontal pathology. Dental extractions, if necessary, should be considered prior to surgery in order to minimize this potential source of bacteremia. Prophylactic antibiotics may be administered before ICD implantation, although their role in reducing the risk of infection has not been evaluated in appropriately controlled studies [11].

Chronic respiratory disease is not a contraindication to surgery unless respiratory function, as assessed by pulmonary function tests, is so significantly impaired that it makes unlikely successful weaning from respiratory support postoperatively. Care should be given to maximizing pulmonary toilet and treating any concomitant infections. Patients with previous amiodarone-induced pulmonary toxicity may be at increased risk of life-threatening postoperative pulmonary complications [12]. To that extent some investigators have recommended discontinuation of amiodarone for several weeks before surgery if possible [12]. In patients whose respiratory status precludes the use of general anesthesia, a nonthoracotomy system may be indicated. A transdiaphragmatic approach using epidural anesthesia has been used with some success in a small number of patients [13].

Chronically elevated liver function tests may be seen in patients as result of low cardiac output states. As long as they do not signify active infection or significant hepatic failure, they do not preclude surgical intervention. Patients with chronic hepatitis who have a prolonged life expectancy may be considered for ICD implant, but patients with or approaching end-stage liver disease are not candidates for ICD implantation. A careful assessment should be performed in patients with underlying liver dysfunction in whom it is anticipated that hepatically metabolized drugs will be required.

Acute renal insufficiency should be stabilized and preferably reversed prior to surgery. Chronic renal insufficiency is not in itself a contraindication to ICD surgery. Patients on hemodialysis may be at increased risk of arrhythmia, given the rapid changes in electrolyte concentrations and volume status. In addition, they may have chronic mineral deficiencies. The above-mentioned considerations in terms of hepatically metabolized drugs apply here as well. The perioperative management should concentrate in optimizing the patient's fluid and electrolyte status. Dialysis should be performed close to the time of surgery and postoperatively as indicated.

The appropriateness of ICD implantation in patients with hematological disorders and malignancy should be addressed on an individual basis. Given the wide spectrum of these disorders, clinical judgment is of paramount importance. For instance, the patient with prostate carcinoma in remission, who may have a life expectancy of several years and is troubled by ventricular tachycardia (VT) refractory to medications, may be considered for an ICD. On the other hand, patients with a depressed immune response would be increasingly vulnerable to infectious complications and may have a markedly reduced life expectancy, making them poor candidates for ICD therapy.

Patients with neurological impairment must have a rather individualized evaluation with regard to their candidacy for ICD treatment. Most important, care should be exercised in minimizing hypotension and volume changes in patients with significant cerebrovascular disease. Patients with carotid bruits or transient neurological symptoms should have noninvasive evaluation of their cerebral circulation. Some young patients with muscular dystrophies are at risk for sudden death because of myocardial involvement [14]. If they are candidates for ICD implant, the potential for bradycardias must be considered during selection of the device.

II. CARDIOVASCULAR RISKS

As with other cardiac and noncardiac surgery, coronary artery disease, valvular heart disease, and congestive heart failure increase the risk of the procedure. Some additional risks inherent to the ICD population include the previous or anticipated use of antiarrhythmic medications. These are often necessary to suppress unsustained VT or to change the VT characteristics to render it pace-terminable or better tolerated hemodynamically [15]. Antiarrhythmic drugs may potentially render ICD surgery less successful by increasing defibrillation thresholds. Although the data in this regard are scant, there are experimental [16] and clinical reports [17–23] which suggest that this is an important consideration. Moreover, it has been suggested that defibrillation thresholds may increase over time. Thus, in patients who are to be started on antiarrhythmic medications, it may be prudent to test defibrillation thresholds after the drug has been initiated [15,17]. Amiodarone therapy in particular may be associated with this problem [17,22,23].

Another potential risk associated with amiodarone use is the development of postoperative respiratory failure and longer stay in the intensive-care unit [24,25]. The risk appears to be reduced by discontinuation of the drug prior to surgery [26]. Abnormal pulmonary function tests, length of amiodarone therapy greater than 300 days, or a total preoperative dose of greater than 100 g were associated with postoperative complications. Postoperative adult respiratory distress syndrome was seen even after a short course of amiodarone therapy in a recent series [25].

Cessation of amiodarone therapy in an attempt to reduce the incidence of postoperative complications requires hospital admission, as these patients would be at high risk for the development of lethal arrhythmia during the washout phase. Most important, a number of patients have ICD treatment prescribed precisely because of pulmonary disease secondary to amiodarone toxicity. These patients are at a particularly high perioperative risk [12]. Unilateral pulmonary infiltrates as a possible postoperative manifestation of amiodarone pulmonary toxicity have been described [27]. Low intraoperative fractions of inspired oxygen (FIO_2) have been suggested in order to minimize amiodarone pulmonary toxicity, as high FIO_2 appear to be a common denominator in postoperative deaths from respiratory failure [28]. Other reported complications have included perioperative atropine/isoproterenol-resistant bradycardia in a patient treated with amiodarone [29]. In addition, a myocardial depressant effect is feared in these patients as well [30]. Intraoperative hemodynamic instability has been noted by some authors [29,30]. It may be attributed to bradycardia or to vasodilatory or negative inotropic effects. Because amiodarone has calcium antagonist properties, it has been suggested that preoperative calcium levels be normalized. Moreover, cardiopulmonary bypass may be associated with significant changes in total ionized calcium [30].

Many patients being considered for ICD therapy have a history of previous myocardial infarction. Although immediate periinfarction arrhythmias would not require long-term treatment, many of these patients develop significant late arrhythmias which eventually lead to electrophysiological studies, antiarrhythmic drugs, surgery, and/or ICD implantation. If arrhythmia surgery is needed, there is a somewhat higher risk to the operative procedure based on the recent myocardial infarction [31]. This risk is probably tempered, however, by detailed knowledge of the patient's coronary anatomy prior to the procedure and the possible beneficial effect of concomitant revascularization.

III. CARDIAC EVALUATION

Given the fact that ventricular tachyarrhythmias are the end manifestation of a large number of disease processes, essentially all diagnostic modalities used in clinical cardiology are valuable in the diagnostic evaluation. Obviously, different techniques have different strengths and applicability, depending on the disease entity involved. Moreover, they all contribute to the overall assessment of patients and their perioperative risk. Some of the test results will aid in the diagnosis, whereas some will serve as preoperative baseline.

The *surface electrocardiogram* (ECG) is most helpful initially in suggesting the etiology of the underlying cardiac disease. For instance, a low-voltage ECG may suggest an infiltrative cardiomyopathy, such as amyloidosis or sarcoidosis, while Q waves and giant T waves are suggestive of hypertrophic cardiomyopathy. Long QT syndromes as well as some metabolic abnormalities may be detected by ECG as well. Previous myocardial infarction is suggested by the presence of Q waves, while short PR interval and delta waves are diagnostic of preexcitation syndromes. Perhaps most important, a 12-lead ECG of the tachycardia may suggest the site of origin of the ventricular tachycardia in patients with or without coronary artery disease [32]. Tachycardias with a fascicular or right ventricular focus may display characteristic patterns. Specifically, bundle branch reentry VT with typical LBBB ECG pattern may be seen in patients with idiopathic dilated cardiomyopathy, and repetitive monomorphic (catecholamine-sensitive) VT with a characteristic LBBB/inferior axis morphology may occur in the absence of organic heart disease. Importantly, both these types of VT are now amenable to catheter ablation with use of radiofrequency energy. In patients with right ventricular dysplasia, VT typically has an LBBB morphology, but in addition, characteristic ECG abnormalities are also present during sinus rhythm, including incomplete RBBB, inverted T waves in V_1–V_3, and occasional "ripples" in the ST segment in V_1 and V_2 (epsilon waves).

The *signal-averaged ECG* and body surface mapping have their greatest utility as risk stratification instruments. These may sway the diagnostic process toward invasive electrophysiological studies and yet by themselves are of limited preoperative value. Signal-averaged ECG has limited usefulness in patients with bundle branch block or intraventricular conduction delay. Frequency domain analysis may be more helpful in these circumstances. Interestingly, there is evidence that the signal-averaged ECG will normalize postoperatively in patients who have undergone subendocardial resection [33]. In patients who undergo implantation of an ICD, the signal-averaged ECG is usually not predictive of postoperative occurrence of ICD shocks [34].

Echocardiography is useful in assessing the presence and severity of valvular disease which may need surgical intervention. In addition, estimates of pulmonary arterial systolic pressure may be obtained if tricuspid regurgitation is present. Assessment of regional wall motion abnormalities and estimates of overall ventricular function are very useful. In terms of specific disease entities, hypertrophic cardiomyopathy, mitral valve prolapse, and right ventricular abnormalities may be readily detectable. The myocardial texture may give clues to infiltrative disease, such as amyloidosis. Cardiac and pericardial malignancies may become evident [35]. Other arrhythmogenic abnormalities may be diagnosed by the echocardiogram, such as tetralogy of Fallot, although in general the diagnosis of these is made during infancy. The presence of a dilated coronary sinus may be a clue to a persistent left-sided superior vena cava. This is most important if placement of an endocardial lead is anticipated either for sensing/pacing or defibrillation purposes, particularly if a coronary sinus configuration is being considered.

Radionuclide ventriculography is particularly useful in providing quantitative assessment of ventricular function, including measuring excess ejection fraction as an estimate of nonaneurysmal left ventricular wall motion. This may be especially important in predicting outcome in patients with markedly diminished left ventricular ejection fraction in the presence of an aneurysm [36]. The presence of dyskinetic areas in both ventricles can be readily ascertained. In addition, experienced observers may be able to detect subtle abnormalities in right ventricular function, including global decrease in wall motion or localized dysfunction of the outflow tract. In patients in whom ventricular reconstruction is anticipated, serial radionuclide ventriculograms can provide a convenient comparison of pre- and postoperative ventricular function. The preoperative left ventricular ejection fraction has prognostic implications in patients who will undergo ICD implant. The benefit, in terms of prolonging survival, appears to be greatest for patients with both moderate and severely depressed function [37].

Exercise radionuclide scans provide very useful information, which can be employed as both a diagnostic parameter and as a branching point for management decision. The exercise portion of the test provides direct information on exercise-induced/ischemia-mediated, or noncoronary artery disease/catecholamine-sensitive ventricular tachycardia. ST segment analysis, as well as an abnormal blood pressure response, may indicate the severity of the ischemic component of the disease. The radionuclide images may suggest significant left ventricular dysfunction when lung uptake is present. In the context of coronary artery disease and ischemia, this may favor revascularization if at all possible.

The most significant contribution to the assessment of myocardium at risk comes from the thallium or sestamibi images, especially in those patients whose baseline abnormalities render ECG changes nondiagnostic. The use of 24-h delayed images [38], or reinjection with thallium [39], may identify areas of viable myocardium which can appear to be areas of infarction if only traditional stress and rest images are used [40] (Fig. 2). Approximately 40% of fixed defects may become reversible upon reinjection. This approach has been expanded and validated using positron emission tomography (PET) scanning with ^{18}F-fluorodeoxy-glucose as a standard test for myocardial viability [41]. In patients in whom exercise is not a practical possibility, resting scans may be used instead.

Myocardial viability is a truly significant issue, especially in the subset of patients with previous myocardial infarction and markedly diminished left ventricular function. Many of these patients will actually have improved ventricular function postoperatively if revascularization is effected. Thus the patient with borderline left ventricular function for coronary artery bypass surgery may actually have a significant improvement in ventricular function and functional status following the surgery. The experience with isotopes other than thallium, such as sestamibi, suggests a correlation with thallium data but remains to be validated [42,43].

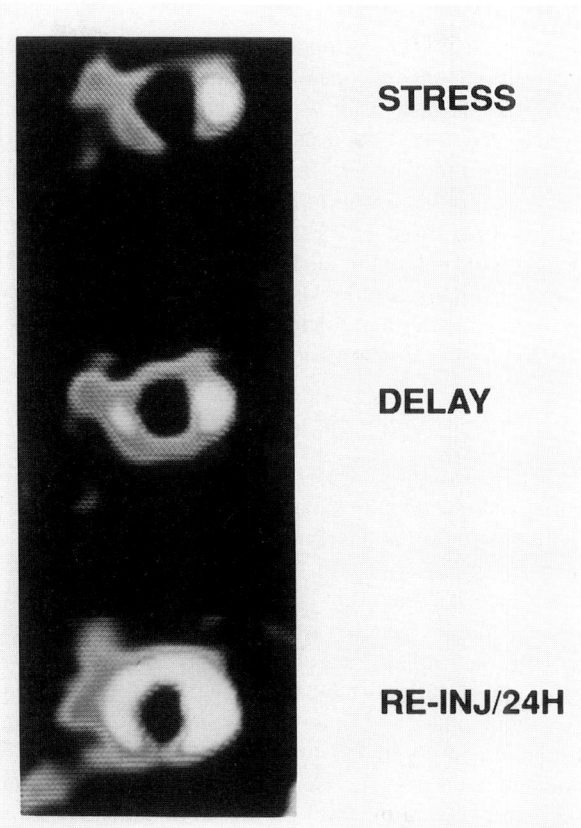

Figure 2 Stress-thallium imaging using the 24-h/reinjection technique. The left ventricle is seen in cross section. The stress image shows evidence of anterior wall and septal ischemia. During the standard delay image there is some improvement of the defect in the inferior septum, suggesting a small area of reversibility. The reinjection/24-h image demonstrates complete reversibility of the defect in the anterior and anteroseptal walls, suggesting myocardial viability of a large territory. (Courtesy of Udelson.)

Computed tomography and magnetic resonance imaging (MR) are nearly always useful in determining pericardial disease and the presence of malignancy in a small number of patients who have this as the cause of their ventricular arrhythmia. MR scans may provide early clues to the diagnosis of arrhythmogenic right ventricular disease as it may be heralded by fatty infiltration.

IV. CARDIAC CATHETERIZATION

Right and left heart catheterizations should be performed routinely in patients undergoing evaluation for ventricular tachycardia. A distinct emphasis is placed in obtaining biplane left ventriculograms to assess motion of all ventricular wall segments. This has obvious advantages in more accurately determining the preoperative left ventricular ejection fraction. Most important, in patients who are candidates for subendocardial resection and/or left ventricular aneurysmorrhaphy, biplane images assessing the location and extent of the aneurysm as well as nonaneurysmal segmental wall motion provide the surgeon with invaluable information in terms of risk stratifying and planning an operative strategy. Moreover, the location of the aneurysm and VT origin in the inferoposterior wall has prognostic implications in terms of postoperative arrhythmia recurrence [44,45]. In patients in whom right ventricular abnormalities are suspected and certainly in those under 40 years of age, biplane right ventriculography is performed as well. This may provide useful information in terms of right ventricular dysplasia or right ventricular outflow tract disease.

Coronary angiography will outline the anatomical need for revascularization. In addition, the presence of anomalous coronary arteries as the possible cause for ventricular arrhythmias must be ruled out. In patients in whom coronary artery bypass surgery is anticipated, it is advantageous to visualize both internal mammary arteries.

V. PREOPERATIVE ELECTROPHYSIOLOGICAL STUDIES

Several specific aspects of electrophysiological (EP) testing should be emphasized. The inducibility of VT at electrophysiological studies may have prognostic implications in some patient populations [46,47]. Noninducibility at baseline EP studies in patients surviving cardiac arrest does not imply a benign prognosis [48–50]. Outcome is significantly poorer in patients in whom the left ventricular ejection fraction is decreased [50–52]. As with any test, the sensitivity and specificity of EP studies depends on the population being studied. It has less predictive accuracy in patients with dilated cardiomyopathy than in those with coronary artery disease [53]. Nonetheless, these patients have a high incidence of sudden death [54,55]. Thus, patients with dilated cardiomyopathy who are cardiac-arrest survivors may benefit from ICD therapy regardless of noninducibility at EP studies. These limitations of EP studies have been recognized by governmental agencies. The Health Care Financing Administration does not require inducibility of arrhythmia in order for a patient to be considered for ICD implantation.

EP-guided pharmacological suppression of ventricular arrhythmias has been shown to be predictive of an improved outcome [49–51]. Even in this group, however, some have argued that ICD therapy is so effective in treating recurrent arrhythmia that it may be worthwhile comparing both therapies prospectively [50]. The case for ICD implantation has been further made for specific subgroups. For instance, it has been suggested that some therapeutic failures in patients rendered noninducible by antiarrhythmic drugs may be due to catecholamine-mediated effects. Adjunctive ICD therapy was offered to patients rendered inducible by isoproterenol challenge in a recent series [56]. In this small sample, those patients were found to be at an increased risk for recurrent arrhythmia. In one series [57], patients whose presenting arrhythmia was ventricular fibrillation had similar arrhythmia-free survival regardless of suppression at the time of EP studies, although most nonsuppressed patients were treated with empiric amiodarone, which would theoretically reduce their risk. This suggested that EP-guided drug therapy may not be as useful in this population as compared to patients presenting with monomorphic ventricular tachycardia. The inability of one antiarrhythmic drug to control ventricular tachycardia is predictive of failure to respond to medical therapy. Studies evaluating the efficacy of serial drug testing have concluded that after failure to respond to two drugs, attempts at suppression by yet a third drug combination are generally unsuccessful [58]. Thus, recently there has been a clear trend toward fewer drug trials, based in part on these latter findings but also on the better long-term outcome with ICD therapy as compared to EP-guided drug therapy. Patients with right ventricular disease may constitute a distinct subgroup with regard to their response to specific drugs. In a recent series [59], the most effective regimen in this population was sotalol. The authors suggested that patients with inducible ventricular tachycardia who are refractory to sotalol treatment should be considered for nonpharmacological therapy. In general, the availability and efficacy of nonpharmacological therapy with ICD implantation, with its consequent low morbidity and mortality, has shifted the focus of the evaluation toward earlier institution of ICD therapy [59–63]. Moreover, this trend may be further fueled as devices become more cost-effective and no thoracotomy is required.

It is of paramount importance to assess the actual mechanism of the ventricular tachycardia at the time of diagnostic EP study, regardless of the suppression of the arrhythmia by drugs. A careful investigation may reveal tachycardia mechanisms which are amenable to relatively simple, nonpharmacological cures. For instance, bundle branch reentrant tachycardia may be eliminated by radiofrequency ablation of the right bundle. Right ventricular outflow-tract ventricular tachycardia may also be responsive to radiofrequency ablation [64]. Verapamil-sensitive VT may be missed and subsequently be refractory to other pharmacological interventions.

Patients being considered for nonpharmacological therapy are generally refractory or intolerant to medical treatment, which, though as already mentioned, there is currently a tendency to limit to two or three drug studies, the exception to this rule being, of course, patients with cardiac arrest whose arrhythmias are noninducible in the EP laboratory. The issue in this group is the lack of endpoints for medical therapy in a population at high risk. Nonetheless, in patients with inducible arrhythmia, the electrophysiological study should be geared to more than the assessment of noninducibility by electropharmacology. Indeed, several other objectives should be considered. Among these, an assessment should be made of the effect of medical therapy in diminishing the amount and ease of inducibility of ventricular tachycardia. This is especially important in patients with very frequent episodes or incessant tachycardia. The goal is to decrease the amount of ICD intervention while allowing for protection against sustained VT and ventricular fibrillation in a population that is not suppressible by medications alone. In addition, if antiarrhythmic drug therapy is anticipated, VT characteristics, especially tachycardia cycle length, must be studied in order to allow for optimal programming of the device. Patients with incessant VT will have their baseline studies performed while on medications, such as intravenous procainamide, as the washout phase is poorly tolerated. It may thus be impossible to obtain a drug-free EP study.

Evaluation of the native conduction system is especially important, as a subgroup of patients may be at risk for atrio-ventricular block. A prolonged HV interval is associated with progression to complete atrio-ventricular block, and treatment with a permanent pacemaker may eventually be required [65]. Most important, in patients who will undergo ICD implantation in whom it is anticipated that antiarrhythmic medications will be used, the conduction system must be reevaluated in the presence of these agents, especially in patients with borderline or already prolonged HV intervals during the baseline EP study, as antiarrhythmic drugs may frequently exacerbate conduction abnormalities. In those with abnormally prolonged conduction, selection of a device with antibradycardia pacing capability is preferred.

In patients who need to be electrically cardioverted at the time of their EP study, it is important to note the need for postshock bradycardia pacing, as this may also affect device selection. Postdefibrillation bradycardia requiring pacing, although infrequent, may be life-threatening [66,67]. It may occur intraoperatively, yet it is difficult to predict on clinical grounds [68]. Patients with permanent pacemakers should be carefully evaluated for potential pacemaker/ICD interactions. In particular, unipolar pacing units will need to be explanted prior to ICD implantation. These are considered a contraindication to ICD implant, as they may induce failure to detect ventricular fibrillation [69–71]. Potential pacemaker/ICD interactions include transient pacemaker dysfunction after ICD discharge [70,72]; oversensing of the pacing artifact by the ICD, leading to double counting [73]; reprogramming of the pacemaker by the ICD [71]; antitachycardia pacing leading to ICD discharge [71,72]; and oversensing during permanent pacemaker magnet tests [74]. Steps to minimize such potential interactions have been outlined by the above-mentioned authors and others [75]. Patients with congestive heart failure or low left ventricular ejection fraction who may require dual-chamber pacing for hemodynamic reasons ought to have both a dual-chamber pacemaker and an ICD implanted, as the present generations of pacemaker/ICD afford ventricular pacing only. Newer ICDs with dual-chamber pacing capabilities may be developed and be especially useful in patients with cardiomyopathy who are prone to both tachyarrhythmias and conduction abnormalities.

The presence of pace-terminable VT must be established. This is of obvious importance in making feasible antitachycardia pacing therapy, which in turn would reduce patient discomfort by decreasing the number of shocks per patient in a given period of time. An interesting issue is that patients occasionally become pace-terminable only while on medications. Thus, pharmacological therapy may be required for optimal use of nonpharmacological options. If an arrhythmia is pace-terminable, it may be worthwhile determining the mode of pacing which affords termination. Some devices may offer burst (fixed-rate) pacing only, while other units may have ramp (incremental) pacing or other combinations as options [76]. In addition, the cycle length of the tachycardia may preclude antitachycardia pacing by certain devices. For example, some patients with tachycardia cycle lengths between 200 and 250 ms may be pace-terminable, yet some devices may not allow the short coupling intervals required to perform successful antitachycardia pacing in these circumstances. Alternatively, medications may increase the tachycardia cycle length to the range in which antitachycardia pacing therapy may be effective. Antitachycardia pacing needs to be tested and the appropriate pacing mode needs to be established separately in each individual case. This pacing mode of therapy is preferred over shock therapy, as it does not cause discomfort to the patient, avoids precipitation of supraventricular tachyarrhythmias, and hardly affects device longevity. The status of the left ventricular function, the rate and hemodynamic tolerance of VT, and the proarrhythmic potential of the pacing technique will influence the selection of a suitable therapeutic program. Relatively slow and hemodynamically stable VTs are amenable to this mode of termination, whereby a success rate of about 80% may be expected.

It is occasionally impossible to perform or complete preoperative electrophysiological studies on certain high risk patients because of unstable angina, congestive heart failure, or prohibitive coronary anatomy such as severe left main or three-vessel disease [77–79]. In these patients, prophylactic patches may be considered at the time of cardiac surgery; although, now with the availability of non-thoracotomy lead ICD systems, there will be no need for such practice any longer. In a retrospective series of 22 such patients undergoing myocardial revascularization and patch implantation, 61% had postoperative VT [78]. In terms of VT surgery, certain patients who have a left ventricular aneurysm and cannot be safely studied or mapped preoperatively may still be considered for intraoperative mapping and resection.

VI. PREOPERATIVE EVALUATION FOR CONCOMITANT SURGERY

A. Revascularization

It has been shown that most cardiac arrests occur in the setting of coronary artery disease [80]. The incidence of sudden cardiac death is decreased after myocardial revascularization (CABG) [81]. Most ICD candidates have coronary artery disease as their arrhythmia substrate [11,15]. Electrophysiological studies should be performed preoperatively in as many sudden-death survivors as possible, prior to undergoing coronary artery bypass graft surgery. The EP testing characteristics of cardiac-arrest survivors also improve after revascularization [79,82], with positive EP studies decreasing postoperatively [79,82,83]. Perhaps most importantly, the survivors of cardiac arrest may have an improved prognosis after revascularization [84,85]. Nonetheless, the majority of cardiac-arrest survivors remain inducible postoperatively [79,83,85]. Moreover, patients who are noninducible postoperatively may still be at risk for recurrent sudden cardiac death [83].

Patients with ventricular fibrillation as a presenting arrhythmia have a less reliable outcome with EP-guided therapy [57]. Thus they may benefit from earlier ICD treatment without prolonged preoperative electrophysiological testing. It has been suggested that ventricular fibrillation in the setting of ischemia may more likely be controlled by CABG surgery [86]. Induction of ventricular fibrillation at preoperative EP study in sudden-death survivors has been reported to predict arrhythmia noninducibility postoperatively [85]. However, other studies have reported conflicting results [87].

In conclusion, revascularization alone is associated with a high postoperative incidence of arrhythmias; thus survivors of cardiac arrest with significant coronary artery disease and ventricular arrhythmias will likely require medical treatment, ICD implantation, or both. Preoperative electrophysiological evaluation can be used to direct ICD treatment during CABG, and thus simultaneous ICD/CABG can be performed at an acceptable risk.

As mentioned above, until recently and before nonthoracotomy ICDs were available, patients who were at high risk for arrhythmia recurrence, yet could not undergo preoperative EP studies because of critical left main coronary artery disease, or unstable angina, might have had prophylactic patches implanted at the time of CABG [77]. Postoperative testing could be performed and an ICD implanted accordingly without the need for repeat thoracotomy. Once the decision to undergo revascularization has been made, several issues in the preoperative assessment should be addressed. During cardiac catheterization it may be advantageous to visualize the internal mammary arteries. This is especially important in patients who have undergone coronary bypass surgery with saphenous vein grafts in the past. The surgical approach for bypass surgery using a median sternotomy was most appropriate for patch placement.

Some patients with ischemia and ventricular tachyarrhythmia may have lesions which are amenable to coronary angioplasty, in addition to requiring ICD therapy. In these patients, angioplasty should be preferably performed prior to ICD implant.

B. Valvular Surgery

These patients should undergo the usual preoperative evaluation for valvular disease. If critical aortic stenosis is present, the patient may not be able to tolerate electrophysiological testing. Again, patches or an ICD could be implanted prophylactically at the time of surgery, but now more appropriately a nonthoracotomy ICD system can be implanted postoperatively.

Mitral valve replacement may be required during VT surgery if the focus of ventricular tachycardia is found to involve the papillary muscles. Cryoablation techniques have rendered this generally unnecessary [88–91]. Conversely, adjunctive cryoablation may be considered if indicated in patients who are to undergo mitral valve replacement for hemodynamic purposes.

C. Subendocardial Resection, Aneurysmectomy, and Left Ventricular Reconstruction

The role of ICD as adjunctive therapy to VT surgery is evolving. In addition, the decision whether to implant ICD patches and/or device was sometimes made intraoperatively, depending on the mapping results, as surgical success is related to the percentage of tachycardias mapped [91].

Moreover, practice patterns and strategy will vary from center to center. The initial experience with VT surgery was one of moderate success and great promise. Twenty to 30% of patients had recurrent VT or sudden cardiac death [90]. This led to proposing adjunctive ICD implantation in all patients with coronary artery disease undergoing these procedures [92]. The limitation to this approach is the cost of the device and the fact that up to 75% of patients may not need an ICD. Surgical success was increased by using sequential map-guided resection [93]. An intermediate approach with implantation of ICD patches depending on pre- and intraoperative mapping results had been advocated [77,94]. With prophylactic patches being implanted in most patients, one-third of these would receive ICDs postoperatively. More recent series have reflected on the notion that clinical success, that is, the response to surgery plus medications, is very high [88,91]. Based on a clinical success rate of 96% in his series, Cox rejected the idea of prophylactic patch implantation. He advocated patches if non-EP-guided surgery is anticipated, or if map-guided surgery is performed under cardioplegic arrest, given the high rate of postoperative inducibility [95]. In summary, the use of ICD/patches as adjunctive therapy in patients undergoing VT surgery is being redefined. Patient selection and perioperative parameters, including completeness of mapping, will likely play an increasingly important role. The overall trend is moving away from prophylactic ICD/patch implantation as the clinical success of arrhythmia surgery has increased, particularly when new computerized mapping methods and novel techniques of left ventricular reconstruction are employed [96], and as the nonthoracotomy ICDs are now available that can be implanted postoperatively. If the use of ICD patches or device was anticipated, a patient was advised of this possibility and psychologically prepared for this option.

D. Practical Aspects of Catheter Mapping [97–106]

The ideal ventricular tachycardia for mapping is one that is monomorphic, sustained, and well tolerated hemodynamically. In addition, it should be identical to the clinical VT. However, all inducible VT morphologies should be mapped [97]. Preoperative mapping in the EP laboratory generally entails placement of a right ventricular endocardiac electrode catheter in order to induce VT. Multipolar mapping catheters or standard quadripolar catheters may be used in both the right and left ventricles in order to characterize electrograms and to localize the site of earliest activation. Given the fact that most patients referred for subendocardial resection/aneurysmorrhaphy have a left ventricular aneurysm and that significant intracavity catheter manipulation will occur, it is important to know whether there is thrombus present in the aneurysm. This can be readily accomplished using two-dimensional echocardiography and cardiac catheterization. If thrombus is present, the patient should be anticoagulated, at least until such time as the left ventricular thrombus appears to be stable and endothelialized in order to minimize the potential for dislodgement.

The aim of catheter mapping is to define areas of the myocardium which are critical to the tachycardia circuit. Two issues are of paramount importance, having a fixed reference point from which to time the recorded electrograms, and obtaining a three-dimensional assessment of catheter position. At the time of mapping, both endocardial and surface ECG electrograms may be employed as reference points. Catheter position should be evaluated fluoroscopically using multiple projections. Bipolar electrogram recordings are most helpful. Mapping should be performed at the largest number of positions possible [97]. It is often necessary to interrupt the tachycardia because of ischemic symptoms or hemodynamic instability. It is prudent to do so and to reinduce VT in order to obtain as complete a map as possible. Localization of areas of slow conduction has been proposed as an important determination of critical components to the tachycardia circuit [101,102].

Sinus rhythm mapping allows for the identification of areas with abnormal or late endocardial electrograms. These relate to the substrate for reentrant arrhythmias in patients with coronary artery disease. Low-amplitude, fractionated electrograms are indicative of abnormal conduction, which in turn is related to scar and arrhythmogenic tissue [100,103,106]. Thus, localization of these areas may be helpful in preparation for surgery. *Pace mapping*, in which ventricular pacing is used to replicate a 12-lead morphology of the ventricular tachycardia, has been used with success. Unfortunately, it is a time consuming technique which should be considered complementary to mapping of the tachycardia itself, especially as sensitivity and specificity are not optimal. Similar QRS morphologies may be obtained from disparate sites and, conversely, very dissimilar morphologies can originate from adjacent sites [97–99]. Another disadvantage of this approach is the fact that other forms of VT which have not been previously determined by 12-lead ECG may be missed.

Ventricular tachycardia mapping is the most accurate method of identifying critical components of the reentrant circuit [106]. Several characteristics of the electrograms during VT are important, such as the presence of continuous diastolic activity, diastolic bridging suggesting areas of slow conduction, and the site of earliest activation. The site of earliest activation is most important, as it signals the endocardial exit point for the VT circuit. In order to demonstrate the location of the earliest activation site, one must record electrograms from adjacent locations as well, and thus determine that an early electrogram is indeed the earliest in one particular region. Occasionally, early diastolic activity is difficult to distinguish from late or unrelated electrograms. Analysis of the electrogram components during spontaneous oscillations in cycle length, as well as during resetting and entrainment maneuvers, may be used in order to differentiate between early diastolic activity related to the tachycardia circuit and other, unrelated electrograms. Once the site of earliest activation has been identified, the ability subsequently to reposition the catheter and to reproduce similar activation patterns would support the accuracy of three-dimensional localization.

These approaches to mapping have recently been validated by using the same criteria during catheter-based radiofrequency energy delivery as for ventricular tachycardia ablation. Radiofrequency energy has been delivered at the area of slow conduction with resultant elimination of VT [103]. In addition, the earliest activation method has been used to deliver a radiofrequency lesion in order to assist with intraoperative identification of the area [105]. Refinements in both mapping and energy delivery techniques have made catheter ablation a realistic approach to the treatment of some types of VT. Catheter ablation has been considered by some as the therapy of choice for incessant ventricular tachycardia [107]. Nevertheless, a number of patients will undergo crossover therapy to ICD treatment or VT surgery. In these cases, ICD therapy may be viewed as complementary to catheter ablation.

When more than one VT has been observed, the postoperative success for subendocardial resection appears to be related to the ability to map the greatest number of morphologies [32,44,93,100]. As mentioned above, the mapping process may include, in addition to the site of earliest activation during the tachycardia [97], the identification of areas of slow conduction [101,102] and fractionated electrograms [103] during sinus rhythm. Outlining these areas may be helpful at the time of surgery.

In patients who will need intraoperative mapping for subendocardial resection and/or for left ventricular reconstruction, a temporary right ventricular apical pacing catheter may be placed, usually within 24 h prior to surgery, in order to allow for intraoperative induction of VT using programmed stimulation. For this purpose, a four-french bipolar electrode catheter can be introduced via the right subclavian vein under sterile techniques and then sutured to the skin. This constitutes a minimally obtrusive location at the time of median sternotomy or left lateral thoracotomy.

E. ICD as a Bridge to Heart Transplantation

Many patients with class III or IV congestive heart failure are considered for orthotopic heart transplantation. These patients may have long waiting periods until a donor organ becomes available. In addition, patients with cardiomyopathy who have a reasonable functional status and consequently are not on a high-priority list for cardiac transplantation, but nonetheless are at risk for life-threatening tachyarrhythmia, may benefit from device therapy [108]. The DEFIBRILAT trial will attempt to clarify indications for ICD therapy in cardiomyopathy patients. Patients who are being evaluated for cardiac transplantation will have an extensive preoperative evaluation which will include viral antibody titers and an in-depth psychological assessment (see Chapter 33).

F. Other Preoperative Practical Considerations

In patients who require implantation of an endocardial lead for their ICD, this is placed either in the EP laboratory prior to device implantation or in the operating room at the same time. An active fixation lead may be chosen to prevent dislodgement at the time of surgical manipulation. Long leads (100 cm) may be coiled in a small pocket which can be readily accessed in the operating room by the surgeon. Although both right and left approaches are possible, use of the left cephalic or left subclavian vein facilitates tunneling in the operating room. It is advantageous to use leads and ICD which are compatible with the least amount of intervening extenders or connectors. This minimizes potential interface problems.

From the patient's perspective, the scientific issues or statistical need for an ICD may be overshadowed by misconceptions, anxiety, and fear of the device and its attendant surgery. Moreover, ignorance of the complex issues surrounding the recommendation for an ICD only help to exacerbate the above-mentioned feelings. It is thus of paramount importance to educate patients in order to afford them as easy an adjustment as possible to life with their device. In patients undergoing concomitant surgery, the issues of simultaneous ICD implant versus staged procedures must be discussed. If a nonthoracotomy device is recommended, the potential need for thoracotomy must be explained, and the patient must agree to this option prior to implantation of the nonthoracotomy lead. Patients must be aware that ICD therapy should be considered as a control measure rather than a curative procedure. Thus it may be necessary for them to continue receiving antiarrhythmic medications postoperatively.

Some of the complex issues surrounding psychological adaptation to ICDs include the fact that some patients may feel as though they are dependent on a machine for their existence. A clear distinction ought to be made between life-support systems and having a "backup" therapeutic instrument. Many patients are afraid of the potential sensation of an ICD discharge. Analogies can generally be made to previous experiences with defibrillation in the electrophysiology laboratory. An extreme form of anxiety may be associated with the patient's anticipation of sudden cardiac death and/or device failure [109]. It must be emphasized to the patient that although they are at high risk for recurrence of sudden cardiac death, efforts will be made to minimize defibrillator discharges even if antiarrhythmic drug treatment is needed. In addition, because of the possibility of multiple discharges and battery depletion, patients with frequently recurring VT/ventricular fibrillation would not be ideal candidates for ICD implantation. In terms of potential device failure, the excellent success record of ICD therapy should be emphasized.

Most patients adapt to their ICD and many return to usual levels of activity and work [110]. Nonetheless, life after surgery includes several significant limitations, the most significant of which is the patient's inability to drive. Although this is not a law in all states, it is certainly the physician's recommendation in most instances. The significant change in lifestyle that this may imply to a given patient must be understood beforehand. Care should be taken to explain that the reason for not driving is not the device but the condition itself, which, similarly to seizure disorders, predisposes the patient to sudden loss of consciousness. The fear of affecting a spouse at the time of an ICD discharge should be allayed. Patients will often wonder what the outcome will be of receiving an ICD discharge. The potential for loss of consciousness must be explained, as well as clear directions as to the procedure to be followed, such as contacting their physician and local emergency ward, and checking ECGs and electrolyte levels.

Although the anxiety and fear issues stated above are of immediate importance to the patient, some practical long-term implications ought to be considered and discussed with the patient. In particular, the follow-up procedure to be performed routinely after ICD implantation must be described. The frequency of follow-up appointments, capacitor re-formation, and counter checks when appropriate should be discussed, as well as whether a given device will require invasive versus noninvasive follow-up testing. The actual frequency of the follow-up visits may be very important for patients in whom independence from the hospital is an issue. In this regard, the difference between follow-up for standard devices versus investigational devices must be weighed against the potential benefits. Moreover, the accessibility of the follow-up center to the patient must be considered. If long trips are necessary for follow-up of the investigational devices but centers capable of approved-device follow-up are available, this must be discussed with the patient, as it may affect compliance.

All of the above issues imply thorough explanations and discussion with the patient before surgery. In addition, given the amount of information to be given and the fact that patients may not be able to assimilate all of it at once, it is prudent to schedule several sessions in which various members of the team discuss the ICD implant with the patient. In particular, the role of a nurse specialist is extremely important in facilitating questions, answers, and eventual follow-up. Written as well as video-recorded materials are now available for patient review. Support group sessions or conversations with patients who have had ICDs implanted may shed light on significant personal issues of importance to the patient.

Once the patient is prepared to undergo ICD implant, preoperative evaluation by the anesthesiologists and surgeon are most important and complementary to the patient's full understanding of the procedure.

VII. SUMMARY

Implantable cardioverter-defibrillators constitute a very effective therapy in decreasing the incidence of sudden cardiac death in patients with poorly tolerated sustained tachyarrhythmia or sudden-cardiac-death survivors. They may be used singly or as an adjunct to medical or surgical therapy. A thorough preoperative evaluation is of paramount importance in outlining the overall therapeutic approach for the individual patient. During this process the patient's rhythm should be initially stabilized after the clinical event, followed by serial ECGs and cardiac enzymes to rule out myocardial infarction, stabilization and assessment of the general medical status of the patient including evaluation of the neurologic, respiratory, renal, and hepatic function, with further, more specific focus directed to the noninvasive and invasive assessment of the cardiac function and arrhythmia evaluation. This latter and most critical stage includes noninvasive assessment of ischemia with sestamibi or thallium, performance of echocardiography, signal-averaged ECG, cardiac catheterization, and electrophysiological and electropharmacological studies, all in an attempt to evaluate most appropriately the patient's candidacy for ICD therapy, determine the need for concomitant cardiac surgery, and select a suitable ICD device for the individual patient.

REFERENCES

1. Lehmann MH, Saksena S. Implantable cardioverter defibrillators in cardiovascular practice: report of the Policy Conference of the North American Society of Pacing and Electrophysiology. PACE 1991; 14:969–979.
2. Dreifus LS, Fisch C, Griffin JC, Gillette PC, Mason JW, Parsonnet V. Guidelines for implantation of cardiac pacemakers and antiarrhythmia devices. A report of the American College of Cardiology/American Heart Association Task Force on Assessment of Diagnostic and Therapeutic Cardiovascular Procedures (Committee on Pacemaker Implantation). AHA Medical/Scientific Statement. Circulation 1991; 84(1):455–467.
3. Manolis AS, Tan-Deguzman W, Lee MA, et al. Clinical experience in 77 patients with the automatic implantable cardioverter defibrillator. Am Heart J 1989; 118:445–450.
4. Manolis AS, Rastegar H, Estes NAM III. Automatic implantable cardioverter defibrillator: current status. JAMA 1989; 262:1362–1368.
5. Manolis A. Non-pharmacologic management of ventricular tachyarrhythmias: role of the AICD. Hellenic J Cardiol 1991; 32:14–24.
6. Manolis AS. Third generation implantable cardioverter defibrillators. Hellenic J Cardiol 1992; 33:1–7.
7. Ferraris VA, Ferraris SP, Lough FC, Berry WR. Preoperative aspirin ingestion increases operative blood loss after coronary artery bypass grafting. Ann Thorac Surg 1988; 45:71–74.
8. Taggart DP, Siddiqui A, Wheatley DJ. Low-dose preoperative aspirin therapy, postoperative blood loss, and transfusion requirements. Ann Thorac Surg 1990; 50:425–428.
9. Becker RC, Alpert JS. The impact of medical therapy on hemorrhagic complications following coronary artery bypass grafting. Arch Intern Med 1990; 150:2016–2021.
10. Bashein G, Nessly ML, Rice AL, Counts RB, Misbach GA. Preoperative aspirin therapy and reoperation for bleeding after coronary bypass surgery. Arch Intern Med 1991; 151:89–93.
11. Winkle RA, Mead RM, Ruder MA, et al. Long-term outcome with the implantable cardioverter-defibrillator. J Am Coll Cardiol 1989; 13:1353–1361.
12. Nalos PC, Kass RM, Gang ES, Fishbein MC, Mandel WJ, Peter T. Life-threatening postoperative pulmonary complications in patients with previous amiodarone pulmonary toxicity undergoing cardiothoracic operations. J Thorac Cardiovasc Surg 1987; 93:904–12.
13. Shapira N, Cohen AI, Wish M, Weston LJ, Fletcher R. Transdiaphragmatic implantation of the automatic implantable cardioverter defibrillator. Ann Thorac Surg 1989; 48:371–375.
14. Wyse DG, Nath FC, Brownell AKW. Benign X-linked (Emery-Dreifuss) muscular dystrophy is not benign. PACE 1987; 10:533–537.
15. Reid PR, Griffith LSC, Mower MM, Platia EV, Watkins L, Juanteguy J, Mirowski M. Implantable cardioverter-defibrillator: patient selection and implantation protocol. PACE 1984; 7:1338–1344.
16. Fain ES, Dorian P, Davy JM, Kates RE, Winkle RA. Effects of encainide and its metabolites on energy requirements for defibrillation. Circulation 1986; 73(6):1334–1341.
17. Jung W, Manz M, Luderitz B. Effects of antiarrhythmic drugs on defibrillation threshold in patients with the implantable cardioverter defibrillator. PACE 1992; 15, 4(III):645–648.
18. Pinski SL, Vanerio G, Castle L, et al. Patients with a high defibrillation threshold: clinical characteristics, management and outcome. Am Heart J 1991; 122:89–95.
19. Epstein AE, Ellenbogen KA, Kirk KA, et al. Clinical characteristics and outcome of patients with high defibrillation thresholds. Circulation 1992; 86:1206–1216.
20. Kelly PA, Cannom DS, Garan H, et al. The automatic implantable cardioverter-defibrillator: efficacy, complications and survival in patients with malignant ventricular arrhythmias. J Am Coll Cardiol 1988; 11:1278–1286.
21. Marinchak RA, Friehling TD, Kline RA, Stohler J, Kowey PR. Effect of antiarrhythmic drugs on defibrillation threshold: case report of an adverse effect of mexiletine and review of the literature. PACE 1988; 11:7–12.
22. Singer I, Guarnieri T, Kupersmith J. Implanted automatic defibrillators: effects of drugs and pacemakers. PACE 1988; 11:2250–2262.

23. Fain ES, Lee JT, Winkle RA. Effects of acute intravenous and chronic oral amiodarone on defibrillation requirements. Am Heart J 1987; 114:8–17.
24. Tuzcu EM, Maloney JD, Sangani BH, et al. Cardiopulmonary effects of chronic amiodarone therapy in the early postoperative course of cardiac surgery patients. Cleve Clin J Med 1987; 54:491–495.
25. Greenspon AJ, Kidwell GA, Hurley W, Mannion J. Amiodarone-related postoperative adult respiratory distress syndrome. Circulation 1991; 84(III):407–415.
26. Kupferschmid PJ, Rosengart TK, McIntosh CL, Leon MB, Clark RE. Amiodarone-induced complications after cardiac operation for obstructive hypertrophic cardiomyopathy. Ann Thorac Surg 1989; 48:359–364.
27. Herndon JC, Cook AO, Ramsay MAE, Swygert TH, Capehart J. Postoperative unilateral pulmonary edema: possible amiodarone pulmonary toxicity. Anesthesiology 1992; 76(2):308–311.
28. Kay GN, Epstein AE, Kirklin JK, Diethelm AG, Graybar G, Plumb VJ. Fatal postoperative amiodarone toxicity. Am J Cardiol 1988; 62:490–492.
29. Gallagher JD, Lieberman RW, Meranze J, Spielman SR, Ellison N. Amiodarone-induced complications during coronary artery surgery. Anesthesiology 1981; 55:186–188.
30. Perkins MW, Dasta JF, Reilley TE, Halpern P. Intraoperative complications in patients receiving amiodarone: characteristics and risk factors. DICP, Ann Pharmacother 1989; 23:757–763.
31. Yee ES, Scheinman MM, Griffin JC, Ebert PA. Surgical options for treating ventricular tachyarrhythmia and sudden death. J Thorac Cardiovasc Surg 1987; 94:866–873.
32. Miller JM, Marchlinski FE, Buxton AE, Josephson ME. Relationships between the 12-lead electrocardiogram during ventricular tachycardia and endocardial site of origin in patients with coronary artery disease. Circulation 1988; 77(4):759–766.
33. Seale WL, Gang ES, Peter CT. The use of signal-averaged electrocardiography in predicting patients at high risk for sudden death. PACE 1990; 13:796–806.
34. Epstein AE, Dailey SM, Shepard RB, Kirk KA, Kay GN, Plumb VJ. Inability of the signal-averaged electrocardiogram to determine risk of arrhythmia recurrence in patients with implantable cardioverter defibrillator. PACE 1991; 14:1169–1178.
35. Zeigler VL, Gillette PC, Crawford FA, Wiles HB, Fyfe DA. New approaches to treatment of incessant ventricular tachycardia in the very young. J Am Coll Cardiol 1990; 16:681–685.
36. Garan H, Nguyen K, McGovern B, Buckley M, Ruskin JN. Perioperative and long-term results after electrophysiologically directed ventricular surgery for recurrent ventricular tachycardia. J Am Coll Cardiol 1986; 8:201–209.
37. Fogoros RN, Elson JJ, Bonnet CA, Fiedler SB, Burkholder JA. Efficacy of the automatic implantable cardioverter-defibrillator in prolonging survival in patients with severe underlying cardiac disease. J Am Coll Cardiol 1990; 16:381–386.
38. Kiat H, Berman DS, Maddahi J, et al. Late reversibility of tomographic myocardial thallium-201 defects: an accurate marker of myocardial viability. J Am Coll Cardiol 1988; 12:1456–1463.
39. Dilsizian V, Rocco TP, Freedman NMT, Leon MB, Bonow RO. Enhanced detection of ischemic but viable myocardium by the reinjection of thallium after stress-redistribution imaging. N Engl J Med 1990; 323(2):141–146.
40. Dilsizian V, Bonow RO. Current diagnostic techniques of assessing myocardial viability in patients with hibernating and stunned myocardium. Circulation 1993; 87:1.
41. Bonow RO, Dilsizian V, Cuocolo A, Bacharach SL. Identification of viable myocardium in patients with chronic coronary artery disease and left ventricular dysfunction. Circulation 1991; 83:26–37.
42. Coleman PS, Metheral JA, Pandian NG, et al. Predicting enhanced regional function post-revascularization: comparison of thallium-201 and sestamibi in patients with left ventricular dysfunction. Circulation 1992; 86(4)I:I-108.
43. Coleman PS, Metherall JA, Cao Q, et al. Comparison of rest-redistribution thallium-201 uptake with resting sestamibi uptake in coronary artery disease (abstr). J Nucl Med 1992; 33(5):905.
44. Miller JM, Kienzle MG, Harken AH, Josephson ME. Subendocardial resection for ventricular tachycardia: predictors of surgical success. Circulation 1984; 70:624–631

45. Hargrove WC, Miller JM, Vasallo JA, Josephson ME. Improved results in the operative management of ventricular tachycardia related to inferior wall infarction. J Thorac Cardiovasc Surg 1986; 92:726–732.
46. Freedman RA, Swerdlow CD, Soderholm-Difatte V, Mason JW. Prognostic significance of arrhythmia inducibility or noninducibility at initial electrophysiologic study in survivors of cardiac arrest. Am J Cardiol 1988; 61:578–582.
47. Wilber DJ, Olshansky B, Moran JF, Scanlon PJ. Electrophysiologic testing and nonsustained ventricular tachycardia. Circulation 1990; 82:350–358.
48. Roy D, Waxman HL, Kienzle MG, Buxton AE, Marchlinski FE, Josephson ME. Clinical characteristics and long-term follow-up in 119 survivors of cardiac arrest: relation to inducibility at electrophysiologic testing. Am J Cardiol 1983; 52:969–974.
49. Eldar M, Sauve MJ, Scheinman MM. Electrophysiologic testing and follow-up of patients with aborted sudden death. J Am Coll Cardiol 1987; 10(2):291–298.
50. Fogoros RN, Elson JJ, Bonnet CA, Fiedler SB, Chenarides JG. Long-term outcome of survivors of cardiac arrest whose therapy is guided by electrophysiologic testing. J Am Coll Cardiol 1992; 19:780–788.
51. Wilber DJ, Garan H, Finkelstein D, et al. Out-of-hospital cardiac arrest: use of electrophysiologic testing in the predicting of long-term outcome. N Engl J Med 1988; 318:19–24.
52. Kim SG. Management of survivors of cardiac arrest: is electrophysiologic testing obsolete in the era of implantable defibrillators? J Am Coll Cardiol 1990; 16(3):756–762.
53. Poll DS, Marchlinski FE, Buxton AE, Josephson ME. Usefulness of programmed stimulation in idiopathic dilated cardiomyopathy. Am J Cardiol 1986; 58:992–997.
54. Benditt DG, Benson W, Klein GJ, Pritzker MR, Kriett JM, Anderson RW. Prevention of recurrent sudden cardiac arrest: role of provocative electropharmacologic testing. J Am Coll Cardiol 1983; 2(3):418–425.
55. Kuhlick DL, Bhandari AK, Hong R, et al. Effect of acute hemodynamic decompensation on electrical inducibility of ventricular arrhythmias in patients with dilated cardiomyopathy and complex nonsustained ventricular arrhythmias. Am Heart J 1990; 119:878–883.
56. Jazayeri MR, VanWyhe G, Avitall B, McKinnie J, Tchou P, Akhtar M. Isoproterenol reversal of antiarrhythmic effects in patients with inducible sustained ventricular tachyarrhythmias. J Am Coll Cardiol 1989; 14(3):705–711.
57. Poole JE, Mathisen TL, Kudenchuk PJ, et al. Long-term outcome in patients who survive out of hospital ventricular fibrillation and undergo electrophysiologic studies: evaluation by electrophysiologic subgroups. J Am Coll Cardiol 1990; 16:657–665.
58. Kavanagh KM, Wyse G, Duff HJ, Gillis AM, Sheldon RS, Mitchell LB. Drug therapy for ventricular tachyarrhythmias: how many electropharmacologic trials are appropriate? J Am Coll Cardiol 1991; 17:391–396.
59. Wichter T, Borggrefe M, Haverkamp W, Chen X, Breithardt G. Efficacy of antiarrhythmic drugs in patients with arrhythmogenic right ventricular disease. Circulation 1992; 86:29–37.
60. Lehmann MH, Steinman RT, Schuger CD, Jackson K. The automatic implantable cardioverter defibrillator as antiarrhythmic treatment modality of choice for survivors of cardiac arrest unrelated to acute myocardial infarction. Am J Cardiol 1988; 62:803–805.
61. O'Donoghue S, Platia E, Brooks-Robinson S, Mispireta L. Automatic implantable cardioverter-defibrillator: is early implantation cost-effective? J Am Coll Cardiol 1990; 16:1258–1263.
62. Larsen GC, Manolis AS, Sonnenberg FA, Beshansky JR, Estes NAM, Pauker SG. Cost-effectiveness of the implantable cardioverter-defibrillator: effect of improved battery life and comparison with amiodarone therapy. J Am Coll Cardiol 1992; 19:1323–1334.
63. Kuppermann M, Luce BR, McGovern B, Podrid PJ, Bigger T, Ruskin JN. An analysis of the cost effectiveness of the implantable defibrillator. Circulation 1990; 81:91–100.
64. Klein LS, Shih HT, Hackett FK, Zipes DP, Miles WM. Radiofrequency catheter ablation of ventricular tachycardia in patients without structural heart disease. Circulation 1992; 85:1666–1674.

65. Scheinman MM, Peters RW, Sauve MJ, et al. Value of the H-Q interval in patients with bundle branch block and the role of prophylactic permanent pacing. Am J Cardiol 1982; 50:1316–1322.
66. Khastgir T, Aarons D, Veltri E. Sudden bradyarrhythmic death in patients with the implantable cardioverter-defibrillator: report of two cases. PACE 1991; 14:395–398.
67. Edel TB, Maloney JD, Moore SL, et al. Analysis of deaths in patients with an implantable cardioverter-defibrillator. PACE 1992; 15:60–70.
68. Niazi I, Kadri N, Mahmud R, et al. Absence of significant postdefibrillation bradyarrhythmias in patients with automatic implantable defibrillators. Am Heart J 1988; 115:830–836.
69. Kim SG, Furman S, Waspe LE, Brodman R, Fisher JD. Unipolar pacer artifacts induced failure of an automatic implantable cardioverter/defibrillator to detect ventricular fibrillation. Am J Cardiol 1985; 57:880–881.
70. Cohen AI, Wish MH, Fletcher RD, et al. The use and interaction of permanent pacemakers and the automatic implantable cardioverter defibrillator. PACE 1987; 11:704–711.
71. Calkins H, Brinker J, Veltri EP, Guarnieri T, Levine JH. Clinical interactions between pacemakers and automatic implantable cardioverter-defibrillators. J Am Coll Cardiol 1990; 16:666–673.
72. Slepian M, Levine JH, Watkins L, Brinker J, Guarnieri T. Automatic implantable cardioverter defibrillator/permanent pacemaker interaction: loss of pacemaker capture following AICD discharge. PACE 1987; 10:1194–1197.
73. Spontnitz HM, Ott GY, Bigger T, Steinberg JS, Livelli F. Methods of implantable cardioverter-defibrillator-pacemaker insertion to avoid interactions. Ann Thorac Surg 1992; 53:253–257.
74. Kim SG, Furman S, Matos JA, Waspe LE, Brodman R, Fisher JD. Automatic implantable cardioverter/defibrillator: inadvertent discharges during permanent pacemaker magent tests. PACE 1987; 10:579–582.
75. Epstein AE, Kay GN, Plumb VJ, Shepard RB, Kirklin JK. Combined automatic implantable cardioverter-defibrillator and pacemaker systems: implantation techniques and follow-up. J Am Coll Cardiol 1989; 13:121–131.
76. Klein LS, Miles WM, Zipes DP. Antitachycardia devices: realities and promises. J Am Coll Cardiol 1991; 18:1349–1362.
77. Manolis AS, Rastegar H, Estes NAM III. Prophylactic automatic implantable cardioverter-defibrillator patches in patients at high risk for postoperative ventricular tachyarrhythmias. J Am Coll Cardiol 1989; 13:1367–1373.
78. Pinski SL, Arnold AZ, Mick M, Maloney JD, Troham RG. Safety of external cardioversion/defibrillation in patients with internal defibrillation patches and no device. PACE 1991; 14:7–12.
79. Manolis AS, Rastegar H, Estes NAM. Effects of coronary artery bypass grafting on ventricular arrhythmias: results with electrophysiologic testing and long term follow-up. PACE. 1993; 16:984–991.
80. Goldstein S, Landis JR, Leighton R, et al. Characteristics of the resuscitated out of hospital cardiac arrest victim with coronary artery disease. Circulation 1981; 64(5):977–984.
81. Holmes DR, Davis KB, Mock MB, et al., and Participants in the Coronary Artery Surgery Study. The effect of medical and surgical treatment on subsequent sudden cardiac death in patients with coronary artery disease: a report from the Coronary Artery Surgery Study, Circulation 1986; 73(6):1254–1263.
82. Garan H, Ruskin JN, DiMarco JP, et al. Electrophysiologic studies before and after myocardial revascularization in patients with life-threatening ventricular arrhythmias. Am J Cardiol 1983; 51:519–524.
83. Fonger JD, Guarnieri T, Griffith LCS, et al. Impending sudden cardiac death: treatment with myocardial revascularization and the automatic implantable cardioverter defibrillator. Ann Thorac Surg 1988; 46:13–19.
84. Tresch DD, Wetherbee JN, Siegel R, et al. Long-term follow-up of survivors of prehospital sudden cardiac death treated with coronary bypass surgery. Am Heart J 1985; 110:1139–1145.
85. Kelly P, Ruskin J, Vlahakes GJ, Buckley MJ, Freeman CS, Garan H. Surgical coronary revascularization in survivors of prehospital cardial arrest: its effect on inducible ventricular arrhythmias and long-term survival. J Am Coll Cardiol 1990; 15:267–273.

86. Zheutlin TA, Steinman RT, Mattioni TA, Kehoe RF. Long-term arrhythmic outcome in survivors of ventricular fibrillation with absence of ventricular tachycardia. Am J Cardiol 1988;62:1213-1217.
87. Kron IL, Lerman BB, Haines DE, Flanagan TL, DiMarco JP. Coronary artery bypass grafting in patients with ventricular fibrillation. Ann Thorac Surg 1989; 48:85–89.
88. Cox JL. Patient selection criteria and results of surgery for refractory ischemic ventricular tachycardia. Circulation 1989; 79:I-163–I-177.
89. Manolis AS, Rastegar H, Payne D, Cleveland R, Estes NAM. Surgical therapy for drug-refractory ventricular tachycardia: results with mapping-guided subendocardial resection. J Am Coll Cardiol 1989; 14:199–208.
90. Mason J, Stinson EB, Winkle RE, et al. Surgery for ventricular tachycardia: efficacy of left ventricular aneurysm resection compared with operation guided by electrical activation mapping. Circulation 1982; 65(6):1148–1155.
91. Hargrove WC, Miller JM. Risk stratification and management of patients with recurrent ventricular tachycardia and other malignant ventricular arrhythmias. Circulation 1989; 79:I-178–I-181.
92. Platia EV, Griffith LSC, Watkins L, et al. Treatment of malignant ventricular arrhythmias with endocardial resection and implantation of the automatic cardioverter-defibrillator. N Engl J Med 1986; 314:213–216.
93. Haines DE, Lerman BB, Kron IL, DiMarco JP. Surgical ablation of ventricular tachycardia with sequential map-guided subendocardial resection: electrophysiologic assessment and long-term follow-up. Circulation: 1988; 77(1):131–141.
94. Hargrove WC, Josephson ME, Marchlinski FE, Miller JM. Surgical decisions in the management of sudden cardiac death and malignant ventricular arrhythmias. J Thorac Cardiovasc Surg 1989; 97:923–928.
95. Swerdlow CD, Mason JW, Stinson EB, Oyer PE, Winkle RA, Derby GC. Results of operations for ventricular tachycardia in 105 patients. J Thorac Cardiovasc Surg 1986; 92:105–113.
96. Foote C, Wang PJ, Clyne CAC, et al. The role of left ventricular reconstruction in preserving cardiac function in patients undergoing endocardial resection (abstr). PACE 1992; 15:533.
97. Josephson ME, Horowitz LN, Spielman SR, Waxman HL, Greenspan AM. Role of catheter mapping in the preoperative evaluation of ventricular tachycardia. Am J Cardiol 1982; 49:207–220.
98. Waxman HL, Josephson ME. Ventricular activation during ventricular endocardial pacing: I. Electrocardiographic patterns related to the site of pacing. Am J Cardiol 1982; 50:1–10.
99. Josephson ME, Waxman HL, Cain ME, Gardner M, Buxton AE. Ventricular activation during ventricular endocardial pacing. II. Role of pace-mapping to localize origin of ventricular tachycardia. Am J Cardiol 1982; 50:11–22.
100. Miller JM, Vasallo JA, Kussmaul WG, et al. Anterior left ventricular aneurysm: factors associated with the development of sustained ventricular tachycardia. J Am Coll Cardiol 1988; 12:375–382.
101. Stevenson WG, Weiss J, Wiener I, Wohlgelernter D, Yeatman L. Localization of slow conduction in a ventricular tachycardia circuit: implications for catheter ablation. Am Heart J 1987; 114(5):1253–1258.
102. Morady F, Frank R, Kou WH, et al. Identification and catheter ablation of a zone of slow conduction in the reentrant circuit of ventricular tachycardia in humans. J Am Coll Cardiol 1988; 11:775–782.
103. Stevenson WG, Weiss JN, Wiener I, et al. Fractionated endocardial electrograms are associated with slow conduction in humans: evidence from pace-mapping. J Am Coll Cardiol 1989; 13:369–376.
104. Kuck KH, Schluter M, Geiger M, Siebels J. Successful catheter ablation of ventricular tachycardia with radiofrequency current guided by an endocardial map of the area of slow conduction. PACE 1991; 14:1060–1071.
105. Pollak SJ, Stowe CL, Wyndham CRC, Cole M. Intraoperative identification of a radiofrequency lesion allowing validation of catheter mapping of ventricular tachycardia with a computerized balloon mapping system. PACE 1992; 15:854–858.

106. Josephson ME. Clinical Cardiac Electrophysiology: Technique and Interpretations, 2d ed. Philadelphia: Lea & Febiger, 1993.
107. Breithardt G, Borggrefe M, Weithold D, et al. Role of ventricular tachycardia surgery and catheter ablation as complements or alternatives to the implantable cardioverter defibrillators in the 1990's. PACE 1992; 15:681–689.
108. Haverich A, Troster J, Wahlers T, Gieguth H, Klein H. The automatic implantable cardioverter defibrillator (AICD) as a bridge to heart transplantation. PACE 1992; 15:701–707.
109. Frichione GL, Olson LC, Vlay SC. Psychiatric syndromes in patients with the authomatic inernal cardioverter defibrillator: anxiety, psychological dependence, abuse and withdrawal. Am Heart J 1989; 177(6):1411–1414.
110. Kalbfleisch KR, Lehman MB, Stein RT, et al. Reemployment following implantation of the automatic cardioverter defibrillator. Am J Cardiol 1989; 64:199–202.

17

Surgical Techniques for the Implantable Cardioverter-Defibrillator

Hassan Rastegar and Robert M. Bojar

*Tufts University School of Medicine
and New England Medical Center
Boston, Massachusetts*

Recurrent life-threatening ventricular arrhythmias refractory to electrophysiologically-guided medical therapy are a major cause of sudden cardiac death. Although direct, map-guided surgical approaches, such as subendocardial resection, have proven beneficial in ablating ventricular tachycardia (VT) in selected patients, the implantable cardioverter-defibrillator (ICD) is considered a primary therapeutic modality for patients with medically refractory VT who are not suitable candidates for this procedure [1].

I. HISTORICAL PERSPECTIVE

The first clinical implant of an automatic implantable defibrillator (AID) system took place in 1980. This device was capable of detecting and treating ventricular fibrillation (VF) and consisted of a transvenous spring-coil electrode placed in the superior vena cava (SVC) and an epicardial cup or patch placed over the left ventricle. Two years later, the AID-B and AID-BR systems underwent clinical evaluation. The AID-B system was capable of sensing rate and morphology of the electrocardiogram and could deliver shocks in response to VF or VT that exceeded a preset rate. The AID-BR system was a rate-only system.

These two early AID systems initially included right ventricular bipolar electrodes for rate sensing as well as the SVC electrode and patch. One of the drawbacks of these systems was the use of the SVC electrode, which was prone to lead migration, resulting in increasing defibrillation thresholds (DFTs), and occasionally to the development of infection and subclavian vein thrombosis. Subsequently, the lead system was modified to include two epicardial defibrillation patches and two epicardial screw-in sensing electrodes rather than the right ventricular electrodes.

During the past 10–15 years, there have been tremendous advances in ICD technology. These have included incorporation of cardioversion and antitachycardia and bradycardia pacing circuitry into the generator. Extensive research has also been geared toward miniaturization of

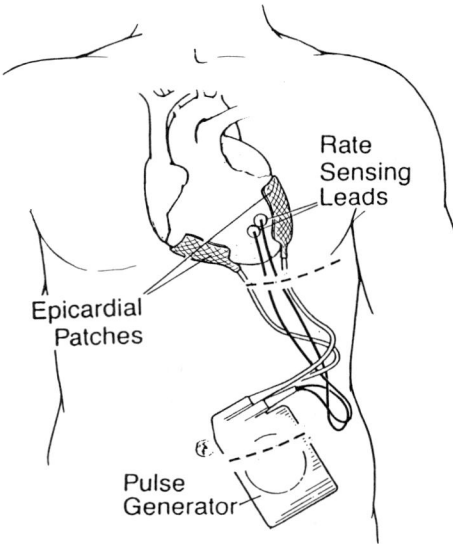

Figure 1 The standard epicardial ICD system consists of two rate-sensing leads placed on the ventricular epicardium, two defibrillator patches placed over the ventricles, either intra- or extrapericardially, and the pulse generator, which is implanted in a subcutaneous pocket.

the devices and evaluating newer modalities of energy delivery. Despite these sophisticated advances, nearly all systems implanted through 1992 required surgical entry into the thorax for implantation. Currently, several clinical trials of nonthoracotomy ICD systems are underway, and these systems should eventually obviate the need for surgically invasive procedures to implant the epicardial systems.

II. STANDARD ICD SYSTEM

The standard ICD system consists of one bipolar electrode pair, a defibrillation lead system, and a generator (Fig. 1). The electrode pair senses the heart rate and provides R-wave synchronization during device discharge for cardioversion. It usually consists of two screw-in electrodes that are placed directly onto the left or right ventricular epicardium. Alternatively, a transvenous electrode placed in the right ventricular apex can be used. The defibrillation lead system senses the electrical waveform and provides defibrillation or cardioversion energy. It consists of a left ventricular and a right ventricular/atrial patch that may be sewn directly onto the heart or placed extrapericardially. An SVC spring electrode can be used instead of the RV patch. The generator weighs about 250 g, contains the battery and electric components housed in a titanium case, and has an epoxy header with four inputs for the lead systems.

The generator is usually housed in a pocket overlying the left upper quadrant of the abdomen. It is positioned either subcutaneously, under the anterior rectus fascia, or under the rectus muscle [2–5]. Placement of the device in the left lower quadrant may be more cosmetically acceptable in young women [6]. Placing the device within the chest wall in the bed of two resected ribs has also been described to prevent protrusion of the device in thin patients [7].

III. GENERAL IMPLANTATION CONSIDERATIONS

The thoracotomy approach was initially used for the implantation of the ICD device, but soon thereafter, median sternotomy, subxiphoid, and subcostal approaches were described for placement of the totally epicardial ICD systems. The selection of an operative approach should be individualized for each patient. Factors that must be taken into consideration include the patient's history of a previous cardiac surgical procedure or plans for concomitant or future cardiac surgery, potential problems with operative exposure, and perhaps most important, the surgeon's experience with various approaches. Other considerations include the selection of the defibrillation system configuration to be used (SVC electrode-one patch versus patch-patch), the size of the patches to be placed and their location (intrapericardial versus extrapericardial), the location of the rate-sensing leads (endocardial versus epicardial-right or left ventricle), and whether implantation will involve only the lead system or include the generator as well. Many surgeons prefer extrapericardial rather than intrapericardial patch placement, because it avoids the potential for constrictive pericarditis and erosion of coronary bypass grafts, facilitates subsequent cardiac surgery, and is easier to use in patients who have had a previous sternotomy. Extrapericardial placement has been demonstrated to have comparable defibrillation efficacy to patch placement directly on the heart [8,9].

The surgical implantation of an ICD device requires the close cooperation of a dedicated team of surgeons, cardiologists, anesthesiologists, and nurses. All operating room personnel must be thoroughly familiar with the nature of the surgical procedure and the requirement for absolute asepsis. Prophylactic antibiotics are given before the procedure and for 48 h afterwards. The appropriate "rescue" equipment must be available, including external and internal defibrillator paddles and self-adhesive external defibrillator pads (R2 pads). The anesthesiologist should be well versed in the appropriate anesthetic agents to use and which ones to avoid, especially those that influence arrhythmia induction and defibrillation thresholds (DFTs). The cardiologist must be a trained electrophysiologist who is knowledgeable in the function of the external cardioverter-defibrillator system to ensure appropriate measurements of DFTs and sensing thresholds.

No matter which surgical approach is used, a systematic plan for ICD implantation and testing should be followed. After the appropriate exposure has been obtained, the rate-sensing leads and patches are placed. The patches should be positioned to include the largest possible ventricular mass between the two patches. They must not touch each other, in order to prevent shunting of the shocking current. The leads are connected to the external cardioverter-defibrillator box for testing of R-wave sensing and DFTs. If DFTs are high, the polarity of the patch leads can be changed, or the patches may be repositioned. Alternatively, an SVC spring-coil electrode or additional patches can be placed [10]. The generator pocket is then created and the leads are tunneled to the pocket and connected to the generator. Defibrillation by the generator is confirmed and the device is implanted. It is generally left inactive at the conclusion of surgery because of the increased risk of arrhythmia development in the immediate postoperative period. Any malignant arrhythmias that occur at this time are treated with standard external defibrillator equipment to avoid depletion of the ICD battery. The ICD is retested and activated in the electrophysiology (EP) laboratory before the patient is discharged from the hospital.

IV. MEDIAN STERNOTOMY

The median sternotomy approach is nearly always used when ICD implantation is performed in conjunction with a cardiac surgical procedure that requires cardiopulmonary bypass (CPB) [2,11,12]. It provides excellent exposure for the placement and/or repositioning of lead systems in nonscarred regions of the ventricle. The patches can be sewn directly on the myocardium or placed extrapericardially. In the unlikely event that DFTs remain high despite patch reconfiguration or reversal of polarity, a transvenous spring-coil electrode can be inserted easily through the subclavian vein without changing the patient's position on the operating room table. Internal and external cardioversion are also performed quite readily. If a permanent transvenous pacemaker is required, the sternotomy approach facilitates the maximum separation between the leads of the two devices to decrease the possibility of device interaction and defibrillator malfunction.

The median sternotomy approach is well tolerated in patients with cardiac dysfunction and pulmonary insufficiency. However, it does create more discomfort than the subxiphoid or subcostal approach, and the hospital stay is slightly longer. Although the risk of infection is no greater than with the other approaches, it may be associated with severe mediastinitis that requires not only explantation of the entire system, but also sternal debridement and muscle flap coverage.

Because a sternotomy approach simplifies establishment of CPB if the patient becomes unstable during ICD implantation and testing, some groups use this approach for nearly all patients undergoing ICD implantation. In reoperative situations, dissection should be limited to the anterior and diaphragmatic surfaces of the heart, to avoid damage or manipulation of coronary bypass grafts that could lead to myocardial infarction [13].

Technique (Fig. 2)

ICD implantation is performed after the cardiac surgical procedure has been completed. The patches and screw-in leads are more easily inserted before CPB is weaned; placement after termination of bypass may require cardiac manipulation that could produce hemodynamic instability. The epicardial screw-in electrodes are placed in a nonscarred region of the left ventricle 1–2 cm apart. Although patches can be sewn to the myocardium, extrapericardial placement is preferable in patients undergoing concomitant coronary artery bypass grafting (CABG) to avoid contact with the grafts that could lead to graft erosion, fibrosis, and occlusion.

The pericardium on either side is retracted medially to expose the mediastinal pleura. The patches are positioned anterior to the phrenic nerves and secured with silk sutures to the external surface of the pericardium. The left patch is placed over the extrapericardial surface of the apical posterolateral aspect of the left ventricle. The right patch is placed over the pericardium such that it apposes the right atrium and ventricle when the lungs are ventilated.

Extrapericardial placement is nearly always required for small hearts. If the DFTs remain unsatisfactory despite several different patch configurations, an intrapericardial right atrial patch folded over the anterior margin of the right ventricle can be placed. Alternatively, an SVC electrode or multiple patches can be used [10].

Cardiopulmonary bypass is weaned once the leads and patches have been positioned appropriately. The leads are then connected to the external cardioverter-defibrillator box for testing of sensing thresholds and DFTs. If the patient is too unstable hemodynamically to tolerate intraoperative testing off CPB, it can be performed on bypass. Alternatively, the leads can be buried in a subcutaneous pocket for subsequent testing in the EP laboratory.

The pocket for the generator is made through a separate transverse incision four fingerbreadths below the left costal margin. It can also be performed by extending the sternal incision and creating a pocket at its left aspect. To prevent lead damage, a chest tube is tunneled from the extraabdominal pocket into the chest incision; the leads are placed within the chest tube, which is then withdrawn through the tunnel. The generator is connected to the lead system and repeat defibrillation testing is performed. The generator is then placed into the pocket, which

Surgical Techniques for the ICD

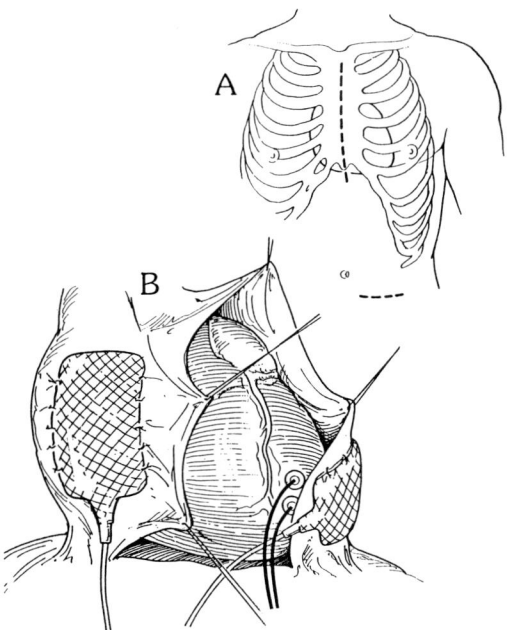

Figure 2 Median sternotomy approach. (A) A midline chest incision is made. An incision is also made in the paraumbilical region for placement of the ICD generator. (B) The defibrillation patches are placed over the posterolateral wall of the left ventricle and over the right atrium/ventricle. In this figure, they are placed outside the pericardium and anterior to the phrenic nerves. The two rate-sensing screw-in electrodes are placed close together in nonscarred regions of the right or left ventricle.

is closed in layers with absorbable sutures. Strict attention to asepsis is imperative during all phases of implantation.

In selected circumstances, it may be decided to place the ICD lead system without the generator. This is often performed in patients with a history of ventricular arrhythmias who undergo coronary bypass grafting without preoperative EP testing because of unstable ischemic syndromes. It is also considered in patients who have undergone endocardial resection in whom there is concern about an increased likelihood of postoperative inducibility of ventricular arrhythmias [14]. After the leads have been tested, they are tunneled to the left upper quadrant just above the rectus fascia. Electrophysiological testing is performed postoperatively and, if the patient is inducible, the generator is implanted. This procedure can be performed under local or general anesthesia using a transverse incision four fingerbreadths below the costal margin, creating a pocket, retrieving the leads deep in the subcutaneous tissue, and connecting them to the generator.

V. ANTEROLATERAL THORACOTOMY

The left anterolateral thoracotomy incision is the approach of choice in most centers for patients requiring isolated ICD implantation, especially if they have undergone a previous sternotomy [2,15]. It allows the operation to be performed through undissected, unscarred tissue and may avoid potential complications associated with a repeat sternotomy. This approach provides

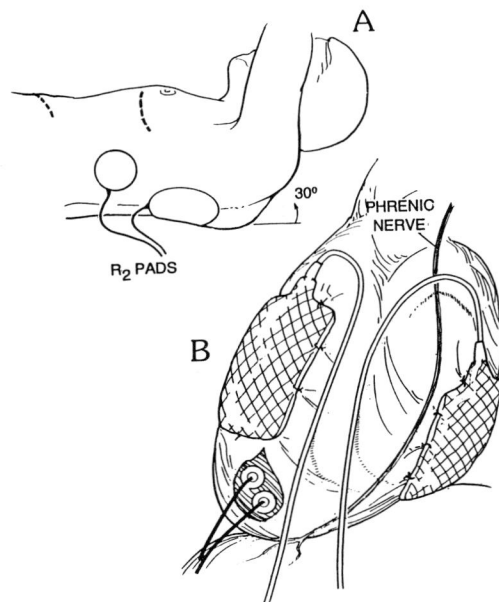

Figure 3 Thoracotomy approach. (A) The patient is positioned with the left side elevated 30°. R2 pads are positioned for external defibrillation. (B) The defibrillation patches are positioned outside the pericardium. One patch is placed behind the phrenic nerve over the posterolateral left ventricle, and the other is placed over the anterior aspect of the left ventricle. The pericardium is opened and two screw-in leads are positioned at the left ventricular apex.

fairly good operative exposure, although it is somewhat limited over the right ventricle and right atrium. It does allow enough flexibility to obtain a variety of defibrillator patch configurations. It is associated with greater postoperative discomfort than any other approach.

Technique (Fig. 3)

A double-lumen endotracheal tube is helpful in improving operative exposure by allowing the left lung to be collapsed. R2 defibrillator pads are placed for external defibrillation, if necessary. The large pad is placed between the shoulder blades and the small pad is positioned at the level of the cardiac apex and the posterior axillary line. The patient's left side is elevated 30°, with the left arm placed on an arm rest. The groins can be prepped and draped into the field for the establishment of CPB if the patient has had a previous sternotomy.

An anterolateral muscle-sparing lateral thoracotomy is made in the left fifth or sixth interspace. A small rib spreader is inserted and opened gradually to avoid rib fractures. Subperiosteal resection of the anterior segments of the fifth and sixth rib with pleural entry through the bed of resected rib may provide slightly better exposure. Adhesions between the lung and pericardium are lysed, and the left lung is gently retracted under a laparotomy pad or collapsed if a double-lumen endotracheal tube is used.

Patch electrodes are usually placed outside the pericardium. This is preferable in patients who have undergone previous cardiac surgery, because it reduces the risk of coronary bypass graft damage or ventricular perforation. It is also beneficial even when there is a free pericardial space in that it will prevent the development of an epicardial reaction and constrictive pericarditis. This should be considered in young patients, in whom cardiac surgery may be anticipated in the future. Extrapericardial patch placement is accomplished by dividing the attachments between the anterior surface of the pericardium and the sternum using electrocautery. Removal of fat from the anterior surface of the pericardium often results in improved DFTs. This should be done with the utmost care in patients with a previous sternotomy to avoid injury to the right ventricle, which is often adherent to the posterior table of the sternum.

The anterior patch usually serves as the anode and is placed as far anteriorly as possible beneath the sternum. The posterior patch, which serves as the cathode, should be located over the apical posterolateral region of the left ventricle posterior to the phrenic nerve. Nonabsorbable sutures are used to fix the defibrillator patches to the pericardium to avoid dislocation and crinkling. If intrapericardial placement of patch leads is desired, it may be necessary to make separate incisions on both sides of the phrenic nerve to improve exposure for fixation of the patches.

The pericardium is then opened and two sutureless myocardial electrodes are positioned 1–2 cm apart in a nonscarred area at the apex or base of the left ventricle. Alternatively, a right ventricular endocardial sensing lead placed through the left subclavian vein can be used. The leads are brought into the left pleural cavity, and all of the electrodes are passed subcostally and tunneled into a subcutaneous pocket in the left upper quadrant of the abdomen.

Warm saline solution is instilled into the chest cavity, and the metal retractor is removed. Defibrillation is performed with the lungs fully inflated, to maximize contact of the patches with the surface of the heart. A 32 Fr chest tube is placed and the ribs are reapproximated with paracostal figure 8 sutures. All incisions are closed in layers with absorbable sutures.

VI. SUBXIPHOID APPROACH

One of the first approaches to ICD implantation was the subxiphoid approach described by Watkins et al. in 1982 [16]. It was initially conceived as a less invasive approach to be used in very sick patients and has subsequently been used very successfully in patients who have not undergone previous open-heart surgery.

The advantage of the subxiphoid approach is that it requires only a very small upper abdominal midline incision with no entrance into the pleural space. If it becomes necessary to establish CPB, the incision can be readily converted into a median sternotomy. Patients develop less postoperative pain, less atelectasis, and fewer pleural effusions than with other approaches. Consequently, it is associated with a faster recovery and a shorter hospital stay. This approach does provide limited exposure, and its successful use requires a learning curve. Difficulty may be encountered in placing the screw-in electrodes and altering patch configurations for high DFTs. Although the patches are generally placed inside the pericardium, they can be positioned extrapericardially if cardiac surgery is anticipated in the future.

Technique (Fig. 4)

Under general endotracheal anesthesia, a short subxiphoid incision is made and the pericardial sac is exposed. The pericardium is opened about 2–3 cm above its attachment to the diaphragm, and the incision is carried down to the diaphragmatic reflection. Using an "upper hand" retractor, the left costal margin is elevated and the pericardial incision is extended laterally to the left to expose the left ventricular apex. A patch is inserted into the pericardial cavity, positioned over the left ventricular apex, and sutured in position to the cut edge of the pericardium.

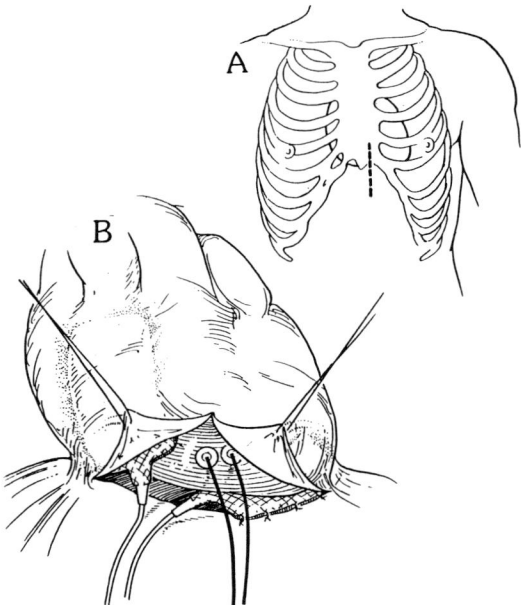

Figure 4 Subxiphoid approach. (A) An incision is made over the xiphoid process. (B) The pericardium is incised vertically and then laterally for placement of the patches. The left ventricular patch is placed over the diaphragmatic surface of the left ventricle. The right ventricular/right atrial patch is positioned over the atrioventricular sulcus. The rate-sensing leads are then placed onto the right ventricle.

Extension of the pericardial incision toward the right facilitates insertion of a second defibrillating patch over the right atrioventricular groove. Care must be taken to avoid folding the patches as they are positioned. If a transvenous right ventricular bipolar electrode has not been used, the two rate-sensing screw-in leads are placed into the right ventricular free wall. A subcutaneous pocket is then developed, either by extending the lower end of the incision or by making a separate incision in the left paraumbilical area. The device may be housed either above the anterior rectus fascia or under the rectus muscle. A chest tube is inserted into the pericardial cavity before closing the incision.

VII. LEFT SUBCOSTAL APPROACH

The left subcostal approach for ICD implantation was first described by Lawrie et al. in 1984 and represented a modification of a technique used previously for placement of epicardial pacemaker wires [17,18]. Only one incision is made for insertion of all leads and the generator. Although this approach produces less pain and atelectasis than the thoracotomy incision, it does create more discomfort than the subxiphoid approach because of division of the rectus muscle and stretching of the rectus sheath. Exposure of the left ventricle may be slightly better than with the subxiphoid approach, but the placement of the screw-in bipolar leads and repositioning of patches for high DFTs can be difficult. This necessitates an adjunctive ''right minithoracotomy'' in about 10–15% of patients to place a patch over the right atrium [19]. Because of the more limited exposure, there is a learning curve to the successful use of this

Surgical Techniques for the ICD

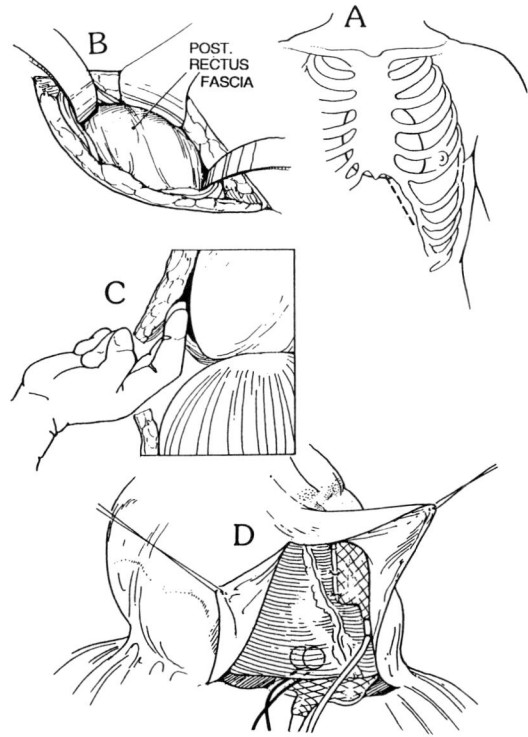

Figure 5 Left subcostal approach. (A) An oblique subcostal incision is made. (B) The rectus sheath is incised and the rectus muscle is split longitudinally, exposing the posterior rectus fascia. (C) Finger dissection is used to divide the costal attachments of the diaphragm and expose the pericardium. (D) The pericardium is incised vertically with lateral extension. One patch is placed along the inferior aspect of the heart and the other is positioned anteriorly over the left ventricle. The two screw-in electrodes are placed onto the right ventricle.

approach. In contrast to the subxiphoid approach, the subcostal incision can be used in patients who have had previous open-heart operations [20].

Technique (Fig. 5)

The patient is placed in the supine position and general endotracheal anesthesia is used. The chest and abdomen are prepped and draped. If the patient has undergone a previous sternotomy, the groins may also be included in the operative field for prompt establishment of CPB, if necessary. A skin incision is made 1–2 fingerbreadths below and parallel to the left costal margin and is extended the entire width of the rectus sheath (approximately 10 cm). The anterior rectus sheath is divided transversely, and both cut edges are dissected off the rectus muscle for several centimeters. The posterior rectus sheath is exposed by splitting the rectus muscle fibers. A large pocket is created beneath the rectus muscle for later placement of the ICD generator. Subrectus placement minimizes protrusion of the device, which is frequently noted when the device is implanted subcutaneously.

Exposure of the pericardium and dome of the diaphragm is obtained by blunt dissection and upward retraction of the left costal margin. The anterior surface of the pericardium is exposed by dividing the diaphragm at its costal attachments. The pericardium is then opened transversely at its junction with the diaphragm and vertically over the left ventricle (inverted "T"). By compressing the diaphragm downward and retracting the left costal margin upward, the heart is exposed.

The two patches are then positioned intrapericardially over the left ventricle. The first patch is placed posteroinferiorly between the diaphragm and heart, and the second patch is positioned anteriorly over the left ventricle. Both are anchored to the epicardium with 4-0 silk sutures. Care must be taken to avoid injury to cardiac structures, especially the left anterior descending artery and the left atrium. The two screw-in electrodes are placed at the apex of the right or left ventricle. The leads are then tunneled into the subrectus pocket and DFTs are determined.

If the pericardial space has been obliterated by previous heart surgery, it is usually possible to achieve a dissection plane along the diaphragmatic surface of the ventricle and place the posterior patch and screw-in electrodes in this region. The anterior patch is placed extrapericardially by separating the pleural fat from the pericardium over the anterolateral region of the heart. Use of transvenous pacing and sensing electrodes may be preferable to avoid damaging the heart or grafts during dissection of the right ventricle.

If DFTs remain high (>30 J) despite different patch configurations or reversal of polarity, an adjunctive "right minithoracotomy" is performed through the bed of the fourth or fifth rib [19]. The placement of a large extrapericardial right atrial patch usually reduces DFTs substantially. After testing is completed, the generator is placed into the subrectus pocket. The anterior rectus fascia and rectus muscle are closed securely with two layers of nonabsorbable suture (O-polypropylene) to minimize potential pericardial fluid leak or wound infection. Mediastinal and pleural tubes are not required unless bleeding or a pneumothorax is anticipated.

VIII. TRANSDIAPHRAGMATIC IMPLANTATION

A transdiaphragmatic approach was developed in order to avoid the morbidity associated with a thoracotomy, especially in patients with poor pulmonary function. It can also be used in patients who have had previous cardiac surgery. The procedure can be performed using an epidural block without the need for endotracheal intubation. An upper abdominal midline incision is made and the preperitoneal fat is exposed. The xiphoid process is excised and its diaphragmatic attachments are divided. The central tendon of the diaphragm is separated from its attachment to the parietal peritoneum using blunt dissection. The central tendon and pericardium are then incised vertically to expose the heart, while the abdominal viscera are retracted caudally. Screw-in electrodes are secured to the inferior aspect of the right ventricle. The patches are placed anteriorly and inferoposteriorly over the left ventricle. If DFTs are satisfactory, the diaphragm is closed with interrupted sutures and the abdominal incision is reapproximated in several layers. A pocket is made in the left paraumbilical region to house the generator [21].

IX. BILATERAL ANTERIOR THORACOTOMY

This technique was introduced as an alternative to an anterolateral thoracotomy in patients with a previous sternotomy in order to avoid anterior dissection and injury to the heart or bypass grafts. It may also be beneficial in the patient with severe chronic obstructive lung disease. The technique allows optimal exposure and can be performed expeditiously using a two-team

Surgical Techniques for the ICD

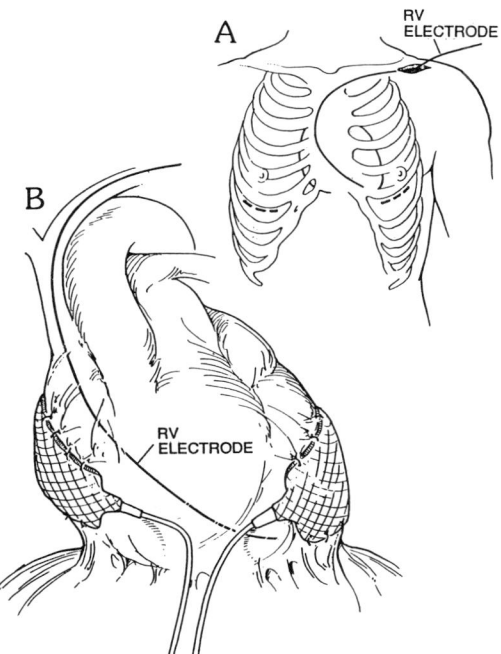

Figure 6 Bilateral anterior thoracotomy approach. (A) A short infraclavicular incision is made to expose the left subclavian vein for placement of the right ventricular endocardial sensing lead. Bilateral anterior thoracotomy incisions are made. (B) The patches are placed extrapericardially over the left ventricular apex and the right atrium.

approach. Short bilateral anterior thoracotomies are made through the fifth intercostal spaces (Fig. 6). The patches are placed extrapericardially with minimal dissection of previously operated regions. Use of transvenous rate-sensing leads minimizes dissection. All leads are then brought into the abdominal pocket and attached to the ICD generator. Bilateral chest tubes are required [22].

X. THORACOSCOPIC IMPLANTATION

Thoracoscopic implantation has recently been developed as a less invasive alternative to a full thoracotomy in high-risk patients (Fig. 7). An examining rigid endoscope (10 mm) is inserted through the sixth intercostal space in the anterior axillary line. Two other 5-mm trocars are inserted into the pleural space through submammary incisions. Through the lower trocars, the pericardium is grasped and incised with a scissors. The leads are passed through one of the lower incisions, positioned with a grasper, and fixated to the pericardium with staples. The leads are then tunneled to an adjacent subcutaneous pocket where the generator is housed [23].

XI. NONTHORACTOMY TRANSVENOUS LEAD SYSTEM

In 1973, Mirowski et al. reported the feasibility of using a transvenous platinum electrode lead system for sensing and defibrillation. This approach was subsequently abandoned because of high energy requirements and unreliable defibrillation [24]. However, ongoing research led to

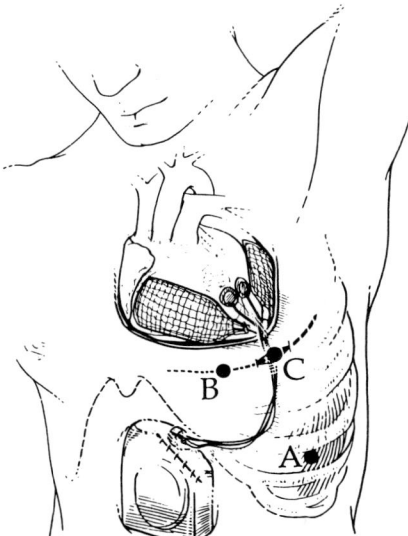

Figure 7 Thoracoscopic approach. Small incisions are made for placement of the trocars. A = 12-mm trocar for the thoracoscope and a chest tube. B = 5-mm trocar for placement of grasper. C = 5-mm trocar for placement of scissors and insertion of leads and patches. (Reproduced with permission from Ref. 23.)

the development of nonthoracotomy endocardial lead systems that could avoid invasive surgical procedures with their attendant morbidity in high-risk patients.

In 1988, Saksena and Parsonnet reported the use of a nonthoracotomy triple-electrode system for defibrillation in a patient with poor ventricular function [25]. This system was based on the theory that two spatially distinct vectors (bidirectional shocks) could reduce defibrillation thresholds (Fig. 8). More than 90% of patients with this system were found to have DFTs within the capability of the standard ICD generator with an electrode configuration that used a right ventricular electrode as a single, common cathode and SVC-right atrial and submuscular patch electrodes as dual anodes [26]. Because of problems with conductor fracture and inadequate long-term performance, measures were taken to improve lead designs as well as to provide two separate catheter defibrillation electrodes for both sensing and pacing capabilities. Clinical trials of these second-generation systems, including the CPI Endotak, Medtronic Transvene, and Telectronics EnGuard systems, were initiated in 1990 and have demonstrated excellent cardioversion and defibrillation capabilities, as well as adequate pacing performance [27–29].

Transvenous DFTs have been found to be comparable to those obtained with epicardial lead systems [30]. In fact, defibrillation efficacy may be superior because of the presence of an endocardial-to-epicardial current vector. In addition, pacing capabilities may be superior to those of epicardial pacing systems. The major problem of transvenous systems is lead dislodgement, which occurs in about 10% of patients.

An occasional patient will demonstrate high DFTs because of difficulty in achieving enough current density across the posterolateral aspect of the left ventricle. To overcome this problem, the SVC electrode can be advanced into the coronary sinus. This will provide higher current densities to the lateral LV and reduce the defibrillation threshold. A coronary sinus electrode used in conjunction with the SVC and RV electrodes can provide satisfactory de-

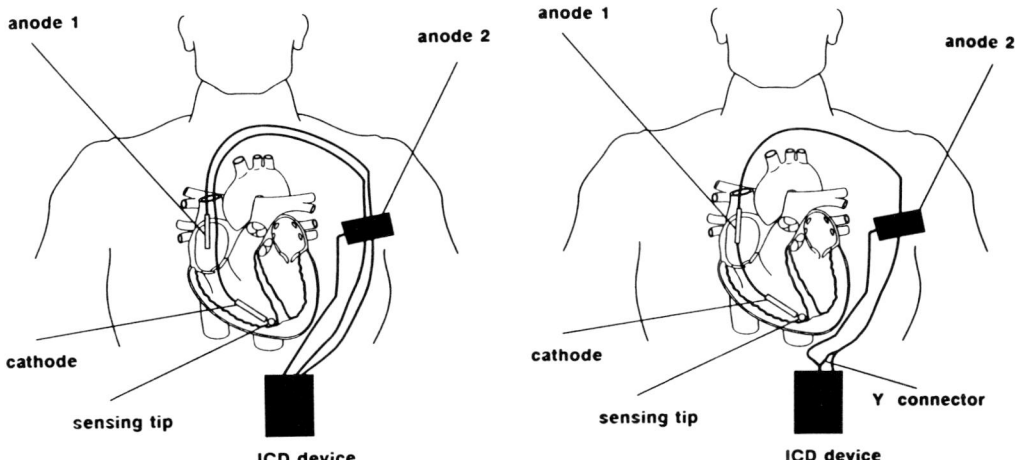

Figure 8 Nonthoracotomy lead systems. (Left) Medtronic Transvene lead system with a tripolar electrode in the right ventricle, a second electrode in the superior vena cava, and a subcutaneous patch. (Right) CPI Entotak system with a triple-electrode lead and a subcutaneous patch. (Reproduced with permission of the Society of Thoracic Surgeons, from Ref. 29.)

fibrillation without the need to implant the subcutaneous patch [31]. Potential problems of coronary sinus electrodes include sinus rupture or thrombosis, lead migration, and inadequate defibrillation efficacy, especially in patients with poor ventricular function.

Technique

The CPI Endotak system consists of one transvenous lead and a subcutaneous chest patch electrode. A 110-cm-long tripolar lead is inserted into the right ventricular apex through the left subclavian or cephalic vein (Fig. 8). This catheter has a distal tip electrode for bipolar rate sensing, a right ventricular spring electrode that serves as a shocking cathode and rate-sensing anode, and an SVC spring electrode, which serves as a defibrillation anode. The Medtronic system consists of two transvenous leads and a subcutaneous patch electrode. The tripolar pace, sense, defibrillation lead (model 6966) is passed into the right ventricular apex. It consists of a cathodal screw-in pacing electrode at its tip and an anodal ring electrode 1.5 cm proximally for bipolar sensing. A platinum-iridium coil electrode proximal to the sensing leads provides for cardioversion and defibrillation. A second transvenous lead (Medtronic model 6963) is placed at the superior vena cava–right atrial junction and can be advanced into the coronary sinus.

If the placement of a subcutaneous patch is necessary, a transverse submammary incision is made along the fourth left intercostal space in the midaxillary line. A large patch electrode (28 cm^2 surface area) is placed beneath the muscles and directly on top of the periosteum of the underlying ribs. All leads are tunneled to a standard anterior abdominal wall pocket, where the pulse generator is housed.

XII. OPERATIVE MORTALITY

Since the initial human implant in 1980, there has been extensive worldwide experience with ICD implantation. The efficacy of the ICD in reducing the incidence of sudden cardiac death caused by malignant ventricular arrhythmias has been well documented. The operative mortality for patients undergoing isolated implantation of the epicardial systems is less than 5%, even though many patients undergoing the procedure have markedly impaired cardiac function. More than 75% of early deaths occur before hospital discharge, usually as a result of intractable tachyarrhythmias or acute myocardial infarction [32–36]. Morbidity is commonly the result of lung complications. Mortality rates for patients undergoing coronary bypass grafting and/or endocardial resection combined with ICD implantation are significantly higher [14,32–36]. This is attributable to the patient's poor left ventricular function and complications of a low cardiac output state, rather than to the additional placement of the ICD device.

Finally, with the advent of nonthoracotomy ICD lead systems the surgical risk and complications of ICD implantation are significantly reduced. Avoidance of thoracotomy accounts for operative mortality rates $\leq 1\%$.

REFERENCES

1. Damiano RJ Jr. Implantable cardioverter defibrillators: current status and future directions. J Cardiac Surg 1992; 7:36–57.
2. Shepard RB, Goldin MD, Lawrie GM, et al. Automatic implantable cardioverter defibrillator: surgical approaches for implantation. J Cardiac Surg 1992; 7:208–224.
3. Watkins L Jr, Taylor E Jr. The surgical aspects of automatic implantable cardioverter-defibrillator implantation. PACE 1991; 34:953–960.
4. Brodman R, Furman S, Waspe LE, Kim SG, Fisher J. Surgical techniques for implantation of the automatic implantable cardioverter defibrillator. Clin Prog Electrophysiol Pacing 1986; 4:292–305.
5. Shahian DM, Williamson WA, Streitz JM Jr, Venditti FJ. Subfascial implantation of implantable cardioverter defibrillator generator. Ann Thorac Surg 1992; 54:173–174.
6. Curiale S, Rosenfeld LE, Elefteriades JA. Cosmetic approach for placement of the automatic implantable cardioverter-defibrillator in young women. Ann Thorac Surg 1991; 52:1340–1341.
7. Hartz RS, Kehoe R, Fredericksen JW, Zheutlin T, Shields TW. New approach to defibrillator insertion. J Thorac Cardiovasc Surg 1989; 97:920–922.
8. Almassi GH, Chapman PD, Troup PG, Wetherbee JN, Olinger GN. Constrictive pericarditis associated with patch electrodes of the automatic cardioverter-defibrillator. Chest 1987; 92:369–371.
9. Lemmer JH Jr, Faber LA, Mariano DJ, Drews TA, Kienzle MG. Pericardial influence on internal defibrillation energy requirements. J Thorac Cardiovasc Surg 1991; 101:839–842.
10. Baerman JM, Blakeman BP, Olshansky B, Kopp DE, Kall JG, Wilber DJ. Use of multiple patches during implantation of epicardial defibrillator systems. Am J Cardiol 1993; 71:68–71.
11. Blakeman BM, Wilber D, Pifarre R. Median sternotomy for implantable cardioverter/defibrillator. Arch Surg 1989; 124:1065–1066.
12. Brodman R, Fisher JD, Furman S, et al. Implantation of automatic cardioverter-defibrillators via median sternotomy. PACE 1984; 7:1363–1369.
13. Blakeman BP, Bakhos M, Foy BK, Calandra D, Pifarre R. Repeat median sternotomy for the automatic implantable cardioverter and defibrillator. Surg Gyn Ob 1992; 174:225–228.
14. Manolis AS, Rastegar H, Estes NAM III. Prophylactic automatic implantable cardioverter-defibrillator patches in patients at high risk for postoperative ventricular tachyarrhythmias. J Am Coll Cardiol 1989; 13:1367–1373.
15. Slater DA, Singer I, Stevens C, Springer MJ, Gray LA Jr. Lateral thoracotomy for the automatic implantable defibrillator. Arch Surg 1991; 126:778–781.
16. Watkins L Jr, Mirowski M, Mower MM, et al. Implantation of the automatic defibrillator: the subxiphoid approach. Ann Thorac Surg 1982; 34:515–520.
17. Lawrie GM, Wright-Hargis H, Lin HT, Nielsen AP, Wyndham CRC. Epicardial implantation of the automatic implantable cardioverter-defibrillator by left subcostal thoracotomy. Clin Prog Electrophysiol Pacing 1986; 4:277–285.

18. O'Neill PG, Lawrie GM, Kaushik RR, Harvill LF, Pacifico A. Late results of the left subcostal approach for automatic implantable cardioverter defibrillator implantation. Am J Cardiol 1991; 67:387–390.
19. Lawrie GM, Kaushik RR, Pacifico A. Right mini-thoracotomy: an adjunct to left subcostal automatic implantable cardioverter defibrillator implantation. Ann Thorac Surg 1989; 47:780–781.
20. Damiano RJ Jr, Foster AH, Ellenbogen KA, et al. Implantation of cardioverter defibrillators in the post-sternotomy patient. Ann Thorac Surg 1992; 53:978–983.
21. Shapira N, Cohen AI, Wish M, Weston LJ, Fletcher RD. Transdiaphragmatic implantation of the automatic implantable cardioverter defibrillator. Ann Thorac Surg 1989; 48:371–375.
22. Karwande SV, Rowles JR. Bilateral anterior thoracotomy for automatic implantable cardioverter defibrillator placement in patients with previous sternotomy. Ann Thorac Surg 1992; 54:791–793.
23. Ely SW, Kron IL. Thoracoscopic implantation of the implantable cardioverter defibrillator. Chest 1993; 103:271–272.
24. Mirowski M, Mower MM, Gott VL, Brawley RK. Feasibility and effectiveness of low energy catheter defibrillation in man. Circulation 1983; 47:79–85.
25. Saksena S, Parsonnet V. Implantation of a cardioverter/defibrillator without thoracotomy using a triple electrode system. JAMA 1988; 259:69–72.
26. Saksena S, Tullo NG, Krol RB, Mauro AM. Initial clinical experience with endocardial defibrillation using an implantable cardioverter/defibrillator with a triple-electrode system. Arch Intern Med 1989; 149:2333–2339.
27. Saksena S, Luceri R, Krol RB, et al. Endocardial pacing, cardioversion and defibrillation using a braided endocardial lead system. Am J Cardiol 1993; 71:834–841.
28. McCowan R, Maloney J, Wilkoff B, et al. Automatic implantable cardioverter-defibrillator implantation without thoracotomy using an endocardial and submuscular patch system. J Am Coll Cardiol 1991; 17:415–421.
29. Hammel D, Block M, Konertz W, et al. Surgical experience with defibrillator implantation using nonthoracotomy leads. Ann Thorac Surg 1993; 55:685–689.
30. Bardy GH, Hofer B, Johnson G, et al. Implantable transvenous cardioverter-defibrillators. Circulation 1993; 87:1152–1168.
31. Yee R, Klein GJ, Leitch JW, et al. A permanent transvenous lead system for implantable pacemaker cardioverter-defibrillator. Nonthoracotomy approach to implantation. Circulation 1992; 85: 196–204.
32. Hammon JW. The role of the automatic implantable cardioverter-defibrillator in the treatment of ventricular tachycardia. Sem Thorac Cardiovasc Surg 1989; 1:88–96.
33. Slater AD, Singer I, Stavens CS, Zee-Cheng C, et al. Treatment of malignant ventricular arrhythmias with the automatic implantable cardioverter defibrillator. Ann Surg 1989; 209:635–641.
34. Mosteller RD, Lehmann MH, Thomas AC, Jackson K, and Participating Investigators. Operative mortality with implantation of the automatic cardioverter-defibrillator. Am J Cardiol 1991; 68:1340–1345.
35. Paull DL, Fellows CL, Guyton SW, Anderson RP. Continuing experience with the automatic implantable cardioverter defibrillator. Am J Surg 1992; 163:502–504.
36. Elefteriades JA, Biblo LA, Batsford WP, et al. Evolving patterns in the surgical treatment of malignant ventricular tachyarrhythmias. Ann Thorac Surg 1990; 49:94–100.

18

Intraoperative Testing

Kenneth A. Ellenbogen, Mark A. Wood, and Bruce S. Stambler

*Medical College of Virginia
and McGuire Veterans Affairs Medical Center
Richmond, Virginia*

> The time is ripe, therefore, to begin to develop a responsible professional mechanism for defining some minimum guidelines for AICD implantation [9].

I. INTRODUCTION

Testing of the implantable defibrillator in the operating room is critical to the appropriate function of the implantable cardioverter defibrillator (ICD). The understanding of defibrillation threshold testing, sensing of ventricular tachyarrhythmias, and specific modes of device functioning are reviewed in detail in this chapter. Intraoperative testing begins with the assembling of equipment and personnel in the operating room.

Successful implantation of an ICD requires a medical and surgical team with skills and knowledge about device testing and implantation. The team should include an electrophysiologist with adequate training and knowledge about preoperative, intraoperative, and postoperative testing and a cardiovascular or thoracic surgeon with experience and interest in ICDs and arrhythmias [1]. The anesthesia team should be experienced in treating patients with heart disease. Access to an open heart team and operating room where the patient can be placed on bypass if necessary should also be available. The electrophysiology personnel should include a nurse and a cardiovascular technician or physician's assistant whose duties include preparation of the patient for intraoperative testing, maintaining and setting up the equipment and connecting the patient to this equipment in the operating room. A cardiovascular technician can perform record-keeping duties and operate the external defibrillator during intraoperative testing.

II. OPERATING ROOM

Prior to the patient's arrival in the operating room, it should be the responsibility of one of the team members to do an equipment and materials check. First, the electrophysiologist must communicate with the surgeon regarding choice of the ICD system and sensing/pacing leads.

If the surgeon is going to attempt to implant a transvenous defibrillation system, the team should have on hand two sets of transvenous defibrillation leads and subcutaneous patches, as well as all the materials for a thoracotomy approach should the defibrillation thresholds be too high with the transvenous system. For patients undergoing defibrillation implantation via a thoracotomy or subcostal, subxiphoid, or median sternotomy approach, two sets of all sizes of patches, epicardial leads, transvenous sensing leads, extra stylets, introducers, and the appropriate connectors or adapters for the ICD should be available in the operating room [2]. The compatibility of connectors and cables to the ICD and external cardioverter defibrillator (ECD) should be confirmed. Proper function of external defibrillators, external cardioverter defibrillator, and physiological recorder should be documented prior to the patient's arrival in the operating room. As the patient is brought into the operating room, extra skin electrodes should be positioned outside the field prior to the patient being prepped. The electrocardiogram (ECG) during intraoperative testing should be available on the physiologic recorder used for marker channels. Alternatively, the ECG may be "slaved" from another monitor.

Prior to or immediately after induction of general anesthesia, a member of the cardiology team should place one or two sets of external defibrillator patches, R2 (R2 Corporation, Skokie, IL) on the patient's chest to defibrillate the patient externally in cases where the maximum output of the external testing equipment is inadequate to convert ventricular fibrillation. Placement of two sets of external patches allows for rapid sequential defibrillation of the patient from two defibrillators, significantly decreasing the time between sequential shocks. The patches should be placed in as orthogonal a configuration as the sterile surgical field allows. In our experience, external defibrillation is necessary in less than 10% of cases. The surgical team should have a defibrillator and internal paddles available for patients in whom defibrillation is unsuccessful with external rescue shocks. Some centers may also have available a backup external cardioverter defibrillator, since despite thorough testing, a failure intraoperatively is always possible. The ICD device to be implanted should also be tested preoperatively, including interrogation and charge time assessment if appropriate. In addition to a backup ICD, some centers also may keep a high-energy generator available for patients with borderline or high defibrillation thresholds. The external testing equipment or ECD must be recharged prior to use in the operating room.

The next step in the setup procedure is to arrange the room for electrophysiological testing (Fig. 1). At the present time, this involves having a physiologic recorder for measuring amplitude and duration of intracardiac signals, as well as an external testing device, in the operating room. The implant support devices or ECDs vary from manufacturer to manufacturer, but are designed to reproduce the function of the ICD and must also be present in the operating room. Prior to the development of these devices, tape recordings of signals for retrospective analysis were the only means of troubleshooting difficulties with ICDs.

Finally, in some cases ventricular tachycardia cardioversion and antitachycardia pacing may be tested intraoperatively. For these patients it will be necessary to bring a programmable stimulator to the operating room.

III. DEFIBRILLATION THRESHOLD TESTING

Defibrillation threshold testing is critical to proper ICD functioning. In a recent study, Epstein and colleagues reported an incidence of 3–18% of patients undergoing ICD implantation with elevated defibrillation thresholds (e.g., >25 J) [3]. Defibrillation efficacy is dependent on the particular waveform delivered by the ICD (e.g., monophasic, biphasic), pulsing technique (e.g., sequential), electrode location and design, and tissue responsiveness (e.g., antiarrhyth-

Intraoperative Testing

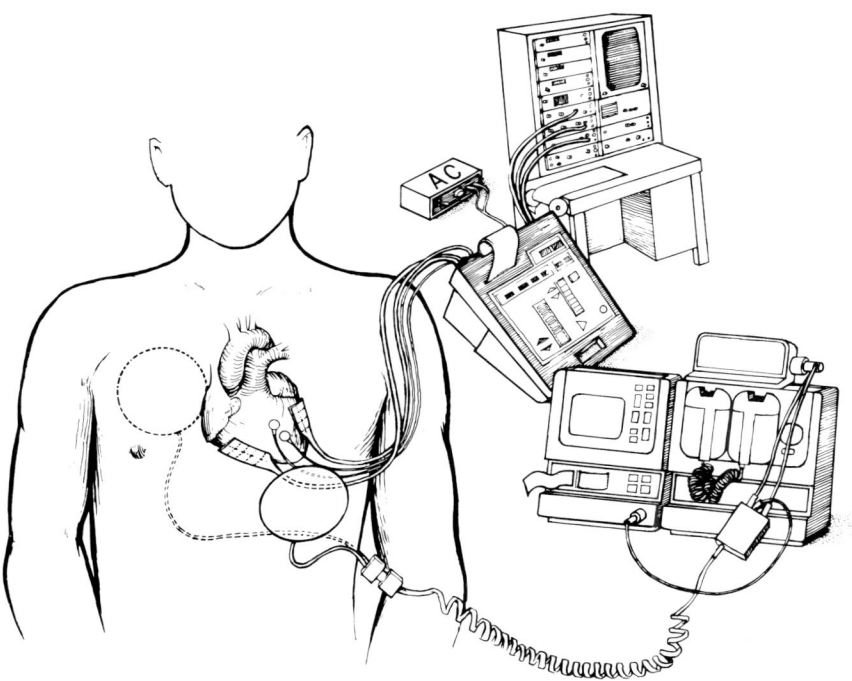

Figure 1 Diagrammatic representation of the operating room setup for defibrillation implantation. Defibrillating and sensing leads are connected to cables that go to the external testing device. The external testing device has outputs to a physiologic recorder and input from either a programmable stimulator or source of alternating current. The patient is monitored through the physiologic recorder and the external defibrillator for "rescue."

mic drugs). Each of these factors is discussed elsewhere in the book. A brief discussion of the physiology of defibrillation threshold testing will be reviewed.

Although the term "defibrillation threshold" is widely used, several investigators have shown that a specific energy level that separates uniformly successful from unsuccessful shocks cannot be demonstrated [4,5]. Defibrillation success is best described by a probability distribution relating the percent of successful defibrillations to delivered energy. The shape of this curve appears to be sigmoidal; increasing or decreasing the energy is associated with a higher or lower chance of successful defibrillation, respectively (Fig. 2). A wide range of energies is associated with an intermediate range of successful defibrillation. In constructing a defibrillation curve in animal models, 30 or more shocks are often required. The underlying mechanism for the statistical nature of defibrillation is not well understood.

In animal experiments, a curve of defibrillation efficacy can be constructed by repeated fibrillation and defibrillation of the animal while constantly stepping up or down to different energy levels until sufficient points are obtained to construct a curve. Since it is not possible to perform 30–40 fibrillation episodes intraoperatively in humans (the minimum number considered necessary to generate a dose-response curve), reasonable estimates of defibrillation thresholds can be made with 10–15 episodes in the majority of patients. In humans, methods for measuring the defibrillation threshold while delivering as few shocks as possible would be ideal. In one set of experiments in pigs, Klein and colleagues demonstrated that the measure-

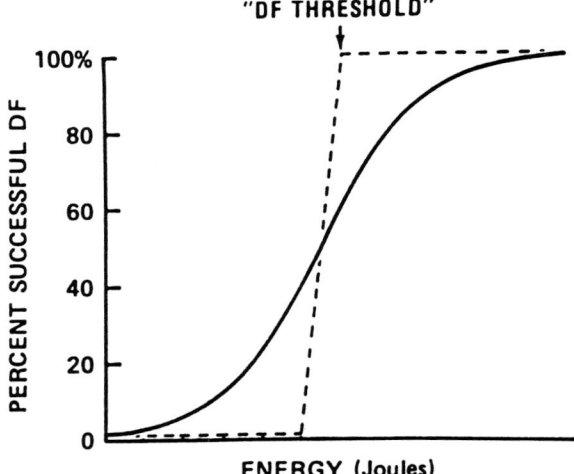

Figure 2 Schematized defibrillation threshold curve emphasizing that there does not exist a specific value separating energies that successfully cause reversion of ventricular fibrillation to sinus rhythm from those that do not. In fact, a wide range of energies is associated with an intermediate chance of successful defibrillation. Defibrillation energy requirement cannot be described by a single value, but rather by a curve that can generally be fit to a sigmoidal shape, and provides energy values associated with selected probabilities of success. In some animal experiments, this curve may, in fact, be more shallow. (Reproduced from Ref. 4, with permission of author and publisher.)

ment of successful defibrillation on three of three trials using a sequential pulse was as accurate an estimate of the defibrillation threshold as that achieved by constructing the entire curve [5–8]. By increasing the number of successful defibrillations at a given energy from one to three, the 95% confidence interval is increased from approximately 60% of animals to almost all animals. The standard clinical practice in most centers is to obtain two or three successful conversions of ventricular fibrillation at a given energy before accepting it as the defibrillation threshold, although guidelines from the North American Society of Pacing and Electrophysiology (NASPE) suggest that the number of fibrillation and defibrillation trials should be individualized [9].

IV. EQUIPMENT FOR DEFIBRILLATION THRESHOLD TESTING

To perform defibrillation threshold testing, there must be an external testing device that delivers shocks of variable energy with a waveform and duration identical to those delivered by the device being implanted. In addition, the physician must have a device that is capable of pacing or delivering alternating current through either an indwelling ventricular catheter, the rate-sensing leads, or the patch leads to induce ventricular fibrillation. In some cases, the external testing device may incorporate a high-output, programmable stimulator that can perform this task. In the currently available devices from several companies, either a source of alternating current or a programmable stimulator with high-energy pacing output is necessary.

All patients undergoing implantation of an ICD should undergo testing of defibrillation threshold regardless of whether their presenting arrhythmia is sustained monomorphic ventricular tachycardia or ventricular fibrillation [1]. Ventricular fibrillation is typically induced by rapid burst pacing through the rate-sensing lead(s). To attain the rapid ventricular rates required for inducing ventricular fibrillation, it is typically necessary to have a stimulator that can pace to a cycle length of 50–200 ms with an output of 30–50 mA and a pulse width of 10–30 ms. Alternatively, ventricular fibrillation can be induced with either direct or alternating current (60 Hz) delivered through a current limited fibrillator (commonly available in operating rooms performing cardiac surgery) or a standard battery-operated fibrillator (with a full-wave rectified output measured as 7 V over a 50-ohm lead) [10]. The alternating current may be delivered through either the epicardial or endocardial sensing leads or through the patch leads. In general, alternating current appears to be more effective at inducing ventricular fibrillation when delivered through the pace/sense leads rather than through the defibrillator's patch leads. Direct current may be used to induce ventricular fibrillation through an endocardial pacing catheter [11].

It was previously thought safer to deliver alternating current through the patch leads, because of concern that the alternating current if delivered through the rate-sensing leads would cause local myocardial necrosis resulting in impaired sensing thresholds [12]. Grubb and colleagues recently examined the acute and chronic pacing threshold, electrogram amplitude, slew rate, and resistance measured before and following at least three inductions of ventricular fibrillation with alternating current delivered through epicardial rate-sensing electrodes [13]. Approximately one-half of these patients had a pulse generator replacement and had these parameters compared to the initial implant values. In all 29 patients, serial serum creatine kinase and MB isoenzyme levels were measured at 8, 16, and 24 h following surgery. Serial creatine kinase and MB measurements demonstrated no evidence of myocardial necrosis in any patient. There was no significant change in pacing threshold, R-wave amplitude, slew rate, or resistance after repeated induction of ventricular fibrillation at the time of ICD implantation. In patients undergoing generator replacement, there was a 154% increase in pacing threshold, as anticipated with chronic epicardial leads, but no significant change in electrogram amplitude. Based on this study, it appears safe to deliver alternating current through either the rate-sensing or patch leads, and the use of a temporary pacing catheter for arrhythmia induction does not appear to be necessary.

A wide variety of external testing or implant support devices are currently being used. Cardiac Pacemakers, Medtronic, Telectronics, Pacesetter-Siemens, and Ventritex all have implant support devices that are used in the operating room to measure defibrillation thresholds. All these devices have at least one feature in common; that is, they all provide a high-voltage output that enables determination of a defibrillation threshold through either patches or a transvenous lead-subcutaneous patch. The high-energy pulse waveform of the implant device is generally identical or programmable to an identical waveform as found in the ICD device. For example, the CPI Ventak 1600 and the CPI Ventak ECD (Model 2805) deliver a monophasic truncated exponential waveform. Other additional features of these devices may include an "emulation mode," which allows one to program a rate and other detection algorithms as additional tachycardia detection criteria and permits the device to automatically sense and deliver a high-energy pulse mimicking the function of the implanted defibrillator. Some devices can also measure amplitude of intracardiac signals during the induced ventricular tachyarrhythmia, energy and current delivered, and transcardiac impedance. Some devices can measure pacing threshold, current, and resistance from the sensing lead(s), without having to have a pacemaker system analyzer also available. Finally, all these devices have the ability to deliver a maximal, high-energy "rescue" shock if the first shock at a lower setting is unsuccessful. With the CPI external testing device, this rescue shock is 40 J.

The currently available ECD produced by Ventritex, the HVS-02 system, includes a cardiac pacing system analyzer, programmable stimulator, and high-voltage cardioverter defibril-

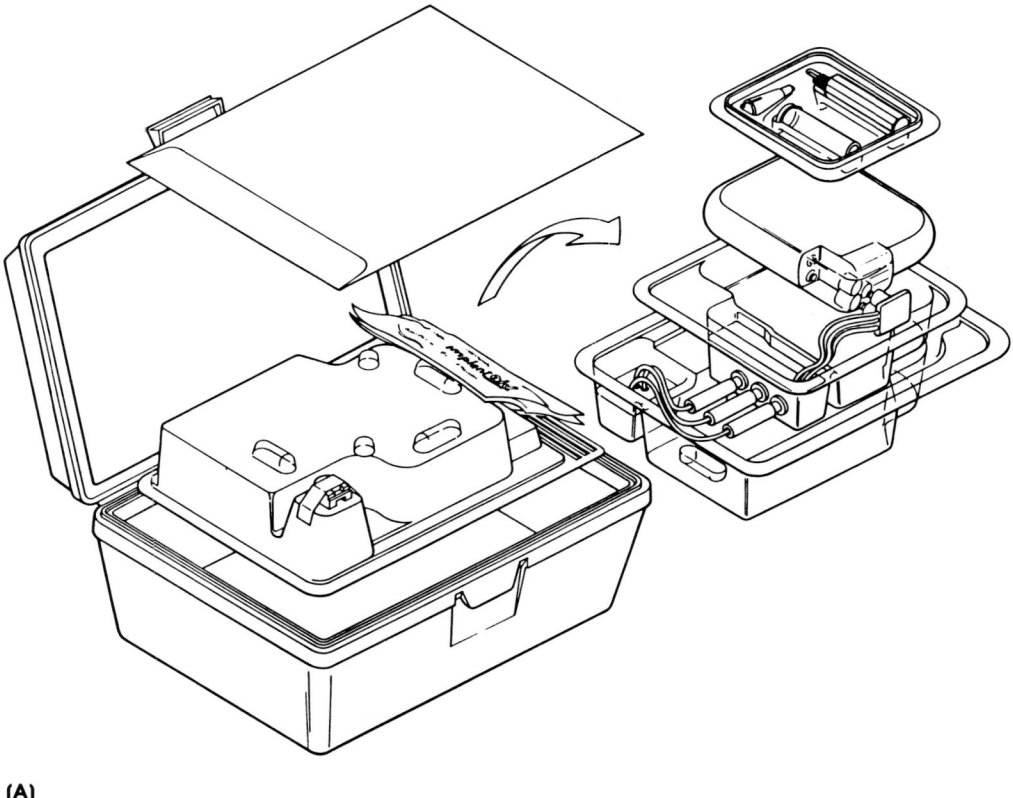

(A)

Figure 3 Schematic diagram of ICD and its connections inside the double blister package (A). Connections of ICD to external cables and patches as well as programmer are shown (B).

lator, and thus is capable of performing all three functions; therefore, additional equipment is not necessary. The cardioverter defibrillator is a dual-channel device that facilitates rapid delivery of shocks by having two separately charged capacitor banks. The waveform of the shock is a truncated exponential waveform that can be programmed to a monophasic, a biphasic single-cycle, or a biphasic 1.5-cycle pulse. The device measures patch or lead impedance and energy delivered as well [14].

A unique solution to defibrillation testing is provided by the Intermedics Res-Q. Intraoperative testing is performed through the ICD package, which is connected to the implanted electrode system through a set of cables. This setup is illustrated in Fig. 3a and 3b. The ICD is contained in a double sterile blister package with heat-laminated Tyvek fabric seals. The electrical connections are made between the header of the ICD through two sterility barriers to a female receptacle located outside the package. Connections between the ICD and the inner blister package are made by spring contacts that are pushed onto the set screws in the device's header [15]. The ICD is programmed to different energy levels or antitachycardia pacing algorithms for testing with the external programmer. A passive switching box may be included in series with the extension cable to allow recording of the cardiac electrograms during ven-

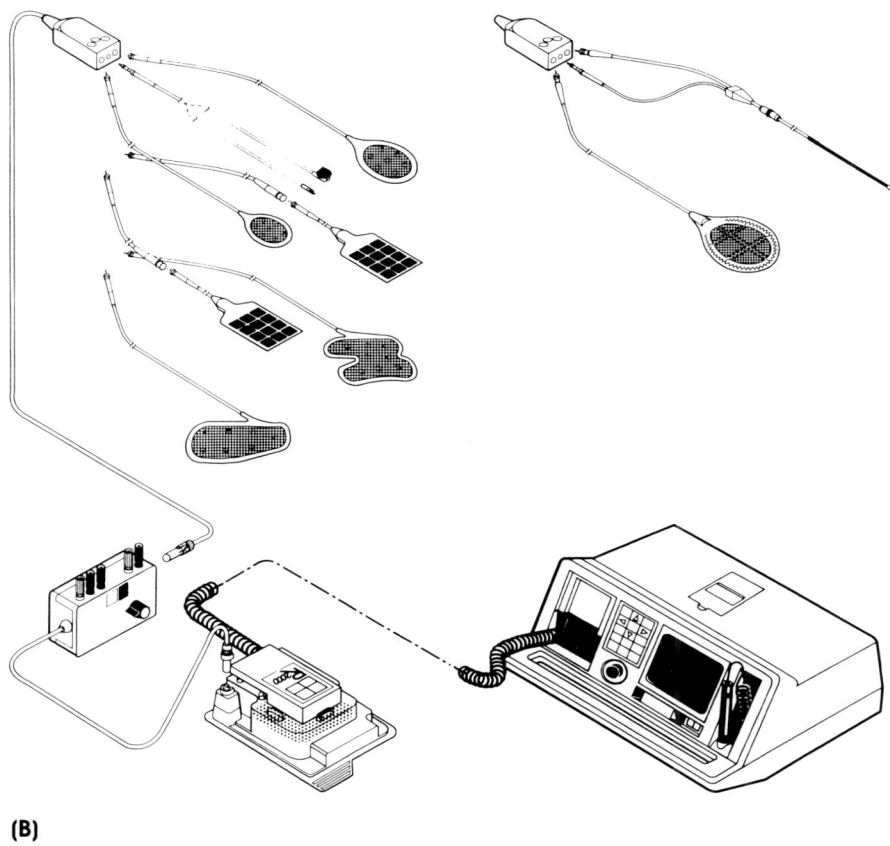

(B)

tricular tachyarrhythmias on a physiologic recorder. Another advantage to this system is that it reduces the hardware required for implantation of an ICD. The time, expense, and education required to use the external testing device or to update it as new waveforms become available are eliminated. A disadvantage of this system is that shocks delivered during defibrillation testing are delivered from the ICD being implanted, and after a lengthy or extensive intraoperative session, the longevity of the ICD being implanted may be significantly reduced.

V. PRACTICAL ASPECTS OF DEFIBRILLATION THRESHOLD TESTING

Defibrillation threshold testing in its simplest form consists of inducing ventricular fibrillation, waiting a variable period of time, and delivering a test shock to terminate ventricular fibrillation. Several guidelines will be suggested here (Table 1), but in general, there is a fair amount of variability in the process of defibrillation threshold testing [9,14].

Defibrillation threshold testing begins with the induction of a ventricular arrhythmia. If ventricular tachycardia (VT) is induced, successful termination of an episode of monomorphic tachycardia is generally accomplished with significantly lower energies than those associated

Table 1 Outline of Intraoperative Testing

I. Preoperative preparations
   A. Supply checklist—Patches, leads, connectors, generator
   B. Equipment checklist—External testing device or implant support device (recharged), ICD programmer, external defibrillator(s) and R2 patches, physiologic recorder, all cables and connectors
   C. Operating room setup Patient attachment to two external (R2) patches; patient ECG attachment to physiologic recorder (ECG)
   D. Equipment setup—Physiologic recorder, external cardioverter defibrillator or testing device, ICD programmer, external defibrillator

II. Intraoperative testing
   A. Defibrillation threshold testing
   B. Sensing evaluation—Sinus rhythm, ventricular fibrillation
   C. Pacing threshold measurement
   D. Cardioversion threshold, if stable

III. ICD device testing
   A. Testing ventricular fibrillation with implanted device
   B. Programming implanted device

with successful termination of ventricular fibrillation [9]. The cardioversion threshold of sustained VT is routinely tested in only about one-third of centers, and induction and successful termination of VT must be considered separately from successful conversion of ventricular fibrillation [9]. Generally, cardioversion thresholds are below those for defibrillation in a given patient. Once ventricular fibrillation is induced, a variable duration of time is measured before the test shock is delivered. Most centers wait 10 s before the delivery of the test shock, with times ranging from 8 to 15 s. About 70% of the centers responding to a NASPE survey began timing after alternating current was stopped. The most important point is that the duration of waiting before a test shock is delivered should closely approximate the sensing and charging time for the particular ICD that is to be implanted.

The duration of ventricular fibrillation before delivery of a test shock has definite clinical importance. Although somewhat controversial, too great a delay in energy delivery during ventricular fibrillation may increase defibrillation energy requirements and potentially result in unsuccessful defibrillation in some cases [16]. Several dog studies have evaluated defibrillation efficacy with an intracardiac catheter or a catheter and patch and have shown either no difference [17,18] or an increase [19,20] in defibrillation threshold between 10 and 40 s or 15 and 30 s. In a clinical study, Bardy and colleagues measured defibrillation thresholds at 10 and 20 s in 10 patients undergoing ICD implantation. The mean defibrillation threshold at 10 and 20 s did not change significantly [21]. In contrast, Winkle et al. studied 22 patients undergoing defibrillator implantation with matched shocks ranging from 5.9 to 24 J after 5 and 15 s of ventricular fibrillation. At higher energies, there was no difference in the efficacy of defibrillation shocks delivered after 5 compared to 15 s of ventricular fibrillation. For 5.9-J shocks, defibrillation was accomplished in 82% of patients at 5 s, but in only 45% of patients when the same energy was delivered after 15 s of ventricular fibrillation [22].

Most centers currently begin defibrillation threshold testing with an initial shock of 15 or 20 J, which would give most patients an adequate safety margin (i.e., 10–15 J less than the maximal output of the device) for defibrillation with the energy level of most currently available devices [9]. In most centers, a 2 to 5-min recovery time is allowed between repeat testing.

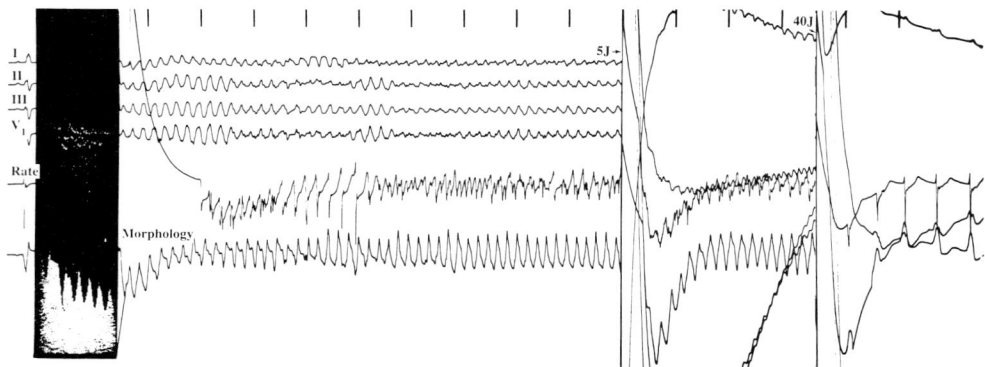

Figure 4 From top to bottom, surface electrocardiographic leads I, II, III, V_1 and rate and morphology electrograms. Ventricular fibrillation is induced with alternating current, and the 5-J shock does not successfully defibrillate the patient. Ventricular fibrillation continues until a 40-J rescue shock is delivered from the external cardioverter defibrillator.

Testing is continued at 15 or 20 J when the first shock is successful, until two or three successful consecutive defibrillations without any failures are noted. If desired, following successful conversions the energy may be decreased by 5 J (or 50–100 V) and the procedure repeated. If the first shock fails to terminate ventricular fibrillation, then a maximal "rescue" shock is immediately delivered followed by additional shocks through either the external R2 patches or internal paddles until sinus rhythm is restored (Fig. 4). Approximately 40% of centers require two successful terminations, with another 40% requiring three successful conversions (without any failures at that energy level) of ventricular fibrillation before an energy level is accepted as the defibrillation threshold. About 20% of centers will stop testing if the lowest successful energy terminating ventricular fibrillation is 10 J, about 50% will terminate testing if the lowest successful energy is 5 J, and another 20% will terminate testing when the lowest successful energy is 1–2 J. Clearly, the end-point for terminating testing will depend on the number of episodes of ventricular fibrillation induced and the patient's underlying heart disease and hemodynamic tolerance of repeated inductions of ventricular fibrillation [23]. The duration of time required for hemodynamic recovery from each episode of ventricular fibrillation is another clinical factor that will determine the number of episodes of ventricular fibrillation that can be tolerated. Defibrillation testing must be individualized so that maximum clinical information can be obtained with the least amount of risk to the patient's clinical stability [24].

VI. ELEVATED DEFIBRILLATION THRESHOLDS

If ventricular fibrillation is not reproducibly terminated by a 20- or 25-J shock, then a number of strategies (Table 2) must be considered [3,25,26]. First, one should check to see that connections to the ICD patches and cables are correct and secure. Next, defibrillation thresholds should be repeated with the patch polarity switched. It is standard practice to test defibrillation thresholds with the posterolateral left ventricular (LV) patch configured as negative (e.g., cathode) and the anterior patch made positive (e.g., anode). In two studies, defibrillation thresholds were measured with each patch polarity (e.g., LV patch negative and then LV patch

Table 2 Evaluation of Patients with High Defibrillation Thresholds

I. Initial troubleshooting
   A. Are lead connections to external cardioverter defibrillator or ICD tight?
   B. Is current being shunted to equipment or metal retractor?
   C. Is air or fluid separating patch from heart? Consider intrapericardial patch placement.
   D. Are patches crinkled or edges touching? Is "right" side of patch touching heart? Have surgeon inspect and palpate patches.
   E. Make sure heart is normothermic, not ischemic.
II. Therapeutic strategies
   A. Try with reversed patch polarity.
   B. Move patches to maximize myocardium between shocking electrodes.
   C. Add a second patch/lead if transvenous shocking system or spring patch not effective. Abandon transvenous defibrillation system.
   D. Add a third patch if two patches already implanted. Consider trying spring lead, if patch-patch configuration fails (optional).
   E. Leave patches, stop antiarrhtymic drugs, and return in 1–2 weeks for testing.
   F. Consider device with higher energy (34–40 J) or biphasic or sequential shock.

positive). Bardy et al. found that 15 of 21 patients had a lower defibrillation threshold when the LV patch electrode was positive, two patients had a lower defibrillation threshold when the LV electrode was negative, and four patients had equal defibrillation thresholds [27]. O'Neill et al. also assessed the effect of patch polarity on defibrillation thresholds and found 19 of 40 patients had a lower defibrillation threshold with the LV patch as the anode and nine patients had a lower defibrillation threshold with this patch as a cathode [28]. In this study, 12 of 40 patients had a 15-J or greater change in defibrillation thresholds with a change in patch polarity.

If alterations in patch polarity do not lead to an adequate defibrillation threshold, then other strategies should be utilized. First, the surgeon should examine the operative field to ensure energy is not being shunted from the heart. For example, energy may shunt to a metal retractor or another metal surgical instrument left in the operative field or chest cavity. Second, if the patches are too big or demonstrate crinkling, it is possible that energy may be shunted between the edges of the patches. This can be corrected by having the surgeon visually and manually inspect the patches to make sure edges are not touching or crinkling. Folding or "crinkling" of a large patch may reduce the surface area for current delivery. If crinkling is a problem, the patch must be repositioned and possibly resutured in a more stable position. If a patch is too large, it can be replaced by a smaller patch. Air or fluid separating the defibrillation leads from the surface of the heart may result in an increased defibrillation threshold as well. Finally, the uninsulated surface of the patch must face the heart.

After these possibilities have been excluded, repositioning of one or more patches is advisable. In addition, if one or more patches are small, and it is felt the heart is large enough to accommodate two large patches, then one or more of the small patches should be replaced by a large patch(es). Troup and colleagues have examined these factors in detail [29,30]. In one study they studied the relationship between echocardiographically determined mass, volume, cavity radius/wall thickness, and defibrillation threshold at the time of intraoperative testing in 10 patients with two large patches. A significant correlation was found between increased LV mass and increased defibrillation threshold ($r = 0.78, p < 0.01$), but the correlations between defibrillation threshold and LV volume and radius/wall thickness were not significant [29]. These authors also observed an excellent correlation between LV weight and defibrillation threshold in dogs. In another study of 41 patients, the authors analyzed the relationship between a number of clinical variables and the defibrillation threshold [30]. The only clinical variable that was statistically significantly associated with higher defibrillation thresholds was amiodarone therapy. The authors were also able to show that the surface area of the defibrillating leads is a critical determinant of defibrillation threshold. The total surface area of defibrillating leads was strongly inversely correlated with the defibrillation threshold. The defibrillation threshold for patch-patch combinations was 9.8 ± 6.5 J compared to 19.1 ± 10.3 J for spring-patch combinations, and the lowest defibrillation thresholds were seen in patients with at least one large patch. This is consistent with a wide body of animal data, as recently reviewed by Ideker and colleagues, who concluded that patches should be placed to cover a maximum amount of myocardium and allow current to flow from the free wall of one ventricle across the interventricular septum to the free wall of the other ventricle [31].

If repositioning and changing patch polarities is unsuccessful, it is our practice to add a third patch usually placed over the anterior right or left ventricle. The additional patch is connected to the right ventricular patch and the two are used as a common anode or cathode in testing against the posterior LV patch. A special high-voltage Y adapter is required and cannot be substituted with a standard pacemaker lead adapter. This allows the entire patch system to cover a larger amount of myocardium and decreases cardiac impedance, allowing more even distribution of the shock voltage across the ventricles. Decreasing the transcardiac impedance will also increase the tilt of a shock waveform delivered from a capacitor, which will also change the peak current required for defibrillation. The additional patch can be small or large, depending on the size and shape of the heart and how easy it is to accommodate without having patch edges touching. Another maneuver to improve defibrillation thresholds is to insert a transvenous superior vena cava (SVC) electrode (e.g., CPI model 0020 SVC lead) and test a combination of the SVC lead and epicardial patches. Again, a high-voltage Y adapter is required. In our experience, addition of the third patch has been helpful in the majority of patients with elevated defibrillation thresholds. In patients with borderline or high defibrillation thresholds, a high-energy device with a maximum output of 35–40 J is recommended. In patients with very high defibrillation thresholds (e.g., 30–40 J), the physician must decide whether to implant a device. This will be a problem in probably less than 1–2% of all implants. Most centers inform patients preoperatively of the possibility of this unlikely outcome.

A final maneuver in the operating room regards the optimal positioning of patches in relation to the pericardium. In one animal study reported by Lemmer et al., there was no significant difference in defibrillation thresholds in dogs between patches placed outside intact normal pericardium and patches placed directly on the epicardium [32]. Defibrillation thresholds were also examined after talc was instilled in the pericardial space to stimulate adhesion formation and pericardial thickening. Thickened, adherent pericardium in this animal model did not increase defibrillation energy requirements, suggesting that placement of patches outside the pericardium in patients should not adversely affect defibrillation efficacy. One of the papers' commentators had an experience where six of 87 patients had patches repositioned from the extrapericardial to the intrapericardial position, to obtain adequate defibrillation thresholds. It is possible that in some patients when patches are moved intrapericardially, more optimal surface contact results and thus provides a lower defibrillation threshold.

This has been the recently reported experience of the group from Columbia University, where 16% of patients had to have patches moved intrapericardially [33].

Alternative pulse sequencing and pulse waveforms are available with devices introduced in 1992 (e.g., sequential pulses with the Medtronic PCD and biphasic pulses with the Ventritex

Cadence, Telectronics Guardian 4211, and CPI Ventak PRx II). In general, both biphasic and sequential shocks may lead to a decrease in the defibrillation threshold in some patients, with the exact magnitude of decrease in the defibrillation threshold being quite variable from patient to patient [34–38]. In the study of Bardy et al., the defibrillation threshold for monophasic and biphasic pulses were compared in 22 patients with epicardial patches [34]. In seven patients, the defibrillation thresholds were unchanged or raised with the biphasic waveform, in 10 patients the defibrillation threshold decreased by <5 J, but in five patients the defibrillation threshold decrease by 5–10 J. Importantly, the three patients with defibrillation thresholds of greater than 14 J had a decrease in defibrillation threshold of 7–9 J. Bardy et al. also compared the defibrillation threshold of the currently available single pulse monophasic waveform to a sequential pulse system using three epicardial patches [35]. There was a decrease in defibrillation energy requirements of 37% with the sequential pulse system. No patient in that study had a defibrillation threshold >14 J with the single pulse, so it is difficult to extrapolate about the utility of this waveform to patients with high defibrillation thresholds. Finally, Bardy and colleagues have also shown that the particular electrode system (e.g., transvenous, transvenous-patch) has an influence on biphasic waveform efficacy for defibrillation [36–38]. If defibrillation thresholds remain elevated despite all these maneuvers, it is worthwhile leaving the patches on the heart and returning for further testing at a later time (see below).

Intraoperative testing of transvenous lead systems also involves testing multiple configurations. The Endotak (CPI) lead system has four possible configurations. These include testing of defibrillation thresholds with the lead tip as the cathode and the spring as the anode, the lead tip and proximal spring as a shocking cathode with the subcutaneous patch as a shocking anode, the lead tip as the shocking cathode and the proximal spring and patch as a common anode, and finally, the lead tip as a shocking anode and the patch as a cathode. Repositioning the patch electrode either posteriorly or anteriorly may improve defibrillation efficacy. Biphasic and sequential shocks will further lower defibrillation efficacy. Other transvenous lead systems currently being investigated include an additional lead in the coronary sinus [36,38].

The influence of cardiopulmonary bypass on defibrillation thresholds has been examined in a series of 10 patients [39]. In this study, the presence of cardiopulmonary bypass did not have a significant effect on defibrillation thresholds. Another study examined the effects of concomitant coronary revascularization and cardiopulmonary bypass in 10 patients [40]. In this study there also did not seem to be any effect on defibrillation threshold from cardioplegia, core cooling, or operative ischemia. Unfortunately, in all these studies only small numbers of patients were included. In contrast, the effects of different anesthetic agents were examined in a dog study, which showed that some anesthetic agents may modify defibrillation thresholds [41]. For example, Dorian noted that fentanyl-anesthetized animals had lower defibrillation thresholds than animals receiving pentobarbital or enflurane. Anesthetics have been shown to affect pacing threshold and ability to induce ventricular arrhythmias, so it is not surprising that they also affect defibrillation thresholds [42–44]. Additionally, since antiarrhythmic drugs seem to be associated with elevated defibrillation thresholds, retesting should be performed off antiarrhythmic drugs, especially if the patient's frequency of arrhythmic episodes is sufficiently low to make the patient's management off antiarrhythmic agents a reasonable possibility [45–48]. Class Ia antiarrhythmic drugs have been shown to variably affect the ventricular defibrillation threshold, either increasing it or causing no change, whereas class Ib antiarrhythmic drugs have been shown to uniformly increase defibrillation thresholds. Class Ic drugs have also been shown to uniformly increase defibrillation thresholds [49,50] and pacing requirements. Finally, the bulk of evidence suggests amiodarone has a variable effect on defibrillation threshold, either increasing it or causing no change [51–54].

Other factors, such as acid-base disturbances and hypothermia, have been shown to adversely affect the defibrillation threshold [55,56]. Ischemia may also influence the defibrillation threshold, with one study showing that the defibrillation threshold following spontaneous ventricular fibrillation with acute coronary occlusion was higher than during induced ischemic ventricular fibrillation [57]. Finally, reports of "threshold creep" relate instances in which after prolonged defibrillation testing and elevated defibrillation thresholds, the patient is returned to the operating room several days later and repeat testing confirms adequate defibrillation thresholds. Apparently, large numbers of defibrillations may increase the defibrillation thresholds during subsequent intraoperative testing. Grubb and colleagues reported six patients in whom adequate defibrillation thresholds were obtained after patch healing when retesting was reperformed 10–15 days after initial intraoperative testing [58,59]. The point at which defibrillation threshold testing becomes dangerous is a clinical judgment that must be made in the operating room based on a number of clinical factors [16].

The importance of testing and the search for the lowest possible defibrillation threshold is emphasized by findings from the studies of Guarnieri et al. and Marchlinski et al. [60,61]. Guarnieri and colleagues measured defibrillation thresholds in 23 patients at the time of generator replacement 24.8 ± 7.5 months from the time of initial implant. All patients had a LV patch and a spring coil lead in the SVC. The defibrillation threshold for the entire group increased from 12.3 ± 4.7 to 16.9 ± 5.9 J and in the patients taking amiodarone, the increase was from 10.9 ± 4.3 to 20.0 ± 4.7 J at replacement. These authors were unable to show any significant change in defibrillation threshold in patients not on antiarrhythmic agents or on class Ia agents, although two of these 12 patients had an increase in defibrillation thresholds of 5 J or more. Another study by Marchlinski et al. examined the relationship between the intraoperative defibrillation threshold and successful postoperative defibrillation judged by the predischarge electrophysiology study [61]. The authors emphasized the importance of attempting to find the lowest possible defibrillation threshold by noting that failure to terminate ventricular fibrillation is not uncommon (27%), when the defibrillation threshold is close to the maximal energy delivered by the ICD.

VII. SENSING

Sensing is the process of turning a continuous electrical signal into a series of sensed events. The process of analyzing a sequence of sensed electrical events by an ICD system must be tested in the operating room. The cardiac rate is by far the most common detection algorithm for classifying and discriminating sinus rhythm from VT, ventricular fibrillation, and asystole.

The first generation of ICDs had excellent sensing during ventricular fibrillation. The true sensitivity and specificity of these devices for detecting ventricular fibrillation is not, however, precisely known because these devices do not have electrogram storage, data logging, or any type of Holter-like function. These devices use an automatic gain control that allows the sensing system to adapt to changes in signal amplitude with different rhythms and requires little or no physician input to set up the system or test it. Signals as low as 0.2–0.3 mV can be sensed with this algorithm. The original automatic gain control is used in the original AID-B from Intec and subsequently Cardiac Pacemakers. Variations in the automatic gain control approach are used by Intermedics, Ventritex, and Pacesetter-Siemens in their devices. The implementation of automatic gain control is different in each device. With the automatic gain control system, the threshold for detection of a signal is a function of the amplitude of the previously sensed signal. The automatic gain control systems may take a significantly long time to adjust to changes in signal amplitude; thus one should wait several seconds after applying alternating current before "turning sensing on" with such a system, because the amplifier is saturated and needs to have time to "gain down." The automatic gain control has been considered the "gold standard" because of its widespread use and clinical efficacy. There are, however, documented limitations, including reports of failure to sense ventricular fibrillation and T-wave oversensing, as well as documented problems of ICD-pacemaker interaction. This is because pacemaker spikes may be identified as ventricular signals because of their large amplitude, and the automatic gain control will then ignore the smaller true ventricular signals [62–64]. The true performance of sensing cannot be adequately measured with earlier models of ICDs (e.g., the CPI AICD models 1520 and 1550) because of the absence of telemetry and data logging. An attempt to evaluate sensing performance using "beep-o-grams" has demonstrated nonspecific over- or undersensing in a study of 27 randomly selected asymptomatic patients without known sensing malfunction [65]. ICD–pacemaker interactions should be studied carefully during intraoperative testing (see Chapter 18).

With fixed-gain devices such as the Telectronics Guardian 4202/4203, programmable sensitivity varies from 0.7 to 5.7 mV. This is the simplest of all sensing systems and is the basic sensing system used in all pacemakers. This is a simple system to design and implement and provides no adjustment to rapidly changing signal amplitude. In a fixed-gain system, effort is required to program the system and decisions must be made about programming the sensitivity. For example, ventricular sensing must be checked during VT and ventricular fibrillation to avoid undersensing [66]. In addition, changes in lead performance and signal characteristics may require reprogramming over time. Another form of sensing, automatic sensitivity adjustment, is employed in the Telectronics Guardian ATP 4210 consisting of two amplifiers, one for low gain and one for high gain. This system has advantages of catering well to smaller signal amplitudes encountered in ventricular fibrillation, allowing for the high-gain amplifier to be optimized, and has good stability and range, allowing for continuous sensing even in the presence of noise. The disadvantages of this approach are: (1) more effort is required to set up the system and (2) it is not possible to sense ventricular fibrillation with relatively small signals if it is not preceded by an arrhythmia that causes a switch from low- to high-gain amplifiers.

Another form of sensing, called automatic sensitivity tracking, is used in the Medtronic PCD II 7216 and PCD III 7217, as well as the Telectronics Guardian ATP II 4211. As in systems with automatic gain control, it is the most sensitive value that determines the system's ultimate ability to correctly sense the low-amplitude ventricular fibrillation. The sensitivity is adjusted continuously and rapidly between each sensed electrogram, which allows this system to deal with rapid change in electrogram amplitude. The disadvantages of this sensing system are that if filtering is optimized for ventricular fibrillation, it may oversense T waves or undersense very-low-amplitude ventricular fibrillation late in the episode.

Routine evaluation of sensing during intraoperative testing consists of several steps. First, the amplitude of the intracardiac electrogram must be measured in sinus rhythm. In one report, Klein and colleagues reported there was a correlation between the amplitude of the cardiac electrogram during sinus rhythm and ventricular fibrillation [67,68]. There is, however, considerable variability between the amplitude of signals during ventricular fibrillation in patients having similar electrogram amplitude during sinus rhythm [69]. In addition, Saksena has argued that the signal characteristics of transvenous sensing leads are better than those of epicardial leads. The change in signal characteristics of these two lead types has not been well studied over time [70,71].

During ventricular fibrillation and sinus rhythm, cardiac electrograms can be measured by comparison to a calibration signal delivered from the external cardioverter defibrillator or im-

Intraoperative Testing

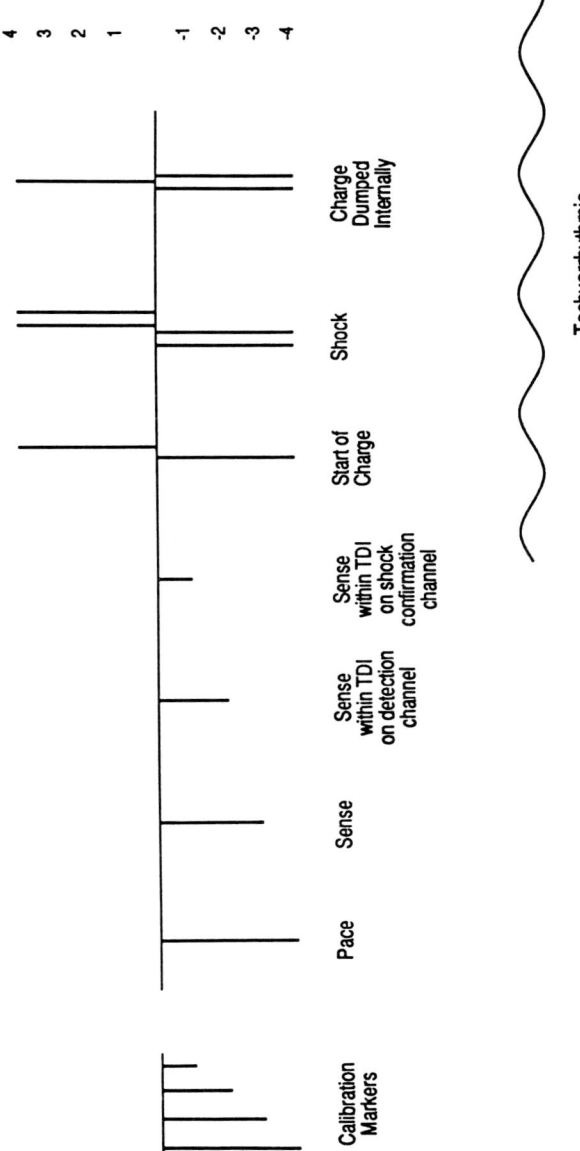

Figure 5 The Telectronics Guardian ATP 4210 is capable of providing telemetry with a number of different markers of sensing and pacing. Most third-generation devices provide bidirectional telemetry and stored electrograms that may be useful for troubleshooting in the operating room during device testing.

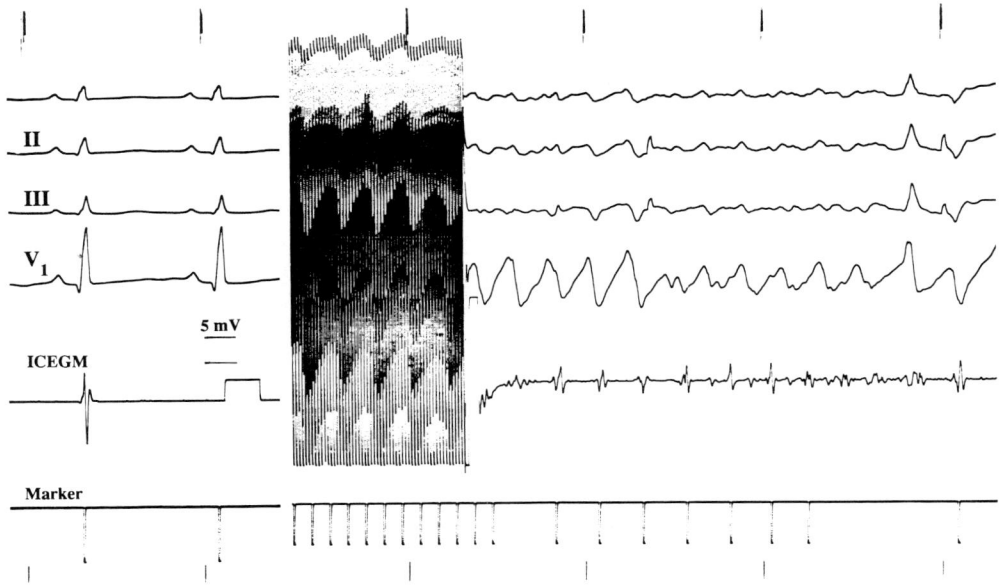

Figure 6 From top to bottom, surface electrocardiographic leads I, II, III, V_1, electrograms recorded from epicardial sensing leads (ICEGM), and marker channel generated from external testing device with a programmed sensitivity of 1.4 mV. A 5-mV calibration signal is shown followed by induction of arrhythmia with alternating current. The full-height downward line on the marker channel denotes sensing of the ICEGM, and signal dropout or undersensing is noted in ventricular fibrillation at this programmed sensitivity. Note the marked variation in ICEGM amplitude.

plant support device and recorded on paper (Fig. 6). The amplitude of the cardiac signal during ventricular fibrillation must be measured and compared to the anticipated programmed sensitivity of the implanted device if it is a fixed-gain sensing device. In some cases, the size of the electrogram measured using a calibration signal may not directly correspond to the size the device senses, owing to differences in filter settings and algorithms used by the device to determine signal amplitude [72].

In addition, some implant support devices have "marker channels" that output a signal to a physiologic recorder that indicates whether the implant support device or external testing device recognizes the signal and how the signal would be treated by an implanted device. For example, in the Telectronics 4210 the marker channel is produced by the implant support device as a result of digital code that relates a sensed signal to an event. There is a unique code for each different event, and these codes are interpreted by the implant support device or the programmer and generate event markers on an analog output, such as a strip chart recorder (Fig. 5). In the Telectronics Guardian ATP 4210 there are different markers for a pacing pulse, sense on low-gain channel above or below the tachycardia detection interval, sense on high-gain channel, start of defibrillator charge, delivery of a shock, internal dump of shock to defibrillator capacitors, and tachycardia present. The marker channels provide information in the intraoperative setting about how an implanted device will function and whether signals are sensed at different programmed sensitivities through the external testing device.

Endocardial leads, especially those that use a right ventricular coil electrode for pacing and sensing as well as delivering a defibrillation shock, are called an integrated bipolar sensing system and appear especially susceptible to substantial decreases in electrogram amplitude after shock delivery [73]. Jung and colleagues studied five patients with such an endocardial lead system and demonstrated failure to redetect ventricular fibrillation after an unsuccessful shock. In their studies, electrogram amplitudes decreased significantly after shock discharge and did not return to baseline for 5 min. In contrast, a true bipolar sensing configuration, where separate electrodes for pacing and sensing are separated from those delivering high-energy shocks, has not been reported to cause undersensing as the possibility of electrode polarization effects is minimized [74].

VIII. TROUBLESHOOTING

If cardiac signals are of inadequate amplitude or significant sensing dropout occurs during ventricular fibrillation, consideration must be given to repositioning the sense/pace lead(s) to a different site and repeating measurements of signal amplitude during ventricular fibrillation and sinus rhythm (Fig. 6). If a transvenous lead is being used for sensing, then repositioning of the lead is necessary with retesting of signal amplitude during sinus rhythm and ventricular fibrillation. In our experience, the vast majority of sensing problems can be treated by replacement of epicardial sensing leads with a tined (e.g., passive fixation) or screw (e.g., active fixation) endocardial sensing lead [69–71]. Low-amplitude epicardial signals may be a particular problem in patients with idiopathic dilated cardiomyopathy or "electrical" heart disease. In addition, epicardial sensing leads are probably more likely to have problems with late sensing following implantation, as there is a greater degree of chronic alteration in pacing and sensing thresholds with epicardial leads [75]. Finally, in patients with sensing problems during intraoperative testing, consideration should be given to implantation of a device with automatic gain tracking rather than fixed sensitivity.

IX. PACING

The general guidelines that are appropriate to the selection of a lead position when implanting a permanent pacemaker apply to assessment of pacing threshold during the implantation of an ICD in the operating room. In general, a pacing threshold of less than 1.5 V with epicardial leads and a pacing threshold of less than 1.0 V with a transvenous sensing lead is desirable. With active fixation transvenous sensing leads, pacing threshold may decrease considerably in the 5–15 min after fixation of the screw. It is often worthwhile to repeat determination of the pacing threshold if it is borderline or modestly elevated.

In patients with a previously implanted, permanent, single- or dual-chamber pacemaker, the interaction of the permanent pacemaker with the sensing of the implantable defibrillator must be thoroughly evaluated. This topic is dealt with in detail in Chapter 29.

X. DEVICE IMPLANTATION AND TESTING

In all patients undergoing implantation of ICDs, the final step in intraoperative testing is to implant the generator and perform further testing. It is our standard procedure to induce at least one episode of ventricular fibrillation and test the ability of the device to sense and ter-

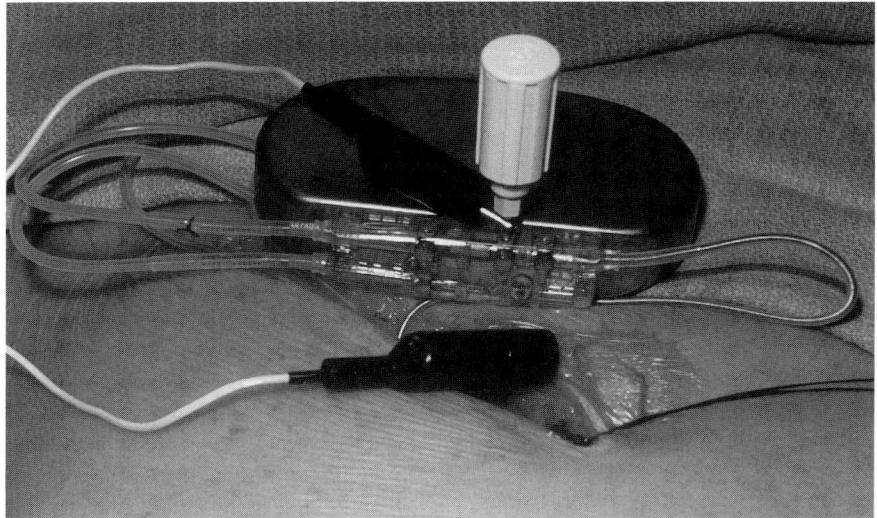

Figure 7 Use of hex wrenches in a CPI Ventak 1700 device connected with alligator clips to a source of AC current to induce ventricular fibrillation in the operating room for device testing.

minate the arrhythmia. In general, the device is interrogated and programmed prior to placement of patches and intraoperative testing. Currently, this involves reforming capacitors and checking a battery charge time and making sure it is within a defined range of its factory specifications. The device is placed in the operative field after adequate defibrillation thresholds and sensing/pacing thresholds are obtained. The device is inactivated prior to transfer to the surgeon. Once the device is connected to the leads, a sterile programming wand is usually used to activate the device.

Implant testing of the device involves assessing features that are specific to each device. With the newer devices currently available from CPI (e.g., Ventak 1600), the device can be programmed to the "EP TEST MODE" in which the device is in a standby mode, allowing the physician to induce the arrhythmia with the device in a "suspended state." Once ventricular fibrillation is induced, the device is reprogrammed to the active mode and the device tracks the number of seconds for detection of the arrhythmia, delay, charging of capacitors, and finally delivery of shock. Ventricular fibrillation may be induced noninvasively by rapid pacing if the device can be coupled to or driven by a programmable stimulator, or by delivering alternating current through a #2 hex wrench inserted into each of the rate-sensing lead set screw sites [76] (Fig. 7). Alternatively, Smith and colleagues have routinely used epicardial wires, placed intraoperatively during a standard midline sternotomy approach, to perform postoperative testing, although these wires can be used for intraoperative testing as well [77]. Sensing is assessed during the ventricular arrhythmia by event markers, as well as markers for charging and termination of the arrhythmia. Confirming appropriate sensing during ventricular fibrillation is critical, but the means of doing this varies according to the type of device implanted. In some devices, sensing can be evaluated with the implant support device or ECG. This is particularly important in devices with programmable sensitivities, as sensing must be verified prior to device implantation. With devices such as the CPI Ventak 1550 and 1600 series, complete beat-to-beat (real-time) sensing data are not provided. Instead, the programmer provides marker channels indicating sensing criteria have been met. For these devices, in particular, it may be more helpful to look at the changing event counter on the programming screen in the EP test mode rather than relying on telemetered marker channels. Finally, the device is reinterrogated to verify proper telemetric functions of the device, and then the device is generally inactivated until the surgeon completes the use of electrocautery for the generator pocket. In some cases the device will be reactivated prior to the patient's transfer from the operating room, but in other cases the device is not activated for 24–48 h, or until the patient is stable.

Proper performance of this stage of the procedure is contingent on a thorough understanding of the functioning of the particular ICD being used. A recent patient we studied emphasizes this point. This patient had routine measurement of defibrillation thresholds and sensing and pacing thresholds. The device was implanted and failed to deliver any shocks despite proper sensing of ventricular fibrillation. The device reported a patch impedance of $>130\ \Omega$ and therefore did not delivery therapy. The device was replaced, and testing of the device revealed a random component failure that may not have been discovered if the device was implanted without testing. Each electrophysiologist must be familiar with the external testing device and programmer for that particular ICD.

XI. SUMMARY

Intraoperative testing prior to ICD implantation is as critical to the long-term proper functioning of implantable defibrillators as is testing the pacing and sensing characteristics of pacing lead(s) at the time of permanent pacemaker implantation. A proper understanding of the limitations of defibrillation threshold testing leads to an organized and safe approach to defibrillation threshold testing in patients. An organized, systematic approach to patients with high defibrillation thresholds will result in the ability to obtain adequate patch positioning or patch configurations in the majority of patients.

REFERENCES

1. Cannom DS, Winkle RA. Implantation of the automatic implantable cardioverter defibrillator (AICD): practical aspects. PACE 1986; 9:793–809.
2. Troup PJ. Lead system selection, implantation, and testing for the automatic implantable cardioverter-defibrillator. Clin Prog Electrophysiol Pacing 1986; 4:260–276.
3. Brooks R, Torchiana D, Vlahakes GJ, Ruskin JN, McGovern BA, Garan H. Successful Implantation of cardioverter–defibrillator systems in patients with elevated defibrillation thresholds. J Am Coll Cardiol 1993; 22:569–74.
4. Davy JM, Fain ES, Dorian P, Winkle RA. The relationship between successful defibrillation and delivered energy in open-chest dogs: reappraisal of the "defibrillation thresholds" concept. Am Heart J 1987; 113:77–84.
5. Jones DL, Irish WD, Klein GJ. Defibrillation efficacy, comparison of defibrillation thresholds versus dose-response curve determination. Circ Res 1991; 69:45–51.
6. Jones DL, Klein GJ, Guiraudon GM, Sharma AD, Yee R, Kallok MJ. Prediction of defibrillation success from a simple defibrillation threshold measurement with sequential pulses and two current pathways in humans. Circulation 1988; 78:1144–1149.
7. Fujimura O, Jones DL, Klein GJ. The defibrillation thresholds: how many measurements are enough? Am Heart J 1989; 117:977–979.
8. Rattes MF, Jones DL, Sharma AD, Klein GJ. Defibrillation threshold: a simple and quantitative estimate of the ability to defibrillate. PACE 1987; 10:70–77.
9. Lehmann MM, Saksena S. Implantable cardioverter defibrillators in cardiovascular practice: report of the policy conference of the North American Society of Pacing and Electrophysiology. PACE 1991; 14:969–979.

10. Mower MM, Reid PR, Watkins L, Mirowski M. Use of alternating current during diagnostic electrophysiologic studies. Circulation 1983; 67:69–72.
11. Weismuller P, Richter P, Binner L, Brossmann G, Hemmer W, Hoher M, Kochs M, Hombach V. Direct current application: easy induction of ventricular fibrillation for the determination of the defibrillation threshold in patients with the implantable cardioverter defibrillators. PACE 1992; 15:1137–1143.
12. Physician Manual for the Automatic Implantable Cardioverter Defibrillator. CPI Document no. 16J 0155, p. 20.
13. Grubb BP, Durzinsky D, Mancini MC, Temesy-Armos P. Serum creatinine kinase activity and sensing characteristics after intraoperative arrhythmia induction using implantable defibrillator rate sensing leads. PACE 1992; 15:9–13.
14. Sweeney MB, Pless BD, Senelly KM. External support equipment for implantable defibrillators. J Electrophysiol 1987; 1:140–143.
15. Haluska EA, Calfee RV. A packaged solution to the problems of testing arrhythmia control devices at implant. PACE 1991; 14:346–351.
16. Vlay SC. Defibrillation threshold testing: necessary but evil? Am Heart J 1989; 117:499–504.
17. Gascho JA, Crampton RS, Cherwek ML, Sipes JN, Hunter FB, O'Brien WM. Determinants of ventricular defibrillation in adults. Circulation 1979; 60:231–240.
18. Babbs CF, Whistler SJ, Yim GKW, Tacker WA, Geddes LA. Dependence of defibrillation threshold upon extracellular/intracellular K^+ concentrations. J Electrocardiol 1980; 13:73–78.
19. Murakawa Y, Gliner BE, Thakor NV. Success rate versus defibrillation energy: temporal profile and the most efficient defibrillation threshold. Am Heart J 1989; 118:451–457.
20. Echt DS, Barbey JT, Black JN. Influence of ventricular fibrillation duration on defibrillation energy in dogs using bidirectional pulse discharges. PACE 1988; 11:1315–1323.
21. Bardy GH, Ivey TD, Allen M, Johnson G. A prospective, randomized evaluation of effect of ventricular fibrillation duration on defibrillation threshold in humans. J Am Coll Cardiol 1989; 13:1362–1366.
22. Winkle RA, Mead RH, Ruder MA, Smith NA, Buch WS, Gaudiani VA. Effect of duration of ventricular fibrillation on defibrillation efficacy in humans. Circulation 1990; 81:1477–1481.
23. Frame R, Brodman R, Furman S, Kim S-G, Roth J, Ferrick K, Hollinger I, Gross J, Fisher JD. Clinical evaluation of the safety of repetitive intraoperative defibrillation threshold testing. PACE 1992; 15(6):870–877.
24. Singer I, Lang D. Defibrillation threshold: clinical utility and therapeutic implications. PACE 1992; 15(6):932–949.
25. Epstein AE, Ellenbogen KA, Kirk KA, Kay GN, Dailey SM, Plumb V. Clinical characteristics and outcome of patients with high defibrillation thresholds: a multi-center study. Circulation 1992; 86:1206–1216.
26. Pinski SL, Vanerio G, Castle LW, Morant VA, Simmons TW, Trohman RG, Wilkoff BL, Maloney JD. Patients with a high defibrillation threshold: clinical characteristics, management and outcome. Am Heart J 1991; 122:89–95.
27. Bardy GH, Ivey TD, Allen MD, Johnson G, Greene HL. Evaluation of electrode polarity on defibrillation efficacy. Am J Cardiol 1989; 63:433–437.
28. O'Neill PG, Boahene KA, Lawrie GM, Harvill LF, Pacifico A. The automatic implantable cardioverter-defibrillator: effect of patch polarity on defibrillation threshold. J Am Coll Cardiol 1991; 17:707–711.
29. Chapman PD, Sagar KB, Wetherbee JN, Troup PJ. Relationship of left ventricular mass to defibrillation threshold for the implantable defibrillator: a combined clinical and animal study. Am Heart J 1987; 114:274–278.
30. Troup PJ, Chapman PD, Olinger GN, Kleinman LH. The implanted defibrillator: relation of defibrillating lead configuration and clinical variables to defibrillation threshold. J Am Coll Cardiol 1985; 6:1314–1321.

31. Ideker RE, Wolf PD, Alferness C, Krassowska W, Smith WM. Current concepts for selecting the location, size and shape of defibrillation electrodes. PACE 1991; 14:227–240.
32. Lemmer JH Jr, Faber LA, Mariano DJ, Drews TA, Kienzle MG. Pericardial influence on internal defibrillation energy requirements. J Thorac Cardiovasc Surg 1991; 101:839–842.
33. Jeevanandam V, Bielefeld MR, Auteri JS, Sanchez JA, Schkel FA, Michler RE, Smith CR, Livelli F, Bigger JT, Rose EA, Spotnitz HM. The implantable defibrillator: an electronic bridge to cardiac transplantation. Circulation 1992; 86(Suppl II):II-276–II-279.
34. Bardy GH, Ivey TD, Allen MD, Johnson G, Mehera R, Greene HL. A prospective randomized evaluation of biphasic versus monophasic waveform pulses on defibrillation efficacy in humans. J Am Coll Cardiol 1989; 14:728–733.
35. Bardy GH, Steward RB, Ivey TD, Graham EL, Adhar GC, Greene HL. Intraoperative comparison of sequential-pulse and single-pulse defibrillation in candidates for automatic implantable defibrillators. Am J Cardiol 1987; 60:618–624.
36. Bardy GH, Ivey TD, Allen MD, Johnson G, Greene HL. Prospective comparison of sequential pulse and single pulse defibrillation with use of two different clinically available systems. J Am Coll Cardiol 1989; 14:165–171.
37. Fain ES, Sweeney MB, Franz MR. Sequential pulse internal defibrillation: is there an advantage to "switched" current pathways? Am Heart J 1989; 118:717–724.
38. Bardy GH, Troutman C, Johnson G, et al. Electrode system influence on biphasic waveform defibrillation efficacy in humans. Circulation 1991; 84:665–671.
39. Klein GJ, Jones DL, Sharma AD, Kallok MJ, Guiraudon GM. Influence of cardiopulmonary bypass on internal cardiac defibrillation. Am J Cardiol 1986; 57:1194–1195.
40. Blakeman BM, Pifarre R, Scanlon PJ, Wilber DJ. Coronary revascularization and implantation of the automatic cardioverter/defibrillator: reliability of immediate intraoperative testing. PACE 1989; 12:86–91.
41. Wang M, Dorian P. Defibrillation energy requirements differ between anesthetic agents. J Electrophysiol 1989; 3:86–94.
42. Natale A, Jones DL, Kim Y-H, Klein AJ. Effects of lidocaine on defibrillation threshold in the pig: evidence of anesthesia related increase. PACE 1991; 14:1239–1344.
43. Zadian JR, Curling PE, Craver JM. Effect of enflurane, isoflurane and halothane on pacing stimulation thresholds in man. PACE 1985; 8:32–34.
44. Hunt GB, Ross DL. Comparison of effects of three anesthetic agents on induction of ventricular tachycardia in a canine model of myocardial infarction. Circulation 1988; 78:221–226.
45. Dorian P, Fain ES, Davy J-M, Winkle RA. Effect of quinidine and bretylium on defibrillation energy requirements. Am Heart J 1986; 112:19–25.
46. Dorian P, Fain ES, Davy J-M, Winkle RA. Lidocaine causes a reversible concentration-dependent increase in defibrillation energy requirements. J Am Coll Cardiol 1986; 8:327–332.
47. Marinchak RA, Friehling TD, Kline RA, Stohler J, Kowey PR. Effect of antiarrhythmic drugs on defibrillation threshold: case report of an adverse effect of mexiletine and review of the literature. PACE 1988; 11:7–12.
48. Echt DS, Black JN, Barbey JT, Coxe DR, Cato E. Evaluation of antiarrhythmic drugs on defibrillation energy requirements in dogs. Sodium channel block and action potential prolongation. Circulation 1989; 79:1106–1117.
49. Hernandez R, Mann DE, Breckinridge S, Williams GR, Reiter MJ. Effects of flecainide on defibrillation thresholds in the anesthetized dog. J Am Coll Cardiol 1989; 14:777–781.
50. Fain ES, Dorian P, Davy J-M, Kates RE, Winkle RA. Effects of encainide and its metabolites on energy requirements for defibrillation. Circulation 1986; 73:1334–1341.
51. Fogoros RN. Amiodarone-induced refractoriness to cardioversion. Ann Intern Med 1984; 100:699–700.
52. Fain ES, Lee JT, Winkle RA. Effects of acute intravenous and chronic oral amiodarone on defibrillation energy requirements. Am Heart J 1987; 114:8–17.

53. Haberman RJ, Veltri EP, Mower MM. The effect of amiodarone on defibrillation threshold. J Electrophysiol 1988; 2:415–423.
54. Huang SKS, Tan de Guzman WL, Chenarides JG, et al. Effects of long-term amiodarone therapy on defibrillation threshold and the rate of shocks of the implantable cardioverter-defibrillator. Am Heart J 1991; 122:720–727.
55. Echt DS, Cato EL, Coxe DR. Ph-dependent effects of lidocaine on defibrillation energy requirements in dogs. Circulation 1989; 80:1003–1009.
56. Mariano J, Faber LA, Lemmer JH, Kienzle MG. Influence of myocardial temperature on internal defibrillation shock efficacy (abstract). PACE 1990; 13:537.
57. Ouyang P, Brinker JA, Bulkley BH, Judgutt BI, Varqese PJ. Ischemic ventricular fibrillation: the importance of being spontaneous. Am J Cardiol 1981; 48:455–459.
58. Grubb BP, Mancini M, Temsey-Armos P, Hahn M, Elliott L. Resolution of high initial epicardial patch defibrillation thresholds following chronic implantation. PACE 1991; 14:149–151.
59. Fain ES, Billingham M, Winkle RA. Internal cardiac defibrillation: histopathology and temporal stability of defibrillation energy requirements. J Am Coll Cardiol 1987; 9:631–638.
60. Guarnieri T, Levine JH, Veltri EP, et al. Success of chronic defibrillation and the role of antiarrhythmic drugs with the automatic implantable cardioverter-defibrillator. Am J Cardiol 1987; 60:1061–1064.
61. Marchlinski FE, Flores B, Miller JM, Gottlieb CD, Hargrove WC III. Relations of intraoperative defibrillation threshold to successful postoperative defibrillation with an automatic implantable cardioverter defibrillator. Am J Cardiol 1988; 62:393–398.
62. Bardy GH, Ivey TD, Stewart R, Graham E, Greene HL. Failure of the automatic implantable defibrillator to detect ventricular fibrillation. Am J Cardiol 1986; 58:1107–1108.
63. Glicksman FL, Zaman L, Huikuri HV, Castellanos A, Myerburg RJ. Reversible failure to sense ventricular tachycardia early after surgical implantation of the automatic implantable cardioverter-defibrillator. Am J Cardiol 1988; 62:833–834.
64. Vlay SC, Moser SA, Seifert F. Sensing aberration by the automatic implantable cardioverter defibrillator during intraoperative testing. PACE 1988; 11:331–335.
65. Ballas SL, Rashidi R, McAlister H, Corbelli R, McCowan R, Wilkoff BL, Castle LW, Morant VA, Simmons TW, Maloney JD. The use of beep-o-grams in the assessment of automatic implantable cardioverter defibrillator sensing function. PACE 1989; 12:1737–1745.
66. Sperry RE, Ellenbogen KA, Wood MA, Stambler BS, DiMarco JP, Haines DE. Failure of a second and third generation implantable cardioverter defibrillator to sense ventricular tachycardia: implications for fixed gain sensing devices. PACE 1992; 15:749–755.
67. Leitch JW, Yee R, Klein GJ, Jones DL, Murdock CJ. Correlation between the ventricular electrogram amplitude in sinus rhythm and in ventricular fibrillation. PACE 1990; 13:1105–1109.
68. Ellenbogen KA, Wood MA, Stambler BS, Welch WJ, Damiano RJ. Measurement of ventricular electrogram amplitude during intraoperative induction of ventricular tachyarrhythmias. Am J Cardiol 1992; 70:1017–1022.
69. Wilber DJ, Poczobutl-Johanos M. Time-dependent sensing alterations in implantable defibrillators: lessons from the Telectronics Guardian 4202/4203. (abstract). PACE 1991; 14:(Pt II):624.
70. Krol R, Saksena S, Tullo N, Karanam R, Gielchinsky I, Saxena A, Holwitt K, Lipsius M. Clinical experience with bipolar epicardial sensing for a combined implantable pacemaker-defibrillator. (abstract). PACE 1990; 14:536.
71. Krol R, Saksena S, Tullo N, Singh S, Saxena A, Karanam R, Gielchinsky I, Burkhardy E, Gordon M, Hibbard D. Optimal pacing and sensing lead systems for implantable hybrid pacemaker cardioverter-defibrillators (abstract). J Am Coll Cardiol 1991; 15(2 Suppl A):55A.
72. Jordaens L. Assessment of the defibrillation threshold and appropriate sensing during cardioverter defibrillator implantation. PACE 1992; 15(4 Pt 3):636–641.
73. Jung W, Manz M, Moosdorf R, Lüderitz B. Failure of an implantable cardioverter-defibrillator to redetect ventricular fibrillation in patients with a nonthoracotomy lead system. Circulation 1992; 86:1217–1222.

74. Bardy GH. Ensuring automatic detection of ventricular fibrillation. Circulation 1992; 86:1634–1635.
75. Williams WG, Hesslein PS, Kormos R. Exit block in children with pacemakers. Clin Prog Electrophysiol Pacing 1986; 4:478–479.
76. Grubb BP, Mancini M. A technique for intraoperative arrhythmia induction during automatic implantable defibrillator placement. PACE 1990; 13:958–960.
77. Smith PN, Schumitsch PA, Seebandt ML, Bores CJ, Weiler ET, Ray JF III, Myers WO, Douglas-Jones JWE, Vidaillet HJ. Usefulness of placement of intraoperative epicardial wires during automatic implantable cardioverter-defibrillator insertion to preclude the need for transvenous catheters at the predischarge electrophysiology study. Am J Cardiol 1991; 68:679–681.

19

Anesthesia for Surgical Placement of Automatic Internal Cardioverter-Defibrillators

George R. Gordon, William S. Panza, and Michael R. England

*Tufts University School of Medicine and
New England Medical Center
Boston, Massachusetts*

I. INTRODUCTION

The therapeutic choices available to the cardiologist in the treatment of a patient with a history of malignant ventricular arrhythmia have increased enormously in recent years. Whereas pharmacological therapy was common and the only option in the past, these patients now frequently come to surgical intervention for therapy. As has been described in other chapters, the procedures include surgical excision of aneurysmal or scarred myocardial regions with electrophysiological mapping, and the intraoperative placement of ICD patches and/or devices. The former requires full cardiopulmonary bypass, while the latter needs a left lateral thoracotomy, or subxyphoid incision.

As with any new technique that is developing in medicine, there is an ongoing learning process regarding the optimal care of these patients. In prior times, these people would rarely surface in the operating room except for surgical correction of a life-threatening noncardiac condition. This was due to the fact that many regarded their underlying arrhythmia history as a contraindication to a successful anesthetic outcome. Fortunately, with improved resources available to evaluate this group of patients more fully, along with a wider range of anesthetic and monitoring choices, it is now felt that these people may safely undergo general anesthesia [1].

The decision to bring a patient to the operating room for placement of an ICD system is one made only after comprehensive evaluation of the patient's cardiovascular and general medical status. Frequently these patients have depressed cardiac output from multiple infarctions and associated impairment of renal and hepatic function [2]. The incidence of underlying pulmonary disease is high in this patient population. It is for these reasons that the management of ICD patients is an anesthetic challenge. This chapter will give an overview of the anesthesia issues relevant to the preoperative evaluation, intraoperative management, and postoperative care of patients undergoing placement of the ICD (see Table 1A and 1B).

Table 1A Preoperative Anesthetic Concerns

History and physical examination
Cardiovascular
   Myocardial infarction
   Congestive heart failure
   Arrhythmia
Pulmonary function
Other organ system dysfunction
Medications

Table 1B Preanesthetic Preparation

NPO
Premedication
Monitoring
   EKG
   Arterial line
   Central venous line vs. pulmonary artery catheter
   Ventilation
Intravenous access
Regional anesthesia
   Epidural vs. spinal

II. PREOPERATIVE EVALUATION

It is imperative that patients scheduled for ICD placement have a thorough preoperative cardiovascular and general medical evaluation. A complete understanding of the nature of the patients's underlying rhythm disturbance, including the spontaneous arrhythmia, the results of electrophysiological testing, and response to medications are essential. Abnormalities of renal, hepatic, and neurological function are common after resuscitation from out-of-the hospital arrest and need thorough preoperative evaluation [1].

One of the greatest risks these patients face is the possibility of a perioperative cardiac event such as a myocardial infarction, pulmonary edema, or atrial or ventricular arrhythmia. Frequently, the patient who has underlying coronary artery disease has had a recent myocardial infarction or an episode of congestive heart failure. Detailed review of the cardiac status of the patient, including review of hemodynamic data and the results of coronary arteriography, is critical. Preoperative adjustment of medications for heart failure, ischemia, hypertension, or arrhythmias can frequently result in improved cardiac status and may lower surgical risk. Diuretics and digitalis are generally held the morning of surgery to avoid hypovolemia, hypokalemia, and arrhythmias from digitalis toxicity (except for those individuals who have atrial fibrillation who would benefit from a slower ventricular rate).

In our institution, most of the ICD implants are done in patients without the need for concomitant cardiac surgery and have been placed via left lateral thoracotomy. This incision postoperatively is painful and intraoperatively requires the deflation of the left lung for improved surgical exposure. This is facilitated by using either a standard double-lumen endotracheal tube or an endobronchial blocker. (The actual technique will be described later in the chapter.) These considerations must be part of the preoperative evaluation; focusing on the status of the pulmonary system will frequently reveal abnormalities. It is our goal to have the patient's respiratory status optimized prior to surgery. Otherwise, the patient may experience hypoxia, hypercarbia, or bronchospasm during surgery. An increase in endogenous catecholamines caused by any of these states could alter intraoperative defibrillation thresholds. After completion of surgery, a patient with poor pulmonary function may develop respiratory failure, requiring prolonged ventilatory support and increased risk for postoperative infection in the face of a freshly implanted foreign body (ICD).

In order to plausibly improve postoperative respiratory function and to make the patient more comfortable, we offer analgesia in the form of neuraxial narcotics and/or ''patient-controlled analgesia'' using intravenous morphine. It is important to inquire about any previous back condition which may preclude, or make it difficult to place, a spinal or epidural needle with or without a catheter. If the patient is anticoagulated with heparin, this should be stopped at least 4 h prior to surgery and an activated clotting time or partial thromboplastin time performed to verify that the effects of heparin have dissipated. Not only will this minimize the risk of an epidural hematoma, it will also minimize intraoperative blood loss.

III. PREPARATION FOR ANESTHESIA

Patients are routinely kept fasting after midnight and frequently are given a dose of an H2 blocker (to minimize the secretion of gastric acid and raise the pH) at bedtime. An appropriate premedication is selected based on their preoperative ejection fraction. It is our experience that a light premedication given sufficiently in advance of surgery is helpful in diminishing anxiety. We give either intramuscular morphine, 0.1mg/kg, with scopolamine, 0.3 mg, or an oral benzodiazepine 1–2 h preoperatively. We do not use a heavy dose of narcotics preoperatively, because this may complicate postoperative ventilation. Patients should also be given an appropriate antibiotic preoperatively as ordered by the surgical team.

Patients are transported to the operating room with the same level of monitoring that they had on the floor. In the preoperative area, intravenous midazolam is frequently used to minimize recall and allay anxiety during line insertion. All patients have an intraarterial catheter placed in the right radial artery to help monitor blood pressure and to follow oxygenation and ventilation intraoperatively. We use lidocaine subcutaneously to decrease the discomfort with line placement; however, large doses should be avoided so as not to attain elevated blood levels and potentially change defibrillation thresholds. It is our practice to have central venous access through an internal jugular vein. This is helpful for vasoactive drug administration [3,4]. The use of a pulmonary artery catheter is reserved for patients who may be at increased risk for developing postoperative cardiac complications. Those who have just recovered from congestive heart failure (and who are taking large doses of diuretics), or who have very depressed ventricular function (ejection fracture 15% or less), may benefit from the use of a pulmonary artery catheter. Generally, their utility is in improving postoperative management rather than intraoperative care.

After the introduction of monitoring catheters, intrathecal or epidural narcotics (with or without bupivacaine) are administered. We have found that it is more efficient to give the patient 10–12 µg/kg of [5] intrathecal (preservation free) morphine in the lumbar region just prior to induction, rather than take the time to place a lumbar or thoracic epidural catheter. These are well-recognized techniques for providing postoperative analgesia, but they require special skills and are more time consuming. It is known that the onset time for spinal morphine may be up to 2 h, therefore, placement prior to induction is optimal.

IV. ANESTHETIC TECHNIQUE

Many factors are considered when arriving at the choice of anesthetic technique, including effects of anesthetics on defibrillation thresholds, hemodynamic side effects, duration of effect, and effects on other organ systems. Prudent choice of anesthetics leads to a smooth intraoperative and postoperative course and a hemodynamically stable patient.

Information on the effects of anesthetics on defibrillation thresholds and inducibility of ventricular tachycardia is sparse. Most of the currently available literature involves animal models, suggesting there is no significant effect [6]. In a small series of human patients, enflurane was found to have no influence on inducibility of ventricular tachycardia [6]. In a ca-

Table 2 Intraoperative Anesthetic Management

Induction	
Intubation	Placement of endotracheal tube
Positioning	(Lateral thoracotomy) Arms padded and not hyperextended
One lung ventilation	Double lumen endotracheal tube
	Univent (TM) tube
	Single lumen endotracheal tube with bronchial blocker
Extubation	(Table 7)
Transport to postoperative ICU	Airway management
	Postoperative analgesia
	Monitoring

nine model of myocardial infarction, both halothane and pentobarbital were shown to decrease significantly the number of dogs in which ventricular tachycardia could be induced. Fentanyl/droperidol/nitrous oxide anesthesia had minimal effects in this same canine model [7,8]. Information on other commonly used anesthetics is currently unavailable. Therefore the choice of anesthetics is made based on the patient's cardiorespiratory status and other coexisting disease states. One concern may be the use of local anesthetics (i.e., lidocaine), used in the epidural space as part of the anesthetic technique. When 2% lidocaine is used with isoflurane, systemic lidocaine levels may be in the therapeutic range, and could have an effect on defibrillation thresholds [9].

Anesthetics can be divided into agents used for induction and agents used for maintaining anesthesia (Table 2). Some drugs may be suitable for both.

A. Induction Agents

Drugs used for induction include ketamine, thiopental, methohexital, propofol, etomidate, narcotics, and benzodiazepines.

Thiopental and methohexital are barbiturate hypnotic drugs used for induction of anesthesia (Table 3). Their effects are terminated by redistribution, and therefore multiple doses may result in a prolonged effect, making them unsuitable for maintenance of anesthesia. Hemodynamically they are potent myocardial depressants and will lower blood pressure, both by depressing cardiac performance and by lowering systemic vascular resistance. Because of this, they may not be suitable agents for use in patients with significantly compromised ventricular function.

Ketamine is a phencyclidine derivative that is used for induction and occasionally for maintenance of anesthesia. It causes sympathetic stimulation with increases in systemic and pulmonary artery pressures, heart rate, and cardiac output.

Etomidate is an imidazole derivative used primarily as an induction agent. Adrenal suppression with prolonged infusions has limited its use as an agent for maintaining anesthesia. It is a hypnotic drug similar to the barbiturates, but the hemodynamic effects differ greatly. A

Table 3 Induction Agents

Barbiturates	Benzodiazepines	Other agents
Thiopental	Midazolam	Ketamine
Thiamylal	Diazepam	Etomidate
Methohexital	Lorazepam	Propofol

bolus of etomidate will cause hypnosis and rarely causes a decrease in blood pressure or a depression of ventricular function. Thus, it is an ideal agent for patients with marked ventricular impairment. It has been advocated as an excellent induction agent for patients undergoing cardiac transplantation.

Propofol, a phenol derivative, is a relatively new agent used for both induction and maintenance of anesthesia. It is a hypnotic drug that is short acting due to rapid metabolism, making it significantly different from the barbiturates. Patients emerge from propofol anesthesia significantly more awake and alert when compared to almost any other anesthetic. Hemodynamically, it causes a decrease in blood pressure similar to that of the barbiturates, but by a different mechanism. One direct comparison of propofol with methohexital showed that with similar decreases in blood pressure and cardiac output, patients receiving propofol showed decreases in filling pressures with maintenance of ejection fraction, while patients given methohexital showed increased filling pressures with a decreased ejection fraction (signifying myocardial depression) [10].

Most anesthetic techniques will include a narcotic as part of the regimen since, except for ketamine, none of the aforementioned drugs has significant analgesic properties. The commonly used narcotics include morphine and the synthetic narcotics fentanyl, sufentanil, and alfentanil (Table 4). Morphine can cause histamine release and vasodilation, especially in high doses. The synthetic narcotics do not cause any significant histamine release and do not cause any myocardial depression. They can cause a decrease in heart rate secondary to their central vagomimetic properties. They differ chiefly in potency and duration of effect. When used in combination with intrathecal or epidural narcotics, we prefer alfentanil, since it has the shortest duration. High-dose narcotic techniques provide exceptional cardiovascular stability and are commonly used for patients undergoing coronary revascularization along with placement of an implantable defibrillator, but use of this technique requires prolonged ventilatory support postoperatively, limiting its use in patients having just ICD placement.

Benzodiazepines are usually used as an adjunct to anesthesia, although they can be used for induction and maintenance of anesthesia. They are usually given to provide sedation for invasive procedures prior to anesthetic induction and to ensure amnesia during surgery. Midazolam has gained great popularity in anesthesia because of its rapid onset, relatively short duration, and water solubility, allowing intramuscular injections and pain-free intravenous administration. The benzodiazepines cause minimal myocardial depression but can cause significant vasodilation, especially when given with narcotics.

B. Maintenance Agents

Anesthesia is commonly maintained with inhalation anesthetics, including nitrous oxide, isoflurane, enflurane, halothane, and recently, desflurane. Nitrous oxide may be used safely but is known to increase systemic vascular resistance and pulmonary vascular resistance (especially if elevated preoperatively). Its potency is quite low, and it must be discontinued during one-lung anesthesia in order to deliver 100% oxygen. The high potency of the halogenated anes-

Table 4 Intraoperative Narcotics

Morphine
Fentanyl
Sufentanil
Alfentanil

Table 5 Commonly Used Neuromuscular Blocking Agents

Blocking agents	Reversal agents
Pancuronium	Neostigmine
Vecuronium	Edrophonium
Pipercuronium	
Atracurium	
Doxacurium	
Succinylcholine	

thetics allows their use when a high FIO_2 is needed. Halothane is used commonly in pediatric anesthesia, but less commonly in adults secondary to concerns of rare but serious liver toxicity; hemodynamically, it causes a decrease in systemic blood pressure, mostly by myocardial depression. Enflurane, another inhalation agent, is free of potential liver toxicity, but is a more potent myocardial depressant and vasodilator than halothane. Isoflurane is the most commonly used inhalation anesthetic. It has minimal negative inotropic effects (in clinically used doses), is a potent vasodilator, and permits a quicker emergence than enflurane. In the past there has been some concern about isoflurane causing "coronary steal" as a result of its vasodilating properties. Several large studies comparing anesthetic techniques for cardiac surgery and looking at patient outcomes have demonstrated that isoflurane is a safe anesthetic in this population and that the incidence of myocardial ischemia does not appear to be increased. Desflurane, the newest potent inhalation agent, has the advantage of rapid onset and elimination compared to the other potent inhalation agents, but its clinical utility still needs to be determined.

Muscle relaxants are commonly used to facilitate intubation, mechanical ventilation, and surgical exposure (Table 5). The depolarizing relaxant succinylcholine is not usually used because of its extremely short duration of action. The intermediate-duration, nondepolarizing types of relaxants are usually used. The choice of relaxant is usually determined by its metabolism and its hemodynamic side effects. Several nondepolarizing relaxants with virtually no hemodynamic effects are available and include vecuronium, pipecuronium, and doxacurium. Vecuronium has a somewhat shorter duration than the latter two. Pancuronium is very commonly used and has a duration of action of about 1 h. It tends to have vagolytic properties and increases heart rate, although this is often attenuated by the vagomimetic effect of concomitantly administered narcotics.

At the end of the procedure, the effects of residual neuromuscular blockade are reversed with a combination of anticholinesterases and vagolytic agents. The anticholinesterase drugs inhibit the enzyme cholinesterase and allow an increase in acetylcholine at the neuromuscular junction to competitively overcome the effects of the nondepolarizing agents. At the same time, a vagolytic agent such as atropine or glycopyrrolate is administered to block the muscarinic side effects of anticholinesterases such as bradycardia and salivation. Neostigmine and edrophonium are the commonly used anticholinesterases.

Monitoring of neuromuscular blockade is accomplished with use of nerve stimulation. The most commonly used nerve is the ulnar nerve in the forearm. The usual pattern of stimulation is four equally spaced stimuli over a period of 2 s, referred to as train-of-four stimulation. Nondepolarizing muscle relaxants will show a decreasing response to each stimulus with increasing neuromuscular blockade. Patients are usually kept with only one of four twitches present during surgery to ensure adequate muscle relaxation. This level of relaxation also ensures the ability to reverse effects of relaxants at the end of surgery as described above.

V. PATIENTS HAVING ICD AND CARDIAC SURGERY

Patients falling into this category have their anesthetic technique and hemodynamic monitoring determined primarily by the type and extent of the cardiac surgery. Commonly this includes a high-dose narcotic anesthetic supplemented by a benzodiazepine and a muscle relaxant. Some period of postoperative ventilatory support is usually necessary.

VI. PATIENTS FOR REVISION OR EXPLANATION OF ICD

The anesthetic considerations for these patients are identical to those having ICD placement, including monitoring and postoperative analgesia.

VII. PATIENTS FOR TRANSVENOUS PLACEMENT OF ICD

The anesthetic considerations for patients undergoing transvenous placement of an ICD differ from those undergoing thoracotomy. Although they still require general anesthesia, invasive monitoring is usually limited to measurement of intraarterial blood pressure. Central venous access is rarely required. One lung ventilation is not necessary so a standard endotracheal tube is adequate. Postoperative pain is easily managed with low doses of systemic narcotics. The more complex methods of postoperative analgesia available for patients undergoing thoracotomy are generally not indicated.

VIII. ONE-LUNG ANESTHESIA

In order to provide adequate exposure to the heart through a left lateral thoracotomy, it is necessary to isolate the left lung (i.e., ventilate the right lung only). There are several ways to accomplish this: most commonly is with a double-lumen endotracheal tube. These are available in left-sided and right-sided versions. The tube has two lumens, one that exits in a mainstem bronchus and one that exits in the trachea, each with its own balloon. Either lung may be isolated utilizing either a right- or left-sided tube. Left-sided endotracheal tubes are considered to be safer and easier to place properly because of the close proximity takeoff of the right upper lobe takeoff to the carina. If a right-sided tube is used, an opening in the tube just proximal to the endobronchial lumen must be aligned with the right upper lobe takeoff. This is not an issue with left-sided tubes, as the left upper lobe orifice is far enough away from the carina that it is generally distal to the endobronchial lumen.

Another way to provide one-lung anesthesia is with the use of bronchial blockers. A small-diameter, balloon-tipped catheter can be placed in the trachea alongside a standard endotracheal tube and placed in either mainstream bronchus to isolate the lung. There is a commercially available tube with a bronchial blocker attached to it (Univent).

The Univent tube has the advantage of having a small lumen in the blocker. Use of this tube means that if postoperative ventilation is necessary, it does not have to be changed (as when a double-lumen endotracheal tube is used for surgery) at the end of the procedure. Correct placement of a Univent tube or separate bronchial blocker requires the use of fiberoptic bronchoscopy. It is possible to place a double-lumen tube without the aid of fiberoptic bronchoscopy by checking auscultation alone; however, we feel that is is far superior management to use a bronchoscope to visualize the correct placement of the tube.

The most common problem seen with one-lung ventilation is arterial hypoxemia. Patients are always placed on 100% oxygen when only one lung is being ventilated. If hypoxemia occurs, one first confirms that placement of the tube is correct. Fiberoptic bronchoscopy is in-

Table 6 Intraoperative Considerations

Hypoxemia
Hypotension
Tachycardia
Ischemia
Defibrillation

valuable in accomplishing this task. If tube position is correct, other interventions must be made to reverse hypoxemia. Delivering continuous positive airway pressure to the lung that is not being ventilated is usually the most successful treatment. Adding positive end expiratory pressure to the lung being ventilated may improve, have no effect on, or even decrease arterial PO_2. Recently, the ability to monitor arterial blood gases (Ph, PO_2, PCO_2) continuously has become available (Puritan Bennet Fox) and may prove to be helpful in monitoring for hypoxia during one-lung ventilation.

IX. INTRAOPERATIVE PROBLEMS

In addition to performing the technical aspects of airway management, the anesthesiologist must be familiar with the sequence of the surgical procedure. This allows one to anticipate and to treat common intraoperative events quickly and appropriately. Patients undergoing ICD surgery represent a challenge for the anesthesiologist, since they frequently have impaired ventricular function and/or may have significant coronary artery disease [1,11] as well as other organ dysfunctions (i.e., lung disease). Those who have coronary artery disease not amendable to surgical revascularization may have end-stage ischemic cardiomyopathy with increased end diastolic volumes and compensatory tachycardia [12]. Successful anesthetic management depends on many factors. Preoperative assessment and anesthetic technique have already been discussed; next we review intraoperative events that may be encountered during anesthesia and surgery for ICD placement. Common intraoperative problems that may occur include hypoxemia, hypotension, ischemia, hypertension, and tachycardia. Rarely, difficult defibrillation or congestive heart failure may occur (Table 6).

A. Hypoxemia

Hypoxemia due to endotracheal tube problems has already been discussed above. Hypoxemia can be quickly recognized by decreasing pulse oximetry saturations. After checking vital signs to rule out hypotension, diagnosis and treatment of hypoxemia must be swift. Arterial blood gas analysis quickly confirms the diagnosis. Auscultation of the lungs bilaterally on 100% oxygen is a first step to help rule out bronchospasm, pulmonary edema, and endotracheal tube malposition. Bronchoscopy is used to confirm proper endotracheal tube position and to suction secretions. A soft-suction catheter should be passed down the endotracheal tube as necessary. Bronchospasm may be treated in a number of ways [13–17]. Changing the depth of anesthesia with additional inhalation agent will decrease airway reactivity and break bronchospasm [16]. One must be mindful that the agents may lower blood pressure [18] (by lowering systemic vascular resistance of myocardial depression). Beta-2 agonists such as albuterol or metaproterenol may be delivered via metered-dose inhaler down the endotracheal tube. Nebulized vagolytic drugs include atropine or glycopyrrolate, or an inhaler of ipratropium bromide may also be delivered through the endotracheal tube. Though available, intravenous infusions of aminophylline, isoproterenol, or epinephrine are rarely required to treat bronchospasm; if they are used, they may precipitate arrhythmias.

The best strategy for congestive heart failure and pulmonary edema is prevention. Those patients who have a history of and are at risk for developing congestive heart failure should be identified during the preoperative assessment. Intraoperative fluid status may be monitored by central venous pressure. Since there are minimal volume shifts (blood loss) during this surgery, urinary drainage from the foley catheter and central venous pressure catheter are sufficient for monitoring volume status in most patients. Care is taken not to give excessive fluids. The anesthesiologist should also consider other causes of congestive heart failure, including ischemia, hypertension, and tachycardia. Rapid treatment includes diuretics, preload/afterload reduction, and narcotics.

B. Hypotension

In an effort to preserve normal organ function, the anesthesiologist should maintain a normal range of perfusion pressures. Moderate degrees of hypotension are not uncommon during anesthesia. A variety of factors predispose these patients to the development of hypotension during anesthesia. These factors may be related to both the intrinsic properties of the anesthetic and to the patient's myocardial disease. Anesthetic agents may act directly to decrease myocardial contractility and reduce vascular sympathetic tone [18,19]. The onset of hypnosis may lead to a loss of sympathetic tone by depriving the patient of sensory stimuli from the surroundings. The effect of decreased sympathetic tone is potentiated by the patient's underlying myocardial disease. Many of these patients have dysfunctional myocardium causing reduced ejection fraction, or congestive heart failure [11]. Treatment of congestive heart failure by fluid restriction and chronic diuresis may lead to intravascular volume contraction. This may make these patients particularly susceptible to the effects of vasodilation. Dysfunctional myocardium may require greater sympathetic stimulation to maintain adequate performance due to downregulation of myocardial adrenergic receptors. Hypotension commonly occurs during induction, after intubation, during the surgical preparation, and during testing of the ICD device. Judicious administration of intravenous fluid to restore volume, along with the addition of vasopressors such as phenylephrine to increase peripheral vascular tone, will usually reverse the hypotension without the need for inotropic support.

More significant hypotension occurs during multiple testing of the patches, when ventricular fibrillation or tachycardia is induced. Systemic blood pressure returns shortly after successful defibrillation. This hypotension rarely requires inotropic support. Occasionally, during prolonged ventricular fibrillation, a phenylephrine infusion is used to support mean blood pressure until pulsatile flow is reestablished after cardioversion. The time to recovery of baseline systemic blood pressure may increase with subsequent episodes of fibrillation and defibrillation. Thus, after each test, the question arises as to when the patient has recovered sufficiently to be retested. Some authors advocate the use of oximetric pulmonary artery catheters to continuously monitor mixed venous oxygen saturations during defibrillation threshold testing [20]. With ventricular fibrillation the mixed venous oxygen saturation decreases. Only after defibrillation and the return of normal blood flow does the mixed venous oxygen saturation rise. They recommend that patients should not have ventricular fibrillation induced until the mixed venous oxygen saturation returns to baseline [20]. There has not been any study to demonstrate a benefit in outcome for patients having an ICD placed using this technology. Disadvantages include the additional cost of an oximetric catheter and specialized cardiac output computer; the risks of placing a pulmonary artery catheter; and the risk of dislodging new endocardial leads. As described under the anesthetic technique, we rarely use pulmonary artery catheters for the anesthetic management of these patients.

Another cause of intraoperative hypotension is hypovolemia. The surgical procedure does not cause major fluid shifts, and there is rarely significant blood loss. However, cardiac tamponade and pneumothorax are two rare causes or relative hypovolemia that may occur. An endocardial lead placed preoperatively could perforate the right ventricular wall. Subsequent filling of the pericardial cavity with blood can cause tamponade. Such hypotension will not respond to volume administration or inotropic agents [22,23]. Rather, drainage of the pericardial cavity will improve the patient's hemodynamic status immediately [21–25]. Frequently, these patients have significant concurrent obstructive lung disease, which puts them at risk for the development of pneumothorax. If a tension pneumothorax develops during airway manipulation, it can cause a decrease in venous return and hypotension. This may occur prior to incision if the peak inspiratory pressure suddenly increases, for instance, during stacked ventilator breaths or coughing. After chest closure, a tension pneumothorax can develop if the chest tubes are not functioning properly. Decompression immediately improves the patient's blood pressure [26].

Occasionally, the administration of medications will cause hypotension. Aside from the anesthetic agents which were discussed previously, frequently used vasoactive drugs may cause unintended hypotension. Infusion of nitroglycerin or sodium nitroprusside could vasodilate the patient more than anticipated. Discontinuation of the infusion and awaiting termination of effect is usually sufficient treatment. Administration of beta-blockers, calcium channel blockers, and some antiarrhythmic agents can lead to unwanted myocardial depression or vasodilation. Of particular concern is the antiarrhythmic, amiodarone. It is a benzofuran derivative that depresses the sinus node, and atrial, atrioventricular nodal, and His-Purkinje conduction. Its antiadrenergic properties may cause bradycardia and hypotension (vasodilation) that is relatively resistant to inotropes, catecholamines, or vasopressors [27]. The bradycardia may be treated by pacing, but the hypotension may be difficult to treat. In our clinical experience, hypotension associated with amiodarone has not been a significant problem. Though its mechanism of elimination is unknown, it has a long half-life, so its side effects may persist for weeks after it is discontinued. Use of amiodarone in the 2 to 3 months preceding general anesthesia was felt to represent a risk factor for postoperative pulmonary complications including adult respiratory distress syndrome. Recent analysis of a large surgical series have not supported this belief [28].

C. Ischemia

Since many patients will have coronary artery disease, the possibility of myocardial ischemia must always be considered as a cause of hypotension. Preoperative antianginal regimens are continued right up until surgery. Intraoperative on-line, multiple-lead EKG monitoring with S-T segment analysis is routinely used in order to allow rapid detection of ischemia. Medications for the treatment of ischemia, such as nitroglycerin, beta-blockers, calcium channel blockers, and narcotics, are all immediately available in the operating room. Many of these patients have depressed ventricular function and a compensatory tachycardia to maintain cardiac output, so negative chronotropic/inotropic agents are used with caution.

D. Hypertension and Tachycardia

During anesthesia, these patients may not tolerate hypertension as well as a younger, healthier population. Hypertension increases myocardial systolic wall tension, thereby increasing myocardial oxygen demand and decreasing subendocardial blood flow, precipitating myocardial ischemia. Many of these patients have other associated cerebral vascular disease, and hypertension may cause aneurysmal bleeding or stroke. Hypertension is commonly seen during stressful parts of anesthesia and surgery from endogenous catecholamine release. Examples include endotracheal intubation, skin incision, retractor placement, skin closure, and emergence from anesthesia. During testing of the patches, multiple defibrillations provide an additional release of stress hormones. Though hypertension is commonly seen at this time and may resolve spontaneously, some anesthetists choose to treat it with a nitroglycerine infusion. This serves to lower systemic blood pressure and vasodilate coronary beds in the patient who is at risk for ischemic heart disease.

Many anesthetic techniques are available to attenuate these responses, including the use of inhalation anesthetics, beta blockers, vasodilators, local anesthetics, and narcotics. Inhalation anesthesia can be used to blunt the response to stimuli such as laryngoscopy [29]; however, in this patient population, the myocardial depressant and vasodilating effects of the inhalation anesthetic may not be tolerated. Halothane may not be a wise choice in patients who are already susceptible to ventricular arrhythmias, because it sensitizes the myocardium to catecholamines [30,31]. Lidocaine has been shown to be effective in decreasing the hemodynamic response to laryngoscopy when used topically or intravenously (1.5 mg/kg) 90 s prior to stimulus [32,33]. Unfortunately it interferes with the testing of the ICD patches and is usually avoided.

Infusion of nitroprusside (0.5–2 µg/kg) or nitroglycerine may be used prophylactically or in response to hypertension [34]. Disadvantages include the development of a reflex tachycardia, and the lack of heart-rate control in response to stimulus. Beta-blockers effectively attenuate the hypertensive and tachycardiac responses; however, negative inotropic effects and changes in pulmonary airway resistance can be problematic. Esmolol, a short-acting beta-blocker, is useful in these situations to avoid a prolonged effect. The major disadvantage of any of these agents is the possibility of overshooting the desired effect with resultant hypotension. This may occur most often when one does not appreciate that these patients have slow circulation time and the drug may have a prolonged effect. Although these agents control blood pressure, they may mask an awake, but still paralyzed patient.

Narcotics provide excellent analgesia and in high enough doses may blunt sympathetic responses to stimuli [35–37]. Unfortunately, at high doses (fentanyl 25–100 µg/kg), patients frequently require postoperative ventilation. The choices of narcotics have previously been discussed. When, on occasion, they do not reduce hypertensive responses, other modalities should be used. The best treatment for hypertension may be to use a mixture of drugs while assuring adequate anesthesia, for example, fentanyl 6–8 µg/kg, isoflurane, esmolol, and nitroglycerin. This will allow the drugs to act synergistically while minimizing the side effects of any one drug.

E. Defibrillation

Since these patients may be defibrillated multiple times, one must ensure the ability to defibrillate. The patient's antiarrhythmic drugs may be discontinued or continued preoperatively based on the assessment of the cardiac service. As a matter of policy, two defibrillator units should always be in the operating room. Prior to induction, R-2 self-adhesive defibrillating pads are placed on the patient's chest for external defibrillation. Sterile internal defibrillator paddles are always available on the surgical field for application directly to the heart. Sterile external paddles are also always available in the operating room. In the case of failed defibrillation, despite multiple electric shocks at increasing energy (joules), reestablishment of systemic flow and adequate perfusion pressure are paramount. Prior to incision, this can be done by external chest compression, cardiopulmonary resuscitation, and pressors such as epinephrine. After incision, open cardiac massage and, if necessary, placement on cardiopulmonary bypass, can be used to restore systemic blood flow. There is one report of the need for a patient to be placed on cardiopulmonary bypass because of inability to defibrillate; successful defibrillation was done on bypass with simultaneous shocks by patches and orthogonally placed internal paddles [38].

X. POSTOPERATIVE CONCERNS

The foundation for postoperative care is laid during the preoperative assessment. The most crucial anesthetic concerns postoperatively are patient monitoring, airway management, and pain management, which should be discussed with the patient and surgical team before the operation.

A. Airway Management

Most patients without preexisting lung disease may be safely extubated in the operating room after thoracotomy for ICD placement. Extubation should be performed only when there is an acceptably low risk of reintubation. The primary reasons for ventilatory failure include: (1) poor gas exchange, due either to airway compromise or to pulmonary parenchymal disease, and (2) poor tissue delivery due to cardiac failure. Anything that increases energy requirements will increase oxygen consumption and carbon dioxide production (i.e., shivering), and can stress the patient's cardiopulmonary status. In order to assure a successful extubation, gas exchange and delivery should be optimized. Prior to extubation, several criteria must be satisfied: (1) The patient must be hemodynamically stable; (2) pulmonary function must provide adequate exchange of carbon dioxide and oxygen, as shown by arterial blood gas, end tidal capnography, or pulse oximetry; (3) the patient should be warm (temperature higher than 35.5°C) in order to avoid postoperative shivering, which may increase oxygen consumption up to 400% [39]; (4) the patient should have the residual effects of neuromuscular blocking agents reversed and demonstrate return of strength either by a blockade monitor or by sustaining a head lift for 5 s [40]. This may assure that the patient will have the stamina to sustain respiration and the strength to clear secretions and avoid atelectasis. Also, this may signify return of the pharyngeal muscle tone necessary to prevent obstruction of the larynx by the tongue, the most common form of airway obstruction. The spontaneous respiratory rate should be between 12 and 24; a lower rate may indicate that the patient is narcotized and is at risk for apnea after extubation. Rates greater than 24 may indicate pain or agitation; at these rates, the patient uses more energy for ventilation and may fatigue. Tidal volumes of 7–10 mL/kg and an inspiratory force of at least 25 cm H_2O should be obtained, indicating that the patient has sufficient strength and effort to avoid having to be reintubated [41]. The patient should be comfortable, permitting deep breaths and coughing, which will avoid airway closure. Most important, the patient should be awake enough to follow simple commands and be able to protect his or her airway from aspiration and obstruction once the endotracheal tube is removed. Though no one criterion will guarantee a successful outcome, the more criteria that are satisfied, the higher are the chances that the patient will stay extubated (Table 7).

Early extubation in the operating room has several advantages. First, if the patient requires reintubation, the equipment, drugs, and personnel are immediately available. Second, removal of the endotracheal tube allows return of normal mucociliary function for clearance of secretions and eliminates a conduit for infection. Third, the endotracheal tube is a potent tracheal

Table 7 Criteria for Extubation

Hemodynamic stability	
Respiratory rate	12–20/min
Tidal volume	7–10 mL/kg
Negative Inspiratory Force	>25 cm/H_2O
Temperature	>35.5°C
Reversal of neuromuscular blockade	
Awake/following commands	

irritant, which could cause tachycardia, hypertension, and coughing. These symptoms may be treated with sedatives, however, extubation removes the stimulus, thus avoiding their use. Fourth, the potential need for exchanging the double-lumen tube to a single-lumen endotracheal tube is eliminated, thus avoiding the risk of losing control of the airway and of further airway trauma. Finally, there is significant cost savings in avoiding the use of a ventilator, and a shorter or nonexistent intensive-care unit stay when the patient is extubated in the operating room.

Patients with an unstable hemodynamic profile, significant lung disease, or combined coronary artery bypass grafting-ICD placement may require prolonged ventilatory support after surgery. When this is anticipated, an anesthetic technique is chosen that will provide sedation well into the postoperative period. A high-dose narcotic technique is an option. If a double-lumen endotracheal tube has been used, it is usually exchanged to a single-lumen endotracheal tube at the conclusion of surgery. The major reason for the change is to avoid endobronchial damage. There have been reports of mucosal damage such as rupture and hemoptysis [42–44]. Long-term pressure on respiratory mucosa could lead to the formation of granulation tissue, and airway stenosis. But these are not usually a problem for short-term tube placement. Tube malposition could lead to bronchial obstruction and lobar collapse [45]. Finally, pulmonary toilet and weaning from a ventilator is easier with a larger-lumen, shorter-length, single-lumen endotracheal tube. There are a variety of ways to change endotracheal tubes. The most frequently used method employs direct laryngoscopy. Under direct vision the double-lumen tube is removed, and a single-lumen tube is replaced. Changing the tube blindly over a stylette or over a bronchoscope has also been discussed in other anesthesia texts, and is more difficult [46]. This procedure is contraindicated when there is a risk of losing control of the airway. For instance, if the initial intubation was difficult, or if there is significant airway edema, and alternatively if extubation is expected within 24 h, one would could consider leaving the double-lumen ETT in place with the bronchial cuff deflated. This would allow even ventilation of both lungs while minimizing the risk of bronchial damage. The same extubation criteria are used in the intensive-care unit as previously described.

B. Postoperative Intensive Care and Monitoring

After surgery, ICD patients are transiently more susceptible to supraventricular and ventricular arrhythmias. These rhythms may trigger the device and discharge its battery. Therefore, the ICD is usually turned off for the first 2 to 3 days postoperatively [1]. After placement of an ICD, all patients should be transported to a postanesthetic-care unit (recovery room) or another intensive-care unit without an interruption of monitoring and with supplemental oxygen. Though some institutions keep their patients in a cardiac intensive-care unit until the ICD is activated [1], we have them stay overnight in the recovery room and then transfer them to a monitored telemetry floor when stable, where the unit is activated. It is imperative to have an

Table 8 Methods of Providing Postoperative Analgesia

Systemic narcotics	Neuraxial narcotics	Local anesthetics	Nonsteroidal anti-inflammatory drugs
Intramuscular	Epidural infusion	Field block	Antiprostaglandin effect
Intravenous infusion	Spinal injection	Intercostal blocks	
Patient-controlled analgesia		Intrapleural catheter	
transdermal			

external cardiac defibrillator readily available. This allows for prompt treatment of sustained arrhythmias. External defibrillation may be performed successfully without damaging the ICD [47]. Placement of the external paddles orthogonally to the implanted patches assures that maximal energy is delivered to the myocardium. Some institutions do not remove adhesive external R2 defibrillator pads postoperatively to assure correct placement of pads in case defibrillation is required [11,48].

Postoperative respiratory monitoring includes frequent arterial blood gases and continuous pulse oximetry. This permits the titration of analgesia necessary to encourage good pulmonary toilet.

C. Postoperative Pain Management

The plan for postoperative pain control is developed preoperatively during the initial assessment of the patient. The goal of postoperative analgesia is patient comfort and a reduction of postoperative complications; postoperative pain may cause tachycardia, hypertension, and muscular splinting of the chest wall (Table 8). Such muscular splinting prevents the patient from breathing deeply. This will reduce functional residual capacity, forced expiratory volume in 1 s, vital capacity, and tidal volume [49,50] Decreased respiratory rate and an inadequate cough predisposes one to a retention of secretions and hypercarbia [51,52]. When the functional residual capacity is less than the closing capacity, atelectasis can develop [53]. Persistent blood flow through atelectatic lung tissue results in shunting and hypoxemia [54]. In order to avoid these problems, postoperative pain may be treated with a combination of narcotics, local anesthetics, and nonsteroidal antiinflammatory drugs. The available routes of administration include systemic applications such as, transdermal, transmucosal (oral, nasal, rectal, sublingual), parenteral (subcutaneous, intravenous, intramuscular), and regional applications, such as neuraxial (intrathecal, epidural).

1. Narcotics

All narcotics produce analgesia by interacting with opiate receptors in the central nervous system. There are many types of opiate receptors (mu-1, mu-2, sigma, delta, kappa). Each type has different locations in the nervous system, and produces a different response when stimulated. Each narcotic has differential affinities for the various classes of opiate receptor. Side effects such as nausea, vomiting, respiratory depression, dysphoria, sedation, pruritus, and urinary retention occur when subsets of receptors in different areas of the central nervous system are stimulated. The most worrisome side effect is the risk of respiratory depression (due to a lack of response to increasing levels of PA CO_2). These side effects can be caused by any narcotic, in any route of administration, if a sufficient dose is given. A balance between quality of analgesia and side effects is the aim of effective postoperative analgesia. Narcotics clinically available include morphine, codeine, meperidine, methadone, oxycodone, levorphanol, hydromorphone, oxymorphone, fentanyl, sufentanil, and alfentanil. The choice of agent depends on the agent's duration of action, planned route of administration, and the clinician's experience with the drug.

Parenteral narcotic administration is the most common form of postoperative pain relief, due to its simplicity and relative safety. It is based on the pharmacokinetic premise that patients require a certain therapeutic blood level of a narcotic to be comfortable; when the blood level falls below this threshold, the patient becomes uncomfortable. Unfortunately, the plasma opioid levels required to achieve adequate analgesia vary widely among patients, and there is no reliable way to predict the dose of narcotic that will be required to achieve adequate pain relief in a particular patient [55,56]. One way to combat pain and stay above the therapeutic threshold would be continuous dosing of narcotic to maintain a target blood level of opioid. Unfortunately, infused narcotic accumulates and eventually reaches a toxic blood level, at which side effects (respiratory depression) become a problem. The goal is to keep the blood level of narcotic between the therapeutic and toxic levels. Intermittent dosing of drug results in peaks and valleys of narcotic blood levels and therefore pain relief. Intramuscular narcotic administration provides a simple, effective way to deposit narcotic for tissue uptake. It avoids a sudden peak of narcotic. However, there is a high degree of variability in response to a single dose of narcotic among patients [56,57]. The peak plasma level and time to reach this peak after a single dose can vary widely among patients [56,57]. Problems associated with intramuscular dosing are unpredictable delivery, which may lead to inadequate pain relief or oversedation. Multiple painful injections are required and may be contraindicated in anticoagulated patients. This method of delivery requires nursing to respond to patient request, and there may be a delay between the time patient encounters the pain and receives pain relief. Intravenous dosing leads to quick onset of action and high peak concentration of drug in the plasma. Intravenous infusions of opioids have been tried to avoid swings in blood levels seen with intermittent dosing. However, as the patient gets further from surgery, the pain and the amount of narcotic required for relief decrease exponentially [58]. Thus the drug may accumulate and cause respiratory depression.

"Patient-controlled analgesia" (PCA) is the self-administration of small doses of narcotic intravenously by patients when experiencing pain. This method attempts to decrease the swings in plasma narcotic concentration by allowing administration of small doses of narcotic immediately as needed [59]. A negative-feedback loop exists to prevent overdosage, since the patient will not dose the PCA when not in pain. The pump incorporates a microprocessor that allows one to set dosage limits, time limits, and bolus dosage to prevent overdosage. This method has been shown to be as safe as the traditional intramuscular route of administration. Several studies have demonstrated comparable rise in arterial carbon dioxide levels and the incidence of respiratory depression to be no greater in either group of patients [60,61]. Advantages of the self-administered route are high quality of analgesia, patient satisfaction since the patient has self-control, no painful intramuscular shots, no delay in response time for delivery of medication, and less nursing time required [58,61,62].

A new approach to the delivery of systemic narcotic is the use of transdermal fentanyl (a semi-synthetic, highly lipid, soluble narcotic) via patches applied to the skin. The patch matrix and transdermal membrane control the rate of opiate delivery [63]. After upper abdominal surgery, use of transdermal fentanyl decreases demand for PCA and improves peak expiratory flow rates [64]. The transdermal system maintains a continuous infusion of opiate without the need for painful injections. The disadvantages include overdosage due to drug accumulation, and slower onset (when compared to the PCA route) [65]. This system is not yet used extensively for postoperative analgesia because it has only recently been approved, most clinicians are unfamiliar with its use, and it is expensive. Oral preparations are initially avoided, because most patients do not eat comfortably immediately after surgery. Though oral formulations are easy to administer, erratic uptake, first-pass hepatic clearance, and gastrointestinal upset can complicate their use [66,67].

In an effort to decrease the total dose of opiate given, and therefore the undesirable side effects of narcotics when given systemically, a newer method of delivering narcotics has become popular. The two methods of delivery are subarachnoid and epidural injection. A small dose of narcotic is delivered to the spinal cord dorsal horn, where it relieves pain without affecting cortical opioid receptors [68]. Despite the much smaller doses, intrathecal narcotic provides better pain relief than systemic narcotic [69–71]. The hydrophilic nature of a narcotic determines its speed of onset, duration of action, and degree of spread [72]. A hydrophilic narcotic such as morphine does not cross membranes easily. Thus it takes longer to diffuse into the nervous tissue or the epidural blood vessels. Therefore it has a slower onset and elimination (longer duration). Since it is in the cerebrospinal fluid longer, morphine will spread a greater distance and has a higher propensity for rostral spread. Fentanyl and its derivatives are hydrophobic (lipid soluble). Consequently, they have a faster onset, shorter duration, and a more localized effect. The side effects of neuraxial narcotics include pruritus, urinary retention, early and late respiratory depression [72]. Pruritus is usually amenable to antihistamines, diphenhydramine, or hydroxyzine. In resistant cases, low-dose naloxone as a 40-µg intravenous bolus or 1 to 4 µg/min intravenous infusion may be necessary [73,74]. Urinary retention is readily relieved by urinary drainage catheter. Early respiratory depression occurs within 90 min of the dose of neuraxial narcotic and is probably a result of systemic absorption of the narcotic. Late respiratory depression is caused by rostral spread of the narcotic [73,74]. It is not seen with fentanyl, but may occur with morphine. This occurs 8 to 24 h after the last opioid dose, but is rarely seen with the low doses of neuraxial narcotic currently used. The risk of respiratory depression necessitates that these patients have hourly respiratory monitoring. To avoid additional risk of respiratory depression, patients who receive neuraxial narcotics should not receive concurrent parenteral opioids.

During intrathecal narcotic administration, a lumbar spinal tap is performed. With evidence of free-flowing cerebrospinal fluid, a dose of preservative-free narcotic (morphine, 10–12 µg/kg, 0.25 to 1 mg) is injected [14]. This single-shot technique is quickly and easily performed. However, it is limited by its single-dosing nature. Spinal catheters are usually not left in place, due to the risk of cerebrospinal fluid leak and contamination. Therefore, repetitive doses are not possible. To overcome this, longer-acting narcotics such as morphine are usually used. Even so, duration of action is limited to about 24 h. Though its risk is much lower in patients over 50, postdural puncture headache is a concern.

The advantage of a catheter technique includes the ability to give additional bolus doses of medication if analgesia is inadequate or to run a continuous infusion to maintain analgesia for several days. If an epidural technique is chosen, the catheter may be placed in either the lumbar or thoracic epidural space. Infusions of narcotic alone, local anesthetic alone, or a combination of dilute local anesthetic (0.125% bupivacaine) and narcotic (fentanyl) are used. Choice of drug regimen depends on the position of the catheter and the qualities of the drugs. The advantage of a thoracic epidural is its location near the incisional dermatomes; however, there is a small risk of spinal cord damage during placement. Lumbar catheters are farther from the incisional site, requiring larger doses of narcotics.

2. Local Anesthetics

Local anesthetics may also be used for the treatment of postoperative pain. They block transmission of nerve impulses by interfering with neuronal sodium channel conductance [75,76]. There are two classes of local anesthetics, esters and amides. Procaine, 2-chloroprocaine, cocaine, and tetracaine are ester derivatives which are metabolized by plasma cholinesterase. The amide derivatives include prilocaine, lidocaine, bupivacaine, mepivacaine, and etidocaine. Amide local anesthetics are metabolized in the liver, so they can accumulate in the plasma if their dose exceeds clearance by the liver.

True allergic reactions to local anesthetics are exceedingly rare [77]. However, allergic reactions to methylparaben, a para-aminobenzoic acid derivative that is used as a preservative for ester-type local anesthetic solutions, may occur [78,79]. Local neurotoxicity may occur when nerves are exposed to high concentrations of local anesthetics [80]. Systemic toxicity may also occur. The symptoms of central nervous system toxicity become more prominent as plasma concentration rises. These symptoms include circumoral numbness, lightheadedness, dizziness, tinnitus, somnolence, slurred speech, visual disturbance, muscular twitching, unconsciousness, and seizures [81]. Cardiovascular toxicity includes myocardial depression, hypotension from vascular smooth muscle relaxation, decreased conduction with refractory arrhythmias, and cardiovascular collapse.

When administered in the subarachnoid space, local anesthetics, unlike narcotics, can be used as sole anesthetics for surgery because they totally block nerve impulses. Local anesthetics placed in CSF have a rapid onset of action (within 5 min). They cause dense sympathetic, motor, and sensory block which is sufficient for surgery, but have a duration of action of 3 to 6 h (bupivacaine). The dense motor block, short duration of action, and hypotension associated with the sympathetic block make the use of spinal anesthetics unsuitable for postoperative analgesia.

However, local anesthetics placed in the epidural space are well suited for postoperative pain relief. At higher concentrations, they also cause a combination (motor and sensory) block that is unsuitable for postoperative pain relief. At lower concentrations patients may develop tachyphylaxis and after a prolonged infusion may develop hypotension from sympathetic blockade and loss of proprioception, leading to imbalance and falling [82]. Therefore, for postoperative pain relief, local anesthetics are rarely used alone like epidural space, but rather in combination with narcotics to reduce the total dose of local anesthetic required and limit tachyphylaxis.

Field blocks can be placed by the surgeon by infiltrating the wound edges with local anesthetic. Epinephrine (1:200,000) is added to the local anesthetic agent to retard systemic absorption and prolong its effect. If 0.5% bupivacaine is used, a field block may last up to 8–12 h. The disadvantage is the one-time nature of the block, without chance for renewal. Placement of a catheter in the incision to continuously infuse local anesthetic has been effective for postoperative relief. However, this may be a portal of entry for infection and may cause local anesthetic toxicity. The catheter may also migrate, reducing its effectiveness.

Intercostal (rib) blocks may be performed with local anesthetic/epinephrine. This block has been shown to improve pulmonary function (forced expiratory volume, forced vital capacity, maximal expiratory flow rate) after thoracotomy [83]. In cholecystectomy patients, improved pulmonary function [70] and a reduction in postoperative narcotic requirement [84] have been demonstrated. Intercostal block can be done under direct vision by the surgeon before closing the wound. Unfortunately, rib blocks require multiple injections sites, which are uncomfortable and time consuming; they risk pneumothorax, infection, bleeding if the intercostal vessels are entered, and local anesthetic toxicity if intravascular injection occurs.

Intrapleural catheters can be placed for the administration of local anesthetic. The local anesthetic most frequently used is bupivacaine, due to its long duration of action. It may be administered through a catheter in an intermittent dosing regimen of 10 to 30 cm^3 of 0.25 to 0.5% concentration every 6 h or by continuous infusion of 0.125 or 0.25% solution [85–87]. The exact mechanism of action is still uncertain. A multiple dermatome intercostal block occurs by diffusion of local anesthetic through the parietal pleura to the intercostal nerves and pleural nerve endings. Blockage of the sympathetic chain with resultant Horner's syndrome has been reported, and blockade of the spinal nerve roots at the paravertebral area could occur [88]. A drawback to using this technique is that the placement of the ICD device in the abdominal wall causes postoperative pain which may not be relieved using an intercostal catheter. Though some studies have shown this to be a good analgesic technique for upper abdominal and thoracic procedures [89,90], other studies have demonstrated inadequate pain relief after thoracotomy [91,92]. Presumably, the chest tubes may drain the local anesthetic from the pleural space before it has had time to act. The large surface area of the pleura readily absorbs local anesthetic, and thus the risk of toxicity is present. The catheter itself is a portal of entry into the pleural space where the patches are located and may increase the risk of a postoperative infection.

3. Nonsteroidal Antiinflammatory Drugs

Though their exact mechanism of pain relief is not known, nonsteroidal antiinflammatory drugs are useful analgesics. They inhibit prostaglandin synthesis by blocking the enzyme, cyclooxygenase, which decreases the amount of tissue prostaglandin available to act at prostaglandin receptors attenuating the inflammatory response. Ketorolac, indomethacin, and ibuprofen are the most commonly used. Ketoralac is the most recently approved agent and, though intended for intramuscular use, it has been given intravenously. The usual loading dose is 30 to 60 mg (IM), with maintenance doses of 15 to 30 mg every 6 h. Intramuscular administration is quite painful, and given orally it produces more gastrointestinal distress than ibuprofen. Ibuprofen is limited to oral use, 600 mg every 6 h, and requires the patient to be able to take oral intake. Rectal indomethacin is quite effective, and avoids the stomach upset associated with oral administration [93]. In the immediate postoperative period, nonsteroidal antiinflammatory drugs may not be sufficient as sole analgesic agents [94,95]. They may serve an adjunctive role in combination with narcotics, by not causing the sedation or respiratory depression associated with opioids [96]. This effect reduces the total narcotic requirement without significantly affecting the quality of analgesia [97,98]. Side effects include antiplatelet action, which may increase the bleeding time [99]. These drugs are frequently avoided in patients with known bleeding tendencies. Irritation of gastric mucosa is dose related and more frequent with the oral route of administration [100].

REFERENCES

1. Deutsch N, Hantler CB, Morady F, Kirsh M. Perioperative management of the patient undergoing automatic internal cardioverter-defibrillator implantation. J Cardiothorac Anesth 1990; 4(2):236–244.
2. Carr CME, Whitley SM. The automatic implantable cardioverter defibrillator. Implications for anaesthetists. Anaesthesia 1991; 46(9):737–740.

3. Lee EM, Carr CME. More on automated cardioverter-defibrillators. Anaesthesia 1992; 47(7):637–638.
4. Cashman JN, Garcia-Rodriguez C, Lamond C. Anaesthesia for transvenous insertion of an automatic implantable cardioverter-defibrillator. Anaesthesia 1992; 47(8):720–721.
5. Cohen E, Neustein S, Ali R, Thys D. Intrathecal morphine reduces Enflurane requirements during thoractomy. Soc Cardiovasc Anesthesiol Abstr 1990; 261.
6. Hief C, Borggrefe M, Chen X, et al. Effects of enflurane on inducibility of ventricular tachycardia. Am J Cardiol 1991; 68:609–613.
7. Denniss A, Richards D, Taylor A, Uther J. Halothane anesthesia reduces inducibility of ventricular tachycardia in chronic canine myocardial infarction. Basic Res Cardiol 1989; 84:5–12.
8. Hunt G, Ross D. Comparison of effects of three anesthetic agents on induction of ventricular tachycardia in a canine model of myocardial infarction. Circulation 1988; 78:221–226.
9. Nishikawa T, Inomata S, Igarashi M, Goyagi T, Naito H. Plasma lidocaine concentrations during epidural blockade with isoflurane or halothane. Anesth Analg 1992; 75:885–888.
10. Lepage J, Pinaud M, Helias J, Cozian A, LeNormand Y, Souron R. Left ventricular performance during propofol or methohexital anesthesia: isotopic and invasive cardiac monitoring. Anesth Analg 1991; 73:3–9.
11. Echt DS, Winkle RA. Management of patients with automatic implantable cardioverter/defibrillator. Clin Prog 1985; 3:4–16.
12. Johnson RA, Palacios, I. Dilated cardiomyopathies of the adult. N Engl J Med 1982; 307:1051–1058.
13. Shnider SM, Papper EM. Anesthesia for the asthmatic patient. Anesthesiology 1961; 22:886–892.
14. Hirshman CA, Edelstein G, Peetz S, et al. Mechanism of action of inhalation anesthesia on airways. Anesthesiology 1982; 56:107–111.
15. Downes H, Gerber N, Hirshman CA. IV lignocaine in reflex and allergic bronchoconstriction. Br J Anaesth 1980; 52:873–878.
16. Heneghan CPH, Bergman NA, Jordan C, Lehane JR, Catley DM. Effect of isoflurane on bronchomotor tone. 1983; 55:248.
17. Kingston HG, Hirshman CA. Perioperative management of the patient with asthma (review). Anesth Analg 1984; 63:844–855.
18. Eger EI. Isoflurane (Forane): A Compendium and Reference. Madison, WI: Ohio Medical Products, 1981:1–110.
19. Roizen MF, Horrigan RW, Frazer BM. Anesthetic doses blocking adrenergic (stress) and cardiovascular responses to incision-MAC BAR. Anesthesiology 1981; 54:390–398.
20. VanRiper DF, Horrow JC, Kutalek SP, Mccormick D, Goldman SM. Mixed venousoximetry during automatic implantable cardioverter-defibrillator placement. J Cardiothoracic Anesth 1990; 4(4):453–457.
21. Shabetal R, Fouilles NO, Gurrsoth WG. The hemodynamics of cardiac tamponade and constrictive pericarditis. Am J Cardiol 1970; 26:480.
22. Reddy PS, Curtiss EI, O'Toole JD, Shaver JA. Cardiac tamponade: hemodynamic observations in man. Circulation 1978; 58:265.
23. Fowler NO, Holmes JC. Hemodynamic effects of isoproterenol and norepinephrine in acute cardiac tamponade. J Clin Invest 1969; 48:502.
24. Kerber RE, Jascho JA, Litchfield R. Hemodynamic effects of volume expansion and nitroprusside compared with pericardio-centesis in patients with cardiac tamponade. N Engl J Med 1982; 306:929.
25. Moller CT, Schoonbee CG, Rosendorff C. Hemodynamics of cardiac tamponade during various modes of ventilation. Br J Anaesth 1979; 51:409.
26. Benumof, JL. Anesthesia for thoracic surgery. Philadelphia: Saunders, 1987:396.
27. AMA Drug Evaluations. 6th ed. Chicago: American Medical Association, 1986.
28. Chelimsky-Fallick C, Kobushigawa J, Stevenson WG, et al. Chronic amiodarone therapy prior to cardiac transplantation does not increase perioperative risk. J Am Coll Cardiol 1991; 17:290A.

29. King BD, Harris LC Jr, Greifenstein FE, et al. Reflex circulatory responses to direct laryngoscopy and tracheal intubation performed during general anesthesia. Anesthesiology 1951; 12:5556.
30. Wood M. Drugs an the sympathetic nervous sytem. In:Wood M, Alistair JJ, eds. Drugs and Anesthesia. Baltimore:Williams & Wilkins, 1982.
31. Maze M, Smith CM. Identification of receptor mechanism mediating epinephrine-induced arrhythmias during halothane anesthesia in the dog. Anesthesiology 1983; 59:322.
32. Stoelting RK. Circulatory changes during direct laryngoscopy and tracheal intubation: influence of duration of laryngoscopy with or without prior lidocaine. Anesthesiology 1977; 47:381.
33. Stoelting RK. Blood pressure and heart rate changes during short duration laryngoscopy for tracheal intubation: influence of viscous or intravenous lidocaine. Anesth Analg 1978; 57:197.
34. Stoelting RK. Attenuation of blood pressure response to laryngoscopy and tracheal intubation with sodium nitroprusside. Anesth Analg 1979; 58:116.
35. Lunn JK, Stanley TH, Eiseele J. High dose fentanyl anesthesia for coronary artery surgery: plasma fentanyl concentrations and influence of nitrous oxide on cardiovascular responses. Anesth Analg 1979; 58:390.
36. Kautto UM. Attenuation of the circulatory response to laryngoscopy and intubation by fentanyl. Acta Anaesth Scand 1982; 26:217.
37. Martin DE, Rosenberg H, Aukburg SJ. Low dose fentanyl blunts circulatory responses to tracheal intubation. Anesth Analg 1982; 61:680.
38. Horrow JC, Pharo G. Successful defibrillation with near-simultaneous orthogonal discharges. Anesthesiology 1991; 75:362–364.
39. Guffin A, Girard D, Kapplan JA. Shivering following cardiac surgery: hemodynamic changes and reversal. J Cardiothoracic Anesth 1987; 1:24.
40. Ali HH, Savarese JJ. Monitoring of neuromuscular function. Anesthesiology 1976; 45:216.
41. Wescott DA, Bendixen HH. Neostigmine as a curare antagonist—a clinical study. Anesthesiology 1962; 23:324–332.
42. Hasan A, Low DE, Ganado AL, Norton R, Watson DCT. Tracheal rupture with disposable polyvinylchloride double lumen endotracheal tubes. J Cardiothoracic Vasc Anesth 1992; 6(2):208–211.
43. Johr M, Sol D, Joos D. Die bronchialruptur. Diagnose und therapie einer seltenen komplikation bei der anwendung von doppellumentuben. Anaesthesist 1991; 40(10):577–579.
44. Strange C. Double lumen endotracheal tubes. Clin Chest Med 1991; 12(3):497–506.
45. McKenna MJ, Wilson RS, Botelho RJ. Right upper lobe collapse with right-sided double-lumen endobronchial tubes: a comparison of two tube types. J Cardiothoracic Anesth 1988; 2(6):734–740.
46. Rusch VW, Freund PR, Bowddle TA. Exchanging double-lumen for single-lumen endotracheal tubes after thoracotomy. Ann Thorac Surg 1991; 51(2):323–324.
47. Cannom DS, Winkle RA. Implantation of the automatic implantable cardioverter defibrillator (AICD): practical aspects. PACE 1986; 9:793–809.
48. Reid PR, Griffith SC, Mower MM, et al. The automatic implantable cardioverter/defibrillator: Patient selection and implantation protocol. PACE 1984; 7:1338–1342.
49. Craig DB. Postoperative recovery of pulmonary function. Anesth Analg 1981; 60:46.
50. Johnson WC. Postoperative ventilatory performance: dependence on surgical incision. Am Surg 1975; 41:615.
51. Egbert LD, Laver MB, Bendixen HH. The effect of site of operation and type of anesthesia upon the ability to cough in postoperative period. Surg Gynecol Obstet 1964; 49:161.
52. Bishop MJ, Cheney FW. Respiratory complications of anesthesia and surgery. Semin Anesth 1983; 2:91.
53. Craig DB, Wahba WM, Don HF, et al. "Closing volume" and its relationship to gas exchange in seated and supine position. J Appl Physiol 1971; 31:717.
54. Ali J, Weisel RD, Layug AB, et al. Consequences of post-operative alterations in respiratory mechanics. Am J Surg 1974; 128:376.
55. Belville JW, Forrest WH, Miller E, Brown BW. Influence of age on pain relief from analgesics. JAMA 1971; 217:1835.

56. Austin KL, Stapleton JV, Mather LE. Relationship between blood meperidine concentrations and analgesic response: a preliminary report. Anesthesiology 1980; 53:460.
57. Austin KL, Stapleton JV, Mather LE. Multiple intramuscular injections: a major source of variability in analgesic response to meperidine. Pain 1980; 8:47.
58. Mathe LE, Owen H. The pharmacology of patient-administered opioids. In:Ferrante FM, Ostheimer GW, Covino BG, eds. Patient Controlled Analgesia. Cambridge, MA: Blackwell, 1990:27.
59. White, PF. Use of patient controlled analgesia for management of acute pain. JAMA 1988; 259:243.
60. Tamsen A, Hartvig P, Fagerlund C, et al. Patient-controlled analgesic therapy: clinical experience. Acta Anaesth Scand 26 (suppl 74): 157. 1982;
61. White WD, Pearce DJ, Norman J. Postoperative analgesia: a comparison of intravenous on demand fentanyl with epidural bupivicaine. Br Med J 1979; 2:166.
62. Johnson LR, Magnani B, Chan V, Ferrante FM. Modifiers of patient controlled analgesia efficacy, locus of control. Pain 1989; 39:17.
63. Caplan RA, Ready LB, Oden RV, et al. Safety and efficacy of transdermal fentanyl for postoperative pain management: a double blind placebo study. JAMA 1989; 261:1036.
64. Rowbotham DJ, Wyld R, Peacock JE, et al. Transdermal fentanyl for relief of pain after upper abdominal surgery. Br J Anaesth 1989; 63:56.
65. Bell SD, Goldberg ME, Lerigani GE, et al. Evaluation of transdermal fentanyl for multi-day analgesia in post-operative patients. Anesth Analg 1989; 68:S22.
66. Boas RA, Holford NHG, Villager JW. Opiate drug choice and drug use. Clin J Pain 1985; 1:117.
67. Sawe J, Dahlstrom B, Paalzow L, et al. Morphine kinetics in cancer patients. Clin Pharmacol Ther 1981; 30:629.
68. Wang JK, Nauss LE, Thomas JE. Pain relief by intrathecally applied morphine in man. Anesthesiology 1979; 50:149.
69. Bromage PR, Camporesi E, Chestnut D. Epidural morphine for postoperative pain relief: a comparative study with intamuscular narcotic and intercostal nerve block. Anesth Analg 1980; 59:473.
70. Rawal N, Sjostrand UH, Dahlstrom B, et al. Epidural morphine for postoperative pain relief: a comparative study with intramuscular narcotic and intercostal nerve block. Anesth Analg 1982; 61:93.
71. Shulman M, Sandler AN, Bradley JW, et al. Postthoracotomy pain and pulmonary function following epidural and systemic morphine. Anesthesiology 1984; 61:569.
72. Cousins MJ, Mather LE. Intrathecal and epidural administration of opioid. Anesthesiology 1984; 61:276.
73. Stenseth R, Sellevold O, Breivil H. Epidural morphine for postoperative pain: experience with 1085 patients. Acta Anaesth Scand 1985; 29:148.
74. Rawal N, Schott U, Dahlstrom B, et al. Influence of naloxone infusion on analgesia and respiratory depression following epidural morphine. Anesthesiology 1986; 64:194.
75. Ritchie JM. Mechanism of action local anesthetic agents and biotoxins. Br J Anaesth 1975; 47:191.
76. Hill B. The common mode of action of three agents that decrease the transient change in sodium permeability in nerves. Nature 1966; 210:1220.
77. Adriani J. Reactions to local anesthestics. JAMA 1966; 196:119.
78. Aldrete AJ, Johnson DA. Allergy to local anesthetics. JAMA 1969; 207:356.
79. Nagel JE, Fuscaldo JT, Fireman P. Paraben allergy. JAMA 1977; 237:1594.
80. Ready LB, Plummer MH, Haschke RH, et al. Neurotoxicity of intrathecal local anesthetics in rabbits. Anesthesiology 1985; 63:364.
81. Wagman IH, de Jong RH, Prince DA. Effects of lidocaine on the central nervous system. Anesthesiology 1967; 28:155.
82. Mogensen T, Hojgaard L, Scott NB, et al. Epidural blood flow and regression of sensory analgesia during continuous postoperative epidural infusion of bupivicaine. Anesth Analg 1988; 67:809.
83. Kaplan JA, Miller ED, Gallager EG. Postoperative analgesia for thoracotomy patients. Anesth Analg 1975; 54:773.
84. Nunn JF, Slavin G. Posterior intercostal nerve block for pain relief after cholecystectomy. Br J Anaesth 1980; 52:253.

85. Rocco A, Reiestad F, Gudman J, McKay W. Intrapleural administration of local anesthetics for pain relief in patients with multiple rib fractures, preliminary report. Reg Anesth 1987; 12:10.
86. Stromskag KE, Reiestad F, Holmqvist ELO, Ogenstad S. Intrapleural administration of 0.25%, 0.375%, and 0.5% bupivicaine with epinephrine after cholecystectomy. Anesth Analg 1988; 67:430.
87. El-Nagger MA, Raad C, Yogaratnam G, et al. Intrapleural intercostal nerve block using 0.75% bupivicaine. Anesthesiology.
88. Sihota MK, Holmblad BR. Horner's syndrome after intrapleural anesthesia with bupivicaine for postherpetic neuralgia. Acta Anaesth Scand 1988; 32:593.
89. Reiestaf F, Stromskag KE. Interpleural catheter in the management of postoperative pain. A preliminary report. Reg Anesth 1986; 11:89.
90. Kambam JR, Hammon J, Parris WCV, et al. Interpleural analgesia for postthoracotomy pain and blood levels of bupivicaine following intrapleural injection. Can J Anaesth 1989; 36:106.
91. El-Baz N, Faber LP, Ivankovich AD. Intrapleural infusion of local anesthetic: a word of caution. Anesthesiology 1988; 68:809.
92. Rosenberg PH, Scheinin BM, Lepntalo MJA, et al. Continuous intrapleural infusion of bupivicaine for analgesia after thoracotomy. Anesthesiology 1987; 67:811.
93. Reasbeck PG, Rice MI, Reasbeck JC. Double-blind controlled trial of indomethacin as an adjunct to narcotic anesthesia after major abdominal surgery. Lancet 1982; 2:115–118.
94. Powell H, Smallman JMB, Morgan M. Comparison of intramuscular ketorolac and morphine in pain control after laparotomy. Anaesthesia 1990; 45:538–542.
95. Power I, Noble DW, Douglas E, Spence AA. Comparison of IM ketorolac tromethamine and morphine sulfate for pain relief after cholecystectomy. Br J Anaesth 1990; 65:448–455.
96. Bravo LJ, Mattie H, Spierdijk J, et al. The effects on ventilation of ketorolac in comparison with morphine. Eur Clin Pharmacol 1988; 35:491–494.
97. Kolker A, Patel U, Shah N, et al. Impact of indocin on postoperative opiod requirement following thoracotomy. Anesthesiology 1989; 71:A670.
98. Gilles GW, Kenny GN, Bullingham BE. The morphine-sparing effect of ketorolac tromethamine. Anaesthesia 1987; 42:727.
99. Spowart K, Greer IA, McLaren M, et al. Haemostatic effects of ketorolac with and without concomitant heparin in normal volunteers. Thrombo Haemostas 1988; 60(3):382–386.
100. Lanza FL, Karlin DA, Yee JP. A double-blind placebo controlled endoscopic study comparing the mucosal injury seen with an orally and parenterally administered new nonsteroidal analgesic ketorolac tromethamine at therapeutic and subtherapeutic doses. Am J Gastroenterol 1987; 82:939.

20

Postoperative Care of the Implantable Cardioverter-Defibrillator (ICD) Patient

David S. Cannom

*Hospital of the Good Samaritan
and UCLA School of Medicine
Los Angeles, California*

The postoperative management of the implantable cardioverter-defibrillator (ICD) patient is not complicated if simple routines are followed. Any hospital which has developed care patterns for the routine coronary artery bypass and valve patient will have no difficulty caring for the ICD patient. However, if carefully planned routines are not carefully followed, the result can be unnecessary patient morbidity or even excessive operative mortality [1] (Table 1).

I. POSTOPERATIVE ROUTINE

Our routine, and that of most implanting centers, is to begin the immediate postoperative care of the ICD patient in the same cardiac surgical unit in which other open-heart patients are recovered. This approach seems clinically logical, as one-third [2] of patients receiving an ICD will have concomitant heart surgery of some type as well. It is advantageous to have such a unit dedicated to the care of cardiovascular cases only. By concentrating ICD patients in one unit, nurses have the opportunity to care for large numbers of ICD patients, which in turn lessens the chance for human error.

Patients in our center leave the operating room with the ICD device turned off. This allows the surgeons to use cautery freely in the OR at the conclusion of the case without affecting device function. Patients are not treated routinely with antiarrhythmic drugs in the early hours and days postoperatively. Once in the cardiac surgical unit, one of the electrophysiology nursing staff carefully documents the device status in the chart. We have used brightly colored stickers (''ICD on''/''ICD off'') on the front of the chart and in the progress notes to alert the nursing staff as to device status.

The care of ICD patients does not differ from the routine postoperative care of the coronary artery bypass graft (CABG) or valve patient. Meticulous management of hemodynamic status is especially important, because the typical ICD patient has a reduced ejection fraction (mean 33%) and is therefore very sensitive to changes in preload. We routinely use a Swan-

Table 1 Postoperative Complications

Atrial fibrillation
Ventricular tachycardia
Pulmonary atelectasis, pneumonia, effusion
Generator hematoma
Pericarditis
Deep venous thrombophlebitis

Ganz catheter to monitor filling pressures and cardiac output. The use of pressors does not differ from that used in other postoperative patients.

It is our routine to extubate the patient the evening of surgery if hemodynamics are stable. We think that this minimizes pulmonary complications and shortens the stay in the cardiac surgical unit. By the second day, most patients are ready for transfer to the cardiac telemetry unit. By then, the patient has been extubated for nearly 24 h, and the chest tubes and the Swan-Ganz catheter have been removed.

On the telemetry floor, the patient is progressively ambulated until ready for the predischarge electrophysiology study (EPS) and home. Predischarge teaching begins as soon as the patient arrives on the telemetry floor. The patient who suffers complications will, of course, stay in the cardiac intensive-care unit until stable for transfer.

The second-generation devices (defibrillator only) are usually activated when the patient moves from the cardiac surgical unit to the telemetry unit (Fig. 1). If the patient has survived a known ventricular fibrillation (VF) arrest, we turn the ICD on with as high a rate cutoff as possible (190–200 beats/min) in order to avoid spurious discharges if the patient develops postoperative atrial fibrillation (AF). If the patient has ventricular tachycardia (VT) rather than VF, we activate the rate cutoff at 10 beats below the clinical VT rate. In patients with multiple VT rates, clinical judgment is required; usually the device rate cutoff which is chosen is less than the slowest clinically relevant VT.

The third-generation devices offer more programming flexibility and other choices. Even in the immediate postoperative period, one can program on the backup brady pacing function and utilize the memory function without programming on any tachycardia therapy. Nurses and doctors can treat ventricular tachycardia and atrial fibrillation with medicines or external cardioversion as they would any immediate postoperative patient without the risk of spurious shocks. Once the patient is moved to the telemetry unit, our practice, and that of many large centers, is to turn on the device initially as a "defibrillator only" (plus backup brady pacing and memory) but with the antitachycardia pacing (ATP) function turned off. We choose the appropriate rate cutoff as if it were a second-generation device. This approach defers sophisticated programming of the antitachycardia pacing function until the predischarge EPS.

There is little risk, however, in turning the antitachycardia pacing functions on shortly after surgery. The overriding goal in many of our decisions is to have the patient avoid unnecessary shocks in the early postoperative period. We prefer that any ATP function have a high likelihood of success. Thus, if postoperatively the patient develops rapid AF which mistakenly the device attempts to pace terminate, it will next deliver defibrillating shocks. This would not occur if a defibrillator-only function with a high rate cutoff had been programmed on.

Within the next 2 or 3 years, the majority of patients in whom an ICD is implanted will have the lead system placed transvenously and thus avoid a sternotomy or thoracotomy [3]. This will change the postoperative care of ICD patients and likely eliminate the need for any time in an intensive-care unit after surgery. We have recovered our transvenous lead system

Postoperative Care of the ICD Patient

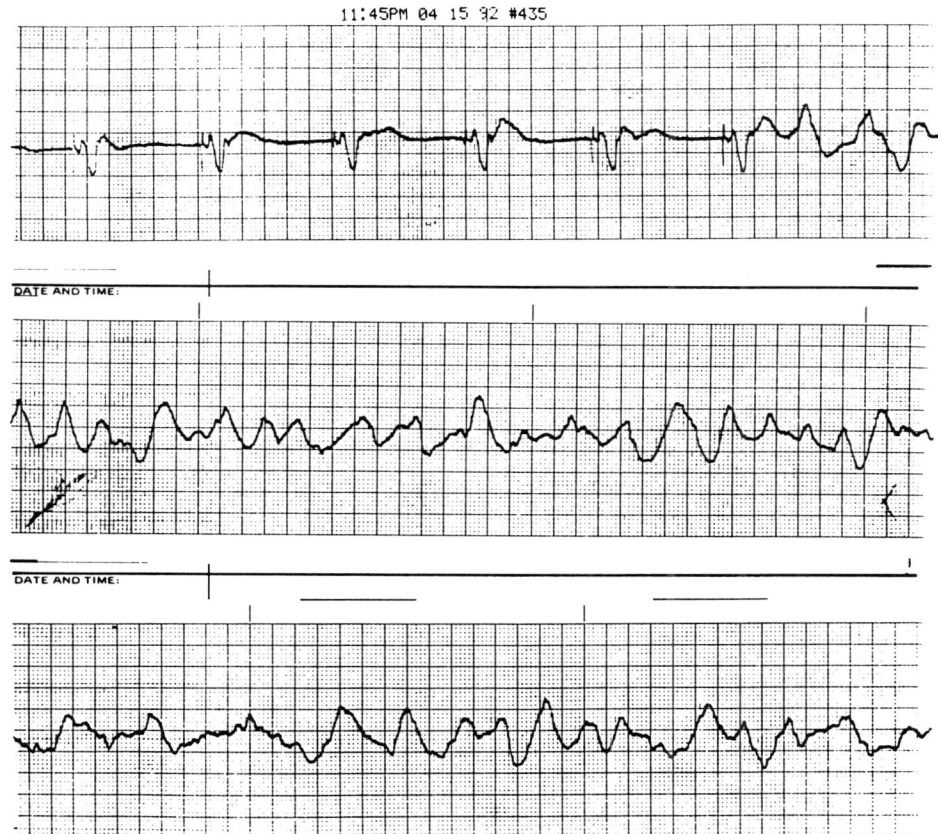

Figure 1 The patient was a SCD survivor who had a third-generation device implanted. He was moved to the telemetry floor on postoperative day 2, but the ICD was not turned on, as is our usual practice. The floor nurses were unaware that the ICD was off. Shown is a continuous telemetry strip with six paced beats which abruptly gives way to a wide complex rhythm. The nurses on the floor waited minutes before initiating CPR, as they thought that the device would treat this rhythm. It also happened on the night shift, which is when such communication breakdowns usually occur.

device patients in the coronary-care unit (CCU) for a few hours or sometimes overnight if still intubated. They are then moved to the telemetry floor and the device is turned on.

The postoperative use of antiarrhythmic drugs is highly variable and subject to physician choice. Some centers begin ICD patients on an antiarrhythmic drug predicted to be effective at the preoperative EPS soon after surgery, while others wait until the postoperative EP study or until the patient first receives a shock. We withhold antiarrhythmic drug treatment unless it seems likely from the postoperative telemetry (which may show high-density ectopy or frequent runs of nonsustained VT) that the patient will receive frequent shocks in the future. If antiarrhythmic drugs are used, they should be started before the postoperative EP test because of their effects on pacing algorithms and defibrillation thresholds (DFTs). The antiarrhythmic drugs employed are those which were judged to be most effective in preoperative EP studies. If no drugs were effective at EPS and an antiarrhythmic is still judged to be needed, amiodarone is usually started in low dose.

It is critical that each center establish its own formula for the safe care of postoperative ICD patients. The principles that assure success include:

1. Thorough in-service training on ICD function for all the intensivists, surgeons, fellows (both EP and surgical), and nurses who will be caring for ICD patients. The night-shift personnel especially must be trained.
2. A system for letting all care providers know whether the ICD is programmed on or off.
3. An established and unwavering clinical-care algorithm for all patients. This is critical to minimize mistakes.
4. A physician, usually the attending electrophysiologist, is designated as "in charge" of postoperative antiarrhythmic drug treatment and device status. Confusion results if the nurses are receiving mixed signals from many sources.

II. POSTOPERATIVE SUPRAVENTRICULAR TACHYCARDIA

Supraventricular tachycardia occurring within the first week after ICD implantation is a relatively common occurrence and is reported to occur in approximately 35% of patients undergoing operation [4]. The most common arrhythmia is atrial fibrillation (30%), although atrial flutter (4%) and paroxysmal atrial tachycardia (1%) occur less commonly. Other series have reported a postoperative incidence of AF varying from 9% [5,6] to 20% [7].

Only a small percentage of patients developing AF had this arrhythmia present before surgery. In the Paulowski data, the mean heart rate during supraventricular tachycardia was 136 + 28 (range 84 to 200) [4]. Nearly all patients had this complication occur by the fourth postoperative day. Postoperative AF developed with equal frequency in patients regardless of patch position (extrapericardial versus intrapericardial), nor was associated CABG a risk factor for the development of AF. However, this complication was noted to occur more frequently in patients who received two patches, in contrast to a superior vena cava spring-one patch configuration [5].

If the device is activated and AF develops, the inappropriate device discharges which result can be serious both medically and psychologically (Fig. 2). This is especially true if the staff is unable to deactivate the device quickly and multiple shocks result.

The frequent incidence of postoperative atrial fibrillation is a strong argument for setting the rate cutoff of the activated device to a high cutoff (greater than 180 beats/min or so) *if* this will not render VT treatment ineffective. Also, the nursing staff must know how to deactivate the device with a magnet if AF results in device discharge. The practice of taping a donut magnet to the end of the bed for use in emergency device deactivation is a sound one.

If the patient develops postoperative AF de novo, then rate control is established with digitalis and, if needed, a calcium channel blocker. If the patient does not quickly revert to sinus rhythm within 24 h, then the patient is usually anticoagulated and a type IA antiarrhythmic agent is started. Each clinician has a preference; we have used either quinidine or procainamide, in conjunction with digitalis, as the preferred agent to pharmacologically convert AF. If an antiarrhythmic drug is successful in converting the patient, then the type IA agent and anticoagulation can be stopped. In this way we are able to perform the final predischarge EP test on the drug regimen on which the patient will go home. If the atrial fibrillation recurs, then we restart the type IA drug, continue to anticoagulate, and commit the patient to at least 3 months of antiarrhythmic therapy. In this latter case, the patient will have his or her predischarge EP study while taking antiarrhythmic drugs.

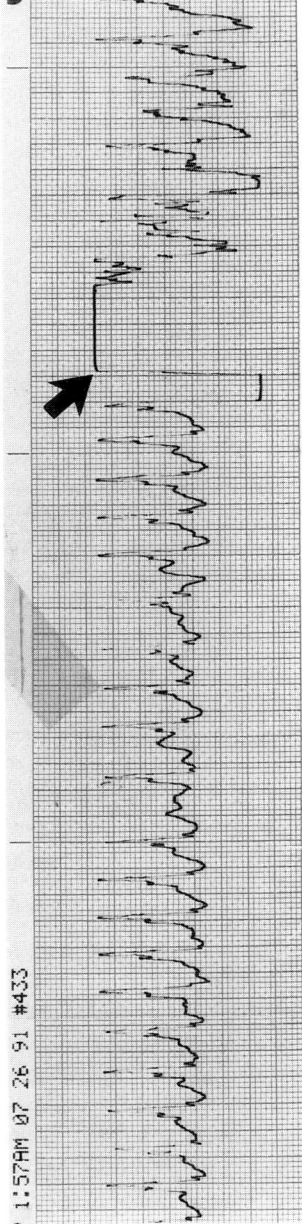

Figure 2 The patient is a SCD survivor who has a dilated congestive myopathy and an EF of 40%. He had a third-generation ICD implanted (two large patches) and was moved to the ward on day 2 with the device activated (rate cutoff 167 beats/min). Later that day he developed rapid AF (>200 beats/min) with hypotension and received multiple discharges before the device could be deactivated. The telemetry strip shows AF with a ventricular response of 180–200 beats/min and ICD discharge at the arrow. Such complications can usually be avoided by intelligent device programming. In this case the rate cutoff should have been higher.

Patients with postoperative atrial fibrillation must have careful attention to their maximal ventricular response with a careful, graded predischarge treadmill stress test. If the maximal-exercise ventricular rate exceeds the rate cutoff of the ICD, then spurious shocks are almost inevitable once the patient goes home. Agents which block AV nodal conduction must be given and the treadmill repeated. On occasion the AV junction must be ablated in patients with fixed AF. By so doing, the clinician assures that the ventricular response in AF will be less than the rate of a clinically significant slow VT and, in turn, the rate cutoff of the device.

A strong case can be made for the prophylactic use of digitalis in patients who are at high risk for the development of atrial fibrillation. This high-risk group includes patients with low ejection fraction (<35%), with an enlarged left atrium, or with a concomitant coronary bypass operation. A calcium channel blocker can be added if there is a history of rapid ventricular response to atrial fibrillation.

III. POSTOPERATIVE VENTRICULAR ARRHYTHMIAS

A significant percentage of patients will develop serious, sustained ventricular tachycardia in the early days after ICD implantation. The incidence of this complication is relatively constant in the literature and has varied from 10% [7] to 17% [8]. Both Wiggins et al. [9] and Kelly et al. [5] reported a postoperative incidence of VT of 13%. The rhythm which develops is typically VT rather than VF. In a small percentage of patients, the VT becomes incessant and of hemodynamic importance.

Wiggins et al. found that the only difference between ICD patients who did and did not develop postoperative VT was increased age in the VT group (71 versus 63 years). There was no difference between the two groups in terms of etiology of heart disease, ejection fraction (31% versus 37%), number of preoperative drug trials (2.3 versus 2.1), or any concomitant surgery [9].

Serious postoperative ventricular arrhythmias usually develop within the first week after surgery. No published series details the development of VT after postoperative day 9. The complication is extremely important clinically, as in all series it conveys a small but real increase in perioperative mortality due to incessant VT (Fig. 3). In a large, multicenter experience, Moeseller et al. [10] reported on the operative mortality in 1545 ICD patients from 17 centers. Of the 35 patients (representing 2.3% of the total) who died within the first 30 days, 8 (22%) deaths were caused by incessant postoperative VT/VF.

Very few patients who have other types of cardiac operations develop postoperative VT. Tam et al. [11] reviewed 2364 patients who underwent heart operations (all types except ICDs) at the University of Pennsylvania. He found that only 16 patients (0.68%) developed unexpected postoperative VT. The clinical rhythm which developed was VT (not VF) and occurred more commonly in patients with a low ejection fraction (most under 30%). It seems then, that the heart operation itself is not the cause of postoperative VT in the ICD patient. The possible causes of postoperative VT in ICD patients include the mechanical irritation of the epicardial screw in electrodes or pericarditis caused by the patches. Kelly et al. [5] found that postoperative VT occurred only in patients who received epicardial sensing leads which are screwed into the heart and not in patients who received endocardial rate-sensing systems. Kim et al. [8] noted that postoperative VT occurred more commonly in patients receiving an ICD alone compared to those receiving both coronary artery bypass and an ICD. There is no clinical evidence that such arrhythmias are caused by ischemia or electrolyte imbalance.

The development of postoperative VT is a serious complication that demands very intensive therapy with antiarrhythmic drugs. The ICD must be turned off and the patient treated in

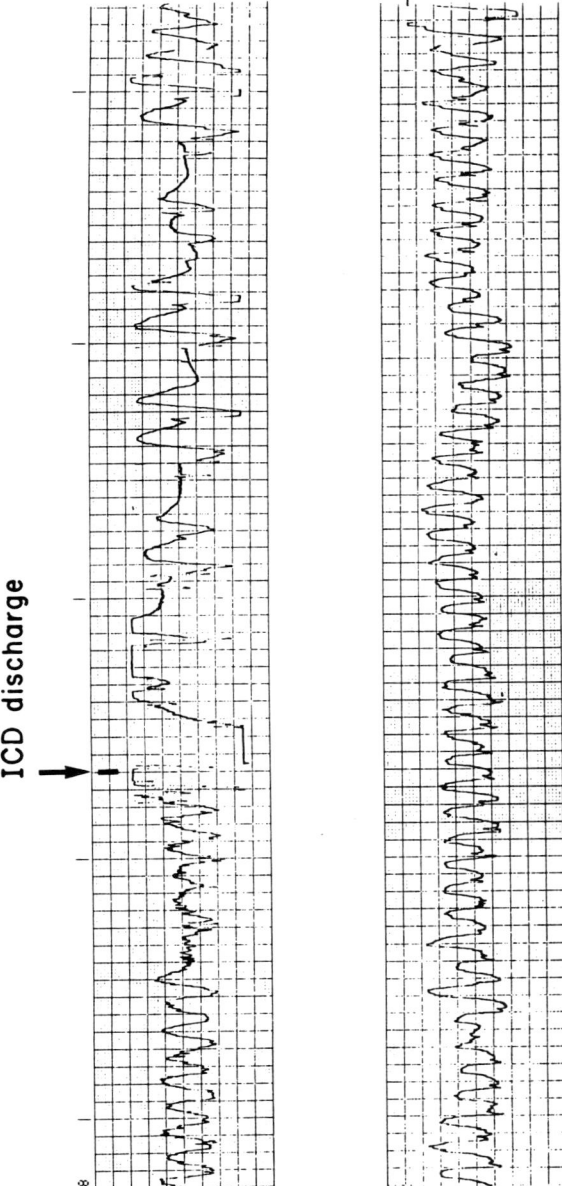

Figure 3 The patient was a SCD survivor with an EF of 25%. He underwent double vessel revascularization and third-generation device implantation. DFTs were 15 J. On postoperative day 3 he moved to the telemetry ward. At 7:00 a.m. on day 4 he felt well and walked to the bathroom, where he had a cardiac arrest which the device sensed but did not treat successfully despite multiple defibrillating shocks of 750 V. A long and ultimately unsuccessful code ensued. At postmortem the grafts were patent and there was evidence of recent infarction involving the septum. The rhythm strip shows sustained VT, a shock (labeled ICD discharge), a few paced beats, then recurrent VT. Some cases of incessant postoperative VT will be fatal. In this case we could develop no changes in our clinical approach that might have prevented this fatality.

a critical-care environment. The full spectrum of antiarrhythmic drugs is often necessary; lidocaine, bretylium, and, at times, intravenous amiodarone are particularly effective. It is also important to give enough magnesium and potassium by vein to keep serum levels in the high-normal range. In rare clinical settings, if intravenous medications fail, the clinician may resort to the intraaortic balloon pump to terminate the VT.

Some patients who develop repetitive, sustained VT and have a third-generation device can use the ATP function to treat VT while drugs are being given. This takes very careful ICD programming and is only a stopgap measure until intravenous drugs take effect.

There are no data to suggest that this complication can be predicted or completely prevented. It is important that the postoperative VT be treated aggressively when it first occurs. Physicians and hospitals implanting ICDs should have experienced staff and equipment available on a 24-hour-per-day basis to treat this important complication. Early and aggressive management of postoperative VT should virtually eliminate death due to incessant VT. On occasion, however, this means that an electrophysiologist needs to be at the bedside for hours, until the VT has stabilized.

IV. PULMONARY COMPLICATIONS

The commonly seen postoperative pulmonary problems include left lower lobe collapse, pneumonia, and left pleural effusion. These complications occurred in 29% of the patients in one series [5] and were related nearly exclusively to the use of an anterolateral thoracotomy approach for patch placement. The use of a midline sternotomy or subxiphoid approach helps to avoid these problems (Fig. 4).

Such problems are resolved with the aggressive use of chest physiotherapy, although antibiotics and bronchoscopy are often needed. The clinical course of such patients is often protracted; this in itself can cause other complications (e.g., deep vein thrombophlebitis), in addition to patient discomfort and added cost.

A syndrome of postoperative adult respiratory distress syndrome (ARDS) has been reported in patients receiving amiodarone who undergo aortocoronary bypass surgery [12]. Similar postoperative complications have been described in postoperative ICD patients on amiodarone. In one series [2], two of four postoperative deaths were related to amiodarone toxicity. This complication is extremely difficult to treat once it occurs, and the best treatment is prevention. We attempt to stop amiodarone preoperatively for days or even weeks before operation if possible. If a patient does go to surgery on amiodarone, we keep intraoperative testing (DFT determination) and systemic hypotension to an absolute minimum, although we cannot prove this to be of benefit.

V. HEMATOMA IN GENERATOR POCKET

Some fluctuation is noted in the pulse generator pocket postoperatively in the majority of patients, but in only a small percentage (2%) [5] is the accumulation of fluid tense or painful enough to require drainage (Fig. 5). The patients in whom this must be done have marked discomfort at the generator site due to the mechanical compression caused by the effusion; virtually all sterile effusions will resolve spontaneously if left alone. If the generator pocket must be tapped for clinical indications, it is done with meticulous sterile technique to avoid infection.

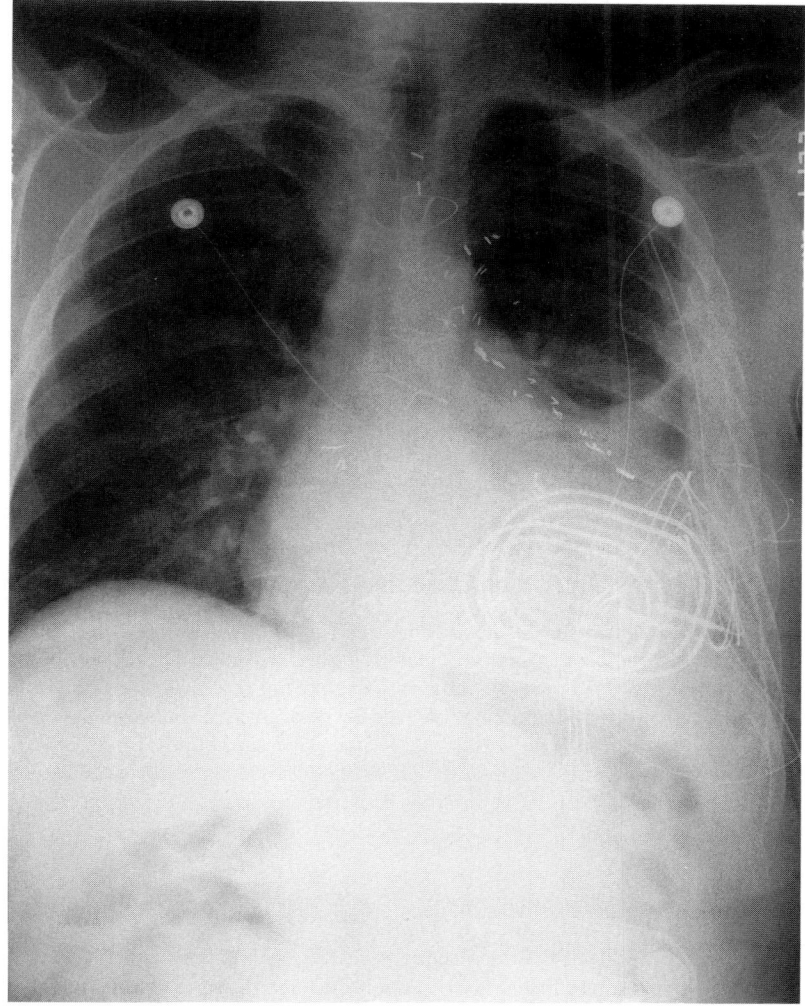

Figure 4 A postoperative chest X-ray (day 3) in a patient who had a Medtronic PCD implanted by a left anterior lateral thoracotomy. This approach was chosen because of prior bypass surgery. The CXR shows cardiomegaly, two patches, a left pleural effusion, and atelectasis. Such pulmonary complications are slow to resolve and delay patient discharge. We prefer a nonthoracotomy approach if possible.

Device infection is usually a late (>6 weeks) complication, is not related to benign postoperative generator effusion, and is covered separately (Chapter 30).

VI. POSTOPERATIVE PERICARDITIS

Many patients develop pericardial friction rubs postoperatively, but in only a small percentage does a clinical syndrome of fever, pleuritic chest pain, and echo evidence of pericardial effusion develop (3%) [5]. Such patients respond to a short course of antiinflammatory drugs.

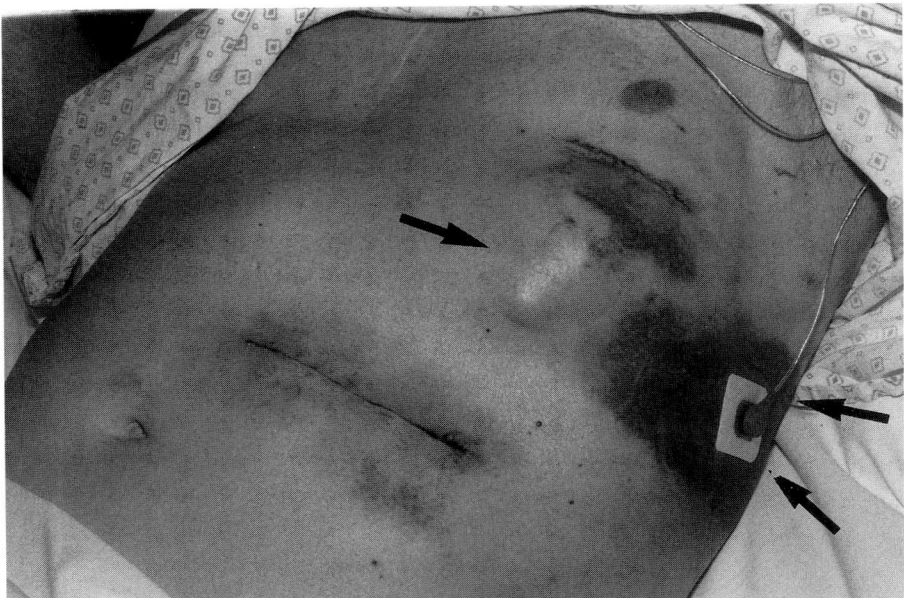

Figure 5 This patient had a transvenous device implanted 1 week earlier. The lead was placed via the left subclavian vein. A subcutaneous patch was placed via the incision under the left nipple. The ICD generator is in the typical left upper quadrant position. A number of potential problems are shown. There is a large hematoma from the subcutaneous patch placement (identified by two arrows). The patch itself is bulging midway between the two horizontal incisions (identified by single arrow). Finally, there is a small to moderate-sized generator effusion. All of these problems resolved without the need for tap of either the patch pocket or the generator pocket. Extreme care must be exercised at surgery to avoid such problems.

VII. DEEP VENOUS THROMBOPHLEBITIS

Deep venous thrombophlebitis occurs infrequently (2%) [5] and is usually seen in patients placed on bed rest for protracted periods of time. The usual preventative measures of early ambulation and prophylactic low-dose heparin can prevent this complication. We have not seen it since we stopped using anterior thoracotomies, which on occasion required long periods of bed rest.

VIII. IMPACT OF THE TRANSVENOUS DEVICES

The transvenous lead system has expanded the number of patients receiving ICDs and will greatly simplify and shorten their postoperative care as discussed in Chapters 45 and 46 [13]. Most of the complications we now see with thoracotomy systems will become historical curiosities.

Nonthoracotomy lead systems have become available for noninvestigational use recently and are now the preferred method of ICD implantation. With this technique, a single or multiple intracardiac leads are transvenously placed with fluoroscopic guidance using the cephalic or subclavian vein. This requires a small (approximately 4 cm) incision in the infraclavicular space, similar to that made for permament pacemaker implantation. Once the leads are placed transvenously, determination of standard pacing parameters such as R wave, threshold, impedance, and slew rate are followed by defibrillation threshold testing. Once these parameters are determined to be adequate, the leads are secured locally and then tunnelled through the subcutaneous space of the left upper quadrant of the abdomen were the ICD is implanted. Current devices in clinical investigation are sufficiently small to allow prepectoralis implants in selected patients, eliminating the need for tunnelling and a separate abdominal incision. It is evident that such lead systems eliminate the need for thoracotomy and dramatically reduce the risk for postoperative pulmonary complication. Furthermore, with elimination of the patches, it is likely that postoperative atrial fibrillation and ventricular arrhythmias will be reduced.

Typically the patient having a nonthoracotomy lead system is extubated in the operating room before being placed in a postanesthesia intensive care unit or recovery room for a period of 2 to 4 hours. Most patients are subsequently able to return to a monitored floor for their postoperative recovery. Selected high risk or unstable patients remain in the postanesthesia recovery area for a longer period of time or are transferred to a postoperative intensive care unit for management. As is discussed in chapter 19, such patients generally have adequate pain control with oral analgesics. Within 24 to 48 hours postoperatively most patients are ambulating and are sufficiently recovered to undergo predischarge electrophysiologic evaluation of the defibrillator. With current third generation devices with the ability to perform noninvasive programmed stimulation, such testing can be done through the device without the need for catheter placement. Most patients are ready for discharge within 48 to 72 hours after nonthoracotomy lead system placement.

IX. IMPACT OF THIRD-GENERATION DEVICES

The enormous flexibility of third-generation devices is a great advantage to patients long term, but their very complexity demands a great deal of time and attention from physicians and nurses alike. If the ATP function is turned on early in the postoperative course, the majority of episodes of VT can be pace-terminated rather than shocked and the telemetry function will accurately diagnose the therapy delivered. Short (3- to 5-s) runs of VT will not be treated with a noncommitted device which does not deliver therapy until the capacitor is charged and VT has been reconfirmed. Backup brady pacing is employed in approximately 10% of third-generation ICD patients and precludes the need for a separate pacemaker.

However, there are programming pitfalls even in the early postoperative period. Many patients with slow VT can achieve sinus rates which exceed the rate of the VT and cause spurious therapies (either ATP or shocks) for sinus rhythm. Antiarrhythmic drugs can further slow the VT rate below the sinus rate, especially with the use of type IA or type IC drugs or amiodarone. The careful use of beta-blockers does not effect the VT rate but does slow the sinus rate and seems the best solution to this problem of overlap between sinus and VT rate [14]. In an occasional patient, AV junctional ablation is necessary to maintain the sinus rate under the VT rate.

X. PATIENT CARE ISSUES

ICD patients and their families are particularly vulnerable to psychological setbacks in the early postoperative period. Often the ICD is placed after a long illness with many studies in the catheterization and EP laboratory, which leaves the patient and family vulnerable and insecure.

For these reasons, it is critical that patients and family be well prepared for what is to occur during the postoperative period. Every center develops its own method of teaching patients and family. We assign a nurse coordinator to each patient to do the teaching and answer questions, but this function could be done by an electrophysiologist, fellow, or EP nurse. Contact with each patient and family twice daily is important to ease anxieties and to assure that the patient goes home on time with all questions answered.

REFERENCES

1. Cannom D, Winkle RA. Implantation of automatic implantable cardioverter defibrillators: practical aspects. PACE 1986; 9(6):793–809.
2. Winkle RA, Mead RH, Ruder MA, et al. Long-term outcome with the automatic implantable cardioverter-defibrillator. J Am Coll Cardiol 1989; 13(6):1353–1361.
3. Cannom D. Implantable cardioverter defibrillator. The promise and perils of an evolving technology. PACE 1992; 15(1):1–4.
4. Paulowski JJ, Joye JD, Fogoros RN, Elson JJ, Bonnet CA, Chenarides JG. Incidence of supraventricular tachycardia after defibrillator implantation. J Am Coll Cardiol 1992; 19(3):123A.
5. Kelly PA, Cannom D, Garan H, et al. The automatic implantable cardioverter-defibrillator: efficacy, complications and survival in patients with malignant ventricular arrhythmias. J Am Coll Cardiol 1988; 11(6):1278–1286.
6. Deutsch N, Hantler CB, Morady F, Kirsh M. Perioperative management of the patient undergoing automatic internal cardioverter-defibrillator implantation. J Cardiothoraci Anesth 1990; 4(2):236–244.
7. Gartman DM, Bardy GH, Allen MD, Misbach GA, Ivey TD. Short-term morbidity and mortality of implantation of automatic implantable cardioverter-defibrillator. J Thorac Cardiovasc Surg 1990; 100:353–359.
8. Kim SG, Fisher JD, Furman S, et al. Exacerbation of ventricular arrhythmias during the postoperative period after implantation of an automatic defibrillator. J Am Coll Cardiol 1991; 18(5):1200–1206.
9. Wiggins S, Wolbrette D, Dougherty AH, Sweeney M, Jenkins M, Naccarelli GV. Is AICD implantation proarrhythmic? Personal communication, July 31, 1992.
10. Mosteller RD, Shuger CD, Thomas AC, Steinman RT, Lehmann MD. Operative (30-day) mortality following implantation of the automatic implantable cardioverter defibrillator. J Am Coll Cardiol 1989; 13(2):122A.
11. Tam SKC, Miller JM, Edmunds LH Jr. Unexpected, sustained ventricular tachyarrhythmia after cardiac operations. J Thorac Cardiovasc Surg 1991; 102:883–889.
12. Nalos PC, Kass RM, Gang ES, Fishbein MC, Mandel WJ, Peter T. Life-threatening postoperative pulmonary complications in patients with previous amiodarone pulmonary toxicity undergoing cardiothoracic operations. J Thorac Cardiovasc Surg 1987; 93(6):904–912.
13. Ehrlich S, for the Endotak Investigator Group. Early survival and follow-up characteristics of 151 patients undergoing transvenous cardioverter defibrillator lead system implantation. J Am Coll Cardiol 1992; 19(3):208A.
14. Paul V, Bashir Y, Anderson M, Ward DE, Camm AJ. Antitachycardia pacing and antiarrhythmics combined: a recipe for misdiagnosis? PACE 1991; 14(II):722.

21

Surgical Complications of Defibrillator Implantation

Connor J. Haugh and Paul J. Wang

*Tufts University School of Medicine
and New England Medical Center
Boston, Massachusetts*

I. INTRODUCTION

Most thoracotomy implantable defibrillator series report a perioperative mortality of 0% to 7% [1–27a] and perioperative complication rates of 10% to 60% (Tables 1 and 2). The perioperative period is typically defined as up to 30 days postoperatively or prior to hospital discharge. The morbidity and mortality of thoracotomy ICD implantation, however, have declined significantly over time. Cohen et al., for example, reported a 50% reduction in both morbidity and mortality between the first and second half of the series [2]. Improvements in surgical technique, intraoperative and postoperative care, and patient selection may all contribute to this decline. As a result of these factors, the current perioperative mortality from ICD implantation is approximately 1% to 3% and in some series less than 1%. Nonthoracotomy systems have resulted in further significant reduction in perioperative complications [28–40]

Numerous factors likely influence the morbidity and mortality of ICD implantation. The significant cardiac and noncardiac co-morbidity present in many recipients is the most potent factor increasing the risk of ICD implantation. Decreased left ventricular function with an ejection fraction of less that 30% may be associated with an increased surgical mortality [41]. These increased risks must be balanced, however, against the benefit of the ICD in patients with a high sudden-cardiac-death mortality [42]. A history of prior myocardial infarction may also be associated with an increased morbidity [7]. Some studies have suggested that concomitant surgery, such as coronary artery bypass graft surgery, increases the morbidity and mortality of ICD placement [8,43], while other studies have not demonstrated this increase [7,16].

Complications of ICD placement via thoracotomy are listed in Table 1 and are reviewed by organ system. Cardiac complications included myocardial infarction, congestive heart failure, cardiac trauma, and pericarditis. Pulmonary complications included pneumonia, respiratory distress syndrome, atelectasis, pneumothorax, and pleural effusions. Trauma, thrombosis, and cerebrovascular accident comprised the vascular complications. Gastrointestinal complications ranged from colonic perforation and ischemic colitis to hepatitis. Infectious complications

Table 1 Reported Complications of Defibrillator Placement

Cardiac	Gastrointestinal
Myocardial infarction	Ischemic colitis
Congestive heart failure	Colonic perforation
Pericarditis	Hepatitis
Trauma	
	Device-related
Vascular	Lead fracture
Superior vena cava thrombosis	Lead migration
Subclavian vein thrombosis	Patch crinkling
Cerebrovascular accident	Fluid accumulation
Trauma	Premature generator failure
Pulmonary embolism	Generator erosion
Infectious	Miscellaneous
Wound infection	Psychiatric
Foreign-body infection	Renal failure
Sepsis	Skin necrosis
Endocarditis	Protamine reaction
	Thoracic nerve injury
Pulmonary	
Pneumonia	
Adult respiratory distress syndrome	
Atelectasis	
Pleural effusions	
Pneumothorax	

Table 2 Summary of Complications Expressed by Series as Percentage of Patients

		Bardy [1]	Cohen [2]	Echt [3]	Edel [4]	Garbry [6]	Gartman [7]	Hargrove [9]	Kelly [10]
Cardiac	Nonfatal		3.6		30.1		23.7	1.2	11.7
	Fatal		6.3	3.7			1.9		2.1
Pulmonary	Nonfatal		5.4				3.9	10.4	29.7
	Fatal		0.9	1.4	0.3		0.9		1.0
Vascular	Nonfatal		10.8				3.9		3.2
	Fatal								
Infectious	Nonfatal					9.0	1.0	4.3	
	Fatal								
Device	Nonfatal		14.4	8.5	2.4	9.0		19.3	13.0
	Fatal								
Other	Nonfatal	2.0		7.1			1.0		
	Fatal		0.9				1.0		
Fatalities		0	8.1	4.2	4.0	0	3.9	3.0	3.2

included sepsis, wound infection, and infection of foreign body. Device and lead-related complications included lead fracture, lead migration, generator failure, patch crinkling, fluid accumulation, and erosion.

II. THORACOTOMY DEVICES

A. Cardiac Complications

1. Congestive Heart Failure

Perioperative congestive heart failure has been reported in 1% to 10% of patients undergoing defibrillator implantation [2-4,7,11,12,14,19,20,22,26] (Tables 3 and 4). This relatively high incidence of congestive heart failure reflects the significantly decreased left ventricular function which is present in the majority of patients undergoing ICD implantation. While many patients also had a history of clinical congestive heart failure, more specific clinical predictors of the development of congestive heart failure postoperatively are not available. The etiologies of postoperative congestive heart failure in these patients may include fluid overload, ischemia, and worsening of left ventricular function following anesthesia and/or cardiopulmonary bypass [2,7,10,11,19]. There is no evidence that ICD patches themselves reduce left ventricular function [44,45], although constriction and restriction have been reported as described below [10,23,46]. In most cases, congestive heart failure is reversible with diuretics and afterload reduction [7,11,26]. Nonfatal hemodynamic collapse, however, requiring intraaortic balloon counterpulsation and pressor support has been reported [4,7]. Congestive heart failure has been reported as the cause in 0% to 11% of deaths [2,3,7,11,12,14,18–20].

2. Myocardial Infarction

Myocardial infarction postoperatively has been reported in 0% to 4% of patients [3,4,10,18,19,22] (Table 4). The risk of myocardial infarction in the subset of patients undergoing concomitant coronary artery bypass graft surgery or valve surgery may be higher. However, since cardiac enzymes typically have not been measured in asymptomatic patients without

Manolis [11]	Marchlinski [12]	Mercando [13]	Mirowski [15]	Olinger [17]	Palatianos [18]	Paull [19]	Porterfield [20]	Tchou [22]	Tresch [24]	Winkle [26]
45.9	3.8			2.1		8.3		2.8	2.3	
	3.8			4.2	0.9		1.3		1.5	0.4
	34.6		0.9		7.2	4.1		2.8	0.8	
							1.3			0.7
	7.6		2.7		0.9			2.8	2.3	2.2
			0.9		0.9			1.4	1.5	0.4
	3.8	2.7	1.8					2.8		0.7
	7.6		6.3		3.6		1.2			4.4
					0.9	4.1				
					0.9					
0	3.8	0	0.9	6.4	2.7	0	2.6	1.4	3.0	1.5

Table 3 Fatal Cardiac Complications Expressed as Percentage of Patients by Series

	Cohen [2]	Edel [4]	Gartman [7]	Kelly [10]	Marchlinski [12]	Olinger [17]	Palatianos [18]	Porterfield [20]	Winkle [26]
Myocardial failure	1.8		1.9			4.3	0.9	1.2	
Ventricular tachycardia/ fibrillation	4.5	1.8		2.1	3.8				0.4
Myocardial infarction		0.3					0.9		
Asystole		0.3							

other evidence of myocardial infarction, the true incidence of myocardial infarction may be significantly higher. In addition, data comparing pre- and postoperative ejection fraction are not available for most series.

3. Pericarditis

Pericardial inflammation, often manifested by a pericardial rub, is felt to be a common consequence of ICD implantation [10,12,47,48]. Symptomatic pericarditis may occur in some patients, usually responding to nonsteroidal antiinflammatory agents or prednisone. In addition, pericardial fluid may be detected radiographically in some patients [10,12,47]. In one series, 8 of 14 asymptomatic patients undergoing CT scanning had evidence of pericardial fluid within the first 2 postoperative weeks [47]. One investigator reported three episodes of pericardial tamponade requiring pericardiocentesis [2]. While some investigators have suggested that fluid collections lasting longer than 4 weeks should prompt consideration of infection, insufficient prospective data are available to make this a general recommendation [47]. Pathologically, intrapericardial placement of the ICD patches results in pericardial remodeling and dense pericardial adhesions [48]. There is very little data regarding extrapericardial ICD patch placement, although it has been suggested that the extrapericardial ICD patch placement may be associated with a decreased incidence of pericardial inflammation compared to intrapericardial location [9]. Randomized data comparing these two approaches are not available.

Table 4 Cardiac Morbidity Expressed as Percentage of Patients by Series

	Cohen [2]	Edel [4]	Gartman [7]	Hargrove [9]	Kelly [10]	Marchlinski [12]	Olinger [17]	Paull [19]	Tchou [22]
Arrhythmia		18.3	19.8		8.5			4.1	
Atrial fibrillation		12.4			8.5			4.1	
Bradycardia		5.9							
Myocardial infarction		0.9			1.1			4.1	2.8
Saphenous vein graft erosion				1.2					
Coronary artery laceration		0.6				3.8	1.1		
Pericarditis							1.1		
Forward output failure	0.9	10.2	3.9		2.1				
Tamponade	2.7								

Constrictive pericarditis has been reported in several patients undergoing ICD patch placement [17,46,47]. The process of pericardial remodeling frequently results in distortion of the ICD patch configuration. In one series examining plain X-rays of the ICD patches, distortion of the patches was seen in 21% of cases [47]. Posterior patches seem to have more than twice the frequency of crinkling compared to anterior patches [47]. Patch crinkling may have several clinical implications. In one series 60% of patients with severe patch crumpling, defined as distortion of at least three edges, experienced increases in defibrillation threshold during follow-up testing [47]. In addition, crumpling may disrupt patch integrity, resulting in detection of noise and inappropriate shocks [49].

4. Cardiac Laceration and Trauma

Coronary artery trauma has been reported as a rare consequence of both patch and lead placement. Patch erosion of a coronary artery and saphenous vein coronary artery graft has occurred [9,17]. In addition, laceration of a coronary artery and of the left atrium have been observed as a consequence of patch placement [4,11,12]. One series reports left ventricular rupture without specific etiology [24].

B. Pulmonary Complications

Pulmonary complications are observed frequently after ICD placement, occurring in 4% to 30% of patients [2,6,7,9–13,19,22] (Tables 5, 6). Such complications have included respiratory failure, pneumonia, atelectasis, pleural effusion, pneumothorax, hemothorax, and pulmonary embolism. Severe respiratory failure requiring mechanical ventilatory support or resulting in death has been reported in 0% to 4% of patients [6,7,10,12,13,20,26]. It has been the cause of 0% to 30% of perioperative deaths [6,7,10,12,13,20,26].

Outstanding pulmonary toilet and incentive spirometry are essential ingredients in postoperative care to minimize the risk of pneumonia, which occurs in 2% to 10% of ICD implants [6,7,10–12]. Most of these episodes of pneumonia are treated successfully without prolonged respiratory support [7,11,12]. Occasionally, a bacterial pneumonia or left-sided empyema may proceed to ICD infection [3]. Aspiration is another etiology of postoperative pneumonia. Prior amiodarone use may be associated with an increased incidence of pulmonary complications. In one series, two-thirds of the fatal and reversible pulmonary complications occurred in patients with prior amiodarone use [18]. The adult respiratory distress syndrome has also been described postoperatively after preoperative amiodarone use [2,4,18,22,24,26].

Pleural effusions occur in 10% to 100% of patients postoperatively [9,12]. Asymptomatic effusions do not require treatment, but respiratory distress or evidence of empyema should prompt consideration of thoracentesis or chest tube placement. Pleurodesis for recurrent symptomatic pleural effusions is only rarely necessary. Pneumothorax can be a consequence of

Table 5 Fatal Pulmonary Complications Expressed as Percentage of Patients by Series

	Cohen [2]	Echt [3]	Edel [4]	Gartman [7]	Kelly [10]	Porterfield [20]	Winkle [26]
Respiratory failure		1.4		1.0	1.1	1.2	0.3
Amiodarone toxicity		1.4					0.3
ARDS			0.3				0.3
Pneumothorax	0.9						

Table 6 Nonfatal Pulmonary Complications Expressed as Percentage of Patients by Series

	Cohen [2]	Gartman [7]	Hargrove [9]	Kelly [10]	Marchlinski [12]	Mirowski [15]	Palatianos [18]	Paull [19]	Tchou [22]
Amiodarone toxicity							3.6		
Respiratory insufficiency		0.9					3.6	4.1	
Atelectasis		0.9			15.3				
Symptomatic Pleural Effusion			10.3		11.5	1.9			
Nonspecific Infiltrate and fever		1.9		28.7					
ARDS	1.8								
Pneumothorax	3.6			1.1	7.6				2.8

transvenous lead placement, bleb rupture, or inadvertent pulmonary puncture during thoracotomy and has been reported as a complication of ICD implantations in 0% to 7% of cases [2,10,12,22,50].

C. Vascular Complications

Superior vena cava perforation during defibrillator lead placement occurs rarely and was the cause of one reported perioperative death [26] (Table 7). Subclavian perforation by a polyethylene catheter also was reported as the cause of one death [15]. Hemothorax has also been observed after central-line access during ICD implantation [2].

Subclavian vein thrombosis due to endocardial lead placement has been described in ICD patients in 0% to 5% of cases. This is generally asymptomatic and does not require therapy. If necessary, it may be treated successfully with long-term anticoagulation [3,6,12,50,51]. Lead fracture and migration seem to be associated with an increased frequency of thrombosis, occurring in up to 25% of such cases [3,10,12,15,23,26]. Improvements in anchoring technique have reduced the incidence of migration and subsequent subclavian vein thrombosis [3]. Superior vena cava thrombosis has only been reported clinically after one ICD placement, and it responded to anticoagulation [14]. However, an autopsy series demonstrated that 17% of patients had thrombus formation associated with superior vena cava leads [48].

Deep vein thrombosis has occurred postoperatively at a frequency of up to 2% [10]. Two cases of deep vein thrombosis occurring 2 weeks after ICD implantation were reported [10]. In some cases, deep vein thrombosis may occur as the result of venous catheterization during diagnostic procedures or immobility postoperatively. Pulmonary embolism has been documented to be a cause of death [18,22,24]. The incidence of asymptomatic pulmonary emboli, however, is not known.

Postoperative cerebrovascular events ranged in frequency from less than 1% to 4% [3,7,10,12–14,26]. In most series hemorrhagic events were not distinguished from ischemic events, and likely etiologies of cerebrovascular events include both hypotension and thromboembolism. In two series multiple episodes of sustained ventricular tachycardia preceded the cerebrovascular events [3,10]. In one case conversion of chronic atrial fibrillation to sinus rhythm was followed by a cerebrovascular event 48 h later [12]. There are not sufficient data to

Table 7 Vascular Complications Expressed as Percentage of Patients by Series

	Cohen [2]	Echt [3]	Edel [4]	Gabry [6]	Gartman [7]	Kelly [10]	Marchlinski [12]	Mirowski [15]	Palatianos [18]	Tchou [22]	Tresch [24]	Winkle [26]
Cerebrovascular accident		1.4	1.8		2.0	1.1	3.8				2.3	0.7
Deep Venous Thrombosis						2.1						
Subclavian Thrombosis	0.9						3.8	0.9				
Subclavian Perforation								0.9				
Vascular insufficiency of ipsilateral arm				2.7								
Superior vena cava thrombosis								0.9				
Hemorrhage	10.0		0.9		2.0			1.8	0.9			0.3
Pulmonary embolism									0.9	1.4	1.5	

Table 8 Infectious Complications Expressed as Percentage of Patients by Series

	Gabry [6]	Gartman [7]	Hargrove [9]	Marchlinski [12]	Mercando [13]	Mirowski [15]	Olinger [17]	Porterfield [20]	Tchou [22]
Wound infection	4.5	1.0		3.8		0.9			2.9
Venotomy		1.0							
Thoracotomy				3.8					
Antecubital						0.9			
Unspecified	4.5								2.9
Fatal Sepsis							2.1	1.3	
Nonfatal sepsis	4.5			7.7	2.7				
Unspecified			4.3			0.9			1.4

compare the incidence of cerebrovascular complication in those patients receiving concomitant coronary artery bypass graft surgery and those without other surgery.

D. Gastrointestinal Complications

Serious gastrointestinal complications are unusual. Postoperative ileus occurs occasionally but it not usually reported as a complication. One patient with a late generator infection was found to have his colon perforated by the ICD leads [52]. Ischemic bowel necrosis was the cause of a postoperative death in one series [11]. Two reports of hepatitis have been noted, one due to non-A non-B virus.

E. Infectious Complications

Nondevice infections occur in 1% to 5% of patients [6,7,9,11,12,14,22,26] (Table 8). Four different series report a total of five episodes of fatal sepsis, one associated with an indwelling catheter [6,11,12,15]. Pulmonary infections have been described previously. Infections may involve the sternum, thoracotomy wound, and antecubital cut-down sites [6,7,12,15,22]. Foreign body material such as central venous lines, chest tubes, and urinary catheters may become infected, and meticulous care must be given to minimize the risk of infection at these sites. Endocarditis is rare but has been described after ICD implantation [24]. Device-related infections are discussed in a separate chapter.

F. ICD Device and Lead Complications

ICD system-related complications are frequent, occurring in 6% to 21% of patients [2,3,6,9,10,12,15] (Table 9). Most of these complications are discussed in other chapters regarding ICD system performance. Lead fracture and migration were the most common device-related complications [3,10,12,14]. Routine radiographic studies are helpful in detecting lead fracture [3,10]. Superior vena cava spring electrodes were initially associated with lead fracture or migration in up to 20% of patients, but subsequent improvements in lead and anchoring technology reduced these rates to approximately 3% to 10% [3]. Insulation breaks have occurred at the site of lead stress, particularly at the sites of anchoring or vessel entry, and at the clavicular-first rib junction. Adaptors in implantable defibrillator systems may be particularly vulnerable to fracture, due to the weight of the device and the twisting which may occur with torso movement.

Surgical Complications

Table 9 Device-Related Complications Expressed as Percentage of Patients by Series

	Cohen [2]	Echt [3]	Edel [4]	Gabry [6]	Hargrove [9]	Kelly [10]	Marchlinski [12]	Mirowski [15]	Porterfield [20]
Lead failure	3.6	8.5				3.2	7.6	6.3	
Fracture		1.4							
Migration		4.2				3.2	3.8	6.3	
Myopotential sensing		1.8			10.3		3.8		
Elevation of DFT									
Premature battery depletion	2.7			4.5		9.0			
							9.8		
Insulation break	2.7			4.5					
No specified cause					9.0				
Pocket erosion	3.6			4.5					1.2
Generator migration									
Nonspecified component failure	4.5								
Defective device			1.2						

Migration or dislodgement of sensing or pacing endocardial or epicardial leads may result in both sensing abnormalities and loss of capture [3,10,13,15]. Anchoring using multiple sleeves at both the generator pocket and lead insertion site may be helpful in decreasing dislodgement and lead stress. Device migration occurs in 0.7% to 1.2% of implants [23]. Implanting the device under the rectus muscle or in a device pouch has been advocated by some surgeons to minimize device migration [53,54].

Some degree of serous fluid accumulation in the generator pocket is present in most patients immediately after ICD implantation. However, fluid accumulation is only rarely associated with pocket infections, and the accumulation may be observed without intervention. Needle aspiration is not indicated and should be avoided [10]. In addition, hematoma has been noted in the pulse generator pocket, particularly in patients anticoagulated immediately after the procedure [26]. The hematomas usually resolve gradually, often over a period of weeks. However, if skin viability is impaired, due to tension produced by the hematoma, surgical evacuation of the hematoma may be urgently required.

Generator erosion is infrequent. One series reported superficial wound break-down progressing to generator exposure in a diabetic patient with prior renal transplantation [17]. Erosion may result from mechanical abrasion resulting, for example, from trouser belt use [6]. Because erosion threatens the entire defibrillator system, the earliest sign of erosion warrants very close observation.

III. NONTHORACOTOMY DEVICES

Based on several recently reported series, the surgical morbidity and mortality of nonthoracotomy defibrillator system implantation are significantly reduced when compared to that of thoracotomy systems [28–40d]. One large series of 751 implants demonstrates a perioperative death rate of 0.3% with nonthoracotomy systems compared to 5.5% with thoracotomy systems [37]. A series reported by Lehmann et al. had a perioperative mortality of 1.6% compared with 4.7% for nonthoracotomy and thoracotomy systems, respectively [34].

Most complications of nonthoracotomy ICD device placement occurred in the initial phase of the series. Bardy et al., for example, reported that most complications were seen in the first third of implants [29]. Similarly, Block et al. noted a reduction in mortality from 3.8% to 0% from the first to the second half of implants [30]. These data suggest that the risk of nonthoracotomy defibrillator implantation may be very low.

Cardiac complications with the use of nonthoracotomy systems are infrequent. Three recent series report a 0% incidence of cardiac complications [28,29,33], and most series report a 0% incidence of myocardial infarction. One series noted a 5.3% incidence of CPK-MB elevation without ECG evolution or hemodynamic alteration [39]. Right ventricular perforation has been reported and may be more likely to occur with nonthoracotomy systems than with thoracotomy systems. While one series of 33 implants reported two deaths from congestive failure [38], most series report a 0% incidence of perioperative congestive heart failure.

Pulmonary complication rates are estimated to be 0% to 3%, with a virtual elimination of pneumonia and atelectasis [28,29,39]. Pneumothorax, pulmonary embolism, and respiratory failure continue to be reported with nonthoracotomy systems [32,33].

Other complications are also uncommon. Reported vascular-related complications include bleeding associated with postoperative heparinization, subcutaneous-patch site hematoma, subclavian thrombosis, and cerebrovascular accident. The reported incidence of infection ranged from 0% to 9% [32,37]. Death due to sepsis was reported in two series [31,40].

Early nonthoracotomy systems were frequently complicated by lead fracture and migration in up to 10% of systems [32,35,37]. Lead-related events have been substantially reduced with improved lead technology and refined implant technique. A recent series of nonthoracotomy implants reported no lead fractures and a 1.2% dislodgement rate [31]. Recent series also report one case of diaphragmatic pacing, one episode of transient long thoracic nerve injury, and one episode of generator migration without lead fracture or displacement [29,31,32].

IV. CONCLUSION

Despite the wide variety of reported complications described (Tables 1–10), the complication rate of ICD placement is relatively low, particularly given the often substantial cardiac and noncardiac morbidity of this patient population. The incidence of complications appears to be declining; further declines have been observed with nonthoracotomy system implantation. Vig-

Table 10 Miscelaneous Complications Expressed as Percentage of Patients by Series

	Bardy [1]	Cohen [2]	Echt [3]	Gartman [7]	Palatianos [18]	Paull [19]
Nonfatal complications						
Psychiatric			7.1			
Renal Failure				1.0		
Skin Necrosis					0.9	4.1
Thoracic nerve injury	2.0					
Fatal complications						
Suicide					0.9	
Protamine feaction				1.0		
Multisystem failure			0.9			

ilant perioperative monitoring, when coupled with a familiarity of anticipated or likely complications, can minimize the incidence of these untoward events.

REFERENCES

1. Bardy GH, Troutman C, Poole JE, et al. Clinical experience with a tiered-therapy, multiprogrammable antiarrhythmia device. Circulation 1992; 85:1689–1698.
2. Cohen TJ, Reid PR, Mower MM, et al. The automatic implantable cardioverter-defibrillator. Arch Intern Med 1992; 152:65–69.
3. Echt DS, Armstrong K, Schmidt P, Oyer PE, Stinson EB, Winkle RA. Clinical experience, complications, and survival in 70 patients with the implantable cardioverter/defibrillator. Circulation 1985; 71:289–296.
4. Edel TB, Maloney JD, Moore S, et al. Six-year clinical experience with the implantable cardioverter defibrillator. PACE 1991; 14:1850–1854.
5. Fogoros RN, Elson JJ, Bonnet CA, Fiedler SB, Burkholder JA. Efficacy of the automatic implantable cardioverter-defibrillator in prolonging survival in patients with severe underlying cardiac disease. J Am Coll Cardiol 1990; 16:381–386.
6. Gabry MD, Brodman R, Johnston D, et al. Automatic implantable cardioverter-defibrillator: patient survival, battery longevity and shock delivery analysis. J Am Coll Cardiol 1987; 9:1349–1356.
7. Gartman DM, Bardy GH, Allen MD, Misbach GA, Ivey TD. Short-term morbidity and mortality of implantation of automatic implantable cardioverter-defibrillator. J Thorac Cardiovasc Surg 1990; 100:353–359.
8. Gohn D, Edel T, Pollard C, et al. Determinants of operative mortality in implantable cardioverter defibrillators. J Am Coll Cardiol 1991; 17:86A.
9. Hargrove WC III, Josephson ME, Marchlinski FE, Miller JM, Edmunds LH Jr. Surgical decisions in the management of sudden cardiac death and malignant ventricular arrhythmias. J Thorac Cardiovasc Surg 1989; 97:923–928.
10. Kelly PA, Cannom DS, Garan H, et al. The automatic implantable cardioverter-defibrillator: efficacy, complications and survival in patients with malignant ventricular arrhythmias. J Am Coll Cardiol 1988; 11:1278–1286.
11. Manolis AS, Rastegar H, Estes NAM III. Automatic implantable cardioverter defibrillator: current status. JAMA 1989; 262:1362–1368.
12. Marchlinski FE, Flores BT, Buxton AE, et al. The automatic implantable cardioverter-defibrillator: efficacy, complications, and device failures. Ann Intern Med 1986; 104:481–488.
13. Mercando A, Furman S, Johnston D, et al. Survival of patients with the automatic implantable cardioverter defibrillator. PACE 1988; 11:2059–2063.
14. Mirowski M, Reid PR, Winkle RA, et al. Mortality in patients with implanted automatic defibrillators. Ann Intern Med 1983; 98(part1):585–588.
15. Mirowski M. The automatic implantable cardioverter-defibrillator: an overview. J Am Coll Cardiol 1985; 6:461–466.
16. Mosteller RD, Lehrman MH, Thomas AC, et al. Operative mortality with implantation of the automatic cardioverter-defibrillator. Am J Cardiol 1991; 68:1340–1345.
17. Olinger GN, Chapman PD, Troup P, Alsmassi GH. Stratified application of the automatic implantable cardioverter defibrillator. J Thorac Cardiovasc Surg 1988; 96:141–149.
18. Palatianos, GM, Thurer RJ, Cooper DK, et al. The implantable cardioverter-defibrillator: clincial results. PACE 1991; 14:297–301.
19. Paull DL, Fellows CL, Guyton SW, Anderson RP. Early experience with the automatic implantable cardioverter defibrillator in sudden death survivors. Am J Surg 1989; 157:516–518.
20. Porterfield JG, Porterfield LM, Bray L. Long-term community hospital experience with the internal defibrillator. PACE 1991; 14:263–266.

21. Saksena S, Poczobutt-Johanos M, Castle LW, et al., for the Guardian Multicenter Investigators Group. Long-term multicenter experience with a second-generation implantable pacemaker-defibrillator in patients with malignant ventricular tachyarrhythmias. J Am Coll Cardiol 1992; 19:490–499.
22. Tchou PJ, Kardri N, Anderson J, Caceres JA, Jazayeri M, Akhtar M. Automatic implantable cardioverter defibrillators and survival of patients with left ventricular dysfunction and malignant ventricular arrhythmias. Ann Intern Med 1988; 109:529–534.
23. Thomas AC, Moser SA, Smutka ML, Wilson PA. Implantable defibrillation: eight years clinical experience. PACE 1988; 11:2053-2058.
24. Tresch DD, Troup PJ, Thakur RK, et al. Comparison of efficacy of automatic implantable cardioverter defibrillator in patients older and younger than 65 years of age. Am J Med 1991; 90:717-724.
25. Tullo NG, Saksena S, Krol RB, Mauro AM, Kunecz D. Management of complications associated with a first generation endocardial defibrillation lead system for implantable cardioverter-defibrillators. Am J Cardiol 1990; 66:411–415.
26. Winkle RA, Mead RH, Ruder MA, et al. Long-term outcome with the automatic implantable cardioverter-defibrillator. J Am Coll Cardiol 1989; 13:1353–1361.
27. Vlay SC. The automatic internal cardioverter-defibrillator: comprehensive clinical follow-up, economic and social impact—the Stony Brook experience. Am Heart J 1986; 112:189-194.
27a. Grimm W, Flores BF, Marchlinski FE. Complications of implantable cardioverter defibrillator therapy: follow-up of 241 patients. PACE 1993; 16:218–222.
28. Aliot E. Sadoul N, Poujois JN, Dodinot B, Pinelli G, Villemot JP. Does the transvenous approach for AICD decrease the risk of complications. Circulation 1992; 86:I-311.
29. Bardy GH, Hofer B, Johnson G, et al. Experience with transvenous defibrillators in 68 consecutive patients. Circulation 1992; 86:I-60.
30. Block M, Hammel D, Isbruch F, Bocker D, Wietholt D, Breithardt G. Three year experience with nonthoracotomy (NTL) defibrillation leads in 120 patients. Circulation 1992; 86:I-58.
31. CPI Endotak Clinical Summary Report Phase II. St. Paul, MN. Cardiac Pacemakers Inc., September 1992.
32. CPI Ventak PRx/Endotak Clinical Summary Report. St. Paul, MN. Cardiac Pacemakers, Inc., November 1992.
33. Herre JM, Bernstein RC, Klevan LR, Szentpetery S, Baker LD. Efficacy, safety and long-term follow-up of nonthoracotomy implantable cardioverter leads in patients with poor left ventricular function. J Am Coll Cardiol 1993; 21:67A.
34. Lehmann MH, Mitchell LB, Saksena S, Sakun V, the Worldwide PCD Investigators. Operative (30-day) mortality with transvenous vs. epicardial ICD implantation: an intention-to-treat analysis. Circulation 1992; 86:I-656.
35. McCowan R, Maloney J, Wilkoff B, et al. Automatic implantable cardioverter-defibrillator implantation without thoracotomy using and endocardial and submuscular patch system. J Am Coll Cardiol 1991; 17:415-421.
36. Moore SL, Maloney JD, Edel TB, et al. Implantable cardioverter defibrillator implanted by nonthoracotomy approach: initial clinical experience with the redesigned transvenous lead system. PACE 1991; 14:1865-1869.
37. Saksena S, Lehmann M, Mithcell LB, Sakun V. Device use and clinical results with a third-generation cardioverter-defibrillator using endocardial or epicardial leads. Circulation 1992; 86:I-60.
38. Suri RS, Woscoboinik JR, Maloney JD, et al. Non-thoracotomy transvenous leads and programmable implantable cardioverter defibrillators: technique, morbidity and outcome. J Am Coll Cardiol 1993; 21:126A.
39. Vendetti FJ, Martin DT, Shahian D. CPI Endotak nonthoracotomy lead system. In: Estes NAM III, Wang PJ, Manolis AS, eds. Implantable Cardioverter-Defibrillators: A Comprehensive Textbook. New York: Marcel Dekker, 1994.

40. Yee R, Klein GJ, Leitch JW, et al. A permanent transvenous lead system for an implantable pacemaker cardioverter-defibrillator: nonthoracotomy approach to implantation. Circulation 1992; 85:196–204.
40a. Trappe HJ, Klein H, Fieguth HG, Kielblock B, Wenzlaff P, Lichtlen PR. Initial experience with a new transvenous defibrillation system. PACE 1993; 16:134–140.
40b. Hauser RG, Kurschinski DT, McVeigh K, Thomas A, Mower MM. Clinical results with nonthoracotomy ICD systems. PACE 1993; 16:141–148.
40c. Frame R, Brodman R, Gross J, Hollinger I, et al. Initial experience with transvenous implantable cardioverter defibrillator lead systems: operative morbidity and mortality. PACE 1993; 16:149–152.
40d. Saksena S and the PCD Investigators and participating institutions. Defibrillation thresholds and perioperative mortality associated with endocardial and epicardial defibrillation lead systems. PACE 1993; 16:202–207.
41. Kim SG, Fisher JD, Choue CW, et al. Influence of left ventricular function on the outcome of patients treated with implantable defibrillators. Circulation 1992; 85:1304-1310.
42. Pinski SL, Sgarbossa EB, Maloney JD, Trohman RG. Survival in patients declining implantable cardioverter-defibrillators. Am J Cardiol 1991; 68:800-801.
43. Troester J, Auricchio A, Trappe HJ, Siclari F, Klein H. Risk and benefit of concomitant coronary artery bypass grafting during cardioverter/defibrillator implantation. PACE 1991; 14:II-718.
44. Trappe HJ, Daniel WC, Klein H, Frank G, Lichtlen P. Evaluation of global and regional left ventricular function using two-dimensional and M mode echo in patients with an automatic implantable cardioverter defibrillator. PACE 1988; 11:1070–1076.
45. Perlmutter RA, Rosenfelf LE, Elefteriades JA, Wackers FJT, Batsford WP. Implanted cardioverter-defibrillator patches do not impair diastolic function. Circulation 1992; 86:I-452.
46. Almassi GH, Chapman PD, Troup PJ, Wetherbee JN, Olinger GN. Constrictive pericarditis associated with patch electrodes of the automatic implantable cardioverter-defibrillator. Chest 1987; 92:369-371.
47. Goodman LR, Almassi GH, Troup PJ, et al. Complications of automatic implantable cardioverter defibrillators: radiographic, CT, and echocardiographic evaluation. Radiology 1989; 170:447-452.
48. Singer I, Hutchins GM, Mirowski M, et al. Pathologic findings related to the lead system and repeated defibrillations in patients with the automatic implantable cardioverter-defibrillator. J Am Coll Cardiol 1987; 10:383-388.
49. Mittleman RS, Mack K, Rastegar H, Manolis AS, Estes NAM III. Inappropriate shocks and elevation of defibrillation thresholds in a patient with automatic defibrillator patch Silastic erosion and titanium mesh fraying. PACE 1991; 14:1452-1455.
50. Lurie AL, Udoff EJ, Reid PJ. Automatic implantable cardioverter-defibrillator: appearance and complications. Am J Roentgenol 1985; 1145:723-725.
51. Becker DM, Philbrick JT, Walker FB IV. Axillary and subclavian venous thrombosis. Arch Intern Med 1991; 151:1934-1943.
52. Krebs TL, Austin JM. Colonic perforation: complication of automatic implantable cardioverter defibrillator placement. Radiology 1989; 172:708.
53. Mancini MC, Grubb BP. A technique for the prevention of automatic implantable cardioverter defibrillator generator migration. PACE 1990; 13:946–947.
54. Shahian DM, Williamson WA, Steitz JM Jr., Vendetti FJ. Subfascial implantation of implantable cardioverter defibrillator generator. Ann Thorac Surg 1991; 54:173-174.

22

Predischarge Testing of the Implantable Cardioverter-Defibrillator

Richard J. Lewis and Enrico P. Veltri

Sinai Hospital of Baltimore
Baltimore, Maryland

I. INTRODUCTION

Many physicians implanting an implantable cardioverter-defibrillator (ICD) perform a predischarge test of all implanted systems, while others retest selected patients only. Several rationales have been offered defending the need and value of predischarge testing. Those clinicians who advocate predischarge testing in all patients include the following arguments: (1) The defibrillation threshold (DFT) may have changed since the time of implant. (2) After lead placement, lead migration or fluid accumulation under epicardial patches may result in less efficient contact with the myocardium, thereby altering either sensing or defibrillating capabilities. (3) Exposing patients to a conscious shock may sensitize them to know "what to expect" and possibly "take the edge off" when they receive spontaneous shocks in the future. (4) Since, at many centers today, the only rhythm tested intraoperatively during ICD implantation is ventricular fibrillation (VF), if a patient's clinical arrhythmia is ventricular tachycardia (VT), the argument is made that all inducible clinical ventricular tachyarrhythmias must be evaluated before discharge, to test VT detection and termination. (5) In cases where VT termination algorithms other than high-energy shock are used, such as antitachycardia pacing or low-energy cardioversion, tiered-therapy efficacy must be confirmed if so programmed.

II. A RATIONAL APPROACH

In the opinion of the authors, the need for predischarge testing in *every* patient may not be necessary. When intraoperative DFT testing provides a "safety margin" of greater than 10 J, and no changes in antiarrhythmic therapy or postoperative complications such as acute myocardial infarction or congestive heart failure (which may alter the cardiac substrate) have occurred, predischarge ICD testing probably provides very little additional benefit. This is especially true if the patient's clinical arrhythmia is VF and the patient had no inducible ventricular tachyarrhythmias during preoperative electrophysiological testing. Similarly, if postoperative radiographs (which should be performed in all patients) reveal satisfactory lead position and no significant change in cardiac silhouette, potential problems such as lead migration, dislodgement, or significant pericardial effusion are extremely unlikely. Notwithstanding, if the device has already been activated, a spontaneous ICD discharge for VT/VF with conversion can serve as a surrogate predischarge test. If, however, antiarrhythmic therapy has been altered (in particular, by the addition of a class IC or class III agent, which may alter DFT or VT cycle length), or the patient has a clinical VT which is inducible and for which the device will be programmed to detect and terminate by either antitachycardia pacing or low-energy cardioversion, then predischarge ICD detection and conversion testing is mandatory [1].

There are few studies evaluating the use of predischarge ICD testing. If intraoperative DFT testing reveals high DFT (with less that a 10-J safety margin between maximum programmed ICD output and the DFT), predischarge testing to reassess defibrillation capability by the device is prudent. Marchlinski et al. have shown that postoperative testing may be unsuccessful in as many as 27% of the latter cases [2]. These investigators, importantly, showed that with a 10-J or greater "safety margin," the chance of successful defibrillation during predischarge testing was essentially 100%. Schamp et al. noted that VF was not reverted in 6 of 83 (7%) of patients in their series [3]. Only one of these patients had a DFT > 20 J. Both of these studies were performed in patients undergoing thoracotomy ICD implantation, and in some patients with concomitant revascularization. Data available from an investigational nonthoracotomy, transvenous ICD (Endotak, Cardiac Pacemakers, Inc.) has shown nonconversion in 3% (12 of 403) and nondetection in 0.7% (3 of 403) of patients at predischarge testing [4]. In our own personal experience with the latter lead system, we have noted 1 of 50 consecutive patients (2%) with nonconversion at predischarge testing. This patient was on amiodarone at postoperative testing; subsequent discontinuation of the drug and retesting confirmed satisfactory function.

III. PREDISCHARGE ICD TESTING PROCEDURE

In patients in whom a predischarge testing procedure has been recommended, the following procedure is suggested. Patients are taken to the electrophysiology laboratory in a fasting, and usually mildly sedated, state. Routine surface ECG leads (1, AVF, V_1, and V_5 in our laboratory) for monitoring and R_2 pads are placed in an anterior-posterior orientation. A donut magnet is used to confirm appropriate baseline rhythm detection in those devices which have this capability. The ICD is programmed to the testing or "EP" mode. A temporary pacing catheter is guided fluoroscopically via venous access to the right ventricle if epicardial pacing leads are not present, or if noninvasive programmed ventricular stimulation via the device is not an option. In several of the latest-generation ICD devices with antitachycardia pacing, built-in noninvasive programmed stimulation protocols may alleviate the need for placement of a temporary pacing catheter. Care must be exercised to avoid dislodgement of recently placed endocardial ICD sensing and defibrillating leads. The tip of the temporary pacing catheter should also be at least 2 cm from these other leads to prevent shunting of current during ICD shocks.

If the ICD has backup bradycardia pacing capability, sensing and capture thresholds should be measured at this time and compared to values obtained during the implantation of the device. Increased pacing thresholds or inappropriate sensing may indicate migration of the lead system, lead fracture, effects of anti-arrhythmic therapy, etc. Routine fluoroscopy of the lead system in the electrophysiology laboratory at this time may be extremely useful. Also, if the patient has a permanent pacemaker, this should be programmed to an asynchronous mode (i.e., VOO or DOO) with maximal outputs for the purpose of ensuring no adverse ICD–pacemaker interaction. Permanent pacemakers can revert to these modes following an ICD shock, so reassessing pacemaker function after conversion testing is also warranted [5].

The ICD should be programmed to desired sensing parameters (heart rate cut off, probability density function, detection delays, committed versus noncommitted mode, and detection enhancements available), as well as to the therapy mode (antitachycardia pacing schemes, low-energy cardioversion outputs, and defibrillation energy). The termination strategy should be clearly defined in the programming of the device, as well as communicated to the electrophysiology laboratory staff, with guidelines as to anticipated response if external intervention is required.

The patient is then informed that arrhythmia induction will commence, and anxiety is allayed. Next, sustained VT or VF is induced using a programmed stimulator or alternating current, and the ICD is reprogrammed from "EP" mode to active mode and given the opportunity to detect and terminate the tachyarrhythmia. If VF is being induced by alternating current, sedation is frequently desired. As many patients may experience temporary apnea postshock, pulse oximetry may be useful in addition to the more routine monitoring. When available, marker channels providing real-time telemetry from the ICD should be recorded, as these may be particularly helpful in troubleshooting. In the authors' experience, up to two defibrillation shocks from the ICD will be permitted before attempting "rescue" with an external defibrillator (starting at 200 J, then 360–400 J if necessary).

With satisfactory detection and conversion testing confirmed, the patient is reassured, the device programmed active to the desired parameters, and the patient discharged shortly thereafter (usually within 24 h). If nondetection or nonconversion emerges, however, troubleshooting the problem using a logical methodology ensues. This is discussed by the authors in Chapter 27.

REFERENCES

1. Lehman MH, Saksena S. Implantable cardioverter defibrillators in cardiovascular practice: report of the Policy Conference of the North American Society of Pacing and Electrophysiology. PACE 1991; 14:969–979.
2. Marchlinski FE, Flores B, Miller JM, Gottlieb CD, Hargrove WC. Relation of the intraoperative defibrillation threshold to successful postoperative defibrillation with an automatic implantable cardioverter-defibrillator. Am J Cardiol 1988; 62:393–398.
3. Schamp DJ, Langberg JJ, Lesh MD, Witherell CL, Scheinman MM, Griffin JC. Post-implant/pre-discharge automatic implantable defibrillator testing: is it mandatory? PACE 1990; 13:510.
4. Endotak FDA Premarket Approval Application, Cardiac Pacemakers, Inc., February, 1992.
5. Calkins H, Brinker J, Veltri EP, Guarnieri T, Levine JH. Clinical interactions between pacemakers and implantable defibrillators. J Am Coll Cardiol 1990; 16:666–673.

23

Antiarrhythmic Drug Use in the Implantable Cardioverter-Defibrillator Patient

Stephanie K. Stevens and N. A. Mark Estes III

*Tufts University School of Medicine
and New England Medical Center
Boston, Massachusetts*

I. INTRODUCTION

The use of the implantable cardioverter-defibrillator (ICD) in patients with serious ventricular arrhythmias is often combined with other treatment modalities, including antiarrhythmic agents and pacemakers. Potential interaction between these modalities has become increasingly important with the introduction and success of the ICD. This chapter will review antiarrhythmic drug use in patients with ICDs, with special emphasis on alteration of defibrillation and pacing thresholds. Conditions that increase defibrillation or pacing thresholds can lead to device failure. Alternatively, device efficacy may improve if these thresholds are reduced.

II. INTERACTIONS BETWEEN PHARMACOLOGICAL AGENTS AND ICDS

A. Introduction

Successful electrical defibrillation of the heart is dependent on many factors, including the type of defibrillating electrodes, the electrical waveform of the defibrillating pulse, the duration of ventricular fibrillation (VF) before a defibrillating pulse is applied, and the presence of antiarrhythmic drugs or substances that alter cardiac electrophysiological properties.

Fifty to 70% of ICD patients require one or more antiarrhythmic drugs. Antiarrhythmic and other cardiovascular agents frequently are necessary for controlling nonsustained ventricular tachycardia (VT), minimizing the frequency of episodes of sustained VT, control of maximum sinus rate, and control of supraventricular tachycardias (SVT) [1,3,4,6]. Table 1 summarizes the pharmacological drug requirements of ICD patients from reports published by Winkle et al. [1], Echt et al., [3], and Huang et al.[4].

Table 1 Concomitant Pharmacological Drug Therapy in ICD patients

Reference Pharmacological agent	[1] Patient (%)	[3] Patient (%)	[4] Patient (%)
Amiodarone	61 (23)	19 (27)	25 (47)
Amiodarone + class I	10 (4)	3 (4)	
Beta-blocker	19 (7)	11 (16)	
Calcium blocker	3 (1)		
Ca^{2+} + beta-blockers	1 (0.4)		
Digoxin	102 (38)		
Digoxin + beta-blocker	11 (4)		
Digoxin + Ca^{2+} blocker	11 (4)		
Disopyramide		1 (1.5)	
Encainide			1 (2)
Flecainide	3 (1)		
Lorcainide	3 (1)	1 (1.5)	
Mexiletine	12 (4)	2 (3)	2 (4)
Mexiletine + class IA	13 (5)	3 (4)	2 (4)
Procainamide	22 (8)	3 (4)	3 (6)
Propafenone	18 (7)	2 (4)	
Quinidine	10 (4)	2 (3)	3 (6)
Quinidine + propafenone			1 (2)
Sotalol	22 (8)		
Tocainide	9 (3)	1 (1.5)	
Other	3 (1)	2 (3)	
Total (antiarrhythmic)	186 (69)	37 (53)	39 (74)
Total (AV blockers)	147 (55)	11 (16)	
Total patients studied	270	70	53

B. Types of Drug Effects on ICD Function

Antiarrhythmic agents can have both beneficial and deleterious influences on arrhythmias and defibrillation energy requirements [7–10]. Class IB and IC antiarrhythmic agents prolong cardiac conduction time with little effect on refractoriness. These agents tend to increase defibrillation energy requirements [8,11–13] and thus have the potential to lead to device failure if the maximum available energy is insufficient for defibrillation. Class III drugs prolong cardiac action potential and refractoriness but do not affect cardiac conduction. These agents tend to decrease defibrillation energy requirements, thus improving device effectiveness [10,14–16].

In addition to alteration of defibrillation energy requirements, antiarrhythmic agents influence other pertinent electrophysiological characteristics of arrhythmias and thus influence ICD efficacy [6,17]. These effects are summarized in Table 2. One example of a deleterious effect is slowing of the VT rate below the rate cutoff of the ICD. Marchlinski reported three patients out of 26 with ICDs who had electrocardiographically documented spontaneous episodes of VT that did not trigger the cardioverter-defibrillator because the rates were below the rate criterion for triggering the device. All three were treated with amiodarone (800 mg/day) for more than 3 months at the time of the tachycardia. One of the three was asymptomatic, but the other two had arrhythmias that caused syncope or increasing heart failure. In one case the amiodarone dose was decreased, and in the other mexiletine was added to prevent recurrence of the slow VT [18].

Table 2 Pharmacological Effects on ICD Function[a]

Beneficial effects	Deleterious effects
Decrease in DFT	Increase in DFT
Decreased frequency of SVT, nonsustained and sustained VT or VF and subsequent device discharge	Double counting of signals due to slowed conduction and ventricular electrogram widening
Control of maximum sinus or SVT rate to prevent satisfaction of rate criteria for device discharge	Change in QRS morphology during SVT, resulting in the satisfaction of PDF criteria for VT
Decreased VT rate to allow successful termination by ATP	Increase in VT cycle length below the rate cutoff
Decreased VT rate to prevent syncope prior to delivery of ICD therapy	Decrease in VT cycle length, resulting in more frequent need for defibrillation rather than ATP
	Increase in the frequency of VT (proarrhythmic effect), resulting in more frequent device discharge
	Change from sustained to nonsustained VT, resulting in inappropriate shocks from committed ICDs during nonsustained VT
	Alteration in postshock excitability, leading to prolonged pauses
	Increase in pacing threshold

[a]ATP = antitachycardia pacing.

C. Defibrillation Threshold (DFT)

The effects of drugs on DFTs has led to a growing field of research. Many studies report conflicting results. These discrepancies are due to a variety of methodological differences, such as different drug dosages; the duration of VF before a defibrillating pulse is delivered; the pulse waveform characteristics; interspecies differences; a variety of both external and internal defibrillating electrode systems; and varying methodologies for measurement of the DFT.

DFT is a concept that characterizes the efficacy of the defibrillation discharge. It implies a clear-cut distinction between uniformly effective and ineffective energies. Defibrillation energy requirements are influenced by numerous variables, including pulse waveform and duration; electrode size, position, and configuration; body and heart weight, impedance; ischemic injury; and drug administration [19].

Numerous methods for defining DFT have been described [9,11,12,19]. Uniform sequential procedures use either decremental (step-down) or incremental (step-up) energy levels and define DFT as the energy that defibrillates the heart. Other investigators use repetitive trials to show uniform success at one threshold value. Another is an averaging method that averages successive threshold determinations. Others use a probability-of-success method that defines DFT as a statistical event where higher energies have greater probability of success. The probability-of-success method expresses data as a sigmoidal dose–response defibrillation curve derived from logistic regression analysis and shows a relationship between a gradual increase in success from 0% to 100% over several energy increments for multiple trials where energy levels are tested in random order.

Although construction of a sigmoidal-shaped dose–response curve is scientifically more precise for animal studies, construction of the curves requires multiple defibrillation trials at various energy levels. Construction of such curves is not only time consuming but is not practical for either human research or as a routine procedure during ICD implantation. Rather, an electrode configuration that provides a high probability of successful defibrillation by 15-J pulses leaves a sufficient safety margin between the DFT and the maximum energy output of the ICD.

Table 3 summarizes the effects of pharmacological agents on DFTs reported by several authors. The disparity among these observations underscores the need for additional study as well as uniform methods of determining energy requirements within species. The way antiarrhythmic drugs influence the electrophysiological properties of arrhythmias and defibrillation energy requirements are important considerations in ICD patients. Furthermore, in patients with marginal defibrillation threshold safety margins, substances that are known to increase the threshold should be avoided. Otherwise, one must check the ICD's ability to terminate an induced arrhythmia.

In addition to pharmacological influences on defibrillation energy requirements, variation in the autonomic state of the heart is an important modulator of cardiac defibrillation threshold. Ruffy et al. [20] demonstrated a decrease in defibrillation energy requirements with beta-adrenergic stimulation of the heart by isoproterenol. This effect is partially blocked by propranolol.

D. Class I Agents

The antiarrhythmic drugs in class I share the dominant electrophysiological property of blocking the fast inward sodium current during depolarization of the cardiac membrane. A reduction in the rate of rise of the action potential or in membrane responsiveness is accompanied by a decrease in conduction velocity together with an increase in the threshold of excitability and in the effective refractory period of the cardiac muscle. In contrast, the action potential duration may either shorten or lengthen, although not to an extent that might alter the absolute refractory period. Table 4 summarizes the data published on the effects of Class I agents on DFTs. The following summarizes selected studies by specific agent.

1. Quinidine

The effect of quinidine on defibrillation thresholds appears to be dose or concentration related, with increases in defibrillation energy requirements only at high plasma or myocardial concentrations and no effect at the concentrations usually achieved in patients treated with quinidine. Babbs et al. [8] reported a marked increase in transthoracic DFT after high doses of quinidine were used in a canine model. In this study quinidine gluconate (50 mg quinidine base/kg) increased threshold peak current by 70% and threshold delivery energy by 172%. The dose of quinidine was sufficient to cause a drop in mean arterial blood pressure from 140 to 73 mmHg [8]. Plasma concentrations were not reported, but these doses are far in excess of therapeutic doses. Likewise, Woolfolk et al. [21] reported that quinidine gluconate (12 to

Table 3 Alteration of Defibrillation Threshold (DFT) by Pharmacological Agents[a]

Agent	Effect on DFT	Reference
Class I		
Quinidine	↑	8,15,21
	↔	9
Procainamide	↔	7,14
N-acetylprocainamide	↓	14
Phenytoin	↑	8
Lidocaine	↑	8,11,14,22–24
	↔	23,24
Mexiletine	↑	25*
Bidisomide	↑	26
Encainide	↑	12
ODE (o-desmethyl encainide)	↑	12
	↔	27
MODE (3-methyl-ODE)	↔	12
Flecainide acetate	↑	13
Propafenone	↑	28
Class II		
Propranolol	↔	7
	↑	20
Class III		
Amiodarone—acute	↔	33,36
	↓	35,38
Amiodarone—chronic	↑	29*,30*,31*,32–34,37
	↔	4*,35,38
Bretylium tosylate	↓	10
	↔	9,23,40
Clofilium phosphate	↓	10,15,39
Sotalol	↓	15,16
Other		
Digoxin	↔	7,50

[a] ↑, increased; ↓, decreased; ↔, no change; *, human study.

40 mg/kg) in pentobarbitol-anesthetized, closed-chest dogs resulted in fewer successful transthoracic defibrillations at a given shock energy. Higher shock energies were necessary to terminate VF after the administration of quinidine. In contrast, Dorian et al. [9], using a canine model, administered quinidine gluconate as two loading and maintenance infusions to achieve mean plasma concentrations usually observed in patients on chronic oral therapy (2.4–2.9 µg/mL). The quinidine had no significant effect on the energy required to achieve 50% and 90% success in defibrillation (E_{50} and E_{90}).

2. Lidocaine

Babbs et al [8] reported that an intravenous bolus of Lidocaine (3 mg/kg) in a canine model raised the maximal elevation of threshold current by 26% and maximal elevation of threshold energy by 48%. A continuous infusion of lidocaine (0.5 mg/kg/min) caused a steady increase in threshold to a maximum of 199% of control energy and 145% of control current after 80 minutes. Mean arterial blood pressure fell from 137 at the beginning to 119 mmHg at the end

Table 4 Effects of Antiarrhythmic Agents on Defibrillation Thresholds (DFT)

Agent	Reference	Dosage	Effect on DFT	Comments
Quinidine	8[1]	50 mg/kg as a single dose	↑ by 172%	VF for less than 30 s; step-down procedure; drug-free controls
Quinidine	21[1]	200 mg; 1–3 doses given	↑	VF for 6 s; compares success at a given energy after each dose
Quinidine	9[1]	10 mg/kg for 2 doses as a loading dose, then 20 or 40 mg/kg/min for maintenance	↔ in E_{50} (6.3→6.2 J); ↔ in E_{90} (8.3→8.3 J)	Dose–response curve; plasma concentration of 2.4–3.0 μg/kL
Quinidine	15[1]	10 mg/kg	↔	Compared with saline controls
Procainamide	7[2]	15 mg/kg	↔	VF for 15 s; step-up procedure; therapeutic levels
Procainamide	14[1]	15 mg/kg plus 5 mg/kg as a loading dose, then 2–3 mg/min for maintenance	↔	VF for 5 and 30 s; dose–response curves; plasma levels 8.5–13 μg/mL
NAPA	14[1]	8.5–68 mg/kg as a sequential loading dose, then 50–400 μg/kg/min for maintenance	↓ in E_{50} (11→8 J); ↓ in E_{90} (15→11 J)	Dose–response curves; class III properties also exhibited
Encainide	12[1]	Titrated for 20–50% widening of the QRS	↑ in E_{50} by 129%; ↑ in E_{80} by 104%	VF for 15 s; dose–response curves; saline controls; DFT returns to baseline E_{50} after 1-h washout
ODE	12[1]	Titrated for 20–50% widening of the QRS	↑ in E_{50} by 76%; ↑ in E_{80} by 46%	VF for 15 s; dose–response curves; saline controls; DFT returns to baseline E_{50} after 1-h washout
MODE	12[1]	Titrated for 20–50% widening of the QRS	↔	VF for 15 s, dose–response curves; saline controls
Flecainide	13[1]	1 mg/kg as a single dose followed by 0.032 mg/kg/min for 50 min, then 0.028 mg/kg/min for 30 min, then 0.021 mg/kg/min	↑ in E_{50} by 75% (6.5→11.4 J); ↑ in E_{80} by 59% (8.1→12.9 J)	VF for 10 s; dose–response curves; saline controls; uniform infusion adjusted to maintain mean plasma levels of 610 ng/mL

Drug	Ref	Dose	Effect	Comments
Propafenone	28[1]	2 mg/kg as a loading dose, then 1 mg/min or 25 μg/kg/min for maintenance	↑ in E_{50} by 75% (8.4→14.7 J); ↑ in E_{80} by 59% (11.1→17.6 J)	VF for 10 s; dose–response curves; Ringer's controls; therapeutic plasma levels
Amiodarone	35[1], 38[1]	10 mg/kg followed by 0.3 mg/kg/min for 10 min as a loading dose, followed by 300 mg b.i.d. for 21 days for chronic therapy	Acute; ↓ in E_{50} by 22% (4.5→3.5 J); ↓ in E_{80} by 20% (5.8→4.6 J)	VF for 15 s; dose–response curves; plasma levels 4.6–9.9 μg/mL
Amiodarone	33[1], 36[1]	5 mg/kg as a loading dose, followed by either 200 or 400 mg q.d. for 9 days	Acute; ↔ after 2 h (10.8→10.8 J); chronic (200 mg/day): ↑ (7.5→15.4 J); chronic (400 mg/day): ↑ (7.5→17.9 J)	VF for 20–80 s, step up procedure
Amiodarone	32[1]	10 mg/kg as a single dose	↑ by 32%	VF for 40 s or less; DFT defined as mid-range value between maximum current that did not defib and minimum current that did defib; DFT determined 15 min after drug given Uniform-sequential procedure
Amiodarone	37[1]	400 mg q.d. for 3 weeks	↑ after 2 weeks and after at least 50 s of VF	
Amiodarone	29[3]	296 g cumulative dose	↑ (11→20 J)	VF for 15 s; step-down procedure; DFT is the lowest energy that terminates VF; compares DFT before and after amiodarone
Amiodarone	30[3]	Not reported	↑ (9→15 J)	VF for 5–10 s; step-down procedure; comparison of patients on amiodarone with drug-free patients
Amiodarone	4[3]	400 mg q.d.	↔ (12→12 J)	VF for 10 s or more; step-down procedure; comparison of patients on amiodarone with drug-free patients

Table 4 (*Continued*)

Agent	Reference	Dosage	Effect on DFT	Comments
Amiodarone	31[3]	1200 mg q.d. for 7 days, then 600 mg q.d.	↑ (10→40 J)	One patient refractory to defibrillation on amiodarone could be defibrillated 3 months after drug was stopped; step-up procedure
Clofilium	14[1]	0.3 mg/kg for 2 doses	↓ in E_{50} (9→8 J; $p<0.05$);	VF for 10 s; dose–response curves
Clofilium	39[1]	100 mg q.d. for 16 days	↓ in E_{50} by 39% within 1 week of therapy	Dose–response curves; compared treated with drug-free dogs
Clofilium	10[1]	0.34 mg/kg as a single dose	↓ by 54%	VF for 30 s; sequential procedure; compared treated with drug-free dogs
Clofilium	15[1]	0.5 mg/kg	↓ by 39% after 1 min	saline controls
Bretylium	9[1]	6 mg/kg or 10 mg/kg	↔ in E_{50} (5.3→6.1 J); ↔ in E_{90} (7.2→8.6 J)	VF for 15 s; dose–response curves
Bretylium	23[1]	5 mg/kg for 2 doses	↔ (60→58 J)	VF for 15 s; step-down procedure; tested at 30 min intervals up to 120 min
Bretylium	40[1]	10 mg/kg or 30 mg/kg	↔ (0.7→0.8 J/kg)	VF from 4–30 s; step-down procedure; tested 1 min after drug given and then at 15 to 30-min intervals up to 5.5 h
Bretylium	10[1]	10 mg/kg	↓ by 31% 15 min after infusion; effect persisted for 3 h	VF for 30 s; sequential procedure

of the lidocaine infusion. Echt et al. [22] also reported an increase in defibrillation energy requirements by lidocaine at normal pH levels. This effect is enhanced with acidosis and reversed by alkalosis.

Dorian et al. [11] showed that lidocaine causes a reversible concentration-dependent increase on the internal defibrillation energy requirement in 20 pentobarbital-anesthetized dogs, before and after treatment. He reported a 61% increase in the mean energy required to achieve 50% success in defibrillation (E_{50}) and a 47% increase to achieve 90% success (E_{90}) at a steady-state lidocaine concentration of 5.6 µg/mL. He also showed that mean energy requirements positively correlated with lidocaine concentration ranging from 1.95 to 9.8 µg/mL, and returned to baseline after drug washout when lidocaine concentration declined to 1.8 µg/mL.

The effects of anesthetic agents on defibrillation threshold are addressed elsewhere, but at least two reports of anesthesia-related differences in lidocaine's effect on DFT were reported by Kerber et al. [23] and Natale et al. [24]. Kerber et al. [23] reported an increase in the energy required for defibrillation by lidocaine, but the effect was dependent on the anesthetic used. In their study, lidocaine (4 mg/kg bolus followed by 0.2 mg/kg/min (first hour) and 0.4 mg/kg/min (second hour) produced a 60% dose-related increase in transthoracic DFT in pentobarbital-anesthetized dogs but no significant change in DFT in chloralose-anesthetized dogs [23]. Lidocaine levels produced by these dosages were in the high therapeutic to toxic range. Similarly, Natale et al. [24] reported no difference in DFT in halothane-anesthetized pigs after lidocaine administration to yield plasma levels considered therapeutic for both humans and pigs. However, a significant increase in DFTs was observed in pentobarbital-anesthetized pigs.

3. Mexiletine

A human case report by Marinchak et al. [25] suggested that mexiletine caused an important increase in DFT after controlling for confounding variables such as hypokalemia and ischemia.

4. Bidisomide

Bidisomide is a new class IA/IB antiarrhythmic agent currently under investigation [26]. In a canine infarct model, therapeutic and supratherapeutic doses of bidisomide increase the energy requirements for successful defibrillation using a modified defibrillation probability curve with decrementing energy levels.

5. Encainide

Fain et al. [12] showed that encainide and its *o*-demethylated metabolite, *o*-demethyl-encainide (ODE) produced large increases in internal defibrillation energy requirements for 50% successful defibrillation (E_{50}) in 25 pentobarbital-anesthetized, open-chest dogs. Encainide, ODE, or another major encainide metabolite, 3-methoxy-ODE (MODE), were infused in loading and maintenance doses (encainide, 100–200 and 50–75 µg/kg/min, ODE 20–35 and 7.5–15 µg/kg/min, and MODE 50 and 20–25 µg/kg/min, respectively) to achieve QRS widening of 20–50%. After administration of encainide and ODE, the E_{50} increased by 129% and 76% and E_{80} increased by 104% and 46%, respectively. These effects were reversible upon drug discontinuation and washout. No significant increase in E50 was observed after administration of MODE. QRS interval prolongation of 20–50% is comparable to that seen in clinical studies examining short-term intravenous and long-term oral encainide. However, in this study the plasma drug concentrations were considerably higher than are normally seen in humans.

Another study reported by Dawson et al. [27] found increased defibrillation energy requirements at high plasma levels of ODE.

6. Flecainide

Hernandez et al. [13] showed that flecainide infusion that produced mean plasma levels of 610 ng/mL increased E_{50} by 75% from 6.5 to 11.4 J and E_{80} by 59% from 8.1 to 12.9 J in an open-chest, anesthetized canine model. These levels were considered to be reasonable and therapeutic in animals and humans.

7. Propafenone

Propafenone exhibits both class IC and class II beta-blocking activity. Peters et al. [28] reported a 75% increase in the energy required for 50% success in defibrillation (E_{50}) and a 59% increase in the energy required for 80% success (E_{80}) when compared with control dogs. Propafenone-treated dogs received a loading dose of 2 mg/kg over 10 min followed by a maintenance dose yielding plasma levels considered in the therapeutic range (1400 ng/mL). No significant blood pressure changes were noted.

E. Class II Agents

Deeb et al. [7] reported that propranolol (0.2 mg/kg) did not alter internal defibrillation energy requirements in dogs. Ruffy et al. [20] reported that larger doses of propranolol (0.2–0.6 mg/kg) raised internal DFT.

F. Class III Agents

Table 4 summarizes the data published on the effects of class III agents on DFTs. The following summarizes selected studies by specific agents.

1. Amiodarone

Amiodarone is a drug with complex pharmacological properties, including prolongation of action potential duration and the refractory periods of all cardiac tissue without changing resting membrane potential (a class III effect) and slowing of cardiac conduction (a class I effect). It also exhibits class II and class IV activity.

Previous observations of patients taking amiodarone at the time of the ICD implantation yield conflicting DFT data. Numerous studies report significant elevation of defibrillation thresholds that decrease the safety margin for successful defibrillation [29–34]. Others have not shown an increase in DFT [4,35,36]. In addition, the extent to which acute intravenous amiodarone loading influences DFTs is less clear.

Frame et al. [33,36] reported dose-dependent increases in internal DFT following chronic amiodarone administration in two groups of dogs that received either 200 or 400 mg daily for 9 days. Oral amiodarone significantly raised the DFT in a dose-dependent manner. No change in DFT was observed within 2 h after intravenous administration of 5 mg/kg amiodarone infused over 10 min.

Fogoros [31] reported a case where a patient chronically treated with amiodarone could not be defibrillated with a 40-J shock during ICD implantation. Internal defibrillation was accomplished with a 10-J shock using the original implanted electrode system 3 months after the drug was discontinued.

Haberman et al. [34,37] also reported an increase in DFT with oral amiodarone. Nine dogs fed amiodarone 400 mg/day for 1, 2, and 3 weeks were compared to three drug-free dogs. DFT was determined in a uniform sequential manner and defined as the lowest successful initial energy level. A statistically significant increase in DFT was found at 2 and 3 weeks when VF was allowed to persist for 50 s prior to defibrillation. Serum and tissue amiodarone levels, desethylamiodarone, and reverse T3 were not predictive of DFTs in that study.

A report by Troup et al. [30] of 41 patients undergoing ICD implantation also found amiodarone to be independently associated with a significantly higher DFT compared with patients not receiving the drug and regardless of lead configuration.

Arrendondo et al. [32] found that amiodarone, 10 mg/kg I.V., elevated DFT by 32%. These investigators also reported a 124% increase in the ventricular fibrillation threshold.

In contrast, Huang et al. [4] reported no difference in the DFT among 28 patients on chronic amiodarone therapy with a mean daily dose of 406 mg (range of 200–800 mg daily) for a mean duration of 6.0 months (range of 1–36 months) when compared to 32 patients not taking amiodarone at the time of ICD implantation.

Fain et al. [35,38] reported a 22% decrease in E_{50} and 20% decrease in E_{80} in dogs after acute administration of amiodarone, 10 mg/kg, as a loading dose and 10 min of a 0.03-mg/kg/min maintenance dose. Chronic therapy (300 mg b.i.d.) had no effect on DFTs after 7, 14, or 21 days of treatment.

2. Clofilium Phosphate

Clofilium is a class III agent that is not currently available for general use. Its properties are similar to those of bretylium tosylate. Tacker et al. [10] showed that canine transthoracic ventricular defibrillation threshold decreased by 54% 15–150 min after a large dose (0.34 mg/kg) of intravenous clofilium.

Dorian et al. [39] studied the effect of clofilium, 100 mg/day, on defibrillation energy requirements and ventricular effective refractory periods in a canine model over 3 weeks using epicardial patch electrodes and fentanyl anesthesia. E_{50} was determined on days 7 (baseline), 14, 21, and 28 after surgery in six clofilium-treated dogs and six control dogs. In the clofilium-treated dogs, long-term oral clofilium lowered defibrillation energy requirements and increased ventricular refractoriness within 1 week of therapy. These effects persisted during the 3-week treatment period.

Dawson et al. [15] reported a significant, 39% decrease in internal defibrillation energy requirements in anesthetized dogs that received intravenous clofilium (0.5 mg/kg) when compared with saline controls.

3. Bretylium Tosylate

Tacker et al. [10] reported substantial declines in canine transthoracic defibrillation energy requirements after 10 mg/kg of bretylium tosylate. Energy requirements decreased by 31% 15 min after infusion. This effect persisted for 3 h.

Despite using similar protocols, Kerber and Koo failed to demonstrate changes with administration of up to 30 mg/kg of bretylium [23,40]. These authors also noted marked changes in heart rate and blood pressure following drug that were not as pronounced in Tacker et al.'s study [10].

Likewise, Dorian et al. [9] showed that 6 and 10 mg/kg of bretylium did not affect the relation between energy and the likelihood of successful defibrillation. The mean energy required to achieve 50% success (E_{50}) or 90% success (E_{90}) in defibrillation was not altered significantly.

4. Sotalol

Sotalol is a unique antiarrhythmic agent with both class II and class III electrophysiological effects. Dawson et al. [15] reported a significant, 29% decrease in internal defibrillation energy requirement in anesthetized dogs treated with d-sotalol (5 mg/kg) when compared to saline controls. Likewise, Wang et al. [16] studied the acute effects of intravenous DL-/ and D-sotalol on the energy requirements for internal defibrillation in 44 anesthetized dogs. Sotalol was administered in a loading bolus of 4 mg/kg over 10 min and a maintenance infusion of 1.5 mg/kg/h to yield mean plasma levels of 4.6 µg/mL. Dose–response curves were measured at 30 min after drug administration. Both DL-/ and D-sotalol significantly lowered the E_{50} (energy requirements for 50% success) by 16% and 25%, respectively. This was accompanied by 22% and 16% increases in ventricular effective refractory period. A decrease in E_{80} was not statistically significant. In addition to lowering the energy requirement for defibrillation, the authors noted that VF became more difficult to induce and, in some instances, reverted spontaneously to normal sinus rhythm.

III. INFLUENCE OF PHARMACOLOGICAL AGENTS AND ICD DISCHARGE ON PACING THRESHOLD

Four to 14% of patients with ICDs also require permanent bradycardia pacemaker support [2,41]. Potential and known adverse interactions between ICDs and pacemakers include: VF nondetection and inappropriate ICD inhibition; oversensing of paced rhythms leading to possible inappropriate ICD discharge; and altered pacemaker function due to defibrillation discharge [3,18,42,43]. Further information regarding these interactions is reviewed elsewhere in this volume. In addition to these interactions, both the ICD discharge and pharmacological agents can alter pacing threshold.

For ICD patients who require pharmacological agents for arrhythmia control and bradycardia pacing support, an increase in pacing threshold with loss of ventricular capture presents a serious clinical problem. Cohen et al. [42] analyzed pacemaker function after 30 episodes of ICD discharge for VT or VF. The immediate rhythm was paced in 10, ventricular in 18, and supraventricular in 2. Lack of ventricular capture was observed in 8 of 22 episodes. The mean duration of lack of capture was 5 s. One patient had no capture for up to 16 s after discharge. Pacemaker waveform analysis revealed no change in the pre- to postdischarge trailing-to-leading-edge ratios or voltage amplitudes, implying that the problem was not in the pacemaker or the lead. No differences in ventricular pacing thresholds were noted 3 min after discharge [42].

Studies by Yee et al. [44] have shown that pacing capture thresholds may double and R-wave amplitudes may halve when electrodes were used for both defibrillation and pacing. In this study, abnormalities persisted for up to 10 min when 5–50 J were delivered. Yee postulated that polarization of the electrodes, gas bubble formation, or electrical injury to the myocardium may be the mechanism of amplitude and threshold changes.

Guarnieri et al. [45] reported a transient loss of ventricular capture during asynchronous ventricular pacing after a 30-J ICD shock was delivered in dogs. The duration of capture loss was related to current strength. During endocardial pacing at threshold current, the time to capture was 5 s, whereas at current levels twice threshold the time to capture from endocardial pacing was 2.2 s. No difference was found between endocardial and epicardial pacing sites in the time to capture.

In contrast, Khastgir et al. [46] studied epicardial ventricular pacing thresholds and time to capture postdefibrillation in humans. In 28 patients with ICDs, no significant difference compared to baseline was found in pacing threshold at 10 s, 60 s, and 3 min after internal defibrillation with 20 J. In addition, no significant difference was seen between drug-free patients and those receiving amiodarone.

Change in pacing threshold has been reported for many pharmacological agents. For ICD patients who require both bradycardia pacing support and antiarrhythmic drug therapy, these interactions are clinically relevant. Furman reviewed this subject and reported that drug administration has little sustained effect on pacing threshold. Even where a pronounced immediate effect occurs, sustained drug administration is accompanied by gradual return to the pretreatment baseline over several hours [47]. In contrast, Hellestrand et al. [48] reported up to a 200% increase in chronic endocardial pacing thresholds in patients receiving oral flecainide. Guarieri et al. [45] noted the time to capture from endocardial pacing was significantly prolonged, 14.9 s at the threshold value and 5.6 s at twice threshold, after an infusion of flecainide yielding mean serum levels of 1.0 mg/L. Hernandez et al. [13] reported that pacing thresholds at cycle length of 300 ms were not significantly different between dogs receiving a flecainide infusion with mean plasma levels of 0.6 mg/mL and saline controls. However, pacing threshold increased after baseline defibrillation determination and flecainide significantly increased pacing threshold (3.10 V versus 6.18 V). Slepian et al. [49] reported a case of failure to capture of a VVI pacemaker in the postshock period during routine ICD DFT testing in a patient on chronic amiodarone for recurrent VT. Lastly, Guarnieri et al. [45] reported that intravenous propranolol (0.13–0.25 mg/kg) had no effect on the time to capture after shock from endocardial pacing.

IV. SUMMARY

Antiarrhythmic agents can have both beneficial and deleterious effects on arrhythmias and defibrillation requirements. Up to 75% of patients with ICDs also require the use of at least one antiarrhythmic agent in order to reduce the frequency of arrhythmia occurrence and subsequent delivery of therapy by the ICD, and to control the maximum sinus rate, especially in patients with poorly tolerated or prolonged slow ventricular tachycardias. Knowledge of the effects of these agents on defibrillation and pacing thresholds is important not only for appropriate selection of agents for specific clinical needs, but also to assure an adequate defibrillation and pacing energy safety margin when programming ICDs and pacemakers. The majority of the studies published report on the effects of various antiarrhythmic agents on the energy required for defibrillation using various canine models. Published reports on human data are much less extensive and are limited to amiodarone. Most studies report either no change or an increase in the energy required for defibrillation in amiodarone-treated subjects. This has important clinical relevance, because amiodarone is used alone or in combination with a class I agent in up to 47% of patients with ICDs [1,3,4]. Unlike amiodarone, other class III agents, such as clofilium phosphate, bretylium tosylate, sotalol, and N-acetylprocainamide, have been reported to decrease the energy requirements for successful defibrillation [10,14–16,38]. Decreasing energy requirements may void device failure in patients with marginal DFTs in the drug-free state and prolong generator life for patients who require frequent cardioversion or defibrillation.

In summary, as patients' antiarrhythmic drug needs change, the risks and benefits of this therapy needs to be weighed carefully. In order to assure proper ICD function, repeat testing to assess defibrillation energy requirements, pacing thresholds, and proper sensing should be performed after significant changes in drug therapy are made and prior to discharge from the hospital.

REFERENCES

1. Winkle RA, Mead RH, Ruder MA, et al. Long-term outcome with the automatic implantable cardioverter-defibrillator. J Am Coll Cardiol 1989; 13:1353–1361.
2. Reid PR, Mirowski M, Mower MM, et al. Clinical evaluation of the internal automatic cardioverter-defibrillator in survivors of sudden cardiac death. Am J Cardiol 1983; 51:1608–1613.

3. Echt DS, Armstrong K, Schmidt P, Oyer P, Stinson EB, Winkle RA. Clinical experience, complications, and survival in 70 patients with the automatic implantable cardioverter/defibrillator. Circulation 1985; 71:289–296.
4. Huang SKS, Tan-deGuzman WL, Chenarides JG, Okike NO, Salm TJV. Effects of long-term amiodarone therapy on the defibrillation threshold and the rate of shocks of the implantable cardioverter-defibrillator. Am Heart J 1991; 122(3 pt 1):720–727.
5. Manolis AS, Tan-deGuzman WL, Lee MA, et al. Clinical experience in seventy-seven patients with the automatic implantable cardioverter defibrillator. Am Heart J 1989; 118:445–450.
6. Winkle RA, Stinson EB, Echt DS, Mead RH, Schmidt P. Practical aspects of automatic cardioverter/defibrillator implantation. Am Heart J 1984; 108:1335–1046.
7. Deeb GM, Hardesty RL, Griffith BP. Thompson ME, Heilman MS, Myerowitz RL. The effects of cardiovascular drugs on the defibrillation threshold and the pathological effects on the heart using an automatic implantable defibrillator. Ann Thoracic Surg 1983; 35:361–366.
8. Babbs CF, Yim GKW, Whistle SJ, Tacker WA, Geddes LA. Elevation of ventricular defibrillation threshold in dogs by antiarrhythmic drugs. Am Heart J 1979; 98:345–350.
9. Dorian P, Fain ES, Davy JM, Winkle RA. Effect of quinidine and bretylium on defibrillation energy requirements. Am Heart J 1986; 112:19–25.
10. Tacker WA, Neibauer MJ, Babbs CF, et al. The effect of newer antiarrhythmic drugs on defibrillation threshold. Crit Care Med 1980; 8:177–180.
11. Dorian P, Fain ES, Davy JM, Winkle RA. Lidocaine causes a reversible, concentration-dependent increase in defibrillation energy requirements. J Am Coll Cardiol 1986; 8:327–332.
12. Fain ES, Dorian P, Davy JM, Kates RE, Winkle RA. Effects of encainide and its metabolites on energy requirements for defibrillation. Circulation 1986; 73:1334–1341.
13. Hernandez R, Mann DE, Breckinridge S, Williams GR, Reiter MJ. Effects of flecainide on defibrillation thresholds in the anesthetized dog. J Am Coll Cardiol 1989; 14:777–781.
14. Echt DS, Black JN, Barbey JT, Coxe DR, Cato E. Evaluation of antiarrhythmic drugs on defibrillation energy requirements in dogs. Sodium channel block and action potential prolongation. Circulation 1989; 79:1106–1117.
15. Dawson AK, Steinberg MI, Shapland JE. Effect of class I and class III drugs on current and energy required for internal defibrillation. Circulation 1985; 72(III):III-384.
16. Wang M, Dorian P. DL and D sotalol decrease defibrillator energy requirements. PACE 1989; 12:1522–1529.
17. Singer I, Guarnieri T, Kupersmith J. Implanted automatic defibrillators: effects of drugs and pacemakers. PACE 1988; 11:2250–2262.
18. Marchlinski FE, Flores BT, Buxton AE, et al. The automatic implantable cardioverter-defibrillator: efficacy, complications, and device failuers. Ann Intern Med 1986; 104:481–488.
19. Davy JM, Fain ES, Dorian P, Winkle RA. The relationship between successful defibrillation and delivered energy in open-chest dogs: reappraisal of the "defibrillation threshold" concept. Am Heart J 1987; 113:77–84.
20. Ruffy R, Schechtman K, Monje E, Sandza J. Adrenergically mediated variations in the energy required to defibrillate the heart: observations in closed chest, nonanesthetized dogs. Circulation 1986; 73:374–380.
21. Woolfolk DI, Chaffee WR, Cohen W, Neville JF, Abildskov JA. The effect of quinidine on electrical energy required for ventricular defibrillation. Am Heart J 1966; 72:659–663.
22. Echt DS, Cato, EL, Coxe DR. pH-dependent effects of lidocaine on defibrillation energy requirements in dogs. Circulation 1989; 80:1003–1009.
23. Kerber RE, Pandian NG, Jensen SR, et al. Effect of lidocaine and bretylium on energy requirements for transthoracic defibrillation: experimental studies. J Am Coll Cardiol 1986; 7:397–405.
24. Natale A, Jones DL, Kim YH, Klein GJ. Effects of lidocaine on defibrillation threshold in the pig: evidence of anesthesia related increase. PACE 1991; 1239–1244.
25. Marinchak RA, Friehling TD, Kline RA, Stohler J, Kowey PR. Effect of antiarrhythmic drugs on defibrillation threshold: case report of an adverse effect of mexiletine and review of the literature. PACE 1988; 11:7–12.

26. Hackett AM, Gardiner P, Garthwaite SM. The effect of Bidosomide (SC-40230), a new class Ia/Ib antarrhythmic agent on defibrillation energy requirements in dogs with healed myocardial infarctions. PACE. In press.
27. Dawson AK, Roden DM, Duff HJ, Woosley RL, Smith RF. Differential effects of o-demethyl encainide on induced and spontaneous arrhythmias in the conscious dog. Am J Cardiol 1984; 54:654–658.
28. Peters W, Gang ES, Okazaki H, et al. Acute effects of intravenous propafenone on the internal ventricular defibrillation threshold in the anesthetized dog. Am Heart J 1991; 122:1355–1360.
29. Guarnieri T, Levine JH, Veltri EP, et al. Success of chronic defibrillation and the role of antiarrhythmic drugs with the automatic implantable cardioverter/defibrillator. Am J Cardiol 1987; 60:1061–1064.
30. Troup PJ, Chapman PD, Olinger GN, Kleinman LH. The implanted defibrillator: relation of defibrillating lead configuration and clinical variables to defibrillation threshold. J Am Coll Cardiol 1985; 6:1315–1321.
31. Fogoros RN. Amiodarone-induced refractoriness to cardioversion. Ann Intern Med 1984; 100:699–700.
32. Arrendondo MT, Guillen SG, Quinteiro RA. Effect of amiodarone on ventricular fibrillation and defibrillation thresholds in the canine heart under normal and ischemic conditions. Eur J Pharmacol 1986; 125:23–28.
33. Frame LH, Hoffman N, Kolenik SA, Sheldon JH. Oral loading with amiodarone increases ventricular defibrillation threshold with implanted electrodes in dogs. J Am Coll Cardiol 1986; 7:82A.
34. Haberman RJ, Veltri EP, Mower MM. The effect of amiodarone on defibrillation threshold. J Electrophysiol 1988; 2:415–423.
35. Fain ES, Lee JT, Winkle RA. Effects of acute intravenous and chronic oral amiodarone on defibrillation energy requirements. Am Heart J 1987; 114(1 pt 1):8–17.
36. Frame LH. The effect of chronic oral and acute intravenous amiodarone administration on ventricular defibrillation threshold using implanted electrodes in dogs. PACE 1989; 12:339–346.
37. Haberman RJ, Veltri EP, Mower MM. Amiodarone has a time-dependent effect on increasing defibrillation threshold. Clin Res 1987; 35:283A.
38. Fain ES, Lee JT, Winkle RA. Effects of acute and chronic amiodarone on defibrillation energy requirements. Circulation 1985; 72:III-384.
39. Dorian P, Wang M, David I, Feindel C. Oral clofilium produces sustained lowering of defibrillation energy requirements in a canine model. Circulation 1991; 83:614–621.
40. Koo CC, Allen JD, Pantridge JF. Lack of effect of bretylium tosylate on electrical ventricular defibrillation in a controlled study. Cardiovasc Res 1984; 18:762–767.
41. Mirowski M, Reid PR, Mower MM, et al. Clinical performance of the implantable cardioverter-defibrillator. PACE 1984; 76(pt II):1345–1350.
42. Cohen AI, Wish MH, Fletcher RD, et al. The use and interaction of permanent pacemakers and the automatic implantable cardioverter defibrillator. PACE 1988; 11:704–711.
43. Kim SG, Furman S, Waspe LE, Brodman R, Fisher JD. Unipolar pacer artifacts induced failure of an automatic implantable cardioverter/defibrillator to detect ventricular fibrillation. Am J Cardiol 1986; 57:880–881.
44. Yee R, Jones DL, Jarvis E, Donner AP, Klein GJ. Changes in pacing threshold and R wave amplitude after transvenous catheter countershock. J Am Coll Cardiol 1984; 4:543–549.
45. Guarnieri T, Datorre SD, Bondke J, Brinker J, Myers S, Levine JH. Increased pacing threshold after an automatic defibrillator shock in dogs: effects of class I and class II antiarrhythmic drugs. PACE 1988; 11:1324–1330.
46. Khastgir T, Lattuca J, Aarons D, et al. Ventricular pacing threshold and time to capture postdefibrillation in patients undergoing implantable cardioverter-defibrillator implantation. PACE 1991; 14(5 pt 1):768–772.
47. Furman S, Hurzeler P, Mehra R. Cardiac pacing and pacemakers IV. Threshold of cardiac stimulation. AM Heart J 1977; 94:115–124.

48. Hellestrand KJ, Nathan AW, Bexton RS, Camm AJ. Electrophysiologic effects of flecainide acetate on sinus node function, anomalous atrioventricular connections, and pacemaker thresholds. Am J Cardiol 1984; 53:30B–38B.
49. Slepian M, Levine JH, Watkins L, Brinker J, Guarnieri T. Automatic implantable cardioverter defibrillator/permanent interaction: loss of pacemaker capture following AICD discharge. PACE 1987; 10:1194–1197.
50. Babbs CF. Alteration of defibrillation threshold by antiarrhythmic drugs: a theoretical framework. Crit Care Med 1981; 9:362–363.

24

Implantable Defibrillator Patient and Family Teaching

Laurie J. Butts and Carol D. Colburn

New England Medical Center
Boston, Massachusetts

Paul J. Wang

Tufts University School of Medicine
and New England Medical Center
Boston, Massachusetts

I. ISSUES IN PATIENT TEACHING

A. Understanding the Patient

Teaching the patient with life-threatening ventricular arrhythmias requires a thorough understanding of the patient's emotional state, coping mechanisms, and his or her medical condition. This process of learning about the patient begins with the admission interview and continues throughout the hospitalization. Informal conversations during daily care and examinations may provide as much information about the patient as special interviewing and teaching sessions. Anxiety and fear may unfortunately impede attempts to educate the patient, and therefore important information must be reinforced during the teaching process. This anxiety may originate from fear of a recurrent life-threatening arrhythmia as well as from uncertainties about the process of arrhythmia evaluation and treatment.

The teaching staff must also understand the patient's emotional and physical limitations in learning about the evaluation and treatment process. Fatigue is an important limiting factor, which much be considered in selecting the pace of the teaching process. For some patients, teaching is best incorporated into daily patient care, with separate teaching sessions used for reinforcement of teaching. For these patients the familiarity of the patient's own room may provide the best setting, while for other patients group instruction in a classroom may be more suitable.

B. The Team Approach to Teaching

The electrophysiology (EP) physician, the EP nurse, and patient's staff nurse, house staff and trainees, and the non-EP cardiologist or internist are important parts of the teaching team. Usually, however, the EP nurse and physician, and to a lesser extent the staff nurse, provide the essential elements of the teaching. Reinforcement by the non-EP physicians is nonetheless crucial in establishing trust and understanding, since they are likely to have had a long-term

Table 1 Teaching plan for ICD Patients

Date of teaching	RN initials	Return verbalization	Topics

			1. Ventricular arrhythmias
			  a. Importance of treatment
			  b. Terminology
			  c. Role of EP testing
			  d. Treatment options
			2. Indications for ICD
			  a. Spontaneous arrhythmia
			  b. Inducible arrhythmias
			2. What is an ICD?
			  a. ICD function
			  b. ICD clinical results
			  c. Demonstration of ICD generator, patches, leads
			  d. Sensation of shock
			  e. Implications for follow-up and lifestyle
			3. ICD procedure and implantation
			  a. Surgical approaches
			  b. Site of generator pocket
			  c. Concomitant surgery
			  d. Risks
			  e. Skin preparation

relationship with the patient. Developing and reviewing a teaching plan (Table 1) [1] with all members of the health-care team is important to make sure that the patient is receiving information which is accurate and appropriate for the patient at the time.

II. PREOPERATIVE TEACHING

A. Discussion of Medical Condition and Diagnostic Evaluation

The complexity of the implantable defibrillator and the underlying arrhythmic process make it essential that the patient and family have a clear understanding of the medical condition. Pre- and postoperative teaching plays a critical role in gaining patient and family acceptance of implantable defibrillator therapy and achieving the long-term compliance which is so critical in the management of ICD patients. Such an understanding enables the patient and family to communicate more effectively with the medical staff and thus to participate more actively in the patient's care.

The first step in the teaching process is educating the patient and family about the nature of the patient's life-threatening ventricular arrhythmia following the initial event. A great deal of time must be spent by the physicians and nurses to teach the patient and the family about the basic concepts of ventricular arrhythmias. Printed materials are particularly important learning tools, since it is common for patients to selectively recall verbal instructions and teaching. Nursing teaching documentation tools with appropriate learning assessment documents may be helpful in ensuring that a better understanding of arrhythmias has been achieved.

Patient and Family Teaching

An important aspect of this initial teaching process is to provide the patient and family with an understanding of the basic medical terminology. A list of basic definitions or a glossary may help the medical staff teach the patient and family to communicate better with the medical staff. Having the patient talk about his or her medical condition using this new terminology may improve the communication process. Initially, it is best not to inundate the patient and family, since additional terminology can be introduced as the process of teaching continues during the patient's hospitalization.

One of the important tasks in patient and family teaching is achieving the delicate balance between allaying patient anxiety while still educating the patient about the life-threatening nature of his or her sustained ventricular arrhythmias. Throughout the medical process, it is important to emphasize to the patient and family that excellent methods of treating ventricular arrhythmias are available. The importance of identifying the best method of treatment and the risks of ventricular arrhythmias without treatment must be emphasized. Such a basic understanding may help the patient and family cope with the complex nature of the therapeutic options and the relatively prolonged hospitalization that is often required. The reaction of individual patients to their initial arrhythmic event varies tremendously. Some patients understand quickly the serious nature of their illness and may develop significant anxiety about the possibility of its recurrence. Reassurance is critical in helping patients to cope with the evaluation and treatment process. Other patients may deny the significant nature of their event and may not acknowledge that their risk of further events is great. Very often they may maintain that they "just passed out" and that the event was due to the specific action that they performed. Instructing patients about the nature of their arrhythmia is critical, and most patients who have been given such teaching will accept the diagnostic and therapeutic plan which is described to them. However, a small subset of patients will continue to deny the severity of their illness and may eventually refuse treatment. For these patients it is particularly important to provide both written and verbal education, documenting that the patient has been informed about the risks of his or her arrhythmia.

A particularly difficult situation arises for the patient who has suffered some degree of anoxic brain damage, resulting in some memory loss. Teaching the patient's family in these cases is of critical importance. A decision will need to be made whether the patient can undergo further evaluation and treatment at the present time. Some patients may benefit from further rehabilitation in a monitored setting, followed eventually by further evaluation and treatment of the arrhythmia.

In addition to the individual teaching by physicians and nurses, an inpatient family support group may be extremely valuable. For example, at our institution two staff nurses who have completed training in arrhythmia education and have experience in leading groups teach a group session designed to discuss issues in arrhythmia management. This allows arrhythmia patients and families to become acquainted and to provide an open arena for questions and answers. It provides an opportunity to correct false information which might be introduced by other well-meaning patients, as well as to discuss some intimate issues which might be brought up by a staff nurse or another patient. It is often extremely reassuring for the patient to realize that the arrhythmia service treats a great number of similar patients on a daily basis.

Since most patients who have life-threatening ventricular arrhythmias will undergo electrophysiologic testing early in their hospitalization, it is important that the patient and family thoroughly understand this diagnostic procedure and its implications for treatment plans. Printed material may be very important in outlining the goals and the nature of the electrophysiologic study. It is important to discuss the purpose of the electrophysiologic study and, in particular, to outline the need to understand and characterize the patient's inducible arrhyth-

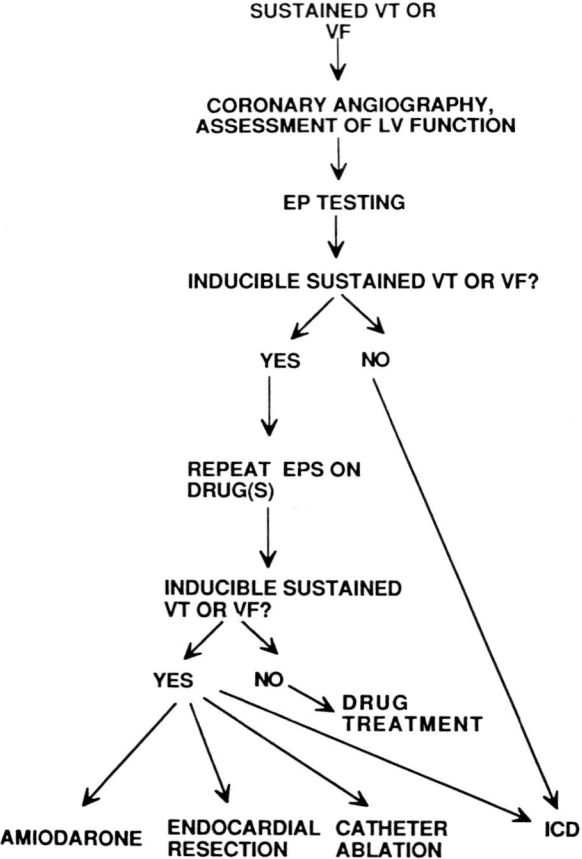

Figure 1 An algorithm for management of patients presenting with sustained ventricular tachycardia or ventricular fibrillation.

mias. This information may be used to stratify the patient's risk for further arrhythmias, to provide a baseline with which to compare results during pharmacological testing, and to select nonpharmacological treatment if needed. Patients need to understand that the electrophysiological test itself is diagnostic and not designed to cure the patient's arrhythmia. In addition, most patients will benefit from understanding that their evaluation and treatment may take a number of days or even up to several weeks. Selected patients may not be able to accept such a full description of the diagnostic and therapeutic plan, and for these patients their medical progress may need to be discussed on a daily basis, one step at a time.

B. Discussion of Treatment Options

Before discussing in detail the individual treatment options, it is very important to stress to the patient and the family that, although the patient may have a life-threatening arrhythmia, the condition has excellent treatment options. For most patients, a discussion of the therapeutic options and a decision algorithm may be useful (Fig. 1). This information, however, has to be given at a time and manner which is appropriate for each patient and family. Most patients want a general assessment of the approach to be taken and some of the therapeutic options but do not seem ready for a detailed discussion of all treatments. Unusually, a patient or family may press to learn about all of these options in detail at the onset. It is important, however, that this additional data be used constructively and not simply to increase their anxiety about their condition and treatment.

If serial drug testing is used to establish the best treatment option, it is important to prepare the patient for the possibility of several electrophysiologic tests. First, it is important to emphasize that selecting a drug empirically is not the best strategy, since life-threatening ventricular arrhythmias occur sporadically and each individual drug may not be effective in preventing a life-threatening arrhythmic occurrence. Thus, an explanation of the utility of EP testing to predict drug response is important. It is also valuable to emphasize that the yield of further drug testing after one or two drug failures is low and that frequently nonpharmacologic therapy is considered at that point.

If the patient has undergone a baseline electrophysiologic study and does not have inducible arrhythmia despite a spontaneous sustained ventricular arrhythmia, many patients will be candidates for implantable defibrillators (see Chapter 12). For this selected population, it is important to describe to the patient the rationale for the need for implantable defibrillators rather than selecting a medication empirically. Such patients may want to know why other patients are being tested on medications while they are being recommended to have an implantable defibrillator immediately.

Selected patients may be candidates for a procedure to attempt to cure them of the ventricular arrhythmia, either surgically or occasionally using radiofrequency catheter ablation. Patients who are felt to be candidates for surgical treatment of ventricular tachycardia should be informed of the advantages and disadvantages of this approach. Because of the differences in both the goals and risks of surgical resection and defibrillator implantation, patient understanding and participation in this decision is appropriate. The goal of surgical treatment of ventricular tachycardia is to completely cure the patient of the arrhythmia. In contrast, the implantable defibrillator is designed to improve overall survival of the patient but will not cure the patient of the arrhythmia itself. The risks for the individual patient should be discussed openly since, typically, the risks of surgical resection are greater than that of defibrillator implantation alone. Patients, upon learning that they will continue to have arrhythmias which may affect their lifestyle, sometimes prefer to have the surgical treatment rather than implantable defibrillator therapy. The importance of concomitant heart surgery such as coronary artery bypass graft surgery also should be discussed with the patient. It may be important to emphasize that both treatments may be required in order to treat the patient's coronary artery disease and arrhythmias.

C. Introduction to the Implantable Cardioverter-Defibrillator

It may be appropriate to introduce some patients to the concept of an implantable defibrillator from the outset of teaching. Initially one may choose to describe it very superficially, even oversimplifying its function. Once electrophysiologic testing has begun, it may be valuable to introduce the concepts of implantable defibrillator function in a stepwise fashion, since a large percentage of such patients may require such a device [1–34]. A more formal presentation of the implantable defibrillator may then be given after the decision to recommend an ICD has been made. Clarifying for the patient the indication for ICD is an important first step. The patient may have had an inducible arrhythmia which could not be suppressed with drug treatment during electrophysiologic testing, or the patient may not have had an inducible arrhythmia despite a spontaneous arrhythmic event. It is important to emphasize that it is a positive point that a device such as an implantable defibrillator can be offered as an option in cases when drug therapy is not feasible or recommended. It may be valuable for the patient to see an ICD video or to read an ICD teaching booklet before the detailed ICD training is started. Patient-teaching ICD videos are available from several ICD manufacturers. Each manufacturer also has a patient-teaching booklet, but it may be useful for each medical center to write a simple ICD booklet as well. During formal ICD teaching, showing the patient an ICD model, patches, and leads may be helpful. This will give the patient an idea about the size and weight of the device.

A discussion of the clinical data regarding the outcome of patients treated with implantable defibrillators is appropriate. It should be emphasized that the defibrillator has been extremely effective in preventing life-threatening consequences of ventricular arrhythmias. Again, it should be emphasized that the implantable defibrillator acts to rescue the patient but does not prevent the arrhythmia itself. It is possible that the patient may feel lightheaded or pass out before the device rescues the patient and converts the rhythm. Thus, one may need to discuss general recommendations of activities to be avoided which might put the patient or others at risk if he or she were to pass out. Typically, this extends to occupational settings such as operating machinery, flying an airplane, or in many cases driving a motor vehicle. Each medical center will need to determine its recommendations regarding driving, as will be discussed in Section III.

It is important to describe the basic function of the implantable defibrillator (Fig. 2), perhaps explaining that the device detects a ventricular arrhythmia and converts it immediately by delivering energy from the ICD patches or leads to the heart or by pacing the heart to terminate the tachycardia. Many patients are familiar with external defibrillation, which they may have seen on television. The analogy of having a rescue squad traveling with the patient is not scientific but may provide a valuable description for some patients. Many patients may have specific questions about how the device can tell when a fast rhythm occurs. They may be concerned about exercising, as will be discussed in Section V.C.

Once it has been determined which model and type of ICD the patient will receive, it is helpful to describe the specific functions of the chosen ICD model. Defibrillators may have four basic forms of treatment or function. All defibrillators have a large battery inside the ICD, which delivers energy to the heart to convert the rhythm back to normal. The patient usually, but not always, experiences this shock as a sudden blow to the chest. Low-energy shocks, particularly those of 1 J or less, may not be felt. The patient may or may not have symptoms of the arrhythmia before the shock. Most ICDs can give a series of four to nine shocks in a row (Fig. 2), with a total capacity of 300 to 500 shocks. The amount of energy necessary to convert the heart rhythm is much less than that required for external cardioversion, since the energy is given directly to the heart muscle. A second form of therapy which is present in some defibrillators is bradycardia pacing. When the heart is beating too slowly, the heart rate is maintained by using small amounts of energy in a manner identical to permanent pacemakers.

The third form of therapy is antitachycardia pacing, which may be available in selected ICDs. In some patients ventricular tachycardia may be interrupted by pacing at fast rates. Since one does not typically feel the antitachycardia pacing, some patients may be asymptomatic and not realize that they are experiencing an arrhythmia. Most commonly, ventricular tachycardia will be converted by the pacing alone, and the patient will not require shock therapy. If the antitachycardia pacing is not successful in interrupting arrhythmia, or if the arrhythmia

Patient and Family Teaching

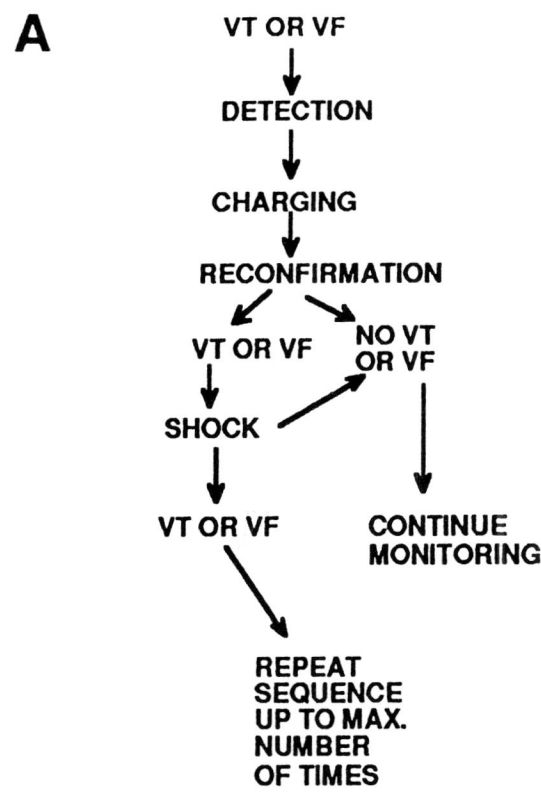

Figure 2 Basic sequence of implantable defibrillator function: (A) device with only shock capability; (B) device with both antitachycardia pacing and shock capability.

rate increases, the ICD will automatically deliver shock therapy (Fig. 2). The fourth function of the ICD may be to keep a memory or record of the arrhythmias which have been treated. It may count the number of times the patient has been shocked, the heart rates which occurred, and the time at which each episode occurred. Many features of these four functions may be adjusted through a process called programming, which changes the parameters noninvasively using a small device called a programmer, which communicates with the defibrillator using radiofrequency waves.

D. The Process of Obtaining Informed Consent

The implanting surgeon in most institutions is responsible for the process of obtaining informed consent. The surgeon will discuss with the patient his or her surgical risks for the ICD implant procedure and any concomitant surgery. However, the surgeon usually relies extensively on the teaching which the electrophysiology staff and other members of the surgical team provide the patient. The amount of information which each patient and family desire or need to make an informed decision regarding implantation of the ICD varies tremendously. However, as discussed above, it is important that the patient understand: (1) the basic purpose of the defibrillator; (2) the basic function of the defibrillator; (3) the risks involved in defibrillator implantation, and (4) the implications for follow-up and lifestyle changes.

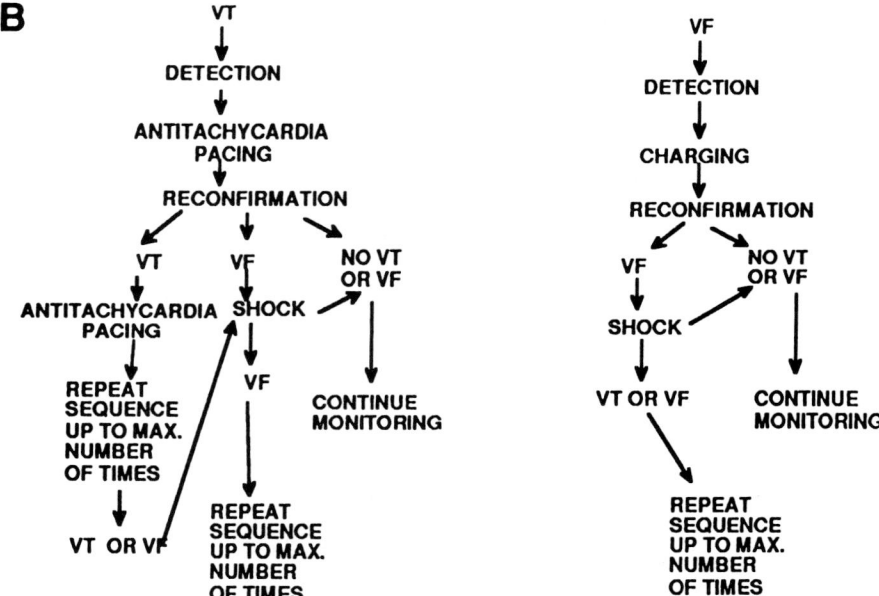

In addition, the patient should understand that very rarely it is not possible to implant the implantable defibrillator because of high defibrillation thresholds at the time of implant (see Chapters 2 and 18). In this case the defibrillator would not be implanted. Similarly, if the patient is planned to have a nonthoracotomy defibrillator lead system, high defibrillation thresholds may prevent it from being implanted. If the patient is to receive an investigational implantable defibrillator, typically a separate consent form is obtained for the investigational device in addition to consent for the ICD implantation procedure.

III. TEACHING REGARDING IMPLANTATION PROCEDURE

A. Preoperative Preparation

Patients should be informed that meticulous attention will be paid to their skin prior to surgery. In many centers a surgical scrub using a bacterial solution is performed three to four times prior to surgery. In addition, patients should be informed that ECG monitoring pads should be positioned so that they are away from any potential incisional approaches to avoid any skin irritation or rash. We inform patients to remind staff that no electrodes should be placed on the anterior or lateral chest wall between the clavicular and the lower rib margins.

Typically, the surgeon will discuss with the patient the type of surgical approach which will be used. Most patients currently receive nonthoracotomy defibrillation lead systems. Other approaches which may be used include: (1) median sternotomy, (2) left lateral thoracotomy, (3) subxiphoid, (4) subcostal. Testing is performed to ensure that the device will work adequately to convert the rhythm. One should describe the ICD implantation site, which is typically in the left lower abdomen and less commonly in the pectoral region. Patients will be particularly interested in learning whether the device may be felt and whether it will move.

B. Patient Recovery Procedure

Patients should be informed that, after the surgical procedure is completed, the patient will usually go to a recovery room or a surgical intensive-care unit, where he or she will be monitored closely. It may be helpful to review with the family the procedure for seeing the patient immediately postoperatively and the mechanism by which the surgeon will contact the patient's family at the completion of the surgery. In some centers a visit to the recovery area or the surgical intensive-care unit is performed postoperatively to allow the family to become familiar with this setting. Many patients receiving nonthoracotomy defibrillator lead systems may be mobilized rapidly. In some centers, lead and generator implantation and defibrillation threshold testing are performed without intubation, further increasing the rate of recovery.

IV. TEACHING DURING THE EARLY POSTOPERATIVE PERIOD

Patient teaching is directed largely toward the need for mobilization, good pulmonary toilet, and pain control. A clear strategy for effective pain control should be discussed with the patient and his or her nursing staff, in order to ensure patient comfort and adequate inspiratory effort to minimize pulmonary infection. In some centers, for patients having thoracotomy or sternotomy approaches, patient-controlled anesthesia is used to achieve optimal patient comfort and permit deep inspiration. The importance of early ambulation should be stressed in the postoperative period.

Education of the nursing staff caring for the patient is particularly important. Dressing changes must be performed meticulously, in order to minimize early device infection. In addition, the exact status and programming of the ICD should be directly available. Frequently, a sign is placed above the patient's bed or outside his or her door stating the ICD model and whether it is activated. Careful arrhythmia monitoring is also performed. In some instances the device is kept inactive because of the possibility of atrial fibrillation or nonsustained ventricular arrhythmia which may result in patient shocks.

V. PREDISCHARGE AND FOLLOW-UP TEACHING

With the rapid recovery of patients having nonthoracotomy defibrillator systems, the predischarge teaching process must be accelerated. The goals of predischarge and follow-up teaching are (1) to continue the education of the patient regarding implantable defibrillator function; (2) to provide emotional support and allay anxiety; (3) to provide detailed instructions regarding immediate postoperative care at home; (4) to provide education regarding patient activity and diet; (5) to educate the patient regarding the need for medications, the amount to be taken, the method of administration, the time of doses, and possible side effects; (6) to review indications for notifying the electrophysiology staff or primary-care physician and the method of contacting these individuals; (7) to review the scheduled follow-up plan, including the dates of the first several visits; and (8) to acquaint the patient with the support systems which have been developed for ICD and other cardiac patients [14]. While each step of the teaching process is very important, predischarge and follow-up teaching is crucial in providing the patient and his or her family with the necessary information and support to function effectively at home after discharge. Education is a key aspect in achieving patient compliance with the treatment plan in continuation of the rehabilitation process [15].

During predischarge teaching, a variety of information sources may be used for patient and family education. It is frequently useful to provide patients with a brief booklet describing their arrhythmia and the defibrillator; an information summary sheet describing their medications, doses, method of administration, time of administration, and possible side effects; information provided from the ICD manufacturer regarding the patient's ICD; and a discharge teaching plan which summarizes the goals of discharge teaching (Table 2). Since ICD patients have follow-up every two to three months, regular office visits are an excellent time to reinforce and continue patient and family teaching.

A. Instructions for Care at Home

In order to minimize the risk of serious infection of the implantable defibrillator, instruction in the care of surgical wounds is critical. The wounds must be inspected carefully for redness, swelling, tenderness, or drainage. Patients should be advised to take their temperature twice daily for approximately 10 days and to report immediately any symptoms of fever, chills, or signs or symptoms of infection to their physician [16]. Specific instructions regarding showering should also be given. At our medical center, for example, showering is avoided for 10 days after the date of surgery. In addition, the patient is instructed to wipe the ICD incision with an iodine-based swab and to change the dressing daily with sterile gauze for 10 days. The swab and the sterile dressing should be given to the patient, or instructions on how to obtain them should be made. The seriousness of an infection of the implantable defibrillator should be emphasized.

B. Medications

Since there may have been many medication changes or additions since the time of the patient's admission, it is very important to clarify what medications the patient should take and what medications which were taken prior to admission should be discontinued. Patients need to know the names of their medications, their actions, their side effects, and their importance. A realistic medication schedule suitable to the patient's lifestyle will improve patient compliance. Instructions about what to do if a medication dose is missed should be made. It is very important to emphasize that medication should not be discontinued without contacting a physician. If antiarrhythmic drugs are used, it may be helpful to describe why they are needed in addition to the patient's implantable defibrillator. Patients often wonder why they continue to require the same medications as taken preoperatively. If some medications should be discontinued after a period of time, for example, warfarin, which should be clearly indicated to the patient on the medication summary sheet (Table 3).

C. Activity

Instructions regarding the patient's activity postdischarge require individualization, since each patient's ability to return to full activity will differ. In general, however, patients should be encouraged to resume the activities of daily living. It is important to review limitations with the patient, explaining that limitations usually are associated with the underlying heart or rhythm disorders rather than with the implantable defibrillator [17]. Many ICD patients will benefit from an outpatient cardiac rehabilitation program, which allows them to gradually increase activity under supervision and gives them the confidence to be active without fear of receiving an implantable defibrillator shock. If the patient has had a median sternotomy, the surgical team will usually advise the patient to avoid activities which might threaten sternal stability for

Patient and Family Teaching

Table 2 Discharge Teaching Plan

Date of teaching	RN initials	Return verbalization	Topics

			1. Precautions:
			  a. Wound care: watch for redness, swelling, or hot to touch; call M.D.
			  b. Take your temperature twice a day for 10 days.
			  c. No lifting for a period of 4–6 weeks as prescribed by M.D.
			  d. No driving or swimming alone.
			  e. Tight clothing may cause discomfort and irritation at the generator site.
			  f. Familiarity with the closest ER.
			    (1) Notification of ER as to patient condition
			  g. Familiarity with the EMT Service in area.
			  h. Carry ID card at all times.
			  i. Wear medic alert bracelet.
			2. Continuation of medications.
			3. Continuation of diet restrictions.
			4. Protocol for countershock follow-up:
			  a. Go to the nearest ER and have an EKG.
			  b. When to activate the emergency medical system.
			  c. Notify ICD clinic of shock.
			5. Discussion of feelings concerning ICD.
			6. Involvement of family/significant other.
			7. Things to avoid:
			  a. Heavy machinery
			  b. Arc welders
			  c. Airport security wands
			  d. Magnetic resonance imaging
			  e. Stereo speakers
			8. Follow-up
			  a. MD appointment to check the device:
			    (1) Initially you are seen week 1, 2, and week 4; then approximately every 2 months.
			  b. Record all events:
			    (1) Record activity before shock.
			    (2) Record feelings of dizziness, diaphoresis, or chest pain.
			    (3) Record number of shocks.

Table 3 Medication Summary Sheet

NAME OF MEDICATION:
Dose:
Why do I need this medication:
Special instructions:
Side effects:
Time to take medication:

NAME OF MEDICATION:
Dose:
Why do I need this medication:
Special instructions:
Side effects:
Time to take medication:

NAME OF MEDICATION:
Dose:
Why do I need this medication:
Special instructions:
Side effects:
Time to take medication:

NAME OF MEDICATION:
Dose:
Why do I need this medication:
Special instructions:
Side effects:
Time to take medication:

NAME OF MEDICATION:
Dose:
Why do I need this medication:
Special instructions:
Side effects:
Time to take medication:

NAME OF MEDICATION:
Dose:
Why do I need this medication:
Special instructions:
Side effects:
Time to take medication:

NAME OF MEDICATION:
Dose:
Why do I need this medication:
Special instructions:
Side effects:
Time to take medication:

Patient and Family Teaching

several months postoperatively. For patients with a nonthoracotomy lead system or a transvenous rate-sensing lead, specific instructions about avoiding vigorous upper extremity exercise for several weeks following implantation may be appropriate.

Prior to discharge, the patient should be given guidelines regarding activities to avoid. For most patients with implantable defibrillators, there remains a potential for loss of consciousness during the period of arrhythmia recognition and capacitor charging [18,19]. Even patients with typically well-tolerated ventricular tachycardia potentially may have a spontaneous rapid ventricular arrhythmias or acceleration after defibrillation or antitachycardia pacing. In addition, symptomatic bradycardias may occur following tachyarrhythmic termination [20,21]. The patient, therefore, should avoid any activity during which syncope would result in injury to the patient or others. Examples of such activities include working at heights, operating large machinery, swimming alone, and driving. In most states, these guidelines are only recommendations and not legal requirements. In some states, driving restrictions may apply to patients with lethal ventricular arrhythmias and not just patients with ICDs [35]. There should be uniformity in the institution's and physician's guidelines to their ICD patients, since inevitably ICD patients will discuss these issues among themselves. In some states there are specific laws regarding driving by patients with implantable defibrillators. However, these laws are far from uniform, and each institution must consult the board of motor vehicles in their state for the current regulations. In addition, often the institution's legal department may have an opinion regarding recommendations for driving.

During the patient's predischarge evaluation or outpatient follow-up, determining the patient's maximal heart rate during exercise may be helpful. This information is useful in setting the ICD detection rate above the maximal sinus rate and below the tachycardia rate, particularly in patients with slow ventricular tachycardia rates. It also may reassure the patient that maximal activity is unlikely to result in ICD shock. In some cases, judicious use of a beta-blocking agent may be necessary. It is extremely important to discuss resumption of sexual activity with the ICD patients and his or her spouse. Both will be afraid of what will happen if the ICD should fire during intercourse. Contact with a person receiving an implantable defibrillator may result at most in a sensation like a static shock received after touching an object after walking across a rug.

D. Implantable Defibrillator Shocks

There is often significant anxiety regarding the sensation of the first spontaneous shock. It may be useful to paraphrase the words which many patients use to describe the sensations they get during the shock, such as "a kick in the chest." It is important to indicate that for most patients this sensation lasts only for several seconds and that each patient feels the shock to a different degree. The energy level at which they may be programmed may be different, but also each patient's sensation of the shock may differ significantly. It is also important to explain to patients with defibrillators that have antitachycardia pacing that this form of therapy may not be felt by the patient. When the patient calls to report a shock, congratulate him or her and make it a positive experience. It is important to let patients know that they haven't done anything wrong and that the device is working properly. Instructions as to what patients should do if they get shocks should be given (Table 4). Many centers suggest that, after the initial shock, patients should go to a local emergency room for follow-up EKG and call the contact person in the electrophysiology laboratory. It is extremely important that patients call immediately if there are multiple shocks, since this may indicate a need for reprogramming or further evaluation of the device. Identifying rhythms such as atrial fibrillation or any sensing abnormalities will be

Table 4 Instructions for Patient Receiving Defibrillator Shock

- If you receive a shock, you should go to the nearest emergency room and have an EKG done and some laboratory work. After the shock we want to make sure that your heart has returned to its normal rhythm and that your lab values are normal.
- If you are alone at home and feel fine after receiving a shock, wait until someone can drive you to the hospital.
- If you are not feeling well after being shocked, dial 911 or activate the Emergency Medical System in your community.
- The ICD clinic should be called by the emergency room doctor or by you.
- We will need to see you in the clinic to read your device.

particularly important [23–25]. After the first one or two shocks, many centers do not ask patients to go to their local emergency room and suggest that they only call the electrophysiology laboratory contact person. However, if at any time, the patient has multiple shocks during a day, immediate attention should be sought. If the patient has persistent dizziness, palpitations, diaphoresis, or shortness of breath, the patient should be instructed to lie down and have an ambulance take him or her to the nearest emergency room. This may represent ventricular tachycardia at a rate below the programmed detection rate, another arrhythmia such as atrial fibrillation, or—much less likely—failure of the device to detect or convert the arrhythmia. Also, it could represent another cardiac event such as a myocardial infarction.

E. Patient Precautions

With most implantable ICDs, magnetic fields should be avoided, since they may inactivate the device. Only a few ICD generators have a programmable response to magnetic fields. With some ICDs, specific device functions may be suspended only while the ICD is in the magnetic field. With some devices, the magnetic field may result in the device being inactivated until it is reactivated using a programmer. Inactivation from inadvertent magnet application is a serious danger, since some patients dying suddenly have been found to have inactive devices. Common forms of magnets in the home include stereo speakers or toy magnets. In the workplace, sources of magnetic fields or electromagnetic interference such as arc welding or industrial magnets should also be avoided. When traveling, it is important that patients notify airport security personnel that they have an implantable defibrillator. It is appropriate to walk through the security gate as instructed. An identification card listing their defibrillator should be shown. They should not allow a hand-held wand to be placed over the device, since these usually contain a magnet. Bingo wands have been shown to contain magnets and should be avoided. Any surgery which is planned should be discussed with the electrophysiology nurse or physician prior to its being conducted. If the surgery involves electrocautery or diathermy, the device may need to be inactivated. ECG monitoring should be used in any surgery in a patient with an ICD, whether the device is active or inactive. Following the surgery, the device will need to be reactivated. In addition, some centers advise patients to have prophylactic antibiotics at the time of surgery. Various diagnostic tests should be discussed with the patient. Routine X-rays or a CAT scan do not present any significant problem. However, magnetic resonance imaging (MRI) should not be performed on an ICD patient [26].

As as precaution, ICD patients should carry their identification with them at all times. They may be instructed to purchase an ICD necklace or bracelet and what information should be included on the medallion. In addition, all patients should be encouraged to know emergency numbers in their town and to place a copy of these numbers by their telephone. The issue

Patient and Family Teaching

of patient/family instruction in cardiopulmonary resuscitation or CPR is controversial. Many centers routinely instruct all patient family members in CPR. They stress that cardiovascular collapse may occur despite the implantable defibrillator. This need may arise due to other changes in the patient's cardiac function, such as an acute myocardial infarction or a refractory arrhythmia, which, though unlikely, might occur. Other centers do not perform CPR instruction routinely and reserve this only for patients at particularly high risk. Some patient families are more reassured after having CPR instructions, while other experience more anxiety.

VI. ICD PATIENT AND FAMILY SUPPORT GROUPS AND ACTIVITIES

Patient support groups have been developed at many centers to provide an ongoing form of support for the ICD patient and family. Goals of the support group are (1) to support the spouses or family members in a group setting, (2) to provide patients and families with information on ICDs, their medications, or their follow-up; and (3) to reduce anxiety by answering questions and correcting misconceptions [27]. Many institutions have one large support group which meets at regular intervals, either monthly or quarterly. Both the patients and their families as well as significant others are invited to attend these meetings. Typically, there will be a socializing and refreshment period, an information period, and a support-group period. Frequently, part of the support-group period enables patients to stand up and speak about their experiences with the ICDs and to share common concerns.

The support group functions to allow patients and their families to realize that they are not alone in having their feelings and anxieties [28]. They often feel less isolated and gain a greater sense of acceptance and belonging. Older members can provide experience, encouragement, and support to the newer members of the support group. Some support groups [29] utilize three facilitators for each support group. This consists of one ICD nurse who sees patients regularly in the clinic, a nurse with experience in group dynamics, and an expert cardiovascular nurse. They emphasize coping skills and expression of feelings about lifestyle changes. A questionnaire may be used to generate areas of interest. Topics for support groups may include cardiopulmonary resuscitation, antiarrhythmic medications, how to handle anxiety, new ICD developments, importance of patient follow-up, issues of travel, and rehabilitation. While data supporting the benefit of ICD support groups is limited, several studies have suggested that support groups for other disorders may be helpful in improving patient attitudes and their sense of well-being [36–43]. These supports groups also provide an important learning experience for the health-care professional. It allows one to see the changes which patients exhibit following ICD implantation as well as identifying patients who may not be coping as well. It allows the members of the ICD team to see their patients in a broader prospective than simply in the hospital or during an office visit. Support can also be provided using smaller group sessions led by several members of the ICD team, including the electrophysiology nurse, the electrophysiology physician, a social worker, or a psychologist or psychiatrist. They may be informal discussions of various issues regarding defibrillators or more formal group therapy sessions.

An important adjunct to further ICD patient support is the "buddy" system, in which a patient having an ICD is paired with a recent ICD recipient. At our institution, this approach has been employed particularly for patients who are having a difficult time adjusting to the idea of having a defibrillator during their postoperative recovery. Often patients will voice particular concerns which are best addressed by a patient who has learned to live with an implantable defibrillator. These are often patients who have had difficult medical or hospital

```
John Smith              Type of Device:              Implant Date:
10 Oak Drive
Boston, MA

Emergency Contact Number Regarding Defibrillator:    970-5138
                                                     Dr. William Doe (EP Physician)

Emergency Contact Number for other Medical Problems: 634-1000
                                                     Dr. Thomas Jones
```

Figure 3. Sample card for emergency phone contacts.

courses themselves and have developed a particularly keen sense of what each patient may be experiencing [28].

Other forms of recreational activity may be planned for defibrillator patients. Recently, a cruise was introduced specifically for ICD patients. Other centers may arrange other recreational or social events designed for this patient group.

VII. EMERGENCY CONTACTS: WHO AND WHEN TO CALL

The patient should have a specific name or telephone number to contact. In many centers this will be an electrophysiology nurse. Alternatively, it may be the electrophysiology physician who is on call for the team. In some cases, it is a general cardiologist who will be able to obtain the necessary information. Each center needs to establish guidelines regarding the procedure to be followed after the patient has received a shock. Most centers, however, continue to request that the patient call one of the electrophysiology staff members. The patient should contact the physician for signs of possible infection, including warmth, redness, swelling, or tenderness at a surgical site. In addition, if the patient develops a fever, he or she should contact an electrophysiology staff member. If the patient is going to have a surgical procedure, this also should be discussed. If the patient is going to travel outside his or her home region, he or she may want to have the name of a physician or hospital to contact.

The patient also should be instructed as to what signs and symptoms require emergency attention. If the patient has dizziness, palpitations, or shortness of breath, an ambulance should be called rather than the electrophysiology team initially. It is extremely important that the patient be taken to the closest emergency room, not necessarily the site at which the ICD follow-up is performed. It is very helpful that the patient have a small card or a piece of paper indicating these emergency numbers (Fig. 3). In addition, the patient should be instructed as when to contact his or her primary physician versus the electrophysiology team. Some centers routinely provide the local emergency medical services with ICD patients' phone numbers and addresses as well as literature about ICDs.

VIII. ASSESSING PATIENT UNDERSTANDING OF ICD FUNCTION AND TEACHING

The assessment of the patient's understanding of the teaching efforts is as important as the teaching itself. The patient should be asked to repeat key items which have been taught and to recall whom to contact in the event of an emergency or specific questions. A teaching assessment tool may be particularly useful in identifying areas which may require repetition and emphasis [1].

REFERENCES

1. Higgins C. The AICD: a teaching plan for patients and families. Crit Care Nurse 1990; 10:69–74.
2. Arato A, Biggs AJ, Williams J. Elderly care. Automatic implantable cardioverter defibrillators. J Gerontol Nurs 1992; 18:15–22.
3. Rankin I. Cardiology update. Implantable defibrillators. Nurs Stand 1992; 6:50–51.
4. Fabiszewski R, Volosin KJ. Refusal of implantable cardioverter defibrillator generator replacement: the nurse's role. Focus Crit Care 1992; 19:97–100.
5. Currier DS, Packa DR. The patient with an implantable cardiac defibrillator: a case study. Focus Crit Care 1992; 19:150–154.
6. Mason P, McPherson C. Implantable cardioverter defibrillator: a review. Heart Lung 1992; 21:141–147.
7. Nichols SK, Wolverton CL. Outcome criteria for patients with implantable defibrillators. Dimens Crit Care Nurs 1991; 10:294–304.
8. Teplitz L. Nursing diagnoses for automatic implantable cardioverter defibrillator patients. Dimens Crit Care Nurs 1991; 10:188–201.
9. Kuiper RA. The automatic implantable cardioverter defibrillator as a therapeutic modality for recurrent ventricular tachycardia: a case study. Prog Cardiovasc Nurs 1990; 5:6–12.
10. Opladen JN. Automatic implantable cardioverter defibrillators. Nursing 1990; 20:64G–64M.
11. Lee BL, Mirabal G. Automatic implantable cardioverter defibrillator. Interpreting, treating ventricular fibrillation. AORN J 1989; 50:1218–1227.
12. Thomas A, Furst E. Automatic Implantable cardioverter-defibrillator. J Cardiovasc Nurs 1988; 3:77–81.
13. Moss PM, Chavez BB, Prostko JM. An implantable defibrillator. Help for ventricular arrhythmias. AORN J 1984; 40(4):551–558.
14. Brannon HB, Johnson R. The internal cardioverter-defibrillator: patient-family teaching. Focus Crit Care 1992; 19:41–46.
15. Cooper DK, Valladares BK, Futterman LG. Care of the patient with the automatic implantable cardioverter defibrillator: a guide for nurses. Heart Lung 1987; 16:640–648.
16. Moser SA, Crawford D, Thomas A. Caring for patients with implantable cardioverter defibrillators. Crit Care Nurse 1988; 8:52–56.
17. Mandalakas N, Butts L, Colburn C, Clyne CA, Wang P, Estes NAM III. Evaluation and management of the ICD patient. Cardio 1991; 45.
18. Cannom DS, Winkle RA. Implantation of the automatic cardioverter defibrillator (AICD): practical aspects. PACE 1986; 9:793–809.
19. Mandalakas N, Stevens SK, Wang PJ, Rastegar H, Estes NAM III. Role of the automatic implantable cardioverter/defibrillator in clinical management of ventricular tachycardia. Intern Med. 1993 Sept. 10–16.
20. Ciccone JM, Saksena S, Shah Y, Pantopoulos D. A prospective randomized study of the clinical efficacy and safety of transvenous cardioversion for termination of ventricular tachycardia. Circulation 1985; 71:S71–S78.
21. Winkle RA, Stinson EB, Bach JM, Echt DS, Ayer P, Armstrong K. Measurement of cardioversion defibrillation thresholds in man by an exponential waveform and an apical patch superior vena cava spring electrode configuration. Circulation 1984; 69:766–771.
22. Schaefer YG, Chicca C, Fisher C. Caring for a patient with an A.I.C.D. Nursing 1992; 22:48–50.
23. Mirowkski M, Reid PR, Mower M. The automatic implantable cardioverter-defibrillator: an overview. J Am Cardiol 1985; 6:461–466.
24. Echt DS, Winkle RA. Management of patients with the automatic implantable cardioverter-defibrillator. Clin Prog 1985; 3:4–16.
25. Mirowski M, Reid PR, Mower M. Clinical performance of the implantable cardioverter defibrillator. PACE 1984; 7:1345–1350.
26. Schuster DM. Patients with an implanted cardioverter-defibrillator: a new challenge. J Emerg Nurs 1990; 16:219–225.

27. Badger JM, Morris PLP. Observation of a support group for automatic implantable cardioverter-defibrillator recipients and their spouses. Heart Lung 1989; 18:238–243.
28. Kuiper R, Nyamathi A. Stressors and coping strategies of patients with automatic implantable cardioverter-defibrillators. J Cardiovasc Nurs 1991; 5:65–76.
29. Teplitz L, Egenes K, Brask L. Life after sudden death; the development of a support group for automatic implantable cardioverter-defibrillator patients. J Cardiovasc Nurs 1990; 4:20–32.
30. Wilson L, Miller P. The automatic implantable cardioverter/defibrillator: a life-saving device. Am J Nurs 1986; 86:1004–1008.
31. Veseth-Rogers J. A practical approach to teaching the automatic implantable cardioverter-defibrillator patient. J Cardiovasc Nurs 1990; 4:7–19.
32. Arteaga WJ, Drew BJ. Device therapy for ventricular tachycardia or fibrillation: the implantable cardioverter defibrillator and antitachycardia pacing. Crit Care Nurs Q 1991; 14:60–71.
33. Moser SA, Crawford D, Thomas A. Updated care guidelines for patients with automatic implantable cardioverter defibrillators. Crit Care Nurse 1993; April:62–73.
34. Bremner SM, McCauley KM, Axtell KA. A follow-up study of patients with implantable cardioverter defibrillators. J Cardiovasc Nurs 1993; 7:40–51.
35. Strickberger SA, Cantillon CO, Friedman PL. When should patients with lethal ventricular arrhythmia resume driving? An analysis of state regulations and physician practices. Ann Intern Med 1991; 115:560–563.
36. Horlick L, Cameron R, Firor W, Bhalerau U, Baltzan R. The effects of education and group discussion in the post-myocardial infarction patient. J Psychosomat Med 1984; 28:485–492.
37. Hackell, T. Group therapy in cardiac rehabilitation. Cardiology 1977; 62:75–84.
38. Baker KG, McCoy PL. Group sessions as a method of reducing anxiety in patients with coronary artery disease. Heart Lung 1979; 8:525–529.
39. Bilodeau CB, Hackett TP. Issues raised in a group setting by patients recovering from myocardial infarction. Am J Psych 1971; 128:73–77.
40. Rahe RH, Tuffli CF, Suchar RJ, Arthur RJ. Group therapy in the outpatient management of post-myocardial infarction patients. Int J Psych Med 1973; 4:77–87.
41. Blanchard E, Miller J. Psychological treatment of cardiovascular disease. Arch Gen Psych 1977; 34:1402–1413.
42. Rahe RH, Ward HW, Hayes V. Brief group therapy in myocardial infarction rehabilitation. Three to four year follow-up of a controlled trial. J Psychosomat Med 1979; 42:229–241.
43. Rahe RH, O'Neil T, Hogan A, Arthur RJ. Brief group therapy following myocardial infarction: eighteen month follow-up of a controlled trial. Int J Psych Med 1975; 6:349–358.

25

Psychiatric Aspects of the Implantable Cardioverter-Defibrillator

Gregory L. Fricchione

*Harvard Medical School and Brigham and Women's Hospital
Boston, Massachusetts*

Stephen C. Vlay

*State University of New York at Stony Brook and University Hospital
Stony Brook, New York*

I. INTRODUCTION

Sudden cardiac death (SCD) has certainly earned its reputation as the major challenge confronting contemporary cardiology [1]. Modern cardiac advances have started to meet this challenge in health care so that survivors of SCD are benefiting from more aggressive interventions which increase their life expectancies. For reasons we will examine in this chapter, the experience of surviving SCD has been accompanied by new psychiatric burdens which offer a challenge to contemporary psychiatry [2].

The electrophysiological accident of ventricular tachycardia-ventricular fibrillation (VT-VF), which is the primary cause of SCD, may be due to transient events. Momentary inputs to the heart may trigger an electrically unstable myocardium into VF [1,3,4]. In this regard, risk factors for VF will include not only physical strains but also stress factors related to CNS activity [4–7]. For this reason research has expanded "from heart as target" to "brain as trigger" [1].

In the past, when a patient survived a cardiac arrest, he or she was evaluated by a cardiologist with a Holter monitor and perhaps a cardiac catheterization and was treated with an antiarrhythmic agent which, while holding out the hope of being antiarrhythmic, might also be proarrhythmic. Patients had to deal with uncertainty about effectiveness of treatment and recurrence of the lethal arrhythmia. However, the treatment approach was essentially familiar and unchallenging. Today SCD survivors face long hospital stays, more invasive investigative procedures, multiple drug trials, and frequently the implantation of a cardioverter-defibrillator. They thus receive an impressive reduction in mortality and medical morbidity, although the potential psychiatric morbidity attendant to the process of evaluation and treatment may also be impressive. Thus medical psychiatrists are more involved in the care and study of patients who survive cardiac arrests. Survivors of cardiac arrests and patients with ventricular arrhythmias are often seen in consultation while they are inpatients undergoing their rigorous and often disturbing evaluations [2]. These patients, particularly those with past psychiatric histories, may develop psychiatric syndromes in reaction to their unique circumstances as they confront death in a concrete way. If they go on to require an implantable cardioverter-defibrillator (ICD), a new series of adaptational tasks emerge, and some patients develop psychiatric sequelae. The adaptational tasks required of the ICD recipient may herald the future challenges patients will face as modern medicine turns increasingly to artificial implantable devices to compensate for organ failures.

In this chapter, after reviewing the neuropsychiatry of cardiac events, we will focus on the experience of the person undergoing electrophysiological studies (EPS) and implantation of the ICD. We will then discuss psychiatric conditions such as anxiety and depressive disorders, grief responses in patients and families, and more rarely, psychosis and delirium in this patient population. Fortunately, successful psychiatric treatments are available for these disorders. At the end of the chapter we will comment on the meaning of this particular illness experience and on the role of the physician as caretaker.

II. THE ROLE OF THE AUTONOMIC NERVOUS SYSTEM AND NEUROTRANSMITTERS

The role of the autonomic nervous system (ANS) in SCD is an extremely important, perhaps primary one. From animal studies it is known that certain, mainly frontal cortical areas may affect cardiovascular function [4,5]. Stimulation in these areas can provoke ventricular premature beats (VPBs). Subcortical areas such as the hypothalamus are even more provocative, capable of igniting ventricular arrhythmias more readily. The incidence of VF in dogs with coronary artery occlusion, whose posterior hypothalamus is stimulated, is 10 times that of occluded dogs without stimulation [7]. The efferent sympathetic pathway arises in the midbrain and quadrigeminal bodies, traverses the C-1 adrenergic neurons to the intermediolateral cell column, and arrives at the heart by means of the stellate ganglia and cardiac sympathetic nerves [4,5,8].

There is substantial evidence implicating heightened sympathetic nervous system (SNS) tone in the predisposition to VT-VF. In animal studies, electrical stimulation of cardiac sympathetic fibers markedly lowers the vulnerable period threshold and, in the presence of myocardial ischemia, may result in VT-VF [4,5]. The left stellate ganglion is the recipient of the majority of the sympathetic fibers and, as such, stimulation here will predispose to VT-VF by virtue of a prolonged QT interval as well as a lowered VT threshold [5,8,9]. Ablation of the left stellate will increase VT threshold by 72% [9]. Recently, more evidence for the importance of the SNS in human arrhythmogenesis has emerged. In some patients it has been shown that VT-VF can be associated with, if not initiated by, a sustained selective increase in cardiac sympathetic activity [10]. Sympathetic activity related to psychological stress would contribute to ventricular arrhythmia risk, not only in patients with structural heart disease, but also in patients without structural disease [11].

A vagal antifibrillatory effect has been noted [3]. By opposing increased SNS tone, vagal stimulation can indirectly lower ventricular vulnerability [5]. This vagal effect is a muscarinic property that can be reversed by atropine. The major terminal for vagal ventricular projection is the His-Purkinje system, a hub for numerous sympathetic fibers as well. A predisposition to VT-VF may reflect an adrenergic-cholinergic imbalance. Talman summarizes the evidence for ANS involvement in SCD as follows: (1) Autonomic stimulation, especially if left side is overactivated can lead to VT-VF. (2) Sympathetic activation reduces VF threshold in normal and particularly in ischemic myocardium. (3) Autonomic activity is closely connected to behavior that is under CNS modulation. (4) Psychological and social-environmental strain can give rise to abnormal autonomic flow. (5) VF threshold can be normalized after stress if the hypothalamus and descending pathways are destroyed. (6) Stress is associated with VT, VF, and SCD in animal studies, as well as with the elevated incidence of SCD in human beings [8].

The indoleamines have also been recently implicated in cardiac disease. While serotonin has a vasodilating effect on normal coronary arteries, it has a vasoconstricting effect on damaged coronaries, thus suggesting a role for serotonin in ischemia-related acute cardiac events [12,13]. Serotonin released after platelet activation may be responsible for myocardial ischemia, thus playing a role in VT-VF threshold.

Atherosclerotic plaques predispose to loss of endothelium-derived relaxant factor [14]. When relaxant factor is unavailable, paradoxical coronary vasoconstriction can be caused by transmitters that normally lead to vasodilatation [14]. In addition to serotonin, acetylcholine is a coronary vasodilator that paradoxically causes vasoconstriction of diseased coronary arteries. In a recent study of eight patients, the angiographic response of coronary arteries to acetylcholine and to mental stress correlated well, suggesting that endothelial damage predisposes to vasoconstriction secondary to mental stress [15].

III. THE ROLE OF PSYCHOLOGICAL STRESS

The question of whether psychological stimuli can increase susceptibility to VT-VF and SCD has been an increasingly important one to cardiologists and behavioral medicine researchers. Until recently, relatively little data was available. In the 1970s, Lown and colleagues demonstrated in dogs with ischemia that repeated exposure to an aversive situation would produce ventricular arrhythmias. Relief of this stimulation by removal to a quiet environment would eradicate them [4,16].

Human studies confirm the importance of stressful situations in the presentation of ventricular irritability [17,18]. Psychiatric intervention has been reported to interrupt VT-VF [19].

Psychological stress has been reported as a risk factor for VT-VF, in patients both with and without structural cardiac illness [11,20,21]. In a recent study of 80 patients presenting with malignant ventricular arrhythmias, Brodsky and his colleagues found six without structural cardiac disease. Of these six patients, five had experienced significant psychological stress. When these five patients underwent EPS, they were demonstrated to have VT related to changes in SNS tone. Four of the five patients had a therapeutic response to monotherapy with a beta-blocking agent [11]. The authors suggest that the mechanism whereby psychological stress predisposes to VT-VF may be through SNS stimulation.

The most striking evidence that SNS activity and stress together can be important in igniting VT-VF is seen in long QT interval syndrome, in which syncope and VT-VF can be seen after emotional and physical stresses [22]. This syndrome is thought to be secondary to an imbalance in sympathetic flow to the heart, with a predominant contribution from the left stellate.

Psychological stress has also been implicated in transient myocardial ischemia [23,24]. Indeed, myocardial ischemia can be induced by mental stress in the laboratory in patients with coronary artery disease who also show exercise-related ischemia [25].

Earlier we alluded to adrenergic-cholinergic relationships and their impact on arrhythmogenesis. Researchers have begun to study sympathovagal interaction during mental stress using spectral analysis of heart rate variability. Pagani and colleagues have found that mental stress does create changes in sympathovagal balance, namely, an increase in sympathetic tone relative to vagal tone [26].

There have been many efforts to characterize individuals at risk for VT-VF and SCD by studying psychological variables. In 1975, Regestein [27] stated that "there is no specific link between a given type of psychological derangement and cardiac arrhythmia." This remains so. Studies have variously shown depression, anger, anxiety, and social alienation to be correlated with ventricular tachycardia-ventricular fibrillation and sudden cardiac death [28–32]. However, six studies [28,29,33–36] have cited a relationship between acute stress and the onset of VT-VF and SCD.

When individuals have experienced sudden-death survival, they often lose the veneer of invulnerability we carry with us as part of our day-to-day denial-like defenses. The ratio of vulnerability to confidence is changed dramatically. Basic anxiety emerges from fear of dying and ultimate separation, while depression arises from a fear of loss of role as "spouse, parent, and citizen" [37]. This emotional strain secondary to having survived SCD will, if anything, increase the risk of recurrence of VT-VF. Indeed, without effective treatment the mortality rate is 26% at 1 year and 36% at 2 years [1]. As a result of their confrontation with their own mortality, survivors of SCD face the possibility of becoming psychiatric casualties, often with the development of maladaptive illness behavior. On the other hand, many patients face the challenge of prescient separation with the development of a mature wisdom. On occasion this wisdom is bolstered in an individual by his or her having had a near-death experience (NDE) [38]. Sequelae from these experiences are mostly positive. Fear of death is reduced, a sense of purpose and destiny emerge, and religious feeling may increase.

We can see from the above discussion that patients who come to EP study alone, and those that subsequently require implantation of the ICD, share to a large extent a common pathophysiology that is neuropsychiatric as well as cardiac in origin. In keeping with the central psychosomatic hypothesis, external and internal environmental stimuli will be reflected in neurophysiological brain behavior. Hyperactivity along the sympathetic axis previously described can precipitate ventricular tachyarrhythmia and the electrophysiological accident of SCD, particularly when the substrate serving as the end organ is a heart weakened and scarred by ischemic disease, which itself can be made worse by psychological stress arising from both external and internal stimuli.

IV. THE EXPERIENCE OF THE ELECTROPHYSIOLOGICAL STUDY

In those patients in whom suppression of VT induction is accomplished during programmed electrical stimulation via EPS, the mortality rates at 1 year diminish to 2–10% from 25–40% if no suitable treatment is found [39–41]. This information becomes vitally important to patients in the throes of deciding whether to accept the rigors of EPS as outlined for them by the electrophysiologist-cardiologist. It usually has the power to counteract the prospect of prolonged coronary care or telemetry unit stays during which patients have much time to anxiously consider their fate. The impressive gain in survival rate and nonrecurrence when EPS are performed also balances out the fearsome prospect of having one's lethal arrhythmia purposefully induced in the EP lab.

The patient with VT-VF experiences uncertainty and a sense of loss of control [2]. Anxiety arises as the patient tries to adjust. This anxiety stems from the fear of sudden death, as it does in recent MI victims [37]. The inevitable discussion of the potential for SCD in the patient undergoing EPS makes the intensity even greater [42]. Some patients develop hypervigilance along with what we have called a "time-bomb mentality" [2]. They may feel dependent on their monitors and experience separation anxiety when disconnected. While awake in the EP lab, patients may find it hard to be calm and still, and if they have been inducible on a previous study, they will anticipate "failing the test" again. A sleep disturbance may result from SCD anxiety, with patients often describing a fear of going to sleep lest they never awaken [2,42].

Another fear results from repeated cardioversion. Occasionally this will prevent completion of the EPS. In the EP lab the induced ventricular tachyarrhythmia may be overdrive paced back to sinus rhythm in more than 65% of cases. In the remaining patients, electrical cardioversion will be required. Our practice at Stony Brook is to allow patients to lose consciousness for approximately 10 s before shocking them, enabling them to be amnesic for the event. However, as Kowey points out, in the EP lab, cardioversion of the awake patient is occasionally difficult to avoid without sedation, because the well-tolerated, slower-rate VT that can emerge while on a type 1-C antiarrhythmic trial sometimes cannot be terminated using programmed electrical stimulation or burst pacing [43]. Kowey advocates using intravenous methohexital if the situation becomes urgent and there is not time for an anesthesia consult, although we have found that intravenous lorazepam and morphine can often be helpful as well.

Despite the best efforts of the electrophysiologist, there may be a few rare cases when shocking a patient while still conscious is unavoidable. The individual cardioverted electrically while awake recalls this trauma and is thrust into an aversive conditioning paradigm wherein the very thought of another EPS with possibility of DC countershock may elicit *panic anxiety* disorder, replete with palpitations, racing heart, chest tightness, gastrointestinal symptoms, hyperventilation, sweating, hot and cold flashes, depersonalization-derealization, dizziness, globus hystericus, and the fear of dying or going crazy [2]. Panic states with the above symptomatology need to be monitored for in the EPS/ICD population in general. This can progress to a phobic state, with the patient avoiding and refusing further testing [2]. Most of the patients we have seen who have been countershocked while awake and have subsequently developed psychiatric sequelae will briefly experience the above secondary panic-phobic syndrome as part of their adjustment reaction. Others, however, may be susceptible to a *posttraumatic stress disorder* in that the cardioversion is persistently reexperienced by virtue of intrusive recollections, distressing nightmares, sudden flashbacks, or symbolic reexposures that ignite symptoms of anxiety, insomnia, estrangement, and hypervigilance. This also seems to be the experience of Kowey [43]. In Menza and colleagues' series of 14 consecutive patients undergoing EPS, all the patients experienced anxiety (13 had adjustment disorder with mixed mood, 1 had major depressive disorder), and they all received benzodiazepines [42]. Cardioversion in this series also often led to a fear of its use. Nevertheless, many of the patients who have required DC countershock, even those who did so while awake, do accept follow-up EPS. This acceptance is influenced by the patients' competing fears, especially those attributable to previous VT-VF episodes and survival of SCD. We have found as well that psychiatric care in the context of an arrhythmia team approach is also helpful in maintaining patient alliance and compliance during what can be a harrowing EPS experience.

Depression is also a risk in VT-VF patients. As with other cardiac conditions, the depressed or demoralized mood is often reactive, as in an *adjustment disorder with depressed mood*. Such an adjustment disorder is characterized by a maladaptive reaction within 3 months of a stressor and is accompanied by the assumption that the disturbance will dissipate when the stressor ceases or when a new level of adaptation is reached. Most VT-VF patients referred for consultation have no history of psychiatric illness and present with such an adjustment disorder [44].

All cardiac patients worry about illness impact on their families and about employment and source of income. Will they become dependent on their spouses? What effects will there be on sexual performance? What will become of their children? Will they be able to hold a job again?

These questions and doubts can be dispelled definitely only in time, but they strongly affect these ruminating patients every day.

Patients with VT-VF, like those with other cardiac diseases, must come to terms with certain real and perceived losses. There is loss of security, control, and independence, as well as a potential loss of role. They grieve for these lost qualities and, moreover, for the loss of the veneer of invulnerability that people apply in their everyday lives [2]. Depression may take hold, and with it patients may lose interest, energy, and the ability to focus. They may become irritable and demanding. Dysfunctional sleep and appetite may arise. In the arrhythmia evaluation, many frustrations may await the patient if drug trials fail. A giving up–given-up syndrome is a possible sequela [45].

The symptoms of depression often lift as progress is made toward a viable treatment. Occasionally an autonomous major depression persists, particularly in patients with previous psychiatric morbidity [46]. We know that a poorer medical prognosis characterizes medically ill patients with DSM-III-R *major depression*, constituted by predominant depressed or disinterested mood for 2 weeks accompanied by at least four of the following: sleep dysfunction, anhedonia, hopeless, helpless and worthless sentiments, anergy, distractibility and indecisiveness, anorexia and weight loss, psychomotor change, and morbid thinking and suicidality. It should be noted that mood and cognitive symptoms may be better indicators of major depression than somatic and vegetative ones in the medically ill population. Affective tone and cooperation can often be important markers. It is also known that patients with recurrent VT may be at higher risk for SCD if they are also depressed [30].

Anger is another mood that occasionally surfaces postmalignant arrhythmia. It is of interest that core pathogenetic mechanism in the type A behavior is now thought to be anger or hostility, especially in men [47].

The attention we have paid to the experience of the arrhythmia patient undergoing EPS is essential to our understanding of psychiatric aspects of the ICD recipient. If we travel the path to ICD implantation, we encounter likely premorbid conditions of acute and chronic stress, a reactive state of anxiety and depression after symptomatic VT-VF and SCD survival, and the strain of a long hospitalization with threatening invasive testing. Optimally, a psychiatrist should be involved in the care of all patients undergoing EPS. If this is not feasible, one should be called to see all patients with a history of psychiatric illness; all those experiencing adjustment difficulties, mood changes, changes in reality testing, and confusion; all those who have undergone cardioversion while conscious; and all those who will require ICD placement. A four-pronged approach to the management of these patients has been recommended by us in the past [2,48] (see Table 1).

Table 1 Psychiatric Management of Malignant Arrhythmia Patients

1. The cardiologist provides information optimistically, offering insight into potential frustrations and eventual success via EP study and ICD if needed. Confidence and diminished apprehension are usually achieved.
2. The psychiatrist evaluates the patient's mental status and provides supportive therapy to strengthen coping and cognitive therapy when needed for mood disturbances.
3. The psychiatrist prescribes medications, usually anxiolytics but on occasion antidepressants, for mood disorders. For severe refractory depression, if ventricular arrhythmias are controlled, electroconvulsive therapy can be used.
4. The psychiatrist, nurse, or mental health assistant teaches behavioral techniques such as relaxation or autohypnosis, offering the patient a sense of self-control over stress.

V. THE EXPERIENCE OF THE IMPLANTABLE CARDIOVERTER-DEFIBRILLATOR

When, as a result of EPS, it is finally determined that a person's malignant ventricular arrhythmia is refractory or not adequately suppressed by available antiarrhythmic medications, the ICD will be offered as an effective strategy, with the theme shifting from prevention to prompt treatment [49]. Patients faced with the news that they will need the ICD may feel insecure in the notion that they have an unusual illness requiring a pioneering approach [50], even though there are well over 18,000 ICD recipients in the United States. After informed consent and educational sessions, the patients can usually see the wisdom of accepting the significant protection against dying (<2% annual chance of SCD) that the ICD affords, despite the adjustments it dictates in their personal lives.

Patients first off are required to come to terms with the need to test the device in the operating room before it is implanted. Often the knowledge that the ICD has been tested enhances patient trust [51]. The postoperative course varies with the co-morbid cardiac condition. At the least, most patients receiving an ICD will have an adjustment phase superimposed on the psychiatric status which has emerged from their crisis with malignant ventricular arrhythmia survival, evaluation, and initial management. Coming to terms with incisional and pericarditis pain is another challenge.

Experiencing the shock from the ICD can be quite frightening for patients. It is sometimes described as being like a jolt from an electric socket, or a kick in the chest, and for many it can be quite uncomfortable, although it lasts less than a second. One of our patients had the device discharge while she was asleep, and she reported feeling like she'd been struck by lightening; she fully expected to be smoking when she awoke. In some cases the patient having the ICD go off has fortunately lost consciousness during the lag between arrhythmia and discharge. The ensuing amnesia for the event can be blissful [51,52]. On the other hand, there are cases of inappropriate ICD discharge which occur capriciously and lead to conscious shocks. Thankfully, these are relatively rare occurrences.

The main reaction to being shocked while awake is anxiety. The patient may anticipate repeated firings and internal thumps, and this may shrink his or her range of activity. A version of the same panic-phobic anxiety syndrome we elaborated on for EPS patients who have been externally cardioverted while awake may emerge [52]. Posttraumatic stress features may also be described by ICD patients who have been internally shocked. When familiarity with their situation grows, confidence is rebuilt as vulnerability declines, and patients become less anxious. Another concern for patients with regard to ICD firings is whether people who come in contact with them, particularly their loved ones, will themselves be jolted by the discharge. With reassurance that only a mild electrical sensation, which may surprise but not hurt anyone, can be felt from an ICD patient's skin, most patients' fears will dissipate [51].

Recently, several papers have emerged describing psychological responses to the ICD (see Table 2). Pycha and colleagues found that common problems reported by ICD recipients included fear, depression, mood lability, and sleep difficulty [53]. In the early post-ICD phase, anxiety and depression were commonplace; however, as time progressed, all but one of the 18 patients adjusted, seeing it as a source of physical and psychological security. Cooper et al. focused on ICD quality of life effects, finding fear of lack of shock warnings and of battery failure along with diminished physical and sexual activity as well as decreased social interaction in an appreciable percentage of cases [54]. Tchou et al., reporting in 1989 on the use of ICDs in over 160 patients, described fear of shocks and activity [55]. Patients associated into high-dependency and low-dependency reactions to the ICD. A renewed sense of physical well-

Table 2 Recent Observations on ICD Psychological Effects

Author	Year	Patient #	Tests	ICD effects
Pycha et al.	1986	18	ICD Questions	Anxiety, depression, sleep disturbance during hospitalization; 17 of 18 adjusted well eventually.
Cooper et al.	1986	17	ICD Questions	Fear of lack of shock warning and of battery failure; decreased activity including sexual and social.
Tchou et al.	1989	>160	ICD Questions	Fear of shocks and activity; high- and low-dependency groups noted; low-dependency groups adjusted well, high-dependency more symptomatic. Younger patients may be at more risk for depression.
Vlay et al.	1989	8	ICD Questions State Trait Personality Inventory Symptom Checklist-90	High levels of anxiety and anger in patient population; trait scores unchanged after ICD; anxiety state reduced after ICD while anger state unchanged.
Keren et al.	1991	18	ICD Questions State Trait Anxiety Inventory Beck Depression Inventory	No significant difference in mood in VT-VF patients with or without an ICD; however, 3 of 6 who had ICD firings felt more anxiety as a result.

being characterizes the latter group. In 1989, Vlay and colleagues reported on eight ICD patients who manifested high levels of anxiety and anger compared to normal controls or to other medically ill populations [56]. Trait scores remained essentially unchanged, but, anxiety state was significantly reduced after implantation, while the state of anger remained unchanged. Acceptance of the ICD was high, with patients becoming accustomed to the device after a mean of 3.6 months. All patients stated that they would insist on battery replacement if it ran down. The ICD permitted return to most normal activities [56]. The authors speculate on the possible relationship between decreased anxiety and reduced number of ICD discharges as time goes on. In 1991, Keren and colleagues reported on 18 patients with a history of malignant ventricular arrhythmias [52]. They separated the population into three groups of six. Group I had experienced conscious ICD discharges, group II had the ICD but had not had any firings, and group III had their VT-VF successfully suppressed with medication alone. There were no significant differences in anxiety and depression scores in the three groups studied, nor any significant differences in questionnaire response in group I versus group II. The investigators found that none of the ICD patients would change their decisions to have it implanted, yet two of the six patients who had firing of the device would not recommend it to others. Three of six patients who had ICD firings stated that they felt more anxious as a direct result of their experiences with the device. The authors speculate on possible associations between the experience of conscious shock in the ICD patient and a laboratory-derived conflict model of anxiety in which the desire for a life-sustaining reward is associated with an electrical shock [52,57]. If ICD firings are frequent and random enough, another laboratory-derived paradigm of mood change as a consequence of "learned helplessness" may also be invoked [61]. It is clear from the above review that the ICD experience represents a significant psychiatric challenge to recipients. Several psychiatric syndromes may result, and specialized care will be required in the ICD patient (see Table 3).

As of this writing we have not been faced with the decision whether to withhold implantation of the ICD to a psychotic patient. Clearly, issues of capacity to give informed consent or refusal are of paramount importance here, along with an appraisal of whether the potential ICD recipient will be capable of being compliant with the follow-up management and restrictions such as avoidance of electromagnetic field sources, heights, swimming alone, or performing other actions, such as driving, in which loss of consciousness could lead to self-injury or injury to others [51]. Certainly, a psychiatric evaluation is required for all patients in whom there is a question of ability to manage the ICD. The opinion of the first author, who has experience with psychiatric evaluation of renal transplant recipients, is that similar guidelines can be appropriated for implantation of the ICD [66]. This would mean that ICD implantation should be withheld in cases of active psychosis and of self-destructiveness.

Somatic preoccupation and amplification of bodily sensations can be an outcome of a patient's bout with the life-threatening condition of VT-VF. Differences in this propensity to somatization, which may emerge from differences in cognition, circumstance, attention, and mood, are perhaps responsible for the variability in symptom reporting which may be found among ICD patients [67]. Management of somatization includes an understanding that the individual is seeking care and not cure, that regularly scheduled supportive medical appointments are essential, that nonillness behaviors should be reinforced, and that nonessential diagnostic tests should be limited [68].

The overrepresentation of type A behavior patients in any cardiac population, including ICD recipients, makes it likely that anger may be a mood to reckon with [47]. In our study of eight ICD patients, a high degree of anger compared to normal controls and to other medically ill populations was found [56]. Keren and his colleagues also found subjective anger in ICD patients. Counseling toward a philosophical life-view change and the incorporation of regular relaxation techniques or meditation, along with regular exercise and activity, have been found to alter type A behavior [69].

We have already discussed the origin of anxiety in the ICD patient. On occasion, as a result of the interaction of this anxiety with denial—the lack thereof or an overabundance of it—special syndromes have been described [70]. ICD dependence syndrome occurs when a patient is so preoccupied with VT-VF and SCD that he or she becomes overreliant on the device and reluctant to be active for fear of both ICD discharge and failure. An ICD withdrawal syndrome occurs when the possibility of removal of the ICD results in fear of resuming daily activities or anything that might trigger an arrhythmia. An abuse of the ICD occurs when, sparked by a sense of mistaken invulnerability provided by the presence of the device, patients carelessly disregard instructions, medications, or common sense. A reasonable balance between confidence and vulnerability is aimed for in the treatment of such patients.

Many of the concerns of ICD patients are shared by their families. Often spouses and family members experience similar adaptational crises manifested by anxiety and depression. There may also be angry feelings directed at the patient for changing the "structure" in the family. Guilt often results. As in other chronic illnesses, there is often an alteration in the balance of power between patient and spouse, and changes in family alliances may be forged.

Table 3 Psychiatric Syndromes in the ICD Patient

Syndrome	Presentation [59]	Therapy [2,48]
I. Anxiety disorders		

A. Adjustment disorder with anxious mood	1. Symptoms occur within 3 months of a recognized stressor (e.g., ICD shock).
	2. Expectation of improvement with time out from stressor. Last no longer than 6 months.
	3. Impairment in functioning noted.
	4. Predominant manifestations are nervousness, worry, jitteryness.
		1. Therapy: Supportive sessions: Emmphasize return of confidence and reduction of vulnerability.
		2. Medications:
		  A. Anxiolytics
		    1. Benzodiazepines (BZs): Very safe in ICD population, e.g., Alprazolam
		    2. Buspirone
		    3. Behavioral therapy: e.g., relaxation response, autohypnosis
		    4. Group therapy

B. Panic disorder with or without agoraphobia or other phobic responses	1. Secondary to an aversive stimulus (e.g., ICD shock) with later result in discrete episodes of fear not triggered by situations.
	2. Following symptoms may occur: shortness of breath, dizziness, palpitations, trembling, sweating, choking, GI distress, depersonalization or derealization, paresthesias, hot or cold flashes, chest pain, fear of dying, fear of going crazy. If fewer than four symptoms, may be a limited symptom disorder.
	3. Agoraphobia in ICD population often takes form of fear of leaving home, of being in a place where help is not available, or of being a distance from their hospital. They also may become phobic of situations in which an ICD discharge has occurred.
		1. Therapy:
		  A. Supportive as above
		  B. Cognitive therapy
		2. Medications:
		  A. Anxiolytics
		    1. Benzodiazepines
		      Alprazolam
		      Clonazepam
		  B. Antidepressants: Usually not required. Tricyclics (TCAs): "Start low, go slow" in ICD population after cautious risk–benefit analysis. Monitor for orthostasis conduction defect, reflex tachycardia, arrhythmias; anticholinergic effects. Discontinue other type 1A drugs. Watch for SVT-induced inappropriate ICD firing. Monitor EKG intervals, as

they will increase. To start, can use nortriptyline (safest for orthostasis). Follow levels. Monoamine oxidase inhibitors (MAOIs): e.g., phenelzine. Requires a tyramine-free diet and avoidance of certain drugs to avoid malignant hypertension. Monitor for orthostasis. May suppress appreciation of chest pain, so warn against overexertion in angina patients. Serotonin Reuptake Inhibitors (SRI)

3. Behavioral therapy: As above plus desensitization techniques.

C. Obsessive-compulsive disorder
   1. A rarer response to ICD.
   2. Repetitive thoughts that are intrusive with patient attempting to suppress them (obsessions).
   3. Repetitive intentional behaviors designed to neutralize obsession or dreaded event (compulsions).
   4. To avoid thought of arrest or ICD discharge, patient may develop these symptoms.

   1. Cognitive therapy
   2. Medications:
      A. Antidepressants
         SRI (e.g. Fluoxetine): Monitor for excitement, anxiety. Has been associated with bradyarrhythmias.
         Clomipramine: Has TCA side effects as noted above. Would not be first choice in ICD population.
      B. Benzodiazepines
         Clonazepam
      C. Buspirone
   3. Behavioral therapy

D. Generalized anxiety disorder
   1. May be sequela of chronic adjustment reaction to ICD.

   1. Therapy: See adjustment disorder with anxiety.
   2. Medications: See adjustment disorder with anxiety. Beta-blockers can also be helpful.

E. Posttraumatic stress disorder
   1. Reexperiencing of traumatizing event (e.g., ICD discharge or cardioversion while awake) by recurrent thoughts, nightmares, a sense of reliving the experience.
   2. Avoidance of events or stimuli associated with the trauma.
   3. Increased physiological arousal.

   1. Therapy: See panic disorder.
   2. Medications: See panic disorder.
   3. Behavioral therapies: See panic disorder.

Table 3 continued

Syndrome	Presentation [59]	Therapy [2,48]
II. Depressive states		

A. Adjustment disorder with depressed mood	1. Symptoms occur within 3 months of a recognized stressor (e.g., loss of job, inability to drive).
	2. As with adjustment disorder with anxious mood.
	3. Manifestations: Depressed mood, tearfulness, hopelessness.
		1. Therapy:
		  A. Supportive
		  B. Cognitive
		2. Medications: Alprazolam usually sufficient Antidepressants rarely needed
		3. Group therapy

B. Major depressive disorder (MDD)	1. At least 5 of the following symptoms present during a 2-week period with at least one of the symptoms being depressed mood or loss of interest or pleasure and symptoms not being directly related to medical condition. Symptoms include: depressed mood, loss of interest or anhedonia, change in appetite or weight, change or weight, change in sleep, psychomotor increase or decrease, loss of energy, feelings of worthlessness, indecisiveness, thoughts of death or suicide.	1. Therapy: Cognintive therapy Interpersonal therapy
		2. Medications:
		  A. Fluoxetine Sertraline, paroxetine: New agents, effects not fully known. Bupropion: Monitor for seizures, confusion, psychosis, weight loss.
		  B. TCAs, amoxapine, maprotiline Same considerations as outline above.
		  C. Trazodone: Monitor for orthostasis, ventricular arrhythmias.
		  D. Alprazolam
		  E. MAOI
		  F. Psychostimulants: e.g., methylphenidate. Must monitor for elevated heart rate, blood pressure, and inappropriate ICD discharge.
		3. Electroconvulsive therapy (ECT): For severe MDD, can be used if ICD first deactivated before and reactivated after ECT. Cardiology anesthesiology should be present [55,60].

C. Dysthymia [61]
1. May be sequela of chronic adjustment reaction to ICD.
2. Depressed mood most of the time for at least 2 years, at times accompanied by appetite, sleep, energy, esteem, concentration problems.
   1. Therapy:
      As in MDD
   2. Medication:
      As in MDD
   3. Group therapy

III. Mania
A. Manic-depressive disorder—manic episode
1. Elevated or irritable mood.
2. At least three of the following symptoms: grandiosity, decreased need for sleep, pressured speech, racing thoughts or flight of ideas, distractibility; hyperactivity, excessive pleasurable or reckless activity.
3. ICD recipient with a history of mania may be at risk postimplantation.
   1. Medication:
      A. Lithium: Benign T-wave changes, sinus bradycardia, SA block, AV block, PVCs, and junctional rhythm may rarely occur. Monitor lithium levels.
      B. Carbamazepine: Hypotension, AV block, arrhythmias (similar to TCA effects). Levels can increase with verapamil or. Follow levels.
      C. Valproic acid
      D. Clonazepam
      E. Neuroleptics: Haloperidol preferable to other neuroleptics. Phenothiazines have more TCA-like effects[63,64,65].
      F. Verapamil
   2. ECT: See above.

IV. Delirium
1. May result from anoxia, hypoperfusion, arrhythmia, toxic (lidocaine, other antiarrhythmias, other medications)-metabolic states as well as other etiologies.
   1. Medications:
      A. Neuroleptics: Haloperidol. It can be used intravenously for agitation with close monitoring [63]. Watch for neuroleptic malignant syndrome.

Table 3 continued

Syndrome	Presentation [59]	Therapy [2,48]
	2. Reduced attention, disorganized thinking; at least two of the following: reduced consciousness, perceptual changes, sleep-wake disturbance, psychomotor change, disorientation, memory loss. 3. Abrupt onset, waxing and waning course.	B. Benzodiazepines: Lorazepam can also be used intravenously for agitation. Monitor for respiratory depression [63]. 2. Environmental approaches A. Frequent reorientation, reassurance B. Family visits C. Posey, restraints every 2 h if needed for patient protection. D. Soft nightlight, clock, calendar in room
V. Psychotic disorders: Secondary to a brief reactive psychosis or to mania, depression, or schizophrenia.	1. Delusions, hallucinations, incoherence, loosening of associations, inappropriate affect. 2. Reality testing is lost.	1. Medications: A. Neuroleptics: As above. B. Benzodiazepines: As above. 2. Therapies: Supportive Family
VI. Organic mood, personality, psychotic disorders	1. Every psychiatric symptom may be brought about by an organic etiology.	1. Treat the etiologic state. 2. If target symptoms remain and benefit outweighs risk, can use above strategies for treatment.

Psychiatric Aspects of the ICD

Dependency-independency conflicts may abound. One particularly nettlesome area of contention usually involves the restriction on patient driving. This not only adds considerably to patient anxiety, depression, and anger over loss of control, but it may have similar repercussions on the family. One case we are familiar with involves an ICD patient who got so angry at his wife over her control of the car that he required emergency psychiatric evaluation after having had thoughts of harming her. Another patient, soon after moving to a suburb prior to VT-VF and the need for an ICD, promptly moved back with her husband and children to her family's neighborhood so transportation would be less of a problem. Obvious, less drastic approaches to the problem of not driving include use of alternative means of transportation and car-pooling; however, it remains an extremely difficult adjustment for many ICD patients and is often a topic in therapy sessions with the patient and his or her spouse, wherein ventilation is encouraged and concrete problem solving is attempted. Counseling of family members as well as the patient is essential, particularly at points of crisis in the patient's course.

Among the treatment modalities we have not discussed is group therapy. This can be a particularly helpful approach, not only because of its cost effectiveness, but also because family members, in particular the spouses of ICD patients, may be included. Building on the experience of DeBasio and Rodenhausen, who used group therapy for VT-VF patients, others, including Badger and Morris, have reported on the use of a support group for ICD patients and their spouses [71–73]. Results support the hypothesis that group therapy is an effective treatment approach in the promotion of positive adjustment to VT-VF and the ICD [71]. There are also suggestions that role functioning and psychological status improve in patients attending group sessions.

Although there have been few formal studies of ICD effects on quality of life and these several show mixed results, subjective reports seem to support the impression that the overall effect is positive, perhaps to some extent because there is a decrease in side effects from antiarrhythmic medications at high doses [54,56,72]. Kalbfleisch and her colleagues looked at return to work as a concrete measure of the quality of life experienced by ICD recipients [74]. In their study of 101 ICD patients, more than 60% of the patients employed before ICD implantation returned to work, which is comparable to other treatment strategies for cardiac disease.

An outpatient cardiac rehabilitation program can be helpful in convincing patients they can be active without receiving an ICD shock. It is important, however, that patients know their device's cutoff rate, since a device can misfire for sinus tachycardia past a certain rate. Thus activity and exercise should follow appropriate pulse rate guidelines [51].

The presence of the pulse generator at the left waistline occasionally causes body image concerns, but these are usually short-lived. Patients also find themselves becoming more protective of this area, but this is not often problematic.

Recently, CPI, the manufacturer of the ICD, issued a "recall" advisement involving approximately 18,000 units. The problem involved a faulty diode, which potentially affected the ability to charge and deliver effective cardioversion or defibrillation.

It became necessary to inform ICD patients, in language they could understand, of the specific nature of the problem. Each patient received a personal letter detailing the facts.

Fortunately, in the 65-patient ICD population we follow, only three were concerned enough to call us for more information, and all were able to be reassured. The matter was discussed with each patient individually at the time of the clinic visit, but none showed any excessive anxiety nor displayed an inability to cope with the situation. Many said the device had already saved them, and any extra time they had was a bonus.

Table 4 General Approach to the Cardiac Patient (Hackett and Cassem) [37] with Reference to the ICD

1. Educate the ICD cardiac patient and dispel any damaging myths.
2. Help the ICD patient to anticipate stressors such as fear of being alone or of ICD discharge.
3. Use anxiolytic medication and occasionally antidepressant.
4. Promote activity and physical conditioning and proper nutrition.
5. Teach behavioral therapies such as relaxation exercises and autohypnosis.

VI. SUMMARY

The natural history of the ICD patient is marked by mood-destabilizing experiences such as surviving sudden cardiac death and undergoing long hospitalizations and invasive EPS, which may include DC countershock while he or she is awake [70]. Later they must have a thoracotomy and ICD implantation, and some will go on to experience ICD discharge while awake. Thus it is not surprising to see psychiatric reactions to the ICD, which we have reviewed in this chapter. Careful and concerned treatment and management by the cardiology team and the psychiatrist can help the ICD patient reach a higher level of adjustment and an improved quality of life. More research is needed to investigate the longitudinal psychiatric status of the ICD population and how it can be improved.

The general approach outlined by Hackett and Cassem to help patients cope with cardiac disease can be adapted for ICD patients and centers of five crucial points [37] (see Table 4). This approach can be enhanced by group therapy.

The people who accept implantable machinery inside their bodies are truly pioneers. The ICD experience is clearly the prototype for future internal integration, both physical and emotional, of hardware and human function. The ICD as an object will be ambivalently held, as it provides protection yet serves as an ever-present reminder, especially after discharge, of the recipient's illness and mortality. Caring for these individuals, who are uniquely encountered by our mortal human condition, involves the physician in a special challenge. In the midst of what is essentially a developmental crisis for the patient marked by basic separation anxiety, the physician, by virtue of transitional relatedness, has the power not only to provide the most modern technological expertise but also the primeval human solace that truly constitutes the best of medical care [75].

REFERENCES

1. Lown B. Sudden cardiac death: the major challenge confronting contemporary cardiology. Am J Cardiol 1979; 43:313–328.
2. Fricchione GL, Vlay SC. Psychiatric aspects of patients with malignant ventricular arrhythmias. Am J Psychiat 1986; 143:1518–1526.
3. Lown B, Verrier R. Neural activity and ventricular fibrillation. N Engl J Med 1976; 294:1165–1170.
4. DeSilva R. Central nervous system risk factors for sudden cardiac death. Ann NY Acad Sci 1982; 382:143–161.
5. Schwartz P, Stone H. The role of the autonomic nervous system in sudden coronary death. Ann NY Acad Sci 1982; 382:162–180.
6. Brodsky MA, Sato DA, Iseri LT, Wolff LJ, Allen BJ. Ventricular tachyarrhythmia associated with psychological stress. The role of the sympathetic nervous system. JAMA 1987; 257:2064–2067.
7. Verrier R, Calvert A, Lown B. Effect of posterior hypothalamic stimulation on ventricular fibrillation threshold. Am J Physiol 1975; 228:923–927.
8. Talman W. Cardiovascular regulation and lesions of the central nervous system. Ann Neurol 1985; 18:1–12.

9. Schwartz P, Vanoli E, Zaza A, et al. The effect of antiarrhythmic drugs on life threatening arrhythmias induced by the interaction between acute myocardial ischemia and sympathetic hyperactivity. Am Heart J 1985; 109:937–948.
10. Meredith IT, Broughton A, Jennings GL, Esler MD. Evidence of a selective increase in cardiac sympathetic activity in patients with sustained ventricular arrhythmias. N Engl J Med 1991; 325:618–624.
11. Brodsky MA, Sato DA, Iseri LT, Wolff LJ, Allen BJ. Ventricular tachyarrhythmia associated with psychological stress—the role of the sympathetic nervous system. JAMA 1987; 257:2064–2067.
12. Golino P, Piscione F, Willerson JT, et al. Divergent effects of serotonin on coronary-artery dimensions and blood flow in patients with coronary atherosclerosis and control patients. N Engl J Med 1991; 324:641–648.
13. McFadden EP, Clarke JG, Davies GJ, et al. Effect of intracoronary serotonin on coronary vessels in patients with stable angina and patients with variant angina. N Engl J Med 1991; 324:648–654.
14. Furchgott RF, Zwadzki JV. The obligatory role of endothelial cells in the relaxation of arterial smooth muscle by acetylcholine. Nature 1980; 388:373–376.
15. Yeung AC, Vekshtein VI, Vita JA, et al. Vasomotor responses of coronary arteries to mental stress (abstr). Circulation 1989; 80(suppl II):II-591.
16. Lown B, Verrier R, Rabinowitz S. Neural and psychological mechanisms and the problem of sudden cardiac death. Am J Cardiol 1977; 39:890–902.
17. Taggert P, Gibbons D, Somerville W. Some effects of motor car driving on the normal and abnormal heart. Br Med J 1969; 4:130–134.
18. Taggert P, Carruthers M, Somerville W. Electrocardiogram, plasma catecholamines and lipids and their modification by oxypundal when speaking before an audience. Lancet 1973; 2:341–346.
19. Reich P, Gold P. Interruption of recurrent ventricular fibrillation by psychiatric intervention. Gen Hosp Psychiatry 1983; 5:255–257.
20. Harvey WP, Levine SA. Paroxysmal ventricular tachycardias due to emotion: possible mechanism of death from fright. JAMA 1951; 150:479–480.
21. Reich P, De Silva RA, Lown B, et al. Acute psychological disturbances preceding life-threatening ventricular arrhythmias; JAMA 1981: 246:223–235.
22. Schwartz PJ, Zaza A, Locati E, Moss AJ. Stress and sudden death: The case of the long QT syndrome. Circulation 1991; 83(suppl II):II-71–II-80.
23. Rozanski A, Bairey CN, Krantz DS, et al. Mental stress and the induction of silent myocardial ischemia in patients with coronary artery disease. N Engl J Med 1988; 318:1005–1012.
24. Carpeggiani C, Skinner JE. Coronary flow and mental stress: experimental findings. Circulation 1991; 83(suppl II):II-90–II-93.
25. Rozanski A, Krantz DS, Bairey CN. Ventricular responses to mental stress testing in patients with coronary artery disease: pathophysiological implications. Circulation 1991; 83(suppl II):II-37–II-144.
26. Pagani M, Mazzuero G, Ferrari A, et al. Sympathovagal interaction during mental stress: a study using spectral analysis of heart rate variability in healthy control subjects and patients with a prior myocardial infarction. Circulation 1991; 83(suppl II):II-43–II-51.
27. Regestein Q. Relationships between psychological factors and cardiac rhythm and electrical disturbances. Comp Psychiat 1975; 16:137–148.
28. Greene W, Goldstein S, Moss A. Psychosocial aspects of sudden death. Arch Intern Med 1972; 129:725–731.
29. Reich P, DeSilva R, Lown B, et al. Acute psychological disturbances preceding life-threatening ventricular arrhythmias. JAMA 1981; 246:233–235.
30. Bruhn J, Paredes A, Adsett C, et al. Psychological predictors of sudden death in myocardial infarction. J Psychosom Res 1974; 18:187–191.
31. Orth-Gomer K, Edwards ME, Erhardt L, et al. Relation between ventricular arrhythmias and psychological profile. Acta Med Scand 1980; 207:31–36.
32. Katz C, Martin R, Landa B, et al. Relationship of psychologic factors to frequent symptomatic ventricular arrhythmias. Am J Med 1985; 78:589–594.

33. Meyers A, Dewar H. Circumstances attending 100 sudden deaths from coronary artery disease with coroner's necropsies. Br Heart J 1975; 37:1133–1143.
34. Rissanen V, Romo M, Siltanen P. Premonitory symptoms and stress factors preceding sudden death from ischaemic heart disease. Acta Med Scand 1978; 204:389–396.
35. Cebelin M, Hirsch C. Human stress cardiomyopathy. Hum Pathol 1980; 11:123–132.
36. Trichopoulos D, Katsouyanni K, Zavitsanos X, et al. Psychological stress and fatal heart attack: the Athens (1981) earthquake natural experiment. Lancet 1983; 1:441–443.
37. Hackett T, Cassem N. Coping with cardiac disease. Adv Cardiol 1982; 31:212–217.
38. Greyson B, Stevenson I. The phenomenology of near-death experience. Am J Psychiat 1980; 137:1193–1196.
39. Horowitz LN. Intracardiac electrophysiologic studies for drug selection in ventricular tachycardia. Circulation 1987; 75(suppl III):134–136.
40. Swerdlow CD, Winkle RA, Mason JW. Determinants of survival in patients with ventricular tachyarrhythmias. N Engl J Med 1983; 308:1436–1440.
41. Ruskin J, DeMarco J, Garan H. Out of hospital cardiac arrest: electrophysiologic observations and selection of long-term anti-arrhythmia therapy. N Engl J Med 1980; 303:607–612.
42. Menza MA, Stern TA, Cassem NH. Treatment of anxiety associated with electrophysiological studies. Heart Lung 1988; 17:555–559.
43. Kowey PR. The calamity of cardioversion of conscious patients. Am J Cardiol 1988; 61:1106–1107.
44. Lloyd G, Cawley R. Distress or illness? A study of psychological symptoms after myocardial infarction. Br J Psychiat 1983; 142:120–125.
45. Engel G. Sudden and rapid death during psychological stress—folklore or folk wisdom? Ann Intern Med 1971; 74:771–782.
46. Levenson J, Friedel R. Major depression in patients with cardiac disease: diagnosis and somatic treatment. Psychosomatics 1985; 26:91–102.
47. Dimsdale JE. A perspective on type A behavior and coronary disease. N Engl J Med 1988; 318:110–112.
48. Guze B, Richeimer S, Szuba M. The Psychiatric Drug Handbook. St Louis: Mosby Year Book, 1992.
49. Mirowski M. The automatic implantable cardioverter defibrillator: an overview. J Am Coll Cardiol 1985; 2:461–465.
50. DeBasio N, Rodenhausen N. The group experience. Meeting the psychological needs of patients with ventricular tachycardia. Heart Lung 1984; 13(6):567–602.
51. Veseth-Rogers J. A practical approach to teaching the automatic implantable cardioverter-defibrillator patient. J Cardiovasc Nurs 1990; 4:7–19.
52. Keren R, Aarons D, Veltri EP. Anxiety and depression in patients with life-threatening ventricular arrhythmias: impact of the implantable cardioverter-defibrillator. PACE 1991; 14:181–187.
53. Pycha C, Gulledge AD, Hutzler J, et al. Psychological responses to the implantable defibrillator: preliminary observations. Psychosomatics 1986; 12:841–845.
54. Cooper D, Luceri R, Thurer R, Myerburg R. The impact of the automatic implantable cardioverter defibrillator in quality of life. Clin Prog Electrophysiol 1986; 4:306–309.
55. Tchou PJ, Piasecki E, Gutman M, et al. Psychological support and psychiatric management of patients with automatic implantable cardioverter defibrillators. Int J Psychiat Med 1989; 19:393–407.
56. Vlay SC, Olson LC, Fricchione GL, Friedman R. Anxiety and anger in patients with ventricular tachyarrhythmias. Responses after automatic internal cardioverter defibrillator implantation. PACE 1989; 12:366–373.
57. Geller I, Seifter J. The effects of meprobamate, barbiturates, d-amphetamine and promazine on experimentally induced conflict of the rat. Psychopharmacologia 1960; 1:482–492.
58. Greenberg L, Edwards E, Henn FA. Dexamethasone suppression test in helpless rats. Biol Psychiat 1989; 26:530–532.
59. Diagnostic and Statistical Manual III-R. Washington, DC: American Psychiatric Association, 1987.
60. Fink, M. Personal communication.

61. Akiskal HS. The interface of chronic depression with personality and anxiety disorders. Psychopharm Bull 1984; 20:393–398.
62. Lydiard RB, Gelenberg A. Hazards and adverse effects of lithium. Ann Rev Med 1983; 33:327–0344.
63. Cassem EH, Lake CR, Boyer WF. Psychopharmacology in the ICU. In: Chernow B, ed. The Pharmacologic Approach to the Critically Ill Patient. 2d ed. Baltimore: Williams & Wilkins, 1988.
64. Falk R, DeSilva R, Lown B. Reduction in vulnerability to ventricular fibrillation by bromocriptine, a dopamine agonist. Cardiovasc Res 1981; 15:175–180.
65. Risch SC, Groom GP, Janowsky DS. The effects of psychotropic drugs on the cardiovascular system. J Clin Psychiat 1982; 43(5 sec 2):16–31.
66. Fricchione GL. Psychiatric aspects of renal transplantation. Aust NZ J Psychiat 1989; 23:407–417.
67. Barsky AJ. Amplification, somatization and somatoform disorders. Psychosomatics 1992; 33:28–34.
68. Goldberg RJ, Novack DH, Gask L. The recognition and management of somatization. Psychosomatics 1992; 33:55–61.
69. Friedman M, Thoresen CE, Gill JJ, et al. Alteration of type A behavior and reduction in cardiac recurrences in postmyocardial infarction patients. Am Heart J 1984; 108:237–248.
70. Fricchione GL, Olson LC, Vlay SC. Psychiatric syndromes in patients with automatic internal cardioverter-defibrillator: anxiety, psychological dependence, abuse and withdrawal. Am Heart J 1989; 117:1411–1414.
71. DeBasio N, Rodenhausen N. The group experience: meeting the psychological needs of patients with ventricular tachycardia. Heart Lung 1984; 13:597–602.
72. Badger JM, Morris PLA. Observations of a support group for automatic implantable cardioverter-defibrillator recipients and their spouses. Heart Lung 1989; 18:238–243.
73. Teplitz L, Egenes KJ, Brask L. Life after sudden death: the development of a support group for automatic implantable cardioverter-defibrillator patients. J Cardiovasc Nurs 1990; 4:20–32.
74. Kalbfleisch KR, Lehmann MH, Steinman RT, et al. Reemployment following implantation of the automatic cardioverter defibrillator. Am J Cardiol 1989; 64:199–202.
75. Horton PC. Solace. University of Chicago Press, 1981. Chicago:

26

Follow-up of Patients with Implantable Cardioverter-Defibrillator Devices

Lee A. Biblo, Mark D. Carlson, and Albert L. Waldo

*Case Western Reserve University and University Hospitals of Cleveland
Cleveland, Ohio*

I. INTRODUCTION

As the complexity of implantable cardioverter-defibrillators (ICDs) has increased, so has the management of patients with these devices. The ICDs vary in their detection of and responses to arrhythmias, as well as in the information they telemeter. Older devices were not programmable and telemetered limited information regarding device function (charge time and discharge count). New tiered-therapy ICDs have multiple programmable functions, and telemeter extensive data regarding the patient's heart rhythm and therapy. Thus a thorough understanding of each device is necessary for proper follow-up of the patient with an ICD.

Frequently, patients with an implantable cardioverter-defibrillator have a variety of coexisting medical conditions which require close supervision. The management of the implantable cardioverter-defibrillator in the context of the patient's arrhythmias should not be isolated from the patient's other cardiac and medical problems. The majority of patients have structural heart disease, most often with associated left ventricular dysfunction and coronary artery disease. General medical problems also are remarkably common. In this regard, the extent of non-ICD-related care which will be provided by the electrophysiologist should be made clear to the patient and the primary-care physicians to avoid unintended gaps in appropriate clinical management.

II. ICD CLINIC—NEW IMPLANT

At our institution, all ICD patients are enrolled in the ICD follow-up clinic. In addition, many ICD patients are seen independently by their electrophysiologist. To ensure that necessary follow-up data are collected and organized in a coherent fashion, enrollment in an ICD follow-up clinic is mandatory.

The follow-up program is initiated before the patient is discharged from the hospital. In the hospital, personnel from the ICD follow-up clinic introduce themselves and explain the outpatient program to each ICD patient. Repetition of information presented preoperatively is important, as patients are distracted before surgery. The introductory conversation by the outpatient staff is supplemented by pamphlets or other written or video materials which explain the outpatient program. Materials designed for this purpose are usually provided by the ICD manufacturer and may be sufficient.

Before hospital discharge, necessary data are secured for the ICD follow-up chart: results from all diagnostic studies, such as cardiac catheterizations, electrophysiological studies, echocardiograms, gated blood pool scans, exercise stress tests, and predischarge chest X-rays and electrocardiograms. In addition, the operative report, device/lead warranty data, and the discharge summary complete baseline data for the follow-up chart.

The first follow-up ICD clinic visit routinely occurs at 6 weeks after discharge from the hospital. At this first appointment, the patient is seen jointly by the usual ICD follow-up staff and by the implanting surgeon. In addition to routine ICD follow-up, the surgeon examines all wounds, and the abdominal pocket. In addition, posterior-anterior and lateral chest X-rays are obtained routinely only on this visit.

III. ICD CLINIC OVERVIEW

The ICD clinic is staffed by a nurse coordinator who is a member of the arrhythmia service. At our institution, clinic convenes once per week. Follow-up appointments are scheduled every 2 to 3 months, depending on the type of ICD implanted.

The occasional loss of ICD charts and the inability to locate ICD programmers or software has taught us important lessons. We keep the ICD records in specific ICD clinic charts that are kept in a designated file with access limited to the nurse coordinator. Reports are photocopied when information is needed in locations other than the ICD clinic. All ICD programming equipment is stored in a secure room (Table 1).

Given that the equipment is often needed in several locations, such as in the electrophysiology lab, on the hospital ward, or in the ICD clinic, a central location or multiple programmers are necessary. We have developed two carts in order to transport all necessary equipment to the ICD clinic once a week. Ample extra programmer paper and batteries are stocked in the ICD clinic. Each manufacturer has different programmer paper. Given the nature of ICD patients, adequate resuscitation equipment is necessary. An external defibrillator with quick-look paddles, necessary airway equipment, and a crash cart should be available in the clinic.

An ICD follow-up visit is usually completed in 15 to 20 min, but may be longer if problems are identified. The recording or retrieval of electrograms from certain devices increases the required time in clinic for patients with these devices.

During the clinic visit, the patient interview is critical. All ICD discharges are recorded and classified as being preceded by symptoms or asymptomatic. If discharges have occurred, and are verified by subsequent ICD interrogation, the electrophysiologist is notified and a decision to evaluate further and/or treat to prevent recurrent ICD discharges is made. A review of all current medications is necessary. The potential effects of all new medications on defibrillation threshold (DFT) must be reviewed with the electrophysiologist [1]. New diuretics may prompt review of a serum electrolyte panel with the primary-care physician to ensure adequate potassium replacement. Patient symptoms of cardiac ischemia or failure must be evaluated by the electrophysiologist, referring cardiologist, or primary-care physician.

Blood pressure, pulse, and weight measurements are obtained from each patient. The lungs and heart are auscultated. The ICD pocket is examined for tenderness, swelling, and redness.

The ICD is then interrogated via the programmer. Particular attention is given to the battery life and any therapies that have been delivered since the last visit. Stored electrograms or

Table 1 Equipment Required for Specific ICD Follow-Up

CPI devices
  CPI 2035 Programmer (includes printer)
  Software Modules
    #2820 for 1550 ICD
    #2825 for 1550 or 1555 ICD
    #2830 for 1660 ICD
  Programmer wand—model #6575
  CPI donut magnet—model #6870
Ventritex—Cadence Model V-100
  Ventritex Cadence Programmer
    Light pen—model AC 1010
    Programmer wand—model AC 1000
  Parallel-interface printer
  Output cable—model AC 1020 (to connect to chart recorder for retrieval of electrograms both stored and real time)
Medtronic—PCD
  Medtronic 9710 Programmer (includes printer)
  Software module 7217B
  Blue ECG cable and ECG patches
Telectronics—Guardian 4204 and 4210
  Telectronics 9600 Network Programmer (includes printer)
  Software module 3.82 CE
  Diagnostic output cable 042-068 (to connect to a chart recorder for retrieval of electrograms)

marker channels should be examined in order to determine if the therapies have been delivered appropriately. Again, information about the patient's activities and symptoms surrounding the therapy is helpful in order to determine if therapies have been appropriate. Some ICDs require the capacitors to be reformed at each visit, while others perform this function automatically. The specific interrogation of each device will be discussed later.

The nurse coordinator collects and records all follow-up data in a standardized fashion. Data recorded on paper from ICD programmers is photocopied, because the print from many of the current programmers fades over time. We record patient and ICD information on follow-up forms provided by the manufacturers. These forms are kept in the specific ICD chart for each patient.

If the patient is doing well clinically and the ICD battery life is acceptable, the patient is scheduled for the next follow-up appointment. The responsible electrophysiologist reviews the patient chart later that day. If the patient has had any clinical problems or if battery life is unacceptable, the ICD coordinator immediately notifies the electrophysiologist and subsequent plans are made. Elective hospital admission, arrangements for generator replacement, or calls to the manufacturer are best performed as soon as possible, preferably before the patient goes home. This strategy leaves little to chance.

IV. SPECIFIC DEVICES

The follow-up routine for each clinic visit is determined by the specific device implanted in the patient. The CPI Ventak models 1550, 1555, 1600, Ventritex Cadence, and Medtronic PCD are currently FDA approved and released for use. Telectronics is currently sponsoring clinical trials with the Guardian 4204, 4210, 4211, and 4215 devices. Each manufacturer's ICDs requires

Table 2 Collection of Data at Routine Follow-up

CPI 1550, 1555, and 1600—follow-up frequency every 2 months
1. Monitor the number of shocks delivered through general interrogation.
2. Obtain reading of lead impedance if shock was delivered.
3. Reform the capacitors.
4. Perform a battery charge time after reforming capacitors.
5. Doughnut magnet test to verify audible tones.
6. Final programming, interrogation, and printout.

Ventritex Cadence—follow-up frequency every 2 months for 1 year and then every 3 months
1. Review of diagnostic and therapy sequencing screens.
2. Obtain reading of lead impedance if last therapy delivered was a shock.
3. Retrieval and review of stored electrograms.
4. Measurement of the real-time parameters (including unloaded battery voltage—ERI parameter).
5. Measure pacing thresholds and sensitivities.
6. Final programming, interrogation, and printout.

Medtronic PCD—follow-up frequency every 3 months
1. Interrogate PCD—monitor battery voltage status.
2. Review VT and VF episode count.
3. Condition capacitors.
4. Measure pacing thresholds and sensitivities. Perform P-wave and T-wave tests.
5. Final programming, interrogation, and printout.

Telectronics Guardian—follow-up frequency every 2 months
1. Interrogate Guardian—read the counters.
2. Check the data log, examine snapshots, and examine lead impedance if shock was delivered.
3. Assess the device longevity (ERI).
4. Confirm the intrinsic rhythm—use main timing events.
5. Perform pacing thresholds, calculate the sensing/pacing lead impedance.
6. Final programming, interrogation, and printout.

periodic capacitor reformation. When inactive, capacitors are prone to leak current with dielectric deformation. During these periods, the aluminum oxide layer of the capacitors is reduced, leading to increased current leakage. Reforming the capacitors allows the aluminum oxide layer to reform, thus minimizing current leakage. CPI recommends a manual capacitor reformation every 2 months. Medtronic recommends a manual capacitor reformation every 3 months. The Ventritex Cadence and Telectronics Guardian 4204 and 4210 reform capacitors automatically at 6-month (Cadence) and 2-month (Guardian) intervals, respectively.

The most important data to be obtained at each ICD follow-up visit are the assessment of remaining battery life and a summary of current ICD functions (Table 2). Unfortunately, the determination of remaining battery life is different for each manufacturer. CPI extrapolates the elective replacement indication (ERI), from a charge time obtained immediately after capacitor reformation. Ventritex and Medtronic measure directly the unloaded battery voltage to calculate the ERI. Telectronics does an internal calculation using the unloaded battery voltage and displays the ERI as a percent of longevity remaining.

Programming of ICDs will be covered in other chapters. For the most part, significant programming changes should not be performed in the ICD clinic. Clearly, changes involving low-energy shocks and antitachycardia pacing need to be evaluated in the electrophysiology laboratory and not the ICD follow-up clinic.

A. CPI Series

The early CPI 1400 series devices used a cumbersome procedure involving simultaneous placement of a doughnut magnet and a hand-held probe over the device to calculate the elective replacement indicator, ERI. After simultaneous placement, only the magnet was removed 2–25 s later. The hand-held probe then displayed two digital readouts, the number of pulse discharges delivered to the patient and the charge time. The 8-month battery charge time multiplied by 1.2 became the ERI. Numerous authors documented this to be an extremely conservative strategy [2]. Fortunately, this method of calculating the ERI is largely historical, as very few 1400 series devices remain in use.

The current CPI devices, models 1550, 1555, and 1600, utilize a programmer to determine the charge time. The beginning of life and ERI charge times are printed on the package insert for each device. Therefore each device has its own specific ERI. Before the ERI charge time is calculated, an initial interrogation should be obtained. Of importance in this interrogation, the patch impedance of the last delivered shock should be examined (Fig. 1). The battery charge time should then be measured immediately after the capacitors have been reformed. Capacitor reformation and charge time are measured sequentially using the CPI programmer.

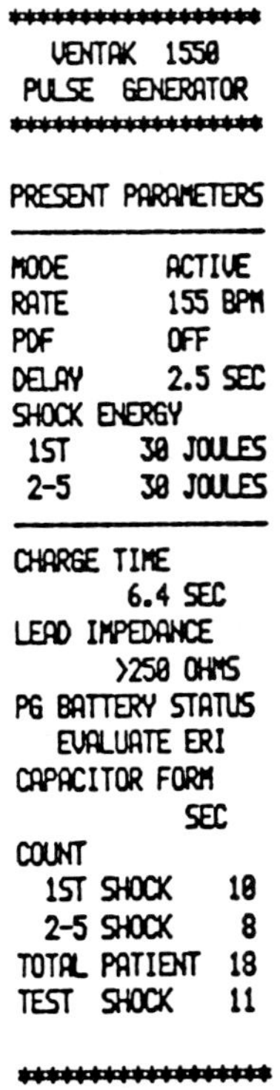

```
*******************
      VENTAK  1550
   PULSE  GENERATOR
*******************

PRESENT PARAMETERS
_____
MODE         ACTIVE
RATE         155 BPM
PDF          OFF
DELAY        2.5 SEC
SHOCK ENERGY
  1ST        30 JOULES
  2-5        30 JOULES
_____
CHARGE TIME
             6.4 SEC
LEAD IMPEDANCE
             >250 OHMS
PG BATTERY STATUS
        EVALUATE ERI
CAPACITOR FORM
                 SEC
COUNT
  1ST SHOCK      10
  2-5 SHOCK       8
  TOTAL PATIENT  18
  TEST SHOCK     11

*******************
```

Figure 1 Interrogation printout from a CPI model 1550 ICD. The charge time of the last shock was 6.4 s. (Of note, the ERI is calculated from the charge time, which is obtained after the batteries have been reformed. Battery reformation is on a different screen.) In this case, a markedly elevated patch impedance occurred with the last shock and should prompt evaluation. The counters revealed a total of 18 delivered shocks.

When the charge time reaches the ERI, plans should be made to replace the generator, as approximately only 3 months of monitoring and ten 30-J shocks remain. As already indicated, CPI recommends that patients be evaluated every 2 months. The rationale for this frequency appears to be the need for capacitor reformation. The every-2-months' follow-up strategy appears extremely conservative but is recommended by the manufacturer. CPI has had a few ICDs which experienced battery depletion at less than 1 year. This failure was determined to arise from a faulty diode component. Such random component failures, which will occur in all devices, emphasize the importance of regular follow-up.

The number of delivered shocks is monitored. Audible tones synchronized to the heart beat are verified with a doughnut magnet which is placed over the ICD for 2–25 s. An audible beep is transmitted with each QRS complex. This audible counting can be used to determine if P waves or T waves are detected. This maneuver is critical in patients who have a permanent pacemaker, where the pacemaker stimulus artifact may be detected by the ICD. If the magnet is left over the ICD for more than 30 s, a continuous tone is emitted which signifies that the device has been deactivated. Reinterrogation of the ICD before the patient leaves the clinic is critical to ensure the device has not been accidentally deactivated by the magnet.

B. Ventritex

The Ventritex Cadence, model V-100, ICD is interrogated using the Cadence programmer. The unloaded battery voltage is used to indicate the need for device replacement, ERI. The unloaded battery voltage is measured on the real-time measurement screen. This, of course, is checked at each patient's follow-up visit (Fig. 2). Of note, after a high-voltage shock, the battery voltage may be lower than its normal value. The unloaded battery voltage of a new pulse generator is approximately 6.0 V. The unloaded battery voltage of 5.1 V is the elective replacement indicator for all Cadence V-100 ICDs. Once the ERI is reached, the battery time remaining is dependent on the frequency of high-energy shocks subsequently delivered and on the pacing requirements. This is usually about 6 months, but with concurrent ventricular pacing at maximum output, this may be only 1 month.

The Ventritex Cadence ICD automatically reforms capacitors at 6-month intervals. This is recorded as a 500-V charge on the device charging history screen. Currently, Ventritex recommends that patients with a Cadence ICD should be seen every 2 months for the first year, and at least every 3 months thereafter. A follow-up visit includes, at minimum: review of the diagnostic summary and therapy sequencing screens; retrieval and review of stored electrograms; and measurement of the parameters on the real-time measurement screen, which will include the unloaded battery voltage. In addition, if the patient is pacemaker dependent, pacing thresholds and sensitivities are measured.

C. Medtronic

The Medtronic PCD is interrogated using the Medtronic 9710 programmer (Fig. 3). The unloaded battery voltage is used to evaluate the ERI. This is found under the DATA screen. Medtronic recommends the following schedule for follow-up frequency. If the unloaded battery voltage is greater than 5.25 V, every 3 months; if < 5.25 V, every month; if ≤ 4.97 V, elective replacement indication; and if ≤ 4.74 V, potential loss of function. If the PCD is accidentally charged before the battery voltage is obtained, the company recommends waiting 30 min before checking the battery voltage. The battery voltage will be artifactually low if it is checked immediately after charging.

Follow-up of Patients with ICD Devices

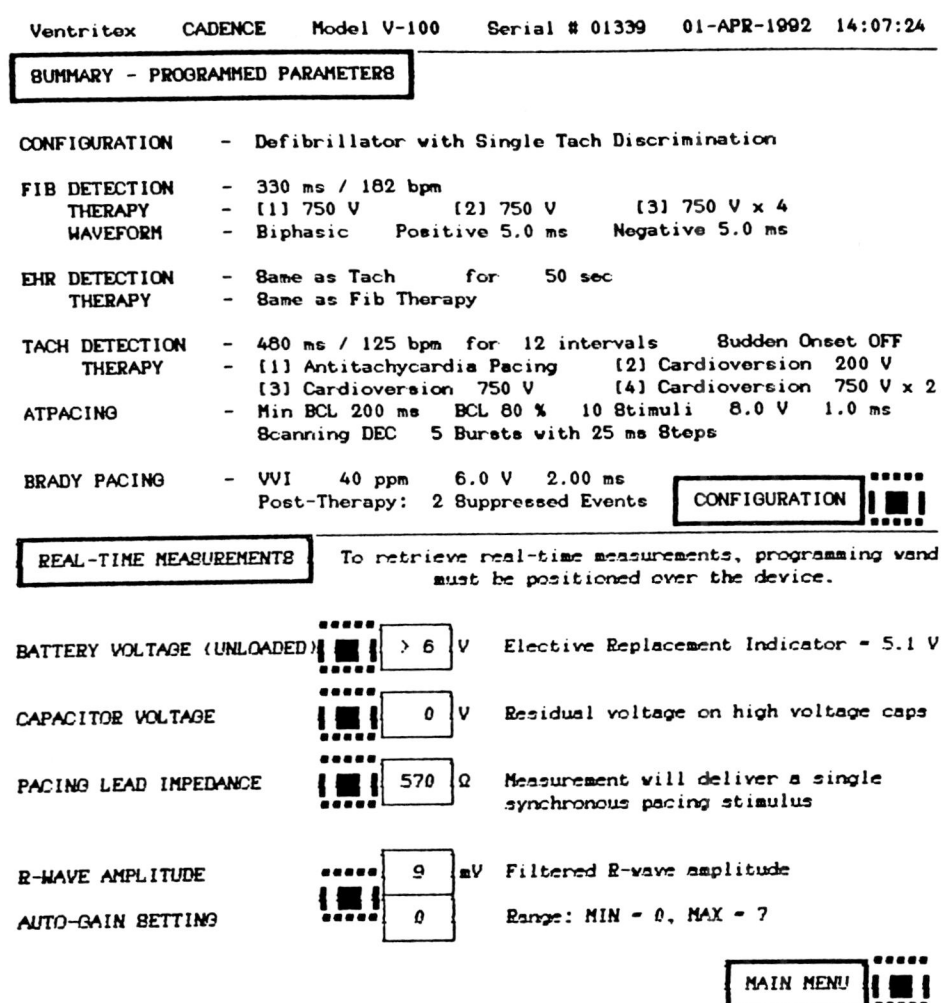

Figure 2 Interrogation printout of programmed parameters and real-time measurements from Ventritex Cadence ICD. This tiered-therapy device was programmed for ventricular fibrillation therapy, ventricular tachycardia therapy, and backup bradycardia pacing. The real-time measurements revealed an unloaded battery voltage of greater than 6.0 V, which was above the ERI. The pacing lead impedance was 570 Ω, and the sensed R wave was 9 mV. (Of note, the patch impedance of the last shock is obtained on a different screen.)

Capacitors must be reformed manually every 3 months. As mentioned earlier, this is performed only after the battery voltage has been obtained. Of interest, VVI pacing is inhibited during charging. Therefore, if the patient is ICD pacemaker dependent, charging should be done in steps of 10, 20, and then 34 J. The total charge time should be less than 11 s. If it is greater than 11 s, Medtronic recommends dumping the charge and determining a new charge time 5 min later. If the charge time is still greater than 11 s, the company is notified immediately. Prolonged charge times indicate impending device malfunction.

```
MEDTRONIC 9710 PROGRAMMER
SOFTWARE REVISION: 9788 - IAQ-1
PCD MODEL 7216/7217
TIME AND DATE:   THU 28 MAY 92 04:32:29 PM

INTERROGATED VALUES:

PACING AND SENSING
------ --- -------
    PACING MODE                      VVI
    PACING RATE                      40 PPM        DATA
    PACING PULSE WIDTH               1.53 MS       ----
    PACING AMPLITUDE                 5.4 V         DEVICE STATUS:
    SENSITIVITY                      0.3 MV          MEMORY RETENTION OK
    REFRACTORY AFTER PACE            320 MS          CHARGE CIRCUIT                 OK
                                                     LAST CHARGE TIME               2.13 SEC
                                                     BATTERY VOLTAGE                6.42 V
                                                     BATTERY OK

VT DETECTION AND THERAPIES                         VT ONSET COUNTER                 0
-- --------- --- ---------
VT DETECT:
    VT DETECTION ENABLE              ON            VT EPISODE AND THERAPY DATA:
    # INTERVALS TO DETECT            16              EPISODE COUNT                  3
    VT DETECTION INTERVAL            400 MS          VT THERAPY #1 SUCCESS COUNT    3
    INTERVAL STABILITY               OFF MS          VT THERAPY #2 SUCCESS COUNT    0
    ONSET CRITERIA ENABLE            OFF             VT THERAPY #3 SUCCESS COUNT    0
    ONSET VALUE (R-R%)               81 %            VT THERAPY #4 SUCCESS COUNT    0
    ONSET COUNTER ENABLE             OFF             # OF VT'S INEFFECTIVE          0
                                                     DEVICE EFFICACIOUS ON LAST VT  YES
VT THERAPY #1:                                       LAST THERAPY USED              #1
    THERAPY TYPE                     RAMP%           #SEQ IN LAST PACE THERAPY      1
    VT THERAPY ENABLE                ON              R-R AVG FOR LAST PACE THRPY    870 MS
    INITIAL # OF S PULSES            5
    FIRST R-S INTERVAL               81 %
    PER PULSE DECREMENT              10 MS
    # OF SEQUENCES                   2
    MINIMUM INTERVAL                 250 MS

VT THERAPY #2:
    THERAPY TYPE            CARDIOVERSION
    VT THERAPY ENABLE                ON
    CV PULSE WIDTH                   3.9 MS
    CV ENERGY (JOULES)               5.0 J
    CV CURRENT PATHWAY               SEQ
```

Figure 3 Interrogation printout from a Medtronic PCD ICD. The pacing and sensing, VT detection and therapies, and data screens are shown. This tiered-therapy device was programmed for ventricular tachycardia therapy, ventricular fibrillation therapy, and backup bradycardia pacing. (The VF detection and therapies screen is not shown.) The battery voltage was adequate. The VT counters revealed three episodes. VT therapy #1 was successful on each occassion.

In addition, the counters which document ventricular tachycardia and ventricular fibrillation episodes are reviewed and then cleared. If the patient is pacemaker dependent, pacing thresholds are obtained. P-wave and T-wave sensing analysis is performed using the marker channel.

D. Telectronics

The Telectronics Guardian 4202 and 4203 models are no longer undergoing clinical trails. Programming and interrogation of these devices was accomplished with a hand-held device which had limited flexibility. Currently, only the 4204 and 4210 ICDs are undergoing clinical evaluation. The 4204 ICD is similar to the 4210, but does not have antitachycardia pacing capability.

Each device is interrogated using a 9600 Telectronic Network Programmer (Fig. 4). The ERI is determined by a function called longevity. Using an internal calculation based on the

Follow-up of Patients with ICD Devices

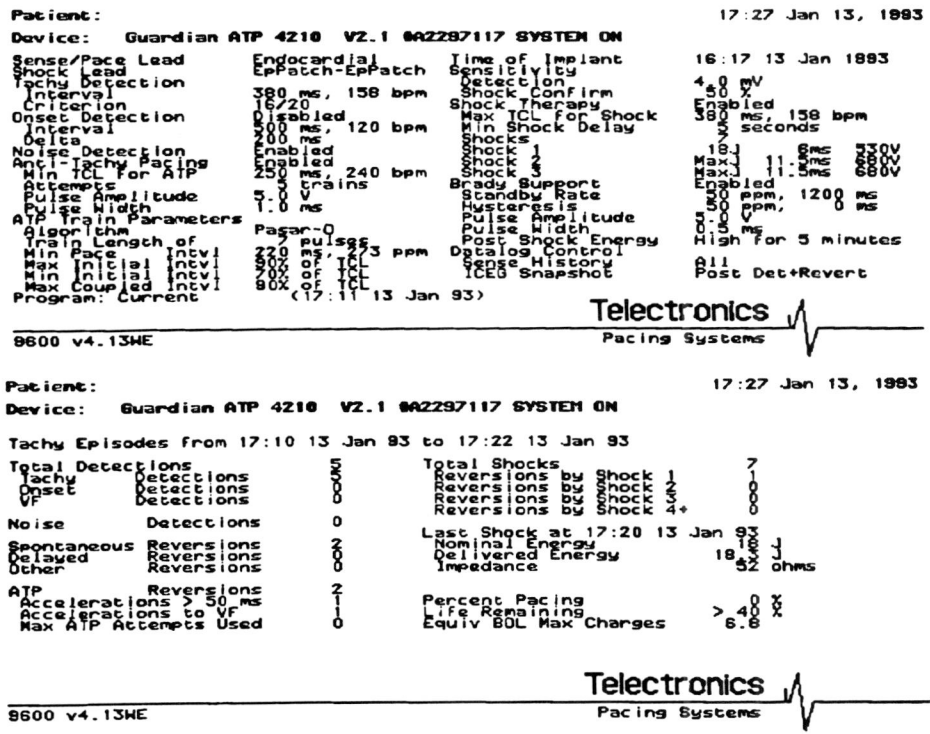

Figure 4 Interrogation printout from a Telectronics Guardian 4210 ICD. In this tiered-therapy device, antitachycardia pacing, shock therapy, and backup bradycardia pacing were all enabled. The ICEG snapshot was enabled. The last shock was delivered on 1-13-93 at 17:20. The patch impedance for that shock was 52 Ω. The remaining battery longevity was greater than 40%.

unloaded battery voltage, remaining battery longevity is calculated by the programmer. The ERI is reached when longevity is 5%. At this point, approximately 25 high-energy shocks remain.

Like the Ventritex Cadence, capacity reformation is automatic. At 60-day intervals, if a charge has not been delivered the device will automatically reform its capacitors. On the 4204 and the 4210 devices, automatic capacitor reformation is not noted on the counters.

In addition, the data log is examined and printed. The data log delineates the time and date of each arrhythmic detection and the sequence of delivered therapy. Snapshots are 1-s samples of intracardiac electrograms with associated markers. Snapshots can be programmed to be obtained as each arrhythmia is detected and/or to follow each delivered therapy. Following examination of the data log and snapshots, the data log is cleared. A marker channel called main timing events (MTE) is used to document appropriate sensing during real time and snapshots. This is examined at each follow-up visit as well.

V. SOCIAL SUPPORT

Perhaps the most difficult facet of care for ICD patients remains their psychological well-being. Loss of control, anticipation of ICD discharge, cosmetic deformities, the inability to drive, and the fear of sudden death all take an immense psychological toll. Most patients require ongoing social support. A few patients require formal psychiatric counseling. The support group has proven to be quite popular among our ICD patients and their families. The support group is an excellent means of reassuring patients that their concerns are quite common [3]. Seeing how other ICD patients cope with these issues provides encouragement to patients with newly implanted ICDs.

At our institution, the clinical nurse coordinator is instrumental in organizing ICD support group meetings. This group of patients, all of whom have ICDs, meets quarterly to discuss issues relevant to their devices. "Elected" or volunteer ICD patients work with the nurse coordinator to plan meeting agendas and distribute a quarterly newsletter. Meetings involving patients from several hospitals are often useful.

VI. FOLLOW-UP ISSUES

The importance of regular follow-up is emphasized to each patient. Occasionally, certain patients consistently miss their follow-up appointments. Special care and counseling are required for these patients. Often, other ICD patients make the best counselors. These counselors can be enlisted at the regular support-group meetings. In addition, an explanation of the necessity for reforming capacitors reinforces the idea that the ICD clinic visit is not just routine.

Patients are advised of the risk of exposure to high magnetic fields. Case reports have documented device deactivation by exposure to stereo speakers [4], magnetized screws [5], and bingo wands [6]. In addition, some workplaces have strong magnetic fields. Company representatives can assist in evaluating specific workplaces for high magnetic fields. Portable meters are available that emit a tone in the presence of a magnetic field that might affect device function.

Exposure to therapeutic doses of radiation for treatment of neoplastic diseases has the potential to damage the ICD. ICD failure appears to be due to increased current leakage [7]. If radiation treatment is necessary, the device is shielded extensively with lead during each session. Currently, manufacturers suggest that the ICD be interrogated after each radiation therapy session.

Patients are counseled to report any erythema, tenderness, discharge, or swelling at the ICD generator site. It is generally accepted that ICD pocket infections appear to occur more frequently following generator replacement than after the initial implant. The infection may become apparent only after hospital discharge.

Tenderness at the generator site after the initial implant is not uncommon. This may be due to generator contact with the lower rib cage. The ICD "settles" over the first few months, relieving this problem. Reassurance to the patient is usually all that is necessary. Patients also report irritation of the generator site by elastic bands or belts. This is often be relieved by wearing suspenders or loosely fitting clothes.

VII. SUMMARY

The ICD follow-up clinic seems to work well when organized by a clinical nurse coordinator who can relate to the needs of the ICD patient and the attending electrophysiologist. Record keeping must be meticulous. ICD patient care issues must be handled expeditiously. In the ICD clinic, the important task of collecting necessary follow-up data is supplemented by acknowledgment of the unique problems ICD patients encounter. As such, ICD patients can continue to function independently with minimal interference in their lifestyles.

REFERENCES

1. Guarnieri T, Levine J, Veltri E, et al. Success of chronic defibrillation and the role of antiarrhythmic drugs with the automatic implantable cardioverter/defibrillator. Am J Cardiol 1987; 60:1061–1064.
2. Epstein A, Shepard R, Kirklin J, McGiffin D. Failure of elective replacement indicator to predict end-of-life of the automatic implantable cardioverter-defibrillator. PACE 1988; 11:569–574.
3. Badger J, Morris P. Observations of a support group for automatic implantable cardioverter-defibrillator recipients and their spouses. Heart Lung 1989; 18:238–243.
4. Karson T, Grace K, Denes P. Stereo speaker silences automatic implantable cardioverter-defibrillator. N Engl J Med 1989; 320:1628–1629.
5. Schmitt C, Brachmann J, Waldecker B, et al. Implantable cardioverter defibrillator: possible hazards of electromagnetic interference. PACE 1991; 14:982–984.
6. Ferrick K, Johnston D, Kim S, et al. Inadvertent AICD inactivation while playing bingo. Am Heart J 1991; 121:206–207.
7. Rodriquez F, Filimonov A, Henning A, Coughlin C, Greenberg M. Radiation-induced effects in multiprogrammable pacemakers and implantable defibrillators. PACE 1991; 14:2143–2153.

27

Troubleshooting Implanted Devices

Richard J. Lewis and Enrico P. Veltri

Sinai Hospital of Baltimore
Baltimore, Maryland

I. INTRODUCTION

An implantable cardioverter-defibrillator (ICD) is an effective treatment modality for sustained ventricular tachyarrhythmias [1,2]. Once it is implanted, however, ICD system problems can arise. These problems can be classified into the following major categories: (1) nonconversion, (2) nondetection, and (3) asymptomatic or inappropriate ICD discharges. Each of these categories and their appropriate troubleshooting strategies will be discussed in detail in this chapter.

In general, each time a patient with an ICD is seen at routine office visit, these potential problems must be screen for. Frequently, the patient may be totally asymptomatic, yet interrogation or magnet testing of the device may elicit abnormal findings. At other times, such as with repetitive ICD discharges, the patient may be very distressed and requires in-hospital observation and evaluation. A thorough history, physical examination, device interrogation and magnet testing (where appropriate), ambulatory electrocardiographic monitoring (Holter or transtelephonic memory loop recording), and radiographic studies are the diagnostic cornerstones of evaluating and troubleshooting an ICD system problem.

II. NONCONVERSION

A number of possibilities exist to explain why an ICD can sense a tachyarrhythmia, charge the capacitors, and deliver a shock to the patient without successful termination of the arrhythmia (even when this was previously successful during ICD implantation and predischarge testing). It is important to realize that the defibrillation threshold (DFT) represents a point on a curve reflecting a "critical mass" of myocardium being depolarized and the statistical probability that a particular energy will successfully terminate ventricular fibrillation (VF) [3]. The first step in troubleshooting this problem requires a review of the patient's operative and intraoperative electrophysiology reports. Did the patient have high or "borderline" DFT during implant? If there was not at least a 10-J "safety margin" between the lowest energy that suc-

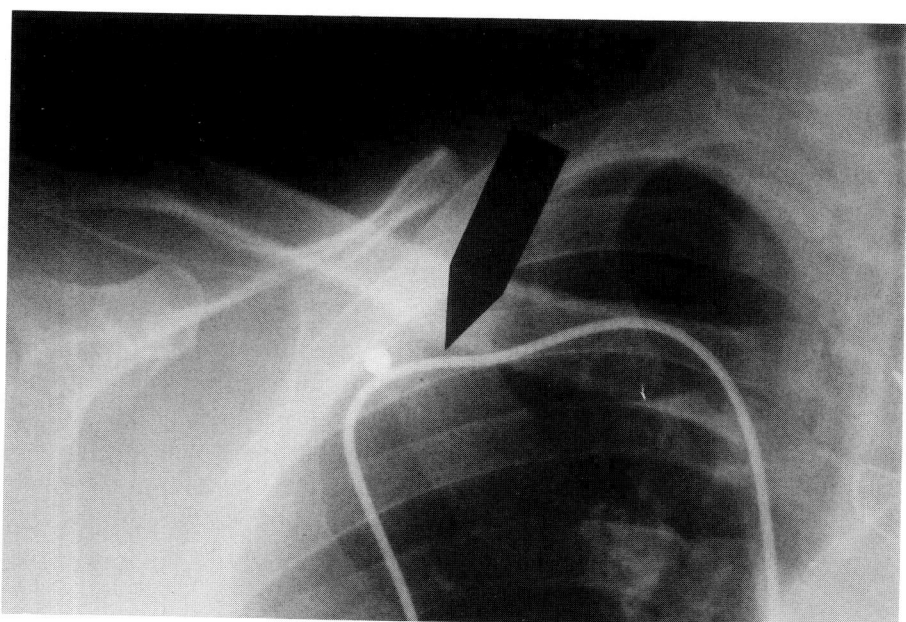

Figure 1 Chest radiograph (right infraclavicular) of a rate-sensing lead fracture. (Reprinted from Ref. 7, with permission from Futura Publishing Co., Inc.)

cessfully converted VF and the programmed ICD shock energy, it should not be surprising that the ICD may not reliably terminate each VF successfully detected. A new lead configuration may be necessary (i.e., change in polarity of leads, biphasic pulse, multiple patches connected with Y-adapters, or additional transvenous or epicardial leads). Under these circumstances, a higher-output ICD generator may also be considered. Before attempting these extreme solutions, however, other explanations for nonconversion should be excluded.

The patient's history since last evaluation must be carefully reviewed, with particular attention to changes in medication. Many pharmacological agents, antiarrhythmic drugs in particular, are associated with elevation in DFT [4,5]. Addition of new drugs can affect the metabolism of other drugs, potentially affecting the DFT as well. Electrolyte abnormalities (especially potassium and magnesium) may be due to changes in diuretic therapy. A deterioration in renal or hepatic function may also be responsible for changes in electrolytes or drug metabolism and elimination. Additionally, progression of underlying cardiac disease such as an interim myocardial infarction or progressive congestive heart failure may change DFT.

Nonconversion may also result from lead migration or dislodgement, poor ICD lead–pulse generator interface (such as a loose set screw), fractured lead, or ICD pulse generator component malfunction. High-quality chest and abdominal radiographs (PA, lateral, and obliques) to identify a potential lead dislodgement, lead fracture, or discontinuity may be helpful when compared to postimplant studies (which should be performed on all patients before being discharged home following the initial ICD implantation). A lead fracture may appear as an obvious discontinuity, or as a new kink or turn in the lead. Figure 1 depicts fracture of an endocardial rate-sensing lead at the right infraclavicular area.

Epicardial patches sewn onto the heart or outside the pericardium (such as subcutaneous or submuscular in current investigational systems) should appear flat and not appear crinkled, crumpled, or folded. A tantalum wire serves as a radiographic marker in many such patches. This wire is not an active part of the electrical circuit, and discontinuities in its path should not be of concern. Radiographs of the ICD pulse generator should be obtained and examined closely. It may be possible to see the lead pins past the connector block set screws. Notwithstanding, a chest radiograph may suggest a new pericardial effusion, explaining the apparent high DFT. An echocardiogram or CT scan may then be used for confirmation.

Interrogation of newer-model pulse generators provides a measurement of the lead impedance during the last shock. A large change in this measured value is good evidence that nonconversion is a problem of lead integrity. Programming a low-energy shock (1–2 J) and testing impedance with a test or "stat" shock can also be considered.

If nonconversion is suspected as being due to a lead problem or ICD pulse generator component malfunction, surgical exploration is required. After opening the ICD pulse generator pocket, the surgeon should visibly inspect the leads as they connect to the pulse generator. Any sutures around leads, whether placed to tack them down or as tags for future identification, can result in insulation fractures, and must be inspected closely. Next, direct visualization of the lead pins in the pulse generator header will serve to ensure that they are past the lead set screws. Gentle tension on the leads, while they are still connected to the pulse generator, can frequently identify a poor or loose connection. While still connected to the ICD pulse generator, morphology/rate-sensing and defibrillating lead electrograms can be measured via the set screws. A discontinuous signal or R-wave amplitude less than 1 mV may confirm a lead problem. The leads can then be disconnected from the pulse generator header. The leads and header should again be inspected visually, and the morphology/rate-sensing and defibrillating lead electrograms should be checked again for a discontinuous signal or small R-wave amplitude. By connecting these leads to a pacemaker system analyzer, the lead impedance can be determined using Ohm's law (dividing the pacing voltage by the current). This is generally performed at 5 V. Comparison with recorded measurements obtained at implant may confirm a lead fracture or dislodgement. If no explanation for nonconversion is identified at this stage, formal reassessment of the DFT must be performed. If DFT is adequate (i.e., ≤20 J reproducibly) the leads should be reinserted into the pulse generator header, the set screws tightened, and, with monitoring leads still in place, ICD conversion testing performed. Only if all the above measures are performed, and still nonconversion is demonstrated, should an ICD component malfunction in the pulse generator be suspected. A new ICD pulse generator can then be implanted and tested. The explanted pulse generator should be returned to the manufacturer, with factory quality assurance analysis performed.

III. NONDETECTION

When a patient has sustained ventricular tachycardia (VT) or VF and no therapy is delivered by the ICD, a finite number of possibilities exist. The problem may be due to inactivation or battery depletion of the device, failure to deliver a shock despite appropriate detection (see previous section), or a failure of the system to detect the tachyarrhythmia. Evaluation of nondetection should begin with an interrogation of the ICD pulse generator. Because strong magnetic fields can deactivate most ICD pulse generators, it should be determined that the system is, in fact, activated, and at preset detection parameters. With newer, more sophisticated devices, it is increasingly likely that interrogation may determine that during the final programming, activation was inadvertently overlooked, or the device was programmed to monitor only.

Actual failure to detect an episode of VT may be due to the VT rate being below the rate detection cutoff. It is important to know the patient's clinical and inducible ventricular tachyarrhythmias, and if any changes in cardiac substrate (infarction, increasing heart failure), electrolytes, or antiarrhythmic drugs may have occurred since last device interrogation. It is for these reasons, as well as the potential to change DFT, that arrhythmia induction and ICD conversion testing is recommended any time a change in cardiac substrate or antiarrhythmic drug therapy occurs. Even without a change in drug therapy, long-term use of certain agents (i.e., amiodarone) can result in slowing of VT rate below programmed rate cutoffs [6]. Noninvasive electrocardiographic monitoring, including 24-h Holter monitoring or memory loop recordings, can be valuable in determining changes in clinical VT rates, or possibly the development of new VT morphologies.

CPI Ventak models 1500, 1510, 1550, 1555, and 1600 have an option for the use of probability density function (PDF) to help discriminate ventricular from supraventricular tachyarrhythmias. If this function has been activated, it is possible for a patient to develop VT above the rate cutoff which may not satisfy PDF criteria due to the "spiky" nature of the ventricular electrogram morphology. In these models, therapy delivery requires satisfaction of both rate as well as PDF criteria. Marker channel recordings (available in Ventak models 1550, 1555, and 1600) while the patient is in VT will clearly document if the rate cutoff and PDF criteria have been satisfied. These marker channels are provided by the ICD pulse generator via the CPI model 2035 hand-held programmer connected to a physiological recorder. When nondetection is due to a failure to meet PDF criteria, it is generally because the morphology-sensing electrograms have R-wave durations less than 100 ms. The intraoperative electrophysiology report should be reviewed to verify the change in this parameter. It should also be noted that intracardiac electrograms can change with electrolyte imbalance and antiarrhythmic drug effects. If failure to detect is due to a failure to satisfy PDF criteria only, this detection parameter should be programmed "off."

Failure to detect VT or VF may be due to fractures in sensing leads (epicardial or endocardial), lead migration or dislodgement (usually endocardial), or loose connection of the lead system to the ICD pulse generator header. As with evaluating for nonconversion (see previous section), radiographs may reveal discontinuities, migration, or inadequate ICD lead–pulse generator connections.

The use of beeping tones and marker channels has been of crucial assistance in troubleshooting these types of problems noninvasively [7]. When a donut magnet is placed over certain implanted, activated ICD pulse generators, soft tones should be heard with each ventricular electrogram. These tones are emitted by a piezoelectric crystal within the ICD pulse generator. The ICD pulse generator will be inactivated after approximately 30 s of continuous magnet application, thus reapplication of the donut magnet over the pulse generator will place the ICD system in the "EP mode," allowing further assessment of detection function. The magnet should be left in place and, with careful attention to beeping tones, correlated to simultaneous surface ECG or rhythm monitoring. One-to-one correlation should be observed, and all beats (including premature atrial or ventricular beats) should be present with a corresponding beeper tone. This test should be performed with the patient lying down, sitting, standing, moving the arms, twisting the trunk, and, if necessary, even while performing ginger exercise on a bicycle.

IV. ASYMPTOMATIC SHOCKS

Approximately 30% to 80% of patients implanted with ICD systems receive shocks from their device [8–10]. In these same patients, a large variation in the number of shocks that are considered clinically appropriate (associated with premonitory presyncope, syncope, cardiac arrest, or electrocardiographic documentation of sustained VT/VF) is also found. One of the most common questions asked is how one determines if an asymptomatic, unmonitored shock was in fact appropriate.

A systematic troubleshooting scheme begins with defining what is appropriate. This seemingly simple question is, in fact, rather complex and dependent to some degree on point of view. For example, a patient, while exercising, experiences a shock from sinus tachycardia above the rate cutoff of the ICD. From the point of view of the ICD system, the shock was appropriate. It correctly sensed a rhythm above the rate cutoff. From the point of view of the patient and clinician, this shock was very inappropriate and unappreciated.

Before ICD implantation and final programming of the ICD pulse generator rate cutoff, a symptom-limited or maximum exercise stress test for the purpose of determining maximum sinus rate is recommended. AV nodal Wenckebach periodicity noted at electrophysiological studies can also be used to approximate maximally conducted ventricular rates; however, catecholamine influences and hemodynamic changes with exercise or stress can result in significant underestimation. Notwithstanding, many patients have atrial fibrillation, thus atrial stimulation is ineffectual. When the patient's clinical VT rate allows, the rate cutoff for the ICD should be at 10–15 beats/min above this maximum sinus rate. In patients who have VT at or below maximal sinus rates, the PDF option available in certain models has occasionally been useful in discriminating ventricular from supraventricular tachycardia. If there are rate-related aberrancy or underlying intraventricular conduction abnormalities, however, PDF is unable to help discriminate. In these patients, beta-blockers are often required to blunt maximum sinus rates. In patients prone to paroxysmal atrial fibrillation, atrial flutter, atrial or AV nodal reentry tachycardias, digoxin and calcium channel blockers also can be useful. Occasionally, these patients may in fact be symptomatic from supraventricular tachyarrhythmia, when the ICD shocks them, it appears appropriate to the patient even though VT or VF was not present. With newer ICD devices programmed to antitachycardia pacing, a supraventricular tachycardia can initiate antitachycardia pacing, thereby provoking VT/VF with subsequent triggering of a shock. Studies reporting on the incidence of spontaneous shocks not accompanied by premonitory symptoms have concluded that a significant proportion of shocks were in fact in response to sustained VT or VF [10].

When a patient presents complaining of an asymptomatic ICD shock, the following evaluation should be routine. Careful history of what the patient's activities were, both at the immediate time of shock and during the moments before the shock, are critical. Interrogation of the ICD pulse generator and comparison of the total number of ICD shocks recorded from previous routine ICD interrogations can confirm or refute the patient's account of an unmonitored ICD shock. An unconfirmed shock, especially if during sleep and causing arousal, is most likely a "phantom" shock.

Patients should undergo repeat magnet testing any time a shock is delivered which was asymptomatic and at rest. As discussed in the previous section, a donut magnet placed over certain ICD pulse generators will cause an audible tone from a piezoelectric crystal within the ICD pulse generator for every R wave perceived by the ICD. Oversensing, whether from myopotentials, multiple counting of P waves, QRS complexes, T waves, or pacemaker artifacts, may be documented by hearing more than one tone per QRS complex seen on a surface ECG

[11]. Ballas et al. have reported on the efficacy of a specially designed "beep-o-gram" or recording device which has two channels, permitting recording of the surface ECG and simultaneous audible tones [12]. A device of this type can be particularly useful when evaluating ICD systems that do not emit a marker channel. As also described in the previous section, magnet-evoked beeper tones or "beep-o-grams" should be obtained with the patient in many positions. Changes in body position may place strain on lead systems, thereby uncovering potential lead fractures or loose connections (elicited by movement of the ICD pulse generator within the pocket). Insulation fractures of the sensing lead system can be documented with use of these audible tones. For example, double (or multiple) counting may be demonstrated only when a patient lifts one arm above the head or stretches it behind the back. Radiographs may also document lead system discontinuities, as detailed previously.

When multiple or erratic counting is demonstrated, once again attention to the patient's surgical implant report and intraoperative electrophysiology report is appropriate. Were sensing lead R waves adequate (i.e., >5 mV)? Was sensing of T waves present? What were the measured slew rates (i.e., $>.75$ V/s)? If any double counting was present at the time of ICD implant, or if marginal R-wave amplitudes and low slew rates were recorded, it is possible that sensing lead revision may be necessary. If new medications have been added to the patient's regimen, especially diuretics which may have altered electrolyte balance, or antiarrhythmic drugs which may have changed the intracardiac electrograms (especially T wave), removal of the drugs or correction of electrolyte imbalance may rectify the oversensing. Pacemakers must never be unipolar systems, and the lowest pacemaker outputs providing reliable capture should be programmed to decrease the likelihood of cross-talk [13,14]. In patients with both an ICD and a pacemaker, post-ICD shocks may reprogram pacemakers, leading to sensing problems and inappropriate shocks [15].

Holter monitoring can be useful following asymptomatic shocks when the history, ICD interrogation, and beeper tones are nondiagnostic. Documentation of paroxysmal atrial fibrillation with rapid ventricular response would be persuasive evidence that this was the culprit arrhythmia. Similarly, documentation of frequent nonsustained VT above the rate cutoff might indicate change in cardiac substrate or inadequate antiarrhythmic drug therapy. These findings should prompt appropriate pharmacological interventions, or reprogramming of the device's detection algorithms. Newer-generation ICD devices have a number of parameters (i.e., reconfirmation and noncommitted modes, detection delays, sudden onset, rate stability, sustained rate duration) which can be considered.

When the above investigative efforts remain nondiagnostic, the use of transtelephonic memory loop ECG recorders appears to be particularly useful in documenting the patient's rhythm at the time of perceived asymptomatic shock [16]. Figures 2 and 3 depict an asymptomatic ICD discharge triggered by nonsustained ventricular tachycardia in a committed device and a symptomatic ventricular tachyarrhythmia, respectively. Many of these devices are activated with ICD discharges and store the electrocardiographic recording before and after the shock. Some investigational monitoring devices also can provide patient-activated transtelephonic "beeper-tone" analyses.

Only infrequently do the above strategies fail to reveal the cause of recurrent asymptomatic ICD shocks. When this does occur, however, there is little choice but to expose the ICD pulse generator pocket and inspect the lead system as detailed in the previous section. Particular attention to the rate-sensing lead parameters (R-wave amplitude, duration, pacing threshold, and resistance) and comparisons to implant measurements are useful. Revision of the sensing leads, if needed, would follow routine implant guidelines. Only if lead integrity is adequate, and no other cause for documented spurious shock is found, would ICD pulse generator replacement and testing be indicated (for suspected pulse generator component malfunction).

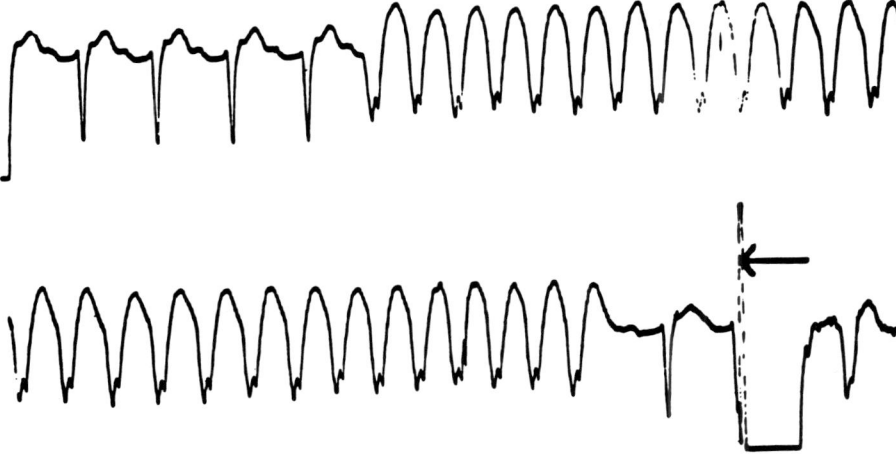

Figure 2 Asymptomatic automatic implantable cardioverter-defibrillator discharge for nonsustained ventricular tachycardia in a committed device. (Reprinted from Ref. 17, with permission.)

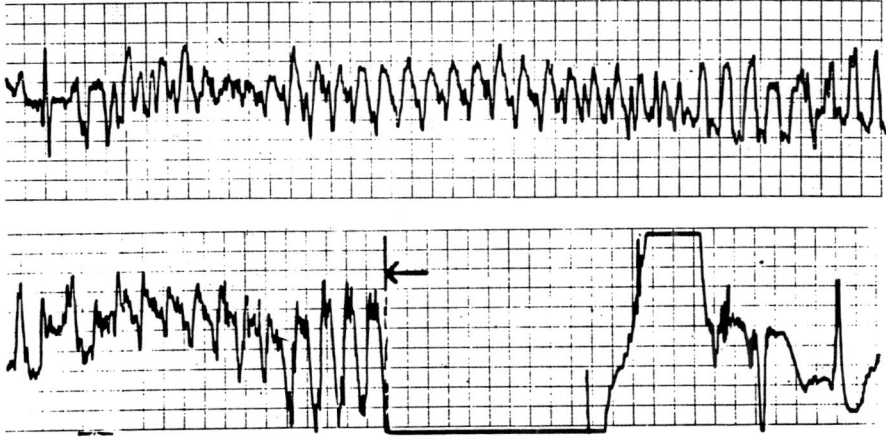

Figure 3 Appropriate automatic implantable cardioverter-defibrillator discharge for sustained ventricular tachyarrhythmia. (Reprinted from Ref. 17, with permission.)

REFERENCES

1. Mirowski M. The automatic implantable cardioverter-defibrillator: an overview. J Am Coll Cardiol 1985; 6:461–466.
2. Winkle RA, Mead RH, Ruder MA, et al. Long-term outcome with the automatic implantable cardioverter-defibrillator. J Am Coll Cardiol 1989; 1353–1361.
3. Davy JM, Fain ES, Dorian P, Winkle RA. The relationship between successful defibrillation and delivered energy in open-chest dogs: reappraisal of the "defibrillation threshold" concept. Am Heart J 1987; 113:77–84.
4. Guarnieri T, Levine JH, Veltri EP, et al. Success of chronic defibrillation and the role of antiarrhythmic drugs with the automatic implantable cardioverter-defibrillator. Am J Cardiol 1987; 60:1061–1064.

5. Singer I, Guarnieri T, Kupersmith J. Implanted automatic defibrillators: effects of drugs and pacemakers. PACE 1988; 11: 2250–2262.
6. Naccarelli GV, Zipes DP, Rahilly GT, Heger JJ, Prystowski EN. Influence of tachycardia cycle length and antiarrhythmic drugs on pacing termination and acceleration of ventricular tachycardia. Am Heart J 1983; 105:1–5.
7. Veltri EP, Mower MM, Mirowski M. Ambulatory monitoring of automatic implantable cardioverter-defibrillator: a practical guide. PACE 1988; 11:315–325.
8. Fogoros RN, Elson JJ, Bonnet CA. Actuarial incidence and pattern of occurrence of shocks following implantation of the automatic implantable defibrillator. PACE 1989; 12:1465–1473.
9. Veltri EP. Letter to the editor. PACE 1989; 12:1964–1967.
10. Maloney J, Masterson M, Khoury D, et al. Clinical performance of the implantable cardioverter-defibrillator: electrocardiographic documentation of 101 spontaneous discharges. PACE 1991; 14:280–285.
11. Singer I, DeBorde R, Veltri EP, et al. The automatic implantable cardioverter defibrillator: T wave sensing in the newest generation. PACE 1988; 11:1584–1591.
12. Ballas SL, Rashidi R, McAlister H, et al. The use of beep-o-grams in the assessment of automatic implantable cardioverter defibrillator sensing function. PACE 1989; 12:1737–1745.
13. Kim SG, Furman S, Waspe LE, Brodman R, Fisher JD. Unipolar pacer artifacts induced failure of an automatic implantable cardioverter/defibrillator to detect ventricular fibrillation. Am J Cardiol 1986; 57:880–881.
14. Epstein AE, Kay GN, Plumb VJ, Shepard RB, Kirklin JK. Combined automatic implantable cardioverter-defibrillator and pacemaker systems: implantation techniques and follow-up. J Am Coll Cardiol 1989; 13:121–131.
15. Calkins H, Brinker J, Veltri EP, Guarnieri T, Levine JH. Clinical interactions between pacemakers and implantable defibrillators. J Am Coll Cardiol 1990; 16:666–673.
16. Steinberg JS, Sugalski JS. Cardiac rhythm precipitating automatic implantable cardioverter-defibrillator discharge in outpatients as detected from transtelephonic electrocardiographic recordings. Am J Cardiol 1991; 67:95–97.
17. Arch Intern Med 1992; 152: 68.

28

Troubleshooting Antitachycardia Pacing in Patients with Implantable Defibrillators

Sergio L. Pinski

Cleveland Clinic Foundation
Cleveland, Ohio

James D. Maloney

Baylor College of Medicine
Houston, Texas

Tony W. Simmons

Bowman Gray School of Medicine
Winston-Salem, North Carolina

Ventricular antitachycardia pacing with backup defibrillation expands the applicability of device therapy to patients who are not ideal candidates for conventional defibrillator therapy. This includes patients with slow, well-tolerated ventricular tachycardia (VT), patients with frequent VT episodes in spite of drug therapy (Fig. 1), and patients with clinically occurring slow as well as rapid VT or ventricular fibrillation (VF). The limitations of conventional defibrillator therapy in these patients can be largely overcome by the very low energy requirements and essentially imperceptible characteristics of antitachycardia pacing, with the fail-safe of defibrillation backup.

Early experience consisted of the combined use of separate antitachycardia pacemakers and implantable cardioverter-defibrillators (ICDs) [1–5]. More recently, devices capable of providing antitachycardia pacing and cardioversion-defibrillation modalities in a tiered or hierarchical arrangement have become available [6–11]. A desirable goal of device therapy should be the complete prevention of sudden death and syncopal VT, with a minimum of high-energy defibrillation shocks, and no (or low-dose) antiarrhythmic drug therapy.

I. GENERAL APPROACH TO THE PROGRAMMING OF ANTITACHYCARDIA PACING IN PATIENTS WITH DEFIBRILLATORS

As a rule, we are conservative at initial programming of antitachycardia pacing in patients with ventricular arrhythmias. Specifically, with tiered-therapy devices, empirical or quasi-empirical programming of antitachycardia pacing as initial therapy in patients whose arrhythmias previously would have been treated with the ICD alone must be avoided (Fig. 2). It is appropriate

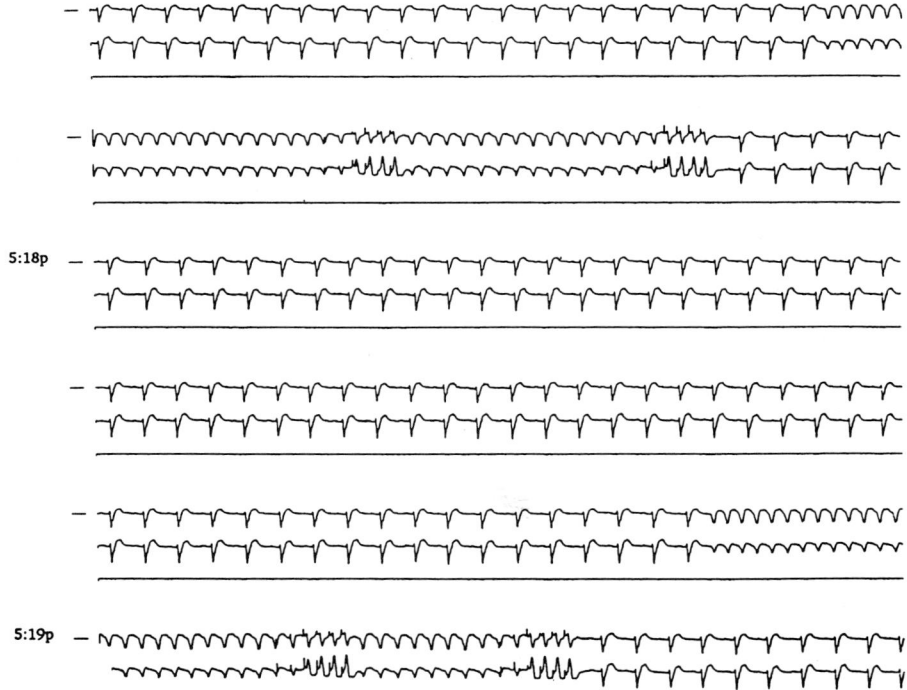

Figure 1 Frequent episodes of VT effectively terminated by a tiered-therapy device. During a 2-min period, two episodes of VT were converted by the scanning algorithm (both in the second attempt), while the patient remained asymptomatic.

to think of therapy in these patients as the interaction of different components. Hardware issues (especially important when using two separate devices), concomitant antiarrhythmic drug therapy, tachycardia detecting algorithms, pacing converting algorithms, and available defibrillation energy all need to be considered when developing the "electrical prescription." An optimal goal can be achieved only through the synergistic working of all these components. *However, it must remain clear that, in terms of preventing sudden death, fail-safe defibrillating function has the highest hierarchy in the system.*

Optimal selection and programming of antitachycardia pacing for VT requires: (1) extensive information about the electrophysiological and hemodynamic characteristics of the tachycardias; (2) complete familiarity with the characteristics and idiosyncracies of the device(s); and (3) investigation of the interactions between the cardiac rhythm and the device(s).

Hemodynamic tolerance of the ventricular tachyarrhythmia is the prerequisite for the selection of patients for antitachycardia pacing. Rate is the most important determinant of the hemodynamic outcome of VT [12], but atrioventricular relationship [13], degree of asynchrony of ventricular contraction, systolic and diastolic ventricular function, presence of myocardial ischemia, and neurohormonal reflexes are also contributing factors [14]. Chronic antitachycardia pacing is feasible mostly for VTs with rates below 200 beats/min. Antitachycardia pacing has a success rate of about 80% in patients with well-tolerated VT, which is similar to success rates with low-energy cardioversion [15,16]. However, antitachycardia pacing has the advantages of better patient tolerance, lower energy consumption, and less likelihood of induction of VF [15-17].

Troubleshooting Antitachycardia Pacing

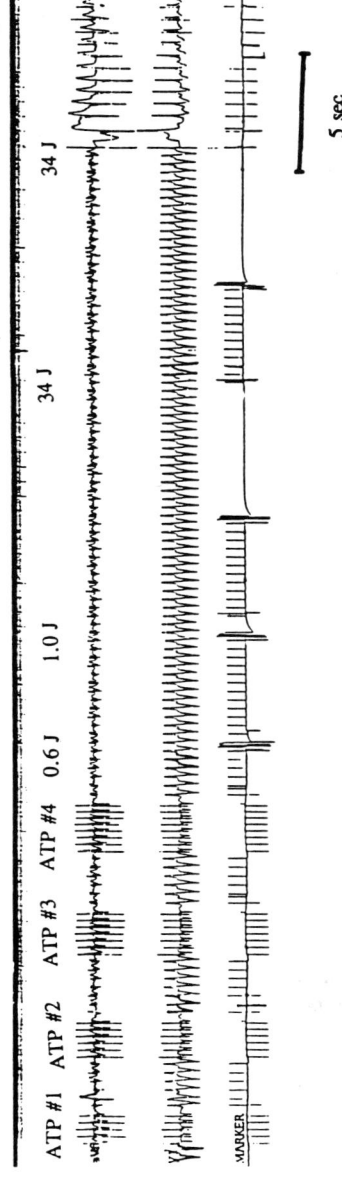

Figure 2 Example of erroneous programming of antitachycardia pacing and low-energy cardioversions in a patient with a tiered-therapy device. Four sequences of antitachycardia pacing and two low-energy shocks are delivered before resorting to high-energy shocks.

A. Follow-up of Patients with Antitachycardia Pacing for Ventricular Tachycardia

Periodic follow-up of patients with antitachycardia devices should be delivered in a setting in which facilities and personnel are focused on this problem ("device clinic") [18]. The capability to perform transtelephonic monitoring can improve follow-up by reducing delay in obtaining data after spontaneous arrhythmic events and decreasing the number of clinic visits [19–21]. Routine follow-up should include a careful history regarding interim symptoms of tachyarrhythmias and defibrillator discharges. Reassessment of antiarrhythmic drug therapy, including dosages, plasma levels, and effects on the electrocardiogram is important. Complete withdrawal of antiarrhythmic drugs is a desirable but not always attainable goal in patients with antitachycardia pacing for ventricular arrhythmias. Many patients require continuing antiarrhythmic drugs to reduce the incidence of tachycardia episodes, slow the tachycardia rate, or treat concomitant supraventricular arrhythmias.

Careful interrogation of the device, including real-time telemetry and retrieval of diagnostic and therapeutic data from the memory, is vital to assess appropriate function of the system. Device malfunction can at times be diagnosed at an asymptomatic preclinical stage. Battery status and pacing lead impedances can be measured in real time by most newer devices. A drop in the battery voltage of a certain magnitude will be an indicator of the need for elective replacement of the unit.

Determination of pacing thresholds should be done routinely in follow-up visits. Confirmation of an adequate safety margin for capture is as crucial as with antibradycardia pacemakers. All newer ICD devices allow for the measurement of the telemetered, real-time, intracardiac signal. This may obviate the need for testing sensing by decreasing the sensitivity to the point of asynchronous pacing. This standard method for evaluating sensing in cardiac pacemakers has more inherent danger in patients with a substrate for VT and VF. Furthermore, as with most devices sensitivity can be programmed down only to 5–8 mV, the assessment of changes in the amplitude of larger electrograms can be done only by monitoring the real-time electrogram. To our knowledge, a direct comparison of these two methods available to assess sensing has not been performed.

B. Use of Information Retrieved from the Device Memory

A major limitation of early defibrillators has been their inability to document the arrhythmia precipitating device discharge. Newer devices store information on the arrhythmias which triggered their intervention and on the results of those interventions, but differ greatly in the extent of their diagnostics capabilities. All devices provide at least data on the total number of interventions for each arrhythmia and more extensive information about the last recorded episode. Some (e.g., CPI PRx, Telectronics Guardian ATP) keep a detailed history of all events detected since the previous interrogation. Digital recordings of RR intervals preceding and following intervention are the more common form of data presentation and have been proven to provide reliable information [22,23] (Fig. 3). The storage of the actual electrograms of the arrhythmias which triggered device intervention further refines follow-up [24]. At the present time only two devices provide for some form of electrogram storage and retrieval. Future devices are expected to have more extensive Holter monitoring capabilities. The Guardian ATP keeps 1-s ECG "snapshots" immediately before and after therapy delivery. The Ventritex Cadence V-100 allows programming for the number and duration of events for which electrograms are stored

Troubleshooting Antitachycardia Pacing

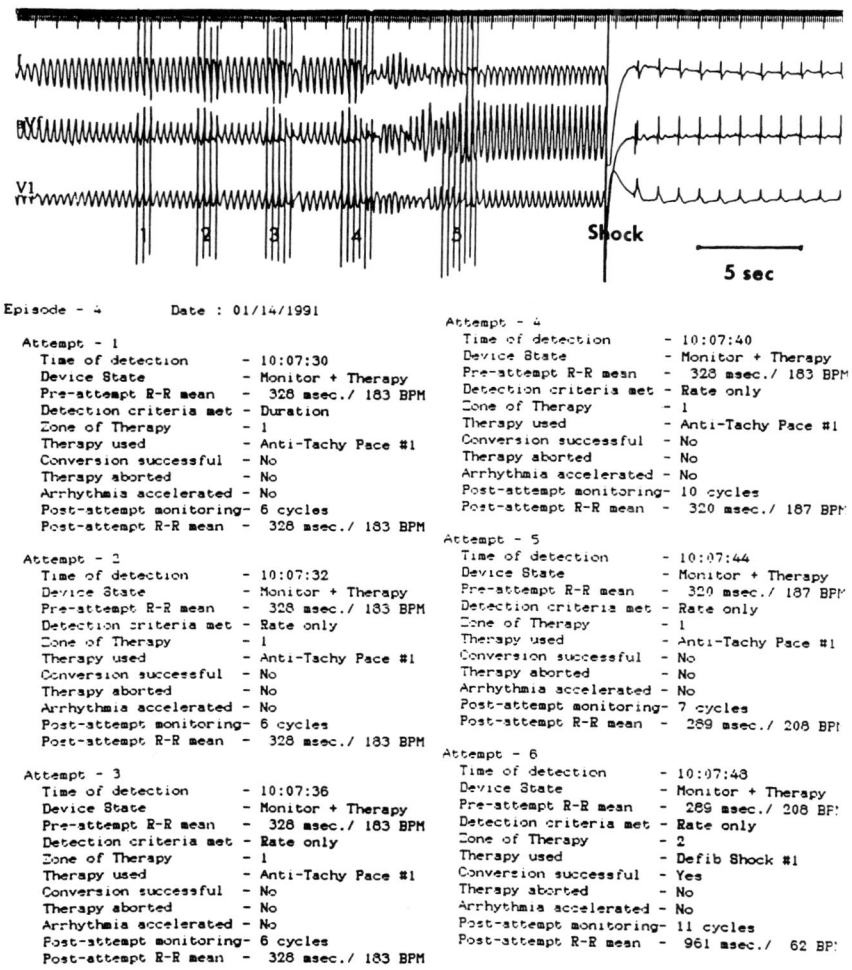

Figure 3 Excellent correlation between an induced arrhythmia and stored information in the CPI PRx device. VT at 180 beats/min was induced via NIPS. Four antitachycardia pacing attempts were unsuccessful in converting the arrhythmia. A fifth sequence resulted in VT acceleration into the VF zone (zone 2). A defibrillation shock was delivered, with restoration of sinus rhythm.

(e.g., one 64-s, three 32-s, or seven 16-s events). The possibility to retrieve and analyze those electrograms is of great clinical value (Fig. 4).

By analyzing the rate, RR interval stability, and configuration of the stored electrograms, a definitive diagnosis of the arrhythmia(s) that triggered device intervention can frequently be established [24]. Electrogram morphology is generally different for beats of supraventricular and ventricular origin. However, they might be identical if the pattern of ventricular activation is similar (e.g., VT arising from the septum in a patient with epicardial sensing leads at a lateral left ventricular site). Supraventricular beats conducted with aberrancy can differ from sinus beats if the conduction disturbance is ipsilateral to the sensing leads [25].

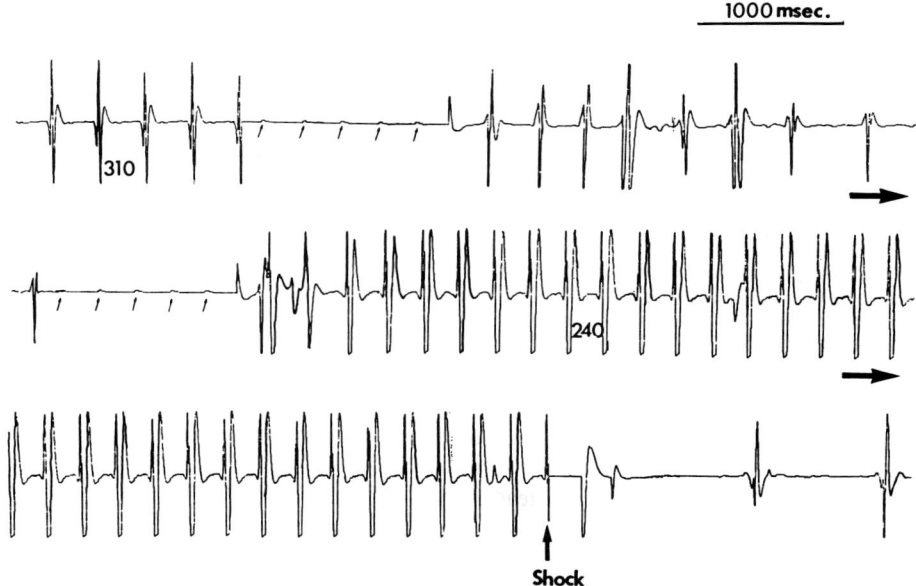

Figure 4 Value of stored electrograms in the assessment of antitachycardia pacing. This patient received a shock preceded by palpitations while at home. Electrograms retrieved from the Ventritex Cadence device showed a VT at a cycle length 310 ms. After the second sequence of antitachycardia pacing (small arrows), the VT was accelerated into the VF zone. A high-energy shock restored sinus rhythm. There is a clear difference in electrogram morphology between sinus rhythm and VT.

II. TROUBLESHOOTING OF ANTITACHYCARDIA PACING SYSTEMS

At times, patients may need a more comprehensive reassessment of antitachycardia pacing. The delivery of more than sporadic defibrillator shocks and the occurrence of syncope or near-syncope are clinical indications for in-depth reevaluation of the correct functioning of the system. Likewise, the finding of frequent aborted defibrillator discharges on interrogation of a noncommitted device (which result in considerable battery drain) should not be ignored [26]. Finally, the initiation of drug therapy that can influence safety or efficacy of antitachycardia device therapy warrants retesting of the tachycardia detection and termination capabilities of the device(s) [27].

Fluoroscopy and flat-plate X-rays are of value when there is a suspicion of lead-related complications. By comparing the follow-up radiograph with the one obtained prior to discharge, the diagnosis of lead migration, fracture, or dislodgment can often be substantiated [28]. Prolonged ambulatory ECG monitoring or in-hospital telemetry are at times the only effective tool to determine the etiology of frequent shocks, particularly with devices without detailed memory functions. Long-term recorders with memory-loop capabilities can also be useful. Formal exercise testing is indicated to assess the ability of the antitachycardia device to discriminate between sinus tachycardia and VT [28].

Repeat electrophysiological study is the mainstay of antitachycardia pacing troubleshooting. This can generally be performed noninvasively, using programmed stimulation features available in most devices (NIPS). The following section addresses in detail the indications, technique, and limitations of noninvasive programmed stimulation. Appropriate use of capabilities available in current devices will limit intraoperative troubleshooting of antitachycardia pacing to cases in which there is strong evidence of hardware malfunction.

A. Noninvasive Electrophysiological Study

Noninvasive electrophysiological studies are technically easy to perform with current antitachycardia devices. However, they must not be taken lightly. All the recommendations regarding personnel and facilities issued for conventional electrophysiological studies remain applicable [29,30]. Noninvasive electrophysiological studies should be performed in the electrophysiological laboratory. Elective performance of programmed ventricular stimulation in other environments cannot be recommended. Physicians, nurses, and technicians participating in the study should be familiar with the intricacies of the different programmers. An external defibrillator should be immediately available; preapplied cutaneous defibrillation patches are recommended. An intravenous line must be initiated before starting the stimulation. Simultaneous display and recording during induced arrhythmias of the telemetered real-time marker channel and at least two surface ECG leads is mandatory for optimal assessment of device function.

Delivery of defibrillator shocks to a conscious patient should be avoided [31]. As energies greater than 1 J are generally perceived as painful [32], we always use medication to decrease any potential discomfort associated with the procedure. Conscious sedation with midazolam will suffice for procedures in which delivery of shocks is unlikely (e.g., patient with well-tolerated VT, known to be pace-terminable). We use short-acting anesthesia with methohexital when shocks are contemplated (e.g., initial testing of antitachycardia pacing, defibrillation threshold testing). Other investigators have used propofol with good results and with minimal demonstrable electrophysiological effects [33]. The presence of an anesthesiologist is not mandatory, but all personnel should be familiar with the use of these drugs and with the management of the airway. The availability of pulse oximetry to guide the administration of supplemental oxygen by mask is valuable. It is our perception that, in some patients, the use of anesthesia may render VT more difficult to induce.

The performance of programmed stimulation itself is simple. With most devices, the desired sequences of extrastimuli are programmed and delivered one at a time. The PRx device can also interact with a standard electrophysiological stimulator in a "slave" mode, further facilitating the study. With a few devices (Cordis Orthocor II, Guardian), noninvasive stimulation is more difficult. The device must be programmed to the VVT mode, and then triggered by cutaneous stimulation. This can generally be achieved with cutaneous pulses of low intensity, and is essentially painless.

Standard stimulation protocols can be used to induce VT [34] (Fig. 5). Unlike regular electrophysiological studies, it is almost always necessary to induce VF during testing of these devices. Rapid decremental ventricular stimulation, although not as effective as direct application of alternating current, will generally induce VF. When using this technique, it is crucial to slowly increment the rate to ensure consistent one-to-one ventricular capture (Fig. 6). Some patients (generally those on amiodarone) require several attempts before VF can be induced, whereas in others very long bursts (which probably induce myocardial ischemia) are needed. The Cadence and the Intermedics Res-Q provide for ultrarapid (20 to 50 ms cycle length) noninvasive ventricular stimulation, which is effective in inducing VF.

When using noninvasive stimulation, only one ventricular site can be paced. In some patients, induction of VT is site-dependent. Some authors have reported a lower inducibility rate

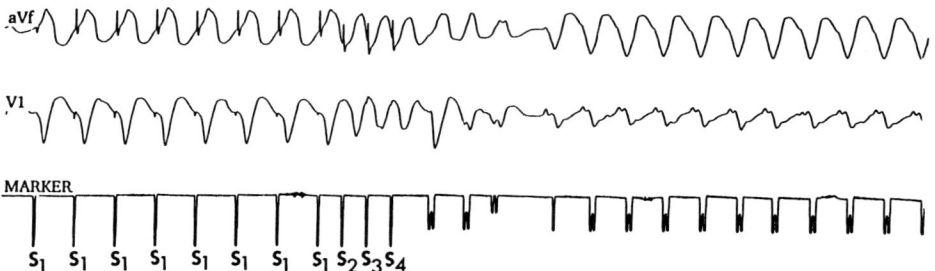

Figure 5 Example of VT induction via noninvasive programmed stimulation in a patient with a Medtronic PCD device. In this case, tachycardia detection began immediately after the delivery of the three extrastimuli.

of VT when using epicardial pacing [35]. Even when using transvenous devices, a rare patient may need a separate temporary transvenous catheter to have a clinical tachycardia induced.

A rather common finding in these patients is the inducibility of multiple morphologies of VT, some of which had not been previously recorded [36]. Some of these tachycardias can, however, occur clinically afterwards [37]. If possible, all inducible tachycardias should be tested for pace termination. Of course, most emphasis should be placed on ensuring adequate detection and termination of clinically occurring tachycardia(s). Ventricular tachycardia should be induced several times, and adjustments should be made until the device is able to terminate induced episodes consistently with one or two bursts of pacing.

B. Troubleshooting Specific Problems

1. Troubleshooting Sensing

Tiered-therapy devices differ greatly in their approaches to sensing. Most devices use the same circuitry for bradycardia and tachycardia sensing, whereas the PRx has two different amplifiers. Sensing can have a programmable fixed gain (antitachycardia pacemakers, Guardian 4202/4203), automatic sensitivity adjustment (Guardian ATP 4210), automatic gain control (Ventak devices, Cadence, Res-Q, Siemens Siecure), or automatic sensitivity tracking (Medtronic PCD). The two latter approaches seem to be more adequate to cope with signals of changing amplitude (e.g., during VF) [38]. A complete understanding of the sensing specifications of each device is necessary for effective troubleshooting of sensing. With some devices, some sensing parameters need to be programmed (Guardian, PCD, Res-Q). With others (Ventak, Cadence), parameters are controlled by the device. This makes setup simpler, but limits the possibilities of noninvasive correction if sensing problems occur.

As sensing is bipolar in all devices [39], oversensing of myopotentials, far-field P waves, or electromagnetic interference rarely results in device intervention, but lead failure (conductor and/or insulation fracture) remains a relatively common cause of false detection of tachycardias. Lead failure might be more common with epicardial leads, although this needs to be prospectively tested. Connectors or adapters can also be a source of problems, and should be avoided whenever possible. Depending on the programmed settings, oversensing may trigger the delivery of antitachycardia pacing (which frequently will then induce VT), shocks, or both. As the electrical noise generated by these fractures is intermittent, shocks will generally be aborted in noncommitted devices. Monitoring of real-time electrograms, marker channels, the beep-o-gram [40], and, when available, stored electrograms allows for correct diagnosis. Pro-

Troubleshooting Antitachycardia Pacing

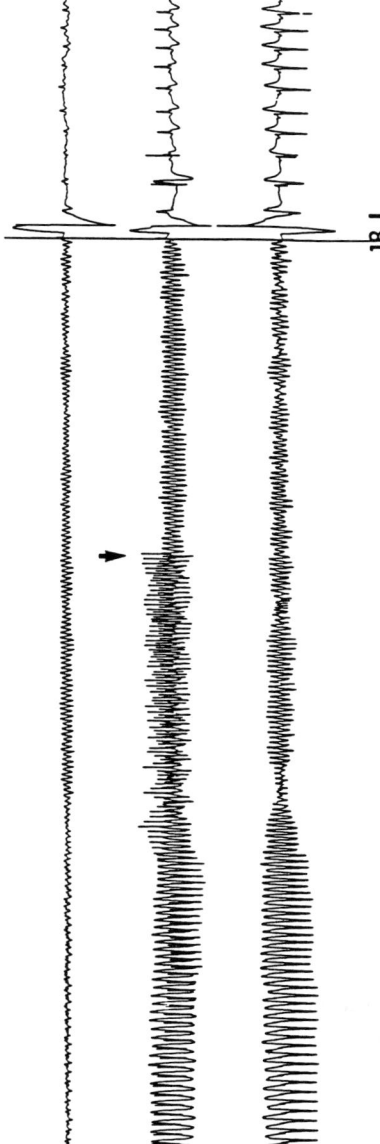

Figure 6 Example of ventricular fibrillation induction via noninvasive stimulation in a patient with a PCD device. Between the arrows, the pacing rate is progressively increased while maintaining 1:1 ventricular capture. The device appropriately detects and terminates the arrhythmia with an 18-J shock.

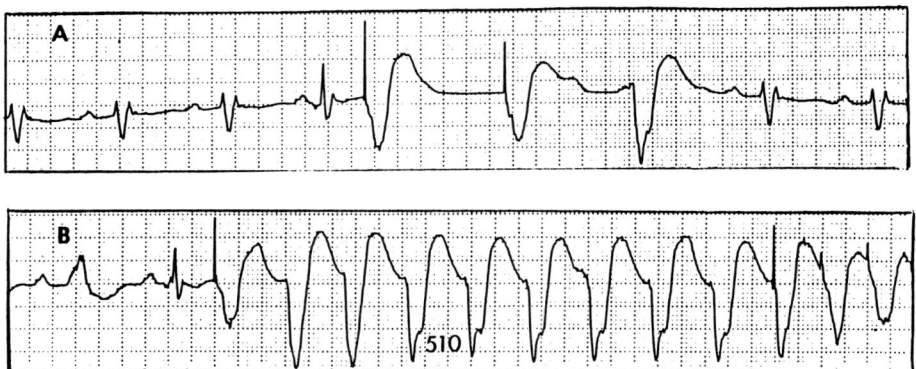

Figure 7 Hazards of intermittent undersensing: (A) a patient with an antitachycardia pacemaker showed undersensing of VPCs, with subsequent VVI pacing at 50 beats/min; (B) a close-coupled asynchronous stimulus induces VT, which the pacemaker then attempts to convert (end of the strip).

vocative maneuvers (manipulation of the generator in the pocket, bending over, straining) are frequently necessary to demonstrate intermittent oversensing. Replacement of the sensing leads (preferably with a transvenous lead) is the rational management. Oversensing due to a loose set screw can present with a similar clinical picture, but the differential diagnosis will be made at time of the operative revision of the system.

Undersensing of tachycardias is uncommon, provided adequate sensing of VF was demonstrated intraoperatively. However, with fixed-gain devices, undersensing of VF can occur in up to 10% of patients during follow-up, and periodic retesting is advisable [41]. When sensitivity is programmable (PCD, Guardian, Res-Q), it should be left at ≤0.7 mV, to ensure a safety margin for detection of VF [42]. Detection of VT does not predict reliable detection of VF, and device evaluation should include testing of both tachyarrhythmias [42].

Intermittent undersensing during sinus rhythm, with the subsequent delivery of asynchronous antibradycardia pacing, may induce VT in patients with arrhythmogenic substrates. Isolated ventricular premature beats or the ensuing sinus beat are more likely to be undersensed (Figs. 7 and 8). When undersensing occurs with separate antitachycardia pacemakers or tiered-therapy devices with two sensing channels, the problem can frequently be corrected by increasing the sensitivity. The problem is more complex when undersensing occurs in devices with a single sensing channel and automatic gain control (e.g., Cadence) [43]. In these devices, undersensing is secondary to spontaneous [44] or amplifier-induced gain changes in signal amplitude after ventricular extrasystoles (Fig. 9). The programming of a shorter escape interval (to preclude the delivery of short coupled ventricular paced beat after a long coupled postextrasystolic sinus beat), has been effective in preventing the occurrence of VT in patients who presented with this problem [43]. To avoid the perils of undersensing during sinus rhythm, antibradycardia pacing should be turned off if not needed, but this is not possible with some devices (e.g., Orthocor, PCD). Furthermore, an occasional patient presents with significant postshock bradyarrhythmias that require backup pacing [45,46]. The capability of programming VVI pacing off, but at the same time providing temporary antibradycardia pacing after delivery of a shock (e.g., PRx) is particularly appealing.

2. Troubleshooting Pacing

The energy required to excite the myocardium rises progressively the earlier one paces in the relative refractory period. During VT episodes, it is necessary to pace at cycle lengths that

Troubleshooting Antitachycardia Pacing

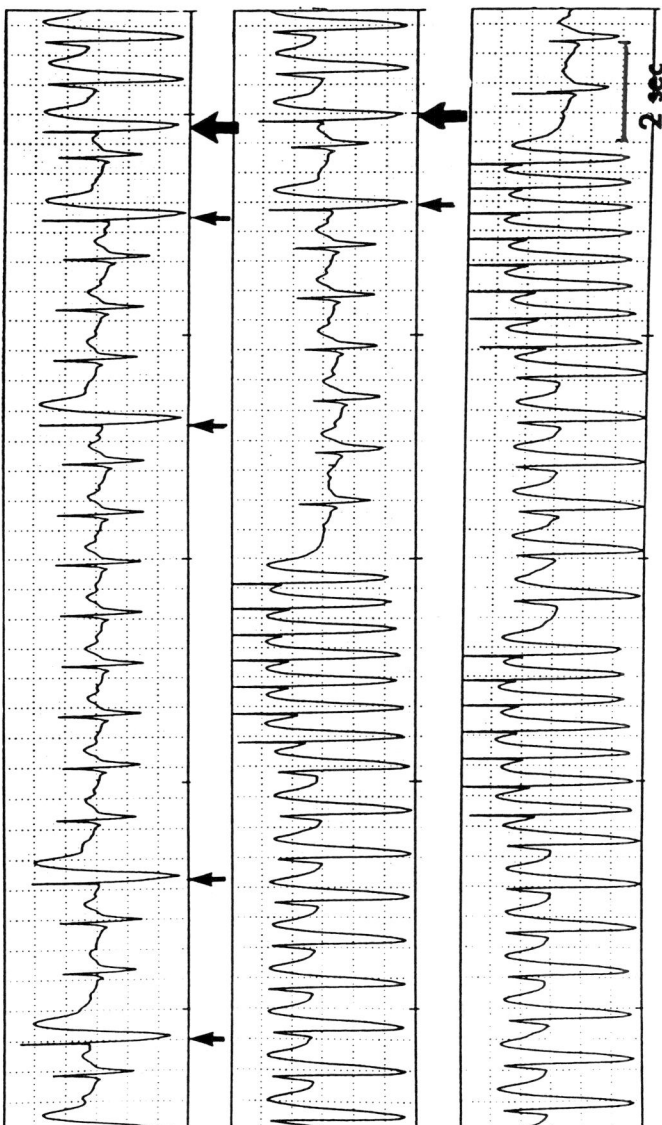

Figure 8 Continuous strips from a Holter monitor in a patient with a PRx device. Intermittent undersensing in the bradycardia channel results in the delivery of asynchronous pulses (arrows). The two with closest coupling intervals (big arrows) trigger episodes of VT, which the device then terminates with antitachycardia pacing.

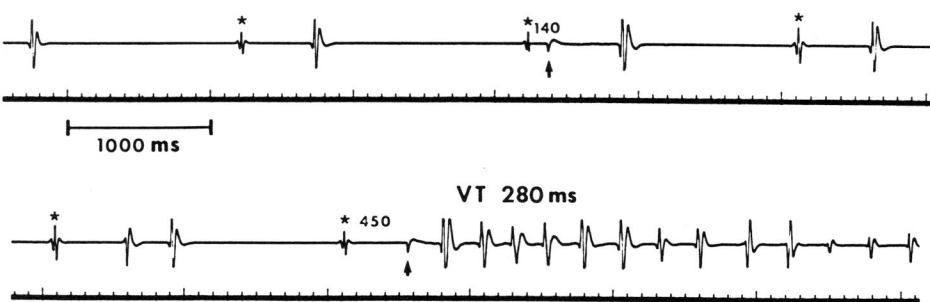

Figure 9 Stored electrograms from an episode of VT induced by bradycardia pacing after a nonsensed sinus beat in a patient with a Cadence device. Sinus rhythm morphology is indicated by the asterisk. The arrow indicates an electrical artifact at the end of the postpacing blanking period, which follows the pacing stimulus by 120 ms. In the bottom panel, the coupling interval of the pacing stimulus (arrow) delivered 310 ms (430 - 120 ms) after a nonsensed sinus beat probably results in ventricular capture and initiation of VT. (From Ref. 43, with permission.)

encroach upon the relative refractory period [47]. The determination of capture threshold at late diastole during sinus rhythm may not reflect the energy required to capture the ventricle during tachycardia. Therefore, a safety margin for output, wider than is customary for bradycardia pacing, is recommended (Fig. 10). The majority of these patients are not pacemaker-dependent. Consequently, issues of battery conservation cannot be allowed to conflict with effective antitachycardia therapy. In patients who require more than infrequent antibradycardia pacing, implantation of a separate, more physiological pacemaker, should be considered.

Transient lack of ventricular capture after a high-energy defibrillation shock is frequently observed, most likely as a result of changes at the tissue–electrode interface [48,49]. This represents an additional reason to program high pacing outputs in these patients.

Thresholds for epicardial pacing are generally higher than for endocardial pacing, and the development of exit block is not uncommon [42,50]. A future preference for endocardial sensing and pacing in antitachycardia devices can be envisioned.

3. Troubleshooting Tachycardia Recognition

In all available devices, tachycardia recognition is based on the measurement of heart rate. The probability density function (PDF), a morphologic criterion available in CPI Ventak devices, is theoretically useful in the prevention of inappropriate discharges for supraventricular rhythms. However, prospective studies have shown that its specificity is low. Therefore, if it is intended to be used, PDF should be tested in the individual patient [51,52]. Assuming correct sensing of the cardiac depolarization signal, a 100% sensitivity for tachycardias above the programmed cutoff rate can be achieved. Occasionally, patients may develop VT below the programmed detection rate, which is consequently not recognized by the device. As these tachycardias are relatively slow and well tolerated, the patient presents to the emergency room or makes a telephone transmission complaining of palpitations. Simple lowering of the detection rate will allow for tachycardia recognition and subsequent therapy delivery.

The major drawback of rate-only detection is its poor specificity. As a result of rate overlap, sinus (Fig. 11) and other supraventricular tachycardias (Fig. 12) often cannot be differentiated for VT. The delivery of ventricular antitachycardia pacing during supraventricular rhythms frequently results in the induction of VT [53]. Two additional rate-related criteria available in most devices can improve appropriate recognition of VT [54,55]. The rate-stability

Troubleshooting Antitachycardia Pacing

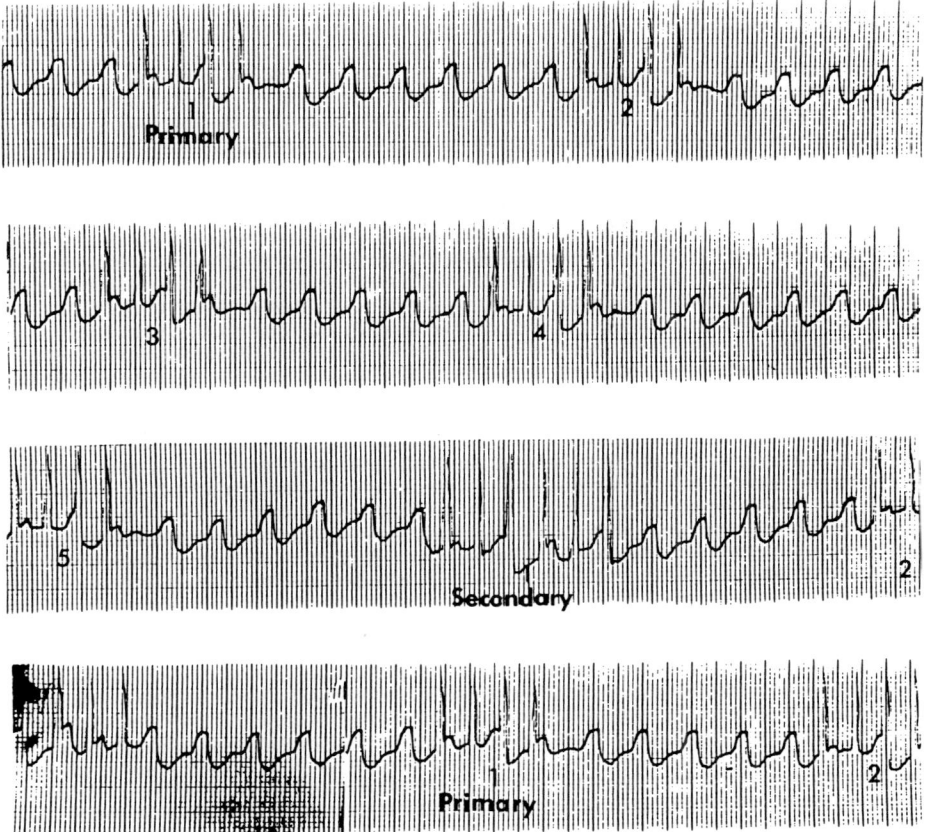

Figure 10 Failure to terminate VT secondary to loss of capture. A patient with an Intertach pacemaker and an ICD made this telephone transmission while complaining of palpitations. VT below the ICD rate cutoff is present; the Intertach appropriately recognized it and delivered all sequences of antitachycardia pacing in the primary and secondary modalities. However, ventricular capture was not achieved. The output of the pacemaker had been decreased 1 week before. After reprogramming the output with a larger safety margin, tachycardia was reliably terminated (not shown).

criterion may be useful to differentiate atrial fibrillation from VT, whereas the sudden-onset criterion is intended to detect and reject sinus tachycardia. Although the underlying concept is similar, different devices implement the criteria differently, and the physician must be familiar with the operation of each feature being programmed. For example, if detection is enabled only after induction of VT by programmed stimulation, the onset criteria will not be met and, consequently, therapy will not be delivered (Fig. 13).

The increased specificity with these "enhancing" criteria can only be attained at the expense of a somewhat decrease sensitivity, and so their routine utilization is not recommended. For example, if VT occurs in the setting of sinus tachycardia (exercise, emotional stress), the change in rate may not satisfy the onset criterion, and so the VT can persist undetected. Therefore, we incorporate the enhancing criteria into the detection algorithm only when there is evidence or clear potential for false detection of tachycardia (e.g., slow VT that overlaps with the maximal sinus rate achieved during exercise). In some patients, pharmacological blunting of

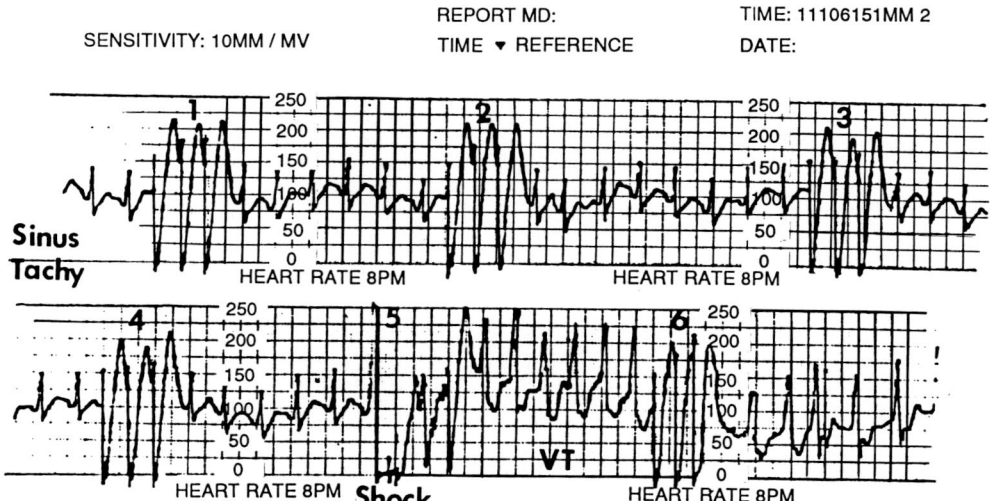

Figure 11 False detection of VT. Holter recording of a patient with an antitachycardia pacemaker and an ICD. Sinus tachycardia above the tachycardia detection rate results in the delivery of scanning sequences of three extraestimuli. The combination of tachycardia and extraestimuli satisfied ICD detection criteria, with delivery of a shock. The shock and the simultaneous fifth sequence of antitachycardia pacing triggered VT, which was then terminated by the sixth burst.

the sinus rate with beta-blockers may be necessary to avoid false recognition of sinus tachycardia [56]. In patients with atrial fibrillation, combined therapy to slow AV conduction is imperative, and catheter ablation of the atrioventricular junction may be considered when the previous maneuvers do not succeed.

At the present time, rate is the only generally available criterion to discriminate between VT and VF and is consequently suboptimal. Difficulties in discriminating fast VT from VF frequently lead to overly aggressive treatment of VT [10]. The turning-point morphology (TPM) is a morphologic criterion that can be programmed in the PRx, and is aimed to discriminate between stable and potentially unstable rhythms. Basically, it examines the shocking lead electrogram during tachycardia, and if its isoelectric time is less than a preset percentage (sinusoidal morphology), it triggers the delivery of maximal shock therapy, regardless of the therapies initially programmed for that rate zone. However, in our small experience in the electrophysiology laboratory, the TPM criterion prompted the delivery of shock therapy for pace-terminable VTs. We believe that further assessment of its clinical performance is needed before it can be recommended. It is our practice to be conservative in programming the rate cutoff between tachycardia and fibrillation. If the fibrillation detection interval is programmed too short, a few undersensed signals during VF could prolong detection or even lead to catastrophic nonrecognition. Therefore, we avoid programming the fibrillation detection rate above 200 beats/min (300 ms). Some patients with slightly faster pace-terminable monomorphic VTs will require further fine-tuning of the detection algorithm (Fig. 14).

Devices differ greatly in the way tachycardia intervals are counted. For example, in the PRx, intervals in a zone are counted in that zone and in all lower zones, but this will not happen in the PCD. Counter resetting is also different among different devices. In the PCD, one interval below the tachycardia detection rate will reset the counter to 0. These device idiosyn-

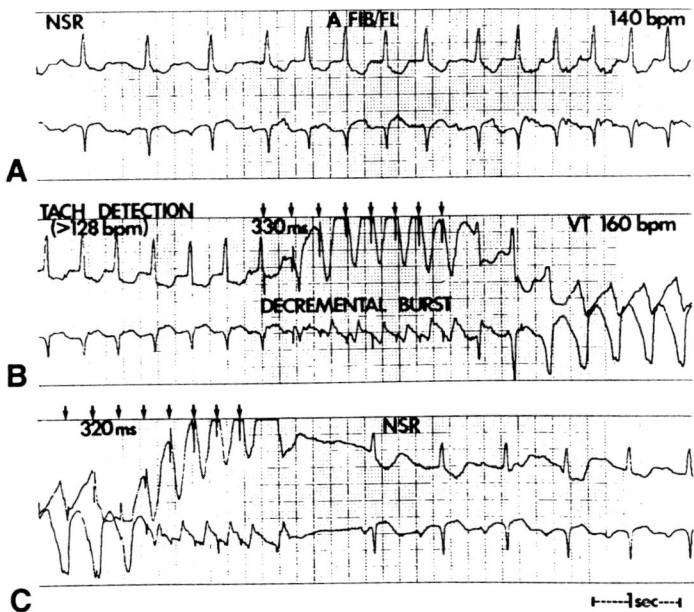

Figure 12 Another example of device diagnostic nonspecificity. Continuous 25-s segment from a Holter monitor recording in a patient with a tiered-therapy device. (A) Atrial fibrillation-flutter with a ventricular response of 140 beats/min began abruptly during sinus rhythm. (B) The criterion for VT detection was satisfied and the device initiated antitachycardia pacing with a decremental burst of eight impulses (arrows). This resulted in the induction of a VT at 160 beats/min. (C) A second successful of burst of antitachycardia pacing was then delivered. (From Ref. 53, with permission.)

cracies can lead to prolonged detection times when the rate of a slightly irregular VT overlaps two different tachycardia zones. For example, when counters in the VF zone are not simultaneously counted in the VT zone, satisfaction of the detection algorithm can be improperly delayed (Fig. 15).

The ability to program a second tachycardia zone amenable to antitachycardia pacing (Res-Q, PRx) may be very helpful in some patients with more than one type of VT. A benign antitachycardia pacing algorithm can be programmed for the treatment of the slower tachycardia, whereas the faster one can be treated with a more aggressive modality. In preclinical studies with the PRx, three tachycardia recognition zones were programmed in 28% of the patients [6] (Fig. 16).

4. Troubleshooting Tachycardia Termination

Attempts to increase efficacy and safety of antitachycardia pacing have spawned a long list of stimulation patterns [57,58]. Unfortunately, there is no agreement on the nomenclature, and different manufacturers often employ diverse names for similar techniques available in their devices.

The clinical design of pacing algorithms for tachycardia termination is based on a trial-and-error approach. In general, termination and acceleration of spontaneously occurring VT with antitachycardia pacing can be predicted from the result of electrophysiological studies. However, in some patients, pacing algorithms which are not 100% effective in terminating induced VT can be effective in terminating spontaneous VT [59]. Patients with frequently re-

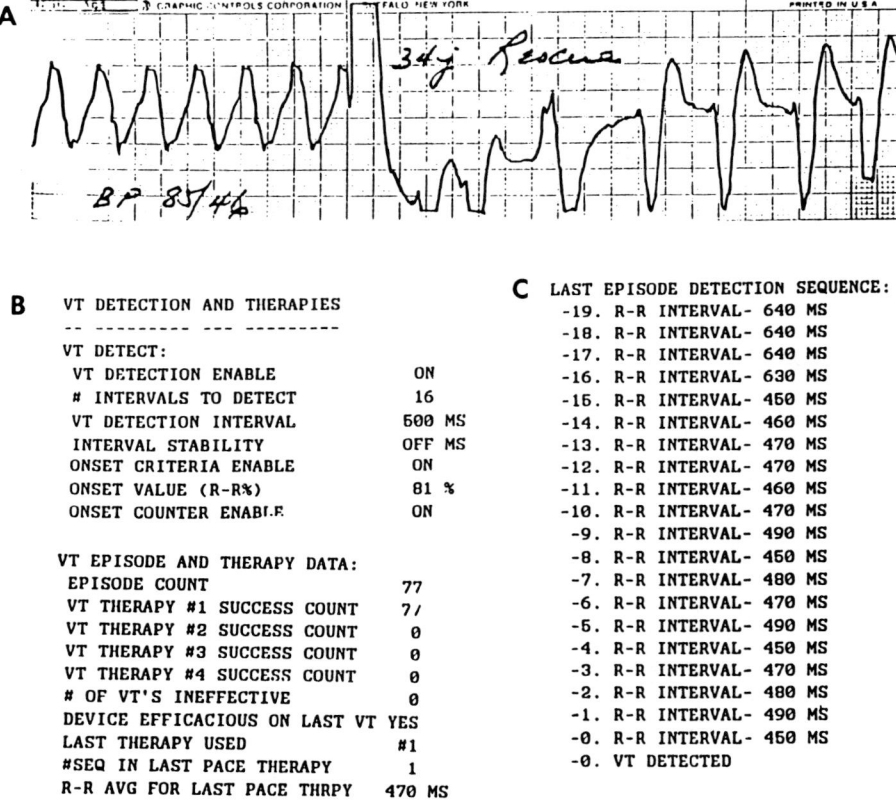

Figure 13 Failure to detect VT during NIPS due to programming of the sudden-onset criterion "ON." (B) VT detection rate was 120 beats/min; onset value was 81%. Seventy-seven episodes have been effectively terminated with antitachycardia pacing. (C) The last episode of VT clearly showed sudden onset, with a change in R–R interval from 630 to 450 ms. (A) However, when VT was induced in the EP laboratory, the PCD device failed to detect it. An emergency rescue shock had to be given. When VT detection was enabled manually after induction, the VT already had a stable cycle length. Its initiation was missed and thus the sudden-onset criterion was not satisfied.

curring sustained VT may be discharged with pacing algorithms which are not invariably effective at electrophysiological study, provided acceleration does not occur. However, programming must be designed to avoid unnecessarily long and fruitless attempts at pacing before resorting to definitive shock therapy. Retesting and reprogramming the antitachycardia pacing algorithm will be frequently necessary in these patients during follow-up [60] (Fig. 17).

Although there is no such thing as an universal antitachycardia pacing algorithm, some recommendations can be provided. Randomized studies did not find significant differences in efficacy or safety of ramp versus burst protocols [61–64], but adaptive (or orthorhythmic) antitachycardia pacing modes have been clearly shown to be more versatile than fixed cycle length modes in terminating VT [65], and should be used preferentially. In adaptive modes, coupling intervals of the first and subsequent stimuli are programmed to occur at a fraction (70 to 90%) of the tachycardia cycle length. This is crucial in patients with multiple VTs, which can occur in a relatively wide range of rates and still be treated with the same

Troubleshooting Antitachycardia Pacing

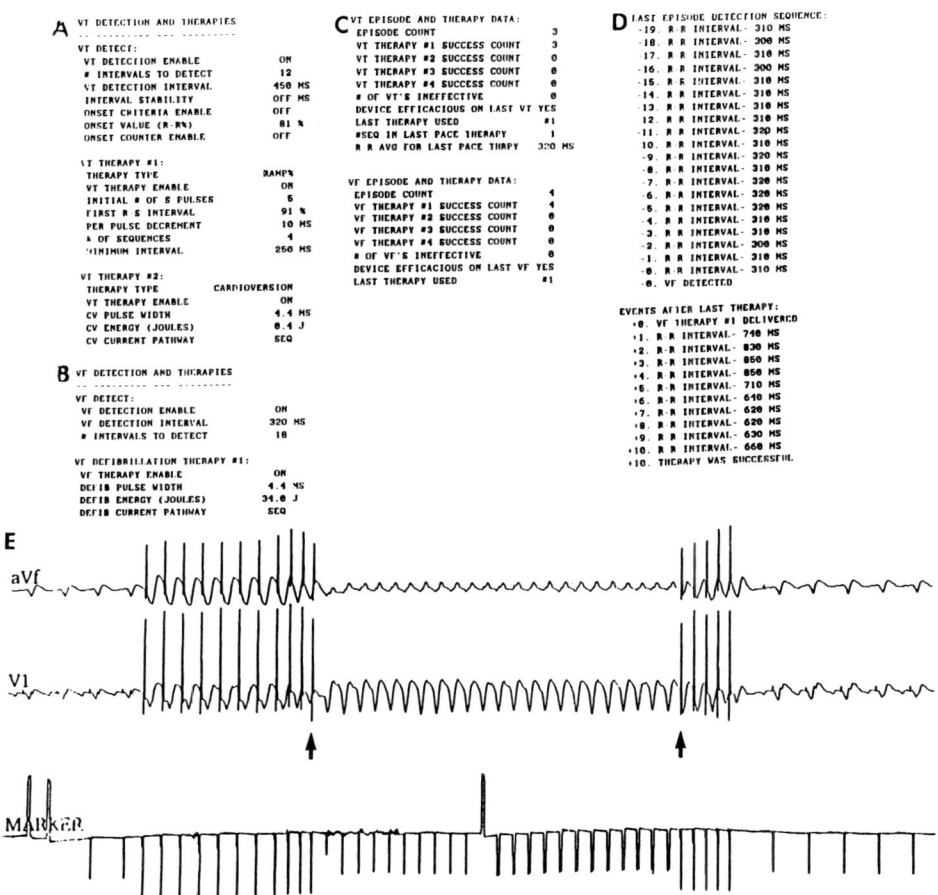

Figure 14 Fine-tuning of TV detection criteria. A patient with a previously pace-terminable VT at 170 beats/min received defibrillation shocks while at home. (A) VT detection rate was 450 ms. (B) VF detection rate was 320 ms. (C) Seven tachyarrhythmic episodes had been treated since last device interrogation. Three were detected as VT and terminated with antitachycardia pacing (average rate for the last one was 320 ms). Four episodes were detected as VF and received shock therapy. (D) The last of these "VF" episodes had an average rate of 310 ms, with R-R intervals overlapping both zones. (E) VF detection rate was increased to 280 ms, and VT at 310 ms was induced via NIPS. Antitachycardia pacing was effective at the first attempt. No further shocks occurred during follow-up, although the device continued to terminate episodes of this fast VT.

algorithm. Furthermore, adaptive algorithms are able to cope with the short- and long-term variations in the tachycardia termination "window" that are secondary to changes in physiological variables. The number of stimuli within a burst should be kept at the minimum that will reliably terminate the tachycardia. Long bursts (>10 stimuli) can reinduce the tachycardia after successful conversion, are more likely to induce tachycardia acceleration, and are often associated with hemodynamic compromise. The total number of allowed pacing attempts is dictated by the hemodynamic tolerance during tachycardia. Typically, if antitachycardia pacing is successful in terminating a given VT, it is so within four to five attempts, and thus the program-

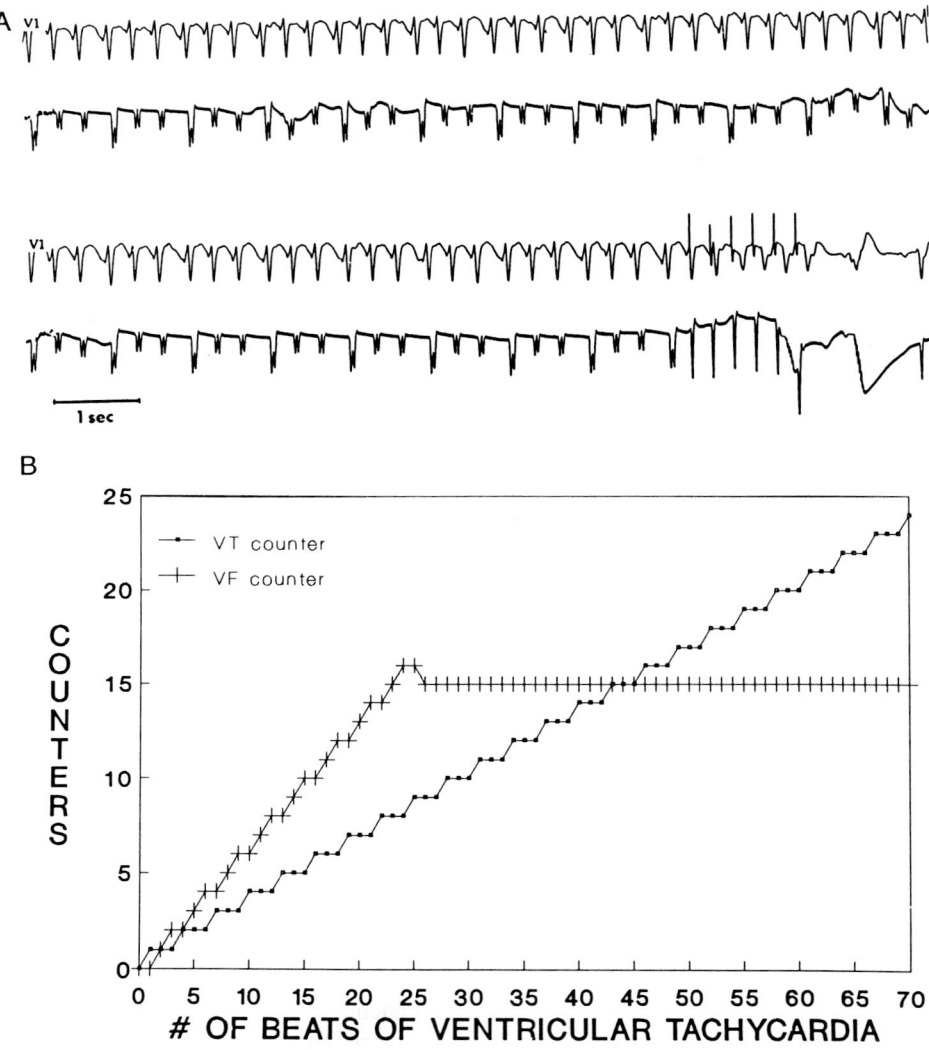

Figure 15 Long detection time for VT in a patient with a PCD device. The detection criteria for VT were 24 intervals at cycle lengths between 450 and 300 ms; VF was to be recognized when 18 of the previous 24 intervals were faster than 300 ms. (A) The slightly irregular tachycardia rate resulted in intervals falling alternatively in the tachycardia zone (larger markers) or the fibrillation zone (smaller markers). Due to the counting algorithms of this particular device, this prolonged detection time. VT was detected and terminated with antitachycardia pacing only after 70 beats. (B) Interpretation of the counters during the episode.

ming of a larger number of trains is not recommended. To avoid hemodynamic compromise in patients who may tolerate antitachycardia pacing for a limited amount of time, several devices allow the programming of an "extended high rate" or "antitachycardia pacing time-out" feature. This consists of a timer that permits antitachycardia therapies to be attempted for a programmable length of time. If the time expires and the tachycardia is still present, the device

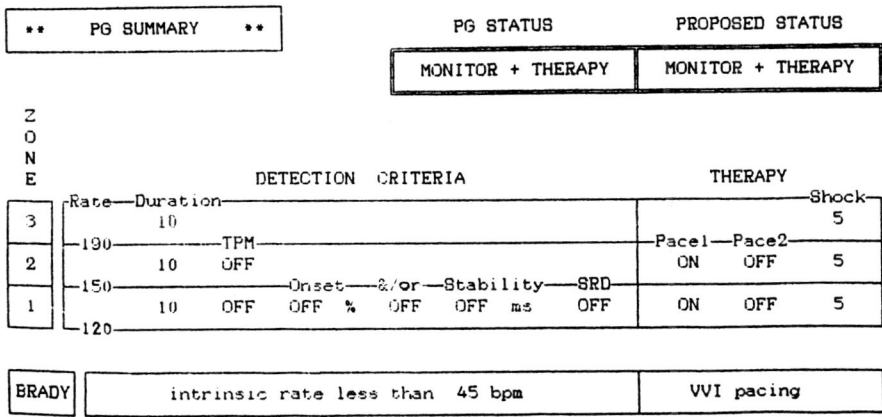

Figure 16 Telemetered data from a PRx device programmed to detect tachycardia in three different rates zones. Tachycardias above 190 beats/min (zone 3) will be treated with high-energy shocks, whereas those with rates between 120 and 149 beats/min (zone 1) and between 150 and 189 beats/min (zone 2) will be first treated with antitachycardia pacing. The device will also deliver antibradycardia pacing at 45 beats/min.

abandons VT therapy and delivers the more aggressive VF therapy. The therapy delivery sequence can be further enhanced in some devices (Intertach, Res-Q, Siecure) by their capability to "remember" previous successful pacing therapies. For each tachycardia class, the Res-Q can be programmed to precede the normal therapy delivery sequence with either the last successful burst, the last successful therapy, or both.

Acceleration of the rate of a previously tolerated uniform VT and degeneration to VF are well-described complications of pacing therapy for VT [66]. The efficacy and safety of antitachycardia pacing techniques are inversely related. A higher incidence of tachycardia termination can be achieved with more aggressive protocols, but often at the price of a high incidence of VT acceleration. When using scanning algorithms, a minimum pacing interval (220–230 ms) should also be programmed to avoid pacing at short cycle lengths and thus diminish the risks of tachycardia acceleration. The incidence of acceleration of spontaneous VT in patients discharged on antitachycardia pacing algorithms proved to be safe at electrophysiological study is acceptably low [7,9,10,60]. Acceleration generally results in a tachycardia rate which falls in an upper zone, with subsequent delivery of an appropriately more aggressive therapy. However, if the programmed tachycardia zone is wide, acceleration can result in a faster tachycardia in the same zone. The PRx allows the programming of an "acceleration percentage" feature. If the rate change exceeds this percentage, maximum energy shocks are delivered, even when the tachycardia remains in the same zone. Devices should always be programmed to deliver progressively more aggressive therapies during an arrhythmic event. This is particularly important when antitachycardia pacing has been programmed for two different VT zones. In the Res-Q, programming of the "ratchet" option will prevent the therapy delivery sequence from moving backward in the event a tachycardia accelerates (e.g., antitachycardia pacing programmed as initial therapy for the faster tachycardia will not be delivered; the next, more aggressive programmed therapy will be delivered instead). In the PRx, if pacing preceded an increase in rate to a higher zone (but the acceleration percentage feature

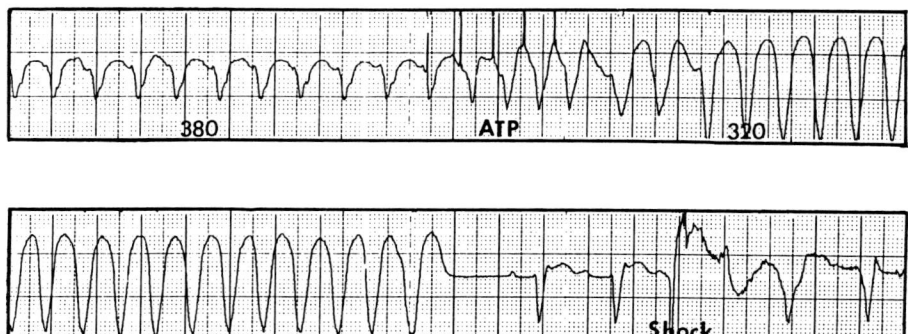

Figure 17 Need to fine-tune the tachycardia termination algorithm in a patient with a tiered-therapy device which is committed for "VF" therapy. Holter recording shows VT at 380 ms. A burst of five pulses of antitachycardia pacing results in transient acceleration to 320 ms before termination. This was enough to satisfy criteria for VF, and a shock is delivered in sinus rhythm.

was not programmed) the next therapy would be the first shock programmed in the higher zone. The Siecure is the only device that will routinely "step down" the level of response if a tachycardia changes or is modified to a less rapid rhythm. The safety of this feature has not been proved, and it is our opinion that it can compromise the safety of defibrillator therapy by delaying the delivery of definitive shock therapy.

Antitachycardia pacing can less frequently slow the rate of a VT without terminating it. This deceleration is generally transient, but at times it can be pronounced and persistent enough to satisfy the sinus rhythm redetection algorithm (Fig. 18). Therefore, when the VT reaccelerates to its baseline rate, it will be interpreted by the ICD as a new arrhythmic episode, precluding the appropriate progression in the therapeutic algorithm.

The site of stimulation may be another variable relevant to the overall success of antitachycardia pacing. In animal models of reentry, tachycardia can be terminated with fewer stimulated beats when stimulation is performed close to the zone of slow conduction [67]. In clinical antitachycardia pacing, however, sites of stimulation are relatively standard and dictated by the operative approach. In some patients, epicardial antitachycardia pacing (with clear ventricular capture in the surface ECG) is ineffective in terminating VT, while endocardial pacing is successful [68]. It is known that, in the setting of chronic coronary artery disease, VT circuits are generally subendocardial. Therefore, it is possible that, as a result of the distance between the site of stimulation and the circuit, an abnormal refractoriness of the interposed tissues, a small size of the excitable gap, and/or the effects of antiarrhythmic drugs (see below), epicardially delivered stimuli might be at times unable to reach and depolarize the critical part of the circuit prematurely enough to permit its termination.

5. Effects of Antiarrhythmic Drugs on Antitachycardia Pacing

Multiple interactions may occur between antiarrhythmic drugs and antitachycardia devices. The combination of antiarrhythmic drugs with antitachycardia pacing may be beneficial by decreasing the number of episodes of tachycardia, facilitating pacing termination of tachycardia, and decreasing the incidence of pacing-induced arrhythmias [69–71].

On the other hand, several deleterious interactions can occur [72]. By changing the conduction properties of the electrical signal, antiarrhythmic drugs could influence electrogram detection. An increase in latency or conduction time can lead to double counting [73]. Slowing

Troubleshooting Antitachycardia Pacing

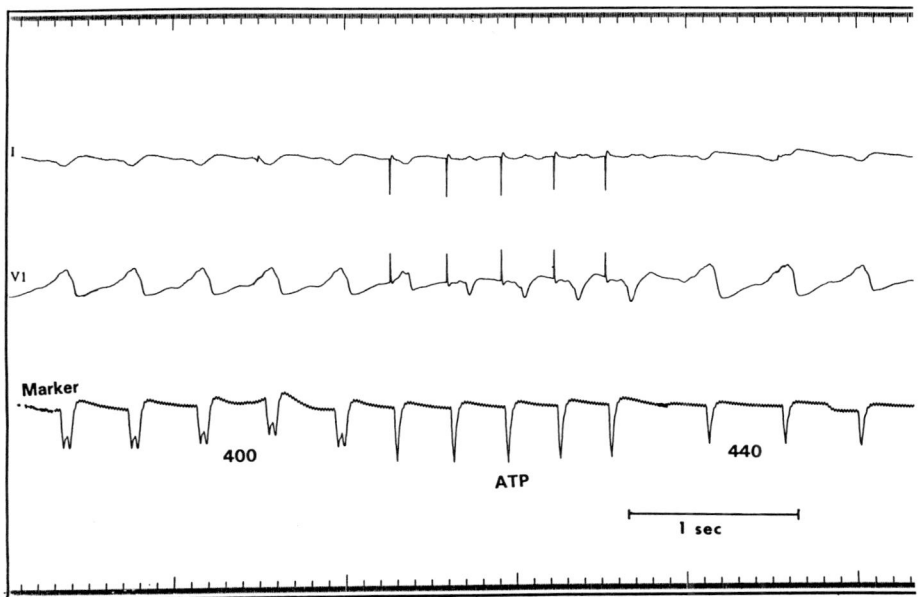

Figure 18 Slowing of VT by antitachycardia pacing. The tachycardia detection interval had been programmed at 420 ms. Successive intervals at 400 ms are detected in the tachycardia zone (double markers) and trigger the delivery of a five-beat burst of antitachycardia pacing. The rate of the VT is decelerated to 440 ms, and subsequent intervals are not detected as tachycardia intervals (single markers).

of the tachycardia rate below the detection rate is a relatively frequent event after the introduction of changes in antiarrhythmic drug therapy [73]. Drug-induced changes in the properties of the reentry circuit (e.g., prolongation of refractoriness with shortening of the excitable gap) might result in more difficult termination of tachycardia by pacing in spite of a slower tachycardia rate. Increases in stimulation thresholds [72], defibrillation thresholds [73,74], or both, can be expected with most antiarrhythmic drugs. Finally, antiarrhythmic agents can have proarrhythmic effects, regardless of the presence of the antitachycardia device [75]. Proarrhythmic responses may turn tachycardia termination by the device difficult if not impossible.

As the occurrence of these beneficial and deleterious effects is generally unpredictable, programmed stimulation to retest detection and termination algorithms is necessary when antiarrhythmic drug therapy is changed [27].

III. USE OF SEPARATE ANTITACHYCARDIA PACEMAKERS AND DEFIBRILLATORS

The combined use of an independent antitachycardia pacemaker and an ICD is cumbersome. The primary design of each device fails to consider the presence of the other one, leaving open the potential for deleterious interactions [4,72,73,76,77]. It should be noted that many of these interactions may also occur when ICDs are used in combination with antibradycardia pacemakers.

Our experience with the use of independent antitachycardia pacemakers and ICDs encompasses 13 patients. We used Intertach I and II and Orthocor II pacemakers, in combination with

AICD/Ventak defibrillators [4,78]. Other investigators have used different antitachycardia pacemakers [1,2,79]. We [4] and others [79] have reported relatively high incidences of total and sudden death in patients with separate antitachycardia pacemakers and defibrillators, whereas other groups reported better outcomes [3,5]. This discrepancy is likely to be due to differences in the approach to patient selection. Patients in our series were severely ill, had depressed left ventricular function, and presented clinically with both rapid and slow recurring VT in spite of drug therapy. In the series by Bonnet et al. [5], patients had better-preserved ventricular function and presented mainly with well-tolerated VT for which antitachycardia pacing was considered as primary therapy; defibrillators were implanted in those patients only as backup. Regardless of the results, all studies have emphasized the occurrence of deleterious interactions between devices and the need for meticulous and time-consuming testing. Therefore, although the combination is clinically feasible in selected patients, it can no longer be recommended. Costs considerations aside, the combination of separate antitachycardia pacemakers and ICDs provides no advantage over tiered-therapy devices.

A. Implantation Protocol

Ideally, the need for antitachycardia pacing will be apparent before defibrillator implantation, and a tiered-therapy device will be utilized. If the need for antitachycardia pacing is apparent only after implantation of a conventional defibrillator and its replacement with a tiered-therapy device is not feasible, then attention to the following guidelines at time of antitachycardia pacemaker implantation will prevent deleterious device-to-device interactions [4,5,76,77, 80]:

  1. *Bipolar pacing and rate-counting ICD electrodes must be distanced as far as possible from each other.* It has been our policy to routinely implant the epicardial sensing leads of defibrillators on the posterolateral left ventricle, in anticipation of the potential later need for a transvenous pacemaker. Alternatively, when an ICD is implanted in a patient with a preexistent pacemaker, the pacemaker stimulus recorded from the defibrillator rate-counting leads should be as small as possible, both in absolute amplitude and relative to the native and paced R waves [77] (Fig. 19). The latency between the pacing stimulus and the local electrogram should be less than the refractory period of the ICD (about 150 ms) [3]. We have been able to successfully implant the sensing/defibrillation lead of nonthoracotomy defibrillator systems in the right ventricular outflow tract in patients with preexistent dual-chamber pacemakers with right ventricular apical leads (Fig. 20).
  2. Active fixation leads are recommended. Our only instance of acute dislodgement following an ICD discharge occurred with a ventricular tined lead.
  3. Optimal pacing and sensing thresholds should be sought.
  4. A comprehensive testing protocol (to detect and avoid potential deleterious device-to-device interactions) must be undertaken. This testing should include:

(a) Programming of the antitachycardia pacemaker to the bipolar mode [76,80].
(b) Establishing the absence of double (or triple) counting [spike(s) plus QRS] by the ICD. Pacing must be initiated above the patient's intrinsic heart rate at maximum energy output for the pacemaker. With early AICD devices, their sensing function was assessed by listening to its audible tone or with a "beep-o-gram" (Fig. 21). Current ICDs provide telemetry of a marker channel to facilitate sensing assessment. *The defibrillator should detect only one event with every paced beat* [76,81].
(c) Reconfirmation of the optimal pacing protocol for terminating VT. This is done by placing the defibrillator in a standby mode and then inducing the patient's VT on several occasions.

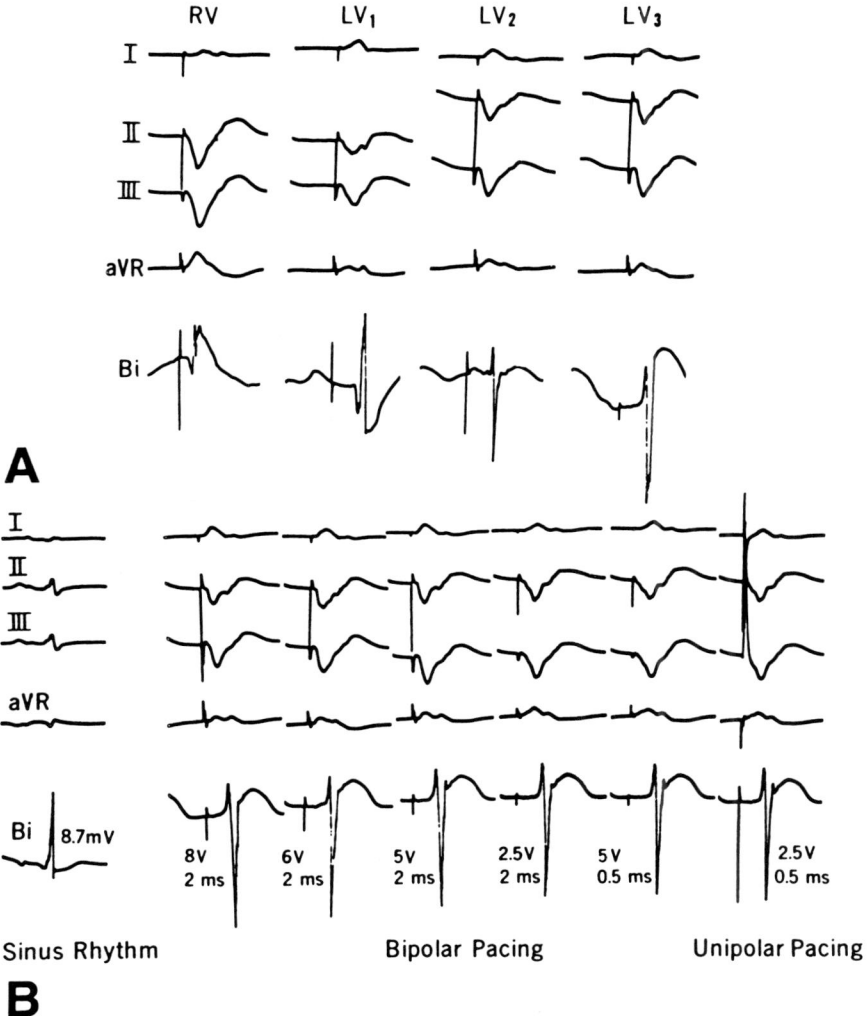

Figure 19 Meticulous testing at defibrillator implantation to avoid cross-talk with a previously implanted pacemaker at the right ventricular apex. Shown are four surface ECG leads and the electrogram recorded from the AICD bipolar epicardial leads (Bi). The gain for all recordings is identical. (A) Epicardial recordings from one right ventricular (RV) and three left ventricular (LV) sites are shown during pacing at high stimulus amplitude (8 V) and duration (2 ms). The pacemaker stimulus artifact is extremely large close to the apex of the RV and at LV sites 1 and 2. LV site 3 is the location where the AICD bipolar sensing electrodes were implanted. Here, the pacemaker stimulus artifact has a modest amplitude and is relatively small compared with the paced R wave. (B) The AICD sensing leads are implanted. The R wave during sinus rhythm is 8.7 mV (left). During bipolar pacing (middle), as the programmed pacemaker stimulus amplitude is decreased, the stimulus artifact similarly decreases as recorded in the AICD electrodes. During unipolar pacing (right), when the pacing stimulus amplitude is only 2.5 V, the stimulus artifact amplitude is larger than that at any bipolar pacing output. (From Ref. 77, with permission.)

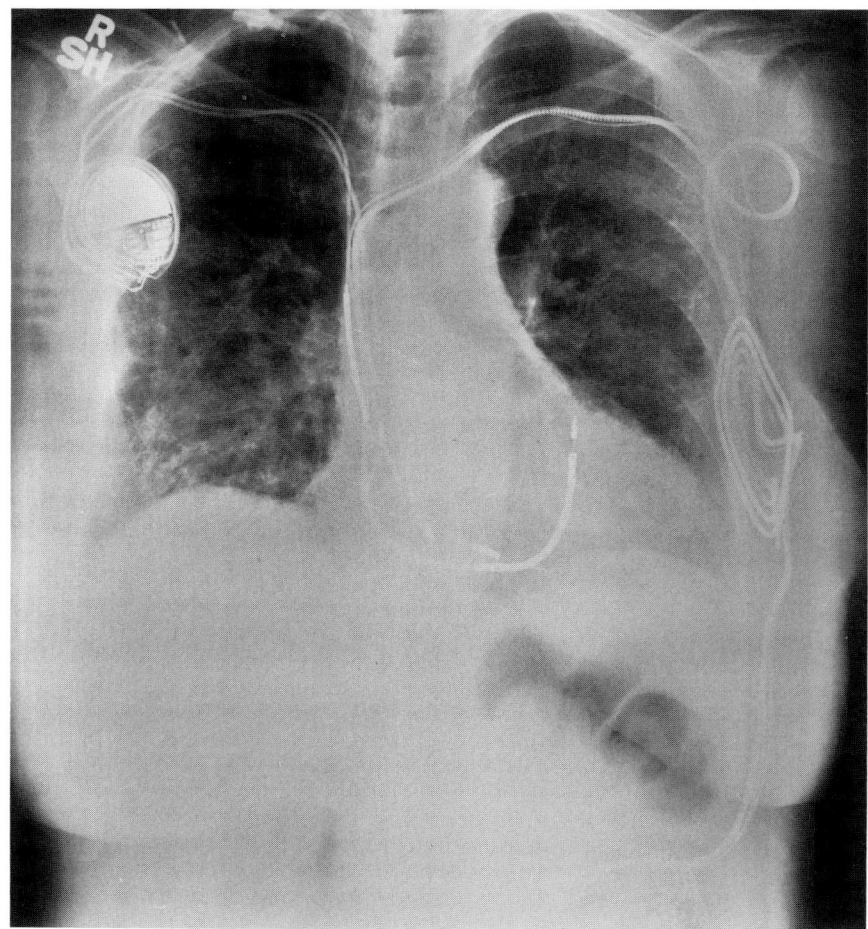

Figure 20 Avoidance of device-to-device interaction between a dual-chamber pacemaker and a nonthoracotomy defibrillator system. A pacing lead had been previously implanted at the right ventricular apex from the right subclavian vein. The defibrillator leads were implanted from the left subclavian vein. The tripolar screw-in pacing-defibrillation lead was positioned in the right ventricular outflow tract. During extensive testing, no evidence of device "cross-talk" was present.

5. The antitachycardia pacemaker detection and termination algorithm is then selected. With early, nonprogrammable defibrillators, it was critical to use devices with high (>175 beats/min) cutoff rates [5]. With current devices, the rates can be programmed so that there is no overlap between the detection rates of the antitachycardia pacemaker and the defibrillator. However, it might be impossible to avoid an overlap between the rate of the burst of antitachycardia pacing and the defibrillator detection rate without compromising the response of the ICD to hemodynamically unstable tachyarrhythmias. *Therefore, the time frame encompassed for successful tachycardia termination by the pacemaker should not exceed the time for tachycardia recognition by the defibrillator.* This means that antitachycardia pacing sequences

Troubleshooting Antitachycardia Pacing

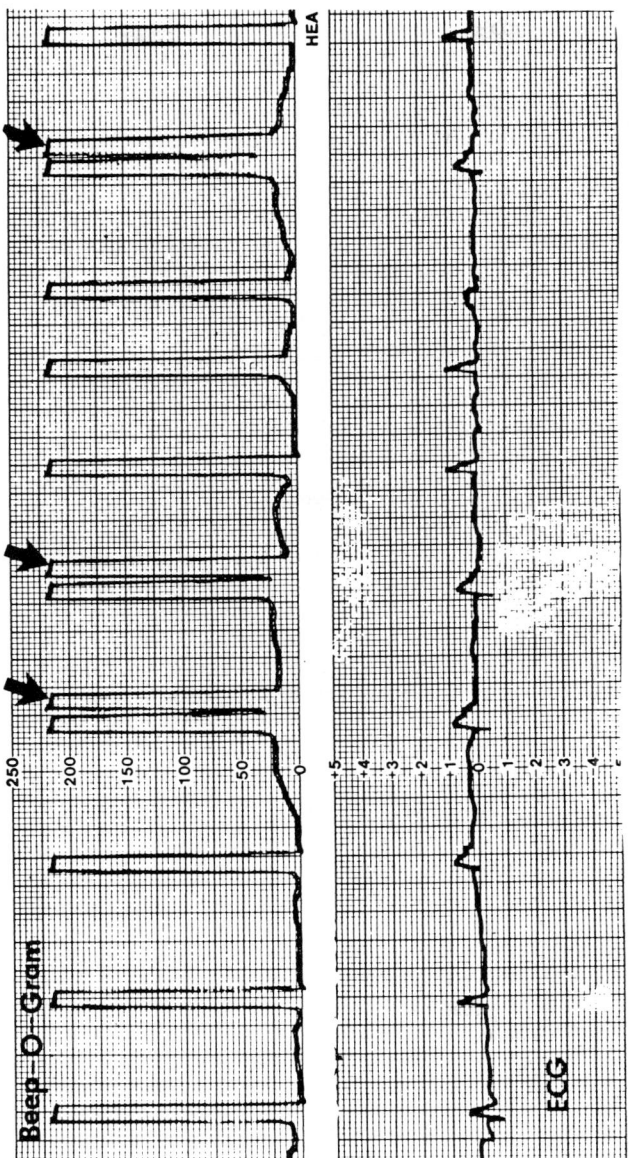

Figure 21 Deleterious interaction between a pacemaker and an ICD. The beep-o-gram (phonocardiographic recording of the tones produced during sensing by the ICD in the standby mode) shows double counting of paced beats (arrows). This could eventually trigger an ICD discharge if the cutoff rate is reached.

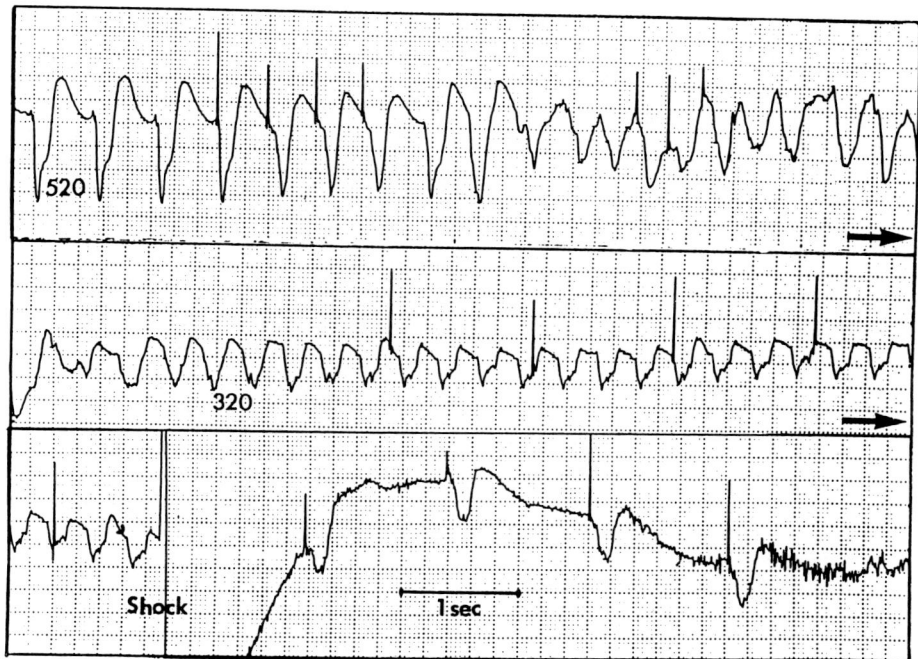

Figure 22 Continuous Holter monitor strip showing a possible deleterious interaction between an antitachycardia pacemaker and an AICD. The pacemaker attempts to terminate a VT below the detection rate of the AICD. The second pacing sequence results in acceleration of the tachycardia above the AICD detection rate. The pacemaker fails to sense this faster tachycardia, and VVI pacing at 50 beats/min is consequently delivered. Because of its automatic gain control, the AICD could misinterpret the pacemaker pulses as QRS complexes and ignore the VT. In this patient, that possibility was adequately explored and ruled out during implant. After capacitor charging, a shock is delivered with restoration of a paced rhythm.

must be limited to 10 beats or less [5]. If the pacemaker provides for a secondary response (Intertach II), it can be programmed more aggressively to trigger the ICD purposefully [3,5].

6. The simultaneous function of both activated devices is then assessed against induced VT. The antitachycardia pacemaker should terminate VT, ideally on its first attempt, without triggering the ICD.

7. *Finally, it is necessary to ensure that pulses delivered by an undersensing pacemaker during VF will not inhibit appropriate arrhythmia detection by the ICD.* In the setting of low-amplitude VF, pacemaker pulses can occur at the escape interval. Due to the automatic gain-control feature, these pulses can be inappropriately sensed as a normal regular rhythm, inhibiting arrhythmia detection. To test for this deleterious interaction, the pacemaker must be programmed to the VOO (or DOO) mode with maximum energy output and VF must then be induced. This "worst-case environment" must not interfere with normal ICD function, which must promptly detect fibrillation (Fig. 22). Again, telemetry of a marker channel is most useful to assess sensing (Fig. 23).

If deleterious interactions are detected during the previous testing steps, the pacing electrode should be repositioned farther from the defibrillator leads and the testing sequence repeated.

Troubleshooting Antitachycardia Pacing

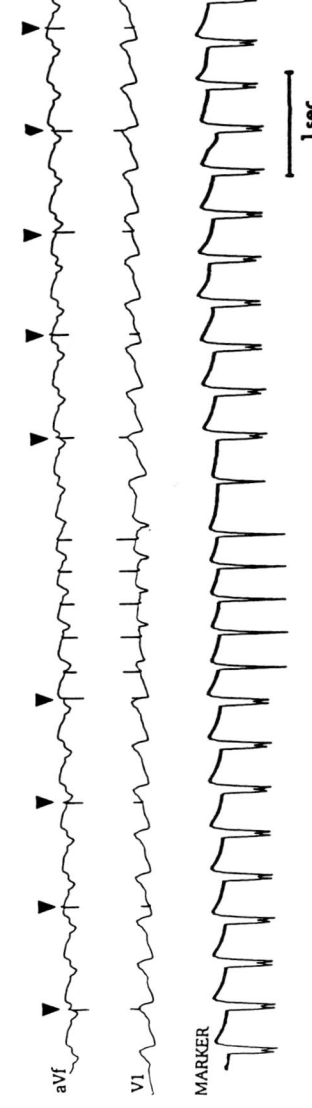

Figure 23 Adequate sensing of VT in spite of pacemaker spikes. This patient with a prior VVIR pacemaker had a tiered-therapy device implanted. The pacemaker was programmed to the VOO mode at maximum output during induced VT. The pacemaker pulses (arrows) did not inhibit tachycardia detection. There is one marker signal for each tachycardia beat.

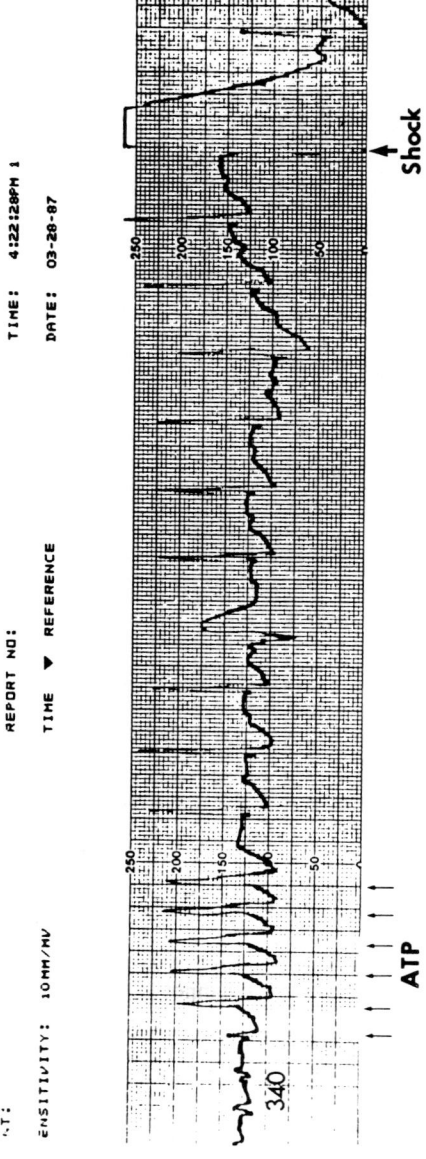

Figure 24 Deleterious interaction between an antitachycardia pacemaker and the committed AICD. VT (three last beats) is terminated by a burst of antitachycardia pacing (ATP, arrows). Nevertheless, the AICD has already begun charging, and a shock is delivered during sinus rhythm (fortunately, without consequences).

B. Special Problems During Follow-up

With careful attention to detail, both devices can work synergistically. In our experience, most potential deleterious device interactions can be avoided. Rarely, the discharge from an ICD may change (reset) the mode of the implanted pacemaker. Resetting to a unipolar pace/sense configuration is particular hazardous. The programming, memory, and telemetry functions of the antitachycardia pacemakers were not affected by discharges from epicardial ICD systems in our patient population, but the resetting of antibradycardia pacemakers after ICD shocks [72,82] has been reported. Lately, we have witnessed several instances of pacemaker resetting by ICD discharges when using concomitant independent pacemakers and transvenous defibrillators.

False-positive shocks due to double or triple counting can be avoided by employing the extensive testing described above. The most difficult interaction to handle is the triggering of ICD discharges by VT previously terminated by the pacemaker (Fig. 24). This may happen even when one tries to set antitachycardia pacemaker recognition and termination time less than the ICD recognition time. The selection of an uncommitted device (e.g., Guardian 4202/4203) should be very helpful in preventing this interaction.

Magnet testing of an implanted pacemaker (with asynchronous pacing) can trigger VT and initiate an appropriate ICD discharge [72,77]. Asynchronous ventricular pacing can also result in ICD discharges when asynchronous pacemaker stimulus artifacts are counted in addition to the native underlying R waves [83]. Furthermore, with CPI devices, a magnetic field generated by a very close magnet and lasting for more than 30 s will result in deactivation of the ICD. For these reasons, many implanting physicians are reluctant to provide magnets to patients with independent pacemakers and defibrillators. Interactions between ICD and pacemaker programmers have also been described [84].

Early in our experience, failure to provide reliable defibrillator backup was implicated in the sudden death of two patients with combined antitachycardia pacemakers and defibrillators [78]. One patient had relatively high initial defibrillation thresholds, which were not retested after the institution of amiodarone treatment. The other patient had infrequent episodes of VT effectively terminated by antitachycardia pacing. This patient's ICD showed early signs of battery depletion, but its replacement was postponed. Postmortem analysis revealed the device to be nonfunctional. The antitachycardia pacemaker memory disclosed one episode of tachycardia at 244 beats/min during the month prior to death. The need to ensure adequate defibrillation backup when using antitachycardia pacing for VT cannot be overemphasized.

REFERENCES

1. Manz M, Gerckens U, Funke HD, Kirchhoff PG, Luderitz B. Combination of antitachycardia pacemaker and automatic implantable cardioverter/defibrillator for ventricular tachycardia. PACE 1986; 9:676–684.
2. Greve H, Koch T. Gulker H, et al. Termination of malignant ventricular tachycardias by use of an automatic defibrillator (AICD) in combination with an antitachycardia pacemaker. PACE 1988; 11:2040–2044.
3. Newman DM, Lee MA, Herre JM, Langberg JJ, Scheinman M, Griffin JC. Permanent antitachycardia pacemaker therapy for ventricular tachycardia. PACE 1989; 12:1387–1395.
4. Masterson M, Pinski SL, Wilkoff B, et al. Pacemaker and defibrillator combination therapy for recurrent ventricular tachycardia. Clev Clin J Med 1990; 57:330–338.
5. Bonnet CA, Fogoros RN, Elson JJ, Fiedler SB, Burkholder JA. Long-term efficacy of an antitachycardia pacemaker and implantable defibrillator combination. PACE 1991; 14:814–822.

6. Herre JM, Xannom DS, Fogoros RN, et al. Initial multicenter clinical experience with a multifunctional implantable pacemaker defibrillator (abstr). Circulation 1991; 84:II-428.
7. Leitch JW, Gillis AM, Wyse DG, et al. Reduction in defibrillator shocks with an implantable device combining antitachycardia pacing and shock therapy. J Am Coll Cardiol 1991; 18:145–151.
8. Saksena S, Stout R, Poliseno M, Krol RB, Mehta D, and Worldwide Guardian 4210 Phase I investigators. Tachycardia detection and treatment with a third-generation implantable cardioverter-defibrillator: an international experience (abstr). J Am Coll Cardiol 1992; 19:286A.
9. Winkle RA, Fain ES, Hardage ML, Senelly KM, and the Cadence® investigators. The value and usage of programmability in a tiered therapy defibrillator (abstr). J Am Coll Cardiol 1992; 19:365A.
10. Bardy GH, Troutman C, Poole JE, et al. Clinical experience with a tiered-therapy, multiprogrammable antiarrhythmia device. Circulation 1992; 85:1689–1698.
11. Sowton E, Sulke N. Clinical experience with Siemens Pacesetter Siecure. J Cardiovasc Electrophysiol 1992; 3:515–522.
12. Hamer AWF, Rubin SA, Peter CT, Mandel WJ. Factors that predict syncope during ventricular tachycardia in patients. Am Heart J 1984; 107:997–1004.
13. Maloney JD, Khoury D, Simmons T, et al. Effect of atrioventricular synchrony on stroke volume during ventricular tachycardia in man. Am Heart J 1992; 123:1561–1568.
14. Krol RB, Saksena S. Hemodynamic effects of tachycardias: B. Ventricular tachycardia. In: Saksena S, Goldschlager N, eds. Electrical therapy for cardiac arrhythmias, Philadelphia: Saunders, 1990:478–488.
15. Saksena S, Chandran P, Shah Y, Boccadamo R, Pantopoulos D, Rothbart ST. Comparative efficacy of transvenous cardioversion and pacing in patients with sustained ventricular tachycardia: a prospective randomized crossover study. Circulation 1985; 72:153–160.
16. Siebles J, Geiger M, Schneider MAE, Kuck K. The automatic implantable cardioverter/defibrillator: does low energy cardioversion offer any advantage over antitachycardia pacing in patients with ventricular tachycardia? (abstr). J Am Coll Cardiol 1991; 17:129A.
17. Bardy GH, Troutman C, Poole JE, Kudenchuk PJ, Dolack GL. A randomized trial of autodecremental pacing vs low energy cardioversion during ventricular tachycardia in man (abstr). Circulation 1991; 84:II-428.
18. Griffin JC. Follow-up techniques for patients with implanted antitachycardia devices. In: Saksena S, Goldschlager N, eds. Electrical therapy for cardiac arrhythmias, Philadelphia: Saunders, 1990: 516–524.
19. Anderson MH, Paul V, Jones S, Ward DE, Camm AJ. Transtelephonic interrogation of the implantable cardioverter defibrillator. PACE 1992; 15:1144–1150.
20. Fetter J, Stanton M, Trsuty J, Benditt D, Collins J. Transtelephonic interrogation and transmission of stored data from an implanted cardioverter defibrillator (abstr). PACE 1992; 15:505.
21. Wolensky L, Gessman L, Hurzeler P, Grant S, Helms B. Transtelephonic defibrillator beepergram follow up of AICD patients: early results and patient acceptance (abstr). PACE 1992; 15:545.
22. Wang PJ, Mandalakas N, Clyne C, et al. Accuracy of rhythm classification using a data log system in implantable cardioverter-defibrillators. PACE 1991; 14:1911–1916.
23. Luceri RM, Puchferran RL, Brownstein SL, Habla SM, David IB, Vardeman LL. Improved patient surveillance and data acquisition with a third generation implantable cardioverter-defibrillator. PACE 1991; 14:1870–1874.
24. Hook BG, Marchlinski FE. The value of ventricular electrogram recording in the diagnosis of arrhythmias precipitating electrical device therapy. J Am Coll Cardiol 1991; 17:985–990.
25. Sarter BH, Hook BG, Callans DJ, Marchlinski FE. Effect of bundle branch block on local electrogram morphology: potential cause of arrhythmia misdiagnosis (abstr). PACE 1992; 15:562.
26. Hurwitz JL, Hook BG, Callans DJ, et al. Importance of abortive shock capability with electrogram storage in cardioverter-defibrillator devices (abstr). Circulation 1991; 84:II-427.
27. Zipes DP, Akhtar M, Denes P, et al. Guidelines for clinical performance of cardiac electrophysiologic studies. A report of the American College of Cardiology/American Heart Association Task

Force on assessment of diagnostic and therapeutic cardiovascular procedures. J Am Coll Cardiol 1989; 14:1827–1842.
28. Veltri EP, Mower MM, Mirowski M. Ambulatory monitoring of the automatic implantable cardioverter-defibrillator: a practical guide. PACE 1988; 11:315–325.
29. Gettes LS, Zipes DP, Gilette PC, et al. Personnel and equipment required for electrophysiologic testing. Report of the Committee on Electrocardiography and Cardiac Electrophysiology, Council on Clinical Cardiology, American Heart Association. Circulation 1984; 69:1219A–1221A.
30. Lehmann MH, Saksena S. Implantable cardioverter defibrillators in cardiovascular practice: report of the policy conference of the North American Society of Pacing and Electrophysiology. PACE 1991; 14:969–979.
31. Kowey P. The calamity of cardioversion of conscious patients. Am J Cardiol 1988; 61:1106–1107.
32. Zipes DP, Jackman WM, Heger JJ, et al. Clinical transvenous cardioversion of recurrent life-threatening ventricular tachyarrhythmias: low-energy cardioversion of ventricular tachycardia and termination of ventricular fibrillation in patients using a catheter electrode. Am Heart J 1982; 103:789–794.
33. Mendoza IG, Kleiman RB, Marchlinski FE. Electrophysiologic effects of the anesthetic propofol at postoperative defibrillator testing (abstr). J Am Coll Cardiol 1992; 19:221A.
34. Waldo AL, Akhtar M, Brugada P, et al. The minimally appropriate electrophysiologic study for the initial assessment of patients with documented sustained monomorphic ventricular tachycardia. J Am Coll Cardiol 1985; 6:1174–1177.
35. Kleiman RB, Marchlinski FE. Failure of noninvasive programmed stimulation with third generation defibrillators (abstr). PACE 1992; 15:569.
36. Wilber DJ, Davis MJ, Rosenbaum, Ruskin JN, Garan H. Incidence and determinants of multiple morphologically distinct sustained ventricular tachycardias. J Am Coll Cardiol 1987; 10:583–591.
37. Trappe HJ, Brugada P, Talajic M, Lezaun R, Wellens HJJ. Value of induction of pleomorphic ventricular tachycardia during programmed stimulation. Eur Heart J 1989; 10:133–141.
38. Sperry RE, Ellenbogen KA, Woods MA, Stambler BS, DiMarco JP, Haines DE. Failure of a second and third generation implantable cardioverter-defibrillator to sense ventricular tachycardia: implications for fixed-gain sensing devices. PACE 1992; 15:749–755.
39. Furman S, Bradman R, Panizzo F, Fisher JD. Implantation techniques of antitachycardia devices. PACE 1984; 7:572–579.
40. Ballas S, Rashidi R, McAlister H, et al. The use of beep-o-grams in the assessment of automatic implantable cardioverter-defibrillator sensing function. PACE 1989; 12:1737–1745.
41. Wilber DJ, Poczobutt-Johanos M. Time-dependent sensing alterations in implantable defibrillators: lessons from the Telectronics Guardian 4202/4203 (abstr). PACE 1991; 14:624.
42. Saksena S, Poczobutt-Johanos M, Castle LW, et al. Long-term multicenter experience with a second-generation implantable pacemaker-defibrillator in patients with malignant ventricular tachyarrhythmias. J Am Coll Cardiol 1992; 19:490–499.
43. Callans DJ, Hook BG, Marchlinski FE. Paced beats following single nonsensed complexes in a "codependent" cardioverter defibrillator and bradycardia pacing system: potential for ventricular tachycardia induction. PACE 1991; 14:1281–1287.
44. Callans DJ, Hook BG, Marchlinski FE. Magnitude of R wave amplitude variability in permanent ventricular sensing lead systems (abstr). Circulation 1991; 84:II–608.
45. Platia EV, Veltri EP, Griffith L, et al. Post-defibrillation bradycardia following implantable defibrillator discharge (abstr). J Am Coll Cardiol 1986; 7:73A.
46. Niazi I, Kadri N, Mahmud R, et al. Absence of significant post-defibrillation bradyarrhythmias in patients with automatic implantable defibrillators. Am Heart J 1988; 115:830–836.
47. Waxman HL, Cain ME, Greenspan AM, Josephson ME. Termination of ventricular tachycardia with ventricular stimulation: salutary effect of increased current strength. Circulation 1982; 65:800–804.

48. Slepian M, Levine JH, Watkins L, Brinker J, Guarnieri T. Automatic implantable cardioverter defibrillator/permanent pacemaker interaction: loss of pacemaker capture following AICD discharge. PACE 1987; 10:1194–1197.
49. Guarnieri T, Datorre SD, Bondke H, Brinker J, Myers S, Levine JH. Increased pacing threshold after an automatic defibrillator shock in dogs: effects of class I and class II antiarrhythmic drugs. PACE 1988; 11:1324–1330.
50. Krol RB, Saksena S, Tullo NG, et al. Optimal pacing and sensing lead systems for implantable hybrid pacemaker-cardioverter defibrillators (abstr). J Am Coll Cardiol 1991; 17:55A.
51. Toinoven L, Viitasalo M, Järvinen A. The performance of the probability density function in differentiating supraventricular from ventricular rhythms. PACE 1992; 15:727–730.
52. Martin D, Venditti FJ. Use of events markers during exercise testing to optimize morphology criterion programming of implantable defibrillators. PACE 1992; 15:1025–1032.
53. Johnson NJ, Marchlinski FE. Arrhythmias induced by device antitachycardia therapy due to diagnostic nonspecificity. J Am Coll Cardiol 1991; 18:1418–1425.
54. Warren J, Martin RO. Clinical evaluation of automatic tachycardia diagnosis by an implanted device. PACE 1986; 9:1079–1083.
55. Olson WH, Bardy GH, Mehra R, Almquist C, Biallas R. Comparison of different onset and stability algorithms for detection of spontaneous ventricular arrhythmias (abstr). PACE 1987; 10:439.
56. Fisher JD, Goldstein M, Ostrow E, Matos JA, Kim SG. Maximal rate of tachycardia development: sinus tachycardia with sudden exercise vs. spontaneous ventricular tachycardia. PACE 1983; 6:221–228.
57. Fisher JD, Kim SG, Mercando AD. Electrical devices for the treatment of arrhythmias. Am J Cardiol 1988; 61:45A–57A.
58. De Belder MA, Malik M, Ward DE, Camm AJ. Pacing modalities for tachycardia termination. PACE 1990; 13:231–245.
59. Gillis AM, Wyse DG, Mitchell LB. Discordance among modes of termination for noninvasively-induced or invasively-induced and spontaneous ventricular tachycardias (abstr). Circulation 1991; 84:II-609.
60. Hurwitz J, Flores B, Marchlinski FE. Clinical efficacy of pacing therapy for ventricular tachycardia in combined antitachycardia pacemaker defibrillators confirmed by stored electrograms (abstr). PACE 1992; 15:565.
61. Gillis AM, Leitch JW, Wyse G, et al. Randomized comparative trial of modes of ventricular tachycardia pace termination (abstr). PACE 1992; 15:505.
62. Newman D, Dorian P, Hardy J. A randomized prospective comparison of ventricular antitachycardia pacing modalities (abstr). PACE 1992; 15:506.
63. Klein H, Hoffman R, Troster J, Trappe HJ, Kielblock B. Efficacy of various antitachycardia pacing modes with ICD therapy (abstr). PACE 1992; 15:506.
64. Cook JR, Kirchhofer JB, Fitzgerald TF, Lajzer DA. Comparison of decremental and burst overdrive pacing as treatment for ventricular tachycardia associated with coronary artery disease. Am J Cardiol 1992; 70:311–315.
65. Vharos GS, Haffajee CI, Gold RL, Bishop RL, Berkovits BV, Alpert JS. A theoretically and practically more effective method for interruption of ventricular tachycardia: self-adapting autodecremental overdrive pacing. Circulation 1986; 73:309–315.
66. Fisher JD, Mehra R, Furman S. Termination of ventricular tachycardia with bursts of rapid ventricular pacing. Am J Cardiol 1978; 41:94–99.
67. Restivo M, Gough WB, El-Sheriff N. Antitachycardia pacing: electrophysiologic mechanisms. In: El-Sheriff N, Samet P, eds. Cardiac Pacing and Electrophysiology. 3d ed. Philadelphia: Saunders, 1991: 685–705.
68. Hurwitz J, Marchlinski FE. Epicardial lead location may be inadequate for ventricular tachycardia termination in antitachycardia pacing/implantable cardioverter defibrillators (abstr). PACE 1992; 15:565.

69. Naccarelli GC, Zipes DP, Rahilly GT, Heger JJ, Prystowsky EN. Influence of tachycardia cycle length and antiarrhythmic drugs on pacing termination and acceleration of ventricular tachycardia. Am Heart J 1983; 105:1–5.
70. Keren G, Miura DS, Somberg JC. Pacing termination of ventricular tachycardia: influence of antiarrhythmic slowed ectopic rate. Am Heart J 1984; 107:638–643.
71. Ip JH, Winters S, Tepper D, Hehran R, Gomes JA. Influence of antiarrhythmic drugs in pace termination and acceleration of ventricular tachycardia (abstr). PACE 1992; 15:585.
72. Luceri RM, Brownstein SL, Habal SM, Castellanos A. Device-device and drug-device interaction. In: Barold SS, Mugica J, eds. New Perspectives in Cardiac Pacing. Vol. 2. Mount Kisco, NY: Futura Publishing, 1991: 527–544.
73. Singer I, Guarnieri T, Kupersmith J. Implanted automatic defibrillators: effects of drugs and pacemakers. PACE 1988; 11:2250–2262.
74. Echt DS, Black JN, Babey JT, et al. Evaluation of antiarrhythmic drugs on defibrillation energy requirements in dogs: sodium channel block and action potential prolongation. Circulation 1989; 79:1106–1117.
75. Lamattina T, Larsen L, Pacetti P, Casvant D, Kosowsky B, Haffajee C. The need for and effects of antiarrhythmic drugs in patients with 3rd generation implantable pacer-cardioverter-defibrillator (abstr). PACE 1992; 15:551.
76. Cohen A, Wish M, Fletcher R, et al. The use and interaction of permanent pacemakers and the automatic implantable cardioverter defibrillator. PACE 1988; 11:704–711.
77. Epstein A, Kay N, Plumb V, et al. Combined automatic implantable cardioverter-defibrillator and pacemakers systems: implantation techniques and follow-up. J Am Coll Cardiol 1989; 13: 121–131.
78. Maloney JD, Pinski SL, Masterson M, et al. Clinical experience with the combination of an antitachycardia pacemaker (Orthocor II) and the implantable cardioverter defibrillator in drug-refractory ventricular tachycardia. J Interven Cardiol 1990; 3:269–276.
79. Lüderitz B. The impact of antitachycardia pacing with defibrillation. PACE 1991; 14:312–315.
80. Kim SG, Furman S, Waspe LE, Brodman R, Fisher JD. Unipolar pacer artifacts induced failure of an automatic implantable cardioverter/defibrillator to detect ventricular fibrillation. Am J Cardiol 1986; 57:880–881.
81. Ahern TS, Nydegger C, McCormick DJ, et al. Device interaction: antitachycardia pacemakers and defibrillators for sustained ventricular tachycardia. PACE 1991; 14:302–307.
82. Ching E, Carlblom D, Wilkoff BL, Castle LW. Risk of pacemaker damage induced by implantable defibrillator shocks (abstr). PACE 1991; 14:629.
83. Kim SG, Furman S, Matos JA, Waspe LE, Brodman R. Fisher JD. Automatic implantable cardioverter/defibrillator: inadvertent discharges during permanent pacemaker magnet tests. PACE 1987; 10:579–582.
84. Rogers R, Ellenbogen KA. Letter to the editor. PACE 1990; 13:1687.

29

Permanent Pacemakers and Implantable Cardioverter-Defibrillators: Potential Interactions

Andrew E. Epstein and Richard B. Shepard

*University of Alabama at Birmingham
and University of Alabama Hospital
Birmingham, Alabama*

There are many reasons why a pacemaker may be implanted in conjunction with an implantable cardioverter-defibrillator: sinus node dysfunction, conduction abnormalities, carotid sinus hypersensitivity, postshock bradycardia, and antitachycardia pacing. The latter indication is the subject of another chapter, but many of the potential interactions between pacemakers and implantable cardioverter-defibrillators can occur regardless of whether the pacemaker is implanted for bradycardia support, antitachycardia pacing, or for both indications [1–13]. New-generation implantable cardioverter-defibrillators will make many of the interactions described in this chapter obsolete. However, since many patients have combined device systems at the present time, and since in the future some patients currently with an implantable defibrillator or a pacemaker may need a second device for bradycardia or ventricular arrhythmias, respectively, discussion is warranted.

Implantable cardioverter-defibrillators can affect pacemaker function and vice versa. The purpose of this chapter is to discuss these interactions and to offer suggestions for combined device implantation that may help to avoid possible problems.

I. PACEMAKER EFFECTS ON IMPLANTABLE CARDIOVERTER-DEFIBRILLATORS

There are numerous effects that pacemakers may have on implantable cardioverter-defibrillators (Table 1). One of the first adverse interactions between pacemakers and implantable defibrillators to be recognized was defibrillator sensing of pacemaker stimulus artifacts. [1]. Such sensing may lead to normal rhythms being misinterpreted as ventricular arrhythmias or to inhibition of detection of tachyarrhythmias. During clinical trials of early-generation implantable defibrillators, warning was made that both pacing stimulus artifacts and evoked electrograms could be interpreted by the defibrillator as intrinsic R waves, called ''double counting'' [1]. If the interventricular conduction delay separating the pacemaker stimulus artifact from the local evoked electrogram exceeded the refractory period of the defibrillator, then counting both the signals

Table 1 Pacemaker Effects on Implantable Cardioverter–Defibrillators

1. Multiple counting of pacemaker stimulus artifacts and evoked R waves may lead to multiple counting and inappropriate implantable defibrillator shocks.
2. Sensing of pacemaker stimulus artifacts during ventricular tachycardia or fibrillation may lead to inhibition of arrhythmia detection.
3. Pacemaker programming may cause inappropriate implantable defibrillator shocks due to electromagnetic signals emitted by the pacemaker programmer being sensed by the defibrillator.
4. Pacemaker magnet or threshold testing may lead to shocks by inducing ventricular tachycardia or by causing multiple counting during asynchronous pacing.
5. Magnet application during pacemaker testing may inactivate some implantable defibrillators if care is not taken to avoid the defibrillator.
6. Pacing in any mode at a rate greater than the detection rate of an implantable defibrillator may satisfy the tachycardia detection criteria and lead to a defibrillator shock or shocks. Especially note that rate-responsive pacing or tracking the atrium in the DDD mode may result in implantable defibrillator discharges.

would be interpreted as ventricular depolarizations. If this measured rate then exceeded the detection rate of the defibrillator, a charging cycle would be initiated. In Fig. 1, transcardiac (via the defibrillating leads) and bipolar electrograms (via the sensing leads of the defibrillator) are shown during dual-chamber pacing at a rate of 60 beats/min. If, for example, the patient's implanted defibrillator is programmed to a detection rate of 110 beats/min, and if the defibrillator sensed both the ventricular pacing stimulus artifacts at 60 beats/min and the evoked R waves at 60 beats/min, the interpreted rate would be 120 beats/min and initiate an "inappropriate" defibrillator discharge. In addition, if pacemaker sensing failure occurs (as may happen after defibrillator shock delivery, see below), asynchronous pacing in competition with natural

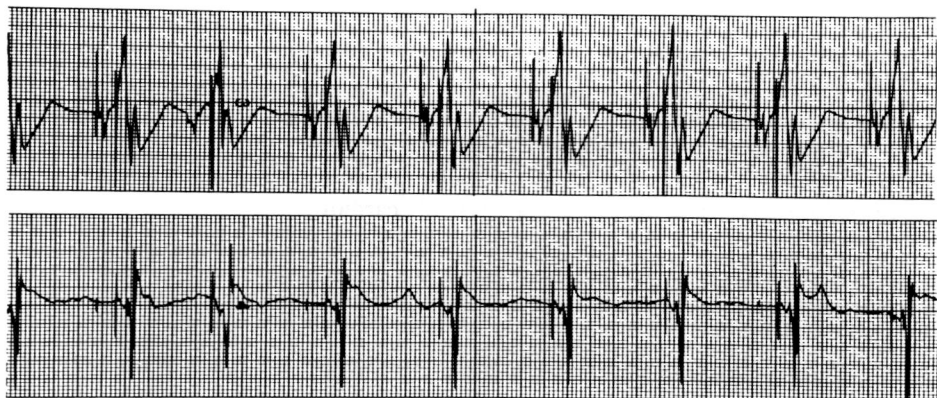

Figure 1 The figure demonstrates the possibility for double counting. The top tracing shows a transcardiac electrogram recorded from the defibrillating leads and the bottom tracing shows the bipolar sensing electrogram from an implanted AID-B system. In the sensing electrogram the interventricular conduction dealy separating the pacemaker stimulus artifact from the local evoked electrogram may exceed the 150-ms refractory period of the AID-B defibrillator, which would lead to counting both signals. If the measured rate exceeds the detection rate of the defibrillator, a charging cycle would be initiated. See text for discussion. (Reprinted with permission from Ref. 1.)

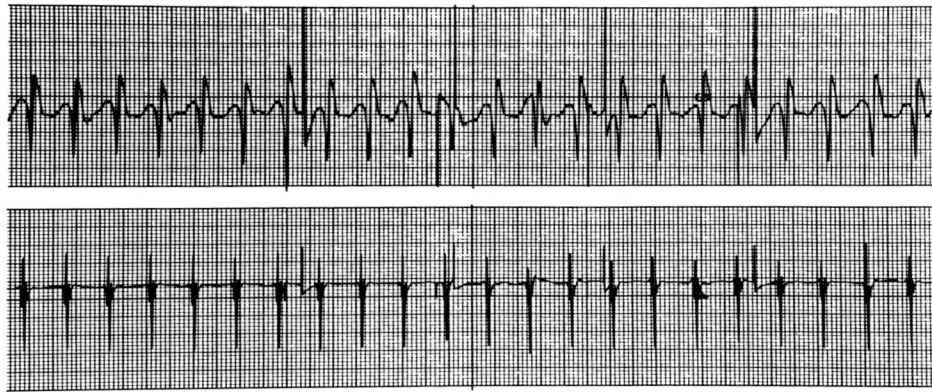

Figure 2 This figure shows pacing during ventricular tachycardia to demonstrate the possibility that pacing may inhibit defibrillator detection of the arrhythmia. As in Fig. 1, the top and bottom tracings are recordings from the defibrillating and bipolar sensing leads, respectively. Since the pacemaker has failed to sense the tachycardia, demand pacing occurs. If the resulting pacemaker stimulus artifacts are large, the defibrillator may ignore the tachycardia signals and base its arrhythmia detection analysis on the stimulus artifact signals thereby inhibiting arrhythmia detection. See text for discussion. (Reprinted with permission from Ref. 1.)

R waves can also lead to counting both the pacemaker stimuli and R waves and shock delivery if the average counted rate exceeds the detection rate [1]. Since unipolar pacing stimulus artifacts as seen by the defibrillator are often significantly larger than bipolar stimulus artifacts, unipolar pacing is contraindicated in patients with implanted defibrillators [1,2,6–8]. Methods for implanting the defibrillator sensing leads to avoid double counting are discussed below [8].

Sensing of pacemaker stimulus artifacts can lead not only to double counting but also to lack of detection (called ''detection inhibition,'' Fig. 2) of ventricular arrhythmias, especially ventricular fibrillation [1,2,6,7]. Since electrograms during ventricular fibrillation are sometimes small and below the sensitivity of pacemakers, pacing may occur during these arrhythmias. Large stimulus artifacts may then reset the automatic gain control of the defibrillator so that the lower-amplitude R waves of the ventricular arrhythmia are not sensed. Kim et al. [2] reported a patient in whom an automatic implantable cardioverter-defibrillator failed to detect ventricular fibrillation (Fig. 3), presumably because large-amplitude pacing stimulus artifacts were interpreted by the defibrillator as intrinsic R waves. Sensing of the large stimulus artifacts led to resetting of the automatic gain control of the implantable defibrillator and lowering of the sensing sensitivity. This resulted in nondetection of the lower-amplitude ventricular fibrillation signals. In contrast, Ruffy et al. encountered no adverse device–device interactions in a patient with both a bipolar dual-chamber pacemaker system and an implantable cardioverter-defibrillator by virtue of lead locations [3]. The pacemaker electrodes were implanted epicardially near the right atrial appendage and over the lateral right ventricular free wall. The sensing leads for the implantable defibrillator were implanted epicardially on the posterobasal left ventricular wall. Absence of device–device interaction was confirmed by listening to beeping tones emitted by the implanted defibrillator during AOO and AV sequential pacing, as well as at postoperative electrophysiological study when polymorphic ventricular tachycardia was induced and sensed.

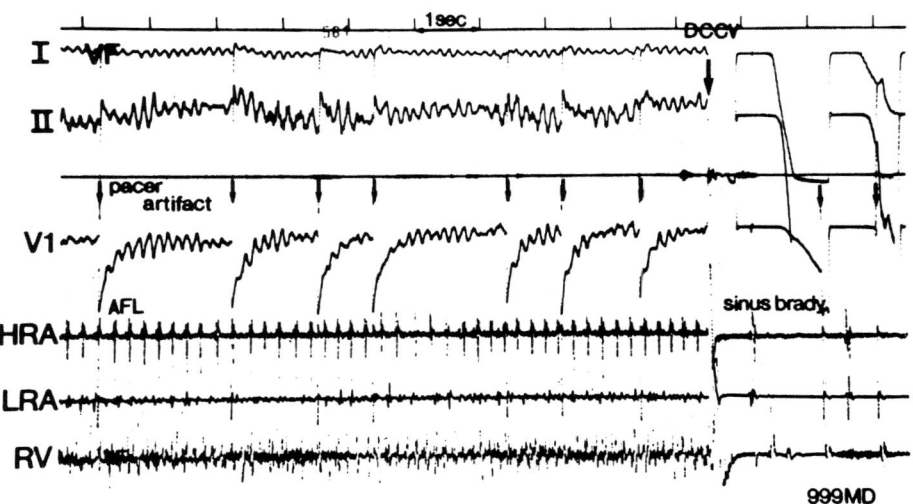

Figure 3 The unipolar ventricular demand pacemaker in this patient with an implantable defibrillator was not totally inhibited during ventricular fibrillation. The large pacemaker stimulus artifacts caused nondetection of the arrhythmia by the defibrillator. Ventricular fibrillation was terminated by external direct-current defibrillation (DCCV). I, II, V1 = surface electrocardiogram leads; HRA = high right atrial electrogram; LRA = low right atrial electrogram; RV = right ventricular electrogram; AFL = atrial flutter, VF = ventricular fibrillation. See text for discussion. (Reprinted with permission from Ref. 2.)

Cohen et al. analyzed 30 episodes of ventricular fibrillation [6]. Failure to sense the arrhythmias appropriately led to pacing during 24 of the episodes. In three patients with unipolar pacemakers, inappropriate pacing led to defibrillator nondetection of the arrhythmia and failure to discharge. In two of these patients who had pacemakers implanted before their implantable defibrillators, the ratios of the pacemaker stimulus artifacts to the evoked R-wave amplitudes in the implantable defibrillator sensing electrograms were 3.5 and 2.1, respectively. For patients with bipolar pacemakers and recordable electrograms, the ratio was 0.2, highlighting the importance of a small pacemaker stimulus artifact being present in the implantable defibrillator sensing electrogram.

One of the first experiences describing device interactions in multiple patients implanted with combined defibrillator-pacemaker systems was reported by Luceri et al. [12] Four important observations were made: First, high-energy shock therapy (25 J) in one patient resulted in prolonged asystole, whereas low-energy shocks produced no bradyarrhythmia. Second, a patient with cardiomyopathy and who was taking amiodarone had failure to capture of an epicardial pacemaker system despite programming the pacemaker to maximal output. Third, one patient expired with electromechanical dissociation and a paced QRS despite having devices implanted to treat both brady- and tachyarrhythmias. Fourth, during pacemaker magnet testing, ventricular tachycardia was induced that was appropriately treated by a defibrillator shock. This latter observation highlights another interaction that pacemakers may have on implanted defibrillators. In fact, we also have witnessed the occurrence of ventricular tachycardia being induced during pacemaker threshold determination in a patient with inducible ventricular tachycardia [8], similar to the case reported by Luceri et al. Sometimes, however, induction of ventricular tachycardia by a pacemaker is desirable. For example, for implantable defibrillators without a noninvasive stimulation mode, pacemakers with the option of triggered ventricular

Table 2 Implantable Defibrillator Effects on Permanent Pacemakers

1. The pacing threshold may increase following implantable defibrillator shocks and lead to pacemaker noncapture.
2. The R-wave signal may deteriorate following implantable defibrillator shocks and cause pacemaker nonsensing.
3. Pacemakers may be reprogrammed by implantable defibrillator shocks.
4. Pacemakers may be damaged by implantable defibrillator shocks.
5. Pacemakers may be reprogrammed by radiofrequency signals from defibrillator telemetry and programming.
6. Magnets placed over implantable defibrillators may influence pacemaker function.

pacing (VVT mode) can be used for ventricular tachycardia induction during implantable defibrillator testing.

Inappropriate defibrillator discharges can result from signals emitted during programming of implanted pacemakers [5]. In a patient with an AID-BR automatic implantable cardioverter-defibrillator (Cardiac Pacemakers, Inc., St. Paul, MN) and a Cordis Multicor II ventricular demand pacemaker, Gottleib et al. reported that impulses generated during programming to the stat VVI mode initiated a defibrillator charging cycle [5]. The explanation for the occurrence was that the implantable defibrillator sensed high-frequency electromagnetic signals lasting only 760 ms sent by the pacemaker programmer during pacemaker programming.

Kim et al. reported the occurrence of shock delivery from an AICD during permanent pacemaker magnet tests [13]. The underlying heart rate was 133 beats/min, and the asynchronous pacemaker rate was 70 beats/min. Presumably, both the native R waves and the pacing stimulus artifacts were sensed leading to "double counting" and the inadvertent shock. Conversely, magnet application during pacemaker testing may result in the inadvertent inactivation of some implantable defibrillators. Thus, special care needs to be taken when any magnets are used. As discussed below, implantation of the pacemaker and defibrillator as far away as possible from one another, often on opposite sides of the body, helps to avoid these undesirable interactions [8].

A rare cause of an adverse pacemaker interaction with an implantable defibrillator was reported by Critelli et al. [14] During esophageal atrial pacing at a rate just above the detection rate for the implantable defibrillator, a charging sequence was initiated. Counting of the stimulus artifact was excluded, since the defibrillator discharged only when the ventricular response exceeded the detection rate of the device. The authors suggested that esophageal pacing could be utilized to assess the potential for the inappropriate discharges secondary to atrial arrhythmias in patients with implantable defibrillators. Although obvious, during rate-responsive pacing and upper rate limit tracking in either the VVIR or DDD(R) mode, the rate detection criterion of defibrillators may be satisfied if pacing occurs above the defibrillator detection rate and lead to unwanted shocks.

II. IMPLANTABLE DEFIBRILLATOR EFFECTS ON PERMANENT PACEMAKERS

Implantable defibrillator shocks can affect implantable pacemakers (Table 2) by increasing the pacing threshold following shocks resulting in pacemaker noncapture [4,6,7,9,12,15,16], causing deterioration of the R-wave signal and nonsensing of native R waves [6,9,15], reprogramming the pacemaker [7,9,10], and potential injury to the implanted pulse generator, al-

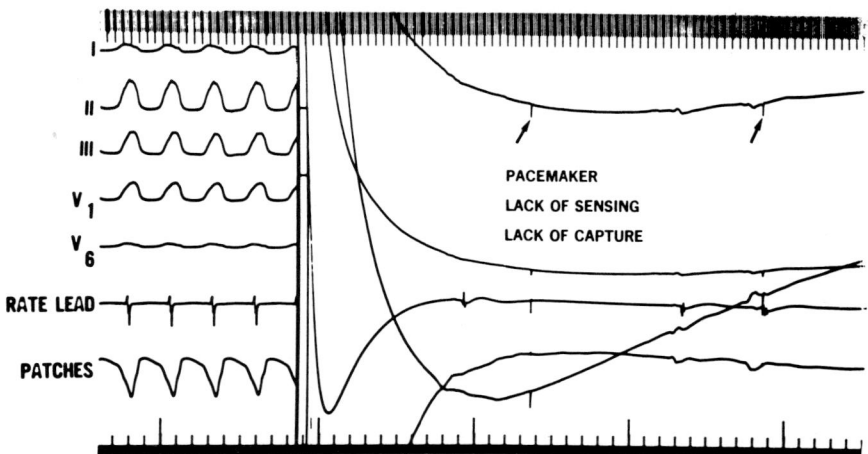

Figure 4. Pacemaker malfunction following a defibrillator shock is illustrated. Following the shock two pacemaker stimuli are shown (arrows) that occur shortly after intrinsic R waves and demonstrate lack of sensing. The first stimulus occurs after the expected ventricular refractory period and also demonstrates failure to capture. I, II, III, VI, and V6 = surface electrocardiographic leads. (Reprinted with permission from Ref. 6.)

though the latter occurrence has not been documented [7]. Some of these interactions can be compounded by drugs that, for example, increase the pacing threshold [7,16–18]. Radiofrequency signals used for defibrillator programming may lead to pacemaker reprogramming [5]. Placement of a magnet over an implantable defibrillator may also affect the implanted pacemaker [19].

Loss of pacemaker capture following defibrillator discharge is shown in Fig. 4 and has been recorded by numerous authors [4,6,7,9,12,16]. The 78-year-old patient reported by Slepian et al. was treated with amiodarone, a ventricular demand (VVI) pacemaker, and an implantable cardioverter-defibrillator [4]. These authors observed that the time of failure to capture was energy-related: The greater the delivered shock energy, the longer failure to capture persisted. Reiter et al. showed that, for longer durations of ventricular fibrillation, the pacing threshold increased postshock [20]. Thus, it appears that the energy level of delivered shocks [4,12] and the duration of arrhythmia before shock therapy [20] are related to both postshock bradycardia [12] and elevation of the pacing threshold following defibrillation [4,20].

Pacemaker function after implantable defibrillator discharge was analyzed by Cohen et al. [6]. Pacemaker nonsensing of ventricular complexes after defibrillation leading to the delivery of inappropriate pacemaker stimuli was observed in 11 of 20 episodes. The mean duration for lack of sensing was 9.1 ± 11.6 s for pacemakers with this problem. Failure of ventricular capture was also observed in 8 of 22 analyzable tracings. The mean duration for lack of capture was 4.9 ± 5.1 s, including one patient who had no pacemaker capture for 16 s following defibrillator discharge.

Yee et al. reported changes in the pacing threshold and R-wave amplitude following transvenous catheter shocks in an animal model [15]. The bipolar R-wave amplitude decreased from 8.3 ± 1.0 mV to 2.0 ± 0.2 mV following shocks ($p < 0.001$). Similarly, the stimulation threshold increased from 1.0 ± 0.1 V to 2.3 ± 0.4 V 15 s after shock delivery ($p < 0.001$). The changes persisted for up to 10 min. Since these R-wave measurements were localized to the defibrillating catheter, a second animal study utilizing five pigs was performed in which the R-wave amplitude was measured distant from the shock-delivery catheter. No significant change in the R-wave amplitude or stimulation threshold was seen at the distant electrode, suggesting that the changes were secondary to local changes at the catheter–myocardium interface.

Not all studies indicate that the pacing threshold remains stable even at catheters separate from the defibrillating catheters. Guarnieri et al. reported not only that there is a finite time to capture due to increases in the pacing threshold following 30-J defibrillator shocks, but also that flecainide makes the increase in time to capture more pronounced [16]. In contrast, Reiter et al. examined the effects of transthoracic defibrillation shocks on the defibrillation threshold in anesthetized dogs and concluded that defibrillation during pacing or within 15 s following initiation of ventricular fibrillation did not increase the pacing threshold regardless of shock energy [20]. However, for episodes of ventricular fibrillation lasting 30 s or longer, the pacing threshold increased [20].

Calkins et al. reported interactions between pacemakers and implantable defibrillators in 30 patients [9]. Interactions were classified into four categories: transient pacemaker dysfunction with failure to sense or capture following defibrillator discharge, oversensing of the pacemaker stimulus by the implantable defibrillator leading to double counting, defibrillator failure to sense ventricular fibrillation due to multiple counting, and pacemaker reprogramming following defibrillator discharge. Pacemaker failure to sense or to capture or both was observed in seven patients. The phenomenon lasted less than 10 s in four patients, from 10 to 35 s in two patients, and for greater than 56 s in one patient. Pacemaker reprogramming by defibrillator discharges was noted in three of the 30 patients. Reprogramming to the pacemaker backup mode occurred in one patient each with a Cordis 415 pulse generator and a Medtronic 7006 pulse generator. A third patient had an Intermedics 262-14 Intertach pulse generator programmed to the ventricular demand pacing mode by a defibrillator discharge. We have seen a similar patient who had an Intermedics device programmed to the backup mode following defibrillator discharge on two occasions. Ahern et al. have described similar observations in patients with antitachycardia pacemaker-defibrillator systems [10]. Defibrillator shocks can potentially irreversibly damage pacemakers, but this occurrence has not been documented.

III. METHODS TO PREVENT ADVERSE DEVICE–DEVICE INTERACTIONS

Implantation techniques to avoid adverse device–device interactions have been described and are highlighted on Table 3 [7,8]. To minimize interaction between pacemaker or defibrillator programmers or magnets, the devices should be implanted as far away from each other as possible [8]. Although we have had satisfactory function when both devices were implanted on the left side of the body (pacemaker in the prepectoral region and the implantable defibrillator in the anterior left upper quadrant of the abdomen), if possible, the devices should even be placed on opposite sides of the body. To avoid adverse device–device interaction, it is usually easier to implant the pacemaker before the implantable defibrillator, as demonstrated below.

A. Defibrillator Implantation in Patients with a Previously Implanted Pacemaker [8]

Although permanent pacemakers, either single- or dual-chamber devices, are usually implanted using transvenous leads, the observations that follow apply to both endocardial and epicardial

Table 3 Methods to Prevent Adverse Device–Device Interactions

1. Implant devices as far away from one another as possible to minimize unwanted interactions with magnets and programmers (opposite sides of the body, if feasible).
2. Implant the pacemaker before the defibrillator, if possible, so that defibrillator sensing-lead position can be optimized. An active-fixation lead may be desirable if cardiopulmonary bypass or other cardiac surgery is contemplated.
3. Defibrillator implantation in patients with previously implanted pacemakers:
    a. Use "worst-case" scenario in the operating room (program pacemaker to highest stimulus amplitude and duration) to maximize the possibility of device–device interaction, since if this can be avoided under these circumstances, the chances of its occurrence are low in clinical setting.
    b. Map epicardial surface to locate site where pacemaker stimulus artifact size is as small as possible.
    c. Maintain electrode tips within 1 cm of each other.
    d. When site is located where pacemaker stimulus artifact is minimal and the R-wave amplitude is large during both ventricular pacing and sinus rhythm, implant the first epicardial lead. Move the second lead circumferentially around the first to find site where pacing stimulus artifact amplitude is the smallest. Implant second electrode at this site.
    e. Test defibrillator sensing during high-output pacing. If a Ventak defibrillator is used, listen for beeps when a magnet is placed over the device, and if more than one beep is heard for each QRS, multiple counting is present and the sensing leads must be moved.
    f. Test function of the implantable defibrillator-pacemaker system in the operating room to assure effective defibrillation and to assess whether pacing occurs during ventricular tachycardia or ventricular fibrillation. Testing worst-case scenario during asynchronous (VOO) pacing at maximal output also useful to assure effective defibrillation if unanticipated pacing were to occur in the future.
4. Pacemaker implantation in patients with a previously implanted defibrillator:
    a. Use standard approach to pacemaker implantation.
    b. Place implanted defibrillator in the standby (EP) mode and advance pacemaker lead to the right ventricle. A pacing system analyzer programmed to maximal output and pulse width is used for pacing and the lead position to find a site where an acceptable pacing and sensing threshold characteristic demonstrable.
    c. Assess defibrillator sensing by listening for beeping tones from the defibrillator, if the device can emit sounds, or observe real-time electrograms or sensing markers by telemetry during pacing.
    d. Implant pacemaker lead where pacing and sensing are satisfactory and where there is no detection of pacing stimuli by the defibrillator.

pacemaker systems. A worst-case scenario is attempted in the operating room to maximize the possibility of device–device interaction, since if this can be avoided under these circumstances, then in the clinical setting, the chances of its occurrence are even lower. Thus, the pacemaker should be programmed to the highest stimulus amplitude and duration so as to maximize the pacemaker stimulus artifact size and increase the possibility of sensing by the implantable defibrillator. The same techniques are used when implanting a defibrillator with an atrial pacemaker, a ventricular pacemaker, or a dual-chamber device.

After calibration of the cardiac electrogram signals, the heart is mapped to locate a site where the pacemaker stimulus artifact size is as small as possible. This can be carried out with the epicardial sensing electrodes of the implantable defibrillator still in their carriers (Fig. 5). They are held in the surgeon's hands and used as mapping electrodes. The tips should be main-

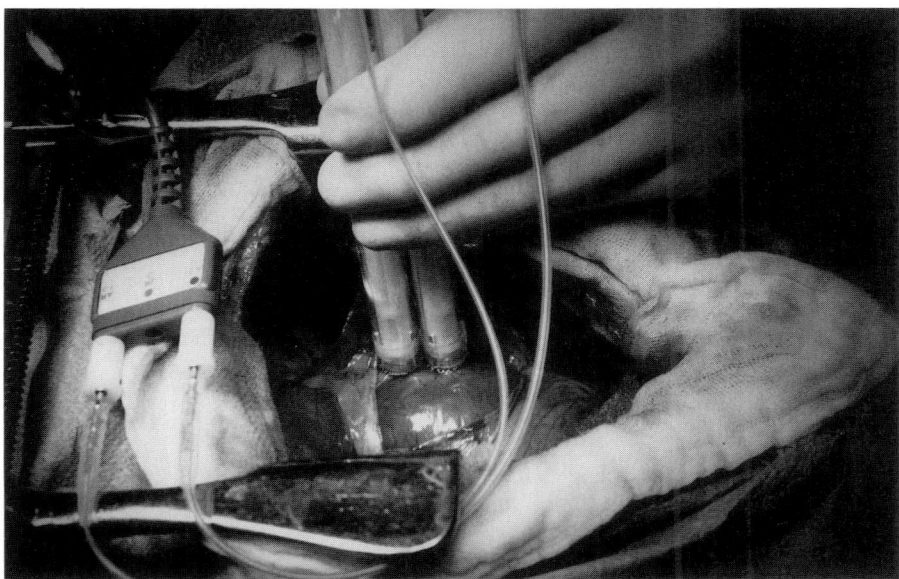

Figure 5 The surgeon holds the bipolar epicardial electrodes in their lead carriers (center) attached to the monitoring cables (left). While held together, the electrodes are applied to the surface of the heart during pacing and the electrogram recordings are analyzed to find a site where the pacemaker stimulus artifact is minimal. At that site the electrodes are implanted. For illustrative purposes, this photograph was made in the animal laboratory. See text for further details. (Reprinted with permission of the American College of Cardiology from Ref. 8.)

tained within 1 cm of each other while the electrode pair is moved to various sites over the epicardium during high-output pacing, so that a site can be identified where the pacemaker stimulus artifact is minimal or is nondetectable (Fig. 6). In our study, R-wave amplitudes during both paced and native rhythms generally exceeded 7 mV. An implantation site where the pacemaker stimulus artifact was < 0.1 mV could generally be obtained. If long stimulus-to R-wave intervals are observed, the bipolar leads should be moved closer to the pacemaker electrode so that the refractory period for defibrillator sensing is not exceeded and the possibility for double counting is decreased. We recommend that mapping be performed before implantation of the defibrillator patches to avoid placing the patches over an optimal sensing site.

When a site is located where the pacemaker stimulus artifact is minimal and the R-wave amplitude is large during both ventricular pacing and sinus rhythm, one of the epicardial leads is implanted. The second epicardial lead is thereafter moved circumferentially around the first to find the site where the pacing stimulus artifact recorded by the electrode pair has the lowest amplitude. Then, at this site, the second electrode is implanted. After sensing-lead implantation, the patches are implanted, followed by cardioversion and defibrillation threshold testing in the usual fashion. After defibrillator implantation, actual sensing by the implantable defibrillator is assessed. If a Ventak device (Cardiac Pacemakers, Inc., St. Paul, MN) is used, this is done by placing a magnet over the pulse generator. If, during high-output ventricular pacing, more than one beep is heard for every QRS response, then double counting is present and the sensing leads must be moved. It is important always to test the function of the implantable defibrillator-pacemaker system in the operating room to assure effective defibrillation, and to

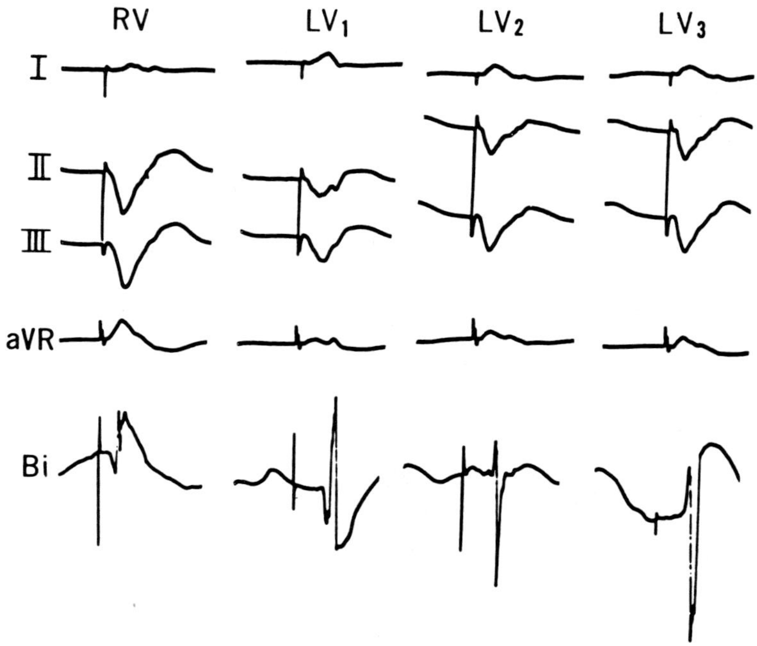

| | RV | LV₁ | LV₂ | LV₃ |

(A)

Figure 6 These recordings were made from a patient with a ventricular demand activity-sensing pacemaker at defibrillator implantation. Surface electrocardiogram leads I, II, III, and aVR are shown on the first four channels. The electrogram recorded from the bipolar sensing leads is labeled Bi. The gain for all recordings is identical. (A) Epicardial recordings from one right ventricular (RV) and three left ventricular (LV) sites during pacing at an 8-Volt output and a 1-ms pulse width. The pacemaker stimulus artifact is large close to the apex of the RV where the pacemaker electrode is implanted, and at LV sites 1 and 2. At LV site 3 the pacemaker stimulus artifact is small compared to the paced R wave and is the site where the leads were implanted. (B) Electrograms recorded after the sensing leads were implanted. The R wave during sinus rhythm is 8.7 mV (left column). During bipolar pacing (middle columns), the pacemaker stimuli amplitudes and pulse widths are shown below the respective stimulus artifacts. As the pacing stimulus amplitude is decreased, the stimulus artifact also decreases. For illustrative purposes, to show the hazard of unipolar pacing, the right column shows unipolar pacing at only 2.5 V, which provides a stimulus artifact larger than at any bipolar output. (C) Recordings from a patient with an atrial demand pacemaker that have virtually no identifiable pacemaker stimulus artifacts in the bipolar sensing electrogram. See text for discussion. (Reprinted with permission of the American College of Cardiology from Ref. 8.)

assess whether pacing occurs during ventricular tachycardia or ventricular fibrillation. It is also worthwhile to program the pacemaker to the asynchronous (VOO) mode at maximal output to stimulate a worst-case scenario and assure that arrhythmia detection occurs, in case pacing occurs in the future during ventricular fibrillation even if pacing was not observed when the pacemaker was programmed to a synchronous mode in the operating room [8]. Electrograms can be easily recorded under these circumstances and later problems potentially avoided (Figs. 7 and 8).

An unusual circumstance is the need for a defibrillator in a patient with a previously implanted epicardial pacing system. Choosing the location for the defibrillator sensing lead(s) will

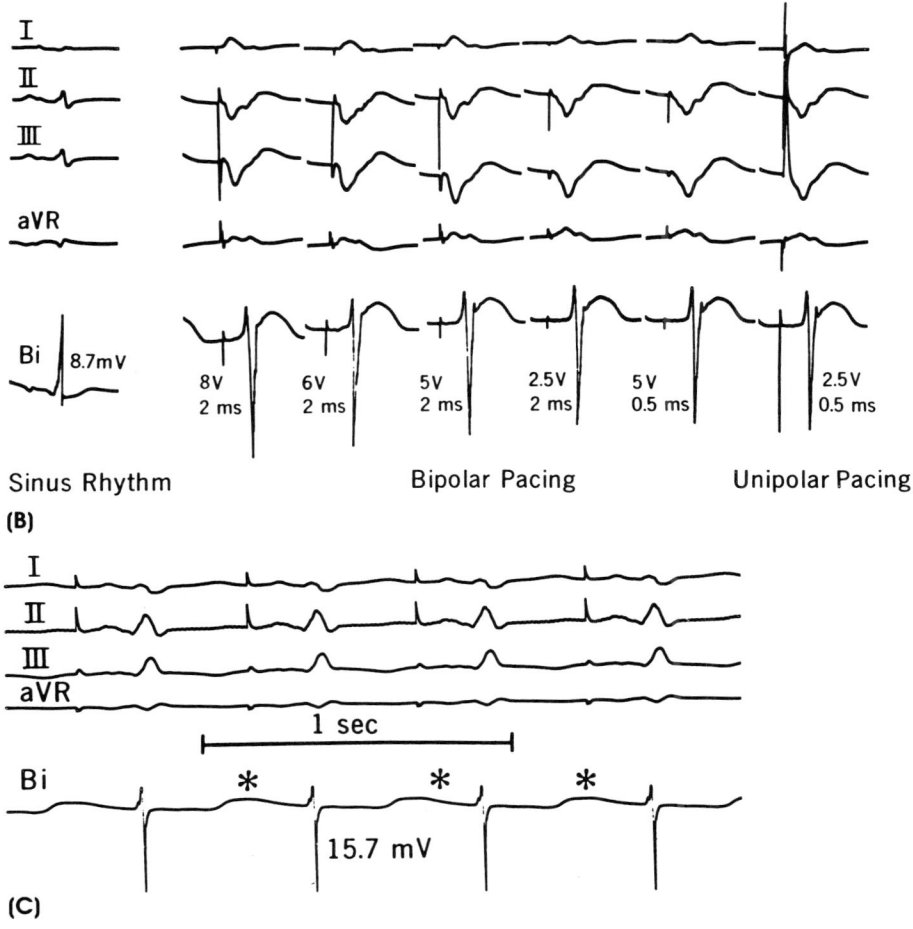

depend on where the epicardial pacing leads were implanted. If the pacing lead system was implanted over the left ventricle, the defibrillator sensing leads may be positioned epicardially over the right ventricle or endocardially in the right ventricle, taking the same measures described above if an endocardial pacing system were present. Whether left lateral thoracotomy, median sternotomy, or a subxyphoid or subcostal approach are used will depend on the location of the epicardial pacing leads and the surgeon's preferences. However, with new technologies available, it may be simpler to use an endocardial defibrillator system and an advanced-generation defibrillator (sometimes incorporating the old pacing lead for pacing and sensing, if satisfactory), rather than combining two devices in the same patient.

B. Pacemaker Implantation in Patients with a Previously Implanted Defibrillator [8]

The standard approach to pacemaker implantation is utilized, usually using a prepectoral incision. For reasons discussed previously, bipolar pacing systems are desirable, and unipolar pacing systems are relatively contraindicated [1,2,6–9,11]. For pacemaker lead implantation, the implantable defibrillator is placed in the standby (EP) mode and the pacemaker lead ad-

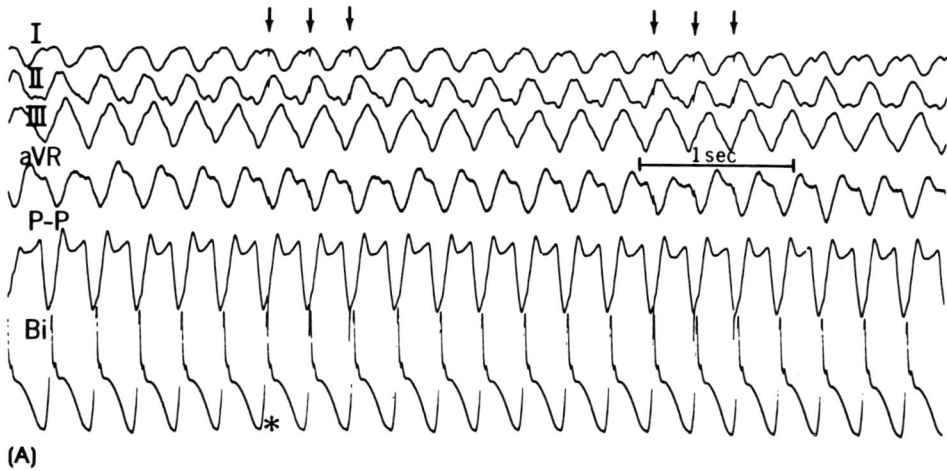

Figure 7 The recordings were made during defibrillation threshold testing at implantation of an implantable defibrillator. Labels are as in Fig. 6 except that P-P refers to electrograms recorded from the two defibrillating patch leads. (A,B) Pacing during (A) ventricular tachycardia and (B) ventricular fibrillation, respectively, in a patient with a previously implanted antitachycardia pacemaker. No pacemaker stimulus artifacts are detectable in the bipolar rate-sensing electrograms (asterisks) during pacing (arrows). In (B), the fourth through sixth impulses are from the antitachycardia pacemaker functioning in the ventricular demand mode. (C) Recordings from a patient with an atrial demand pacemaker. Again, no pacemaker stimulus artifact is detectable in the bipolar rate-sensing electrogram (asterisks) during pacing (arrows). See text for discussion. (Reprinted with permission of the American College of Cardiology from Ref. 8.)

vanced to the right ventricle. A pacing system analyzer is used to identify a site where acceptable pacing and sensing threshold characteristics are demonstrable. Then, with the pacing system analyzer programmed to maximal pulse width and amplitude, sensing of the pacemaker stimulus artifacts by the implantable defibrillator can be assessed by listening for beeping tones from the defibrillator if the device can emit such sounds with each sensed event (devices manufactured by Cardiac Pacemakers, Inc., St. Paul, MN). Some newer-generation implantable defibrillators provide real-time electrograms that can be used to observe the sensing electrogram and see that the stimulus artifacts are small. Use of an active-fixation lead helps to find a site satisfying these criteria by allowing a larger portion of the right ventricle to be potentially usable for lead implantation. Active-fixation leads may also decrease the risk of lead dislodgement following cardiopulmonary bypass or manipulation of the heart during future cardiac surgery if ever needed. The lead and pacemaker are then implanted.

For ventricular pacing, Spotnitz et al. [11] prefer using two unipolar, positive-fixation, screw-in pacing electrodes positioned together in the right ventricular outflow tract or at the anterior right ventricular free wall, rather than a single bipolar lead positioned at the right ventricular apex. The authors recommend using unipolar positive-fixation leads linked with an adaptor because of their increased flexibility in comparison to in-line bipolar leads, which have greater stiffness. The defibrillator sensing leads are placed over the left ventricle. In contrast, we have not had trouble finding satisfactory ICD sensing lead sites when pacing leads are positioned at the right ventricular apex, and we have not had any pacemaker lead dislodgements.

Implanting an endocardial pacing system in a patient with a previously implanted endocardial defibrillator system is difficult, since sensing of pacing stimulus artifacts is enhanced by

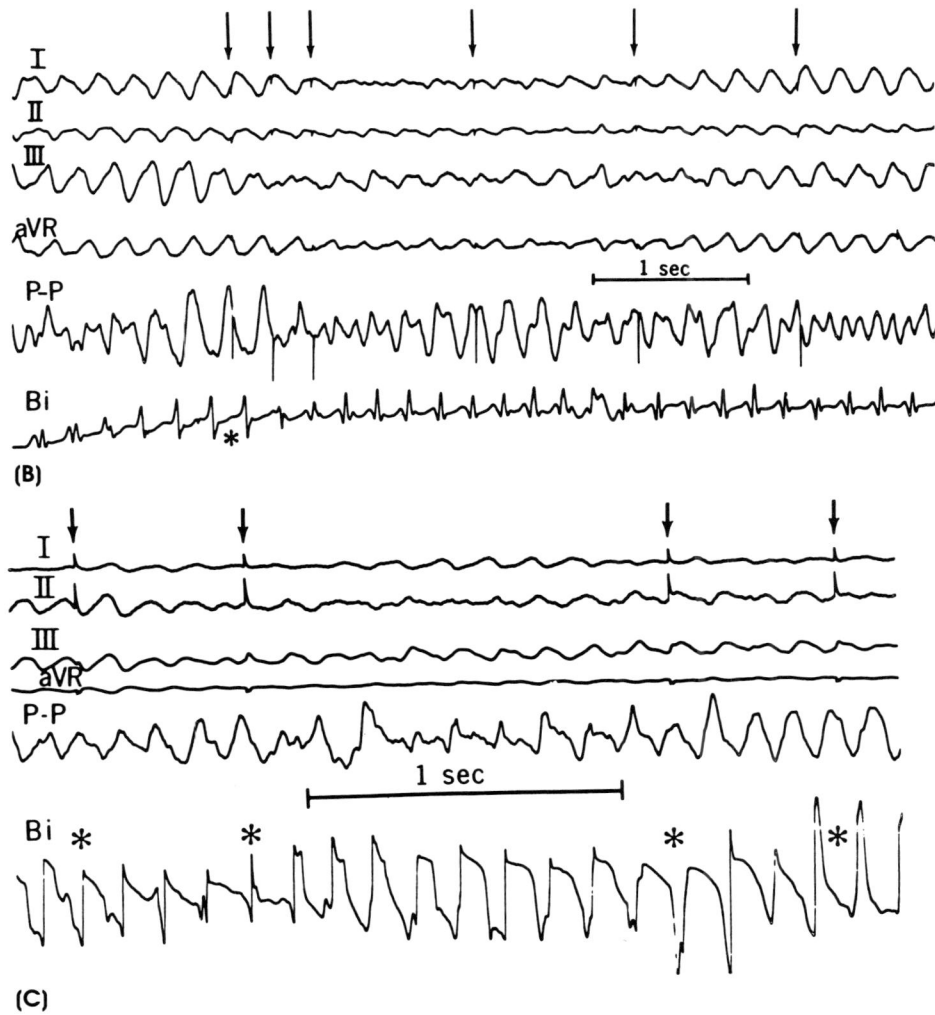

having both the pacing lead of the pacemaker and the sensing lead of the defibrillator in the same cardiac chamber. Using an active-fixation pacing lead increases the area available for implantation at sites distant from the defibrillator sensing lead and at a location where the defibrillator does not sense the stimulus artifacts. Another option, of course, is to upgrade the defibrillator to one with pacing capability in addition to defibrillation and cardioversion functions, whether or not the previously implanted defibrillator uses endocardial or epicardial sensing leads. Often, the old sensing leads function satisfactorily and can be used as the pacing/sensing lead(s) for the new defibrillator-pacemaker device.

C. Postoperative Testing [8]

In patients with combined device systems, it is important always to test the entire system before the patient is discharged from the hospital (Fig. 9). Ventricular fibrillation should be induced to assure that pacing during the arrhythmia does not cause inhibition of detection by the

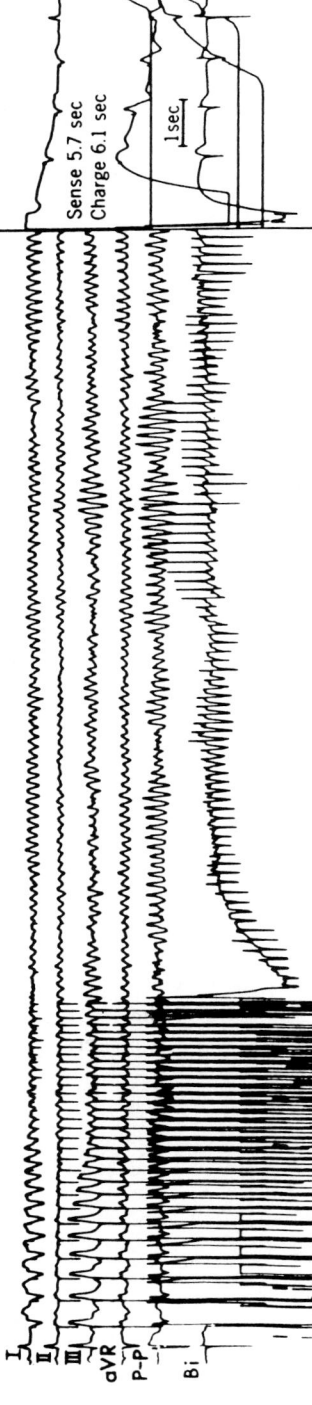

Figure 8 Intraoperative testing of an implantable defibrillator in a patient with a ventricular demand pacemaker. Surface ECG leads I, II, III, and aVR are shown with electrograms from electrograms recorded from the defibrillator patch leads (P-P) and bipolar sensing leads (Bi). After 17.0 s (standby time 4 s, sensing time 5.7 s, charging time 6.1 s, and synchronization time 1.2 s, and 30-J shock restores sinus rhythm. The pacemaker supported the rhythm postshock for bradycardia but did not pace during ventricular fibrillation. (Reprinted with permission of the American College of Cardiology from Ref. 8.)

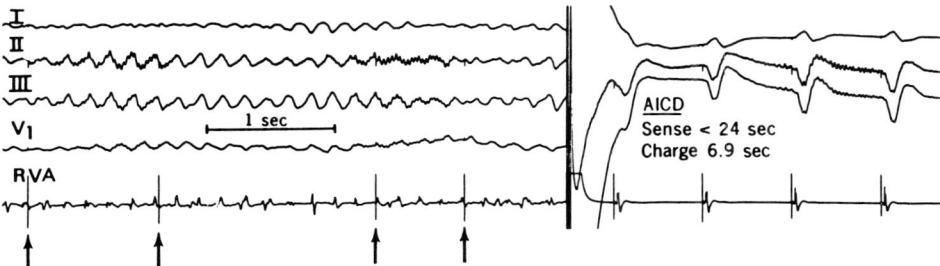

Figure 9 At postoperative electrophysiological study in a patient with an implantable defibrillator and an activity-sensing, rate-adaptive ventricular demand pacemaker conversion of ventricular fibrillation. Surface ECG leads, I, II, III, and V1 are shown with electrograms from a temporary transvenous electrode catheter advanced to the right ventricular apex (RVA) for programmed stimulation. The implanted defibrillator was placed in the standby mode, ventricular fibrillation was induced, and then the defibrillator was activated. Despite ventricular pacing during ventricular fibrillation, the arrhythmia was correctly sensed and converted by the defibrillator. Bradycardia is supported by the pacemaker postshock. (Reprinted with permission of the American College of Cardiology from Ref. 8.)

implantable defibrillator [1,2,6–9]. Also, it is useful to reassess that the pacemaker is not reprogrammed by defibrillator therapy [7,9,10]. In patients with ventricular tachycardia, arrhythmia conversion should also be tested if an antitachycardia pacemaker is implanted or if the implantable defibrillator is used for conversion. The same concerns regarding inhibition of detection hold under these circumstances as for when ventricular fibrillation is present.

IV. SUMMARY

Implantable defibrillators can affect pacemaker function and vice versa. However, with careful attention to minimizing the pacing stimulus artifact in the defibrillator sensing electrogram, many adverse device–device interactions can be avoided. Only bipolar pacemakers should be implanted in conjunction with implantable defibrillators. During defibrillator implantation, the possibility for ventricular demand or antitachycardia pacing need in the future must always be considered. Thus, bipolar rate-sensing electrodes should be implanted over the left ventricle so that if later a pacemaker is required, its lead can be positioned in the right ventricle, far from the defibrillator sensing leads. If the defibrillator epicardial sensing electrodes are placed over the right ventricle, the chances of adverse device–device interactions are increased. For patients with previously implanted pacemakers, mapping of the left ventricle should be undertaken at the time of defibrillator implantation to find a site where the sensing lead records a minimal pacemaker stimulus artifact even when the pacemaker is programmed to maximal output. If a combined device system is contemplated, pacemaker implantation should precede implantable defibrillator implantation whenever possible, since it is easier to map the left ventricle when the permanent pacemaker lead is already in place, to minimize the possibility for pacemaker inhibition of arrhythmia detection by the implanted defibrillator, and to avoid multiple counting by the implantable defibrillator of the pacing stimulus artifacts and evoked R waves. Postoperative electrophysiological study to assure lack of device–device adverse interaction should always be performed before patients are released from the hospital when combined device systems are implanted. Function of the two devices during ventricular fibrillation should always be tested, and during ventricular tachycardia, as appropriate. Late management of these patients is easier and safer when early management has followed these guidelines.

REFERENCES

1. Bach SM, Jr. AID-B cardioverter-defibrillator possible interaction with pacemakers. Technical communication, Intec Systems, August 29, 1983.
2. Kim SG, Furman S, Waspe LE, Broadman R, Fisher JD. Unipolar pacer artifacts induced failure of an automatic implantable cardioverter/defibrillator to detect ventricular fibrillation. Am J Cardiol 1986; 57:880–881.
3. Ruffy R, Lal R, Kouchoukos NT, Kim SS. Combined bipolar dual chamber pacing and automatic implantable cardioverter/defibrillator. J Am Coll Cardiol 1986; 7:933–937.
4. Slepian M, Levine JH, Watkins L, Brinker J, Guarnieri T. Automatic implantable cardioverter defibrillator/permanent pacemaker interaction: loss of pacemaker capture following AICD discharge. PACE 1987; 10:1194–1197.
5. Gottlieb C, Miller JM, Rosenthal ME, Marchlinski FE. Automatic implantable defibrillator discharge resulting from routine pacemaker programming. PACE 1988; 11:336–338.
6. Cohen AI, Wish MH, Fletcher RD, et al. The use and interaction of permanent pacemakers and the automatic implantable cardioverter defibrillator. PACE 1988; 11:704–711.
7. Singer I, Guarnieri T, Kupersmith J. Implanted automatic defibrillators: effects of drugs and pacemakers. PACE 1988; 11:2250–2262.
8. Epstein AE, Kay GN, Plumb VJ, Shepard RB, Kirklin JK. Combined automatic implantable cardioverter-defibrillator and pacemaker systems: implantation techniques and follow-up. J Am Coll Cardiol 1989; 13:121–131.
9. Calkins H, Brinker J, Veltri EP, Guarnieri T, Levine JH. Clinical interactions between pacemakers and automatic implantable cardioverter-defibrillators. J Am Coll Cardiol 1990; 16:666–673.
10. Ahern TS, Nydegger C, McCormick DJ, et al. Device interaction—antitachycardia pacemakers and defibrillators for sustained ventricular tachycardia. PACE 1991; 14:302–307.
11. Spotnitz JM, Ott GY, Bigger JT Jr, Steinberg JS, Livelli F Jr. Methods of implantable cardioverter-defibrillator-pacemaker insertion to avoid interactions. Ann Thorac Surg 1992; 53:253–257.
12. Luceri RM, Thurer RJ, Castellanos A, Stafford W, Saoudi N, Myerburg RJ. Initial experience with automatic defibrillator-implanted pacemaker interactions (abst). PACE 1985; 8:296.
13. Kim SG, Furman S, Matos JA, Waspe LE, Brodman R, Fisher JD. Automatic implantable cardioverter/defibrillator: inadvertent discharges during permanent pacemaker magnet tests. PACE 1987; 10:579–582.
14. Critelli G, Monda V, Scherillo M, Coltorti F, Greco C, Reale A. The automatic implantable cardioverter/defibrillator: transesophageal atrial pacing discloses the potential for erroneous discharges. PACE 1988; 11:419–422.
15. Yee R, Jones DL, Jarvis E, Donner AP, Klein GJ. Changes in pacing threshold and R wave amplitude after transvenous catheter countershock. J Am Coll Cardiol 1984; 4:543–549.
16. Guarnieri T, DaTorre SD, Bondke H, Brinker J, Myers S, Levine JH. Increased pacing threshold after an automatic defibrillator shock in dogs: effects of class I and class II antiarrhythmic drugs. PACE 1988; 11:1324–1330.
17. Salel AF, Seagren SC, Pool PE. Effects of encainide on the function of implanted pacemakers. PACE 1989; 12:1439–1444.
18. Montefoschi N, Boccadamo R. Propafenone induced acute variation of chronic atrial pacing threshold: a case report. PACE 1990; 13:480–483.
19. Hayes DL. Effects of drugs and devices on permanent pacemakers. Cardio 1991 (Jan); 70–75.
20. Reiter MJ, Lindenfeld J, Breckinridge S, Mann DE. Does defibrillation raise the ventricular pacing threshold? (abst). J Am Coll Cardiol 1988; 11:144A.

30

Device Infection: Prevention and Treatment

Susan O'Donoghue and Edward V. Platia

*George Washington University School of Medicine
and Washington Hospital Center
Washington, D. C.*

The development of an infection involving an implanted defibrillator system is one of the most feared and frustrating complications. Appropriate management must include not only treatment of the infection itself, but also consideration of the patient's risk of lethal arrhythmias in case of device explantation. Prolonged hospitalization may be required. Scrupulous attention to the prevention and optimum treatment of such infections clearly has a significant impact on the morbidity and cost effectiveness of device therapy. This chapter will review the incidence and types of device infections, and outline recommended strategies for both prevention and treatment.

I. INCIDENCE

Infections in defibrillator systems can take a variety of forms. Patients who have had implantation of defibrillator leads only at the time of coronary artery bypass graft surgery or other heart surgery may develop infections involving these leads. Such instances may include sternal wound infection with subsequent mediastinitis, or may present primarily as mediastinitis involving the defibrillator leads without preceding sternal wound infection. Alternatively, the capped terminal pin ends of the leads, which are generally coiled subcutaneously in the subxiphoid region if no generator is implanted, may become involved in a localized infection, which may subsequently extend to the mediastinum. Proximity of these coiled leads to a chest tube exiting through the skin could potentiate this mode of infection. Patients who undergo initial implantation of a complete defibrillator system may develop infection involving the lead system and/or the generator pocket. Finally, infections can occur following generator replacement, and usually present as infected pockets.

Data regarding the incidence of device infections are available from a variety of sources. The CPI database, which included over 24,000 device implants as of May 1992, has recorded a 1.2% incidence of generator explantation due to infection. This figure is likely to be less than

Table 1 Incidence of Infections in Defibrillator Systems

Series	n (pts/generators)	Surgical approach[a]	Incidence of infection (%)		
			Leads only	Initial implant	Generator replacements
Mirowski, 1985 [1]	112	Not specified	—	6/112 (5.4)	—
Borbola et al., 1988 [2]	25/33	60% MS 40% LAT	—	5/25 (20)	0/9 (0)
Kelly et al., 1988 [3]	91/109	63% LAT 23% MS 8% SX	—	2/91 (2.2)	0/18 (0)
Olinger et al. 1988 [4]	94	54% MS 46% LAT	4/35 (12)	2/59 (3.4)	—
Winkle et al. 1989 [5]	270/392	30% MS 70% LAT	—	4/270 (1.5)	2/122 (1.6)
Wunderly et al. 1990 [6]	207/263	Not specified	—	4/207 (1.9)	4/56 (7.1)
Siclari et al. 1990 [7]	115/154	100% MS	—	3/115 (2.6)	5/39 (12.8)
Bakker et al. 1992 [8]	70/90	81% MS 19% LAT	—	1/70 (1.4)	0/20 (0)
Platia and O'Donoghue, 1992	292/369	40% MS 39% LAT 21% SX	3/66 (4.8)	4/226 (1.7)	0/77 (0)

[a]MS = median sternotomy, LAT = left anterior thoracotomy, SX = subxiphoid approach.

the actual incidence, due to underreporting; furthermore, it does not reflect infections of lead systems only, or infections which did not result in generator explantation.

There are a number of series in the literature reviewing the overall clinical experience with implantable defibrillator systems. Larger series which include data on infections are tabulated in Table 1. In 1985, Mirowski reported the initial 112 patients receiving implants between 1980 and 1984 [1]. The lead system in this series consisted of transvenous right ventricular rate-sensing and superior vena cava defibrillating leads, as well as an apical patch lead. The latter was positioned via median sternotomy, left lateral thoracotomy, or the subxiphoid approach. Six infections were reported. In four, the primary site was the pulse generator pocket, in one a pervenous catheter placement site, and in one the site was unknown. Explantation of the entire system was required in two cases. No further details are provided in this series.

Borbola et al. reported a 20% incidence of infection in a series of 25 patients, but none were actually device-related infections [2]. This included three patients with diabetes mellitus who underwent median sternotomy, and subsequently developed sternal wound infections which responded to local wound care and systemic antibiotics. One patient had bacteremia due to an intravenous line infection 5 days postoperatively, and responded to intravenous antibiotics. One patient developed pneumonia and pleuropericarditis which responded to antibiotics, antiinflammatory drugs, and thoracentesis. Two additional patients developed pocket seromas which resolved spontaneously. This commonly recognized phenomenon probably does not represent infection. Excluding these last two cases, the infection rate in this series would be 12%, and none of the systems required explantation.

Kelly et al. found a 2.2% incidence of infections involving the implanted defibrillator in a study of 91 patients who received the device [3]. The two infections presented 6 weeks and 6 months following implantation. Both were caused by *Staphylococcus aureus*, and both required

Device Infection: Prevention and Treatment

explantation of the defibrillator generator and lead system. Additionally, nine patients reportedly had postoperative pulmonary complications for which they received intravenous antibiotics. Including these patients, the total incidence of postoperative infection would be 12% in this series. Olinger et al. reported six infections among 94 patients with implanted defibrillator hardware [4]. Importantly, five of the six occurred in patients who underwent concomitant cardiac surgery via a median sternotomy. Four of these patients had the lead system implanted without a generator, and two of these developed sternal wound infections. The sixth patient had the entire defibrillator system placed via left anterior thoracotomy, and subsequently developed an infection of the generator pocket. All defibrillator hardware was explanted in each case, and there were no deaths attributed to these infections, although there were three deaths in the entire series due to other infections.

Winkle et al. presented a 7-year experience involving 392 defibrillator generators used in 270 patients [5]. Device-related infections were reported in six patients. Three occurred following initial implantation, one following lead repositioning, and two following generator replacement. A seventh patient experienced generator erosion with subsequent infection. In six patients the infection was due to *Staphylococcus aureus*. One of these patients died from the infection, and the other five had the entire system removed. The seventh patient, in whom infection was due to *Serratia*, was treated with generator removal and antibiotics, with the lead system left in place. Wunderly et al. found the incidence of infection to be 1.9% among 207 initial defibrillator implantations and 7.1% among 56 generator replacements [6]. Three of these eight infections were initially treated by removing all hardware. In five patients, initial treatment consisted of explanting the generator only. Four of these five had subsequent recurrence of infection, requiring complete explantation. The eighth patient was not considered an operative candidate, and was treated with chronic antibiotic suppression.

Siclari et al. reported infections in three of 115 initial implants, and in five of 39 generator replacements [7]. All patients were initially treated with local antibiotic irrigation alone. This yielded apparent success in just one patient, with 4 months of follow-up. All others required explantation, which included all hardware in five patients, and generator only in one. One patient died of sepsis after refusing device explantation, and two additional patients died of heart failure following explantation, with locally active infection still present. A series of 90 defibrillator implants in seventy patients was presented by Bakker and colleagues [8]. Only one device infection was reported, in a diabetic who had concomitant coronary artery bypass grafting. A *Staphylococcus epidermidis* infection became evident in the generator pocket 18 months postoperatively. Because of severe heart failure, the patient was treated conservatively with intravenous antibiotics, debridement, and continuous irrigation of the pocket. The patient died suddenly 5 weeks later, and postmortem examination revealed purulent material at the site of the posterior patch. Interestingly, previous leukocyte scanning had shown infection only at the generator site.

Our own experience includes 369 implants in 292 patients. Three infections have occurred among the 66 patients who had implantation of leads only during concomitant cardiac surgery. All three patients developed *Staphylococcal* mediastinitis in the early postoperative period, and were treated with removal of the lead system and systemic antibiotics. Among 226 patients who received defibrillator leads and generator, four infections have been encountered. One patient, who had concomitant coronary bypass grafting, developed *Staphylococcus aureus* mediastinitis and pocket infection, and died of overwhelming infection despite removal of all hardware and antibiotic therapy. One other patient developed an infected pocket and subsequent pneumonia due to *Mycobacterium chelonae*, and was treated successfully with removal of the entire system and antibiotics. The two additional patients had superficial infections of the thoracotomy incision and a chest-tube skin site, respectively, without systemic infection or in-

Table 2 Causative Organisms

| Organism | No. of reported cases | Incubation period [1] | Type of surgery[a] | | | | Explanted n (%) [a] | Deaths |
			CABG and leads	CABG and AICD	AICD Gen. LAT	Gen repl.		
Staphylococcus aureus	18	7–180 days	3	1	3	1	14/16 (87)	2
Staphylococcus epidermidis	11	4–30 mos	1			3	4/6 (67)	0
Serratia species	2	5 wks; 30 wks		1			1 (50)	0
Corynebacterium species	2	8 days, 11 mos					2 (100)	0
Torulopsis glabrata	1	13 days			1		1 (100)	0
Candida species	1	7 mos	1				1 (100)	0
Mycobacterium chelonae	1	18 days						0
Pseudomonas aeroginosa	1	—					—	
Negative cultures (gm + cocci on smears)	2	3.5 mos; 18 mos		1		1	2 (100)	0

[a]When specified

volvement of the defibrillator system. Both were treated successfully with local wound care and antibiotics. We have encountered no infections among the 77 patients who have undergone defibrillator generator replacement. In addition to these data, no infections have occurred among 27 patients who have undergone device implantation utilizing transvenous leads and a subcutaneous patch.

II. CAUSATIVE ORGANISMS

Table 2 contains details regarding the various organisms which have been reported to cause infections involving implanted defibrillator hardware. Seventy-one percent of all infections in the literature were caused by *Staphylococcus* organisms. *S. aureus* infections usually present fairly early after device implantation, as would be expected with this virulent organism. The one case with a reported incubation period of 180 days presented as folliculitis and lower-extremity cellulitis followed several days later by fluid in the defibrillator pocket [9]. Thus, this case likely represents hematogenous seeding rather than infection resulting from the initial implantation. Excluding this case, the mean incubation time for *S. aureus* infections was 35 days. It is important to note that both of the fatalities due to device infections were the result of *S. aureus* sepsis.

Staphylococcus epidermidis is the second most common causative organism in defibrillator infections. *S. epidermidis* infections generally occur months or even years after device implantation. Nevertheless, it is likely that these infections are due to contamination by skin flora at the time of surgery. An exopolysaccharide "slime" produced by *S. epidermidis* appears to facilitate adherence of the organism to plastic surfaces, and may also be a factor in resistance to phagocytosis and antibiotic therapy [12]. Two cases have been reported in which gram-positive cocci were seen in infected material, but no organism grew in culture [4,6]. These infections were most likely also due to *Staphylococcus epidermidis*.

Among the other organisms in Table 2, *Serratia*, *Corynebacterium*, *Torulopsis*, *Candida*, and *Pseudomonas* share the propensity to colonize the skin or respiratory tract, and cause opportunistic infections particularly in association with catheters or prosthetic material. We have encountered one defibrillator infection due to *Mycobacterium chelonae*. This patient developed fever and fluid in the generator pocket 18 days following defibrillator implantation. Five days later, left lower lobe consolidation was noted. Both pocket aspirate and sputum grew *Mycobacterium chelonae*. The entire system was explanted, antibiotic therapy was administered, and the patient recovered. *Mycobacterium chelonae* is a rapidly growing acid-fast organism which can be isolated from many sources, including municipal and hospital water supplies. It has been responsible for sporadic infections including prosthetic valve endocarditis [10].

The spectrum of organisms causing infections in defibrillator systems is very similar to that of infections involving permanent pacemakers. In a review of 180 cases of pacemaker infections, Bluhm found 75% to be caused by *Staphylococcus* [11]. *S. epidermidis* infections were more common than *S. aureus*, unlike the distribution reported to cause defibrillator infections.

III. DIAGNOSIS

Early diagnosis of defibrillator system infections is crucial to minimizing morbidity and mortality. It is important to note that low-grade fever and leukocytosis are very common in the first few days following defibrillator implantation, and this observation in the early postoperative period rarely presages infection. Furthermore, there is often serous fluid in the generator pocket early after implantation, and this again generally does not signal infection. Routine aspiration of fluid from the generator pocket is not necessary, especially early after implantation. The aspiration procedure itself would carry some risk of introducing bacteria into the environment of the generator.

Most early infections are due to *Staphylococcus aureus*, and the patient will usually appear ill, with clinical evidence of wound infection, or septicemia. Patients who have had a median sternotomy may have evidence sternal wound infection or of mediastinitis. Fever developing after the first few postoperative days, or any evidence of local infection, is grounds for aggressive evaluation. Blood cultures should be obtained if appropriate. Sputum and urine cultures should be obtained, as well as aspiration of the defibrillator pocket if the incision appears infected or the pocket is warm or fluctuant. Appropriate cultures will identify the majority of infections.

Late infections, usually due to less virulent organisms, may present with local warmth and fluctuance of the generator pocket in an otherwise well-appearing patient; or with fever, weight loss, and other systemic manifestations.

Although the diagnosis of an infected defibrillator system is usually straightforward, confusing clinical presentations and challenges do occur. A variety of diagnostics techniques have been reported to contribute importantly in individual cases. Kelly reported three cases in which a gallium scan demonstrated increased tracer uptake around the generator and electrodes in infections presenting 2 weeks, 5 weeks, and 6 months following implantation [9]. Although the defibrillator infection was not always obvious at the time of initial presentation, all three patients had fluid in the generator pocket by the time the gallium scan was done. Thus, it is not clear whether the scan yielded information that altered patient management.

Almassi et al. encountered three patients in whom computed tomographic (CT) scan of the chest contributed to the diagnosis of late defibrillator infections [12]. All three patients presented with induration of the skin over the generator or leads, without fever or other manifestations of infection. In each case, chest CT showed fluid between the defibrillator patches and the heart. In one patient, CT-directed aspiration yielded infected fluid; in the other two, infection was demonstrated by other means. All patients underwent explantation of defibrillator hardware. A subsequent prospective study from the same institution found that pericardial fluid collections were frequently found by chest CT scans during the first month after surgery in noninfected patients, but were rare thereafter [13]. Echocardiography was noted to be insensitive for detecting these fluid collections, probably because of artifacts created by the metal in the patches. Siclari et al. reported a case in which echocardiography detected a bulging mass in the right ventricle, which at surgery was found to represent a patch infected with *Staphylococcus epidermidis* which had migrated into the right ventricle [14]. Interestingly, this patient had a negative gallium scan.

Finally, indium-111-labeled leukocyte scintigraphy has been used to detect a wide variety of infections, including purulent pericarditis and prosthetic valve abscess [15,16]. This technique may prove to have diagnostic utility in occult defibrillator infections.

IV. TREATMENT

A long-held maxim in medicine states that in cases of infection involving a foreign body, the foreign body must be removed in order to treat the infection successfully. The bulk of experience with infected defibrillator systems reaffirms this concept. Once infection is diagnosed, the entire system is generally removed, and appropriate antibiotic therapy is administered. When infection is suspected but the organism has not yet been identified, vancomycin therapy is generally administered, since it covers even resistant strains of *Staphylococcus*.

There are very limited data demonstrating successful treatment of infection without device explantation. Taylor et al. reported a case of *Staphylococcus aureus* and *Serratia marcesans* infection involving the subcutaneous tissue over the pocket, developing 5 weeks postimplant [17]. There was no fever of leukocytosis, and no fluid or air in the pericardium on chest CT scan. Treatment consisted of open debridement of the pocket and washing of the device with povidone iodine, antibiotic irrigation of the pocket via a closed drainage system for 5 days, 2 weeks of parenteral antibiotics, and 6 months of oral antibiotics. A similar approach has been used to salvage permanent pacemaker pocket infections [18]. However, success without explantation is clearly the exception rather than the rule.

Even when the infection appears to be localized to the generator pocket, explantation of the entire system is likely to be required. Wunderly et al. described four such patients in whom initial therapy consisted of generator explantation and parenteral antibiotics [6]. Three of the four subsequently required removal of the lead system due to ongoing or recurrent infection. It is unclear whether chest CT scan or other scanning techniques might be able to identify patients in whom there is subclinical evidence of lead system involvement when a pocket infection is present. Even in the absence of such findings, however, subsequent lead infection would still be possible, since the leads provide contiguity between chest and pocket. Impending generator erosion due to pressure, when unaccompanied by evidence of infection, generally can be managed successfully by generator explantation and reimplantation in a different location.

V. REUSE OF DEVICES

The cost of the defibrillator generator may contribute to a reluctance to explant the device in cases of infection. However, there is evidence that devices can be successfully sterilized and

Table 3 Prevention of Infection—Defibrillator Implantation

Preoperative
    Hibiclens or Phisohex shower night before and morning of surgery (hospitalized patients)
Operative
    Betadine scrub
    Duraprep scrub
    Betadine-impregnated drape
    Extensive irrigation of pocket
    Surgeon and assistant change gloves prior to handling device
Antibiotic prophylaxis
    Vancomycin or cefazolin immediately pre-op and for 48 h post-op

later reimplanted in the same patient. The Cleveland Clinic experience includes five patients in whom this strategy was employed, with no recurrent infection or device malfunction [6]. Generators were hand scrubbed in betadine, then soaked in 0.005% neomycin solution for 1 h, dried, and sterilized in 90°F ethylene oxide followed by 24 h of aeration. These generators were placed in a new pocket after the patient had received 4 weeks of parenteral antibiotics.

The North American Society for Pacing and Electrophysiology has reviewed the worldwide data regarding permanent pacemaker reuse, and recommended guidelines to encourage reuse in the United States, even between different patients [19]. Adoption of similar policies to allow defibrillator reuse has enormous potential for cost savings.

VI. PREVENTION OF DEVICE INFECTIONS

Patient selection may play a role in the incidence of postoperative infections. Diabetes mellitus, prolonged steroid therapy, and other immunocompromised states clearly increase the risk of infection. However, the majority of defibrillator infections have occurred in patients without any such predisposing condition. While underlying conditions must weigh into the decision for device implantation, in reality they are not variables that can be altered to reduce the incidence of infection. Obviously, all patients must be free of active infection at the time of device implantation.

Antibiotic prophylaxis is widely used and accepted as contributing to the prevention of postoperative infections. Clinical data to confirm this belief are limited. Two large randomized trials of antibiotic prophylaxis for pacemaker implantation have been reported, and the results are discordant. Muers et al. found a 0.9% incidence of infection in the treatment group, compared to 3.6% among the controls, in a randomized study of 431 patients [20]. In contrast, Ramsdale et al. reported no difference in infection rates between treatment and control groups (3.3% and 5.1%, respectively) among 500 patients [21]. An extensive, multiarm prospective trial reported by Bluhm found evidence of benefit from systemic antibiotics for initial pacemaker implants, and from local antibiotic irrigation during generator replacements [11].

It is likely that thorough skin preparation is the single most important measure that can be taken to reduce the incidence of device infections, since most are due to skin contaminants introduced at the time of surgery. Many authors describe a combination of skin cleansing and antibiotic prophylaxis as their standard procedure. Winkle et al. utilized preoperative betadine shower and prophylactic cephalosporin plus vancomycin [5]. The usual protocol followed at our institution for initial defibrillator implantations is outlined in Table 3. Close attention is given to preoperative skin preparation and prevention of intraoperative contamination by skin flora.

Table 4 Protocol for Protection from Infection Associated with Defibrillator Generator Replacement

Preoperative
   Betadine scrub of abdomen the night before and morning of procedure (hospitalized patients)
Operative
   Betadine scrub
   Betadine solution prep
   Plastic adhesive drape
   Copious irrigation of pocket with bacitracin-polymixin solution
Antibiotic prophylaxis
   Cefazolin immediately pre-op and for 24 h post-op

In addition, prophylactic vancomycin and cefazolin are administered immediately preoperatively, and for 48 h postoperatively. There are no controlled trials evaluating specific protocols for the prevention of defibrillator infections.

The literature regarding device infections, as reviewed previously in this chapter, suggests that infections involving defibrillator leads in the chest are relatively more common when the hardware was implanted via sternotomy with accompanying cardiac surgery than by other approaches. Indeed, the incidence of mediastinitis following coronary bypass grafting alone is reported to range from 0.5% to 5% [22]. It is not clear how many device infections in this group of patients are truly device-related, as opposed to those which began as sternal wound infections and mediastinitis unrelated to the device itself. In any case, the issue raises caution regarding concomitant defibrillator and cardiac surgery, particularly for "prophylactic" lead placement. The availability of nonthoracotomy lead systems may alter the equation regarding this last procedure. Finally, there are no data available as to whether infections are more common when device implantation as the sole procedure is performed via median sternotomy versus left anterior thoracotomy or the subxiphoid approach. However, median sternotomy is generally not necessary from a technical standpoint for defibrillator implantation.

Some data show that the incidence of infection is higher following defibrillator generator replacement than following initial device implantation (see Table 1) [6,7]. Concern has been raised as to whether this is because replacements were performed in the electrophysiology laboratory rather than the operating room. However, the organisms responsible for infections following generator replacements comprise the same distribution of various skin flora and pathogens as with initial infections. Thus, it seems unlikely that the operative environment per se is the source of infection. Data from the pacemaker literature consistently shows a higher infection rate postgenerator replacement compared to initial implantation [23]. It is postulated that the avascular environment of an old pocket may reduce the effectiveness of systemic antibiotics and the body's own response to bacterial contamination. As with initial device implants, rigorous skin preparation and sterile technique are likely of paramount importance. Local antibiotic irrigation may play a particularly important role during device replacement procedures [11]. Our own protocol for prevention of infection associated with defibrillator generator replacement is shown in Table 4.

Finally, the issue of antibiotic prophylaxis for dental and other procedures must be addressed with reference to patients with defibrillators. There are no controlled data as to the risk of device infection related to subsequent procedures. The vast majority of defibrillator infections appear to relate to contamination at the time of device implantation. The American Heart Association does not currently specifically recommend endocarditis prophylaxis for patients with pacemakers or defibrillators. Nevertheless, roughly 30–60% of cardiologists and surgeons surveyed recommend prophylaxis for such patients [24].

VII. SUMMARY

In summary, infection is one of the most dreaded complications following implantation of defibrillator hardware. The incidence of infection is similar to that associated with permanent pacemakers. Most infections are due to contamination by skin flora or colonizers at the time of device implantation. Very few fatalities have been reported due to device infections, possibly because prompt removal of all hardware is the norm. Physical examination and appropriate laboratory studies are sufficient to identify the majority of infections. Generator sterilization and reimplantation appears to be a viable and cost-saving approach. Local skin preparation and sterile technique are likely the most important preventive measures. Local and systemic antibiotics are probably also beneficial. The role of endocarditis prophylaxis for subsequent procedures, as recommended for patients with prosthetic valves, has not been established for patients with implanted defibrillators.

REFERENCES

1. Mirowski M. The automatic implantable cardioverter defibrillator: an overview. J Am Coll Cardiol 1985; 6:461–466.
2. Barbola J, Denes P, Ezri MD, Hauser RG, Serry C, Goldin MD. The automatic implantable cardioverter defibrillator. Clinical experience, complications, and follow-up in 25 patients. Arch Intern Med 1988; 148:70–76.
3. Kelly PA, Cannom DS, Garan H, et al. The automatic implantable cardioverter-defibrillator: efficacy, complications and survival in patients with malignant ventricular arrhythmias. J Am Coll Cardiol 1988; 11:1278–1286.
4. Olinger GN, Chapman PD, Troup PJ, et al. Stratified application of the automatic implantable cardioverter defibrillator. J Thoracic Cardiovasc Surg 1988; 96:141–149.
5. Winkle RA, Mead RH, Ruder MA, et al. Long-term outcome with the automatic implantable cardioverter defibrillator. J Am Coll Cardiol 1989; 13:1353–1361.
6. Wunderly D, Maloney J, Edel T, McHenry M, McCarthy PM. Infections in implantable cardioverter defibrillator patients. PACE 1990; 13:1360–1364.
7. Siclari F, Klein H, Troster HJ. Infectious, complications after AICD implantation (abst). PACE 1990; 13:547.
8. Bakker PFA, Hauer RNW, Wever EFD. Infections involving implanted cardioverter defibrillator devices. PACE 1992; 15(III):654–648.
9. Kelly PA, Wallace S, Tucker B, et al. Postoperative infection with the automatic implantable cardioverter defibrillator: clinical presentation and use of the gallium scan in diagnosis. PACE 1988; 11:1220–1226.
10. Kuritsky JN, Bullen MG, Broome CV, et al. Sternal wound infections and endocarditis due to organisms of the *mycobacterium fortuitum* complex. Ann Internal Med 1983; 98:938–939.
11. Bluhm G. Pacemaker infections. A clinical study with special reference to prophylactic use of some isoxazolyl penicillins. Acta Med Scand Suppl 1985; 669:1–62.
12. Almassi GH, Olinger GN, Troup PJ, Chapman PD, Goodman LK. Delayed infection of the automatic implantable cardioverter defibrillator. Current recognition and management. J Thorac Cardiovasc Surg 1988; 95(5):908–911.
13. Goodman LR, Almassi GH, Troup PJ, et al. Complications of automatic implantable cardioverter defibrillators: radiographic, CT, and echocardiographic evaluation. Radiology 1989; 170(2):447–452.
14. Siclari F, Klein H, Troster J. Intraventricular migration of an ICD patch. PACE 1990; 13:1356–1359.

15. Greenberg ML, Niebulski HI, Linetsky BF. Occult purulent pericarditis detected by indium-111 leukocyte imaging. Chest 1984; 85:701–703.
16. Oates E, Sarno RC. Detection of a prosthetic aortic valvular abscess with indium-111-labeled leukocytes. Chest 1988; 94:872–874.
17. Taylor RL, Cohen DJ, Widman LE, Chilton RJ, O'Rourke RA. Infection of an implantable cardioverter defibrillator: management without removal of the device in selected cases. PACE 1990; 13:1352–1355.
18. Hurst LN, Evans HB, Windle B, et al. The salvage of infected cardiac pacemaker pockets using a closed irrigation system. PACE 1986; 9:785–792.
19. Boal BH, Escher DJW, Furman S, et al. Report of the policy conference on pacemaker reuse sponsored by the North American Society of Pacing and Electrophysiology. J Am Coll Cardiol 1985; 5:808–810.
20. Muers MF, Arnold AG, Sleight P. Prophylactic antibiotics for cardiac pacemaker implantation. A prospective trial. Br Heart J 1981; 46:539.
21. Ramsdale DR, Charles RG, Rowlands DB, Singh SS, Gautam PC, Faragher EB. Antibiotic prophylaxis for pacemaker implantation: a prospective randomized trial. PACE 1984; 7:844.
22. Sarr MG, Gott VL, Townsend TR. Mediastinal infection after cardiac surgery. Ann Thorac Surg 1989; 38:415–423.
23. Kennelly BM, Piller LW. Management of infected transvenous permanent pacemakers. Br Heart J 1974; 36:1133–1140.
24. Vlay SC. Prevention of bacterial endocarditis in patients with permanent pacemakers and automatic internal cardioverter defibrillators. Am Heart J 1990; 120:1490–1492.

31

Radiology of the Implantable Cardioverter-Defibrillator

Caroline Breckwoldt Foote and Antonis S. Manolis

*Tufts University School of Medicine
and New England Medical Center
Boston, Massachusetts*

After a cardioverter-defibrillator (ICD) is implanted, radiography plays an important role in the routine evaluation as well as the troubleshooting of these devices. This chapter will provide the reader with a systematic approach to the interpretation of radiographs of ICD systems. The application of computerized tomography, echocardiography, and radionuclide imaging will also be discussed.

I. RADIOGRAPHY

Initially in the immediate postoperative period, antero-posterior chest radiographs will be available for patients with newly implanted ICDs, but prior to hospital discharge both postero-anterior (PA) and lateral chest projections (Fig. 1) as well as abdominal films should be obtained. These will provide baseline radiographs of the ICD system that can be compared with subsequent films. Chest radiographs should be evaluated systematically, looking at the boney structures, cardiac silhouette, great vessels, trachea, lung, and diaphragm before evaluating the ICD and other "hardware," especially as atelectasis, pleural effusions, infiltrates, and pneumothoraces are frequently seen immediately postoperatively (Fig. 2) [1]. If the main purpose of the radiograph is to look at the ICD leads and patches, then this should be communicated to the radiology technician, as an overpenetrated film allows the hardware to be visualized better, especially in the presence of pulmonary infiltrates or effusions.

A. Sensing/Pacing Lead System

The ICD system is best evaluated by identifying and assessing its components separately. As discussed in other chapters, the ICD system consists of a sensing/pacing lead system, a cardioverting/defibrillating lead system, and the pulse generator [2]. The sensing/pacing lead system is a bipolar system, either transvenous endocardial or epimyocardial. Typically, the distal tip of a transvenous bipolar sensing lead sits at the right ventricular apex, while the proximal

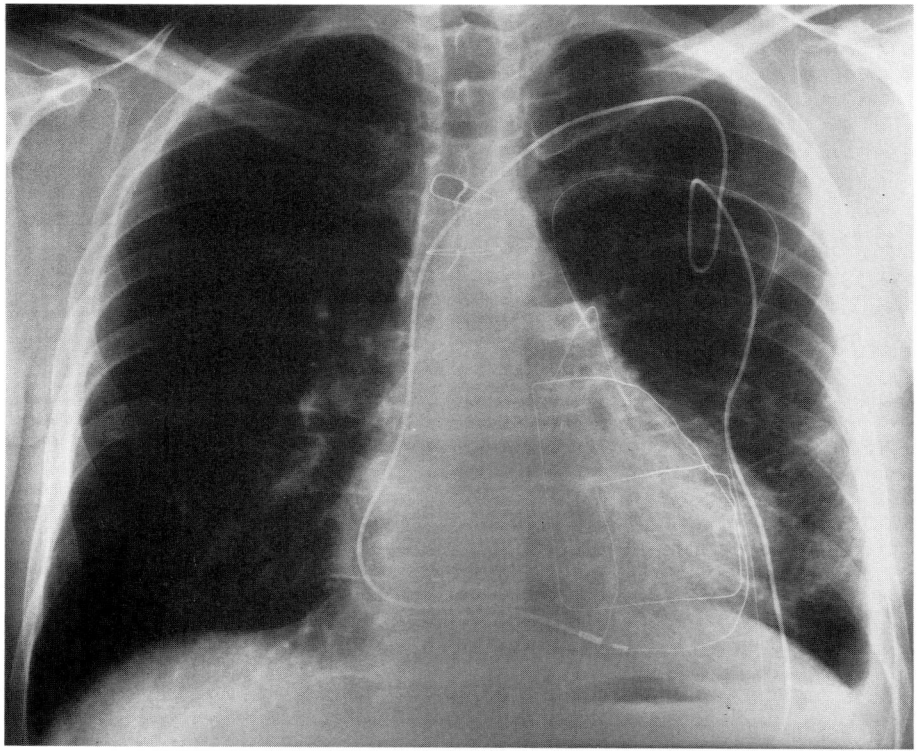

(A)

Figure 1 The normal radiographic appearance of the endocardial right ventricular sensing/pacing ICD lead is demonstrated in this patient. The postero-anterior (PA) projection shows the lead entering the venous system under the left clavicle through the subclavian vein and traveling medially into the superior vena cava before entering the right atrium, where it courses inferiorly, forming a gentle curve along the lateral wall (A). The lead then crosses the tricuspid valve, and within the ventricle there is a gentle concave down curve with the tip lying at the right ventricular apex. The lateral projection shows the lead traveling anteriorly and caudally (B), confirming placement of the lead tip in the right ventricular apex. The two epicardial defibrillating patches are also appreciated.

end exits either the left or right subclavian vein and travels subcutaneously to the abdomen (Fig. 1). On the PA projection of a radiograph, the distal tip of the sensing lead will appear between the vertebral column and left heart border. There should be a gentle curve along the right atrial lateral wall before the lead crosses the tricuspid valve to the right ventricular apex, with another gentle curve within the ventricular chamber, this time concave inferiorly, to ensure both proper position and lead fixation. On the lateral projection, the lead will be directed anteriorly and caudally, differentiating it from a coronary sinus position, where the lead is directed posteriorly (Figs. 1–3).

Redundancy within the cardiac chamber is usually abnormal, although prior to generator implantation the proximal portion of the lead can normally be seen coiled in an infraclavicular subcutaneous pocket after it exits the subclavian vein. Once the pulse generator is implanted, this coil is no longer appreciated, and the lead should appear radiographically continuous as it

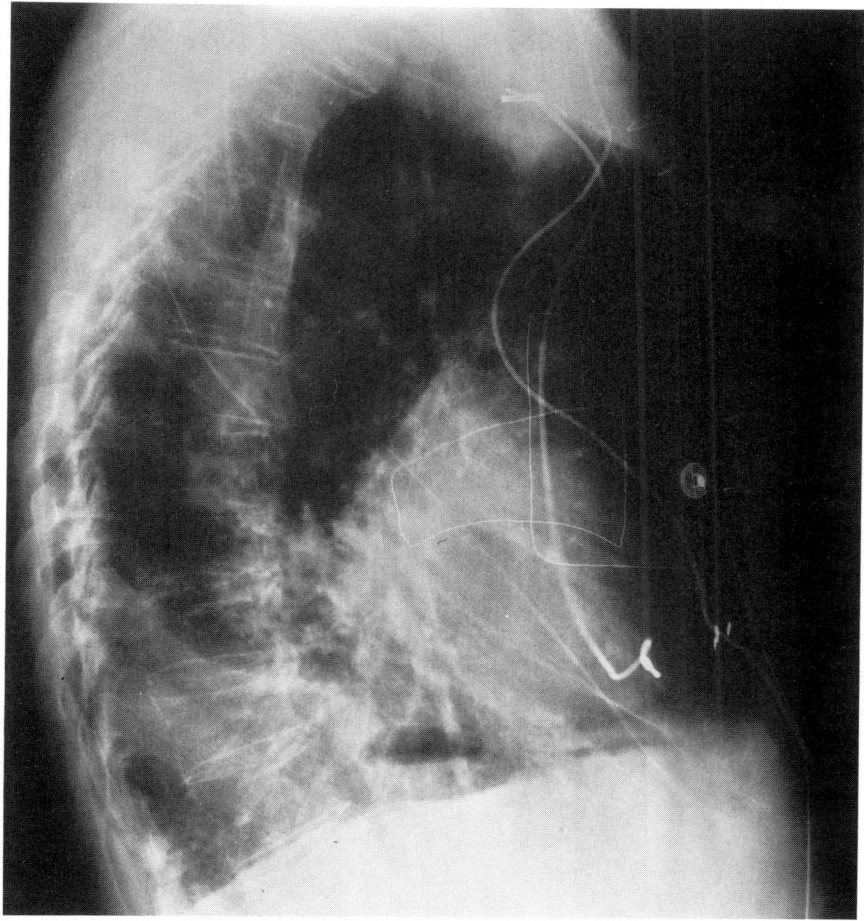

(B)

traverses the chest wall and connects to the generator in the abdomen, usually the left paraumbilical area (Fig. 4). Alternatively, a short transvenous right ventricular lead can be used that requires a connector to complete the circuit to the generator (Fig. 5).

The sensing/pacing system can also be a pair of epimyocardial leads placed during thoracotomy, usually onto the surface of the left ventricle (Fig. 6). These leads appear as ''coils'' overlying the left lateral cardiac silhouette on the PA projection of the chest radiograph, with leads traversing inferiorly to the abdomen (Fig. 6). Combined sensing and defibrillating leads have also been developed; their radiographic appearance will be described in the next section.

If the sensing/pacing lead system malfunctions, PA and lateral chest and abdominal radiographs should be obtained to inspect the leads for continuity and position. Lead fractures may be evident (Fig. 7), especially at stress points, although insulation breaks will not show discontinuity. ''Pseudo-fractures'' at connector sites have also been described, although they have no clinical significance [3] except when they are mistaken for true fractures (Fig. 8). Lead dislodgement may be obvious if the lead migrates to the right atrium or great vessels (Fig. 9), but careful comparison to the original postimplantation films should be made, as a ventricular

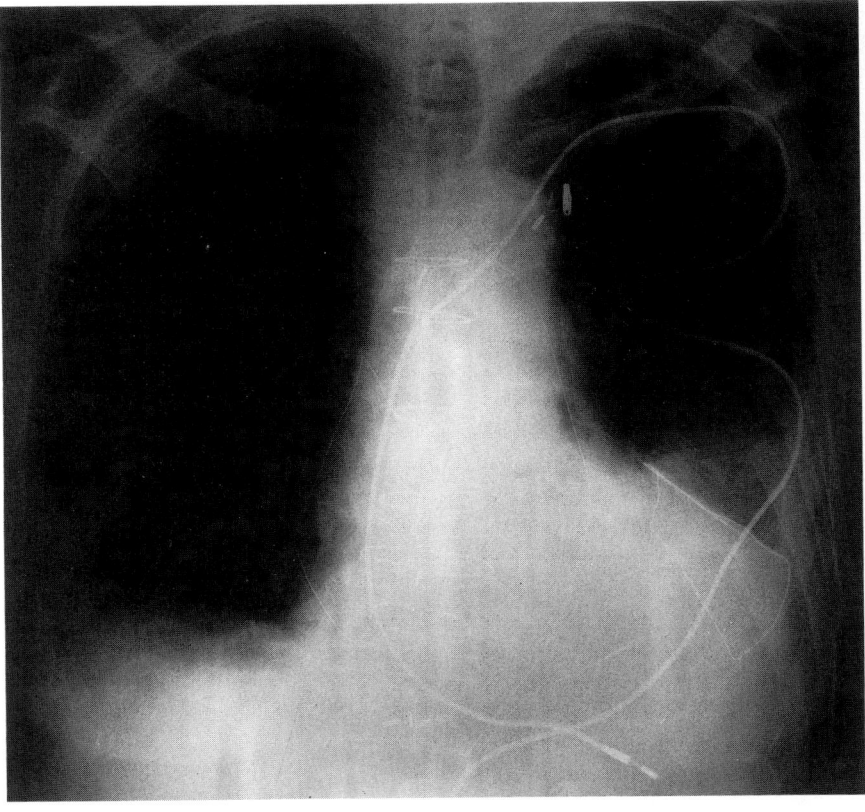

(A)

Figure 2 This set of postoperative radiographs (A and B) also demonstrates normal placement of the right ventricular sensing/pacing lead. In addition, a large left pleural effusion is present; this common postoperative finding resolved over the following few weeks.

lead dislodgement may be subtle if the distal tip remains in the ventricular cavity. *Fluoroscopy* and *cinematography* can also be helpful in checking for fixation of the lead within the right ventricular cavity or looking for abnormal movement suggesting penetration into the pericardium or left ventricle. In certain cases, cinematography may be preferred over fluoroscopy as, although both can provide continuous visualization of the lead system throughout its course, the former images are permanent and usually of sharper resolution (Fig. 8).

B. Cardioverting/Defibrillating Lead System

The cardioverting/defibrillating lead system is usually also a bipolar system, although tripolar configurations are occasionally employed, especially in nonthoracotomy systems. Most bipolar thoracotomy systems consist of either left and right epicardial (intra- or extrapericardial) ventricular patches or a single left ventricular patch with a transvenous "spring" electrode at the junction of the superior vena cava and right atrium. The radiographic appearance of the ventricular patch varies depending on the manufacturer. Cardiac Pacemakers, Inc. (CPI), patches are rectangular titanium mesh electrodes covered with silicone elastic and are radiographically

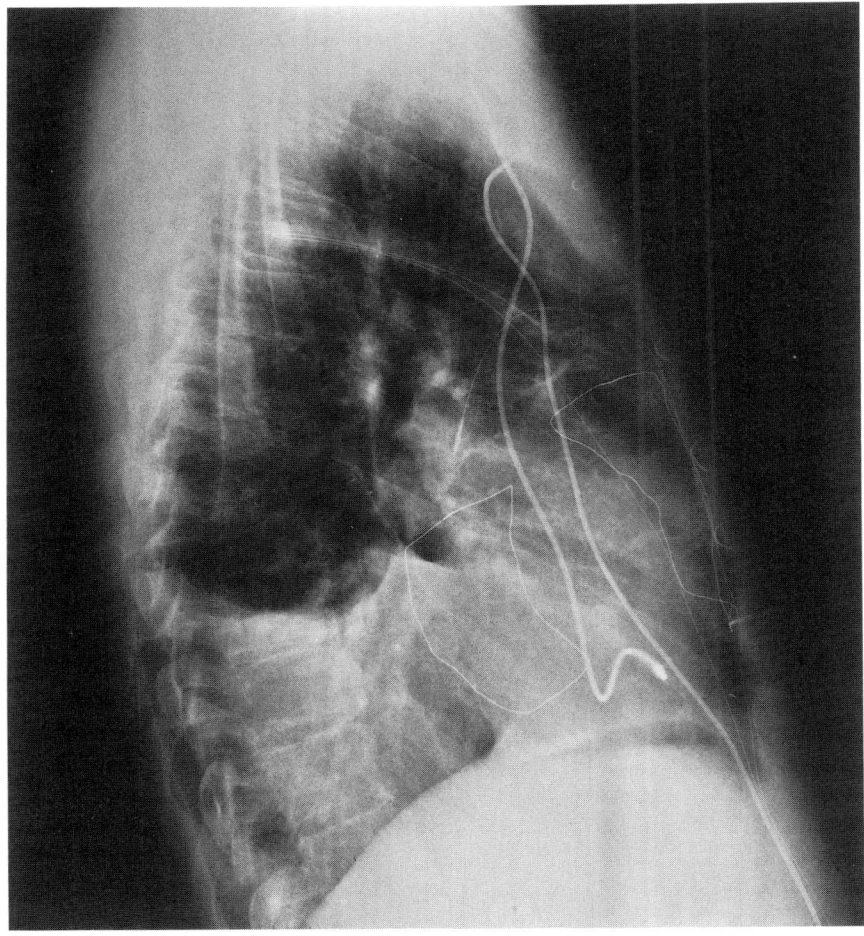

(B)

invisible except for the stainless steel wire that is used to mark the perimeter (Fig. 6). The wire not only identifies placement but also allows for assessment of configuration of the patch. However, it should be remembered that the wire is simply a marker and not part of the electronic circuitry, so any radiographic breaks are inconsequential. Between the patch's stainless steel marker and the patch's lead body, a connector "gap" of 1–2 cm is usually noted on radiographs; this is a normal radiolucent area of the patch as it attaches to the lead, and again it does not have clinical significance (Fig. 6) [2].

The Medtronic epicardial defibrillating leads are oval-shaped patches which come in three sizes. All Medtronic patches have concentric coil construction and increasing coil pitch from inside to outside coils (Fig. 10). The Telectronics patches are rectangular titanium mesh electrodes, the Ventritex patches are oval-shaped titanium mesh electrodes, while the Intermedics patches are titanium electrodes of two types, either elliptical or contoured to fit the shape of the right and left ventricles, both types having a tantalum wire in the periphery for X-ray visualization.

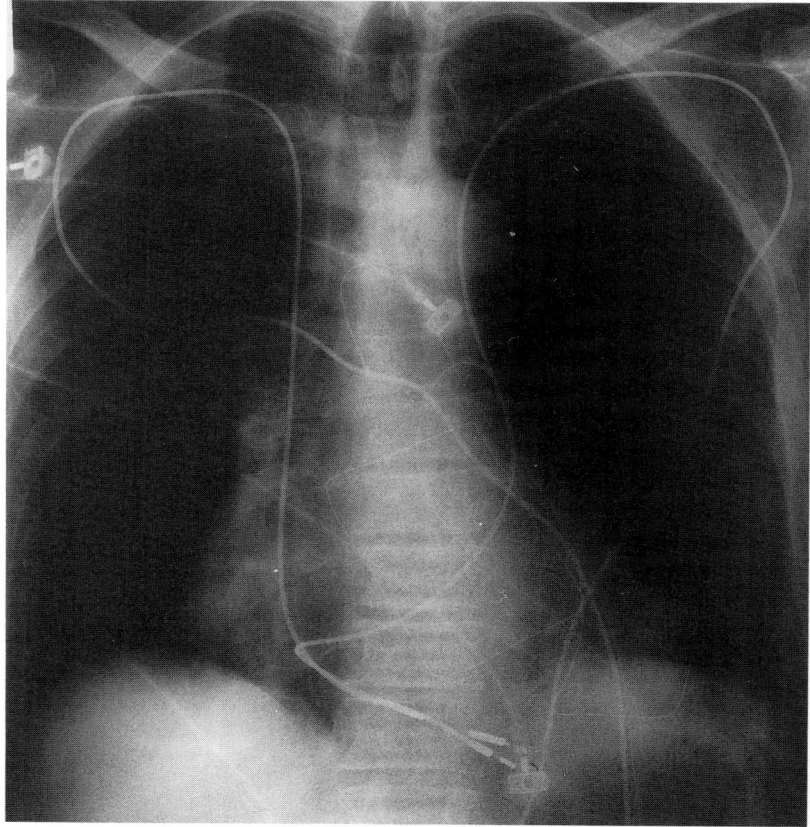

(A)

Figure 3 This patient has two sensing/pacing leads. The first lead was placed using a right subclavian approach, but due to lead malfunction, this lead was capped and replaced by a second right ventricular sensing/pacing lead approximately 1 year later. The second lead was inserted on the contralateral side using a left cephalic approach. On the PA projection, this second lead remains left of midline before traversing the cardiac silhouette, suggesting the presence of a persistent left superior vena cava that drains into the coronary sinus, which subsequently drains into the right atrium (A). This anatomical variant is confirmed by the lateral projection (B), where the second lead is found to travel along the posterior aspect of the cardiac silhouette (i.e., through the coronary sinus) before entering the right atrium, crossing the tricuspid valve, and resting at the right ventricular apex.

Crumpling of the epicardial patches can be assessed on radiographs (Fig. 11). Although patch crumpling can be asymptomatic, this phenomenon has been associated with defibrillator malfunction with both the development of inappropriate shocks and high defibrillation thresholds [4,5]. Infection and fibrosis have been identified as the etiologies of the crumpling and computerized tomography can better assess this (see below).

Endocardial defibrillation leads or "spring" electrodes are transvenous leads with helical coils at the distal end. Classically, in a bipolar system this type of lead replaces the right ven-

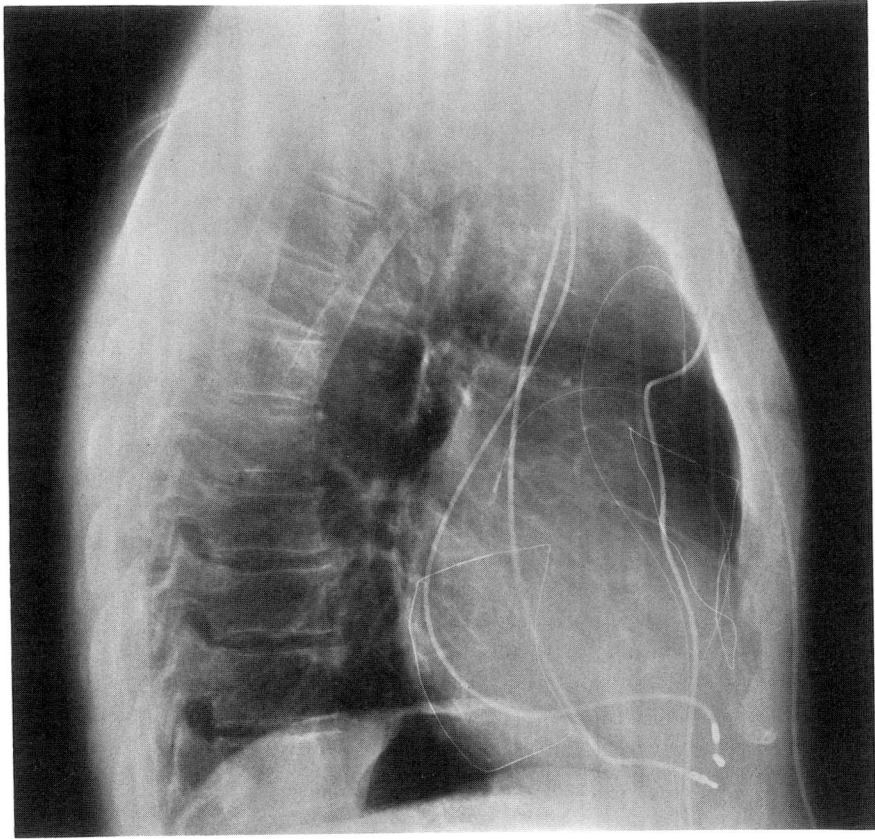

(B)

tricular epicardial patch and the coil sits at the junction of the superior vena cava and right atrium (Fig. 12). As there is no intracardiac fixation with this lead, migration can occur (Fig. 13); this occurred not uncommonly prior to the addition of a "butterfly" sleeve to the spring electrode, a device used to anchor the lead [6]. Like the endocardial sensing lead, the proximal lead exits the subclavian vein and is tunneled subcutaneously inferiorly across the chest wall to the generator in the abdomen. The lead is most commonly introduced via the left subclavian vein ipsilateral to the implantation site of the ICD pulse generator (left paraumbilical pocket).

With the advent of *nonthoracotomy systems*, endocardial electrode systems have become more sophisticated. Bipolar and tripolar systems using individual or combined superior vena cava, right atrial, or coronary sinus and right ventricular defibrillation leads have been implanted, with the right ventricular lead also having sensing and/or pacing capabilities (Figs. 14–18) [7–10]. Proper positioning of the coronary sinus defibrillation leads is best visualized with lateral radiographs showing these leads along the posterior surface of the heart [9,10]. Nonthoracotomy ICD systems can also employ a combination of endocardial leads and submuscular or subcutaneous patches or electrode arrays that appear lateral to

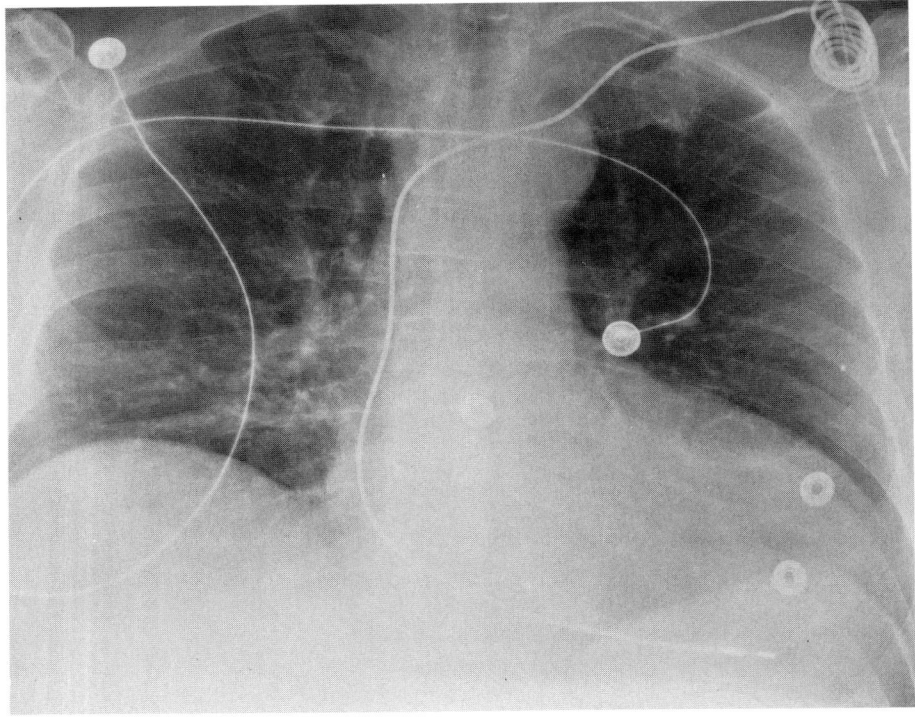

Figure 4 The first radiograph (A) was requested to confirm good positioning of a right ventricular sensing/pacing lead inserted a day prior to surgical implantation of the ICD pulse generator and defibrillating patches. Note the coiled distal end of the lead under the left clavicle. The second radiograph (B) was taken after the system was totally implanted, at which time the coil was unwound and the distal tip was tunneled under the subcutaneous tissue to the abdomen, where it was connected to the generator. ICD defibrillating patches were also implanted.

the left heart border and outside the rib cage on the PA and lateral projections [7–10] (Figs. 14–19).

C. Pulse Generators

Generally, abdominal radiographs will confirm that the pulse generators are located subcutaneously or submuscularly, most commonly in the left abdomen, with the leads exiting laterally. Occasionally, generators will be implanted on the right side of the abdomen, often due to prior surgery or previous device explantation secondary to infection. Abdominal films will also be helpful in evaluating the lower portion of the ICD lead systems and their connections, including any adaptors which attach the lead systems to the pulse generator (Fig. 8). If lead system integrity is being questioned and the leads and/or adaptors are partially obscured by an overlapping device, then manual manipulation of the device during fluoroscopy or cinematography together with lateral projections may minimize the overlap and maximize exposure of the entire ICD system, facilitating better images (Fig. 8).

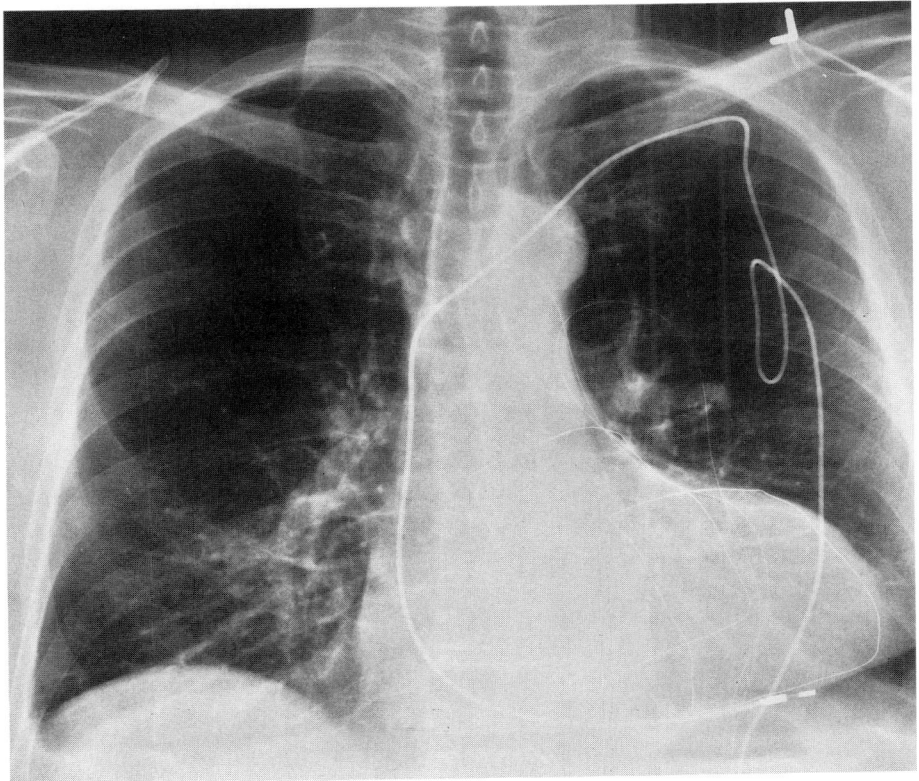

(B)

Rotation of ICD pulse generators has been reported [11], and although this can often be appreciated by abdominal palpation, fluoroscopy and/or radiography will confirm a clinician's suspicion. Usually the rotation occurs within the plane of the generator, but rare cases of rotation about the device's long axis have also occurred [12]. Therefore, it has been recommended that radiography or fluoroscopy be used to troubleshoot a device if an unexpected error code is encountered upon interrogation [12]. Migration of the pulse generator has been described in the literature [13]. This can be annoying and painful for a patient, so if migration is clinically suspected, an abdominal radiograph can confirm this. Abdominal radiographs can also be used to identify specific devices, by their shape, internal circuitry appearance, and identification code (Fig. 20). Potentially, this could be important and perhaps life-saving if an unresponsive or critically ill patient arrived for emergency care.

II. COMPUTED TOMOGRAPHY

Computed tomography (CT) of the chest is especially helpful in the assessment of the ICD epicardial patches, as it allows for visualization of not only the patches but also the pericardium and the mediastinum. Although application of this modality is usually reserved for assessment of suspected patch infection or patch crumpling, a recent prospective analysis of asymptomatic

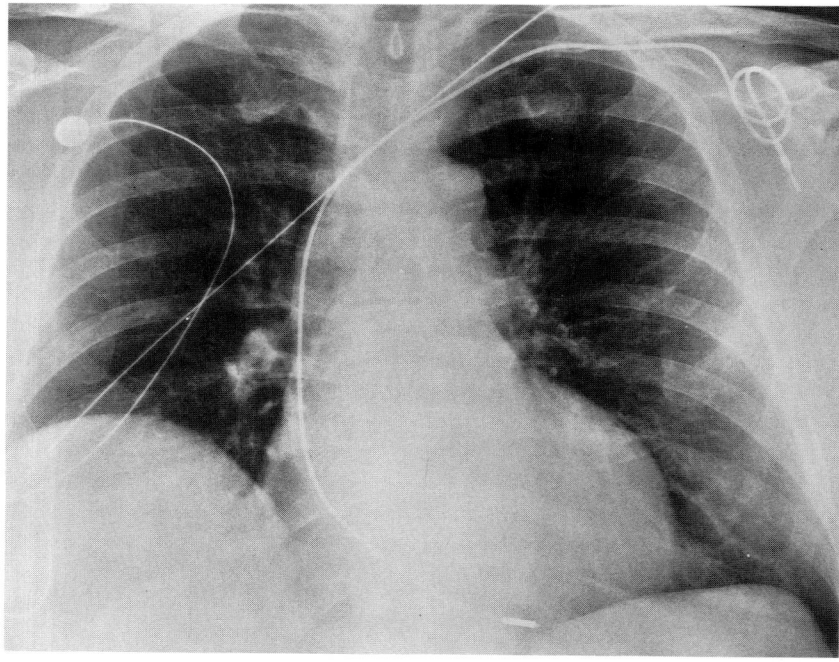

(A)

Figure 5 This radiograph shows a right ventricular sensing/pacing lead that was placed 1 day prior to implantation of the ICD generator in the abdomen. Although it is difficult to appreciate as the proximal pole overlies the spine, this is a bipolar lead with active fixation as evidence by the screw-in tip. The distal tip lies in the right ventricular cavity and the proximal end is coiled in a subcutaneous infraclavicular pocket after exiting the cephalic vein (A). At surgery, a connector (arrow) is tunneled through the thoracic subcutaneous tissue and attached to the right ventricular lead proximally and the pulse generator distally (B). A lateral projection better delineates both the endocardial and subcutaneous course of the lead and its connector (C).

patients having undergone epicardial patch placement demonstrated the ''normal'' CT appearance postoperatively [5]. Scans done within 2 weeks postoperatively frequently show pericardial fluid collections, usually adjacent to the patch, although the fluid can be distinct from the patches. Tiny air bubbles within the fluid can occasionally be appreciated, as well as fluid in the anterior mediastinum. Chest CT scans done later after surgery rarely show pericardial fluid, but fibrosis adjacent to the patches is not an infrequent finding and is associated with patch crumpling.

Computed tomography is also useful in suspected pericardial infections associated with ICD patches. In the same study, Goodman and associates retrospectively analyzed the CT scans of four patients with proven pericardial infections associated with ICD patches; all scans demonstrated fluid adjacent to both patches [5]. Other reports have confirmed these CT scan findings in similar patients [14]. Therefore, as nearly all pericardial fluid collections resolve between 2 and 4 weeks postoperatively, pericardial fluid demonstrated on CT scans done after this initial postoperative period in patients with epicardial patches and suspected ICD infections is strongly suggestive of pericardial infection (Fig. 21). CT-guided aspiration can also be

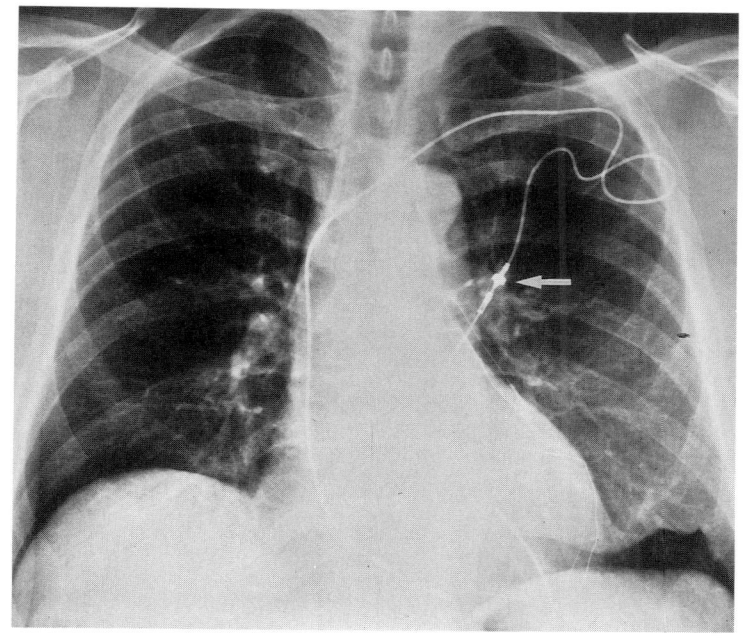

(B)

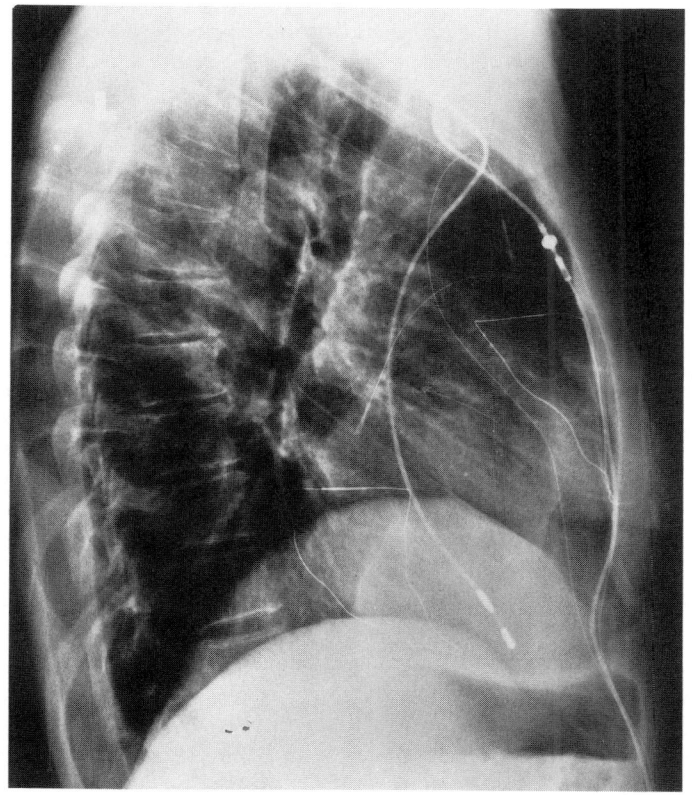

(C)

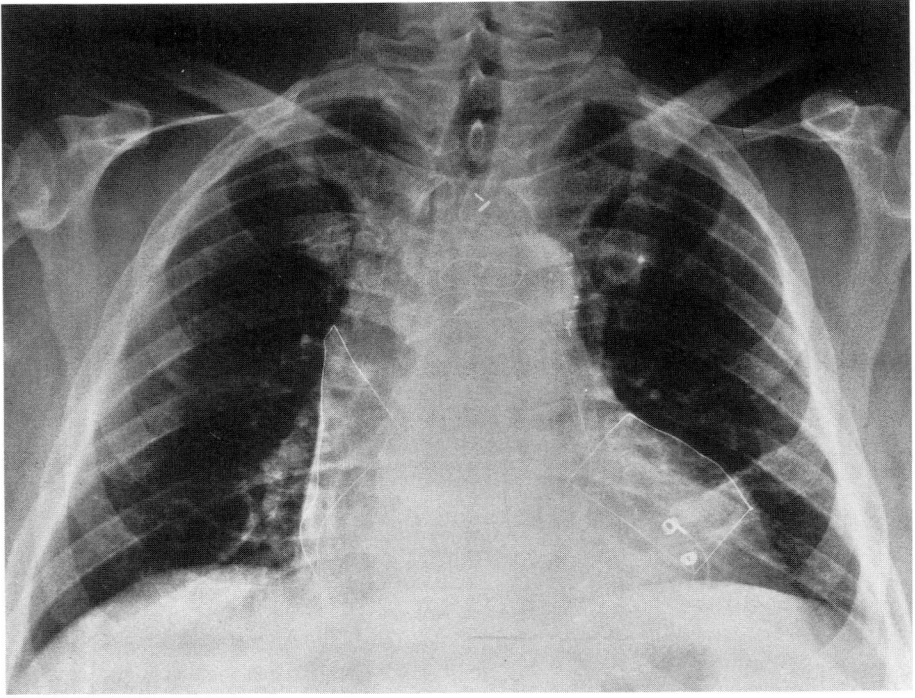

(A)

Figure 6 These PA (A) and lateral (B) projections show proper positioning of the two epimyocardial rate sensing leads with their tips (spiral coils) placed 1 cm apart onto the left ventricle. Also shown here are the two epicardial defibrillating patches placed over the left and right ventricles. A gap (better seen on the lateral projection) exists between the stainless steel wire marking the perimeter of the patch and the cable of the defibrillating lead; this is a normal phenomenon owing to the radiolucency of the titanium mesh of the patch [2].

performed prior to surgical removal of the device if preoperative culture-directed antibiotic therapy is desired.

Another application of computed tomography is further assessment of epicardial patch crumpling demonstrated by chest radiographs. CT scans will not only confirm patch crumpling, but will also demonstrate the extent of fibrosis or pericardial effusion, usually associated with this phenomenon (Fig. 22) [5]. Often patch crumpling secondary to fibrosis is asymptomatic, but it can be associated with high defibrillation thresholds [4]. A case report of constrictive pericarditis believed to be secondary to ICD epicardial patches has also been described in the literature [15]. In this case, CT scan demonstrated mild pericardial thickening with associated inferior vena cava dilation.

It should be remembered that CT scans can provide a three-dimensional reconstruction of the heart and great vessels such that patch placement can be determined more accurately than with chest radiographs. Clinically, this allows qualitative assessment of patch placement and provides answers to important questions. Are the patches overlying the great vessels or atria? Is there adequate ventricular mass between patches? In addition, CT has been used as an investigational tool to understand better the relationship of ventricular mass encompassed by epi-

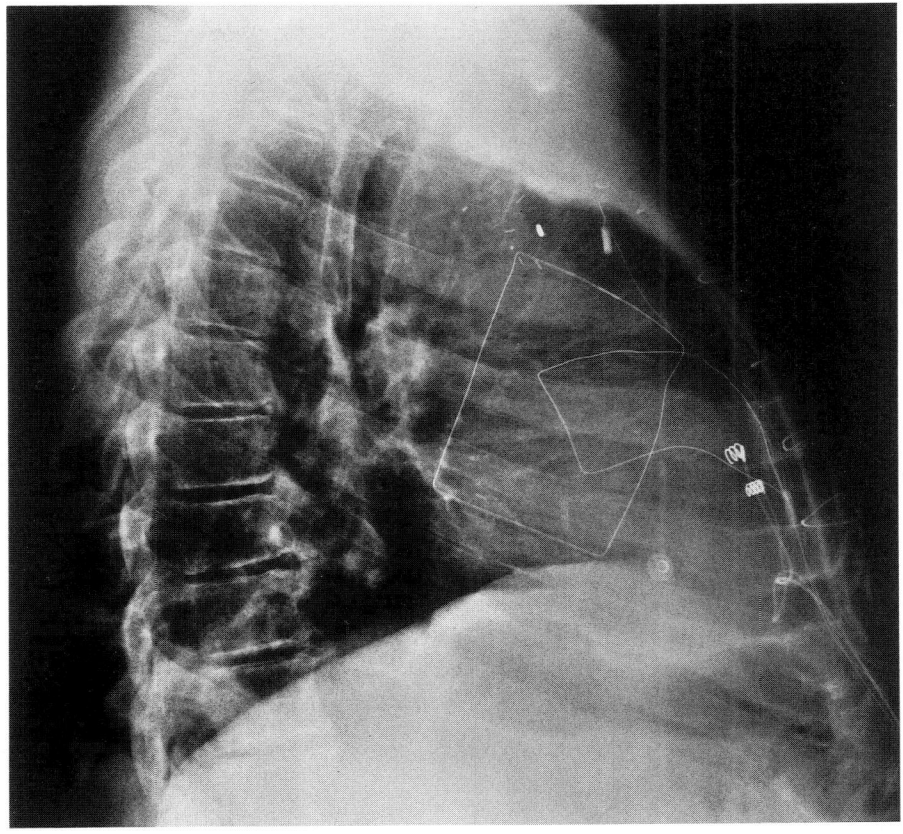

(B)

cardial patches and the defibrillation threshold. As both the septum and free wall can be visualized, CT can provide insight into the individual and additive contributions of both to threshold determination [16].

Abdominal CT scans provide little information about the generator, as there is a lot of scatter caused by the device. This not only limits assessment of the generator's subcutaneous pocket, but may interfere with assessment of surrounding structures. Thus, information from CT scans may at best be limited to confirming the presence or absence of fluid in the pocket.

III. ECHOCARDIOGRAPHY

Little has been published regarding echocardiography and ICDs, as most believe CT is the preferable imaging modality for these devices. While occasionally echocardiography allows visualization of pericardial effusions associated with ICD patches (Fig. 23), usually the patch and pericardium are not well delineated. In Goodman's study, only one of nine CT-documented patch-associated postoperative pericardial effusions in asymptomatic patients was visualized by echocardiography [5]. The sensitivity of echocardiography in symptomatic patients with infections has yet to be studied, however. There is a case report of transesophageal echocardiography demonstrating a large right ventricular mass in a patient with a suspected

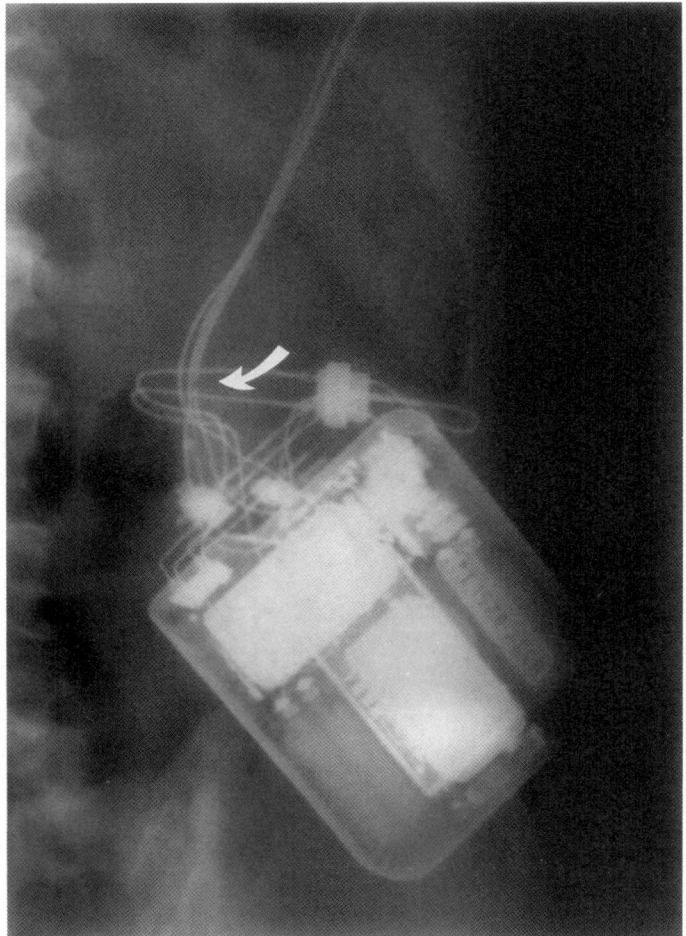

Figure 7 Discontinuity in one of the leads (arrow) shortly before it connects to the header of the generator represents a lead fracture in this abdominal radiograph. (Courtesy of CPI.)

ICD system infection [17]. Several months earlier, CT and gallium scans were reported to be unremarkable, but at surgery the mass was an infected pericardial ICD patch that had perforated the right ventricle [17].

IV. NUCLEAR IMAGING

Both gallium-67 imaging and indium-111-labeled leukocyte scanning have been used to aid in the diagnosis of ICD system infections [18,19]. Marked increase in tracer uptake in the region of the pulse generator and/or its leads suggests the presence of infection with both imaging modalities. A possible problem with gallium scanning is the potential for false-positive results, as gallium accumulates in any area of inflammation including noninfected healing surgical wounds [20]. Therefore, although no studies have been published that compare the two imaging

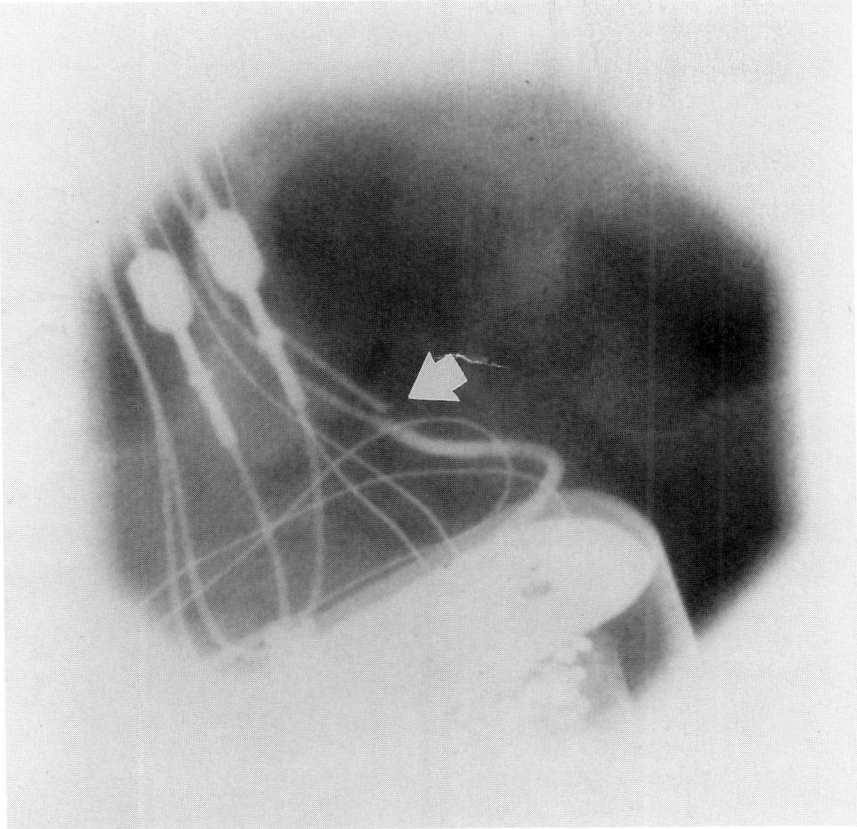

Figure 8 A lead connector "fracture" (arrow) is visualized radiographically in a patient with documented multiple spurious ICD shocks [3]. However, this is the normal radiographic appearance of this Telectronics Y-connector, and if this is not known a priori, it can be easily mistaken for a true fracture. Internal circuitry malfunction of the pulse generator was confirmed as the cause of oversensing with resultant inappropriate shocks in this particular patient [3].

modalities directly, theoretically indium-labeled leukocyte imaging might be preferable in the early postoperative period.

V. MAGNETIC RESONANCE IMAGING

Finally, the discussion would not be complete without mention of magnetic resonance imaging (MRI), which should not be performed in the patient with an ICD. If the need for an MRI can be anticipated, the patient should have this done prior to ICD implantation, as the metallic content of the device is a contraindication to having an MRI. Using a simulated model of a heart with both epicardial screw-in sensing leads and defibrillating patches, Stanton and colleagues determined that MRI generates voltages on defibrillator lead systems of sufficient strength to induce ventricular fibrillation even without a device connection [21]. In addition, there would be the potential for irreversible damage and/or reprogramming of the device given the strong magnetic field.

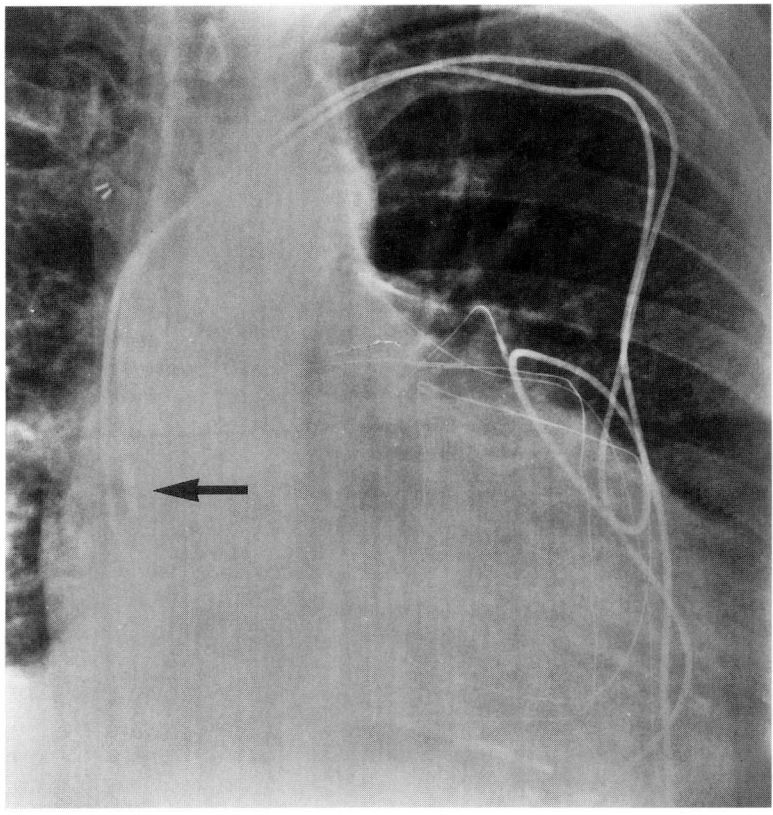

(A)

Figure 9 These radiographs (A and B) were taken after pacing thresholds were found to exceed programmable values and ventricular capture was not obtainable at a routine ICD clinic visit. The patient has two sensing/pacing leads. The original lead, whose tip is located at the right ventricular apex, had been abandoned and capped after an insulation break had been suspected. A second lead had subsequently been implanted and incorporated into the ICD system, and this is the lead that has migrated form the right ventricle to the right atrium (arrow), explaining the loss of pacing capture.

VI. SUMMARY

This chapter has stressed the importance of baseline postoperative radiographs of ICD systems and their systematic interpretation. The radiological appearance of several different systems has been shown, and the application of radiography and its limitations in troubleshooting the malfunctioning ICD system have been discussed. Radiography can be complemented by fluoroscopy and cinematography in certain cases, whereby additional information can be derived. CT has been shown to be a useful modality, especially in patients with suspected infections and patch crumpling. Echocardiography has had limited application, as neither the lead system nor the pericardium is visualized adequately. Radionuclide imaging has been shown to confirm suspected infections of ICD system, but the sensitivity, specificity, and preferred radioisotope for imaging of ICD systems have yet to be determined. Lastly, an ICD is a contraindication to MRI imaging, due both to the metallic content and the potential for irreversible damage to the device.

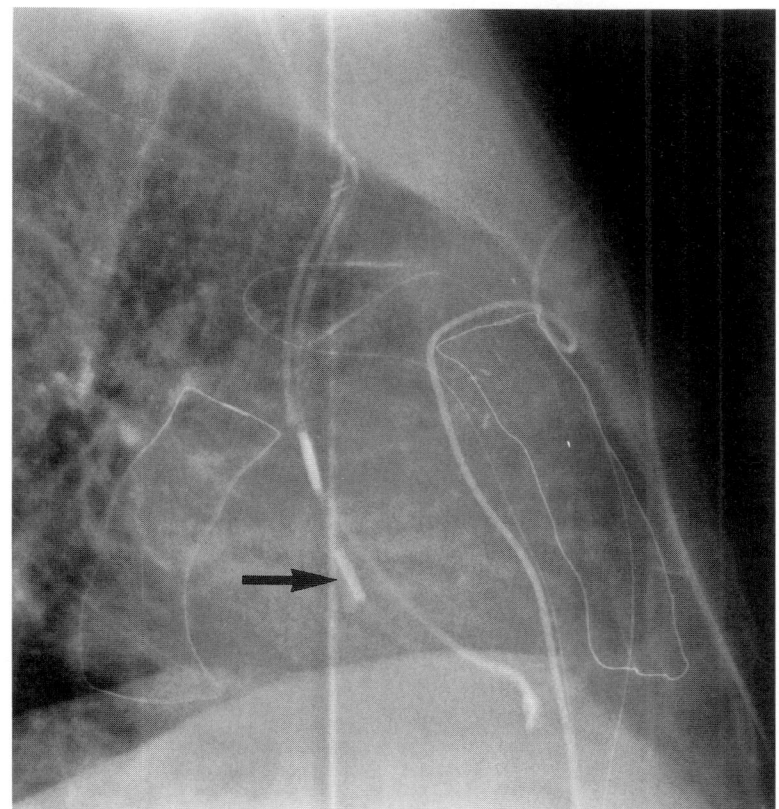
(B)

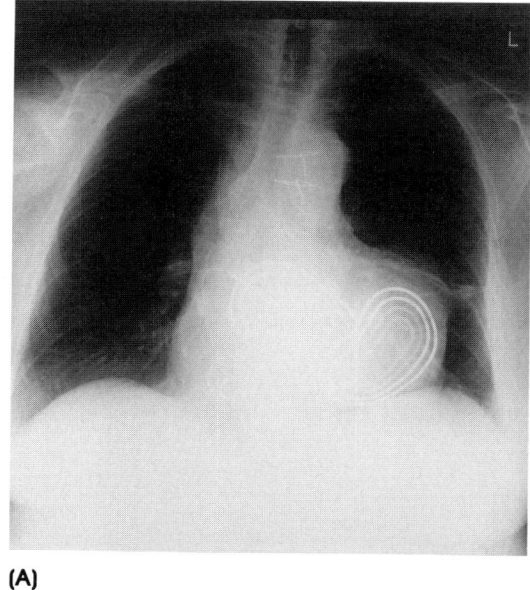

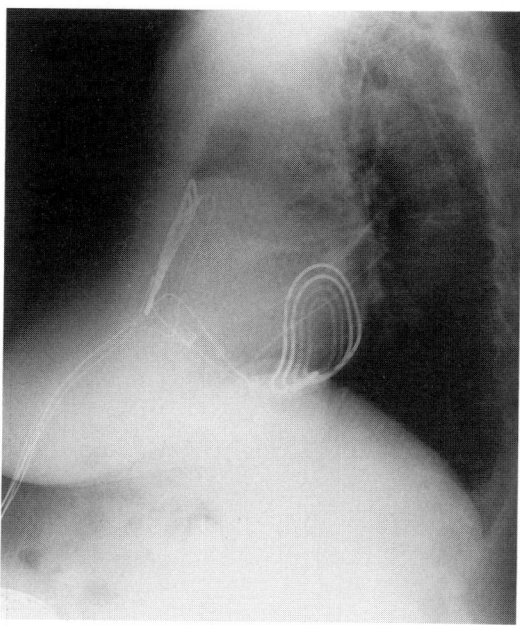

Figure 10 These radiographs demonstrate the normal appearance of Medtronic's oval-shaped epicardial patches with concentric coil construction. Both a bipolar (A and B) and tripolar (C and D) defibrillation

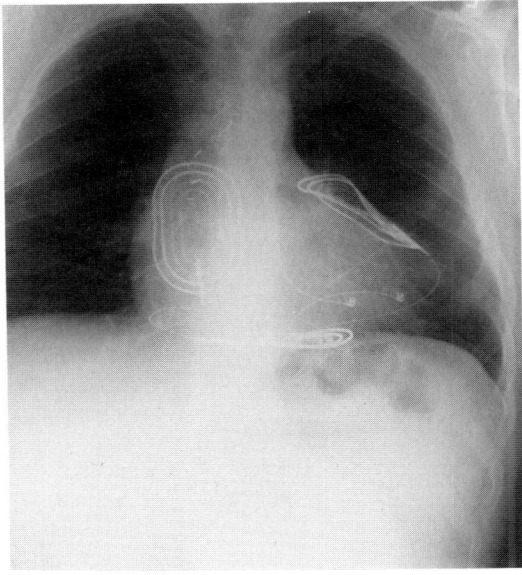

(C)

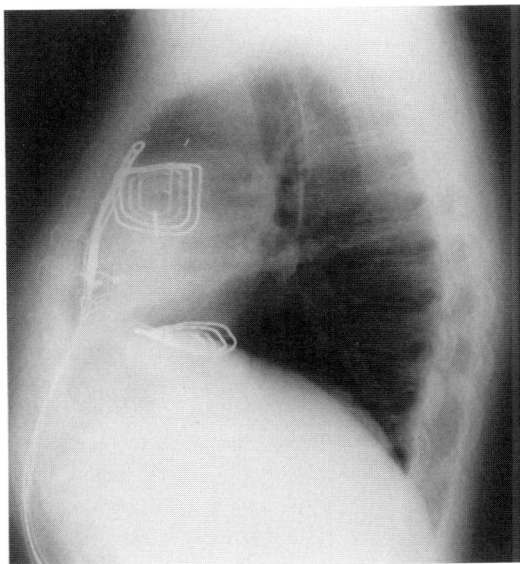

(D)

system are possible with these patches. Screw-in epicardial leads are used for the sensing system in both patients. (Courtesy of Medtronic.)

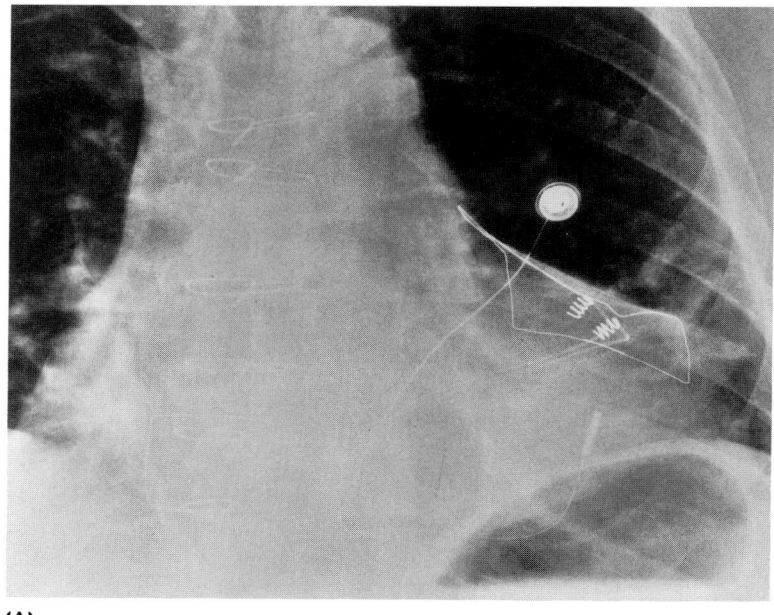

(A)

(B)

Figure 11 Postero-anterior and lateral projections of epicardial patches were obtained shortly after ICD implantation (A and B). Four years later, high defibrillation thresholds developed and chest radiographs showed development of severe patch crumpling, indicated by the tortuosity of the stainless steel markers

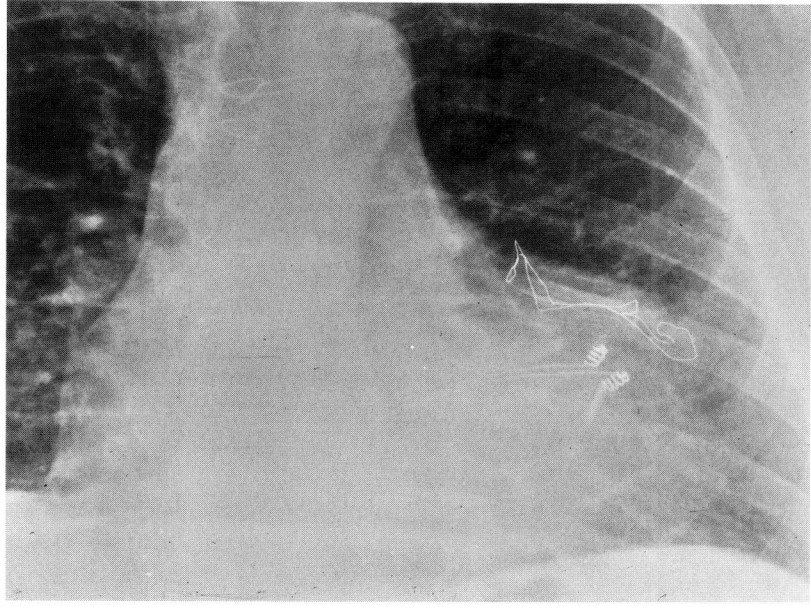

(C)

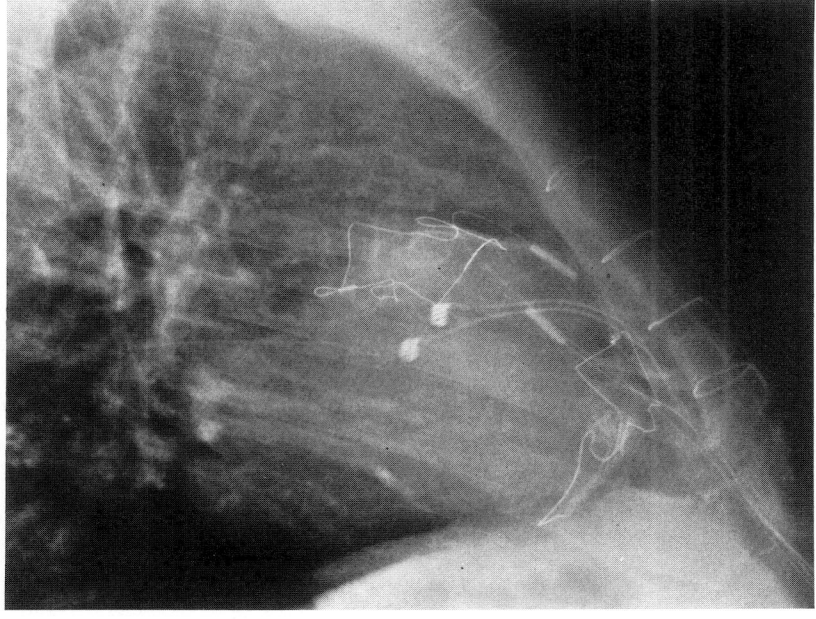

(D)

(C and D). Note is also made of the screw-in epicardial sensing leads, as well as the normal "gaps" between the patches and their cables.

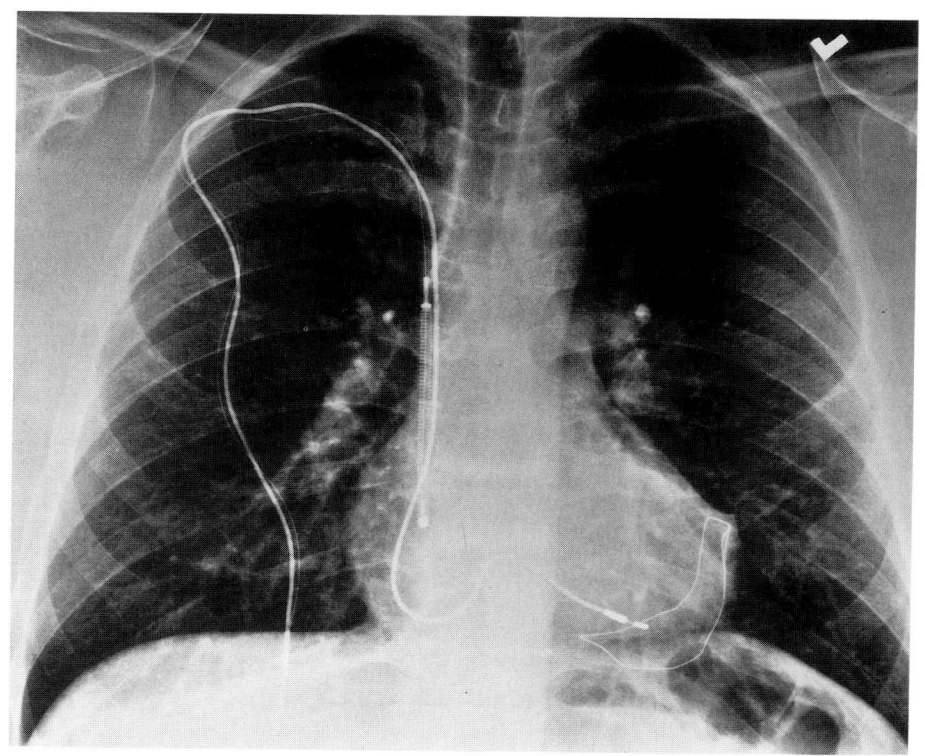

(A)

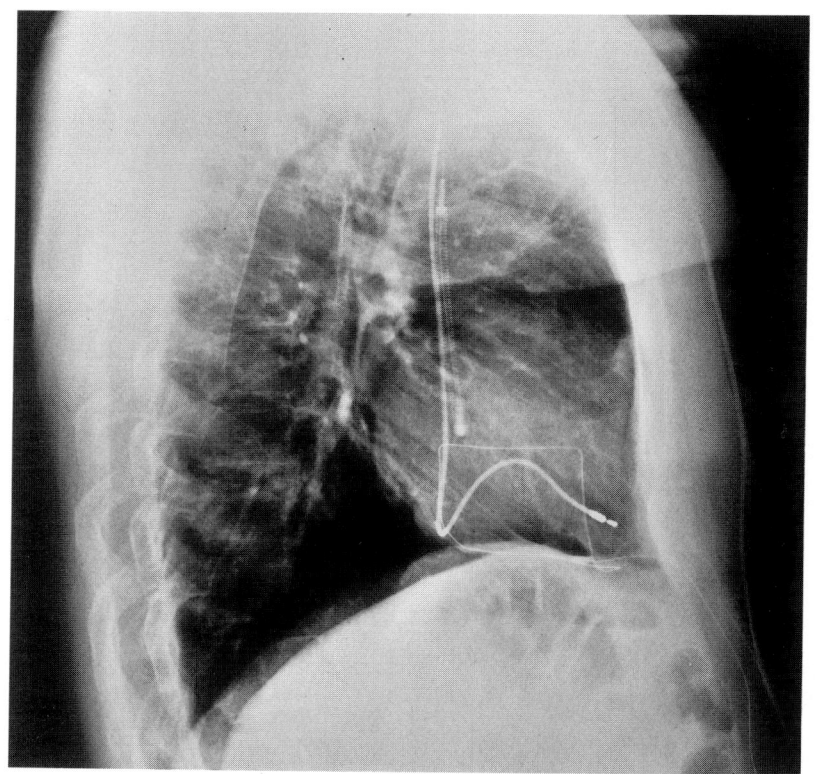

(B)

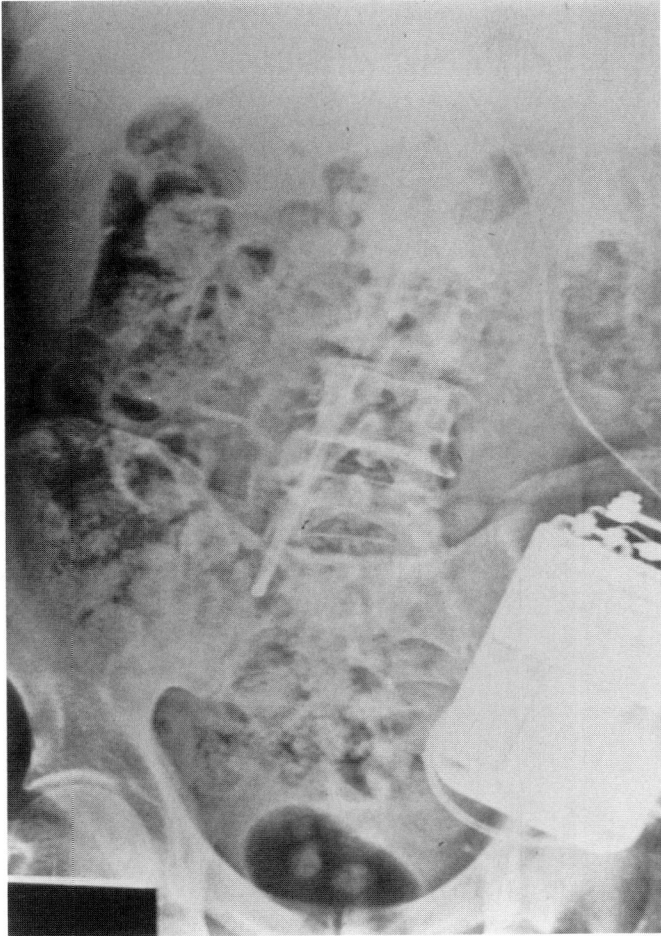

Figure 13 This abdominal radiograph revealed migration of a superior vena cava lead through the inferior vena cava to the right iliac vein. (Courtesy of CPI.)

Figure 12 A combined superior vena cava ("spring" electrode) and single epicardial left ventricular patch defibrillating lead system was used in this patient. The spring electrode is positioned at the junction of the superior vena cava with the right atrium. For rate sensing, a bipolar endocardial lead at the right ventricular apex was utilized. PA (A) and lateral (B) projections are shown.

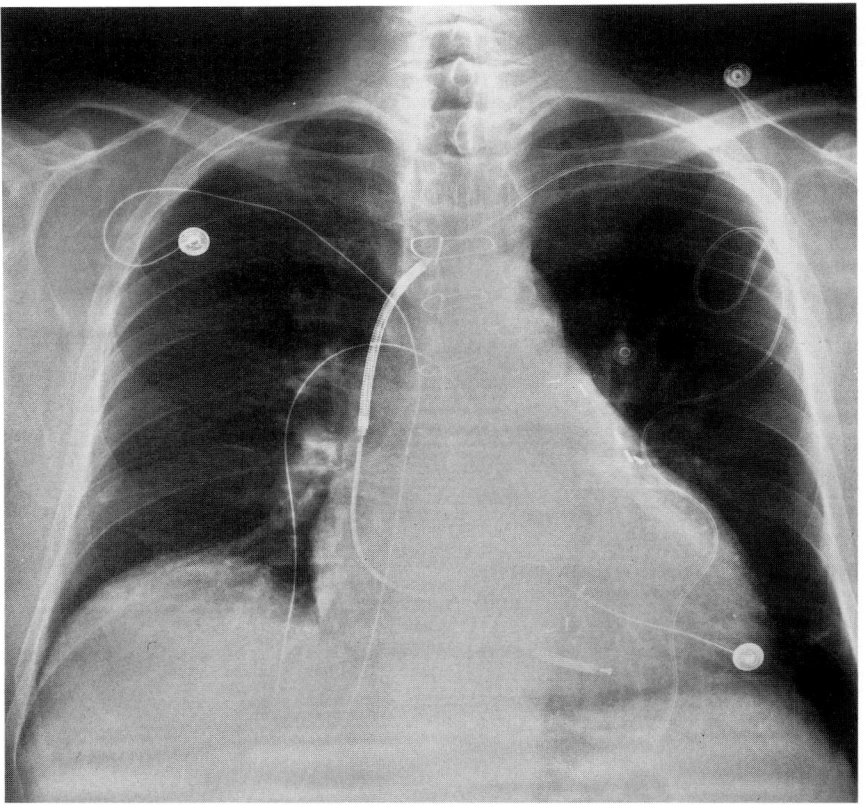

(A)

Figure 14 A nonthoracotomy ICD system was implanted in this patient, who had previous coronary artery bypass surgery. His radiographs, PA (A) and lateral (B) projections, demonstrate proper positioning of a combined defibrillating/pacing/sensing lead (Endotak C, CPI). The lead enters the left subclavian vein through the cephalic vein under the left clavicle and travels medially to the superior vena cava before coursing inferiorly, where it forms a gentle curve along the right atrial lateral wall. The lead then crosses the tricuspid valve and forms a curve concave down, with the tip anchored in the right ventricular apex. The lead is anchored proximally at the entry site (left infraclavicular area), where for that purpose a loop is formed and sewn to the fascia or muscle over a sleeve. The defibrillating system is a bipolar system consisting of a coil in the superior vena cava and a coil in the right ventricular apex (pure transvenous ICD system). The pacing/sensing system is also located in the distal portion of this lead in the right ventricular apex.

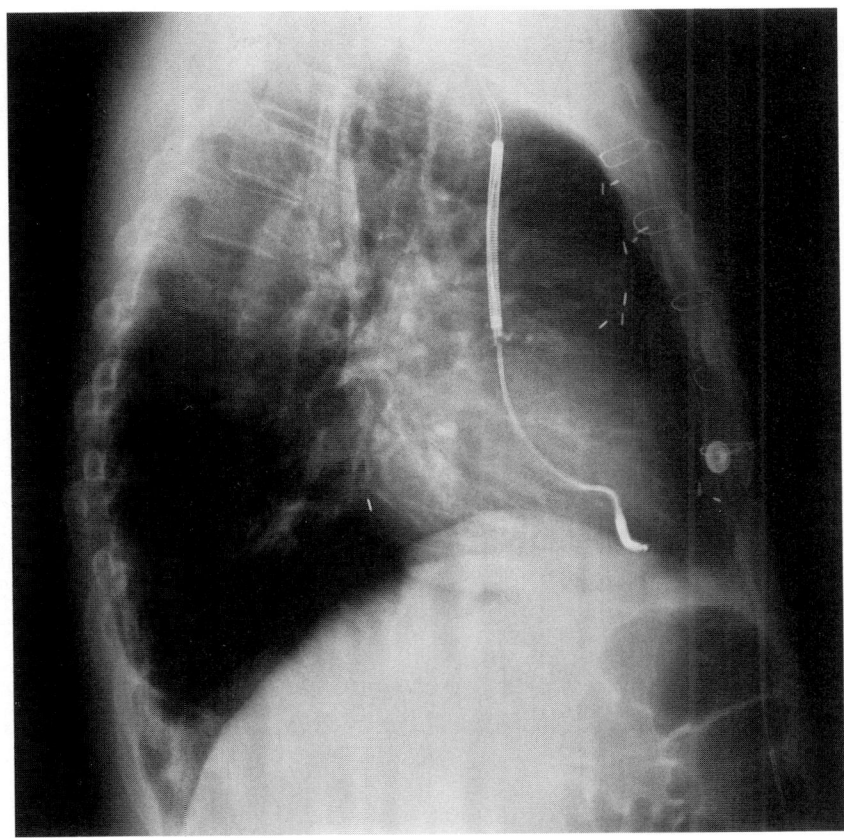

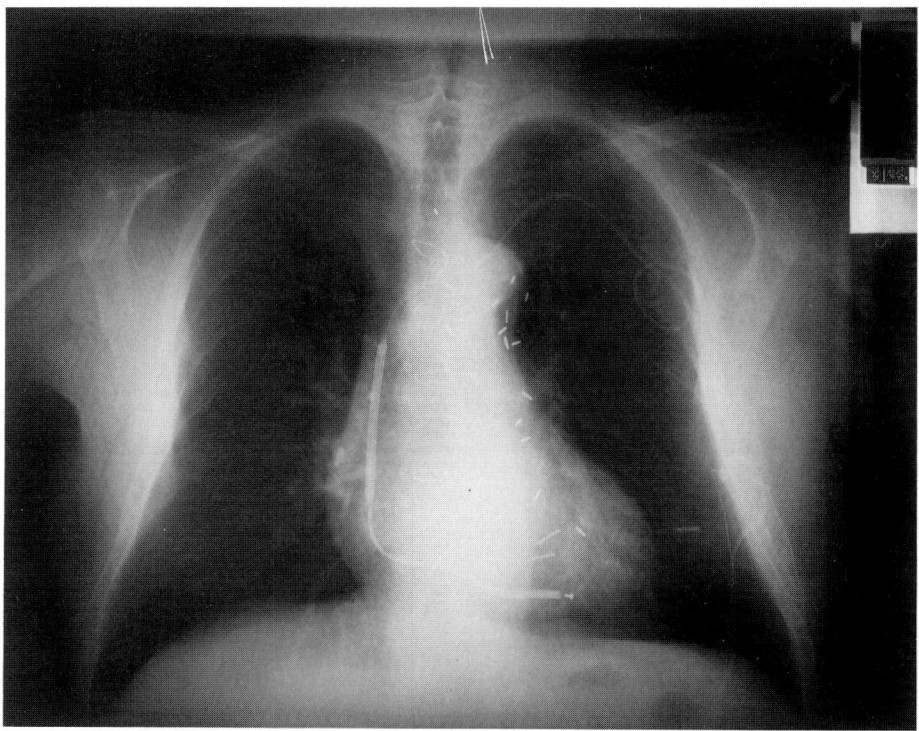

(A)

Figure 15 This is another nonthoracotomy ICD system using a transvenous lead similar to that in Fig. 14. In this case, defibrillation threshold was unacceptably high with the transvenous-only, bipolar configuration, so a subcutaneous patch was placed along the posterolateral portion of the left chest wall outside the rib cage, allowing for a tripolar defibrillating configuration. PA (A) and lateral (B) projections are shown. (Courtesy of CPI.)

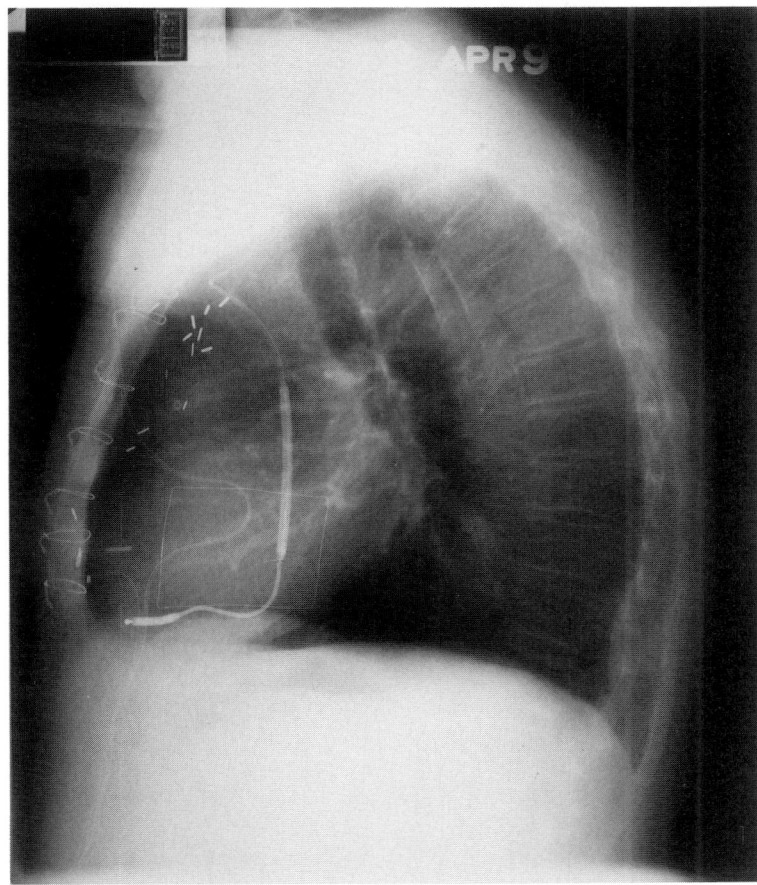
(B)

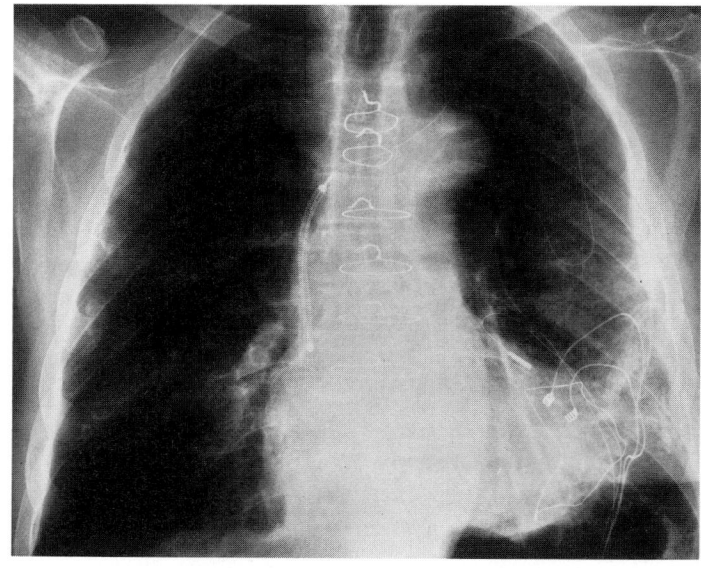

(A)

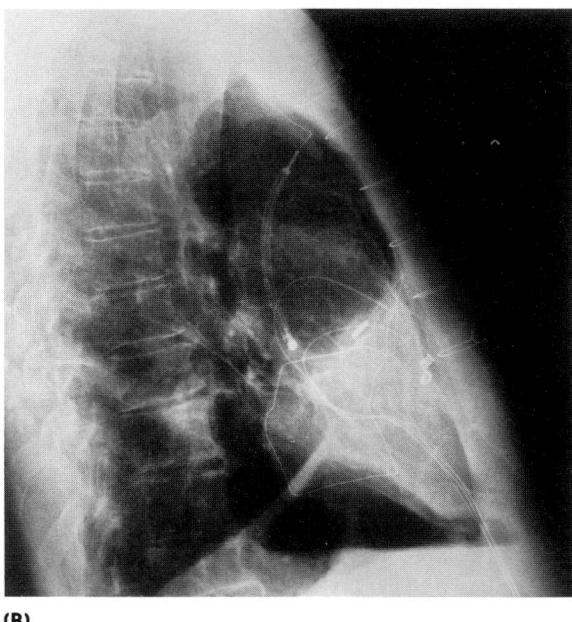

(B)

Figure 16 This patient's initial ICD system consisted of an epicardial patch over the left ventricle with a superior vena cava (SVC) lead, two epimyocardial screw-on sensing leads, and a pulse generator (A and B). This system became infected, necessitating the removal of the entire ICD system except for the SVC lead, which was cut and capped as its removal was felt to pose a high risk of vascular damage. After completion of intensive antibiotic therapy, this patient received a second ICD system, and due to previous surgical procedures, chronic lung disease, and general poor health, the patient underwent implantation of

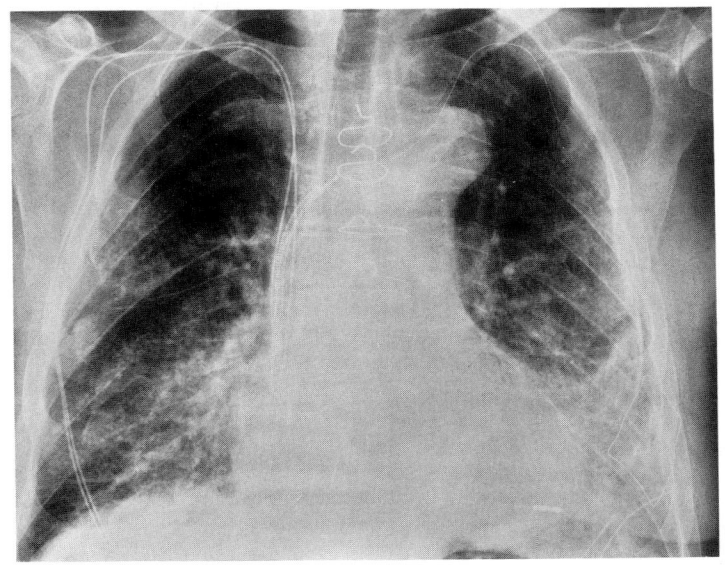

(C)

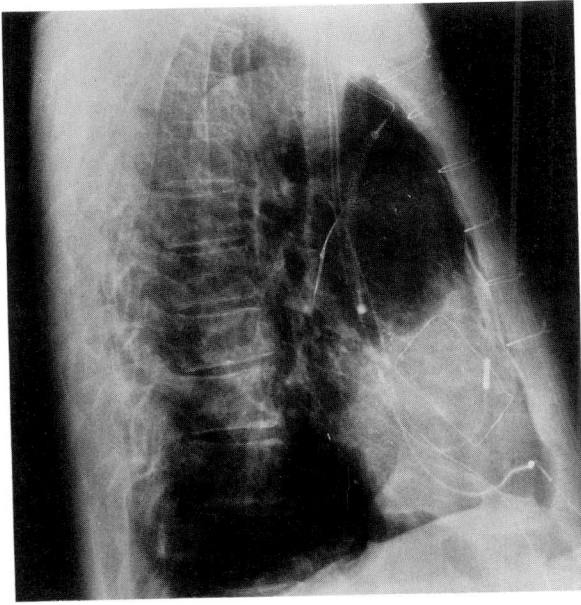

(D)

a nonthoracotomy system (C and D). This tripolar defibrillating system consists of a submuscular patch that lies outside the rib cage paired with the right atrial lead (placed at the right atrial appendage) forming the anode and the right ventricular lead forming the cathode (EnGuard system, Telectronics). The right ventricular lead is also the sensing/pacing lead. Note that the transvenous leads were placed via the right subclavian vein and were tunneled to the right side of the abdomen, as the new pulse generator was implanted on the contralateral side because of the previous infection.

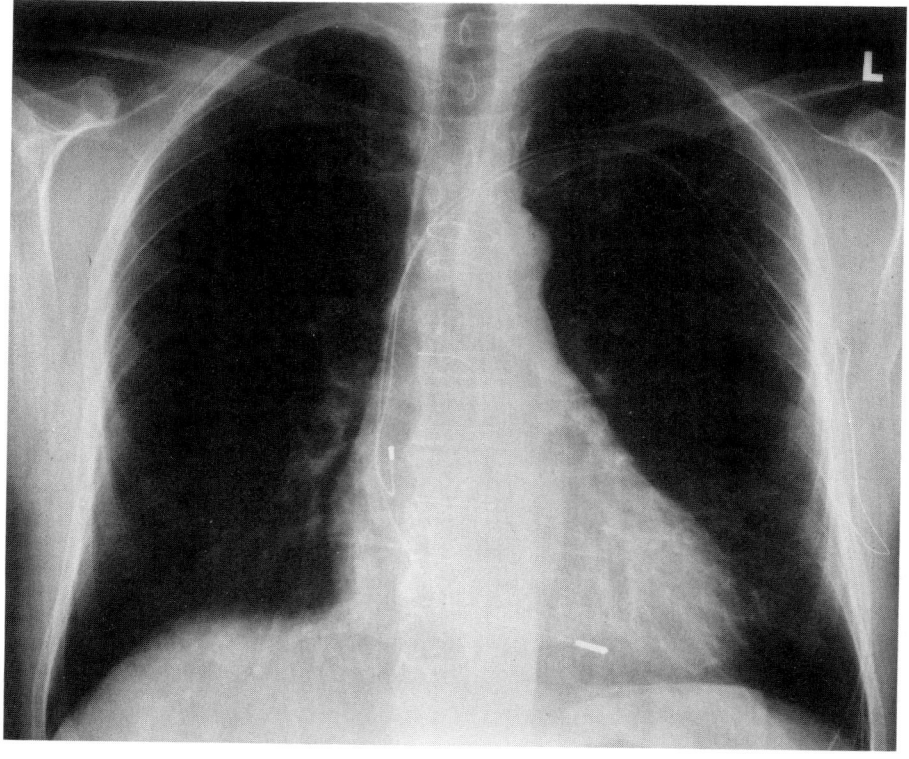

(A)

Figure 17 This is another example of a nonthoracotomy system similar to that in Fig. 16. PA (A) and lateral (B) projections are shown. (Courtesy of Elena Hugo.)

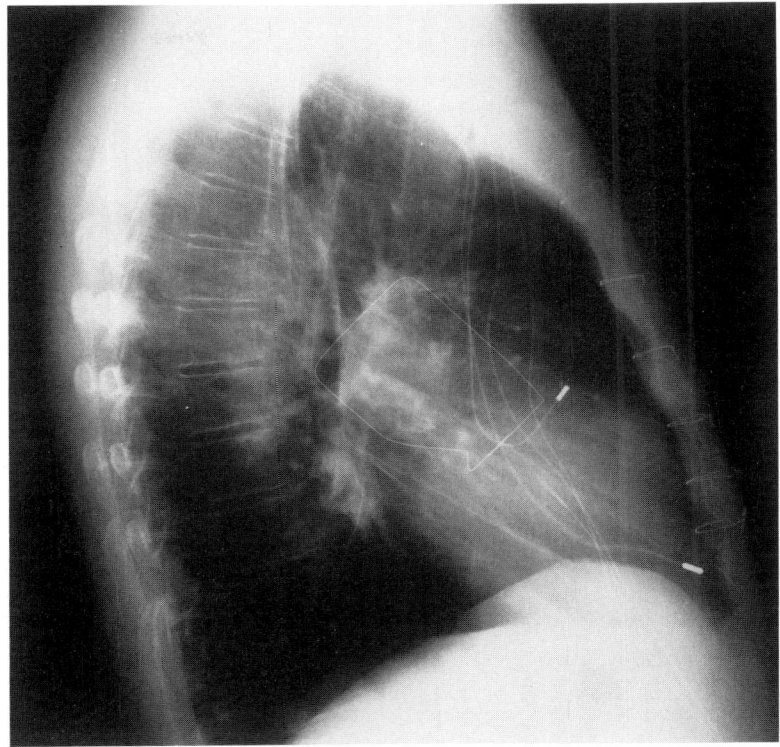
(B)

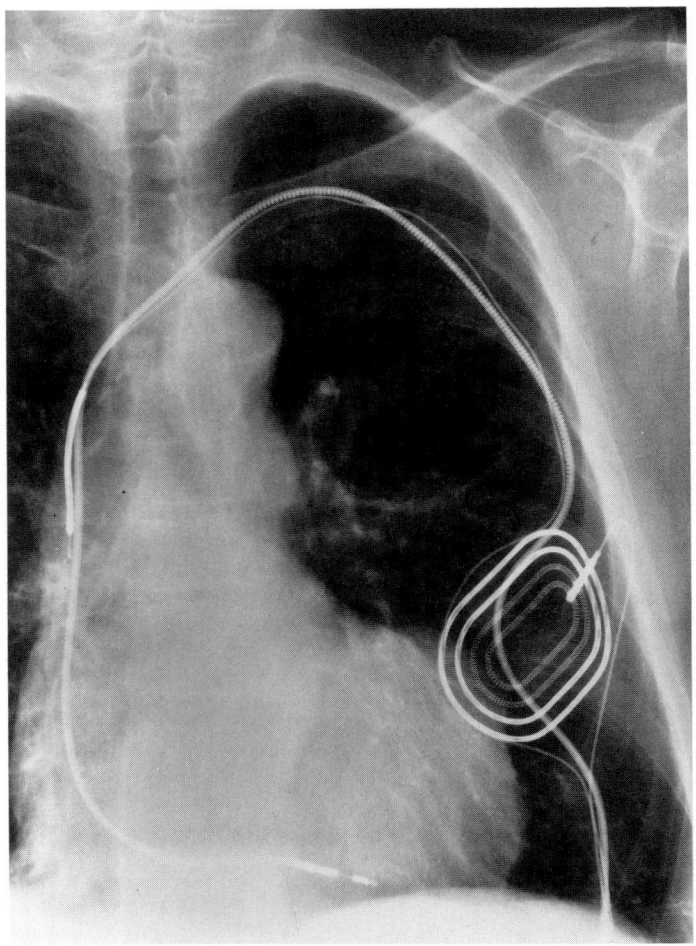

Figure 18 This radiograph shows proper positioning of transvenous leads and subcutaneous patch for another nonthoracotomy system (Transvene, Medtronic). In this system, the superior vena cava (SVC) lead is a defibrillating lead separate from the ventricular lead, which has combined defibrillation and pacing/sensing function. (Courtesy of Medtronic.) The SVC lead may alternatively be placed in the coronary sinus [10].

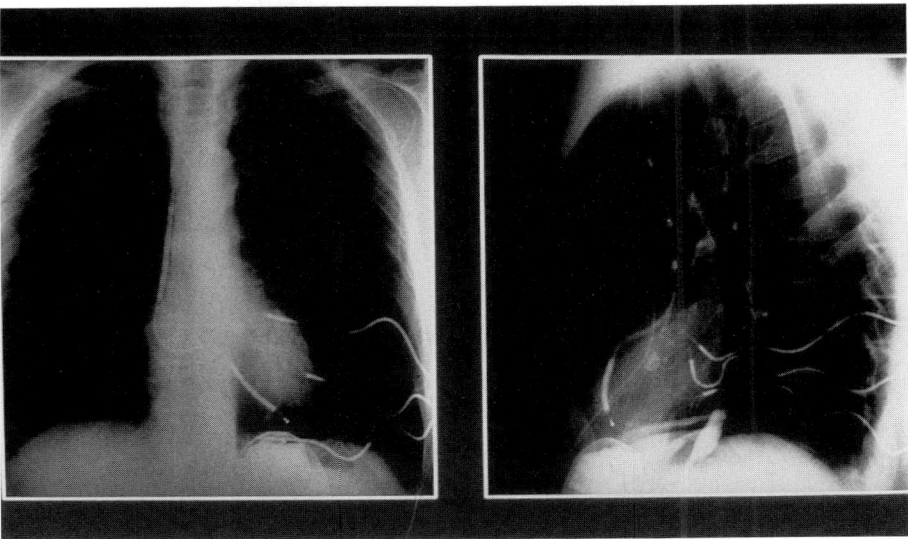

Figure 19 This radiograph shows the endocardial Endotak C lead combined with a new subcutaneous lead system (SQ-Array, CPI) consisting of three electrically common multifilar coil elements comprising one electrode. PA (left) and lateral (right) projections are shown. (Courtesy of CPI.)

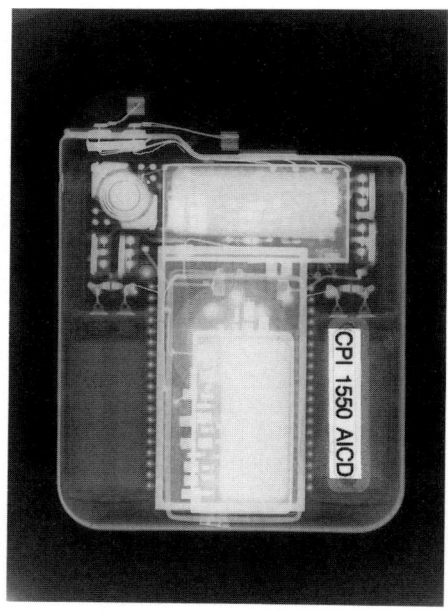

(A.1)

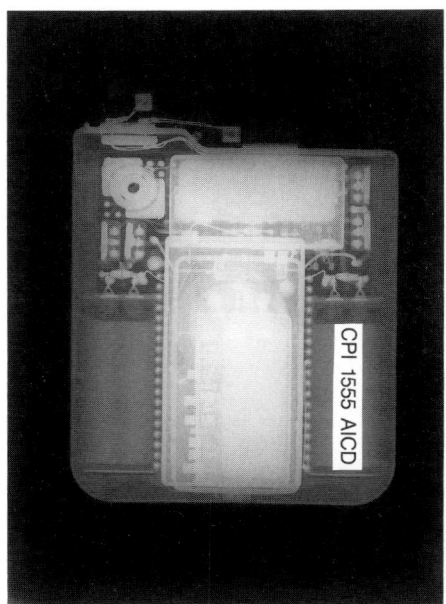

(A.2)

Figure 20A Pulse generator identifier radiographs. (Courtesy of CPI): A1, CPI Ventak 1550; A2, CPI Ventak 1555; A3, CPI Ventak P 1600; A4, CPI Ventak P2 1625; A5, CPI Ventak PRX 1700.

Radiology of the ICD

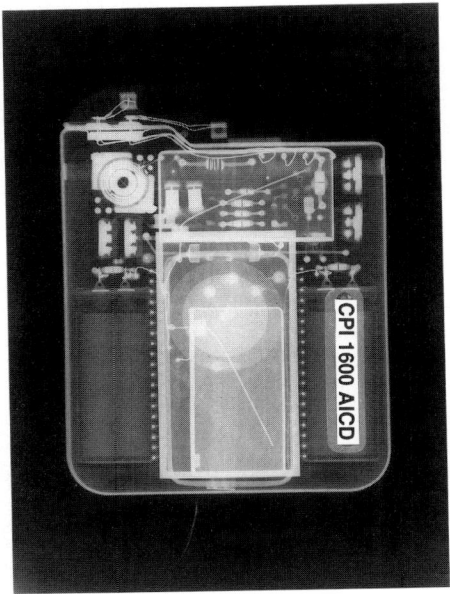

(A.3)

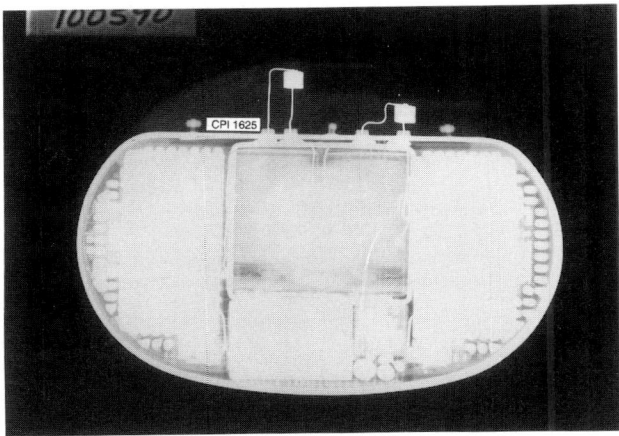

(A.4)

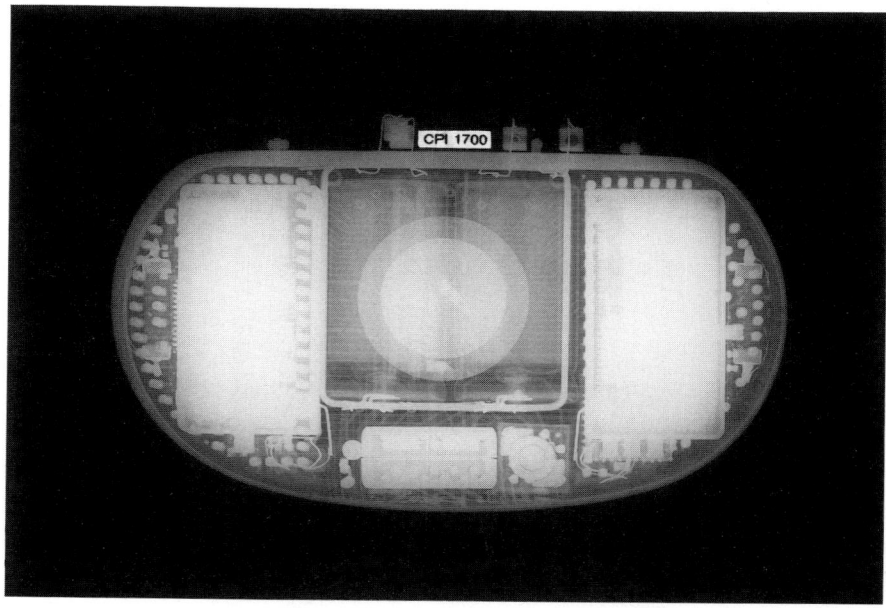

(A.5)

Radiology of the ICD

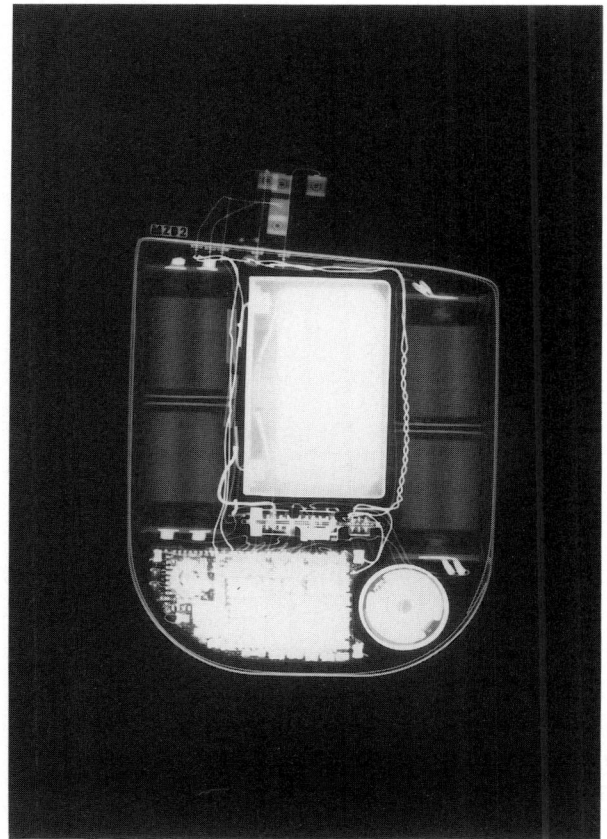

Figure 20B   Medtronic PCD 7217B. (Courtesy of Medtronic.)

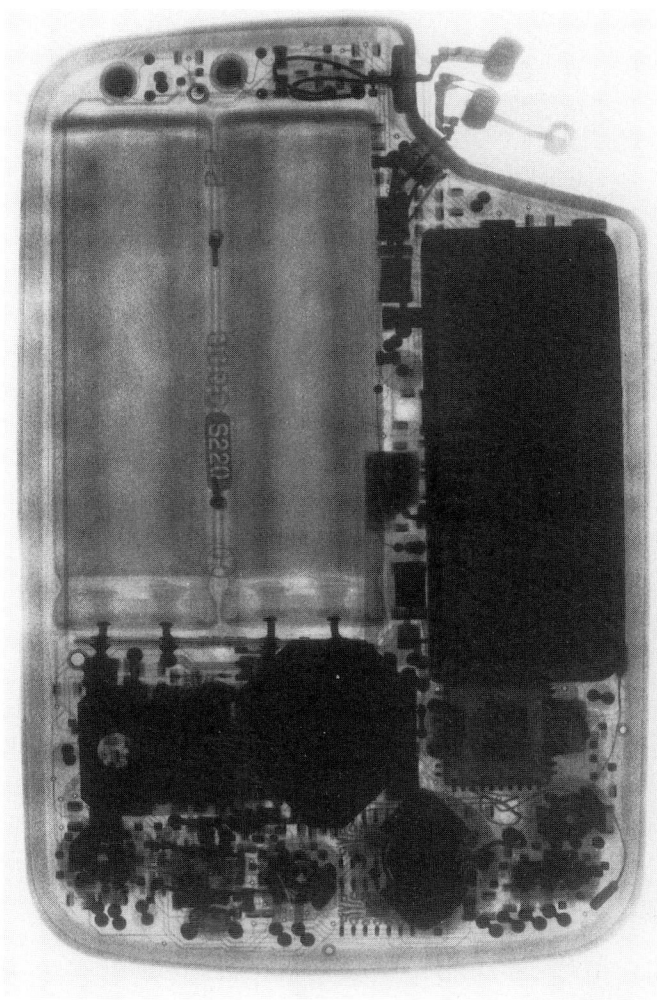

Figure 20C Pacestter Siecure 2120. (Courtesy of Pacesetter.)

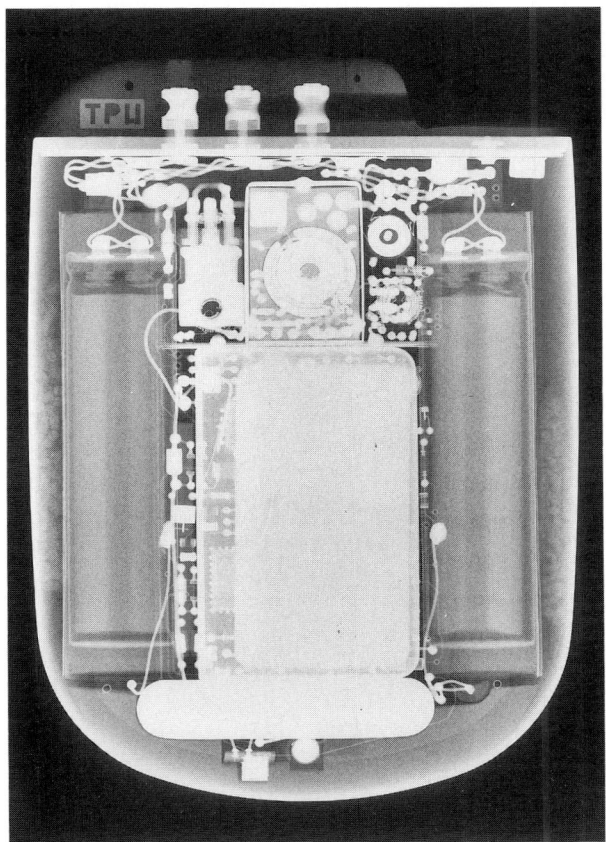

Figure 20D (Courtesy of Telectronics): D1, Telectronics Guardian 4203; D2, Telectronics Guardian 4204; D3, Telectronics Guardian 4210; D4, Telectronics Guardian 4211; D5, Telectronics Guardian 4215; D6, Telectronics Guardian 4310.

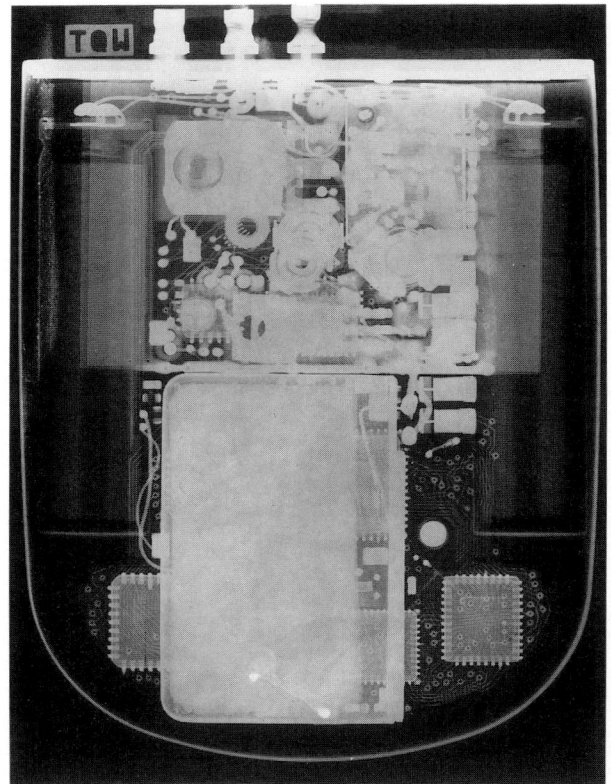

(D.2)

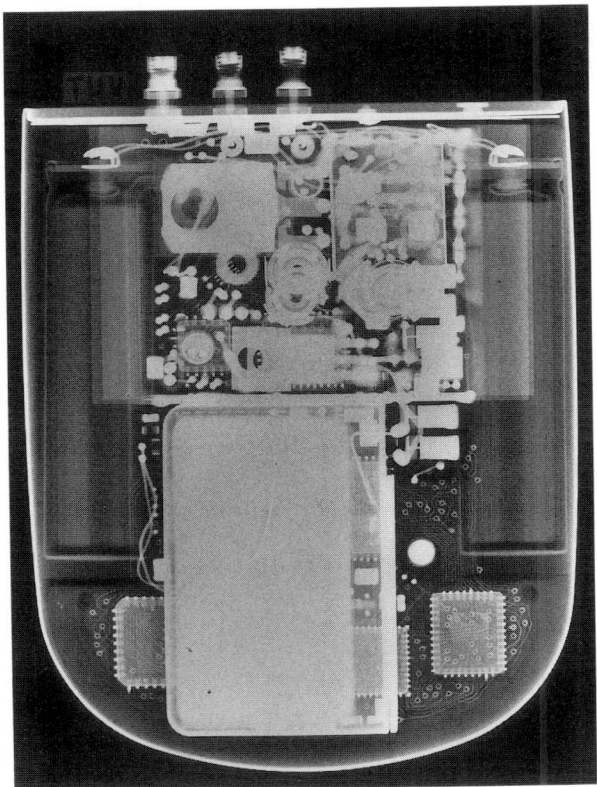

(D.3)

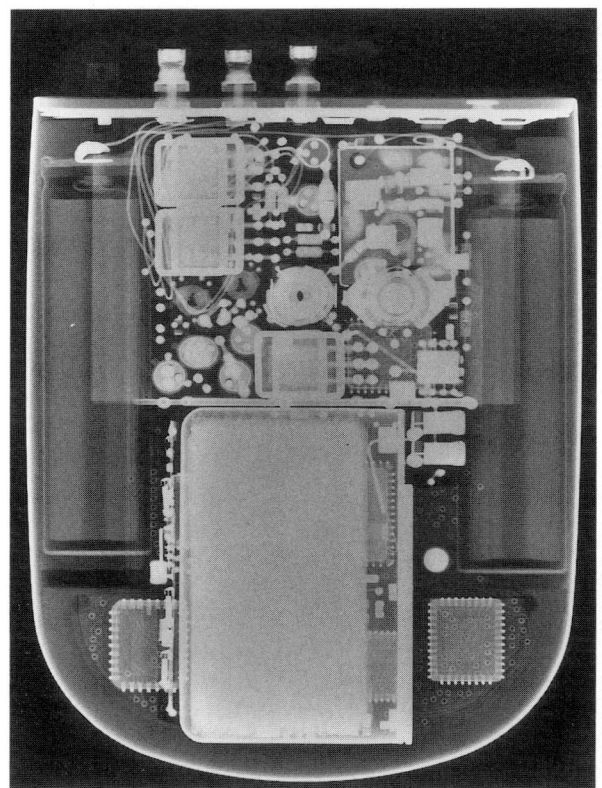

(D.4)

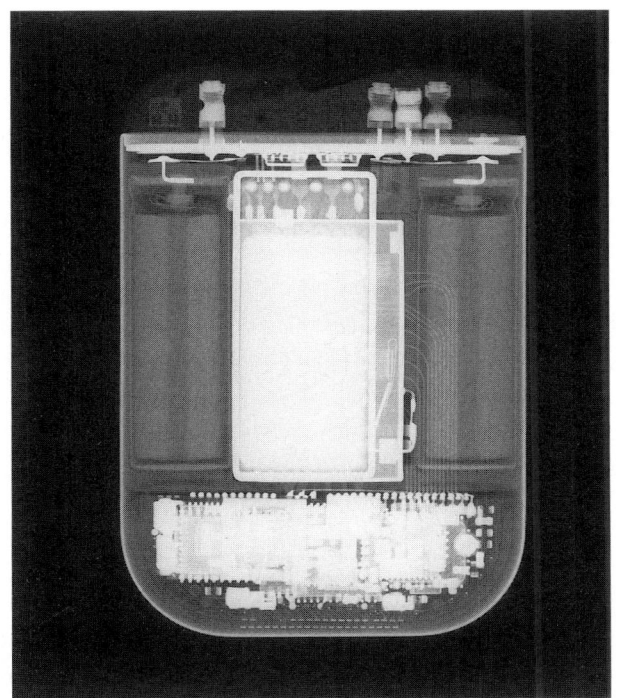

(D.5)

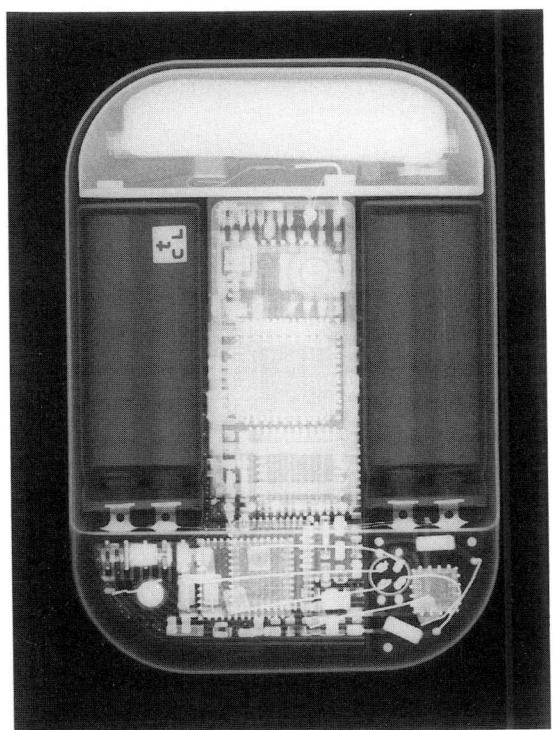

(D.6)

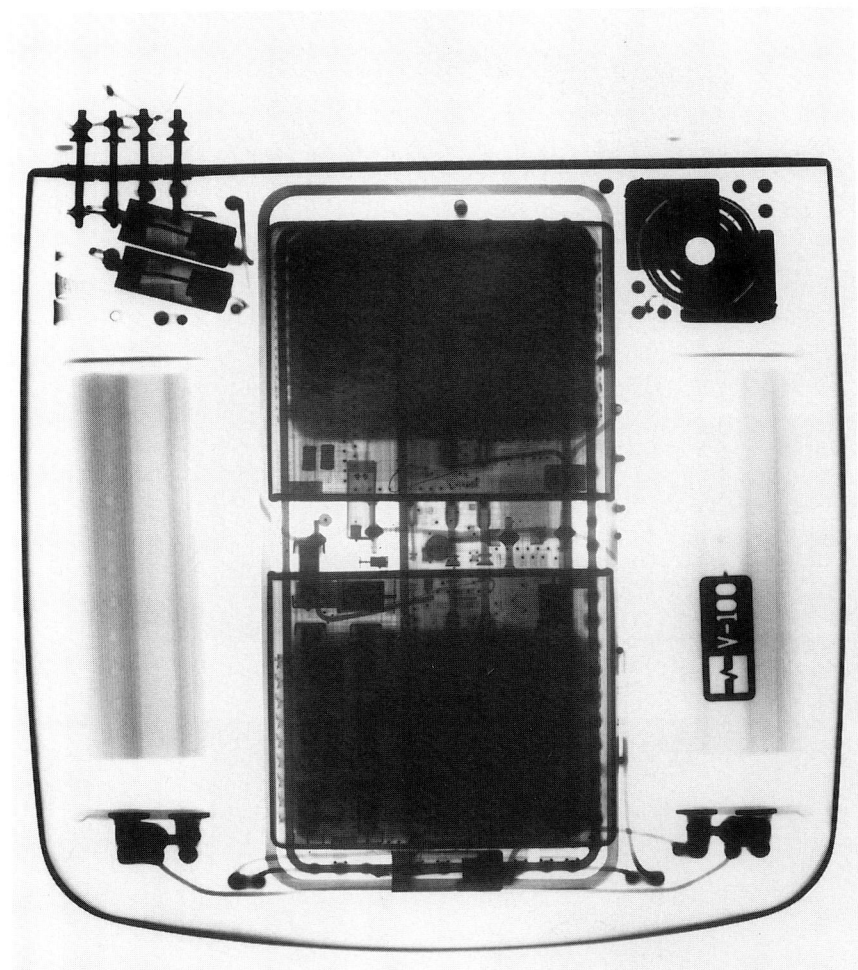

Figure 20E Ventritex Cadence V-100. (Courtesy of Ventritex.)

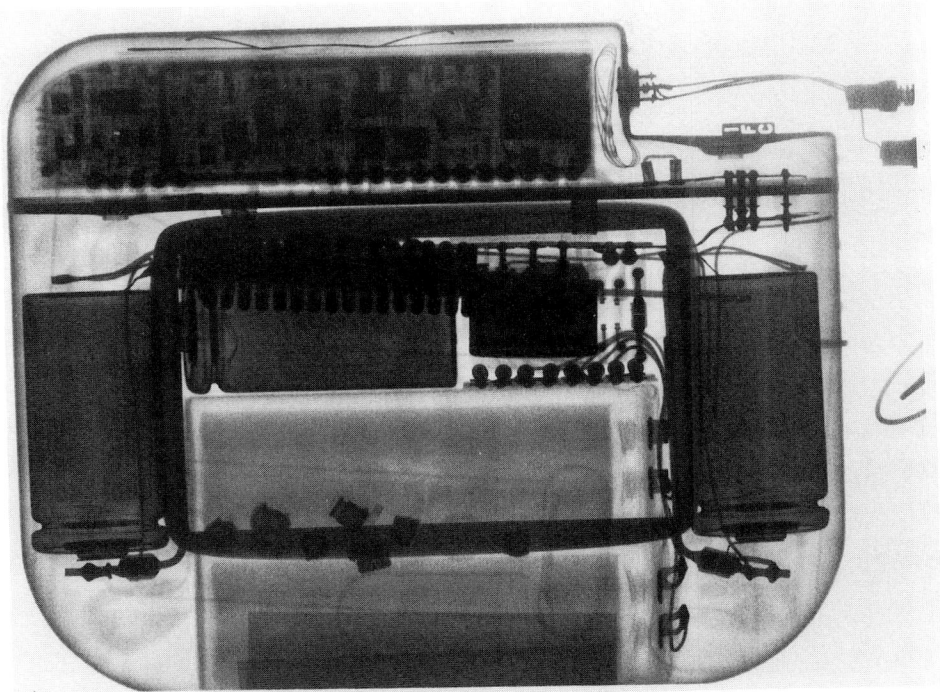

Figure 20F Intermedics Res-Q 101-01. (Courtesy of Intermedics.)

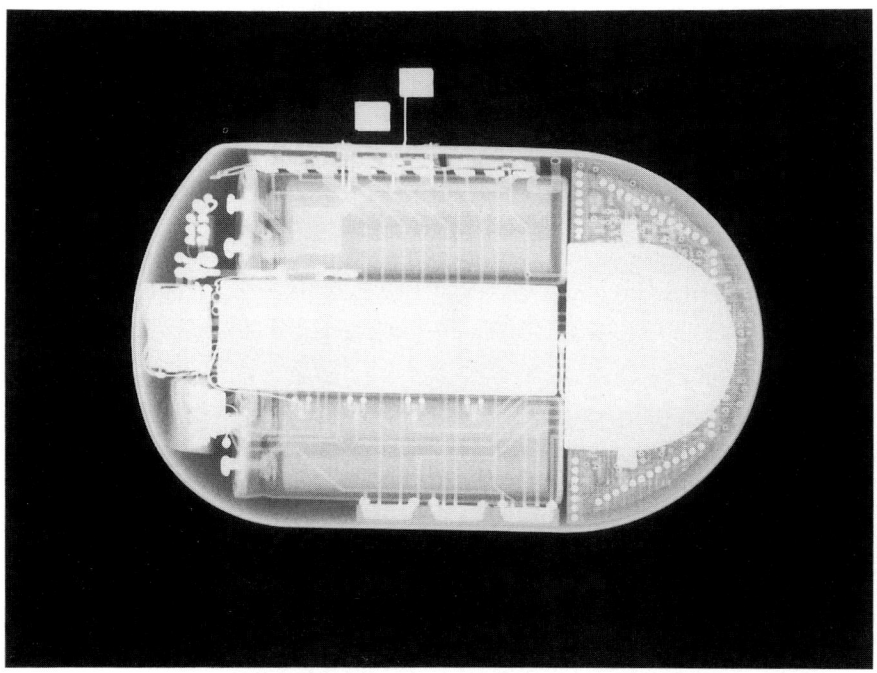

Figure 20G AngeMed Sentinel 2001. (Courtesy of AngeMed.)

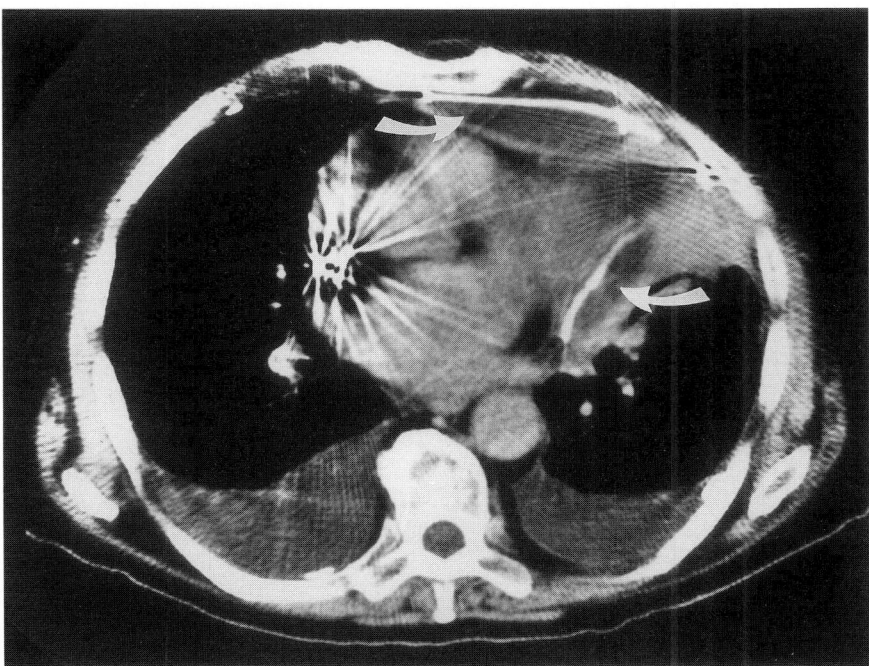

Figure 21 This CT scan was done on a patient with a suspected ICD infection who developed fever several weeks after implantation of a defibrillator system. Pericardial fluid is demonstrated beneath the right ventricular patch and above the left ventricular patch (arrows). Although pericardial fluid is a normal postoperative finding following epicardial patch placement, the fluid should resolve over a 2- to 4-week period. After this time, the demonstration of pericardial fluid adjacent to the ICD patches is practically diagnostic of an ICD infection, especially in a febrile patient [5]

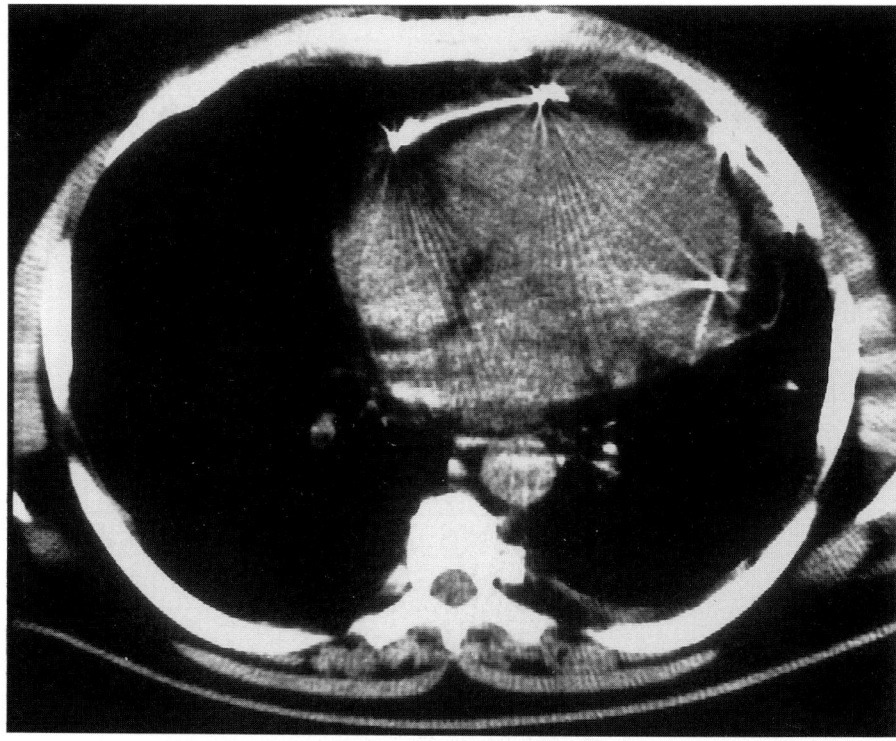

(A)

Figure 22 This CT scan was performed on the same patient whose radiographs are pictured in Fig. 11. Shortly after implant, the first CT scan (A) was performed. Note that the patches appear as straight bright lines. Four years later, another chest CT scan was done (B). Now the right ventricular patch has a crumpled appearance with a soft tissue density surrounding it, compatible with fibrosis. The left ventricular patch is not visualized as well.

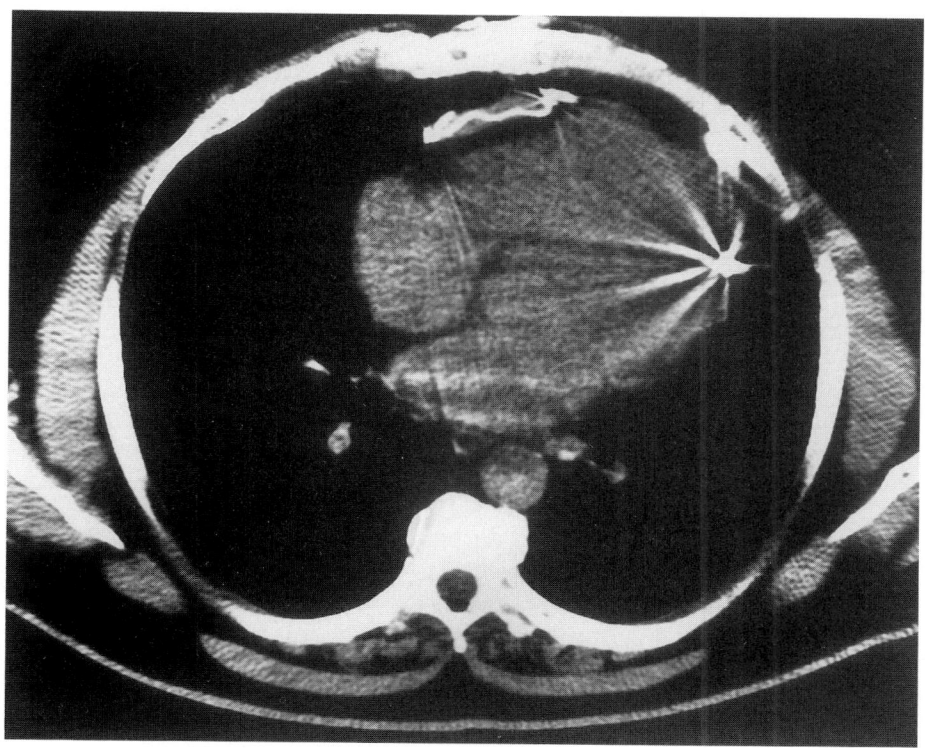

(B)

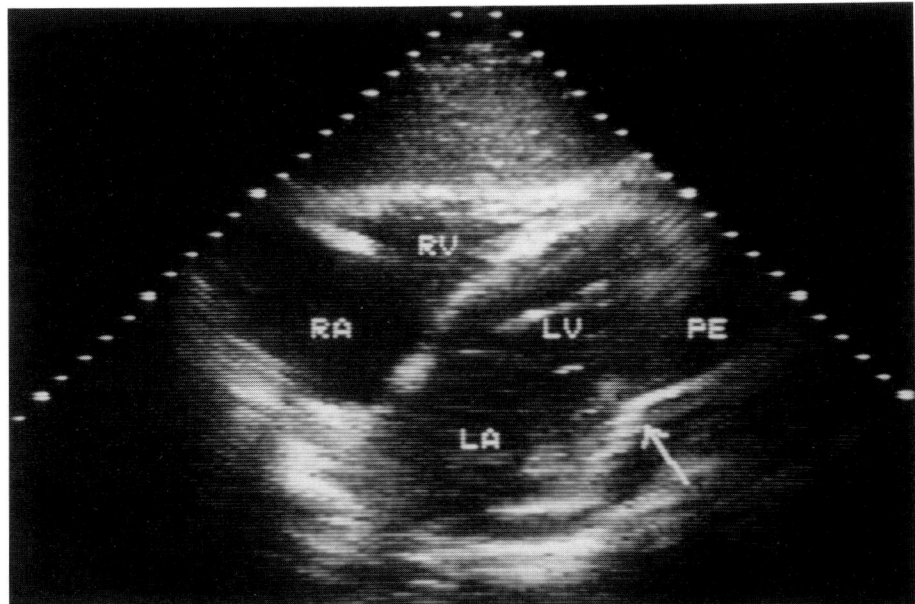

Figure 23 An echocardiogram was performed on the patient described in Fig. 21. Although rarely are ICD patches seen by cardiac echo, this echocardiogram demonstrates the bright (echo-dense) left ventricular patch fairly clearly (arrow) probably due to the dark (echo-free) sizable pericardial effusion surrounding it. LA = left atrium; LV = left ventricle; PE = pericardial effusion; RA = right atrium; RV = right ventricle.

REFERENCES

1. Lurie AL, Udoff EJ, Reid PJ. Automatic implantable cardioverter-defibrillator: appearance and complications. Am J Radiol 1985; 145:723–725.
2. Goodman LR, Troup PJ, Thorsen MK, Youker JE. Automatic implantable cardioverter defibrillator: radiographic appearance. Radiology 1985; 155:571–573.
3. Manolis AS, Makos G, Katsaros C, Olympios CD, Koulizakis N, Cokkinos DV. Initial experience in Greece with the implantable cardioverter defibrillator systems. Hellenic J Cardiol 1992; 33:182–194.
4. Mittleman RS, Mack K, Rastegar H, Manolis AS, Estes NAM. Inappropriate shocks and elevation of defibrillation thresholds in a patient with automatic defibrillator patch silastic erosion and titanium mesh fraying. PACE 1991; 14:1452–1455.
5. Goodman LR, Almassi GH, Troup PJ, et al. Complications of automatic cardioverter-defibrillators: radiographic, CT, and echocardiographic evaluation. Radiology 1989; 170:447–452.
6. Kelly PA, Cannon DS, Garan H, et al. The automatic cardioverter defibrillator: efficacy, complications and survival in patients with malignant ventricular arrhythmias. J Am Coll Cardiol 1988; 11:1278–1286.
7. McCowan R, Maloney J, Wilkoff B, et al. Automatic implantable cardioverter defibrillator implantation using an endocardial and submuscular patch system. J Am Coll Cardiol 1991; 17:415–421.
8. Saksena S, Mehta D, Krol R, et al. Experience with a third generation implantable cardioverter defibrillator. Am J Cardiol 1991; 67:1375–1384.
9. Yee R, Klein GJ, Leitch JW, et al. A permanent transvenous lead system for an implantable pacemaker cardioverter defibrillator. Circulation 1992; 85:196–204.

10. Bardy GH, Hofer B, Johnson G, et al. Implantable transvenous cardioverter defibrillators. Circulation 1993; 87:1152–1168.
11. Veltri EP, Mower MM, Reid PR. Twiddler's syndrome; a new twist, PACE 1984; 7:1004–1009.
12. Gering LE, Ruskin JN, Garan H. Modified magnet test for a reversed automatic implantable cardioverter defibrillator. PACE 1989; 12:1838–1840.
13. Mancini MC, Grubb BP. A technique for the prevention of automatic implantable cardioverter defibrillator generator migration. PACE 1990; 13:946–947.
14. Almassi GH, Olinger GN, Troup PJ, Chapman PD, Goodman LR. Delayed infection of the automatic implantable cardioverter defibrillator. J Thorac Cardiovasc Surg 1988; 95:908–911.
15. Almassi GH, Chapman PD, Troup PJ, Wetherbee JN, Olinger GN. Constrictive pericarditis associated with patch electrodes of the automatic implantable cardioverter defibrillator. Chest 1987; 92:369–371.
16. Oeff M, Abbott JA, Scheinman ED, Yee ES, Scheinman MM, Griffin JC. Determination of patch position for the internal cardioverter defibrillator by cine computed tomography and its relation to the defibrillation threshold. J Am Coll Cardiol 1992; 20:210–217.
17. Siclari F, Klein H, Troster J. Intraventricular migration of an ICD patch. PACE 1990; 13(I):1356–1359.
18. Kelly PA, Wallace S, Tucker B, et al. Postoperative infection with the automatic implantable cardioverter defibrillator: clinical presentation and use of gallium scan in diagnosis. PACE 1988; 11:1220–1225.
19. Bakker PFA, Hauer RNW, Wever EFD. Infections involving implanted cardioverter defibrillator devices. PACE 1992; 15:654–658.
20. Littenberg RL, Taketa RM, Alazraki NP, Halpern SE, Ashburn WL. Gallium-67 for localization of septic lesions. Ann Intern Med 1973; 79:403–406.
21. Stanton MS, Stahl W, Gray JE. Interaction between magnetic resonance imaging and implantable defibrillators (abst). J Am Coll Cardiol 1992; 20:243A.

32

Prediction and Prevention of Sudden Cardiac Death

J. Thomas Bigger Jr.

*Columbia University
and The Presbyterian Hospital in the City of New York
New York, New York*

The high sudden death rate in the United States and other Western countries and the low salvage rates for out-of-hospital cardiac arrest provide intense motivation for the effort to identify high-risk patients so that everything possible can be done to prevent sudden death. In this chapter we will discuss strategies and tests used to identify patients at high risk for sudden cardiac death. Also, we will discuss efforts going on to define better the potential benefit of using implantable cardioverter-defibrillators prophylactically to prevent sudden cardiac death in high-risk subgroups.

I. RISK STRATIFICATION

A. Overview of Risk Stratification in Cardiovascular Diseases

1. Purposes of Risk Stratification

During the past 20 years, there has been intense effort to identify, among patients with cardiovascular disease, those who have increased risk for death or nonfatal morbid events, e.g., malignant ventricular arrhythmias or heart failure. Most investigators study samples of patients who present with an index event or symptom complex, e.g., myocardial infarction, unstable angina, heart failure, syncope, or cardiac arrest. A baseline evaluation, often including special tests, is done to characterize the patients at the time of recruitment and, then, they are followed for months or years to count the outcome events. Risk predictors often suggest the pathophysiology leading to death or cardiovascular morbid events. Mechanistic interpretations of the deaths or other events provide a rationale for intervention trials aimed at interrupting harmful mechanisms and reducing morbidity and mortality. Of course, hypotheses derived from mechanistic interpretations should be tested in randomized clinical trials before becoming accepted in clinical practice. A striking example of a hypothesis that did not prove true was the ventricular premature complex (VPC) hypothesis: Since frequent VPC predict death, suppressing

VPC with antiarrhythmic drugs will reduce mortality. The Cardiac Arrhythmia Suppression Trial (CAST) showed this hypothesis to be false; encainide and flecainide suppressed ventricular arrhythmias, but increased mortality [1,2]. In clinical practice, risk stratification suggests diagnostic and therapeutic approaches for individual patients. One cost-saving result of risk stratification has been the early identification of a large subgroup of low-risk patients who can be discharged early after myocardial infarction and subjected to a minimum of diagnostic studies or treatments.

2. Identifying Patients at Risk of Sudden Death Specifically

Although promising leads have appeared very recently, no variables have been shown definitively to identify specifically those persons at substantially greater risk for sudden than for nonsudden death. Part of the problem may lie with the mechanistic classification of deaths as sudden, arrhythmic, ischemic, or hemodynamic. None of these mechanistic classifications has been validated. For example, left ventricular ejection fraction predicts sudden cardiac deaths as well as it predicts heart failure deaths. Similarly, spontaneous ventricular arrhythmias predict nonsudden cardiac death as well as they predict sudden death [3]. Multiple and competing risks after myocardial infarction may contribute importantly to the difficulty in finding a relationship between baseline risk assessment and the mechanism of death. Patients with coronary heart disease usually have multiple functional deficits as they approach death. Many have both arrhythmias and heart failure, and about half have either angina pectoris or recurrent myocardial infarction in the last few weeks of life. Many have subtle dysfunction of the autonomic nervous system as well. How these four important mechanisms interact pathophysiologically to lead to death is almost impossible to determine. Because several pathophysiologic factors often contribute to death in coronary heart disease, it was difficult to link baseline indicators, i.e., left ventricular dysfunction, arrhythmias, or ischemia to the mechanism of death. A postinfarction patient who has frequent and repetitive ventricular arrhythmias in a baseline 24-h ECG recording and good left ventricular function may have a second myocardial infarction and die after of myocardial failure. If the death is classified as due primarily to heart failure or ischemia, the relationship between functional risk and mechanism of death is obscured; i.e., although arrhythmic risk dominated the baseline assessment, the death was due to heart failure. Had the fatal infarct not occurred, the patient may have died in arrhythmic death at some later point in time, but this can never be known.

II. TESTS TO PREDICT HIGH RISK OF CARDIOVASCULAR DEATH

In this section we will discuss briefly the tests used to identify high-risk patients. Much of the work has been done in samples of patients with recent myocardial infarction. We will discuss tests that identify the presence of risk in the categories of left ventricular dysfunction, ventricular arrhythmias, and abnormal function of the autonomic nervous system (see Table 1). Discussion of myocardial ischemia is omitted.

A. Left Ventricular Dysfunction

1. Clinical Variables

Many clinical variables that can be assessed in the coronary-care-unit (CCU) phase of acute myocardial infarction predict death during the acute phase of infarction and after discharge from hospital [4–9]. Most of the CCU predictor variables reported in the literature reflect

Table 1 Tests to Identify Patients at High Risk for Cardiac Death

---
Left ventricular dysfunction
    Clinical heart failure (NYHA functional class)
    Left ventricular ejection fraction
Ventricular arrhythmias
    24-h ECG recording
    Signal-averaged ECG
    Electrophysiological study
Abnormality of the autonomic nervous system
    RR variability in 24-h ECG recordings
    Baroreflex sensitivity

---

marked left ventricular dysfunction, e.g., shock, low blood pressure, rales, increased heart rate, increased respiratory rate, and pulmonary venous congestion or cardiomegaly on chest X-ray. Prognostic indices derived from these data, such as the Norris and Peel indices [10,11], indicate extensive myocardial damage at the time of infarction and predict long-term outcome as well as hospital mortality. The impressive and quantitative predictive value of rales detected during the CCU phase of acute myocardial infarction has been shown in two large prospective studies. In the Multicenter Post Infarction Program study, rales, graded as none, bibasilar, greater than bibasilar but less than one-third up the posterior thorax, and greater than one-third up the posterior thorax, was associated with 6%, 11%, 25%, and 35% mortality during 2 to 4 years of follow-up (average follow-up 31 months) [12–14]. Rales in the CCU was one of the best predictors of death in the first 6 months, reinfarction, and high-frequency ventricular arrhythmias in 24-h ECG recordings [14,15]. These findings were confirmed in the Multicenter Diltiazem Post Infarction Trial [16]. Pulmonary congestion on a chest X-ray taken in the CCU has almost identical long-term predictive value [14,16]. Rales or pulmonary congestion on a CCU chest X-ray probably reflect ischemic risk as well as risk of heart failure and death [13].

2. Infarct Size

In coronary heart disease, infarct size importantly determines left ventricular dysfunction which, in turn, is a prime determinant of sudden, arrhythmic, and total mortality early and late after myocardial infarction. Studies that quantified infarction size using serial changes in serum creatine kinase (CK) activity [17–19] have shown that infarction size is an excellent predictor of death early and late after myocardial infarction [19–22].

3. Noninvasive Evaluation of Left Ventricular Function

Radionuclide ventriculograms, echocardiography, and dye angiograms are three commonly used methods for quantifying ventricular function after myocardial infarction. The most common measure of ventricular function is the left ventricular ejection fraction (LVEF). Radionuclide methods or dye angiography have been used more commonly in clinical practice and clinical trials, but two-dimensional echocardiographic methods are gaining wider acceptance. Radionuclide ventriculograms probably have greater accuracy and precision than echocardiographic and angiographic methods, but LVEF is such a strong risk predictor that small measurement errors have little practical significance. Next to rales heard in the CCU or pulmonary vascular congestion on a chest X-ray in the CCU, LVEF is the strongest predictor of death after myocardial infarction [12]. In Table 2, the mortality rates for patients with LVEF < 0.40 are

Table 2 Left Ventricular Ejection Fraction (LVEF) and All-Cause Mortality After Myocardial Infarction

Study	LVEF < 0.40		LVEF ≥ 0.40		Relative risk
	No. of patients	Mortality rate	No. of patients	Mortality rate	
MPIP	256	21.5%	510	7.1%	3.02
MILIS	181	23.7%	352	6.5%	3.63
MDPIT placebo	278	19.2%	677	7.7%	2.49
UCSD SCOR	185	22.7%	564	8.5%	2.68

compared to the mortality rates for patients with LVEF ≥ 0.40 in four large studies [23–26]. Overall, 30% of the patients have a LVEF < 0.40, and the mortality rate is 21.5% in this group during several years of follow-up, compared to 7.6% in the group with LVEF ≥ 0.40, a relative risk of nearly 3.0. The relationship between LVEF and all-cause mortality is a hyperbolic curve; risk does not increase until the LVEF falls below 0.40. Below LVEF values of 0.40, mortality rate increases sharply as LVEF falls (see Fig. 1). LVEF and rales are weakly associated, but each predicts all-cause mortality independently of the other in the years after acute myocardial infarction. LVEF predicts deaths occurring in the first 6 months after myocardial infarction better than deaths occurring later [23]. Also, LVEF predicts readmission for heart failure and sustained arrhythmias, but is not a good predictor of early recurrent myocardial

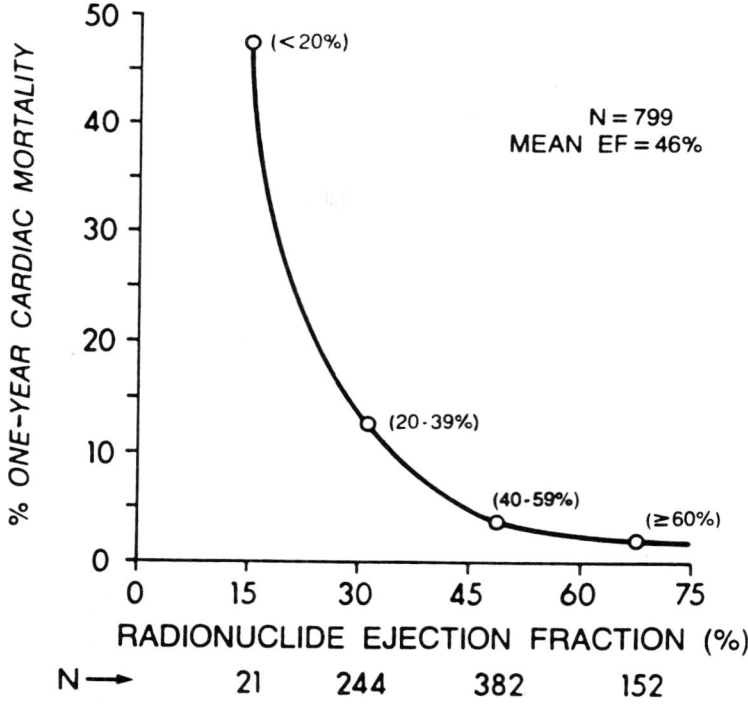

Figure 1 Prediction of 1-year cardiac death by LVEF. Note that the mortality rate rises sharply at LVEF < 0.36. From Ref. 12.

infarction [15]. Radionuclide methods have been best validated for an association with death during long-term follow-up after myocardial infarction. However, in chronic coronary heart disease, patients with reduced LVEF measured using contrast angiography have high mortality rates during long-term follow-up [27].

B. Ventricular Arrhythmias

1. Spontaneous Ventricular Arrhythmias After Myocardial Infarction

a. VPC Frequency as a Predictor of All-Cause Mortality. Data from four large studies that analyzed 24-h ECG recordings made about 10 days after myocardial infarction are shown in Table 3 [23–26]. The frequency of ventricular premature complexes (VPC) is not high at the time of discharge from hospital, more than half the patients have fewer than 1.0 VPC per hour. Only 15% to 20% have $\geq$ 10 VPC per hour (Table 3). The 41% figure given for the University of California San Diego represents the prevalence of Lown grade $\geq$ 2. Multiform VPC (Lown grade 3) is responsible for the high prevalence of ventricular arrhythmias in this study [28]. The relationship between VPC frequency and mortality rate during follow-up is an S-shaped curve (see Fig. 2). More than half of the patients have an average VPC frequency $<$ 1 per hour and have a 2-year mortality rate of about 5%. The curve rises steeply between 1 and 10 VPC per hour to mortality rates over 20% [12,23,29]. As VPC frequency rises another two orders of magnitude, mortality rates do not increase very much. Overall, mortality rates are about 2.5 times as great for patients with 10 or more VPC per hour in a 24-h ECG recording as for patients with lower VPC frequencies (Table 3). The cut point that gives the highest relative risk for death is about 3 VPC per hour [23]. The strength of the association between VPC frequency and death is about the same as between left ventricular ejection fraction $<$ 0.40 and death.

b. Repetitive VPC as a Predictor of All-Cause Mortality. Previous studies have suggested that "complex" VPC features are at least as important as frequency, i.e., have as strong an association with death during follow-up. Early studies proposing this concept used short ECG recordings and polyvalent definitions of complex ventricular arrhythmias [30,31]. Two large postinfarction studies analyzed 24-h ECG recordings to evaluate the relationship between complex VPC features and mortality and concluded that repetitive ventricular arrhythmias, i.e., pairs or runs of VPC, are very important predictors of subsequent mortality [23,28,29]. Using

Table 3 Frequency of Ventricular Premature Complexes (VPC) and All-Cause Mortality After Myocardial Infarction[a]

Study	VPC $\geq$ 10/h		VPC $<$ 10/h		Relative risk
	No. of patients	Mortality rate[b]	No. of patients	Mortality rate[b]	
MPIP	150	21.5%	616	9.6%	2.25
MILIS	78	29.5%	455	9.4%	3.12
MDPIT placebo	163	20.7%	792	9.1%	2.27
UCSD SCOR	308	18.5%	441	7.4%	2.48

[a]MPIP = Multicenter Post Infarction Program; MILIS = Multicenter Investigation of the Limitation of Infarct Size; MDPIT = Multicenter Diltiazem Post Infarction Trial; UCSD SCOR = University of California San Diego, Special Center of Research. The values of MPIP and MDPIT are 24-month Kaplan-Meier estimates of mortality rates. The values for MILIS are crude mortality rates with average follow-up of 18 months. The values for UCSD are 12-month Kaplan-Meier estimates of mortality rates.
[b]UCSD arrhythmia data are categorized as Lown grade $<$ 2 and $\geq$ 2.

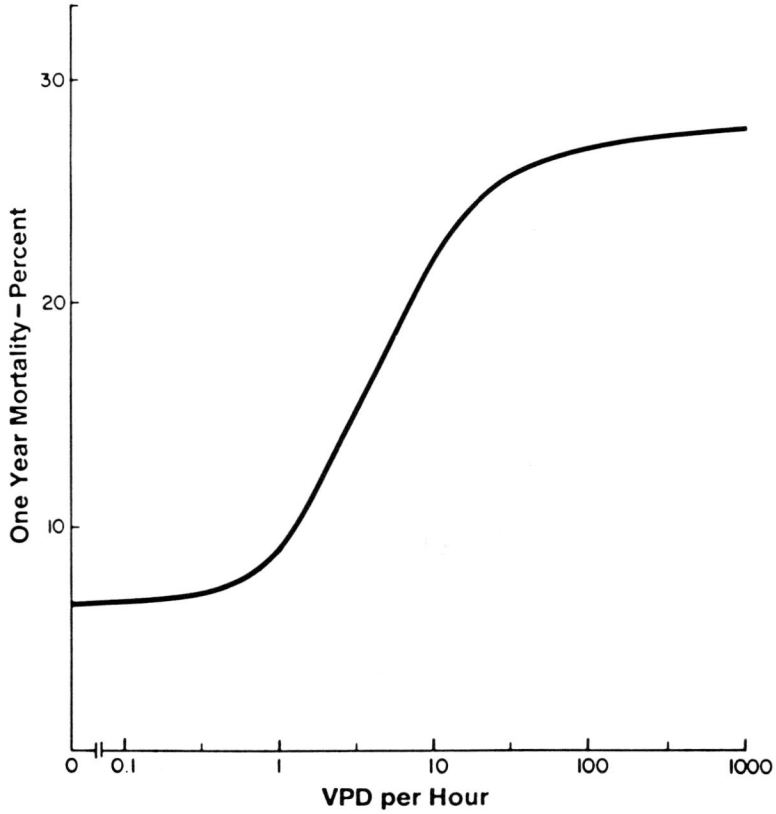

Figure 2 Prediction of 2-year all-cause mortality by frequent VPC. Note that the mortality rate rises sharply between 1 and 10 VPC/hour. From Ref. 14.

multivariate statistical techniques, both studies found that repetitive VPC are associated with death independent of VPC frequency [23,28]. An increasing degree of repetitiveness is associated with a corresponding decrease in survival over 3 years of follow-up. Unsustained VT occurring in a predischarge 24-h ECG recording has a very strong relationship with subsequent mortality (odds ratio = 4.2) but occurs relatively infrequently, i.e., in about 10% of the patients [23,29,32,33].

c. The Relationship Between Left Ventricular Dysfunction and Ventricular Arrhythmias After Myocardial Infarction. Four large, multicenter studies have evaluated the relationships among left ventricular dysfunction, ventricular arrhythmias, and mortality in a total of more than 3000 postinfarction patients (see Table 4). [23–26]. There was a weak but statistically significant association between left ventricular dysfunction and ventricular arrhythmias after myocardial infarction. On average, patients with LVEF < 0.40 were 1.6 times as likely to have ventricular arrhythmias as patients with left ventricular ejection fraction ≥ 0.40 (the range among the relative risks for this relationship for the four studies was 1.49 to 2.08). There was no statistical interaction between ventricular arrhythmias and left ventricular ejection fraction with respect to their ability to predict mortality; i.e., these two factors each predict risk independent of the other (see Fig. 3) [34]. When both of these important risk factors are present,

Table 4 Relationship Among Ventricular Arrhythmias, Left Ventricular Dysfunction, and Mortality After Myocardial Infarction[a]

Study	Total number of patients	Left ventricular ejection fraction < 0.40					Left ventricular ejection fraction ≥ 0.40				
		VPC < 10/h		VPC ≥ 10/h			VPC < 10/h		VPC ≥ 10/h		
		N	Mortality rate	N	Mortality rate	Relative risk	N	Mortality rate	N	Mortality rate	Relative risk
MPIP	766	184	17.3%	72	32.2%	1.87	432	6.3%	78	11.7%	1.84
MILIS	533	141	19.1%	40	40.0%	2.09	314	5.1%	38	18.4%	3.61
MDPIT (placebo)	955	203	15.2%	75	30.2%	1.99	589	7.0%	88	12.6%	1.81
UCSD SCOR[b]	749	84	17.9%	101	26.7%	1.50	357	5.0%	207	14.5%	2.87

[a]MDPIT = Multicenter Diltiazem Post Infarction Trial; MILIS = Multicenter Investigation of the Limitation of Infarct Size; MPIP = Multicenter Post Infarction Program; UCSD SCOR = University of California San Diego, Special Center of Research in Ischemic Heart Disease; VPC = ventricular premature complexes. Values for MPIP and MDPIT are Kaplan-Meier estimates of mortality rates at 24 months of follow-up; values for MILIS are crude mortality rates after an average follow-up of 18 months.
[b]The UCSD SCOR arrhythmia data are partitioned, not by VPC value of 10/h, but by grade < 2 and ≥ 2 from the Lown grading system for ventricular arrhythmias (many patients in the ≥ 2 group have infrequent VPC and no repetitive ventricular arrhythmias). The mortality values are crude rates at the end of 12 months of follow-up.

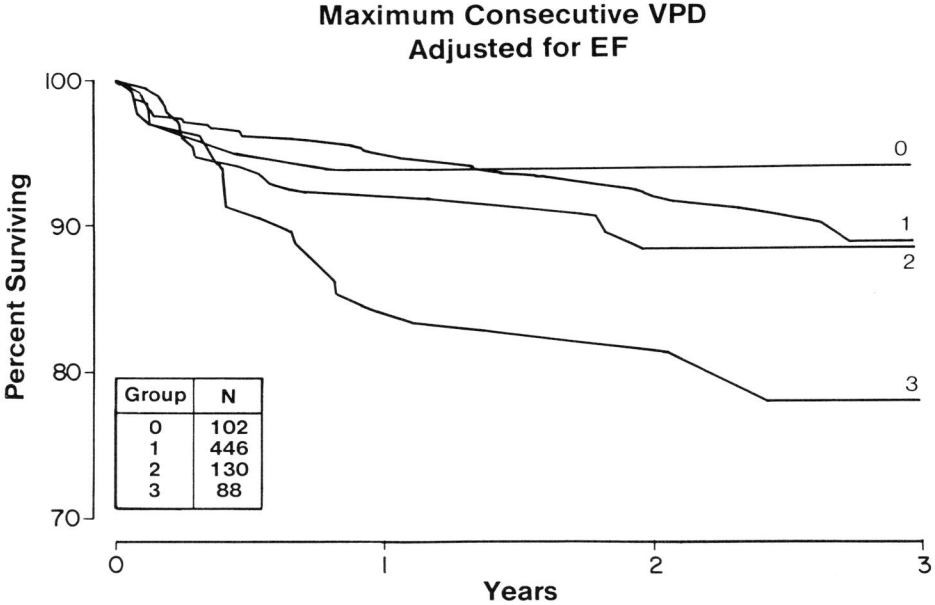

Figure 3 Prediction of all-cause mortality by LVEF and VPC: group 0 = LVEF ≥ 30, VPC <10/h; group 1 = LVEF ≥ 30, VPC ≥ 10/h; group 2 = LVEF < 30, VPC ≥ 10/h; group 3 = LVEF < 0.30, VPC ≥ 10/h. From Ref. 34.

their relative risks can be multiplied to obtain the combined risk (e.g., 2.84 × 2.32 = 6.59-fold increase in risk).

d. The Rationale for Suppressing Unsustained Ventricular Arrhythmias. The four large studies that indicate an independent and reasonably strong association between ventricular arrhythmias and subsequent mortality provided a strong scientific rationale for a large-scale clinical trial to determine if suppression of ventricular arrhythmias after myocardial infarction will reduce sudden cardiac death. However, there is a serious missing link in the chain of information linking ventricular arrhythmias to sudden cardiac death. The mechanism of the spontaneous, unsustained, asymptomatic ventricular arrhythmias found after myocardial infarction is unknown. Also, it is unknown how these arrhythmias relate to the sustained arrhythmias that cause sudden cardiac death. If this important gap in our understanding of the pathophysiology could be filled, we would have a clearer view of how to proceed to prevent sudden cardiac death. Our lack of understanding of the genesis and significance of unsustained ventricular arrhythmias in coronary heart disease is underscored by the finding in CAST that suppression of ventricular arrhythmias with encainide or flecainide increased mortality [1,2]. Another new finding from CAST with important implications is that patients whose arrhythmias were suppressible on the first dose of the first drug had better survival than those whose arrhythmias were not suppressible (both groups were followed without encainide or flecainide treatment) [35]. As a group, patients who are suppressible on the first dose of the first drug had less heart failure and better left ventricular function than those who are not. However, the suppressible group still had a better survival experience after adjusting for differences between the suppressible and nonsuppressible groups, suggesting that suppressibility is an independent predictor of

Table 5 Relationship Between Signal-Averaged ECG (SAECG) and Mortality After Myocardial Infarction

Study	Total no. of patients	Percent with positive SAECG	Arrhythmic event rate (%)[a]		Relative risk
			Positive SAECG	Negative SAECG	
Breithardt et al. [36]	132	44.7	16.9	4.1	4.12
Gomes et al. [37]	102	44.1	26.5	4.2	6.37
Kuchar et al. [38]	200	39.0	15.4	0.8	18.77
Denniss et al. [39]	306	26.1	18.8	3.5	5.30
Cripps et al. [40]	159	23.9	26.3	0.8	31.84
Steinberg et al. [41]	182	39.0	15.7	4.5	3.49
Farrell et al. [42]	416	21.4	18.0	2.4	7.35
Overall	1497	30.7	19.8	2.8	7.17

[a]Sudden cardiac death (55%) or sustained ventricular tachycardia or ventricular fibrillation (45%).

arrhythmic death or cardiac arrest. There are a number of important implications of this new finding. First, it is clear, because of the controlled nature of the CAST experiment, that suppressibility of spontaneous ventricular arrhythmias after myocardial infarction is a strong indicator of outcome. This means that patients who are treated with antiarrhythmic drugs that have class I action in routine clinical practice are likely to do well even though drug therapy increases their mortality rate. Only the patients whose ventricular arrhythmias are suppressed by antiarrhythmic drugs and also tolerate them will be treated chronically. Practitioners do not treat patients if their arrhythmias are not suppressed or if they cannot tolerate the drugs. Suppressible patients have low mortality rates without treatment compared to patients whose ventricular arrhythmias are not suppressed by antiarrhythmic drugs or who do not tolerate them. Without a randomized control group, the harm done by antiarrhythmic drug treatment could not be detected. It is not clear whether this finding applies to other classes of antiarrhythmic drugs or to other methods of assessment, e.g., cardiac electrophysiological studies. Clearly, however, this is an important finding to pursue. Further explorations should lead to a better understanding of how to use this new information to predict and prevent sudden cardiac death.

2. The Signal-Averaged ECG to Predict Arrhythmic Events After Myocardial Infarction

Late potentials in the signal-averaged ECG are thought to represent late activation of portions of the ventricles due to slow conduction. Thus, late potentials in the signal-averaged ECG identify patients with an increased likelihood of sustained ventricular arrhythmias. Table 5 displays data from seven relatively small postinfarction studies that related the signal-averaged ECG to arrhythmic events during follow-up [36–42]. In all the studies together, there were 1497 patients. Most of the patients in these studies had a signal-averaged ECG done during the first 3 weeks after the acute myocardial infarction and were followed for an average of 12 to 18 months. All studies used sudden cardiac death or cardiac death and sustained ventricular arrhythmias as the endpoint. Overall, 30.7% of the patients had a positive signal-averaged ECG, each using slightly different criteria. The overall predictive accuracy of a positive test was 19.8%, and the overall predictive accuracy of a negative test was 97.2%. The pooled relative risk was 7.2; i.e., patients with a positive signal averaged ECG were 7.2 times as likely to experience an arrhythmic event as patients with a negative signal-averaged ECG. There was no interaction between a positive signal-averaged ECG and either LVEF or VPC frequency with

Table 6 Significance of Programmed Ventricular Stimulation Early After Myocardial Infarction

	Richards et al. [45]	Breithardt et al. [36]	Roy et al. [46]	Denniss et al. [39]	Bourke et al. [47]
Number of patients	165	132	150	306	1,209
Mean time between infarction and electrophysiological study (days)	10	22	12	12	11
Stimulus amplitude (mA)	<2,20	<2	<1.5	<2,20	<2,20
Prevalence of inducible VT-s[a]	23%[b]	21%	11%	20%	6%
Follow-up (months)	8±4	15±11	10±5	12±6	12±1
Number of deaths	17	8	5	22	77
Mortality rate					
With inducible VT-s[a]	26%[b]	3%	3%	22%	20%
Without inducible VT-s[a]	6%[b]	8%	4%	5%	5%
Relative risk	4.33	0.38	0.75	4.40	3.66
Spontaneous VT-s during follow-up with inducible VT-s[a]	11%	25%	3%	8%	13%

[a]VT-s = sustained ventricular tachycardia.
[b]Sustained ventricular tachycardia or ventricular fibrillation.

respect to predicting subsequent arrhythmic events [41]. Although the total experience with the signal-averaged ECG is still small, the estimated magnitude of increase in risk in these preliminary studies is impressive. The relative risk for patients with a positive signal-averaged ECG is about twice as large as the relative risk for patients who have reduced LVEF or spontaneous ventricular arrhythmias. Definitive studies that permit comparison of the signal-averaged ECG with other predictors still have not been reported, but such studies are underway and will be available in the near future.

C. Electrophysiological Studies After Myocardial Infarction

The utility of electrophysiological studies to assess risk early after acute myocardial infarction has been controversial. Patients with complicated or uncomplicated myocardial infarction have been studied using programmed ventricular stimulation [36,39,43–47], but most of the studies are small, done on biased samples, and, therefore, may not be generalizable. The best estimate of the prevalence and significance of inducible ventricular arrhythmias after myocardial infarction is provided by five studies that include more than 100 patients each (see Table 6) [36,39,45,46].

1. Prevalence of Inducible Ventricular Tachycardia

The prevalence of inducible, unsustained or sustained VT after acute myocardial infarction varies with arrhythmia definitions, selection of the patients, and the stimulation protocol. In reporting results of programmed ventricular stimulation, authors often combine unsustained and sustained VT or sustained VT and ventricular fibrillation. Combining responses to programmed ventricular stimulation can obscure prognostic significance, because different responses are associated with different event rates during follow-up. The group of patients selected for study is an important determinant of the prevalence of inducible ventricular arrhythmias as well. Denniss et al., from the Westmead Hospital in Australia, studied this relationship in 403 patients an average of 12 days after uncomplicated myocardial infarction [39]. All electrophysiological studies were done off antiarrhythmic drugs. They found that infarct size and arrhythmia markers had a substantial influence on the likelihood of inducing sustained ventricular arrhythmias. Patients with left ventricular ejection fraction < 0.40 were about 10 times as likely (52% versus 5%) to have sustained VT induced by programmed ventricular stimulation [39]. Bourke et al., also from Westmead Hospital, studied 1209 patients 11 ± 4 days after uncomplicated myocardial infarction [47]. Patients with clinical ischemia that needed treatment, heart failure, or spontaneous, sustained ventricular arrhythmias were excluded from the study; i.e., a low-risk group was recruited. Sustained VT with a cycle length ≥ 230 ms and lasting > 10 s was induced in 6.2% ($n = 75$) of the patients. There were 423 of these patients who had ventricular stimulation done and a LVEF measured. Patients with LVEF < 0.40 were 3.48 times as likely to be inducible with programmed ventricular stimulation as patients who had LVEF ≥ 0.40. A positive signal-averaged ECG and ventricular arrhythmias detected by Holter recordings also increased the likelihood of inducing sustained VT by programmed ventricular stimulation; exercise ST depression did not.

2. Stimulation Protocol Determines Prevalence of Positive Responses

Denniss et al. also found that stimulation characteristics were important determinants of the prevalence of inducible sustained ventricular arrhythmias [39]. Stimulus amplitude twice diastolic threshold was compared to a stimulus amplitude of 20 mA. The endpoint for the protocol was VT lasting ≥ 10 s. Sustained VT was induced in 20% and ventricular fibrillation in 14%. The prevalence of VT or ventricular fibrillation was about half as great for stimulation at twice diastolic threshold as for stimulation with 20-mA pulses. Bourke et al. compared a protocol that used up to four premature stimuli at an amplitude twice distolic threshold with the protocol used by Denniss et al. in 324 patients and found the protocol with up to four stimuli was twice as sensitive as the high-energy stimulation protocol (46% versus 23%) [47]. Also, the predictive value of a positive test was greater for the protocol using more premature stimuli (20% versus 14%). The predictive value of a negative test was about the same for the two protocols (98% versus 97%).

3. Prediction of Mortality by Programmed Ventricular Stimulation Early After Myocardial Infarction

Data from the five studies that enrolled more than 100 patients are summarized in Table 6. In the 1983 Westmead Hospital report [45], patients with ≥ 10 s of VT or ventricular fibrillation had a 1-year mortality rate of 26%, contrasted with 6% for patients who did not have one of these arrhythmias induced (relative risk 4.33, $p < 0.01$). In inducible patients, 80% of the deaths were instantaneous, and ventricular tachyarrhythmias were documented in 63%; none of the uninducible patients died instantaneously. In 1986, the same group reported another study in which 22% of those with inducible sustained VT early after myocardial infarction developed spontaneous sustained VT, ventricular fibrillation, or instantaneous death by 2 years of follow-up, compared to 5% in those without inducible sustained VT (relative risk 4.40, $p < 0.01$) [39]. Ventricular fibrillation induced by a programmed stimulation during the first month after myocardial infarction did not predict spontaneous sustained VT, ventricular fibrillation, or death during follow-up. In the study by Roy et al. [46], the incidence of spontaneous sustained VT and sudden cardiac death during follow-up did not differ between the groups with and without inducible ventricular tachyarrhythmias; however, the event rate was very low (two sudden cardiac deaths and two sustained VTs in 10 months of follow-up). With such a low event rate, the power to detect a threefold difference between the two groups is less than 50%. Bourke et al. found that patients with inducible sustained VT (cycle length ≥ 230 ms and lasting > 10 s) had an arrhythmic event (spontaneous VT, ventricular fibrillation, or witnessed instantaneous death) rate of 20% (15/75) in the first year of follow-up versus a rate of 5% (62/1134) for patients who were not inducible [47].

4. Ventricular Fibrillation Induced by Programmed Ventricular Stimulation Is a Poor Predictor of Arrhythmic Events

Much of the controversy about postinfarction electrophysiological studies may be attributable to the lack of association of inducible ventricular fibrillation with subsequent death. Nearly all of the smaller studies that did not find an association between inducible ventricular arrhythmias and death used VT and fibrillation as a combined endpoint. In patients who had inducible, sustained VT less than 1 month after myocardial infarction, the factors that predicted death were: anterior myocardial infarction, left ventricular ejection fraction < 0.30, presence of ventricular aneurysm, increased QRS duration in the signal-averaged ECG, and slower induced VT rates [45]. Studies are not available to show whether treating inducible sustained VT decreases the rate of death or spontaneous sustained ventricular arrhythmias. Such studies are badly needed.

D. Variability of RR Intervals

1. Standard Deviation of Normal RR Intervals (SDNN) to Predict Mortality of All Causes After Myocardial Infarction

Ventricular fibrillation is promoted by increased sympathetic activity [48–50] and by decreased vagal activity [51–53]. In 1987, Kleiger et al. reported a strong association between the standard deviation of the normal RR intervals (SDNN) calculated over 24 hours and all-cause mortality in the Multicenter Post Myocardial Infarction Program (MPIP) [54]. For the 808 patients in the study, the standard deviation of all normal RR (NN) intervals during a 24-h continuous ECG recording, the SDNN, was < 50 ms in 15.5% of the patients, and this subgroup had a mortality rate of 34.4% compared to 12.3% for patients with SDNN ≥ 50 ms, a relative risk of 2.8. SDNN was weakly correlated with age, heart rate, and measures of left ventricular function, but not with ventricular arrhythmias. Of all the Holter variables, SDNN had the strongest association with all-cause mortality. After adjusting statistically for other risk predictors (age, New York Heart Association functional class, rales in coronary-care unit, LVEF, and ventricular arrhythmias), SDNN was still significantly associated with all-cause mortality over the next 4 years. This is an important result because of the large group of representative patients enrolled ($n = 808$) and the 127 deaths that occurred during follow-up, permitting precise estimation of death rates.

2. Power Spectral Measures of RR Variability and All-Cause Mortality or Arrhythmic Death

SDNN measures both slow and fast oscillations in RR interval and does not, therefore, provide specific information on the vagal or sympathetic modulation of RR intervals. However, its independence from left ventricular function and ventricular arrhythmias does suggest that it provides information about a different lethal force, probably information about the autonomic nervous system. To examine the contribution of autonomic nervous activity to prediction of all-cause and cause-specific (cardiac and arrhythmic) death, Bigger et al. reanalyzed 715 24-h ECG recordings from MPIP [55]. Digitized 24-h ECGs were analyzed to compute the power spectra for the entire 24-h period and power in four frequency bands was calculated: (1)

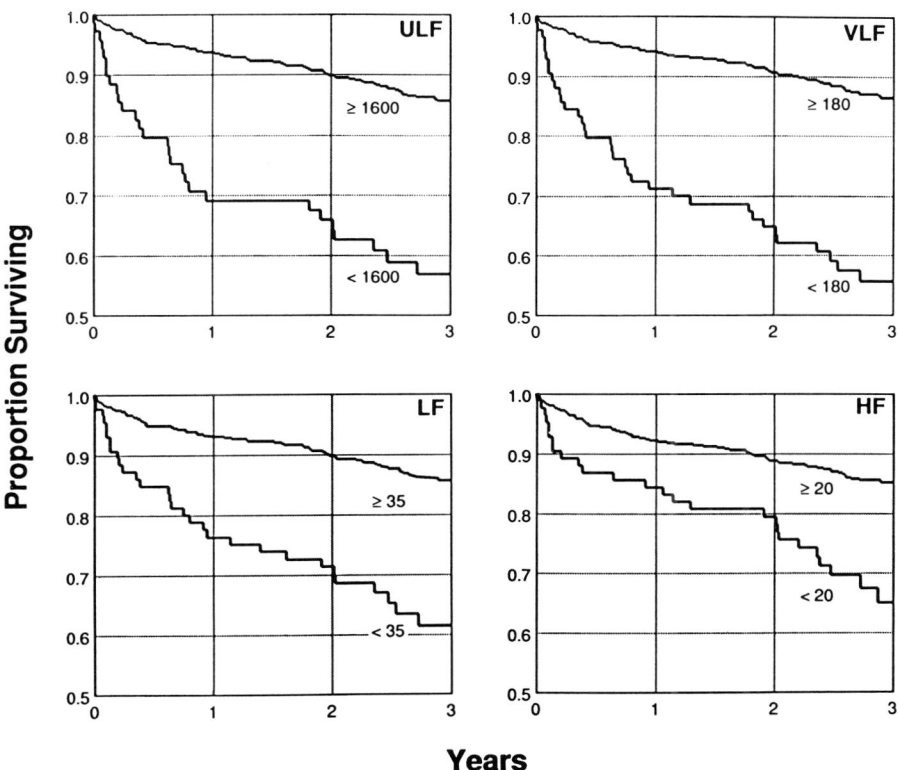

Figure 4 Prediction of mortality by frequency domain measures of RR interval variability. From Ref. 55.

<0.0033 Hz, ultralow-frequency power; (2) 0.0033 to <0.04 Hz, very-low-frequency power; (3) 0.04 to 0.15 Hz, low-frequency power; and (4) 0.15 to 0.40 Hz, high-frequency power. Also, total power (≤ 0.40 Hz) and the ratio of low- to high-frequency power were calculated. Each measure of RR variability had a significant and at least moderately strong univariate association with three mortality endpoints: all-cause mortality, cardiac death, and arrhythmic death (see Fig. 4). This study estimates mortality rates and relative risks with considerable precision because there were 119 deaths that occurred during 31 months of follow-up, with 88 of these classified as cardiac and 68 as arrhythmic. After adjustment for important covariates (age, New York Heart Association functional class, rales in the CCU phase of acute myocardial infarction, left ventricular ejection fraction, and ventricular arrhythmias) using a Cox regression model, ultralow- and low-frequency power remained strongly and significantly associated with death. Low- and high-frequency power were not strongly associated with death after adjustment for the same covariates. Very-low-frequency power was more strongly associated with arrhythmic death than all-cause mortality or cardiac death, before and after adjustment for other risk predictors. Combining measures of RR variability with left ventricular ejection fraction or ventricular arrhythmias identified small subgroups of postinfarction patients with a 2.5-year mortality rate greater than 50%. This study suggested that slower cycling variability was

a stronger predictor than the high-frequency variability that reflects vagal tone. The physiological mechanism for ultralow-frequency modulation of RR intervals is not known.

3. Correlations Among Time and Frequency Domain Measures of RR Variability After Myocardial Infarction

Bigger et al. explored the correlations between the most commonly used time domain and frequency domain measures of heart period variability using the MPIP sample [56]. There were three natural clusters among the time and frequency domain variables: (1) total power, ultralow-frequency power, SDNN, and SDANN index (the standard deviation of the average RR interval for each 5-min period in a 24-h ECG recording); (2) very-low-frequency power, low-frequency power, and SDNN index; and (3) high-frequency power, r-MSSD (the root-mean-squared successive difference), and pNN50 (the proportion of adjacent NN intervals that differ by 50 ms or more). All of the time domain measures of RR variability were significantly associated with all-cause mortality, but SDANN index and SDNN index had the strongest univariate associations with death. After adjusting for other risk predictors, only SDNN, SDANN index, and SDNN index were significantly associated with all-cause mortality. These findings are quite similar to the findings for the corresponding frequency domain variables in this same data set [55].

4. Heart Rate Variability Index, All-Cause Mortality, and Arrhythmic Events

Odemuyiwa et al. [57] studied 385 survivors of myocardial infarction to compare the sensitivity and specificity of left ventricular ejection fraction and heart rate variability index, a time domain measure derived from the distribution of normal RR intervals in a 24-h ECG recording that is dominated by ultralow-frequency information. Endpoints were all-cause mortality ($n = 44$), arrhythmic events (sudden death or symptomatic, sustained VT) ($n = 26$), and sudden death ($n = 14$). For all-cause mortality, heart rate variability index and left ventricular ejection fraction had similar sensitivity and specificity (75% and 50%). For arrhythmic events, heart rate variability index of ≤30 units had a sensitivity of 75% and a specificity of 76%, while left ventricular ejection fraction ≤ 0.40 had a sensitivity of 42% and a specificity of 75%. For sudden death, when sensitivity was set at 75%, heart rate variability index had a specificity of 75% compared to a specificity of 47% for left ventricular ejection fraction. These findings suggest that heart period variability predicts arrhythmic events better than nonarrhythmic events.

5. The Correlation Between Heart Rate Variability Index and Spontaneous Ventricular Arrhythmias or the Signal-Averaged ECG

Farrell et al. studied 416 survivors of myocardial infarction to investigate the prognostic value of heart period variability in combination with ventricular arrhythmias found in a 24-h ECG recording or a positive signal-averaged ECG [58]. Thrombolytic therapy was given to 48% of these patients, and 24% had coronary artery bypass graft surgery or percutaneous transluminal coronary angioplasty. The continuous 24-h ECG recording and signal-averaged ECG were done 5 to 7 days after infarction. A heart rate variability index < 20 ms (a measure of ultralow-frequency RR variability) was found in 113 (27%) of the 416 patients. Ventricular premature complex frequency >10/h was found in 84 (20%) patients, and repetitive ventricular premature complexes were found in 86 (21%). Also, 110 (26%) of the patients had a left ventricular ejection fraction < 0.40, and 210 (50%) had a positive exercise test. Heart rate variability index was positively correlated with average normal RR (NN) interval ($r = 0.56$) and LVEF ($r = 0.30$), and inversely correlated with age ($r = 0.22$). Heart rate variability index was significantly associated with a positive signal-averaged ECG (odds ratio, 3.0). The signal averaged ECG was abnormal in 89 (21%) of the 416 patients. A positive signal-averaged ECG was associated significantly with age > 65 years, ventricular ectopy, and low values (< 20 ms) of the RR variability index (odds ratio = 3.0, $p < 0.001$), but not with left ventricular ejection fraction, positive exercise test, or site of myocardial infarction.

6. Heart Rate Variability Index, Mortality, and Arrhythmic Events

During a mean follow-up of 612 days, there were 47 cardiac deaths and 24 arrhythmic events. The best univariate predictor of cardiac death were heart rate variability (relative risk = 7; 95% confidence interval, 4–12). The best univariate predictors of arrhythmic events (arrhythmic deaths using the Cardiac Arrhythmia Pilot Study definition) or sustained ventricular tachyarrhythmia) were heart rate variability index (relative risk = 32; 95% confidence interval, 8–138), followed by signal-averaged ECG (relative risk = 7; 95% confidence interval, 3–15) and repetitive ventricular premature complexes in the Holter recording (relative risk = 5; 95% confidence interval, 2–11). Left ventricular ejection fraction and Killip class were weaker predictors of arrhythmic events. In a Cox regression analysis, the best combination of predictors for arrhythmic events was: heart rate variability index < 20 units, a positive signal-averaged ECG, and repetitive ventricular premature complexes. After these three variables were in the model, heart rate, LVEF, and positive exercise test did not add significantly to the prediction of arrhythmic events. Heart rate variability index did not predict nonfatal myocardial infarction.

7. Specificity of the Heart Rate Variability Index for Predicting Arrhythmic Events

These results suggest that heart rate variability index has some specificity for predicting arrhythmic events, i.e., it predicts arrhythmic events better than cardiac death or nonfatal reinfarction. Even though heart rate variability index is significantly associated with a positive signal-averaged ECG, these two risk predictors each have substantial predictive power independent of the other. The prediction of arrhythmic events by heart rate variability index also seems to be independent of spontaneous ventricular arrhythmias, LVEF values, and positive exercise tests.

E. Baroreflex Sensitivity (BRS)

1. BRS and Ventricular Fibrillation with Ischemia During Exercise

BRS usually is measured by quantifying how much the RR intervals increase when blood pressure increases. The study by Schwartz et al. [59] definitively demonstrated that depressed BRS was associated with susceptibility to ventricular fibrillation in dogs with healed experimental myocardial infarction. This animal model of sudden death incorporates three features often implicated in human sudden death: (1) healed myocardial infarction (created by ligation of the left anterior descending coronary artery); (2) a transient episode of myocardial ischemia; and (3) physiologically increased sympathetic nervous activity. One month after experimental myocardial infarction, the dogs ran on a treadmill. When their heart rate reached the target rate of 220 beats/min, the left circumflex coronary artery was occluded for 2 min with a previously implanted balloon occluder. More than half the dogs develop ventricular fibrillation during this ''exercise/ischemia test.'' The response to the test is very reproducible. Susceptible dogs have high values for BRS and are incapable of responding to acute myocardial ischemia with vagally mediated reductions in heart rate. BRS measurement before the exercise/ischemia test accurately predicted the occurrence of ventricular fibrillation. Moreover, measurement of BRS before the experimental infarct predicted the BRS after infarction and the response to the exercise/ischemia test. Exercise training of dogs with low BRS after infarction increased the BRS and converted dogs from susceptible to resistant to ventricular fibrillation.

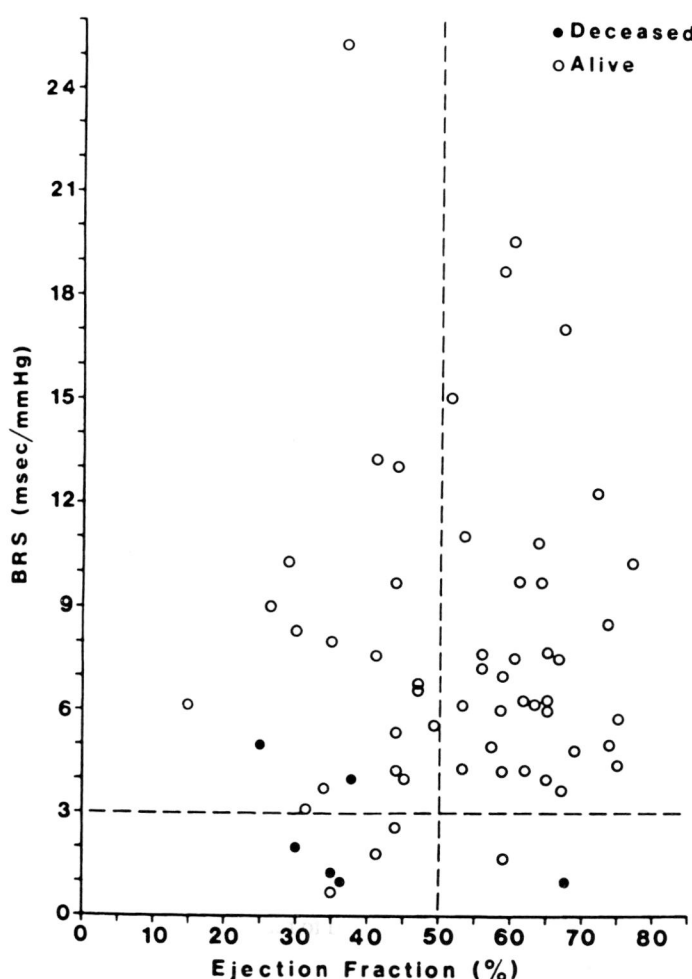

Figure 5 Relations among baroreflex sensitivity (BRS), left ventricular ejection fraction, and cardiovascular mortality. Broken lines indicate the arbitrary limits for reduced LVEF (<50%) and for markedly reduced BRS (<3 ms/mmHg). BRS improves the prediction of death in patients with depressed left ventricular function. From Ref. 60.

2. Preliminary Studies of BRS After Myocardial Infarction in Man

On the basis of the experimental studies conducted by Schwartz and colleagues, La Rovere et al. evaluated BRS in 78 low-risk patients 1 month after myocardial infarction [60]. All were men who had survived for 30 days after their first myocardial infarction, were below age 65, and were all able to perform a maximal exercise stress test off all drugs. The 2-year mortality for this selected group was low, 9%. This study documented that BRS is not correlated with LVEF ($r = 0.07$), so that a depressed BRS must provide prognostic information independent of LVEF (see Fig. 5). During 2 years of follow-up, seven patients died, four of them suddenly. The BRS was markedly lower in the 7 patients who died than in the 71 survivors (2.4 ± 1.5 versus 8.2 ± 4.8 ms/mmHg) ($p < 0.005$). Patients with BRS < 3.0 ms/mmHg (i.e., 1 standard deviation below the mean for the entire group) had a mortality rate of 50%, versus 3% for those with BRS ≥ 3.0. These rates should be viewed with caution, because the small number of patients who died ($n = 7$) make these estimates of mortality rates imprecise. Nevertheless, the difference in BRS values between those who survived and those who died is impressively large.

3. BRS and Arrhythmic Events After Myocardial Infarction

The initial results of La Rovere et al. were confirmed in a study by Farrell et al. in 122 patients who had myocardial infarction 7–10 days earlier [61]. During 1 year of follow-up, there were 13 deaths and 10 documented arrhythmic events (five sudden deaths and five sustained VTs requiring hospital admission). The BRS of the patients who had major arrhythmic events was substantially lower than those who did not (1.73 ± 1.49 versus 7.83 ± 4.50 ms/mmHg) ($p < 0.0001$). However, the relative risk for arrhythmic events was 23 (95% confidence interval, 7.7–69.2), comparing patients with BRS < 3.0 to those with BRS ≥ 3.0. This relative risk was greater than that for either depressed LVEF (relative risk = 10.4; 95% confidence interval, 3.3–32.6) or reduced heart rate variability index (relative risk = 10.1; 95% confidence interval, 5.6–18.1).

4. Is RR Variability or BRS the Better Predictor of Sudden Death or Arrhythmic Events?

Even though these two studies are too small to permit definite conclusions, they suggest that BRS is a powerful predictor of arrhythmic death in patients with recent myocardial infarction. The data suggest that BRS is superior to RR variability as a predictor of arrhythmic events. A natural history study, ATRAMI (Autonomic Tone and Reflexes After Myocardial Infarction), is underway to determine the relative merits of RR variability and BRS. This prospective epidemiological study, involving over 20 enrolling centers in Europe, the United States, and Japan, is designed to test the prognostic value of baroreflex sensitivity and of RR variability in a large population of patients with a myocardial infarction; left ventricular ejection fraction, and the presence of late potentials also will be determined. ATRAMI began recruitment in the summer of 1990 and is scheduled to reach its target sample size of 1200 by the end of 1994.

F. Combinations of Risk Predictors

Risk predictors found to have moderate positive predictive accuracy for total, cardiovascular, or arrhythmic death individually often perform much better when combined with other risk predictors. Examples include low left ventricular ejection fraction combined with frequent or repetitive ventricular arrhythmias in 24-h continuous ECG recordings, which increases the positive predictive accuracy from about 15% to 25% [23,55]. Another example is a positive signal-averaged ECG combined with low left ventricular ejection fraction or ventricular arrhythmias, which increase the positive predictive accuracy from about 20% to 35% [41]. Also, ultralow-frequency power in the heart period power spectrum combined either with LVEF or ventricular arrhythmias gives positive predictive accuracies of about 50% [55]. Combining heart rate variability index, a positive signal-averaged ECG, and repetitive ventricular premature complexes also yielded a positive predictive accuracy of about 50% [58]. To be used together, variables must have modest associations at most with each other. Combining variables not only has the benefit of increasing positive predictive accuracy, but also has the adverse effect of decreasing the size of the group subject to treatment.

G. Future Needs in Risk Stratification

There still is a great deal of work to do to improve risk stratification after myocardial infarction and in chronic heart diseases. Progress has been substantial in recent years, and hopefully rapid progress will continue during the next few years.

H. The Importance of Randomized Clinical Trials to Evaluate Therapy

Even after risk stratification has developed to the point of providing a positive predictive value of 50%, treatments that are hypothesized to be of benefit will have to be evaluated in randomized, controlled clinical trials. It would be easier to select treatments to interrupt harmful pathophysiological sequences if we had a better understanding of the mechanisms that lead to death in various cardiovascular diseases. Modification of risk predictors does not ensure a beneficial effect on survival. We have learned that suppressing ventricular arrhythmias with class I drugs increases mortality rates, and that treating patients with heart failure with inotropic drugs can increase mortality rates. We probably will never understand the pathophysiological mechanism and the treatments well enough to circumvent randomized clinical trials.

III. TREATMENT OF HIGH-RISK PATIENTS TO PREVENT FATAL ARRHYTHMIAS AFTER MYOCARDIAL INFARCTION

Beta-adrenergic blocking drugs are the only treatment that is established as safe and effective for reducing the risk of arrhythmic events after myocardial infarction. Angiotensin-converting enzyme inhibitors have recently been shown to be associated with a modest decrease in total mortality rates in patients who have heart failure after myocardial infarction [62–64]. The CONSENSUS trial suggested that converting enzyme inhibitors had no detectable benefit for sudden cardiac death [62]. The evidence is conflicting on whether prophylactic use of converting enzyme inhibitors in patients with left ventricular dysfunction, but no clinical heart failure, will improve survival. SOLVD and CONSENSUS II showed no benefit [65,66], while SAVE did [64]. Furthermore, our confidence in antiarrhythmic drug therapy for ventricular arrhythmias has been shaken by the adverse effects of two drugs with class IC antiarrhythmic action in CAST I, i.e., encainide and flecainide [1,2] and by the lack of efficacy of a drug with class IA antiarrhythmic action in CAST II, i.e., moricizine [67]. Other small randomized clincal trials tend to support the findings of the larger trials.

A. Amiodarone for Prophylaxis of Ventricular Arrhythmias

Currently, amiodarone is indicated only for treatment of sustained, symptomatic ventricular arrhythmias. In an unusual move, the Food and Drug Administration permitted amiodarone to be marketed for this indication without any randomized controlled clinical trials [68]. Encouraging uncontrolled experience with amiodarone and the discouraging experience with antiarrhythmic drugs that have class I action have raised considerable interest in extending the use of amiodarone to unsustained, but prognostically important, ventricular arrhythmias. Ongoing clinical trials are examining the advisability of prophylactic amiodarone treatment for unsustained ventricular arrhythmias.

1. Amiodarone Prophylaxis After Myocardial Infarction

There are at least two large randomized clinical trials underway to evaluate the use of amiodarone for patients with recent myocardial infarction. The Canadian Myocardial Infarction Amiodarone Trial (CAMIAT) is an ongoing randomized, placebo-controlled clinical trial to evaluate amiodarone treatment (a drug with class I, II, III antiarrhythmic action) in patients with prognostically significant, but asymptomatic, ventricular arrhythmias after myocardial infarction [69]. A ventricular premature complex frequency of $\geq 10/h$ is required to qualify for CAMIAT. Patients do not have to have a low ejection fraction or clinical heart failure to qualify for amiodarone treatment in CAMIAT. The European Myocardial Infarction Amiodarone Trial (EMIAT) is evaluating amiodarone treatment in patients with left ventricular ejection fraction < 0.40 after myocardial infarction. Ventricular arrhythmias are not required to qualify for EMIAT.

2. Amiodarone Prophylaxis for Ventricular Arrhythmias in Patients with Heart Failure

In addition to the postinfarction studies, the Veterans Administration Cooperative Studies Program is conducting a randomized, double-blind, placebo-controlled clinical trial that is enrolling in 25 clinical centers to determine whether patients with heart failure and frequent VPC have improved survival when treated with amiodarone. To qualify for the VA study, which is called CHF STAT, patients must have class III or IV congestive heart failure, defined as: (1) dyspnea at rest or with minimal exertion, (2) left ventricular internal diastolic dimension $\geq$ 55 mm by echocardiogram or a cardiothoracic ratio > 0.50 by chest X-ray, and (3) LVEF $\leq$ 0.40 by radionuclide ventriculogram. In addition, patients must have an average of $\geq$ 10 VPC/h on a 24-h continuous ECG recording. CHF STAT plans to enroll about 700 patients and follow them for a minimum of 2 years. Patients will be randomized to placebo or amiodarone. The amiodarone doses will be (1) 800 mg/day for 14 days, (2) 400 mg/day for 50 weeks, and (3) 300 mg/day until the end of the study. All patients are treated with enalapril if it is tolerated. If enalapril is not tolerated, they are treated with captopril or hydralazine and isosorbide dinitrate.

B. Randomized Clinical Trials of ICD Prophylaxis

Other randomized clinical trials are evaluating prophylactic treatment with implantable cardioverter-defibrillators (ICD) [70,71]. This is a bold step, since there is no evidence from randomized clinical trials that ICDs improve survival in patients who have malignant (i.e., sustained and hemodynamically important) ventricular arrhythmias. Although sudden death rates have been reported to be as low as 5% at 5 years after implantation [72], such optimistic results have been questioned [73]. First, sudden cardiac death is a judgmental diagnosis, i.e., subject to interpretation. Second, the low non-sudden death rates in ICD follow-up studies suggest a selection bias favoring ICD therapy. Since the ICD is a treatment of last resort, it is often used a relatively long time after the presenting event. As a result of delay, the sickest patients may die before an implant can be done, making the mortality rate for ICD therapy lower than for historical controls. Even if sudden death were totally eliminated by ICD treatment, it might not reduce the all-cause mortality rate much. Patients dying of malignant ventricular arrhythmias usually have other risks as well as arrhythmic risk, e.g., chronic multivessel coronary disease and left ventricular dysfunction. ICD treatment might not prolong survival very much, because death from ischemia or heart failure may cancel the benefit of eliminating arrhythmic deaths.

1. ICD Therapy for Malignant Ventricular Arrhythmias

We will never know how much ICD treatment improves survival compared to no therapy in patients who have survived an episode of cardiac arrest or sustained VT. However, three studies will be done to compare ICD therapy to drug therapy in patients with malignant ventricular arrhythmias: the Canadian Implantable Defibrillator Study (CIDS), the Cardiac Arrest Study of Hamburg (CASH), and the NHLBI trial Antiarrhythmics versus Implantable Defibrillators (AVID). CIDS, CASH, and the NHLBI study cannot estimate accurately the benefit of ICD treatment, because each has or plans to have a positive control group; i.e., ICD treatment is being compared to drug therapy. For example, in the CIDS, no difference between ICD and amiodarone therapy could result if both treatments have little effect, or if both have beneficial or harmful effects of similar magnitude. A large difference in favor of ICD treatment could indicate a substantial benefit of ICD therapy or a modest benefit coupled with a harmful effect of amiodarone. Nevertheless, if these trials show a better outcome for patients assigned to ICD treatment, it will provide important support for ICD treatment and prophylaxis.

2. The Rationale for Prophylactic Treatment of Patients with Unsustained Ventricular Tachycardia

A meta-analysis was done by Kowey et al. for the 12 studies that reported results of programmed ventricular stimulation in 926 patients with heart disease and unsustained VT [74]. The mean age was 61 years, 80% were male, 88% had coronary heart disease, and 72% had previous myocardial infarction. One-third ($n = 302$) of the patients had sustained ventricular arrhythmias induced by programmed ventricular stimulation. The studies that enrolled only patients with LVEF < 0.40 had higher percentages of positive tests, about 45%. During an average follow-up of 19.4 months, 100 arrhythmic events occurred: 60 sudden cardiac deaths, 39 episodes of spontaneous, sustained VT, and 1 episode of syncope attributed to VT. The arrhythmic event rate was 17.9% for the inducible patients and 7.4% for noninducible patients, a relative risk of 2.4. Programmed ventricular stimulation had a positive predictive accuracy, 18% and a negative predictive accuracy, 93%. There is no convincing evidence that antiarrhythmic drug therapy guided by results of programmed ventricular stimulation improves survival in patients with left ventricular dysfunction and unsustained VT. However, the high risk in this group for arrhythmic events makes it a prime target for randomized controlled trials to evaluate treatment effects on survival.

3. The Multicenter UnSustained Tachycardia Trial (MUSTT)

MUSTT will test the hypothesis that electrophysiologically guided antiarrhythmic therapy will reduce the risk of arrhythmic death or cardiac arrest in patients with unsustained VT and left ventricular dysfunction (see Table 7) [70,71]. MUSTT started in October 1991 with 25 clinical centers in North America participating. MUSTT plans to enroll patients with coronary heart disease who are age < 80 years, have a left ventricular ejection fraction < 0.41, and have asymptomatic, or minimally symptomatic, unsustained VT (duration, 3 complexes to 30 s, rate, ≥ 100/min). Patients who are anticipated to need coronary artery bypass graft (CABG) surgery or angioplasty are not enrolled. Patients who qualify and consent have an electrophysiological study, and those who are not inducible will be followed on no therapy. About 900 patients who have inducible, sustained ventricular arrhythmias will be randomized. Half will be followed on no antiarrhythmic treatment and half will have antiarrhythmic treatment guided by serial electrophysiological studies. Seven drugs (procainamide, quinidine, disopyramide, mexiletine, propafenone, acebutalol, and amiodarone) will be used. Two drug failures are required before amiodarone can be used, and three drug failures are required before ICD therapy can be

Table 7 Design Features of ICD Prophylaxis Trials in Patients with Coronary Heart Disease[a]

	MUSTT	MADIT	CABG Patch II
Stratification variable(s)	Center	Center, Time after MI	Center, LV ejection fraction
Eligibility criteria	Coronary heart disease	Q-wave MI	CABG surgery
	Age < 80	Age < 75	Age < 80
	LVEF < 0.41	LVEF < 0.36	LVEF < 0.36
	Unsustained VT	Unsustained VT	SAECG positive
	Inducible VT	Inducible VT, fail procainamide	
Primary endpoint	Sudden death, cardiac arrest	Death from any cause	Death from any cause
Minimum follow-up (mo.)	24	6	24
Average follow-up (mo.)	36	26	40
Event rate			
Control group	15.0% (24 mo.)	30.0% (26 mo.)	36.5% (40 mo.)
ICD group	10.0% (24 mo.)	16.3% (26 mo.)	27.0% (40 mo.)
Percent reduction	33.3%	46.0%	26.0%
Alpha	5.0%	5.0%	5.0%
Power (1-beta)	80.0%	85.0%	85.0%
Drop-in rate	Not estimated	<5.0%	10.0%
Drop-out rate	Not estimated	<5.0%	6.0%
Sample size (each group)	450	140	400

[a]VT = ventricular tachycardia.

chosen. Early results suggest that about 35% to 40% of MUSTT patients will be inducible and that about 40% of these will fail a series of antiarrhythmic drugs and be offered ICD therapy.

a. What Will We Learn from MUSTT? MUSTT should determine whether patients with LVEF < 0.41 and unsustained VT are significantly benefited by prophylactic drug treatment guided by electrophysiological studies. MUSTT will not give a definitive answer about which drugs are more efficacious, better tolerated, or safer, although trends may develop that generate hypotheses. Similarly, MUSTT cannot estimate definitively the benefit of ICD therapy relative to no treatment or drug treatment, because only about 100 patients will receive ICDs and there will be no randomized comparison of the ICD group with any other group. MUSTT will provide precise estimates of how good electrophysiological testing is for assessing risk and, for the first time, will determine the outcome of uninducible and inducible patients without the confounding effects of antiarrhythmic drug treatment.

4. The Multicenter Automatic Defibrillator Implantation Trial (MADIT)

MADIT is testing the hypothesis that implantation of an ICD in patients with coronary heart disease, left ventricular dysfunction, and unsustained VT will result in a significant reduction in all-cause mortality when compared to "conventional" pharmacological therapy [75]. MADIT began enrolling in the fall of 1990 in 24 hospitals in the United States and Europe. MADIT is enrolling patients who have had a Q-wave myocardial infarction, who are < 75 years of age, have a left ventricular ejection fraction < 0.36, and have asymptomatic, unsustained VT (3 to 30 complexes, rate ≥120/min). Patients who are anticipated to need CABG surgery or angioplasty are not enrolled. Patients who enroll have an electrophysiological study, and those with sustained, inducible ventricular arrhythmias that do not respond to an intravenous procainamide infusion are randomized to conventional pharmacological therapy (ranging from no treatment to amiodarone treatment) chosen by the patients' private physician or to ICD implantation. MADIT expects to enroll about 280 patients, but has a sequential design, and will be stopped when the difference in all-cause mortality between the two groups crosses a boundary indicating that the ICD group is significantly better or worse than conventional therapy.

a. What Will We Learn from MADIT? MADIT should clarify whether prophylactic treatment with an ICD significantly improves survival in patients with left ventricular dysfunction, unsustained ventricular tachycardia, and inducible, sustained ventricular tachycardia. This information will be a valuable addition to medical science. However, MADIT cannot estimate definitively the effect size of ICD therapy relative to no treatment or to any particular drug therapy. Some of the patients in the control group will not be treated at all, while others will be treated with drugs, many with amiodrarone. Interpretation of the mortality rate in the ICD group will be governed by the profile of treatment in the control group.

5. The CABG Patch Trial

The CABG Patch Trial will test the hypothesis that implantation of an ICD in high-risk patients who are having CABG surgery will improve survival [76]. A pilot study began in September 1990; the full-scale trial began in March 1993. The CABG Patch Trial is enrolling patients with coronary heart disease who are having elective CABG surgery, are <80 years of age, have a left ventricular ejection fraction < 0.36, and have a positive signal-averaged ECG. Patients are randomized to ICD therapy or to a control group that receives no additional therapy except for their routine CABG surgery. The CABG Patch Trial expects to randomize about 800 patients in 30 centers and follow them 2 to 5 years.

a. What Will We Learn from the CABG Patch Trial? The CABG Patch Trial will determine whether ICD prophylaxis will improve survival of high-risk patients (LVEF < 0.36 and positive signal-averaged ECG) having CABG surgery. It will clarify the magnitude of benefit of ICD therapy on mortality of all-causes. Since the control group is not being treated, the CABG Patch Trial will be able to estimate precisely the magnitude of the effect of ICD therapy on survival of coronary heart disease patients; it is the only ICD trial underway or contemplated that can do this. This trial is not confounded by antiarrhythmic drug therapy. The CABG Patch Trial will not be confounded by the effects of thoracotomy or by ischemic events either, since both the ICD-treated group and the control group have thoracotomy and complete surgical revascularization. The effect of thoracotomy can be factored out to estimate the efficacy of nonthoracotomy ICD systems. Since the treatment employed in the CABG Patch Trial addresses only tachyarrhythmic deaths and the control group gets no treatment that will cloud the issue, the trial should clarify the extent to which currently used mechanistic classifications of death are valid. Finally, the CABG patch Trial is well positioned to provide new insights into the pathophysiology of sudden cardiac death.

6. The German Dilated Cardiomyopathy Study (GDCMS)

The German Dilated Cardiomyopathy Study is testing the hypothesis that implantation of an ICD in patients with dilated cardiomyopathy will result in a significant reduction in all-cause mortality when compared to no antiarrhythmic treatment [77]. The German Dilated Cardiomyopathy Study began a pilot study in 1991 in eight German hospitals, enrolling patients who have noncoronary dilated cardiomyopathy, who are 18–70 years of age, have a left ventricular ejection fraction ≤ 0.30, and have class II or III congestive heart failure. Patients who have symptomatic ventricular arrhythmias or coronary heart disease are excluded. Baseline studies include 24-h continuous ECG recordings, a signal-averaged ECG, exercise testing, and an electrophysiological study. After baseline studies, patients are randomized to no antiarrhythmic therapy or to ICD implantation via the transvenous approach, if possible. The ICD group and the control group will be treated aggressively for heart failure with digitalis, diuretics, and angiotensin-coinverting enzyme inhibitors. After recruitment and follow-up of 100 patients, the accumulating data will be examined and a decision will be made to continue or discontinue the study. If the study is continued, the German Dilated Cardiomyopathy Study ultimately expects to enroll about 720 patients based on the expectation that a 30% one-year mortality rate in the control group will be reduced to 24%.

a. What Will We Learn from the German Dilated Cardiomyopathy Study? The German Dilated Cardiomyopathy Study should clarify whether prophylactic treatment with an ICD significantly improves survival in patients with dilated cardiomyopathy and heart failure. This study can estimate definitively the effect size of ICD therapy relative to no treatment in this high-risk group. Also, the German Dilated Cardiomyopathy Study will provide valuable information on the natural history of a homogeneous group of noncoronary cardiomyopathy patients who have well-defined left ventricular dysfunction and functional capacity, but who have not had sustained or symptomatic ventricular arrhythmias.

7. Should ICD Prophylaxis Be Used in Conventional Practice?

There is no significant evidence that ICD therapy reduces all-cause mortality. Therefore, there is no scientific justification for ICD prophylaxis at the present time. Recent experience in cardiovascular clinical trials has taught us that hopes for therapeutic benefit often are not realized in practice. The cost and quality of life issues surrounding ICD therapy dictate that substantial scientific evidence for benefit accumulate from randomized clinical trials before ICD prophylaxis is recommended. It is hoped that practicing physicians and surgeons, clinical trials scientists, device manufacturers, and the National Heart Lung and Blood Institute will cooperate to gather the critical information needed to evaluate the value of ICD prophylaxis in patients who are at high risk for sudden cardiac death. We hope that either amiodarone or ICD therapy will show benefit in ongoing studies, because a therapy capable of preventing sudden death is sorely needed for high-risk cardiac patients.

ACKNOWLEDGMENTS

This work was supported in part by NIH grants HL-41552, HL-48120, and HL-48159 from the National Heart, Lung, and Blood Institute, Bethesda, MD, and RR-00645 from the Research Resources Administration, NIH; and by funds from Cardiac Pacemakers, Inc., The Bugher Foundation, The Dover Foundation, and Mrs. Adelaide Segerman, New York, NY.

REFERENCES

1. The Cardiac Arrhythmia Suppression Trial (CAST) Investigators. Effect of encainide and flecainide on mortality in a randomized trial of arrhythmia suppression after myocardial infarction. N Engl J Med 1989; 321:406–412.
2. Echt DS, Liebson PR, Mitchell LB, et al., and the CAST Investigators. Mortality and morbidity in patients randomized to receive encainide, flecainide, or placebo in the Cardiac Arrhythmia Suppression Trial. N Engl J Med 1991; 324:781–788.
3. Marcus FI, Cobb LA, Edwards JE, et al., and the Multicenter Post-infarction Research Group. Mechanism of death and prevalence of myocardial ischemic symptoms in the terminal event after acute myocardial infarction. Am J Cardiol 1988; 61:8–15.

4. Rutherford BD, McCann WD, O'Donnovan TPB. The value of monitoring pulmonary artery pressure for early detection of left ventricular failure following myocardial infarction. Circulation 1971; 43:655–666.
5. Ratshin RA, Rackley CE, Russell RO. Hemodynamic evaluation of left ventricular function in shock complicating myocardial infarction. Circulation 1972; 45:127–139.
6. Forrester JS, Diamond GA, Swan HJC. Correlative classification of clinical and hemodynamic function after myocardial infarction. Am J Cardiol 1977; 39:137–145.
7. Weber KT, Janicki JJ, Russell RO, Rackley CE. Identification of high risk subsets of acute myocardial infarction. Derived from the Myocardial Infarction Research Units Cooperative Study Data Bank. Am J Cardiol 1978; 41:197–203.
8. Shell W, Peter T, Mickle D, Forrester JS, Swan HJC. Prognostic implications of reduction of left ventricular filling pressure in early transmural acute myocardial infarction. Am Heart J 1981; 102:334–340.
9. Cohn JN, Franciosa JA, Francis GA, et al. Effects of short term infusion of sodium nitroprusside on mortality rate in acute myocardial infarction complicated by left ventricular failure. N Engl J Med 1982; 306:1129–1135.
10. Norris RM, Brandt PWT, Caughey DE, Deeming LW, Scott PJ. A new coronary prognostic index. Lancet 1969; 1:274–278.
11. Peel AAF, Semple T, Wang I, Lancaster WM, Dall JLG. A coronary prognostic index for grading the severity of infarction. Br Heart J 1962; 24:745–760.
12. Multicenter Post-Infarction Research Group. Risk stratification after myocardial infarction. N Engl J Med 1983; 309:331–336.
13. Greenberg H, McMaster P, Dwyer EM Jr, the Multicenter Post-Infarction Research Group. Left ventricular dysfunction after myocardial infarction: results of a prospective multicenter study. J Am Coll Cardiol 1984; 4:867–874.
14. Bigger JT Jr. Risk stratification after myocardial infarction. Zeitschr Kardiol 1985; 74 (suppl 6):147–157.
15. Dwyer EM Jr, McMaster P, Greenberg HM, and the Multicenter Postinfarction Research Group. Non-fatal cardiac events and recurrent infarction in the year following acute myocardial infarction. J Am Coll Cardiol 1984; 4:695–702.
16. The Multicenter Diltiazem Post-Infarction Trial Research Group. The effect of diltiazem on mortality and reinfarction after myocardial infarction. N Engl J Med 1988; 319:385–392.
17. Shell WE, Kjekshus JK, Sobel BE. Quantitative assessment of the extent of myocardial infarction in the conscious dog by means of analysis of serial changes in serum creatine phosphokinase activity. J Clin Invest 1971; 50:2614–2625.
18. Roberts R, Sobel BE, Parker CW. Radioimmunoassay for creatine kinase isoenzymes. Science 1976; 194:855–857.
19. Geltman EM, Ehsani AA, Campbell MK, Schechtman K, Roberts R, Sobel BE. The influence of location and extent of myocardial infarction on long-term ventricular dysrhythmia and mortality. Circulation 1979; 60:805–814.
20. Roberts R, Henry PD, Sobel BE. An improved basis for enzymatic estimation of infarct size. Circulation 1975; 52:743–754.
21. Marmor A, Sobel BE, Roberts R. Factors presaging early recurrent myocardial infarction ("extension"). Am J Cardiol 1981; 48:603–610.
22. Roberts R. Non-transmural myocardial infarction. Council on Clin Cardiol Newsl 1985; 11:1–17.
23. Bigger JT Jr, Fleiss JL, Kleiger R, Miller JP, Rolnitzky LM, and the Multicenter Post-Infarction Research Group. The relationship among ventricular arrhythmias, left ventricular dysfunction and mortality in the 2 years after myocardial infarction. Circulation 1984; 69:250–258.
24. Mukharji J, Rude RE, Poole KE, et al., the MILIS Study Group. Risk factors for sudden death after acute myocardial infarction: two-year follow-up. Am J Cardiol 1984; 54:31–36.
25. Coromilas J, Bigger JT Jr, Kleiger RE, Rolnitzky LM, Fleiss JL, and the MDPIT Research Group. Relations among left ventricular dysfunction, ventricular arrhythmias, and mortality after myocardial infarction. Circulation 1989; 80 (suppl II): 48.

26. Nicod P, Gilpin E. Dittrich H, Henning H, Ross J Jr. Prognostic significance of complex ventricular arrhythmia for cardiac death during the first year after myocardial infarction. J Electrophysiol 1987; 1:93–102.
27. Hammermeister KE, DeRouen TA, Dodge HT. Variables predictive of survival in patients with coronary disease. Selection by univariate and multivariate analyses from the clinical, electrocardiographic, exercise, arteriographic, and quantitative angiographic evaluations. Circulation 1979; 59:421–430.
28. Bigger JT Jr, Weld FM. Analysis of prognostic significance of ventricular arrhythmias after myocardial infarction. Shortcomings of Lown grading system. Br Heart J 1981; 45:717–724.
29. Bigger JT Jr, Weld FM, Coromilas J, et al. Prevalence and significance of arrhythmias in 24-hour ECG recordings made within one month of acute myocardial infarction. In: Kulbertus H, Wellens HJJ, eds. The First Year After a Myocardial Infarction. Boston: Martinus Nijhoff, 1983:161–175.
30. Moss AJ, Davis HT, DeCamilla J, et al. Ventricular ectopic beats and their relation to sudden and nonsudden cardiac death after myocardial infarction. Circulation 1978; 60:998–1003.
31. Bigger JT Jr, Rolnitzky LM, Merab JP. Epidemiology of ventricular arrhythmias and clinical trails with antiarrhythmic drugs. In: Fossard HM, Haber E, Jennings RB, Katz AM, Morgan HE, eds. The Heart and Cardiovascular System: Scientific Foundations. Boston: Martinus Nijhoff, 1986:1405–1449.
32. Bigger JT Jr, Weld FM, Rolnitzky LM. The prevalence and significance of ventricular tachycardia detected by ambulatory ECG recording in the late hospital phase of acute myocardia infarction. Am J Cardiol 1981; 48:815–823.
33. Bigger JT Jr, Fleiss JL, Rolnitzky LM, The Multicenter Post-Infarction Research Group. Prevalence, characteristics and significance of ventricular tachycardia detected by 24-hour continuous electrocardiographic recordings in the late hospital phase of acute myocardial infarction. Am J Cardiol 1986; 58:1151–1160.
34. Bigger JT Jr. Relation between left ventricular dysfunction and ventricular arrhythmias after myocardial infarction. Am J Cardiol 1986; 57:8b–14b.
35. Goldstein S, Pawitan Y, Kennedy H, Daly J, Lee JT, CAST Investigators. Ventricular arrhythmia suppression predicts survival in the Cardiac Arrhythmia Suppression Trial (CAST). Circulation 1990; 82:III-198.
36. Breithardt G, Borggrefe M, Haerten K. Role of programmed ventricular stimulation and noninvasive recording of ventricular late potentials for the identification of patients at risk of ventricular tachyarrhythmias after acute myocardial infarction. In: Zipes DP, Jalife J, eds. Cardiac Electrophysiology and Arrhythmias. New York: Grune & Stratton, 1985:553–561.
37. Gomes JA, Winters SL, Stewart D, Horowitz SL, Milner M, Barreca P. A new noninvasive index to predict ventricular tachycardia and sudden death in the first year after myocardial infarction: based on signal averaged electrocardiogram, radionuclide ejection fraction and Holter monitoring. J Am Coll Cardiol 1987; 10:349–357.
38. Kuchar DL, Thorburn CW, Sammel NL. Prediction of serious arrhythmic events after myocardial infarction: signal-averaged electrocardiogram, Holter monitoring and radionuclide ventriculography. J Am Coll Cardiol 1987; 9:531–538.
39. Denniss AR, Richards DA, Cody DV, et al. Prognostic significance of ventricular tachycardia and fibrillation induced at programmed stimulation and delayed potentials detected on the signal-averaged electrocardiograms of survivors of acute myocardial infarction. Circulation 1986; 74:731–745.
40. Cripps TR, Bennett ED, Camm AJ, Ward DE. High gain signal averaged electrocardiogram combined with 24-hour monitoring in patients early after myocardial infarction for bedside prediction of arrhythmic events. Br Heart J 1988; 60:181–187.
41. Steinberg JS, Regan A, Sciacca RR, Bigger JT Jr, Fleiss JL. Predicting arrhythmic events after myocardial infarction: results of a prospective study and a meta-analysis using the signal-averaged electrocardiogram. Am J Cardiol 1992; 69:13–21.
42. Farrell TG, Bashir Y, Cripps T, et al. Risk stratification for arrhythmic events based on heart rate variability, ambulatory electrocardiographic variables and the signal-averaged electrocardiogram. J Am Coll Cardiol 1991; 18:687–697.

43. Hamer A, Vohra J, Hunt D, Sloman G. Prediction of sudden death by electrophysiologic studies in high risk patients surviving acute myocardial infarction. Am J Cardio 1982; 50:223–229.
44. Marchlinski FE, Buxton AE, Waxman HL, Josephson ME. Identifying patients at risk of sudden death after myocardial infarction: value of the response to programmed stimulation, degree of ventricular ectopic activity and severity of left ventricular dysfunction. Am J Cardiol 1983; 52:1190–1196.
45. Richards DA, Cody DV, Denniss AR, Russell PA, Young AA, Uther JB. Ventricular electrical instability: a predictor of death after myocardial infarction. Am J Cardiol 1983; 51:75–80.
46. Roy D, Marchand E, Theroux P, Waters DD, Pelletier GB, Bourassa MG. Programmed ventricular stimulation in survivors of an acute myocardial infarction. Circulation 1985; 72:487–494.
47. Bourke JP, Richards DAB, Ross DL, Wallace EM, McGuire MA, Uther JB. Routine programmed electrical stimulation in survivors of acute myocardial infarction for prediction of spontaneous ventricular tachyarrhythmias during follow-up: results, optimal stimulation protocol, and cost-effective screening. J Am Coll Cardiol 1991; 18:780–788.
48. Verrier RL, Lown B. Sympathetic-parasympathetic interactions and ventricular electrical stability. In: Schwartz PJ, Brown AM, Malliani A, Zanchetti A, eds. Neural Mechanisms in Cardiac Arrhythmias. New York: Raven Press, 1978:75–85.
49. Schwartz PJ, Vanoli E. Cardiac arrhythmias elicited by interaction between acute myocardial ischemia and sympathetic hyperactivity: a new experimental model for the study of antiarrhythmic drugs. J Cardiovasc Pharmacol 1981; 3:1251–1259.
50. Schwartz PJ, Priori SG. Sympathetic nervous system and cardiac arrhythmias. In: Zipes DP, Jalife J, eds. Cardiac Electrophysiology. From Cell to Bedside. Philadelphia: Saunders 1990:330–343.
51. Kolman BS, Verrier RL, Lown B. The effect of vagus nerve stimulation upon vulnerability of the canine ventricle: role of the sympathetic-parasympathetic interactions. Circulation 1976; 52:578–585.
52. Vanoli E, De Ferrari GM, Stramba-Badiale M, Hull SS Jr, Foreman RD, Schwatz PJ. Vagal stimulation and prevention of sudden death in conscious dogs with a healed myocardial infarction. Circ Res 1991; 68:1471–1491.
53. De Ferrari GM, Vanoli E. Stramba-Badiale M, Hull SS Jr, Foreman RD, Schwartz PJ. Vagal reflexes and survival during acute myocardial ischemia in conscious dogs with healed myocardial infarction. Am J Physiol 1991; 261:H63–H69.
54. Kleiger RE, Miller JP, Bigger JT Jr, Moss AJ, and the Multicenter Postinfarction Research Group. Decreased heart rate variability and its association with increased mortality after acute myocardial infarction. Am J Cardiol 1987; 59:256–262.
55. Bigger JT Jr, Fleiss JL, Steinman RC, Rolnitzky LM, Kleiger RE, Rottman JN. Frequency domain measures of heart period variability and mortality after myocardial infarction. Circulation 1992; 85:164–171.
56. Bigger JT Jr, Fleiss JL, Steinman RC, Rolnitzky LM, Kleiger RE, Rottman JN. Correlations among time and frequency domain measures of heart period variability two weeks after acute myocardial infarction. Am J Cardiol 1992; 69:891–898.
57. Odemuyiwa O, Malik M, Farrell T, Bashir Y, Poloniecki J, Camm J. Comparison of the predictive characteristics of heart rate variability index and left ventricular ejection fraction for all-cause mortality, arrhythmic events and sudden death after acute myocardial infarction. Am J Cardiol 1991; 68:434–439.
58. Farrell TG, Bashir Y, Cripps T, et al. Risk stratification for arrhythmic events based on heart rate variability, ambulatory electrocardiographic variables and the signal-averaged electrocardiogram. J Am Coll Cardiol 1991; 18:687–697.
59. Schwartz PJ, Vanoli E, Stramba-Badiale M, De Ferrari GM, Billman GE, Foreman RD. Autonomic mechanisms and sudden death. New insight from the analysis of baroreceptor reflexes in conscious dogs with and without a myocardial infarction. Circulation 1988; 78:969–979.
60. La Rovere MT, Spechia G, Mortara A, Schwartz PJ. Baroreflex sensitivity, clinical correlates and cardiovascular mortality among patients with a first myocardial infarction. Circulation 1988; 78:816–824.

61. Farrell TG, Odemuyiwa O, Bashir Y, et al. Prognostic value of baroreflex sensitivity testing after acute myocardial infarction. Br Heart J 1992; 67:129–137.
62. The CONSENSUS Trial Study Group Effects of enalapril on mortality in severe congestive heart failure: results of the Cooperative North Scandinavian Enalapril Survival Study (CONSENSUS). N Engl J Med 1987; 316:1429–1435.
63. The SOLVD Investigators. Effect of enalapril on survival in patients with reduced left ventricular ejection fractions and congestive heart failure. N Engl Med 1991; 325:293–302.
64. Pfefer MA, Braunwald E, Moye LA, et al., on behalf of the SAVE Investigators. Effect of captopril on morality and morbidity in patients with left ventricular dysfunction after myocardial infarction. N Engl J Med 1992; 327:669–677.
65. The SOLVD Investigators. Effect of enalapril on mortality and the development of heart failure in asymptomatic patients with reduced left ventricular ejection fractions. N Engl J Med 1992; 327:685–691.
66. Swedberg K. Held P, Kjekshus J, Rasmussen K. Ryden L, Wedel H, in behalf of the CONSENSUS II Study Group. N Engl J Med 1992; 327:678–684.
67. The Cardiac Arrhythmia Suppression Trial II Investigators. Effect of the antiarrhythmic agent moricizine on survival after myocardial infarction. N Engl J Med 1992; 327:227–233.
68. Winkle RA. Amiodarone and the American way. J Am Coll Cardiol 1985; 6:822–824.
69. Cairns JA, Connolly SJ, Gent M, Roberts R. Post-myocardial infarction mortality in patients with ventricular premature depolarizations. Canadian Amiodarone Myocardial Infarction Arrhythmia Trial Pilot Study. Circulation 1991; 84:550–557.
70. Bigger JT Jr. Future studies with the implantable cardioverter defibrillator. PACE 1991; 14 (part II): 883–888.
71. Bigger JT Jr. Should defibrillators be implanted in high risk patients without a previous sustained ventricular arrhythmia? In: Naccarelli GV, Veltri EP, eds. Implantable Cardioverters/Defibrillators. Cambridge, MA: Blackwell, 1993, pp 284–317.
72. Winkle RA, Mead RH, Ruder MA, et al. Ten year experience with implantable defibrillators (abst. Circulation 1991; 84:II-426.
73. Connolly SJ, Yusuf S. Evaluation of the implantable cardioverter defibrillator in survivors of cardiac arrest: the need for randomized trials. Am J Cardiol 1992; 69:959–962.
74. Kowey PR, Taylor JE, Marinchak RA, Rials SJ. Does programmed stimulation really help in the evaluation of patients with nonsustained ventricular tachycardia? Results of a meta-analysis. Am Heart J 1992; 123:481–485.
75. MADIT Executive Committee. Multicenter Automatic Defibrillator Implantation Trial (MADIT): design and clinical protocol. PACE 1991; 14 (part II): 920–927.
76. The CABG Patch Trial Investigators and Coordinators. The Coronary Artery Bypass Graft (CABG) Patch Trial. Prog Cardiovas Dis 1993; 36:97–114.
77. The German Dilated Cardiomyopathy Study Investigators. Prospective studies assessing prophylactic therapy in high risk patients: the German Dilated Cardiomyopathy Study (GDCMS)—Study Design. PACE 1992; 15 (part III):697–700.

33

Use of the Implantable Cardioverter-Defibrillator in Patients Awaiting Heart Transplantation

John J. Smith, James E. Udelson, Marvin A. Konstam, and Deeb Salem

*Tufts University School of Medicine
and New England Medical Center
Boston, Massachusetts*

I. INTRODUCTION

Orthotopic heart transplantation (OHT) has become an accepted treatment modality for selected patients with symptomatic congestive heart failure (CHF) and a limited life expectancy due to left and/or right ventricular systolic dysfunction. The actuarial survival in recent cohorts of patients after OHT ranges from 80 to 90% at 1 year and 60 to 70% at 5 years [1]. We are now completing the first decade of heart transplantation in the cyclosporine era and should soon have reports of 10-year survival rates in a group of patients with an original prognosis limited to months at time of consideration for transplantation. The clinical success of heart transplantation has led to a number of new challenges. The recent trend has been to transplant patients from two groups that were formerly excluded from consideration—older patients and those with comorbidities such as diabetes mellitus. The relaxation of these contraindications has resulted in considerable increases in both the number of candidates and the waiting period for heart transplantation. Less than half of the patients waiting for OHT in a given year actually have the operation during that year. The ratio of transplanted patients to listed patients continues to fall yearly [2]. Many of these patients succumb to the complications of left ventricular dysfunction—progressive heart failure and sudden death.

The implantable cardioverter-defibrillator (ICD) has proven to be an effective therapeutic option in selected patients with life-threatening ventricular arrhythmias who are awaiting OHT. These devices can be implanted in very ill patients with acceptable risk and may provide a "bridge" to the more definitive therapeutic intervention—the transplant. This chapter will review the current indications for OHT, review the pretransplant patient profile, and finally discuss therapeutic options, focusing particularly on the role of the ICD in these patients.

II. THE POPULATION AT RISK

The indications for OHT have not changed significantly in the 25 years since the first procedure was performed. Current indications for cardiac transplantation include (1) cardiac pathology, either primary or secondary, which is not amenable to correction or compensation with conventional medical or surgical therapy; (2) symptomatic congestive heart failure, New York Heart Association (NYHA) class III or IV despite optimal medical therapy; (3) a prognosis that is limited only by the cardiac pathology or its reversible systemic complications; and (4) absence of significant contraindications such as "advanced age," irreversible major organ failure, psychiatric disease, or medical noncompliance (Table 1) [3]. These criteria define a population of relatively young individuals who have an extremely poor prognosis. In these patients, the 1-year survival rate is approximately 55%—similar to that observed in the Cooperative North Scandanavian Enalapril Survival Study (CONSENSUS) enalapril limb [4]. This is contrasted with an expected 1-year survival of 80–90% and 5-year survival of 60–70% with orthotopic heart transplantation (OHT) [1]. The promise of improvement in functional capacity and prognosis is not realized by all patients awaiting heart transplantation. Unfortunately, the supply of donor hearts has not kept pace with the expanding waiting list. In 1988, only 48% of the 3390 patients registered with the United Network for Organ Sharing (UNOS) were transplanted during that year. In the following year, the percentage transplanted fell to 42% of the 3915 patients listed. During 1988 and 1989, 527 and 650 patients, respectively, died while waiting. Forty-six percent of these patients died from progressive congestive heart failure, and 29% died suddenly. Most sudden deaths in this population can probably be attributed to dysrhythmia. Additionally, a number of patients equal to the number dying are removed from the waiting list, often due to the development of contraindications. A significant proportion of these "inactivated" patients also succumb to the complications of CHF and dysrhythmia without being relisted for transplantation.

Finally, with a constantly expanding waiting list and a relatively constant resource (donor heart supply), the waiting time has lengthened considerably. The waiting time for patients in an intensive care unit was 10.7 days in 1985, increasing to 50.3 days in 1989. The proportion of patients who are in an intensive care unit prior to transplantation continues to grow, as we now consider patients who were formerly thought to be too ill to survive the surgery and perioperative period. [2] Conversely, there are patients who survive longer than expected while awaiting transplantation. Some of these patients may be well enough to be delisted until such time as they become more symptomatic. [5] Stevenson and co-workers recently estimated that if current trends continue, all donor hearts available for transplantation will be utilized by urgent candidates [6]. Currently, the waiting time for outpatients is exceeding 1 year for patients

Table 1 Contraindications to Heart Transplantation

1. Severe pulmonary hypertension (calculated pulmonary vascular resistance > 6 Wood units)
2. Irreversible hepatic, renal, or pulmonary dysfunction
3. History of medical noncompliance, substance abuse, or psychiatric illness that would prevent patient from following a complex medical regimen
4. Insulin-dependent diabetes mellitus with end organ damage
5. Active infection, including active myocarditis
6. "Advanced age"
7. Symptomatic or severe peripheral vascular disease
8. Absence of psychosocial support

in blood group O in some regions of the country. It is this population of unmonitored, ambulatory patients who are at particularly high risk for fatal ventricular tachyarrhythmias and bradyarrhythmias.

III. SUDDEN DEATH AND CONGESTIVE HEART FAILURE

Sudden cardiac death, secondary to dysrhythmia, has long been considered one of the leading mechanisms resulting in the premature demise of patients with CHF [7]. There are difficulties in the classification of "sudden death," particularly in cohorts of patients with CHF. All patients have a dysrhythmia at the time of death. The death of a patient with moderate but compensated CHF is often unexpected and thus classified as "sudden," whereas in the patient with advanced CHF, death is expected and therefore more likely classified as "pump failure." Ventricular tachycardia detected by ambulatory electrocardiographic monitoring is commonly seen in patients with left ventricular dysfunction (see Chapter 32). Mechanisms leading to the genesis of ventricular arrhythmias include electrolyte disturbance (particularly decreased potassium, and decreased magnesium), neurohumoral activation, myocardial scarring and hypertrophy, and ischemia as well as the medications used to treat the condition itself, such as diuretics and inotropes. A survey of the literature by Bigger in 1987 revealed that the annual mortality rate of patients with NYHA class III or IV CHF was approximately 40% per year, with about 50% of those deaths being classified as sudden [8]. In most investigations, the presence of nonsustained VT on ambulatory monitoring is positively associated with mortality, although ventricular ectopy has not emerged as an independent predictor of mortality in any of these studies [9]. In a subset of these series, nonsustained ventricular tachycardia (VT) was identified on ambulatory monitoring in 25–80% of patients, averaging about 50%. In each of these studies, patients with VT were more likely to die during the follow-up period.

The high prevalence of complex ventricular arrhythmias with advancing NYHA class of CHF may not necessarily translate into a higher incidence of sudden death. In the patient with advanced CHF, complex ventricular arrhythmias may serve only as a marker of severe LV dysfunction. Stratification of sudden death risk and classification of mechanism of death in this group is therefore difficult. Given the high mortality risk in all groups with CHF, ventricular tachyarrhythmias associated with hemodynamic collapse should be assessed by formal electrophysiological evaluation.

IV. THERAPEUTIC IMPLICATIONS

The implication of the above discussion is that the population awaiting heart transplantation is continuing to grow and is waiting longer but maintains a high risk of sudden death. Treatment of these patients includes optimization of their medical regimen of vasodilator therapy and diuretics and treatment of their underlying cardiac disease where applicable. Approximately 60% of patients awaiting transplantation have an ischemic basis for their cardiomyopathy. Beta-adrenergic receptor blocking agents can be safe and effective in patients with coronary artery disease-associated cardiomyopathy, both in reducing recurrent ischemia and in blocking the arrhythmogenic effects of the sympathetic nervous system activation which accompanies advanced congestive heart failure [10]. They must be used with caution, as the use of beta-blocking agents can occasionally lead to worsening of symptoms. Nitrates are also useful for treatment of ischemia in this population and are generally tolerated without hemodynamic compromise.

The utility of vasodilator therapy in this population cannot be overemphasized. Data from the CONSENSUS [4], Studies of left ventricular dysfunction (SOLVD) [11], and Vasodilator-

Heart Failure Trial (V-HEFT)-II [12] trials all favor angiotensin-converting enzyme inhibitors (CEI) as first-line therapy for patients' left ventricular dysfunction and symptoms, regardless of functional limitation. This conclusion is also supported by the Survival and Ventricular Enlargement (SAVE) study, where captopril was initiated soon after hospital admission for acute myocardial infarction [13]. The combination of hydralazine and isosorbide dinitrate was also shown to prolong survival when compared to placebo in the V-HEFT-I study [14], but was inferior to enalapril in V-HEFT-II [12]. Interestingly, the V-HEFT-II investigators reported a reduction in sudden death in the population randomized to enalapril when compared to the hydralazine-isosorbide dinitrate combination. This reduction in sudden death was not observed in the SOLVD treatment trial when enalapril was compared with placebo. It is conceivable that the apparent reduction of sudden death observed in the V-HEFT-II study may have been due to a mild proarrhythmic effect in the hydralazine-isosorbide dinitrate treatment arm, balanced by the benefit on pump function. Vasodilators may reduce the substrate for ischemia by reducing left ventricular wall tension. These data, taken together, all favor the CEIs as first-line therapy in all patients with left ventricular systolic dysfunction.

Treatment with intravenous inotropic agents in patients with advanced heart failure is commonplace but should be reserved for clinical decompensation refractory to conventional medical therapy. Long-term therapy with milrinone in patients with advanced CHF has been associated with a significant increase in mortality and sudden death when compared to conventional therapy in the "Prospective, Randomized Milrinone Survival Evaluation" or PROMISE study [15]. Treatment with nondigitalis, positive inotropic agents should be employed in a hospital setting with effective rhythm monitoring, as the commonly used inotropic agents are associated with a high incidence of frequent and complex ventricular arrhythmias. Even the oldest available therapy for CHF—namely, digoxin—has yet to prove its long-term safety and is currently the subject of a randomized, placebo-controlled trial [16].

Pharmacological therapy for ventricular dysrhythmias would be an attractive treatment strategy if therapy were successful in reducing symptomatic ventricular arrhythmias and effective in reducing the incidence of sudden death, and if such therapy had an acceptable side-effect profile. Currently there are no data suggesting that nonselective use of antiarrhythmic therapy in patients with CHF offers any protective effect, and such therapy may cause more harm from the proarrhythmic effects. The only randomized, placebo-controlled trial of antiarrhythmic therapy in patients with CHF was performed by Nicklas and co-workers using amiodarone [17]. There was a significant reduction of spontaneous ectopy seen on ambulatory monitoring in the amiodarone group, with no significant change in those randomized to placebo. Patients were followed a mean of 357 days postrandomization. The 1-year actuarial mortality was 19% in the placebo group and 31% in the amiodarone group (p = NS). Patients with a >75% reduction of ambient ectopy with amiodarone therapy had a 1-year mortality rate of 31% compared with 17% in patients with less suppression of ventricular ectopic activity (p = NS). A higher NYHA class was associated with a higher mortality rate, suggesting that ectopy was a marker of severe left ventricular impairment. There have been some concerns regarding the safety of amiodarone in patients who eventually undergo transplantation, but these concerns have been refuted by more recent data showing that the drug is not associated with a higher incidence of pulmonary complications following transplantation [18]. Unfortunately, there are no other randomized trials of antiarrhythmic therapy in patients with CHF with data available at this time. Most series of patients with cardiomyopathy contain patients who are selected to receive antiarrhythmic therapy, usually a type I agent. The definition of clinical efficacy varied in these studies, as did the modality by which efficacy was defined (ambulatory monitoring versus programmed electrical stimulation). There are no clinically meaningful conclusions that one can draw from these studies.

The class II agents, namely, beta-adrenergic blocking drugs, may provide a favorable impact on survival, as suggested by the small, nonrandomized studies performed over the past two decades. [19] Clinical trials empowered to test the effect of these drugs on survival in patients with CHF when added to conventional therapy are underway or in the planning stages. In summary, at the present time there are no data from prospective randomized trials which demonstrate that chronic administration of any antiarrhythmic drug impacts favorably on survival of patients with advanced heart failure from left ventricular systolic dysfunction.

V. USE OF THE IMPLANTABLE CARDIOVERTER-DEFIBRILLATOR IN PATIENTS AWAITING TRANSPLANTATION

The success of the ICD in patients with symptomatic or life-threatening arrhythmias has prompted Lehmann and co-workers to propose a randomized trial (DEFIBRILAT—*Defi*brillator as a *Bri*dge to *La*ter *T*ransplantation) of ICD implantation in potential cardiac transplantation recipients with inducible ventricular arrhythmias and coronary artery disease [20]. To initiate this investigation, these investigators surveyed the clinical activity of 11 transplant centers occurring between January 1, 1988, and December 31, 1989, and found that 26% of patients awaiting OHT in these programs died prior to receiving a donor organ. Of the deaths, 41% were classified as sudden, with most of these deaths occurring in patients with NYHA class III symptoms.

There is a limited literature on the risks of ICD surgery in pretransplant patients (Table 2). Siegal et al. recently reviewed the Medical College of Wisconsin experience in the implantation and use of ICD in patients awaiting OHT [21]. Of 91 patients accepted for OHT at this center, 15 patients required ICD implantation. Eleven patients were found to have symptomatic ventricular tachycardia (VT) not controlled by conventional therapy, and 4 patients had VT and were noninducible at baseline electrophysiological study. The NYHA functional class of this group was not reported. Of the patients undergoing ICD implantation, two developed reversible postoperative acute renal failure, and one developed an ICD patch infection necessitating removal. This patient died suddenly before another device could be implanted. Nine patients had what were classified as "appropriate" ICD discharges. Of those having ICDs implanted, 10 patients were transplanted and 2 were still waiting at the time of the report. One patient died

Table 2 Comparison of Studies of ICD use in Pretransplant Patients[a]

Reference	No. of patients	Year	Perioperative mortality (ICD)	Patients with ICD discharges	Follow-up (months)
Siegel [21]	15	1992	7%	9	N/A
Haverich[b] [22]	18	1992	0	14[c]	9
Haverich[b] [22]	38	1992	3%	31[c]	19

[a]ICD, implantable cardioverter-defibrillator; N/A, data not available.
[b]Patients were stratified by result of transplant evaluation (see text).
[c]ICD discharge not classified as "appropriate" or "inappropriate."

of progressive CHF and one patient was removed from consideration for unreported reasons. One point underemphasized in this report was the fate of those patients who did not have ICDs implanted (76 patients). Nine of these patients died suddenly prior to OHT. This study demonstrated that ICD implantation can be performed with acceptable risk in these very will patients, but also underscored our inability to identify prospectively all patients at risk for sudden death. The uncertainty complicates the decision as to when to place a patient on the search list for a donor heart.

Haverich et al. recently reviewed the experience of the medical school of Hannover (Germany) with the use of ICDs in patients referred for cardiac transplantation [22]. Of the 556 patients initially accepted for transplantation evaluation, 138 patients died and 322 patients were considered too well for transplantation. Follow-up data were available from 217 patients in the "too well" group, of which 38 patients were referred with malignant ventricular ectopy and underwent ICD placement. In general, these patients had less severe CHF as classified by symptoms. Mean follow-up was 19 months, ranging from 3 to 54 months. Survival at mean follow-up was 78.4%. One patient died in the perioperative period, and 7 patients died "late." Of the 37 patients surviving surgery, 31 experienced ICD discharges in the follow-up period. Of the 7 patients dying, 5 were classified as having a "cardiac death," but only one of these deaths was "sudden." These investigators reported the follow-up of a second subgroup of 45 patients found to have VT or ventricular fibrillation but who were felt not to have sufficient symptoms to warrant OHT at the time of evaluation. Eighteen of these patients underwent ICD placement, nonrandomized. There was no perioperative mortality in this group, and 14 of these patients subsequently experienced ICD discharges. There were 5 "nonclassified" deaths after a mean follow-up period of 9 months. These nonrandomized data indicate that ICDs can be implanted in patients with advanced CHF with acceptable morbidity and mortality. The broader issue of risk and benefit must await larger randomized studies.

VanVeldehuisen and co-workers compared the outcome of a group of patients waiting for OHT with a group considered "too well" for transplant based on symptoms and peak oxygen consumption measured with symptom-limited exercise testing. [23] This strategy was effective in predicting which patients were at risk of dying of progressive CHF. Nine of 53 patients in the "good prognosis" group died suddenly in the 2-year follow-up period. These data again suggest that the less symptomatic patients are a considerable risk for sudden death, whether they are waiting for a donor or are waiting to become "sick enough" to warrant transplantation.

There is little doubt that ICD implantation would provide a "bridge," allowing some patients to survive the longer waiting periods for heart transplantation. If implementation of the technology were inexpensive and risk-free, widespread application would be warranted. This, unfortunately, is not the case, as 20% of the patients in Siegal's small series experienced complications related to ICD implantation. Patients in the Hannover series had fewer complications from ICD surgery but were, in general, healthier. Routine ICD implantation in patients suspected to be at very high risk for sudden death will carry a substantial financial cost as well. Data from the prospective, randomized trials planned or in progress, may help answer these difficult questions.

Sudden death in patients with CHF itself is not consistent in mechanism. Considerable attention has been given to ventricular tachyarrhythmias as the cause of the majority of sudden deaths in patients with CHF. This conclusion was supported by the common observation of ventricular arrhythmias in patients with advanced heart failure. Consideration must be given to the other potential causes of sudden death in patients with CHF. Luu and co-workers reviewed the records of 20 hospitalized patients with advanced CHF who had died suddenly [24]. Many of these patients had been admitted for OHT evaluation, and this experience probably does not represent what would be observed in an ambulatory population. All patients were continuously monitored at time of cardiopulmonary arrest. Interestingly, 62% of the sudden deaths were classified as being due to electromechanical dissociation or bradyarrhythmias. In this series 38% of the arrests were in the setting of ventricular tachyarrhythmias. Only 50% of patients experiencing VT/ventricular fibrillation and 45% of patients with bradyarrhythmias were resuscitated successfully, despite a rapid response. The two patients experiencing electromechanical dissociation at the time of arrest both expired, both patients having acute myocardial infarction. There are several points that can be gleaned from this investigation. First, prompter initiation of therapy (such as can be provided by an ICD) may have resulted in a better survival rate. Second, devices with pacing capabilities would be highly desirable in this patient population; and third, despite the rapid implementation of appropriate therapy, it is not likely that the risk of sudden death can be completely eliminated in this population.

Newer-generation ICDs with backup bradycardia pacing and nonthoracotomy ICD systems may be more effective than currently available units in reducing the incidence of total and sudden death in patients with CHF. There will presumably be fewer perioperative deaths from the less invasive nature of the implantation procedure. Deaths from bradycardia or asystole may be preventable with the pacing capability that these units will have incorporated into their design. Current or third-generation ICDs will not prevent deaths due to the complications of cardiomyopathy, particularly stroke, liver, renal and respiratory failure, or recurrent myocardial infarction. Prevention of these complications is within the realm of cardiac transplantation.

VI. FUTURE DIRECTIONS: THE NEED FOR RANDOMIZED DATA

The review presented above emphasizes that current medical therapy reduces the mortality in patients with congestive heart failure but that even with optimal treatment, a large percentage of patients still die before a donor heart becomes available. The available data do not support the routine use of standard antiarrhythmic drug therapy in these patients. Data from the upcoming or in-progress beta-blocker trials in CHF as well as the proposed DEFIBRILAT trial should help in decision making in the patient with ventricular ectopic activity and no symptoms. In patients with symptomatic ventricular arrhythmias and CHF, we would recommend formal invasive electrophysiological study if the patients' heart failure symptoms are sufficiently compensated by medical therapy such that the majority of their pretransplant wait will be spent outside the hospital. Most of these patients will likely require ICD implantation, which can be accomplished with a mortality rate of 5% or less. Patients who will remain hospitalized until transplantation probably do not require invasive study for several reasons. This group of patients has a high frequency of ventricular ectopic activity but a smaller percentage of patients dying suddenly. In-hospital monitoring and rapid initiation of therapy for life-threatening arrhythmias should be adequate. These patients are usually too ill to consider ICD surgery. The group which is the subject of the most concern is the patients who are compensated enough to wait for transplantation at home. This is also the largest group, comprising >70% of those waiting for a donor organ. This population is the target of the DEFIBRILAT trial, which is proposed to begin in the next year [20].

In the future, the newer transvenous and nonthoracotomy ICD systems may be particularly appropriate for patients awaiting transplantation. These devices would offer several advantages over currently available systems. The major advantage would be the avoidance of major surgery in patients with advanced CHF. These very ill patients are probably more likely to have complications requiring prolonged hospitalization than patients without symptomatic CHF. These complications may render the patient too ill for transplantation, requiring their temporary or permanent removal from the waiting list. The presence of scarring from the ICD implant thoracotomy can prolong cardiectomy at the time of transplantation, possibly interfering with the timing of implantation and potentially prolonging ischemic time of the graft.

The issue of cost effectiveness must also be considered. The current ICD technology requires a minimum 7–10 days of hospitalization, including thoracotomy and intensive care monitoring added to the cost of the device. Many of these devices would then be explanted weeks to months later when the transplant is performed. It would be short-sighted to amortize the cost of ICD implantation over the short period in which the unit is actually in place. This cost must be considered in the context of total pre-/ and posttransplant care. Nonthoracotomy or transvenous ICDs may be cost effective in that they would not put the patient at risk for thoracotomy-related complications and would shorten the in-hospital recovery period. Even with these potential cost savings, routine application of this technology would add to the already considerable cost of OHT. There are other potential areas where this technology could reduce the total cost. For patients with advanced but compensated heart failure who are unlikely to survive because of life-threatening ventricular dysrhythmias, the effective protection afforded by the ICD may allow these patients to remain off the waiting list until such time as their symptoms and exercise capacity warrant transplantation. In patients whose symptoms are advanced enough to require transplantation, ICD implantation may allow them to safely wait at home, reducing hospitalization costs. Unfortunately, the paradox of this treatment strategy is that this therapy, which effectively prolongs the lives of those waiting for heart transplantation, increases the total number of patients waiting and prolongs the average waiting period. Assessment of the direct and indirect cost of therapy should be included as part of any prospective randomized trials of this therapy [25].

The major limitation of heart transplantation today is the tenuous supply of donor organs, a problem which will continue well into the 1990s. We consider the death of a patient waiting for transplantation to be due to complications of heart disease, but in reality, most of these patients expire because they do not receive a donor organ in time to delay death. All the therapies discussed above do nothing to improve the availability of donor hearts. By reducing the risk of sudden death, we may do no more than to increase the proportion of patients classified as dying of pump failure without actually affecting total number of deaths. The current allocation system for donor organs favors patients with CHF requiring intensive care, as it is assumed that these patients are the closest to death and have the most to gain from transplantation. Widespread ICD implantation may serve only to increase the number of hospitalized patients in relation to the small, relatively fixed number of donor hearts available. This approach may only reduce the proportion of patients dying suddenly, without reducing total mortality. On the other hand, concomitant strategies to reduce mortality in patients awaiting heart transplant as well as to increase donor availability would produce the optimal result. Refinement of this overall strategy will ideally result from carefully controlled clinical trial results as well as refinement, by society as a whole, of an approach to the complex ethical issues involved.

REFERENCES

1. Kreitt J, Kaye MP. The registry of the International Society for Heart and Lung Transplantation, 8th annual report—1991. J Heart Lung Transplant 1991; 10:491–498.
2. McManus RP, O'Hair DP, Beitzinger J, et al. Patients who die awaiting heart transplantation. J Heart Lung Transplant 1992; 11(2):191.

3. Copeland JG, Emery RW, Levinson MM. Selection of patients for cardiac transplantation. Circulation 1987; 75:2–9.
4. CONSENSUS Study Group: Effects of enalapril on mortality in severe congestive heart failure—report of the Cooperative North Scandanavian Enalapril Survival Study (CONSENSUS). N Engl J Med 1987; 316:1429–1435.
5. Kermani M, Stevenson LW, Chelimsky-Fallick C, et al. Importance of serial exercise testing after evaluation for cardiac transplantation. J Heart Lung Transplant 1992; 11(2):191.
6. Stevenson LW, Warner SL, Kobashigawa JA, Drinkwater D, Laks H. All donor hearts will soon be required for urgent candidates. J Heart Lung Transplant 1992; 11(2):191.
7. Kjekshus J. Arrhythmias and mortality in congestive heart failure. Am J Cardiol 1990; 65:42–48.
8. Bigger JT. Why patients with congestive heart failure die: arrhythmias and sudden cardiac death. Circulation 1987; 75(IV):28–35.
9. Francis GS. Development of arrhythmias in the patient with congestive heart failure: pathophysiology, prevalence and prognosis. Am J Cardiol 1986; 57:3B–7B.
10. Cohn JN, Levine B, Olivari MT, et al. Plasma norepinephrine as a guide to prognosis in patients with chronic congestive heart failure. N Engl J Med 1984; 311:819–823.
11. The SOLVD Investigators. Effect of enalapril on survival in patients with reduced left ventricular ejection fractions and congestive heart failure. N Engl J Med 1991; 325:293–302.
12. Cohn JN, Johnson G, Ziesche S, et al. A comparison of enalapril with hydralazine-isosorbide dinitrate in the treatment of chronic congestive heart failure. N Engl J Med 1991; 325:303–310.
13. Pfeffer MA, Braunwald E, Moye LA, et al. Effect of captopril on mortality and morbidity in patients with left ventricular dysfunction after myocardial infarction—results of the Survival and Ventricular Enlargement Trial. N Engl J Med 1992; 327:669–677.
14. Cohn JN, Archibald DG, Ziesche S, et al. Effect of vasodilator therapy on mortality in chronic congestive heart failure. Results of a Veterans Administration cooperative study. N Engl J Med 1986; 314:1547–1552.
15. Packer M, Carver JR, Rodeheffer RJ, et al., for the PROMISE study research group. Effect of milrinone on mortality in severe chronic heart failure. N Engl J Med 1991; 325:1468–1475.
16. Gheorghiade M, Zarowitx BJ. Review of randomized trails of digoxin therapy in patients with chronic heart failure. Am J Cardiol 1992; 69:48G–63G.
17. Nicklas JM, McKenna WJ, Stewart RA, et al. Prospective, double blind, placebo-controlled trial of low dose amiodarone in patients with severe heart failure and asymptomatic frequent ventricular ectopy. Am Heart J 1991; 122:1016–1021.
18. Chelimsky-Fallick C, Kobashigawa J, Stevenson WG, et al. Chronic amiodarone therapy prior to cardiac transplantation does not increase the perioperative risk. J Am Coll Cardiol 1991; 17:290A.
19. Eichhorn EJ. The paradox of beta-adrenergic blockade for the management of congestive heart failure. Am J Med 1992; 92:527–538.
20. DEFIBRILAT Study Group. Actuarial risk of sudden death while awaiting cardiac transplantation in patients with atherosclerotic heart disease. Am J Cardiol 1991; 68:545–546.
21. Siegel R, McManus RP, Cinquegrani M, Chapman P, Schweiger J, Beitzinger J. Results of automatic implantable cardio defibrillator in patients awaiting cardiac transplantation. J Heart Lung Transplant 1992; 11:206.
22. Haverich A, Troster J, Wahlers T, Fieguth HG, Klein H. The automatic implantable cardioverter defibrillator (AICD) as a bridge to heart transplantation. PACE 1992; 15:701–707.
23. van Veldhisen DJ, van den Brock SAJ, Hillige H, Crijns HJ, van Gilst WH, Lie KI. Mode of death in patients eligible for cardiac transplantation; should an AICD be implanted. J Heart Lung Transplant 1992; 11:206.
24. Luu M, Stevenson WG, Stevenson LW, Baron K. Walden J. Diverse mechanisms of unexpected cardiac arrest in advanced heart failure. Circulation 1989; 80:1675–1680.
25. Nisam S, Thomas A, Mower M, Hauser R. Identifying patients for prophylactic automatic implantable cardioverter defibrillator therapy: status of prospective studies. Am Heart J 1991; 122:607–612.

34

Analyzing the Costs and Cost Effectiveness of the Implantable Cardioverter-Defibrillator

Greg C. Larsen

*Oregon Health Sciences University
and Portland Veterans Affairs Medical Center
Portland, Oregon*

Stephen G. Pauker

*Tufts University School of Medicine and New England Medical Center
Boston, Massachusetts*

I. INTRODUCTION

By any standard, the implantable cardioverter-defibrillator (ICD) is an expensive device. For example, the first generation of FDA-approved generators cost $15,500 each, the sensing lead system costs $750, and a pair of defibrillator patches cost $1600. In addition, the defibrillator is costly to implant, requiring the skills of many highly trained physicians, nurses, and others in a technically sophisticated hospital setting. Hospital charges generated for patients undergoing initial defibrillator implantation have averaged $45,000 to $50,000 in the past [1,2]. The newer, nonthoracotomy devices are more expensive: a generator costs approximately $18,000, and the patch and lead system range in cost from approximately $3400 to $7000, but the costs of implantation should be somewhat lower.

Balanced against these costs must be the benefits which accrue to patients who receive defibrillators. Intuitively, if society "gets what it pays for" when a patient receives a defibrillator, then the expense, even if it is a large expense, can often be justified. Unfortunately, "getting what one pays for" can be an elusive concept, hard to define explicitly and to quantify. This chapter will attempt to define the clinical and methodological underpinnings necessary to understand the costs and the benefits of implantable defibrillators, and how these can be compared to the costs and benefits of other medical treatments.

II. PERSPECTIVES OF ANALYSIS

A. The Payment-Benefit Perspective

Assessing the costs and benefits of defibrillator implantation depends importantly on the analyst's perspective. Several such perspectives can be considered: that of the patient; the hospital; the insurance company, health maintenance organization, or government funding agency responsible for payment; or of society in general. Although each perspective is valid, analyses from different perspectives may produce strikingly different results. For example, consider a patient who has complete financial coverage for all inpatient and outpatient services through his health maintenance organization, save a $100 deductible annual copayment for hospitalization. From his perspective, the financial cost of defibrillator implantation is $100; the benefit is the extended life expectancy the device provides. For the hospital, the immediate costs of the patient's care may be zero or even negative (to the extent that they are borne by the insurer and to the extent that reimbursement may exceed true costs), but the benefits may be complex, including maintaining the hospital's continuing financial viability and its ability to provide services to the community, and enhancing its prestige. For the insurer, the bill for the patient's device and hospitalization (both present and future) must be paid. The benefit to the insurer is likewise complex: It can be a satisfied patient, a full portfolio of services, and the intrinsic value of helping its clients to live longer and better lives. But there may be no financial benefit: The patient's monthly premiums may never offset the huge charges incurred in the care of his ventricular arrhythmia. In fact, if the patient were to die sooner, his medical costs may be lower. From the societal perspective, treatment with the implantable defibrillator yields a balance of financial costs and survival benefits. In order for our society as a whole to judge the ultimate value of a complex therapy such as the implantable defibrillator, we must compare it to other worthy programs. Because the societal perspective is the broadest and most generally relevant one, it is the most commonly used perspective in published cost-effectiveness analyses.

B. The Time Horizon

Cost-effectiveness analyses are usually performed with limited data collected over a limited period of time. For this reason, some analyses restrict their time horizon to the length of time for which observational data are available (from 1 to 10 years, typically). The strength of these analyses is that they make no assumptions about outcomes beyond those observed in clinical studies. The weakness of this approach is, however, that for many chronic conditions, major benefits (and costs) of therapy may not be realized until many years after treatment begins. If the time horizon of analysis is arbitrarily restricted to the relatively short period of data collection, the longer-term costs and benefits of therapy will never be considered. For this reason, many analyses project the results of therapy far into the future, much further than the duration of observation in any clinical study and often for a patient's lifetime. No consensus has been reached about the optimal time horizon for cost-effectiveness analyses.

III. EXPENSES

A. Charges Versus Costs

One way to define the expense of an implantable defibrillator is to total up the hospital bills and the physician fee statements sent to the patient. These represent the *charges* billed to the patient. This definition of expenses has simplicity as its main virtue. Charges are relatively easy to obtain, but hard if not impossible to interpret. Given the often competitive climate in which today's hospitals do business and the complex regulations (both historical and current) which govern billing patterns, what a hospital administrator may decide to charge for a patient's room and board, laboratory tests, operating room time, nursing services, and equipment may relate only loosely to the actual cost to supply them to a patient. In addition, what physicians may choose to charge for their services may not closely reflect their actual time and effort, although this may change with the advent of the Resource Based Relative Value Scale (RBRVS) for determining the financial value of physicians' work.

For these reasons, it is customary to define expenses in terms of actual costs (direct and indirect) [3, p. 21]. The *direct costs* associated with a treatment, drug, or service are those expenses specifically required to supply it. Direct costs can be of three types: *variable* direct costs, *fixed* direct costs, and *average* direct costs. *Variable direct costs* are the costs required to provide one additional unit of treatment and exclude costs of developing new programs or facilities. They vary with each treatment. For example, the variable direct cost of an oral dose of procainamide includes the cost to the hospital pharmacy of that pill plus the cost of the pharmacist's time (i.e., the amount of salary) needed to dispense the pill. The variable direct cost of a cardiac catheterization includes the purchase price of the catheters, contrast medium, ECG leads, gowns, gloves, masks, and other disposable supplies used, as well as the time expense (i.e., salary) of the catheterization laboratory technicians required to complete the procedure. *Fixed direct costs* are those which are required to establish or maintain the program or hospital as a viable entity, but which do not vary with an additional single unit of service. Examples include building or equipping a cardiac catheterization laboratory or an operating room. These "costs of doing business" are "fixed," and would be present even if the additional patient were not being treated. In analyses that identify both variable and fixed direct costs, sometimes only variable direct costs are counted because fixed direct costs accrue whether or not one more patient is treated. Therefore, fixed costs do not reflect the explicit costs of that particular treatment. Of course, if a given treatment represents a very large fraction of a facility's total business or if the treatment requires very expensive equipment used only for that treatment, then *average direct costs* (including both fixed and variable components) may be a better measure. But for relatively infrequent procedures (especially those that do not require investment in special equipment), variable costs seem most appropriate. Such would seem to be the case for defibrillator implantation.

Indirect costs include facility costs such as lighting, heat and air conditioning, cleaning and maintenance, and mortgages, bonds, and tax payments. If one takes the patient's perspective (rather than that of society, third-party payor, or health maintenance organization), costs borne by patients and their families may be relevant. For example, time missed from work to receive medical treatment, the expenses of travel to and from the hospital, of special modifications to the home, or of special foods, could be included as indirect costs of the treatment being evaluated. In the analyses so far performed on the implantable defibrillator, these costs have not been considered.

B. Valuing Future Costs: Discounting

Many illnesses occur and resolve rapidly. Treatment are instituted and outcomes may be assessed in days or weeks. Examples include common bacterial infections, appendicitis, and simple fractures. For these ailments, all benefits and costs can be represented at their current values. However, most common cardiovascular diseases are chronic. Life spans are measured in years or decades, and the costs associated with treatment stretch far into the future. When such treatments are formally evaluated, a long time horizon is usually chosen. In such analyses it is often assumed that benefits, such as potential years of life saved far into the future, or the future dollars required to pay for such benefits, should not be valued as highly as the year of life we are living now or the current costs we incur to preserve it. In addition, with analyses which use a long time horizon, treatments which extend future survival may also incur additional future costs as a result of their success in extending life expectancy. Discounting provides a way to compare current with future costs and health benefits.

In evaluating the implantable defibrillator, one must compare present and future health costs and benefits fairly. Not all expenses associated with implantable defibrillator therapy occur initially; in fact, most occur after the device is implanted. Defibrillator battery replacements, recurrent hospitalizations, clinic visits and laboratory tests, and the costs associated with them all continue long after therapy has begun. These expenses are all paid for with "future" dollars when considered from today's frame of reference. As a general tenet of economic analysis, future dollars are valued less than present ones, because present dollars not used to buy immediate (present) benefits can be invested productively. The return on these investments should allow even more future benefits to be purchased and delivered. Thus, costs incurred in the future are "discounted" relative to the same costs incurred today [3, p. 29; 4, p. 248]. The discount rate is roughly equal to the noninflationary rate of return on low-risk, long-term investments; a value of 5% per year is used in many analyses of medical therapies. Thus, a dollar spent or gained in the future loses 5% of its value each year. For example, a $1000 expense incurred next year is actually $1000/1.05 or $952, whereas a $1000 expense incurred 10 years from now is actually $1000/(1.05)^{10}$ or $614.

A thornier problem arises when one considers the net "value" of future medical benefits [5]. Are the future years of life saved by a life-extending therapy, such as the implantable defibrillator, of equal value to one's current year of life, or should future years be discounted as having less intrinsic value? There is no unanimity on this issue. Each patient's unique personal circumstances dictate different answers to such a question. However, if costs are to be discounted, then in order to maintain proportional symmetry between the values of future dollars and future survival benefits, many decision analysts and economists believe it methodologically appropriate to discount both future costs and future years of life saved. If such matched discounting is not done, then logic would argue for displacing most health care programs as far into the future as possible, because the costs will be lower (discounted) while equal benefits will be achieved. In other words, failure to discount both cost and benefits would make any program appear more and more cost effective the longer its implementation is delayed [6]. Using this logic, no new program would ever be started, no matter how beneficial!

IV. BENEFITS

A. Choice of Benefit

All useful medical therapies provide some benefit, usually to the individual patient treated, but often to society as well (for example, treatment of disease by vaccination). These benefits must be explicitly defined to establish the true worth of the therapy. Patient benefits may be of several types: an increase in survival (measured increasingly often as a change in life expectancy), a reduction in pain, an increase in functional capacity, or a reduced frequency of unwanted events (e.g., myocardial infarction or stroke). As has been suggested in several uncontrolled reports, the implantable defibrillator appears to increase life expectancy substantially over that afforded by various antiarrhythmic drug regimens in similar patients [7–9]. Thus, additional years of life is the appropriate measure of benefit to compare the implantable defibrillator to other medical strategies.

B. Quality of Life

It can be argued that life spent in different health states should be valued differently. For example, quality of life in constant pain is not likely to be valued as highly by most people as life in robust health. Even if extended survival is the benefit measured in evaluations of the implantable defibrillator, then the quality of that survival, relative to other therapies, may also be important in determining the overall "value" of the defibrillator. No study has measured empirically the quality of life or health status of patients with an implantable defibrillator. However, it is possible to evaluate quality of life with a defibrillator relative to that with another therapy, to assess the importance of quality of life on the relative value of defibrillator therapy. For example, many cardiologists with experience using both the implantable defibrillator and drugs such as amiodarone believe that most patients experience a higher quality of life with the defibrillator.

V. METHOD OF ANALYSIS

At least two methods have been used in economic analyses of health practices. *Cost-benefit analysis* compares the relative value of different programs with different kinds of outputs (for example, a program of postmastectomy reconstructive surgery for breast cancer compared to an immunization program for preschool children). It requires that all benefits, including years of life, be accounted in monetary terms. Once both benefits and costs have been converted to financial terms, the net benefit of the program is the difference between the two. The major disadvantage of cost-benefit analyses is that years of life and quality of life must be translated into a dollar value. Cost-benefit analyses address the net effects of a program, either positive or negative. Comparisons among programs are typically only with respect to total cost, not with respect to cost per benefit obtained.

In contrast, *cost-effectiveness analysis* is a method used to maximize the usefulness of scarce (usually financial) resources by comparing the output (health effectiveness) of a program per unit of input (cost) required. Costs are still accounted in dollars, but health benefits are not. They can be represented in many different ways, such as years of life saved, number of complications avoided, or number of diseased patients identified. A program's effectiveness compared to an alternative program is represented as a *marginal cost-effectiveness ratio*, defined as additional dollars spent per additional year of life saved. Alternative programs can then theoretically be ranked using this ratio to define their relative values, and scarce resources can then be allocated starting with the most cost-effective programs and descending the list until available resources are exhausted. The major limitation of cost-effectiveness analyses is that programs with different outputs (breasts reconstructed versus children immunized, for example) cannot be compared unless a common outcome metric (e.g., quality-adjusted life years) is found.

Evaluation of the Implantable Defibrillator

In isolation, the implantable defibrillator may be seen as an expensive therapy, if we ignore its therapeutic efficacy, or as an effective therapy, if we ignore its expense. However, the defibrillator does not exist in a therapeutic vacuum. Antiarrhythmic drug treatment guided by electrophysiological testing represents the therapeutic standard against which a new therapy must be evaluated. Cost-effectiveness analysis can be used to make this comparison [3,4,10]. The difference in marginal costs between medical therapy and the defibrillator is divided by the increased years of survival provided by the defibrillator.

The optimal way to assess the cost and mortality differences between defibrillator and drug therapy for malignant ventricular arrhythmias would be a randomized clinical trial, in which the costs and clinical outcomes of the different strategies are collected prospectively. Such a trial has been initiated in the Netherlands, but no results have yet been announced [11]. However, even clinical trials have their problems. As mentioned earlier, patients are not followed over a lifetime of care, so the time horizon is relatively short. Also, because patients in a clinical trial are followed so closely, their survival is usually better than that of comparable patients receiving "usual" care. Trials frequently recruit only a carefully selected subset of patients, so that the results of the trial may not be generalizable to the majority of patients. Furthermore, the costs of care in a trial (even if they are measured) may not predict the costs of usual care, because these patients are often followed more closely in a trial. Finally, trials are often extremely expensive to conduct. In any event, currently published studies of the cost effectiveness of the implantable defibrillator have used models to simulate the potential outcomes of medical or defibrillator therapy and their costs. These models derive their estimates of survival from the medical literature and their estimates of costs from a variety of sources.

VI. LITERATURE REVIEW

Among the few published studies evaluating the costs and benefits of the implantable defibrillator, methodologies vary widely. Only two formal cost-effectiveness analyses have been performed [2,12]. Two other studies have examined more selective aspects of defibrillator costs [1,13]. The basic methods and results of these four studies are summarized in Table 1.

A. Formal Cost-Effectiveness Analyses

The studies by Kuppermann and colleagues [2] and Larsen and colleagues [12] were very different in methodology but had strikingly similar results. Kuppermann and colleagues used a computer model which estimated survival time and costs over a lifetime of care for patients with defibrillators and compared them to patients treated with a variety of (unspecified) antiarrhythmic drugs [2]. A societal perspective of analysis was adopted. Medicare payments were used to estimate expenses, represented in 1986 dollars. Survival with and without defibrillator treatment was estimated from mortality rates reported in the literature. Of special note, nonsudden mortality was assumed to be the same for both medical and defibrillator patients. Expenses and survival were both discounted 5% per year. Defibrillator battery replacement was assumed to occur every 24 months. Initial hospitalization charges for patients receiving defibrillators were almost $50,000, and lifetime treatment charges were estimated to be $120,000 at a mean estimated survival of 5 years. Compared to drug therapy, the additional cost of defibrillator treatment was estimated to be $17,000 per year of life saved. In anticipation of improved technology, a second scenario was evaluated in which battery life was 5 years, and implantation did not require a thoracotomy. Under these assumptions, the projected marginal cost effectiveness of the defibrillator fell to $7400 per year of life saved. No adjustments were made for variations in quality of life.

In a somewhat different study, Larsen and colleagues used a computer model to estimate the lifetime cost effectiveness from a societal perspective of the implantable defibrillator compared to amiodarone therapy [12]. Amiodarone therapy was chosen for comparison because, prior to the availability of the implantable defibrillator, it was considered to be the most effective treatment for prevention of recurrent sudden cardiac death among these patients. Actual direct variable costs (valued in 1989 dollars) for a group of patients treated at the New England Medical Center were used in the analysis. Survival was estimated from the literature. In contrast to Kuppermann's study, nonsudden cardiac mortality rates were modeled explicitly, 9% per year for amiodarone-treated patients but only 5.5% per year for defibrillator patients, based on rates reported in prior studies. The difference reflects, in part, the benefits of myocardial revascularization achieved with the bypass surgery which is often performed during the thoracotomy for defibrillator implantation. Both costs and survival were discounted at 5% per

Table 1 Studies Examining the Costs of the Implantable Defibrillator[a]

	Kuppermann et al. [2][b]	Larsen et al. [12]	Anderson and Camm [13]	O'Donoghue et al. [1]
Type of analysis	Computer model, marginal cost effectiveness	Computer model, marginal cost effectiveness	Simple cost-outcome description of ICD use in various subgroups	Cost analysis by direct comparison of patient groups
Expenses measured	Charges (from Medicare data)	Variable direct costs from 64 hospital patients	Total direct costs over 3-year follow-up	Charges from one hospital stay
Monetary value used	1986 dollars	1989 dollars	1991 British pounds	1985–1988 dollars, uncorrected
Benefits measured	Lifetime survival, from literature-derived mortality rates	Lifetime survival, from literature-derived mortality rates	Lives saved over 3 years compared to medical therapy, from literature-derived mortality rates	Reduced charges from early ICD implant and shorter hospital stay
Quality adjustment	No	Yes	No	No
Discounting	5%	5%	No	No
ICD compared with:	Unspecified medical therapy	Amiodarone therapy	Not compared to other therapies	Unspecified medical therapy
Index admission hospital expenses	$49,830	$36,915	$31,730[c]	$17,200–$73,400
ICD patient lifetime treatment expenses	$121,500	$89,600		
Average ICD patient life expectancy	5.1 years	6.1 years		
Baseline C/E ratio	$17,400	29,200	Variable: $44,800[c] for "combined high-risk" group	
C/E ratio assuming a 5-year ICD battery life	$7,400 nonthoracotomy device)	$16,500 (thoracotomy device)		

[a] ICD, implantable cardioverter-defibrillator; C/E ratio, cost/effectiveness ratio.
[b] Numbers in parentheses refer to study reference number.
[c] Converted from British pounds at 1 pound = $1.90.

year, and quality of life was reduced for time in the hospital and for recovery from surgery. The analysis showed that, compared to amiodarone therapy, defibrillator treatment required an additional $29,200 in variable direct costs per year of life saved. If defibrillator battery life was assumed to be 5 years, the cost-effectiveness ratio dropped to $16,500 per year of life saved.

Larsen and colleagues also evaluated the impact of quality of life on implantable defibrillator cost-effectiveness ratios. When quality of life on amiodarone was assumed to be worse than quality of life with the implantable defibrillator, there was an incremental gain in quality-adjusted life expectancy with the defibrillator relative to amiodarone, and the marginal cost-effectiveness ratio for the defibrillator dropped. If quality of life on amiodarone fell below 40% of that with the defibrillator, the marginal cost-effectiveness ratio for the defibrillator ($14,000/QALY) actually fell below that for amiodarone therapy ($17,000/QALY), making the defibrillator the preferred choice for the investment of scarce resources.

Conversely, if one assumes that quality of life with the implantable defibrillator is *less* than that on amiodarone, the marginal cost-effectiveness ratio for the defibrillator compared to amiodarone quickly rises. For example, if defibrillator quality of life falls to only 70% of that on amiodarone, its marginal cost-effectiveness ratio rises from a baseline of $29,200 to $190,000 per quality-adjusted year of life saved. If quality of life with the defibrillator falls below 65% of that on amiodarone, then quality-adjusted life expectancy with the defibrillator becomes lower than with amiodarone and there would be no rational reason to select defibrillator therapy over amiodarone. In this instance amiodarone therapy is said to *dominate* therapy with the implantable defibrillator, because it is both more effective and less expensive.

B. Other Analyses

In a novel report from Great Britain, Anderson and Camm compared the relative cost per life year saved of the implantable defibrillator in patient populations with varying sudden-cardiac-death risks, including several subsets of sudden-cardiac-death survivors, myocardial infarction survivors, patients with nonsustained ventricular tachycardia, and patients awaiting cardiac transplantation [13]. This study is not strictly a cost-effectiveness analysis, because no attempt was made to compare the incremental increase in costs of the defibrillator over the costs of conventional therapy. In addition, a relatively short time horizon of 3 years was used. Thus, the simple *total* of all defibrillator costs over 3 years was divided by the 3-year *difference* in mortality produced by the defibrillator over medical therapy. This "total cost per incremental life year saved" ratio was then calculated for the various defibrillator candidate populations listed above. Of note, no battery replacement costs were included in the analysis, and no nonsudden cardiac mortality rates were incorporated. These "omissions" are not insignificant. Both assuming the cost of conventional medical therapy is zero and neglecting the nonsudden death rate associated with the implantable defibrillator tend to overestimate the marginal cost-effectiveness ratio of the device. Omitting battery replacement costs tends to underestimate it. Also, omitting the cost of other therapies may produce quite different effects in different subsets of patients. Nevertheless, their results (converted from 1991 pounds sterling) showed that defibrillator treatment *in Great Britain* would cost $108,000 per life year saved if applied to all sudden-cardiac-death survivors, but only $43,000 per life year saved if applied selectively to those with ejection fractions less than 30% who failed electrophysiological testing while on antiarrhythmic drug therapy. If applied to all noninducible sudden-death survivors with low ejection fractions plus all who remain inducible after drug treatment (the "combined high-risk" group), the cost would be $45,000 per life year saved. Anderson and Camm estimate that strategies now being tested in clinical trials for defibrillator treatment of patients with nonsustained ventricular tachycardia would yield costs of $45,000 to $81,000 per life year saved. They predict that prophylactic defibrillator implantation in myocardial infarction survivors at high risk for sudden cardiac death would cost $69,000 to $84,000 per life year saved, depending on the definition of "high risk."

Because their analysis is not a true marginal cost-effectiveness analysis, Anderson and Camm's results cannot be compared to other studies. The main strength of their work is to show how important patient selection criteria are in determining the overall value of a new therapy and to suggest for which defibrillator patient subgroups the allocation of scarce funds might yield the greatest life expectancy gains.

Finally, work by Susan O'Donoghue and colleagues has attempted to show the cost savings possible with "early" defibrillator implantation in survivors of sudden cardiac death or sustained ventricular tachycardia [1]. This is a pure "cost analysis," since survival differences were not measured. The study was a retrospective review of 39 patients. Seven patients were noninducible at baseline electrophysiological study and underwent defibrillator implantation without further testing. Their mean hospital length of stay was 12.6 days, with accumulated charges of $40,000 (including defibrillator hardware). The other 32 patients underwent serial drug testing, had a mean hospital length of stay of 20 days, and accumulated $49,000 in charges. Of these 32, only 12 (38%) were suppressible with antiarrhythmic drugs, requiring 12 hospital days and $17,000 in charges. The other 20 failed all drug trials and went on to defibrillator implantation, requiring 26 hospital days and $73,000 in charges (including the cost of electrophysiology testing, drug trials, defibrillator hardware, and implantation). The authors conclude that ". . . defibrillator implantation as an early intervention is not more costly and indeed may be cost-effective [sic] compared with serial electrophysiologic testing. As antitachycardia devices become more versatile, longer lived and easier to implant, earlier implantation is likely to compare even more favorably to drug therapy."

VII. LIMITATIONS OF PUBLISHED ANALYSES

Several important issues are inadequately addressed by the few published analyses reviewed above. First, no study has fully explored the important impact which the nonsudden cardiac death rate has in determining the overall efficacy of the implantable defibrillator. For example, if the defibrillator were to be implanted only in patients whose nonsudden mortality rate was much greater than their malignant arrhythmia mortality rate, the defibrillator would not prevent the majority of deaths, even if it were 100% effective in preventing sudden death. In that case, the defibrillator would be less cost effective, because fewer years of life would be saved. On the other hand, the expense of implanting and following up the defibrillator cohort could also drop, because the patients would live less long.

The impact of changes in the nonsudden cardiac death rate can be illustrated. Using the model of Larsen and colleagues [12], if all parameters remain at baseline except that nonsudden death rates are doubled for all groups, survival is shortened significantly. As a consequence, costs for battery replacements and follow-up care also drop. On balance, however, the cost of the defibrillator to save a year of life rises by approximately 7.5%, because survival drops relatively more than costs. Similarly, if nonsudden death rates are reduced to one-half their baseline values, the cost of the defibrillator to save a year of life falls by approximately 3%, because survival improves relatively more than costs rise. Of course, this is a very artificial illustration: Sudden death rates and operative mortality probably do not remain constant, and nonsudden death rates may well increase in patients who are revascularized when the defibrillator is implanted. If the cardiac nonsudden death rate doubles every 5 years after defibrillator implantation until it equals the rate in patients treated with conventional therapy, then the cost to save a year of life increases by 40%.

Second, the electrophysiological evaluation of lethal arrhythmias has tended to become shorter and simpler over time. Fewer failed drug trials are in general required before a patient is considered a candidate for an implantable device; thus hospital stays (and probably hospital costs) have declined. These reductions have not been reflected in any of the published analyses to date. Their impact is hard to judge, since the overall cost of the implantable defibrillator is determined by a complex interaction of initial hospital and device costs, costs of follow-up, and survival rates, which are in turn influenced by patient selection criteria.

Third, the impact of newer, nonthoracotomy devices has not been fully accounted for. Kuppermann and colleagues [2] evaluated a "future scenario" in which nonthoracotomy devices with longer battery lives were implanted, resulting in lower initial hospitalization costs and fewer battery replacements, leading in turn to lower cost per year of life saved. However, literature review has suggested that open-chest defibrillator implantation, perhaps as a result of concomitant coronary bypass grafting or left ventricular aneurysmectomy, has resulted in a lower nonsudden cardiac mortality than that seen in medically treated patients [12]. This "hidden" benefit of defibrillator implantation may be lost if all patients receive nonthoracotomy devices in the future.

We extended our prior model [12] to estimate how much a nonthoracotomy device might change the baseline cost-effectiveness ratio of the open-chest implantable defibrillator. We assumed that the nonsudden cardiac death rate for defibrillator and amniodarone-treated patients would be the same, i.e., that the "hidden" benefit of open-chest implantation would be lost. We also assumed that the extra hospital costs and all surgeons' fees associated with defibrillator implantation surgery would not be incurred, but that a much smaller physician fee for nonthoracotomy device implantation would be charged instead and that the cost of the nonthoracotomy device and its leads would be some 33% higher. We assumed no change in device battery life. These assumptions are simplistic but were designed to illustrate the general effects of using nonthoracotomy devices. Acknowledging these limitations, the new analysis demonstrates that the cost-effectiveness ratio for a nonthoracotomy device strategy compared to amiodarone increases from an original baseline estimate of $29,000 per year of life saved to $55,000 per year of life saved, an increase of almost 90%. This increase largely reflects a substantial decrease in life expectancy because the "hidden benefit" of revascularization will not occur.

Perhaps more likely than the above scenario, however, is one in which some patients continue to have open-chest defibrillator implantation in association with other cardiac surgery, while others receive nonthoracotomy devices. If so, the cost-saving impact of the nonthoracotomy device will be blunted but the reduction in nonsudden cardiac mortality associated with open-chest implantation will be partially preserved. The interplay of these factors has not been accounted for in any analysis to date.

VIII. SUMMARY

Few analyses have been performed examining the costs and benefits obtained from implantable defibrillator therapy. In those which have, methods vary widely, making direct comparisons between studies difficult or impossible. Two formal cost-effectiveness analyses done so far have shown, however, that the cost-effectiveness ratio of the implantable defibrillator is comparable to a variety of other therapies for cardiovascular disease, including intravenous thrombolytic therapy for a large myocardial infarction [14], coronary bypass surgery for two-vessel coronary artery disease [15], treatment of mild to moderate (diastolic blood pressure 94–104) hypertension [15], therapy with nifedipine for mild to moderate hypertension [16], and electophysiological testing to determine appropriate therapy for syncope in patients with chronic bifascicular heart block and preserved left ventricular function [17]. As technology improves, costs of the device will continue to decline. On the other hand, current interest in implanting defibrillators in patients with lower mortality risks than those in whom the devices were originally implanted, such as patients with nonsustained ventricular tachycardia or patients who are noninducible after cardiac arrest, may lead to increased costs per life year saved, depending on length of hospital admission and number of drug tests performed before device implantation. This issue is the focus of at least one ongoing clinical trial.

REFERENCES

1. O'Donoghue S, Platia EV, Brooks-Robinson S, Mispireta L. Automatic implantable cardioverter-defibrillator: is early implantation cost-effective? J Am Coll Cardiol 1990; 16:1258–1263.
2. Kuppermann M, Luce BR, McGovern B, Podrid PJ, Bigger JT Jr, Ruskin JN. An analysis of the cost effectiveness of the implantable defibrillator. Circulation 1990; 81:91–100.
3. Drummond MF, Stoddart GL, Torrance GW. Methods for the Economic Evaluation of Health Care Programmes. Oxford: Oxford Medical Publications, 1987.
4. Weinstein MC, Fineberg HV. Clinical Decision Analysis. Philadelphia: Saunders, 1980.
5. Robinson JC. Philosophical origins of the social rate of discount in cost-benefit analysis. Milbank Quart 1990; 68:245–265.
6. Keeler EB, Cretin S. Discounting the life saving and other non-monetary effects. Management Sci 1983; 29:300–306.
7. Manolis AS, Tan-DeGuzman W, Lee MA, et al. Clinical experience in seventy-seven patients with the automatic implantable cardioverter defibrillator. Am Heart J 1989; 118:445–450.
8. Winkle RA, Thomas A. The automatic implantable cardioverter defibrillator: the U.S. experience. In: Brugada P, Wellens HJJ, eds. Cardiac Arrhythmias: Where to Go from Here? Mount Kisco, NY: Futura, 1987.
9. Winkle RA, Mead RH, Ruder MA, et al. Long-term outcome with the automatic implantable cardioverter-defibrillator. J Am Coll Cardiol 1989; 13:1353–1361.
10. Detsky AS, Naglie GI. A clinician's guide to cost-effectiveness analysis. Ann Intern Med 1990; 113:147–154.
11. Wever EFD, Hauer RNW. Cost-effectiveness considerations: the Dutch prospective study on the automatic implantable cardioverter defibrillator as first-choice therapy. PACE 1992; 15(part III):690–693.
12. Larsen GC, Manolis AS, Sonnenberg FA, Beshansky JR, Estes NAM, Pauker SG. Cost-effectiveness of the implantable cardioverter-defibrillator: effect of improved battery life and comparison with amiodarone therapy. J Am Coll Cardiol 1992; 19:1323–1334.
13. Anderson MH, Camm AJ. Implications for present and future applications of the implantable cardioverter defibrillator resulting from the use of a simple model of cost-efficacy. Br Heart J. In Press.
14. Laffel GL, Fineberg HV, Braunwald E. A cost-effectiveness model for coronary thrombolysis/reperfusion therapy. J Am Coll Cardiol 1987; 10:79B–90B.
15. Weinstien MC, Stason WB. Cost-effectiveness of interventions to prevent or treat coronary heart disease. Ann Rev Public Health 1985; 6:41–63.
16. Edelson JT, Weinstein MC, Tosteson ANA, Williams L, Lee TH, Goldman L. Long-term cost-effectiveness of various initial monotherapies for mild to moderate hypertension. JAMA 1990; 263:408–413.
17. Beck JR, Salem DN, Estes NAM, Pauker SG. A computer-based Markov decision analysis of the management of symptomatic bifascicular block: the threshold probability for pacing. J Am Coll Cardiol 1987; 9:990–935.

35

Implantable Cardioverter-Defibrillator Lead Systems

Antonis S. Manolis

*Tufts University School of Medicine
and New England Medical Center
Boston, Massachusetts*

The entry of other manufacturers in the field and the world market of implantable cardioverter-defibrillator (ICD) devices, previously and until recently dominated by the pioneering company (Cardiac pacemakers, Inc., CPI), has spawned new competition and has led to the development of various ICD lead systems. In this chapter a general and, whenever possible, a specific description of the currently available ICD lead systems will be presented (Tables 1–17).

I. DEFIBRILLATION LEADS

The initial lead system which was used with the first defibrillator device that was implanted in a patient, employed a spring coil lead in the superior vena cava and an epicardial cup/patch electrode for both sensing and defibrillating [1]. This was a single pair of electrodes used for detecting and treating ventricular fibrillation only. It quickly became obvious, however, that ventricular tachycardia was very common and not reliably detectable by the shocking electrodes, while accurate rate counting could not be easily obtained by using such a lead system. Separate rate-sensing and defibrillating lead systems were, therefore, subsequently introduced and have since been utilized, at least with the epicardial ICD systems. The defibrillation electrodes now include patch leads of various sizes for epicardial or extrapericardial (and recently for subcutaneous or submuscular) placement and a spring electrode for endocardial insertion (superior vena cava lead). For defibrillation, the combination of two patches or one patch and a spring electrode can be used. Either electrode system can also be used for arrhythmia morphology sensing in the CPI devices.

The patch electrodes are designed to be sewn onto the heart and can be placed on the epicardium or sutured to the pericardium by means of a thoracotomy procedure [2], either during implantation of the full ICD system or with initial intraoperative placement of prophylactic patches during a staged procedure (3–6). When combined with a superior vena cava lead, the patch is placed at the apex of the left ventricle. When two patches are employed, one is usually sewn on the posterolateral side of the left ventricle or the apex and the other on the right ventricle and/or right atrium, attempting to include the maximal myocardial mass between the two electrodes [7]. Caution is exercised during extrapericardial placement of the patches to avoid phrenic nerve damage. The patch is sewn with the active (mesh) side of the electrode against the heart and the insulated side facing out. If a patch covers part of the atrium, it may be advisable to sew the patch to the inside or outside of the pericardium rather than the thin atrial myocardium, to avoid perforation and bleeding.

Selection of the appropriate defibrillation lead combination, position, and size is made intraoperatively based on the size of the patient's heart, the surgical access used, and the electrical testing that yields a satisfactory defibrillation threshold (DFT) (usually $\leq$ 15–20 J). The lowest DFT has been reported with the use of two large patches [8]. Most clinical implants of ICDs have been done with use of two epicardial patches. In addition to CPI, other manufacturers have now developed their own patch electrodes with different shapes, sizes, and other specifications (Tables 1–5). The CPI and Telectronics patches are rectangular titanium mesh electrodes, the Medtronic patches are oval-shaped platinum alloy helical-coil electrodes, the Ventritex patches are oval-shaped titanium mesh electrodes, and the Intermedics patches are contoured titanium mesh electrodes (Figs. 1–4).

In the design as well as the placement of these electrodes, several important aspects have been considered. It has been suggested that a *minimum* and even (similar in all parts of the ventricles) potential gradient (5–6 V/cm for a 14-ms low-tilt or 10-ms high-tilt truncated exponential waveform) generated by the shock is necessary for effective cardiac defibrillation [9–11]. This potential gradient is affected and thus determined by the voltage of the shock and the electrode configuration [12]. It has also been suggested that a *maximum* potential gradient (10- to 13-fold higher than the minimum) also exists and that, beyond this value, deleterious electrophysiological and mechanical effects may occur, such as new arrhythmias, myocardial necrosis, or contractile dysfunction [9,10]. Biphasic waveforms may be less deleterious than monophasic waveforms with a higher safety factor (lower minimum gradient necessary for defibrillation and higher maximum gradient causing deleterious effects). For a higher potential gradient and more even shock field, the surface area of the electrodes is large. Materials with

Table 1 CPI Patch Lead Specifications

Models	0040/0041	0063 (Endotak SQ)	0048 (Endotak SQ lead array)
Compatibility	PG with 6.1-mm pulse output connectors	PG with 6.1-mm connectors	PG with 6.1-mm connectors
Length	67 cm	69 cm	70 cm
Electrode material	Titanium mesh	Titanium mesh	Platinum-clad titanium
Surface	14 cm^2 (0040) 28 cm^2 (0041)	28 cm^2	NA[a]
Conductor	Drawn-brazed-stranded (DBS) wire (silver and stainless steel)	DBS wire Teflon coated	DBS wire
Insulation	Silicone rubber	Silicone rubber	Silicone
Lead body diameter	3.3 mm	3.3 mm	3.3 mm
Lead resistance	1 Ω	1 Ω	< 1 Ω
Connector size	6.1 mm	6.1 mm	6.1 mm

[a]Electrode surface depends on the spatial arrangement of the array, covering an area up to 128 cm^2.
PG = pulse generator; SQ = subcutaneous

Table 2 Telecronics Defibrillator Patches[a]

Models	040-105	040-106	040-107	040-125 NTL	040-126 NTL	040-127 NTL
Size	Small	Standard	Large	Small	Standard	Large
Compatibility	ICD PG with HV.1 (3.2-mm) top caps	HV.1	HV.1	HV.1	HV.1	HV.1
Length	53 cm	53 cm	53 cm	53 cm	53 cm	53 cm
Electrode material	Titanium	Titanium	Titanium	Titanium	Titanium	Titanium
Surface	15 cm^2	28 cm^2	40 cm^2	15 cm^2	28 cm^2	40 cm^2
Lead body diameter	3.2 mm	3.2 mm	3.2 mm	3.2 mm	3.2 mm	3.2 mm
Lead resistance	1 Ω	1 Ω	1 Ω	1 Ω	1 Ω	1 Ω
Connector size	3.2 mm	3.2 mm	3.2 mm	3.2 mm	3.2 mm	3.2 mm
Number of mesh windows	6	12	20	6	12	20

[a]ICD, implantable cardioverter defibrillator; NTL, nonthoracotomy lead (subcutaneous patch); PG, pulse generator.

Table 3 Medtronic Patch Leads

Models	6897S/6921S	6897M/6921M	6897L/6921L	6895/6999 (subcutaneous)
Size	Small	Medium	Large	Medium
Compatibility	ICDs with 3.2/6.5-mm connectors	ICDs with 3.2/6.5-mm connectors	ICDs with 3.2/6.5-mm connectors	ICDs with 3.2/6.5-mm connectors
Length	50 cm	50 cm	50 cm	50 cm
Electrode material	Platinum alloy (coil)	Platinum alloy	Platinum alloy	Platinum alloy
Surface	30 cm^2	45 cm^2	60 cm^2	45 cm^2
Coils	3	4	5	4
Connector size	3.2/6.5 mm	3.2/6.5 mm	3.2/6.5 mm	3.2/6.5 mm

Table 4 Ventritex Defibrillation Leads[a]

Models	DP-5019	DP-5038
Compatibility	ICDs with 5-mm connectors	ICDs with 5-mm connectors
Size	small	large
Surface area	19 cm^2	38 cm^2
Length	64 cm	66 cm
Electrode material		
Mesh	Grade CP1 titanium	Grade CP1 titanium
Backing	Dacron-reinforced medical-grade silicone rubber sheet	Dacron-reinforced medical grade silicone rubber sheet
Conductor material	Teflon-coated DBS 316LVM stainless steel/silver composite	Teflon-coated DBS 316LVM stainless steel/silver composite
Insulation	Medical-grade silicone rubber	Medical-grade silicone
Radiographic marker	90/10 platinum/iridium wire	90/10 platinum/iridium wire
Resistance	1 Ω	1 Ω
Connector size	5 mm	5 mm

[a]Intended for use with the Ventritex Cadence defibrillator, models V-100 and V-100B. Ventritex defibrillation lead adapter, model LA-6450, can be used to connect the CPI defibrillation leads (6.4 mm) to the Ventritex Cadence device (5 mm), model V-100. However, new Cadence model V-100C accepts CPI or similarly sized defibrillation leads (6.1 mm). The Cadence model V-100B accepts 5-mm defibrillation leads and 5-mm pace/sense leads.

Table 5 Intermedics Patch Leads[a]

Models	497-01	497-02	497-11	497-12
Shape	Elliptical	Elliptical	Contoured (RV)	Contoured (LV)
Surface area	16 cm^2	32 cm^2	48 cm^2	48 cm^2
Material	Titanium	Titanium	Titanium	Titanium
Insulation	Silicone rubber	Silicone rubber	Silicone rubber	Silicone rubber
Length	50 cm	50 cm	50 cm	50 cm
Lead body diameter	2.5 mm	2.5 mm	2.5 mm	2.5 mm
Resistance	≤ 3.5 Ω	≤ 3.5 Ω	≤ 3.5 Ω	≤ 3.5 Ω
Connector	4 mm	4 mm	4 mm	4 mm

[a]LV, (to fit shape of) left ventricle; RV, (to fit shape of) right ventricle.

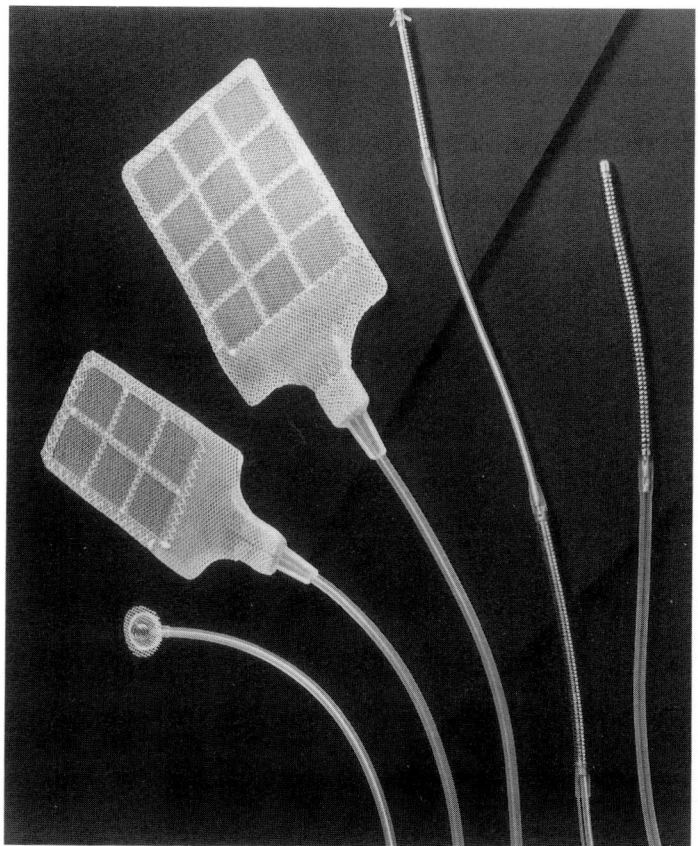

Figure 1 Four types of CPI leads are displayed from left to right: epimyocardial rate-sensing lead, small (14 cm^2) and large (28 cm^2) defibrillating patches, endocardial pace/sense and defibrillation lead with two coil electrodes (Endotak C lead), and the superior vena cava (spring electrode) lead (Tables 1,6,9). (Courtesy of CPI.)

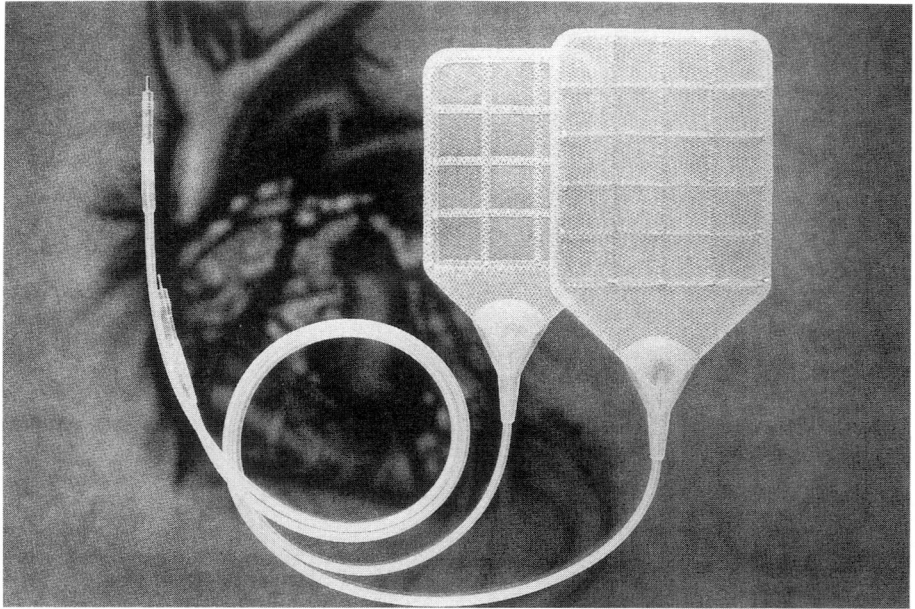

Figure 2 Two different-sized Telectronics patch leads (small, 15 cm^2; and standard, 28 cm^2) are displayed which are used with the epicardial ICD systems. Telectronics also make a large-size (40-cm^2) patch for epicardial use, and three different-sized subcutaneous/submuscular patches as well, for use with nonthoracotomy systems (15 cm^2, 28 cm^2, and 40 cm^2) (Table 2). (Courtesy of Telectronics.)

low impedance are generally used. Large electrodes also have lower impedance, which allows the delivery of more voltage during the shock to the ventricles beyond the electrode–tissue interface, generating a higher potential gradient field in the heart and resulting in successful defibrillation with lower energy.

Increased electrode surface area results in reduction in DFT attributed to a decrease in impedance and an increase in current density [13]. However, at a critical patch surface area no further DFT reduction is noted, even though the impedance may continue to decrease. It has also been suggested that the shape of the patch may affect threshold, with large contoured electrodes having a lower DFT as compared to flat ones, probably as a result of better contact [14]. On the other hand, the large size of the defibrillating electrodes may cause some problems that have to be taken into account, such as interference with wall motion and overall left ventricular function, difficulty in fitting hearts of various sizes, greater pericardial irritation and thus incidence of pericarditis and/or atrial arrhythmias or focal bleeding, or heart insulation with resultant increase in energy required or even failure to defibrillate the heart with an external transthoracic shock [15]. During implantation of the defibrillating electrodes an attempt is made to include most of the ventricular myocardium between the two electrodes to create a maximal potential gradient, while at the same time the electrode borders are kept equidistant and apart as far as possible to avoid shunting of current between the edges. The position chosen for the two electrodes, with one on the right ventricle and the other on the left ventricle, is usually such that the current flow traverses the intraventricular septum for highest defibrillating efficacy [7,16] and at the same time placement over the major epicardial coronary arteries is avoided, to prevent possible vessel injury or spasm [9].

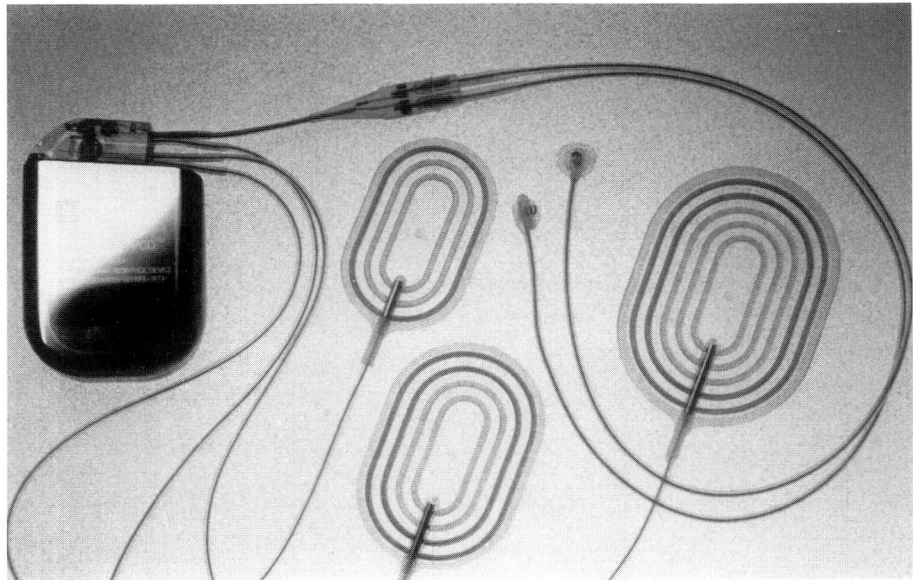

Figure 3 Two epicardial sense/pace leads and three epicardial patch leads of different sizes from Medtronic, Inc., are shown. Note the difference in design and shape of these patch leads as compared to the ones shown previously. Medtronic makes patches of three different sizes (small, 30 cm^2; medium, 45 cm^2; large, 60 cm^2) for epicardial ICD systems, and one patch of medium size (45 cm^2) for subcutaneous implantation and use with the nonthoratomy systems (Tables 3,8,11). See text for discussion. (Courtesy of Medtronic, Inc.)

Not infrequently, however, one is faced with high DFT despite using two patches of various sizes in different positions, and the need arises for use of multiple (three or four) patches in an attempt to improve the defibrillation energy requirements [17–19]. If three or more smaller electrodes are used, to avoid some of the drawbacks of larger electrodes, it is suggested that two of them be connected in parallel as a common anode or cathode to deliver sequential and not simultaneous shocks in order to avoid low potential gradients within the heart [9]. Placement and connection of multiple patches is made possible with use of Y connectors (CPI, Ventritex, Medtronic, Intermedics) and/or defibrillator systems having three-patch ports (Medtronic) [20]. The three-port system of the Medtronic device (PCD) allows a greater number of available programmable options, such as bidirectional and sequential shocks [21]. Potential problems with multiple patches, though, have to be taken into account. Among these, the likelihood of impairing ventricular function, developing constrictive pericarditis, occurrence of current shunting or tissue injury, and the difficulty of effective external defibrillation need to be considered [17]. Furthermore, the expectation of lower DFT with the triple epicardial electrode system is not always realized [21].

Another effective way to reduce DFT in either thoracotomy or nonthoracotomy ICD systems is the use of biphasic rather than monophasic shocks [22–24]. Sequential monophasic or biphasic shocks with certain intershock interval may also have similar effect [25–27]. Switching patch polarity and/or including the right side of the heart and left ventricle during patch positioning may lower the DFT in an individual patient [7,28,29]. Lead patch configurations that include the septum (right atrium-left ventricle or right ventricle-left ventricle) provide bet-

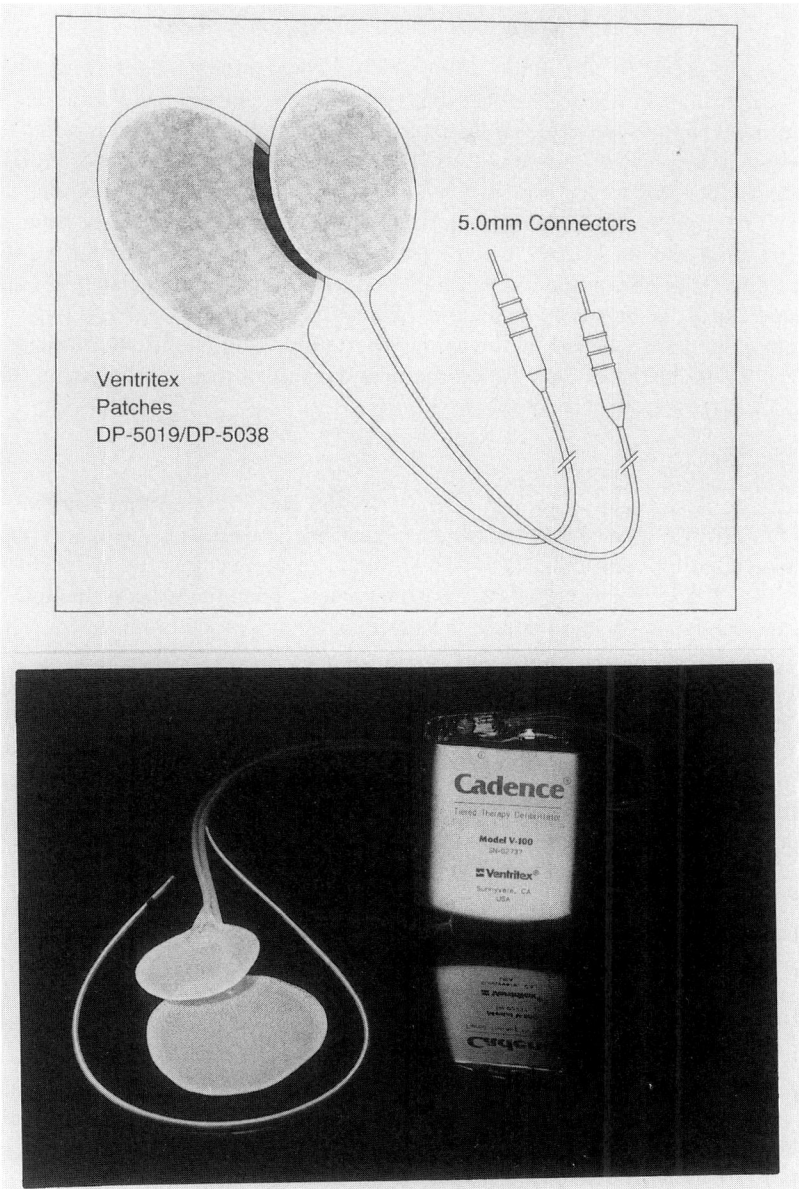

Figure 4 A drawing (upper panel) and a photograph (lower panel) of the two Ventritex patch leads: small, 19 cm^2, and large, 38 cm^2 patches, used with the Cadence ICD device (Table 4). (Courtesy of Ventritex.)

ter defibrillating efficacy than those confined to either side of the septum (e.g., left ventricle-left ventricle) [7].

Titanium and steel, or alluminum alloy are the conventional materials used in the construction of defibrillation leads. The electrodes are usually constructed of titanium, except the Medtronic models, which are made of platinum alloy coils, while the lead conductors are commonly made of drawn-brazed-stranded (DBS) stainless steel/silver composite with the back of the electrode and the conductor insulated with silicone or polyurethane. New material such as carbon fibers, or new electrode designs such as porous disk electrodes, have been proposed as means of lowering the impedance and thus the energy required for effective defibrillation [30,31]. In general, defibrillation can be improved by designing better patches with large area and contoured shape, and/or using sequential orthogonal pulses and biphasic pulses [14,19,26,27,32]. Finally, the consequences of device programming, with an initially unsuccessful shock causing a rise in defibrillation energy requirement during subsequent shocks, need to be considered and discerned from lead problems [33].

A. Complications

In the immediate postoperative period, lead-associated complications may include acute pericarditis due to friction incurred by the patches, further causing atrial tachyarrhythmias or occasionally exacerbating ventricular tachyarrhythmias, focal bleeding due to mechanical causes related to the leads and their sutures, patch displacement, pneumothorax or hemothorax during subclavian vein puncture for insertion of the superior vena cava lead [4,34–38]. In addition, in patients having devices programmed to rely on the morphology criterion for arrhythmia detection, reversible failure to sense the arrhythmia has been observed postoperatively, attributed to inflammatory and reactive tissue-patch interactions [39].

Patch crumpling [40], lead fracture [41], infection [42,43], constrictive pericarditis [44], patch erosion [45], and patch dislodgement [20] have all been observed as long-term complications with the defibrillation leads. Spring lead migration has also occurred, especially before the availability of the "butterfly" anchoring device [35,36]. In patients with prophylactic patches, the concern has been raised of potential failure of external defibrillation due to insulation of the heart [15]; however, this has not been the case in humans for at least the combination of a small and a large patch [46]. Lead-related complications occur with equal frequency (up to about 8–10% for both patch and sense/pace leads) in first-, second-, or third-generation ICD systems [21,35–38].

Computed tomography is helpful in assessing patch position and evaluating for the presence of patch crumpling or fluid collection [16,40]. When prophylactic patches are implanted, usually together with the epicardial rate-sensing leads, the wire terminals are placed subcutaneously in the area where the pocket for the pulse generator will be fashioned in case the device is needed later. Retrieval of these wires is not always easy, and extensive dissection of the excessive fibrotic tissue that has grown locally is usually required, with the risk of possible seroma formation and, more important, wire damage. To facilitate such wire retrieval, a silicone pouch has been used by some to protect the leads [47].

Pathology reports in patients with ICD leads include localized fibrosis around the patch (probably as a result of acute pericarditis with subsequent progressive changes), thrombi associated with the superior vena cava and right ventricular electrodes, and asymptomatic pulmonary emboli [48]. The localized myocardial injury confined under the patch was observed more frequently in patients who had received multiple defibrillations. The clinical significance of some of these findings has been questioned [49]. It seems that the intensity, rapidity of ICD discharges, and the electrode size are important factors determining the degree of myocardial injury, with reduced damage noted with fewer, less frequent defibrillations and larger-size electrodes. Cardiac enzyme release has not been reported to be significantly different with extrapericardial or intrapericardial patch placement.

B. Nonthoracotomy Lead Systems

A nonthoracotomy defibrillation lead system could have major advantages over the epicardial lead systems by reducing the morbidity, mortality, and cost of thoracotomy procedures, as long as defibrillation is effected using transvenous and/or subcutaneous/submuscular electrodes. Such lead systems currently available for clinical or investigational use in the United States and in Europe include the Endotak lead system (CPI), the Enguard system (Telectronics), and the Transvene system (Medtronic) (Tables 6–8) [50–54]. These systems may extend the indications for ICD implantation to patients unable to withstand a thoracotomy procedure, and make ICD therapy available at a lesser cost and lower risk [55]. These systems may also make feasible and affordable prophylactic ICD use in high-risk patients [56]. The major remaining problem with these systems is that of high defibrillation thresholds, which have been observed in as many as 17–30% of patients having nonthoracotomy systems implanted. Use of amiodarone and low ejection fraction is probably predictive of such a problem. With the availability of sequential and/or biphasic shocks, DFTs may improve [22,23,57–59]. The results and data accumulated thus far from testing various combinations of nonthoracotomy defibrillating lead systems suggest that no single technique or system tested is clearly superior, but that an efficacious defibrillation method can be found individually during testing, which will obviate the need for thoracotomy in the majority of patients. Some of these defibrillation lead combinations are described below. To select the best method for an individual patient, various combinations of defibrillating leads, defibrillation technique, and current pathways need to be tested during implantation of these systems [60]. Also, different devices used with these electrode systems now provide multiple options for defibrillation, rendering such electrical testing feasible. With the experience accumulated thus far, systems providing wider spatial distribution of current flow through the myocardium are favored [55].

1. Combined Transvenous-Subcutaneous/Submuscular Leads

Saksena et al. used a triple electrode system, including two transvenous catheter defibrillating electrodes (mounted on a single tripolar catheter with a tip-sensing electrode) and a submuscular patch [61]. Several problems were identified with this original system, which was subsequently revised [50,51,53]. A chest (subcutaneous or submuscular) patch or electrode array has been used in various combinations with right ventricular/coronary sinus electrodes as a two- or three-electrode system in an attempt to improve DFTs [60]. The effect of position of the cutaneous patch on the DFT has not been adequately explored [13]. Single, sequential and/or simultaneous pulse defibrillation techniques have been utilized, but not always can major differences in DFTs be proven clinically [13,62]. Rather, the method with the lowest DFT could be determined in each individual patient only after testing of all available options. However, when different pulse waveforms are tested, such as monophasic, biphasic symmetric or biphasic asymmetric, and triphasic waveforms, it appears that most studies show a significant DFT reduction with use of biphasic shocks, with preference placed on the asymmetric biphasic pulses requiring only one capacitor as compared to symmetric pulses utilizing two capacitors [13,18,23,58,63].

2. Transvenous Lead Systems

As early as in 1971 a transvenous two-electrode catheter was developed and tested in dogs by Schuder et al [64]. Following the success of the epicardial ICD system, efforts at transvenous

Table 6 CPI Endocardial Defibrillation/Rate-Sensing/Pacing Leads

Models	0020 (SVC lead)	0060, 0062, 0064 [Endotak CJ][a]	0070, 0072, 0074 [Endotak CJ][a]	0010 (tined)	0056 (screw-in) with adapter (59 cm)
Function	Defibrillation	Defib/sense-pace	Defib/sense-pace	Sense-pace	Sense-pace
Length	100 cm	100 cm	100 cm	100 cm	59 cm
Electrode size	4.1 mm (diameter) 82 mm (helical coil)	3.95 mm (14 Fr)[b] 3.1 mm (lead body)	3.95 mm (14 Fr)[b] 3.1 mm (lead body)	2.2 (10 Fr)[b]	2.2–2.6 mm(9Fr)[b]
Electrode material	Titanium	Platinum-iridium	Titanium (shock) Steel (rate-sensing)	Platinum-iridium	Platinum-iridium
Surface	70 cm^2	29.5 cm^2 (distal spring) 61.7 cm^2 (proximal spring) 0.9 cm^2 (tip)	37.9 cm^2 (distal spring) 61.7 cm^2 (proximal spring) 0.9 cm^2 (tip)	8 mm^2 (distal) 52 mm^2 (proximal)	10 mm^2 (distal) 35 mm^2 (proximal)
Conductor	DBS wire	DBS	DBS	DBS	DBS
Insulation	Silicone rubber	Silicone rubber	Silicone rubber	Silicone	Silicone
Lead resistance	2 Ω	5.2 Ω	5.2 Ω	300 Ω (bipolar)	180 Ω
Connector size	6.1 mm	6.1 mm (2) (shock) 4.75 mm (2) (sense)	6.1 mm (2) 4.75 mm (1)	4.75 mm	3.2 mm (1) adapter: 4.75 mm (2)
Distance between electrodes	NA	10 cm (0060) 13 cm (0062) 16 cm (0064)	11.7 cm (0070) 14.7 cm (0072) 17.7 cm (0074)	10 mm	11 mm
Fixation	NA	Tines	Tines	Tines	Screw-in

[a]Nonthoracotomy system.
[b]Suggested size of introducer sheath.
NA = not applicable

Table 7 Telectronics Endocardial Defibrillation/Rate-Sensing/Pacing Leads

Models	Accufix: 330-201 (ventricular), 330-801 (atrial "J")	EnGuard PFX: 040-068[a] (Ventricular)	EnGuard PFX: 040-069[a] (Atrial "J")
Function	Pacing	Pace/sense and defibrillation	Defibrillation (pace/sense: not used)
Fixation	Active	Passive	Passive
Length (cm)	58 ventricular, 48 atrial	100	90
Electrode material	Platinum	Titanium/platinum-iridium	Titanium/platinum-iridium
Surface	10.2 mm^2 (tip) 57.2 mm^2 (ring)	distal 8.8 mm^2 braid 60 cm^2	distal 8.8 mm^2 braid 60 cm^2
Conductor	MP35N inner and outer quadrifilar	inner: quadrifilar MP35N (cobalt-nickel) helical coil; outer: MP35N alloy heptafilar	inner: quadrifilar MP 35N helical; outer: MP35N alloy heptafilar
Insulation	Polyurethane	Polyurethane	Polyurethane
Lead body	2.2 mm, max 2.8 mm (distal) (9 Fr)	2.0 mm (12 Fr)	2.0 mm (12 Fr)
Lead resistance	55–95 Ω (201), 45–165 Ω (801)	braid 5 Ω, inner 95 Ω	braid 5 Ω, inner 95 Ω
Connector type/size[b]	Pace/sense: bipolar VS.1 (3.2 mm)	Bifurcated: pace/sense bipolar VS.1; high-voltage unipolar 3.2 mm (HV)	Bifurcated: pace/sense bipolar VS.1; high-voltage unipolar 3.2 mm (HV)
Helix penetration	1.9 ± 0.2 mm	NA	NA
Electrode distance	29 mm (201), 17 mm (801)	18 mm	8.5 cm

[a]Nonthoracotomy system (revised, 1993)
[b]Pace/sense connectors for all Guardian models are VS.1B (bipolar).
NA = not applicable

Table 8 Medtronic Endocardial Defibrillation-Sense/Pace Leads and Subcutaneous Patch (Transvene System)

Models	6966 (RV)	6968 (RV)	6963 (SVC/CS)	6999 (SQ Patch)
Function	Defib-sense/pace	Defib-sense/pace	Defib	Defib
Polarity	Tripolar	Tripolar	Unipolar	Unipolar
Length	110 cm	110 cm	110 cm	50 cm
Electrode material	Platinum alloy	Platinum alloy	Platinum alloy	Platinum alloy
Insulation	Polyurethane	Polyurethane	Silicone	Silicone
Lead diameter	3.3 mm (spring)	3.3 mm	2.3 mm	2.5 mm
Surface area (coil)	426 mm^2	426 mm^2	90 mm^2	660 mm^2 (4 coils)
Connector size	6.5 mm (defib: unipolar)	3.2 mm (pace: bipolar)	6.5 mm	6.5 mm
Fixation	Screw-in	Tines	None	Sutures
Chamber	Ventricle	Ventricle	SVC/CS	NA
Introducer	11 F	11 F	8 F	NA

CS = coronary sinus; NA = not applicable; RV = right ventricle; SQ = subcutaneous; SVC = superior vena cava.

defibrillation were renewed over the past few years, and various transvenous electrode systems have been tested in animal and clinical studies. One simple two-electrode system involves a right ventricular and a superior vena cava electrode [65] or a right ventricular and a right atrial electrode [66]. A coronary sinus and right ventricular electrode system has also been tested [67]. A three-electrode system has been used and involves right ventricular, superior vena cava, and coronary sinus electrodes [68,69]. Concerns about thrombosis and/or perforation of the coronary sinus or easier lead migration or dislodgement have been raised [13,68] but not substantiated. Thus the option to include a coronary sinus catheter for effective defibrillation during implantation of nonthoracotomy systems has been heralded as safe and reliable [69].

The easiest and most convenient way for the implantation of a fully transvenous system is, indeed, the use of only one endocardial lead with both sense/pace and defibrillation capabilities. One such lead is the Endotak C (CPI) lead, which is a tripolar, tined, endocardial lead featuring a porous tip electrode (placed in the right ventricular apex) that serves as the cathode for intracardiac right ventricular electrogram rate sensing, and two spring electrodes, with the distal one serving as the anode for rate sensing and as the cathode for morphology sensing and defibrillation while the proximal spring (seated in the superior vena cava) functions as the anode for defibrillation [50,52] (Figs. 1 and 5, Table 6). If no satisfactory DFTs are obtained with the single catheter, a cutaneous patch can be used as well. The first Endotak lead system underwent clinical trials from March 1988 to January 1989, but it was withdrawn due to lead fractures requiring several revisions. In May 1990 in Europe and in September 1990 in the United States, the redesigned and revised system reentered clinical investigation [50]. The revisions included change in the high-energy conductor of the endocardial lead, the patch, and the Y adaptor from coiled wire to Teflon-coated braided flexible cable; change in the platinum screen mesh of the patch to titanium; and change to a closed lead system [53]. The Endotak lead system was finally approved by the FDA for clinical use on August 27, 1993.

Other transvenous leads with combined sence/pace and defibrillation function are the EnGuard PFX lead (Telectronics), and the Transvene lead (Medtronic), which are positioned at the right ventricular apex; the EnGuard lead is a passive fixation lead with tines, while the Transvene lead is an active-fixation (screw-in) lead. The Transvene system has an additional separate transvenous lead for defibrillation that is permanently placed in the superior vena cava or the coronary sinus (Fig. 6) [52,54,68,69]. The EnGuard system also has a separate bifur-

ICD Lead Systems

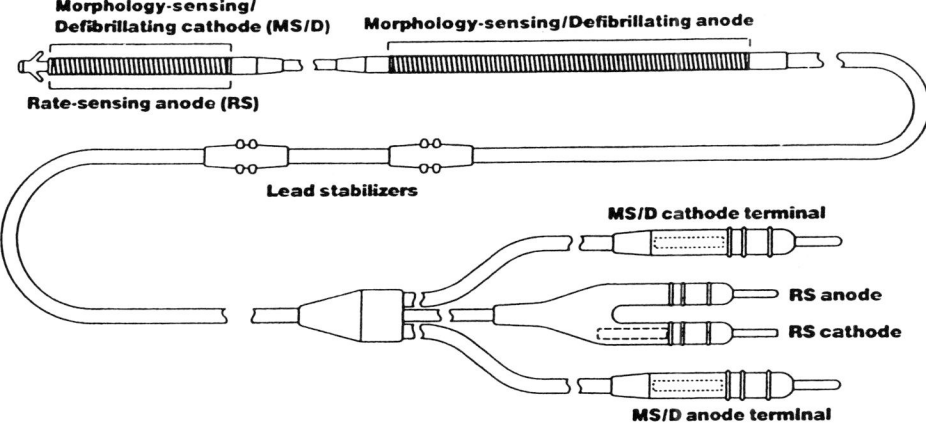

ENDOTAK C Lead Components

Figure 5 Component diagram of the single sense/pace and defibrillation lead (Endotak C, CPI) designed for use with pure transvenous or mixed (transvenous-subcutaneous) nonthoracotomy ICD systems. (Courtesy of CPI.)

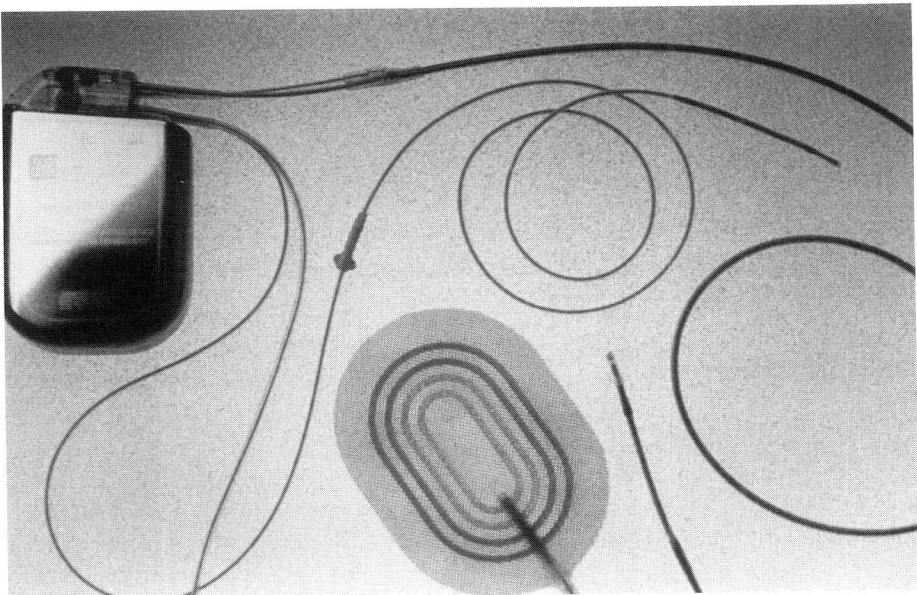

Figure 6 The Medtronic nonthoracotomy lead system includes the sense/pace and defibrillation lead (right-hand corner), placed at the right ventricular apex; a second endocardial defibrillation lead (top loop), placed at the superior vena cava or the coronary sinus; and the subcutaneous/submuscular patch (bottom center). (Courtesy of Medtronic, Inc.)

cated, J-shaped, tined, atrial pacing and defibrillation lead for placement in the right atrial appendage (see Chapter 46). Additionally, a subcutaneous or submuscular patch placed in the lateral chest wall can be used with either system (Fig. 6) [52]. The Transvene system was recently (December 9, 1993) approved by the FDA for clinical use. Most recently, Ventritex developed its own nonthoracotomy ICD lead system (Cadence TVL) (Table 17).

3. Thoracoscopic Lead Systems

Preliminary reports on thoracoscopic implantation of ICD leads suggest that this may be a feasible option in the future for patients who are poor candidates for thoracotomy and who have high defibrillation thresholds through transvenous or other nonthoracotomy lead systems [70]. Thoracoscopy is performed with the use of three trocars and a video-linked system. It can provide adequate exposure for ICD lead placement, accommodating the passage and placement of both ICD lead types (defibrillation and sense/pace leads). Bleeding is controlled with the use of electrocautery. Pediatric defibrillator paddles have been proposed for use through the thoracoscopic incision for rescue defrillation if ever needed [70]. This technique of ICD lead insertion minimizes postoperative pain and other thoracotomy-related complications.

4. Complications and Limitations of Nonthoracotomy Lead Systems

A significant number of lead system complications were reported with the early nonthoracotomy ICD systems [54,71]. Among these, there were observed lead fractures that were asymptomatic in some patients but in others resulted in high pacing thresholds, oversensing, inappropriate shocks or inability to defibrillate and sudden death [71,72]. These major lead problems with the early systems of Endotak (CPI) and EnGuard (Telectronics) leads led to interruption of investigational trials of these systems. Trials of leads with improved design were subsequently resumed [54]. With the newer generation lead systems, especially when combined with ICD devices capable of delivering biphasic shocks, the number of pure transvenous ICD implants (without the need for a cutaneous patch) is growing (92% among 38 nonthoracotomy ICD implants according to our own experience).

Endocardial leads used for both defibrillation and rate sensing have been reported to suffer from technical inadequacies that may pose significant risk to the patient. Endocardial electrograms obtained from such integrated sense/pace-defibrillating leads have been shown to be affected after shock delivery, with their amplitude decreasing to such a significant degree that arrhythmia redetection is dangerously compromised [73]. As already mentioned above, obtaining adequate defibrillation thresholds has been a major problem with the nonthoracotomy systems. Thromboembolism related to transvenous spring defibrillation lead has also been observed [54].

II. SENSE/PACE LEADS

Reliable sensing and detection of the ventricular tachyarrhythmia is of paramount importance in all ICD systems. Although device sensing and arrhythmia detection circuits are critical in this regard, the sensing leads used to obtain suitable electrocardiographic signals are equally important. Furthermore, with the development of newer-generation devices providing antibradycardia and antitachycardia pacing, major attention is now paid intraoperatively to establishing both adequate sensing and pacing thresholds via the implanted sense/pace electrodes. In the early version of the ICD, VF or sinusoidal VT sensing was derived from the shocking leads. In all subsequent ICD models, however, a separate sensing lead system was utilized [74]. For this purpose, either two epimyocardial leads or a bipolar endocardial right ventricular lead have been employed.

ICD Lead Systems

Table 9 CPI Epicardial Rate-Sensing/Pacing Leads[a]

Models	4312[b]	4313[c]	4320	4321	4322
Length	54 cm	35 cm	54 cm	54 cm	35 cm
Electrode material	Platinum-iridium	Platinum-iridium	Platinum-iridium	Platinum-iridium	Platinum-iridium
Electrode surface	10 mm^2	10 mm^2	10 mm^2	10 mm^2	10 mm^2
Resistance	44 Ω	29 Ω	41 Ω	41 Ω	27 Ω
Type	Unipolar	Unipolar	Unipolar	Unipolar	Unipolar
Lead body diameter	3 mm	3 mm	1.8 mm	1.8 mm	1.8 mm
Connector size	4.75 mm	4.75 mm	4.75 mm	3.2 mm (pm)	3.2 mm (pm)
Penetration depth	3.5 mm	3.5 mm	3.5 mm	3.5 mm	3.5 mm
Insulation material	Silicone	Silicone	Silicone	Silicone	Silicone

[a] pm, pacemaker compatible. There is also a 4316-25 lead with 25-cm length for use in infants.
[b] 4316-54 model is IS-1 compatible (3.2 mm).
[c] 4316-35 model is IS-1 compatible (3.2 mm).

A. Epicardial Leads

Most commonly, epicardial leads have been used with an ICD system for rate sensing, and a separate procedure to implant endocardial leads is thus avoided. Two screw-on epimyocardial leads are frequently employed (Tables 9–13, Figs. 1 and 3). They are placed at about 1 cm apart to obtain acceptable bipolar signals with an R wave of at least 5 mV in amplitude and less than 100 ms in duration. However, when one is unable to obtain satisfactory lead signals with the

Table 10 Telectronics Epicardial Rate-Sensing/Pacing Leads[a]

Models	033-571/572	030-574/575	325-452 (Encor)
Type	Unipolar, screw-in	Unipolar, screw-in	Unipolar, porous-surfaced
Length (cm)	35/54	35/54	52
Electrode material	Platinized platinum	Platinized platinum	Platinum-iridium
Electrode surface	10 mm^2	10 mm^2	6 mm^2
Lead body diameter	1.8 mm	1.8 mm	2.25 mm
Connector type/size	VS.1/3.2 mm	5 mm	3.2 mm, upsizing 5/6 mm
Helix penetration	3.5 mm	3.5 mm	N/A
Insulation material	Silicone	Silicone	Polyurethane
Number of turns	2.25	2.25	N/A

[a] N/A = not applicable.

Table 11 Medtronic Epicardial Pacing Leads

Model	6917T	6917AT	4951P
Length	53 cm	53 cm	53 cm
Electrode material	Platinum-iridium	Platinum-iridium	Platinum-iridium
Fixation	Screw-in (three turns)	Screw-in (two turns)	Barb
Type	Unipolar	Unipolar	Unipolar
Connector size	5.0 mm	5.0 mm	5.0 mm

Table 12 POSSIS Epicardial Pacing Leads

Models	1111	1112	1211	1212
Length	35 cm	54 cm	35 cm	54 cm
Electrode material	Platinum/iridium	Platinum-iridium	Platinum-iridium	Platinum-iridium
Anode			Titanium	Titanium
Conductor	Nickel cobalt multifilar coil			
Surface	10 mm^2	10 mm^2	10 mm^2	10 mm^2
Anode surface			62 mm^2	62 mm^2
Resistance	27 Ω	41 Ω	27 Ω cathode 46 Ω anode	27 Ω cathode 46 Ω anode
Type	Unipolar	Unipolar	Bipolar	Bipolar
Connector size	3.2 mm	3.2 mm	3.2 mm	3.2 mm
Penetration depth	3.5 mm	3.5 mm	3.5 mm	3.5 mm
Insulation material	Silicone	Silicone	Silicone	Silicone
Number of helix turns	$2\frac{1}{4}$	$2\frac{1}{4}$	$2\frac{1}{4}$	$2\frac{1}{4}$

epicardial leads, or when newer-generation devices with pacing capabilities are used and thus more reliable sense/pace electrodes are needed, bipolar endocardial leads are implanted.

The epicardial leads are usually implanted on the left ventricle, but also on the lateral right ventricle or the right ventricular outflow tract. Care is taken to place the leads in areas of healthy-appearing myocardium. Caution is exercised when the myocardium is infarcted, thin-walled, or infiltrated with fatty or fibrotic tissue. Various arrhythmic substrates (scarred, fibrotic, or hypertrophied myocardium) may present different sensing or pacing difficulties [75]. Particular attention is paid during ICD lead placement in patients with permanent pacemakers [76]. Most adverse interactions between the two devices can be avoided by implanting the ICD sensing leads at a location that minimizes the amplitude of the pacemaker artifact, as observed in recorded electrograms obtained from the external test/support equipment. Also, in patients

Table 13 Intermedics Epicardial Pacing Leads

Model	439-04 (Epicardial)	439-07 (Myocardial)
Length	45 cm	35 cm
Electrode		
Material	Platinum (90%)-iridium (10%)	Platinum (90%)-iridium (10%)
Base	Medical-grade silicone rubber	
Anchoring		Polyester mesh
Surface	21 mm^2	8 mm^2
Resistance	65 Ω	40 Ω
Type	Unipolar	Unipolar
Connector size	3.2 mm (VS.1)	3.2 mm (VS.1)
Penetration depth	NA	3.4 mm
Insulation	Polyurethane	Silicone rubber
Lead body diameter	1.7 mm	2.5 mm
Number of helix turns	NA	2

NA = not applicable

ICD Lead Systems

anticipated to need future pacemaker implant or rather routinely in all patients, as suggested by some, implanting the rate-sensing leads high on the lateral left ventricle, 1–2.5 cm below the atrioventricular groove, avoids potential problems with device interaction should a permanent pacemaker become necessary in the future.

B. Endocardial Leads

Bipolar endocardial leads are more frequently used for rate sensing and pacing during ICD implants when the third-generation devices are used. Usually a bipolar lead is inserted either through the cephalic or the subclavian vein and positioned at the right ventricular apex with use of fluoroscopy as for permanent pacemaker implants (Tables 6–8). When no concomitant surgery is planned, a passive-fixation lead may be used, but when some additional procedure is going to be performed, such as coronary bypass or aneurysmectomy or valve surgery, then due to risk for lead dislodgement with manipulation of the heart, an active-fixation lead is preferred. The endocardial lead may be placed separately in the catheterization or electrophysiology laboratory before the ICD implant, or it can be inserted in the operating room with use of a fluoroscopy bed. The lead will need to be long enough to allow for tunneling to the abdominal pocket, or a lead extender will be required. The lead should be carefully secured at the intravenous entry site to avoid dislodgement during tunneling, after which it should be retested to confirm satisfactory pacing and sensing thresholds and thus evaluate for possible lead damage during the tunneling procedure. Endocardial ventricular leads should be used with extreme caution in patients with tricuspid valve prostheses.

C. Combined Defibrillation-Sense/Pace Leads

For pure transvenous or mixed (transvenous-subcutaneous) ICD systems, as already described earlier, there are now integrated endocardial lead systems combining defibrillation and sense/pace functions on a single endocardial lead (Endotak C lead, CPI; EnGuard PFX lead, Telectronics; Transvene lead, Medtronic; and Cadence TVL, Ventritex) (Tables 6–8, 17) [50–54]. The lead may have an active- or passive-fixation mechanism for placement at the right ventricular apex. It includes a dual electrode system for sensing and pacing, with the tip electrode as the cathode and the distal defibrillation (coil) electrode as the anode. The lead is bifurcated and has two connectors, one in-line bipolar or bifurcated pace/sense terminal connector, and one defibrillation terminal connector, which may be in-line unipolar if the lead has only one defibrillation electrode intended for use in combination with another endocardial lead-EnGuard PFX/Transvene or a subcutaneous patch (Telectronics/Medtronic), or bifurcated if the lead has two defibrillation electrodes (CPI).

D. Complications

Complications similar to those occurring with defibrillating leads are also observed with sense/pace leads, although their frequency may be lower, at least for the epicardial systems [36]. Among these, lead fractures, migration, dislodgement, or infection may occur and require reintervention for management. Sense/pace lead fractures or insulation breaks may cause oversensing, which can subsequently trigger inappropriate ICD shocks [77]. Problems similar to those associated with pacemaker leads occur in patients receiving transvenous ICD leads, including pneumothorax, hemothorax, air embolism, cardiac perforation, tamponade, arrhythmias, subclavian vein thrombosis, lead dislodgement, fracture, migration, or infection. In patients with pacemaker/ICD devices, other particular problems related to the sense/pace leads, such as high pacing thresholds or even exit block, may develop. Finally, sense and/or pace failure may develop in a rare patient with Twiddler's syndrome [78]. Various devices have different means of noninvasively assessing sensing lead problems, including the use of "beep-o-gram" systems and telemetric transmission of intracardiac electrograms and/or main timing events, which are extremely useful for troubleshooting [21,79].

Some have alleged that epicardial pacing and sensing may be problematic in the long term, with deterioration of sensing during sinus rhythm and ventricular fibrillation, and rising pacing thresholds [21]. Thus reprogramming may be needed, but lead replacement and/or repositioning or revision to an endocardial lead may also be required. For this reason it has been suggested that endocardial leads for pacing and sensing be preferably implanted in newer-generation devices incorporating pacing capabilities.

Adverse effects of defibrillation shocks have been reported on subsequent cardiac pacing and sensing thresholds. These effects are not related to the pace/sense electrodes per se but to the myocardial tissue itself. Thus an increase in pacing threshold and a decrease in R-wave amplitude that persist for up to 10 min after a shock have been observed [80]. As a matter of fact, mechanical function, pacing, and defibrillation thresholds may deteriorate immediately after high-energy shocks [33]. This assumes critical importance in patients with endocardial leads of combined sense/pace and defibrillation function, where failure of arrhythmia redetection after a shock may have dire consequences [73].

III. LEAD SIGNAL EVALUATION AND DEFIBRILLATION THRESHOLD TESTING

A pacemaker system analyzer (PSA) is used intraoperatively to check pacing and sensing thresholds of the pace/sense leads. The capture threshold is determined, which should be ≤ 1.5 V at 0.5 ms for the epicardial leads and ≤ 1 V at 0.5 ms for the endocardial leads. The impedance usually ranges from 300 Ω to 1000 Ω. The R-wave amplitude should be ≥ 5 mV during sinus rhythm. A slew rate of ≥ 0.75 V/s is also sought. During pulse generator replacement, the acceptable chronic thresholds should measure ≤ 3 V for the capture threshold, ≥ 3 mV for the R wave, and ≥ 0.5 V/s for the slew rate with same range of impedance (300–1000 Ω). Alternatively or additionally, certain external cardioverter defibrillator testing devices used intraoperatively for DFT testing also have the capability to provide measurements of lead signals. For example, amplitude and duration of lead signals can be measured with the CPI external device (ECD) for both the rate-sensing and defibrillation leads using a strip-chart recorder. Certain ICD systems use one of the defibrillating leads together with one epicardial lead for antibradycardia pacing, and thresholds should therefore also be measured using this specific lead combination. Some external devices used for intraoperative testing have in-built PSA function (e.g., Ventritex and Telectronics devices) and can thus be used for all measurements and electrical tests. During measurement of the lead signals (R-wave amplitude and duration), one should avoid measuring the voltage potential of the current of injury that may be induced acutely during lead implantation.

After obtaining satisfactory signals from the implanted leads, arrhythmia conversion testing is undertaken to demonstrate successful conversion of VF with energy that ensures adequate safety margin [81–83]. For the majority of cases the defibrillation threshold, despite its variability, should be at least 10 J lower than the maximum energy the device can deliver. Although test protocols vary, most implanting physicians aim for a DFT ≤ 15 J. Measurement of DFT is accomplished with induction of VF with use of an alternating-current fibrillator device or by rapid pacing via a programmed stimulator or via certain external testing devices with

Table 14 Telectronics Defibrillator Adaptors

ICD model[a]	Adaptors/connectors
Guardian 4202	040-054/Telectronics 3.2 mm HV
(HV connector: 5/6 mm)	040-053/Medtronic 3.2 mm
	040-045/CPI 6 mm
Guardian 4203/4204	Direct fit/Telectronics 3.2 mm HV
(HV connector: 3.2 mm)	040-055 /Medtronic 3.2 mm
	040-047/CPI 6 mm
Guardian ATP 4210/4211/4215	Direct fit/Telectronics 3.2 mmHV
(HV connector: 3.2 mm)	040-055/Medtronic 3.2 mm
	040-047/CPI 6 mm

[a]Pace/sense connectors for all Guardian models are VS.1B (in-line bipolar).

in-built fibrillation-inducing function. At least three successful conversions of VF are performed with successively decreased energies. To minimize the potential for variability dependent on the arrhythmia duration, an attempt is made to maintain consistent VF duration (10–15 s) during DFT testing. Among the various factors affecting DFT, the most important appear to be the type of defibrillating lead system, the size, position, and polarity of patches, the pulse waveform and duration, arrhythmia duration, and antiarrhythmic drug effects. In addition to DFT testing, ventricular tachycardia conversion is also evaluated intraoperatively in patients whose clinical arrhythmia is ventricular tachycardia, although usually this is better assessed during predischarge testing in the electrophysiology laboratory.

During arrhythmia conversion testing, attention is also directed to evaluation of lead signals recorded through the external testing device. Also, the patch lead impedance can be measured during DFT testing. This represents an important measurement for assessing patch lead integrity. Arrhythmia recognition depends on the characteristics of the sensed electrograms. In most devices the rate, as detected by the sensing electrodes, remains the main detection criterion. Some devices may combine rate with morphology characteristics (e.g., probability density function or turning-point morphology in CPI devices) assessed from the electrogram recorded via the defibrillating leads. Thus the adequacy of arrhythmia detection should be assessed and is of particular importance for devices without the capability for automatic sensitivity adjustment (e.g., Guardian-4210). For purposes of proper sinus rhythm sensing and antibradycardia pacing as well as effective tachycardia detection and therapy, satisfactory sens-

Table 15 CPI Adaptors[a]

ICD models	Adaptor/connector
Ventak 1550/1555/1600/1705	6016, 3.2 mm, unipolar/(5 mm) (4.75)
(two rate-sensing ports, each 4.75 mm;	6015, 6 mm (5.38), unipolar/(5 mm) (4.75)
two HV ports, each 6.1 mm)	6516, 6 mm (5.38), unipolar/(5 mm) (4.75)
	[30-cm lead extender]
(Endotak lead system)	6836-Y connector (6.1 mm) (6.1 mm)/(6.1 mm)
Ventak PRX 1700	6021, bifurcated 3.2 mm/(3.2 mm)
(one 3.2-mm in-line bipolar rate-sensing/	6029, 6 mm in-line bipolar/(IS.1)
pacing lead port; two 3.2-mm HV ports)	

[a]CPI also has a lead tunneler (model 6888) made of stainless steel.

Table 16 Medtronic Lead Adaptors and Sizing Sleeves

Models	5866-23	6886	5866-24	5866-24M	6920
Type	Sizing sleeve	Adaptor	Adaptor	Adaptor	Sizing sleeve
Leads	Patch leads/connector	Pace/patch lead	Pace leads	Epicardial sense/pace leads	Patch leads
Function	3.2 mm to 5.0 mm	two 5.0-mm to one 3.2-mm bipolar	two unipolar 5.0-mm to one 3.2-mm bipolar	two 5.0-mm unipolar to one IS-1 bipolar	3.2-mm to 6.5-mm

Table 17 Ventritex Nonthoracotomy Lead System (Cadence TVL Lead System)

Models	RV-1101	SV-1101	SQ-701
Function	Defib-sense/pace	Defib	Defib
Polarity	Bipolar	Unipolar	Unipolar
Length	110 cm	110 cm	70 cm
Electrode material	Platinum iridium	Platinum iridium	Platinum iridium
Insulation	Silicone	Silicone	Silicone
Lead diameter	3.5 mm (11 Fr)	2.67 mm (8.5 Fr)	NA
Surface area, coil	470 mm^2	550 mm^2	39 cm^2
Connector size	3.2 mm	3.2 mm	3.2 mm
Fixation	Tines	None	Sutures
Location	Right ventricle	Superior vena cava	Subcutaneous/submuscular chest wall

NA = not applicable.

ing and electrogram characteristics during both sinus rhythm and VT/VF should be confirmed at the time of intraoperative electrical testing. Electrocardiographic or event markers are used to monitor and check proper sensing and arrhythmia detection during intraoperative testing, initially via the external testing equipment and finally via telemetry from the ICD device itself.

In patients with high defibrillation thresholds, observed at an estimated frequency as high as 4–5% of ICD implants [84], vigorous testing to optimize patch location, use of devices allowing sequential and/or biphasic shocks, and adjustments in antiarrhythmic drug therapy are some important measures to consider. In some patients DFTs may improve after patch healing occurs when retesting is performed 10–15 days postoperatively. Patients with persistently high DFTs who receive an ICD remain at high risk for arrhythmic death and alternative therapy, if at all possible, needs to be considered [84].

IV. FUTURE DIRECTIONS

Lead systems that incorporate dual-chamber sensing and pacing with capability for hemodynamic monitoring need to be developed in the future that will render current ICD devices more adaptable, physiological, and selective in the type of therapy they provide to patients with hemodynamically stable or unstable tachyarrhythmias who have concomitant bradyarrhythmic problems and varying degrees of myocardial dysfunction [85–87].

New technology that includes the use of multiconductor tubing may reduce the size and stiffness of leads used with the ICDs [88]. Further research and advances in electrode design, with development of electrodes that can convert arrhythmias with lower energy, will probably lead to smaller and longer-lasting ICD devices with more simplified nonthoracotomy implantation techniques [89]. Efforts should concentrate on developing lead systems that would implement improved arrhythmia detection via more sophisticated algorithms, hemodynamic monitoring and dual-chamber pacing, all applied through pace/sense endocardial leads, perhaps with endocardial electrode arrays [90]. However, there should be no need for special leads that would modify the implantation technique or exacerbate the problem of lead removal should explantation become necessary.

REFERENCES

1. Mirowski M, Reid PR, Mower MM, et al. Termination of malignant ventricular arrhythmias with an implanted automatic defibrillator in human beings. N Engl J Med 1980; 303:322–324.
2. Flaker G, Boley T, Walls J, Curtis JJ. Comparison of subxiphoid and traditional approaches for ICD implantation. PACE 1992; 15(I):1531–1533.
3. Manolis AS, TanDeguzman W, Lee MA, et al. Clinical experience in seventy-seven patients with the automatic implantable cardioverter defibrillator. Am Heart J 1989; 118:445–450.
4. Manolis AS, Rastegar H, Estes NAM III. Automatic implantable cardioverter defibrillator: current status. JAMA 1989; 262:1362–1368.
5. Manolis AS. Nonpharmacologic management of malignant ventricular tachyarrhythmias: role of the automatic implantable cardioverter defibrillator. Hellenic J Cardiol 1991; 32:14–24.
6. Manolis AS, Rastegar H, Estes NAM III. Prophylactic automatic implantable cardioverter defibrillator patches in patients at high risk for postoperative ventricular tachyarrhythmias. J Am Coll Cardiol 1989; 13:1367–1373.
7. Tedder M, Wharton JM, Anstadt MP, Revishvili AS, Hegde SS, Lowe JE. Optimal defibrillator patch configurations include the right side of the heart and left ventricle. Am J Cardiol 1993; 71:349–350.
8. Troup PJ, Chapman PD, Olinger GN, Kleinman LH. The implanted defibrillator: relation of defibrillating lead configuration and clinical variables to defibrillation threshold. J Am Coll Cardiol 1985; 6:1315–1321.

9. Ideker RE, Wolf PD, Alferness C, Krassowska W, Smith WM. Current concepts for selecting the location, size and shape of defibrillation electrodes. PACE 1991; 14(I):227–240.
10. Ideker RE, Hillsley RE, Wharton JM. Shock strength for the implantable defibrillator: can you have too much of a good thing? PACE 1992; 15:841–844.
11. Wharton JM, Smith WM, Wolf PD, Ideker RE. Mechanisms of electrical defibrillation. In: Luderitz B, Saksena S, eds. Interventional Electrophysiology. Mount Kisco, NY: Futura, 1991: 361–376.
12. Tang ASL, Wolf PD, Afework Y, Smith WM, Ideker RE. Three-dimensional potential gradient fields generated by intracardiac catheter and cutaneous patch electrodes. Circulation 1992; 85:1857–1864.
13. Mehra R, DeGroot PJ, Norenberg MS. Energy waveforms and lead systems for implantable defibrillators. In: Luderitz B, Saksena S, eds. Interventional Electrophysiology. Mount Kisco, NY: Futura, 1991:377–394.
14. Dixon EG, Tang ASL, Wolf PD, et al. Improved defibrillation thresholds with large contoured epicardial electrodes and biphasic waveforms. Circulation 1987; 76:1176–1184.
15. Walls JT, Schuder JC, Curtis JJ, Stephenson HE, McDaniel WC, Flaker GC. Adverse effects of permanent cardiac internal defibrillator patches on external defibrillation. Am J Cardiol 1989; 64:1144–1147.
16. Oeff M, Abbott JA, Scheinman ED, Yee ES, Scheinman MM, Griffin JC. Determination of patch electrode position for the internal cardioverter defibrillator by cine computed tomography and its relation to the defibrillation threshold. J Am Coll Cardiol 1992; 20:210–217.
17. Baerman JM, Blakeman BP, Olshansky B, Kopp DE, Kall JG, Wilber DJ. Use of multiple patches during implantation of epicardial defibrillator systems. Am J Cardiol 1993; 71:68–71.
18. Fain ES, Sweeney MB, Franz MR. Sequential pulse internal defibrillation: is there an advantage to "switched" current pathways? Am Heart J 1989; 118:717–724.
19. Jones DL, Klein GJ, Guiraudon GM, Sharma AD. Sequential pulse defibrillation in humans: orthogonal sequential pulse defibrillation with epicardial electrodes. J Am Coll Cardiol 1988; 11:590–596.
20. Fromer M, Brachmann J, Block M, et al. Efficacy of automatic multimodal device therapy for ventricular tachyarrhythmias as delivered by a new implantable pacing cardioverter defibrillator. Results of a European multicenter study of 102 implants. Circulation 1992; 86:363–374.
21. Saksena S, Mehta D, Krol RB, et al. Experience with a third generation implantable cardioverter defibrillator. Am J Cardiol 1991; 67:1375–1384.
22. Wyse DG, Kavanagh KM, Gillis AM, et al. Comparison of biphasic and monophasic shocks for defibrillation using a nonthoracotomy system. Am J Cardiol 1993; 71:197–202.
23. Saksena S, An H, Krol RB, Burkhardt E. Simultaneous biphasic shocks enhance efficacy of endocardial cardioversion defibrillation in man. PACE 1991; 14(II):1935–1942.
24. Fain ES, Sweeney MB, Franz MR. Improved internal defibrillation efficacy with a biphasic waveform. Am Heart J 1989; 117:358–364.
25. Johnson EE, Alferness CA, Wolf PD, Smith WM, Ideker RE. Effect of pulse separation between two sequential biphasic shocks given over different lead configurations on ventricular defibrillation efficacy. Circulation 1992; 85:2267–2274.
26. Jones DL, Klein GJ, Guiraudon GM, Yee R. Biphasic versus sequential pulse defibrillation: a direct comparison in humans. Am Heart J 1993; 125:405–409.
27. Bardy GH, Ivey TD, Allen MD, Johnson G, Greene HL. Prospective comparison of sequential pulse and single pulse defibrillation with use of two different clinically available systems. J Am Coll Cardiol 1989; 14:165–171.
28. Bardy GH, Ivey TD, Allen MD, Johnson G, Greene HL. Evaluation of electrode polarity on defibrillation efficacy. Am J Cardiol 1989; 63:433–437.
29. O'Neill PG, Boahene KA, Lawrie GM, Harvill LF, Pacifico A. The automatic implantable cardioverter defibrillator: effect of patch polarity on defibrillation threshold. J Am Coll Cardiol 1991; 17:707–711.

30. Alt E, Theres H, Heinz M, Albrecht K, Georg H, Bloemer H. A new approach towards defibrillation electrodes: highly conductive isotropic carbon fibers. PACE 1991; 14(II):1923–1928.
31. Rubin L, Rosenberg D, Parsonnet V, Villaneuva A, Ferrara-Ryan M. Comparison of titanium mesh and porous disc electrodes for epicardial defibrillation. PACE 1991; 14(II):1860–1864.
32. Irnich W. The fundamental law of electrostimulation and its application to defibrillation. PACE 1990; 13(I):1433–1447.
33. Bardy GH, Ivey TD, Johnson G, Stewart RB, Greene HL. Prospective evaluation of initially ineffective defibrillation pulses on subsequent defibrillation success during ventricular fibrillation in survivors of cardiac arrest. Am J Cardiol 1988; 62:718–722.
34. Saksena S, Mehta D, Krol RB, et al. Experience with a third generation implantable cardioverter defibrillator. Am J Cardiol 1991; 67:1375–1384.
35. Kelly PA, Cannom DS, Garan H, et al. The automatic implantable cardioverter defibrillator: efficacy, complications and survival in patients with malignant ventricular arrhythmias. J Am Coll Cardiol 1988; 11:1278–1286.
36. Winkle RA, Mead RH, Ruder MA, et al. Long-term outcome with the automatic implantable cardioverter defibrillator. J Am Coll Cardiol 1989; 13:1353–1361.
37. Echt DS, Armstrong K, Schmidt P, Oyer PE, Stinson EB, Winkle RA. Clinical experience, complications, and survival in 70 patients with the automatic implantable cardioverter defibrillator. Circulation 1985; 71:289–296.
38. Saksena S, Poczobutt-Johanos M, Castle LW, et al. Long-term multicenter experience with a second generation implantable pacemaker defibrillator in patients with malignant ventricular tachyarrhythmias. J Am Coll Cardiol 1992; 19:490–499.
39. Glicksman FL, Zaman L, Huikuri HV, Castellanos A, Myerburg RJ. Reversible failure to sense ventricular tachycardia early after surgical implantation of the automatic implantable cardioverter defibrillator. Am J Cardiol 1988; 62:833–834.
40. Goodman LR, Almassi GH, Troup PJ, et al. Complications of automatic implantable cardioverter defibrillators: radiographic, CT, and echocardiographic evaluation. Radiology 1989; 170:447–452.
41. Bardy GH, Gregg MG, Johnson G, Greene HL, Ivey TD. Intraoperative identification of lead fracture during automatic implantable cardioverter defibrillator replacement. J Electrophysiol 1989; 3:75–80.
42. Wuderly D, Maloney J, Edel T, McHenry, McCarthy PM. Infections in implantable cardioverter defibrillator patients. PACE 1990; 13(I):1360–1364.
43. Bakker PFA, Hauer RNW, Wever EFD. Infections involving implanted cardioverter defibrillator devices. PACE 1992; 15(III):654–658.
44. Almassi GH, Chapman PD, Troup PJ, Wetherbee JN, Olinger GN. Constrictive pericarditis associated with patch electrodes of the automatic implantable cardioverter defibrillator. Chest 1987; 92:369–371.
45. Mittleman RS, Mack K, Rastegar H, Manolis AS, Estes NAM III. Inappropriate shocks and elevation of defibrillation thresholds in a patient with automatic defibrillator patch silastic erosion and titanium mesh fraying. PACE 1991; 14:1452–1455.
46. Pinski SL, Arnold AZ, Mick M, Maloney JD, Trohman RG. Safety of external cardioverison defibrillation in patients with internal defibrillation patches and no device. PACE 1991; 14:7–12.
47. Cilley JH, Cernaianu AC, Libby JA, Baldino WA, DelRossi AJ. Silicone pouch for protection of automatic implantable cardioverter defibrillator leads. Am Thorac Surg 1991; 51:504–505.
48. Singer I, Hutchins GM, Mirowski M, et al. Pathologic findings related to the lead system and repeated defibrillations in patients with the automatic implantable cardioverter defibrillator. J Am Coll Cardiol 1987; 10:382–388.
49. Avitall B, Port S, Gal R, et al. Automatic implantable cardioverter defibrillator discharges and acute myocardial injury. Circulation 1990; 81:1482–1487.
50. Hauser RG, Mower MM, Mitchell M, Nisam S. Current status of the Ventak PRx pulse generator and Endotak nonthoracotomy lead system. PACE 1992; 15(III):671–677.

51. McCowan R, Maloney J, Wilkoff B, et al. Automatic implantable cardioverter defibrillator implantation without thoracotomy using an endocardial and submuscular patch system. J Am Coll Cardiol 1991; 17:415–421.
52. Jordaens L, Trouerbach J-W, Vertongen P, Herregods L, Poelaert J, Van Nooten G. Experience of cardioverter-defibrillators inserted without thoracotomy: evaluation of transvenously inserted intracardiac leads alone or with a subcutaneous axillary patch. Br Heart J 1993; 69:14–19.
53. Moore SL, Maloney JD, Edel TB, et al. Implantable cardioverter defibrillator implanted by nonthoracotomy approach: initial clinical experience with the redesigned transvenous lead system. PACE 1991; 14(II):1865–1869.
54. Block M, Hammel D, Isbruch F, et al. Results and realistic expectations with transvenous lead systems. PACE 1992; 15(III):665–670.
55. Saksena S. Endocardial lead systems for implantable cardioverter defibrillators: uncertain progress beyond base camp. PACE 1992; 15:123–125.
56. The German Dilated Cardiomyopathy Study Investigators. Prospective studies cardiomyopathy study (GDCMS)-study design. PACE 1992; 15(III):697–700.
57. Saksena S, An H, Mehra R, et al. Prospective comparison of biphasic and monophasic shocks for implantable cardioverter defibrillators using endocardial leads. Am J Cardiol 1992; 70:304–310.
58. Kavanagh KM, Tang ASL, Rollins DL, Smith WM, Ideker RE. Comparison of the internal defibrillation thresholds for monophasic and double and single capacitor biphasic waveforms. J Am Coll Cardiol 1989; 14:1343–1349.
59. Jones DL, Klein GJ, Guiraudon GM, et al. Internal cardiac defibrillation in man: pronounced improvement with sequential pulse delivery to two different lead orientations. Circulation 1986; 73:484–491.
60. Bardy GH, Allen MD, Mehra R, Johnson G. An effective and adaptable transvenous defibrillation system using the coronary sinus in humans. J Am Coll Cardiol 1990; 16:887–895.
61. Saksena S, Tullo NG, Krol RB, Maura AM. Initial clinical experience with endocardial defibrillation using an implantable cardioverter defibrillator with a triple electrode system. Arch Intern Med 1989; 149:2333–2339.
62. Wetherbee JN, Chapman PD, Bach SM, Troup PJ. Sequential shocks are comparable to single shocks employing two current pathways for internal defibrillation in dogs. PACE 1988; 11:696.
63. Saksena S, Scott SE, Accorti PR, Boveja BK, Abels D, Callaghan FJ. Efficacy and safety of monophasic and biphasic waveform shocks using a braided endocardial defibrillation lead system. Am Heart J 1990; 120:1342–1347.
64. Schuder JC, Stoeckle H, West JA, Keskar PY, Gold JH, Denniston RH. Ventricular defibrillation in the dog with a bielectrode intravascular catheter. Arch Intern Med 1973; 132:286–290.
65. Winkle RA, Bach SM, Mead RH, et al. Comparison of defibrillation efficacy in humans using a new catheter and superior vena cava spring left ventricular patch electrodes. J Am Coll Cardiol 1988; 11:365–370.
66. Saksena S, An H. Clinical efficacy of dual electrode systems for endocardial cardioversion of ventricular tachycardia: a prospective randomized crossover trial. Am Heart J 1990; 119:15–22.
67. Bardy GH, Allen MD, Mehra R, et al. Transvenous defibrillation in humans via the coronary sinus. Circulation 1990; 81:1252–1259.
68. Yee R, Jones DL, Klein GJ, Sharma AD, Kallock MJ. Sequential pulse countershock between two transvenous catheters: feasibility, safety, and efficacy. PACE 1989; 12:1869–1877.
69. Yee R, Klein GJ, Leitch JW, et al. A permanent transvenous lead system for an implantable pacemaker cardioverter defibrillator. Circulation 1992; 85:196–204.
70. Ely SW, Kron IL. Thoracoscopic implantation of the implantable cardioverter defibrillator. Chest 1993; 103:271–272.
71. Tullo NG, Saksena S, Krol RB, Mauro AM, Kunecz D. Management of complications associated with first generation endocardial defibrillation lead system for implantable cardioverter defibrillators. Am J Cardiol 1990; 66:411–415.

72. Jugo ES. EnGUARD Defibrillation Lead System. Telectronics Pacing Systems, Inc., Communication, July 31, 1992.
73. Jung W, Manz M, Moosdorf R, Luderitz B. Failure of an implantable cardioverter defibrillator to redetect ventricular fibrillation in patients with a nonthoracotomy lead system. Circulation 1992; 86:1217–1222.
74. Winkle RA, Bach SM, Echt DS, et al. The automatic implantable defibrillator: local ventricular bipolar sensing to detect ventricular tachycardia and fibrillation. Am J Cardiol 1983; 52: 265–270.
75. Grubb BP, Durzinsky, D, Temesy-Armos P, Hahn H, Elliot L. Tachycardia sensing failure of an implantable cardioverter defibrillator in a patient with hypertrophic cardiomyopathy. PACE 1992; 15:845.
76. Epstein AE, Kay GN, Plumb VJ, Shepard RB, Kirklin JK. Combined automatic implantable cardioverter defibrillator and pacemaker systems: implantation techniques and follow-up. J Am Coll Cardiol 1989; 13:121–131.
77. Chapman PD, Troup P. The automatic implantable cardioverter defibrillator: evaluating suspected inappropriate shocks. J Am Coll Cardiol 1986; 7:1075–1078.
78. Mehta D, Lipsius M, Suri RS, Krol RB, Saksena S. Twiddler's syndrome with the implantable cardioverter defibrillator. Am Heart J 1992; 123:1079–1082.
79. Ballas SL, Rashidi R, McAlister H, et al. The use of beep-o-grams in the assessment of automatic implantable cardioverter defibrillator sensing function. PACE 1989; 12:1737–1745.
80. Yee R, Jones DL, Jarvis E, Donner AP, Klein GJ. Changes in pacing threshold and R wave amplitude after transvenous catheter countershock. J Am Coll Cardiol 1984; 4:543–549.
81. Lehmann MH, Steinman RT, Schuger CD, Jackson K. Defibrillation threshold testing and other practices related to AICD implantation: do all roads lead to Rome? PACE 1989; 12:1530–1537.
82. Singer I, Lang D. Defibrillation threshold: clinical utility and therapeutic implications. PACE 1992; 15:932–949.
83. Jordaens L. Assessment of the defibrillation threshold and appropriate sensing during cardioverter defibrillator implantation. PACE 1992; 15(III):636–641.
84. Epstein AE, Ellenbogen KA, Kirk KA, et al. Clinical characteristics and outcome of patients with high defibrillation thresholds. Circulation 1992; 86:1206–1216.
85. Sharma AD, Bennett TD, Erickson M, Klein GJ, Yee R, Guiraudon G. Right ventricular pressure during ventricular arrhythmias in humans: potential implications for implantable antitachycardia devices. J Am Coll Cardiol 1990; 15:648–655.
86. Mirowski M, Mower MM. Hemodynamic sensors for implantable defibrillators. J Am Coll Cardiol 1990; 15:656–657.
87. Ellenbogen KA, Lu B, Kapadia K, Wood M, Valenta H. Usefulness of right ventricular pulse pressure as a potential sensor for hemodynamically unstable ventricular tachycardia. Am J Cardiol 1990; 65:1105–1111.
88. AICD Advances, Cardiac Pacemaker, Inc., 2nd quarter, 1989.
89. Santel DJ, Kallock MJ, Tacker WA. Implantable defibrillator electrode systems: a brief review. PACE 1985; 8:123–131.
90. Pannizzo F, Mercando AD, Fisher JD, Furman S. Automatic methods for detection of tachyarrhythmias by antitachycardia devices. J Am Coll Cardiol 1988; 11:308–316.

36

Overview of the Implantable Cardioverter-Defibrillator

N. A. Mark Estes III

*Tufts University School of Medicine
and New England Medical Center
Boston, Massachusetts*

I. INTRODUCTION

Since the initial report of a human implantation of an implantable cardioverter-defibrillator (ICD) in 1980, there has been remarkable evolution of the features and capabilities of these devices [1]. The early devices were designed to recognize only ventricular fibrillation and to treat it with high-energy shock therapy [1]. It became evident that a device capable of recognizing ventricular tachycardia as well as ventricular fibrillation was essential for prevention of arrhythmic death. From the early, nonprogrammable, committed devices with no telemetry capabilities, the ICD's arrhythmia recognition and therapy capabilities have been refined. Currently, programmable, tiered-therapy, noncommitted devices incorporate bradycardia pacing, antitachycardia pacing, cardioversion capability with low-energy shock, defibrillation shock therapy, noninvasive programmed stimulation, data logging, and telemetry [1–15]. Eight separate manufactures have over 20 devices which have undergone human implantation. Programmable shock waveforms in some devices allow for individualization of the most effective cardioversion or defibrillation [16–24]. Devices now have the capability of telemetering extensive data from memory regarding device function as well as stored electrograms from the time of arrhythmia detection [15,25–27]. Enhancement for arrhythmia detection such as sudden onset, rate stability, sustained high rate, or probability density function are incorporated to optimized sensitivity and specificity of arrhythmia classification [27]. Most devices currently are using an automatic gain control or automatic sensitivity adjustment to allow sensing down to a minimum of 0.2–0.3 mV. The ability to noninvasively induce arrhythmias with VOO or VVT pacing, slaved programmed electrical stimulation (PES), or noninvasive programmed stimulation (NIPS) allows for assessment of antiarrhythmic drug effects on ventricular tachycardia, and adequacy of programming for arrhythmia detection and termination with antitachycardia pacing, shock therapy, or defibrillation.

First-generation devices were not programmable and were capable only of arrhythmia recognition and termination with maximal shock therapy [1,6]. Devices with minimal programmability which have bradycardia pacing capability are known as second-generation devices [1,6]. Many of these devices also have limited telemetry, such as number of shocks delivered. ICDs with bradycardia pacing, antitachycardia pacing, cardioversion, and defibrillation capability with more extensive programmability and telemetry are known as third-generation devices [6]. With the addition of antitachycardia pacing and low-energy shock capabilities, progressive therapy defined by tachycardia rate and lack of success of prior therapy, known as tiered therapy, has been incorporated. Devices with tiered therapy may be programmed to deliver antitachycardia pacing, which if unsuccessful may be followed by low-energy shock therapy before going on to a maximum shock. Immediately before delivery of therapy, third-generation devices reconfirm the presence of an arrhythmia. These ''noncommitted'' devices have the advantages of eliminating shocks for self-terminating arrhythmias. Automatic gain control or automatic sensitivity adjustment supplemented by detection enhancements are being incorporated in all third-generation devices to optimize arrhythmia classification. The telemetry, data logging, memory capability, and storage of electrograms have proven to be extremely useful for analysis of therapy or troubleshooting the devices [13–15]. Finally, the ability to induce the arrhythmias with noninvasive programmed stimulation allows for confirmation of appropriate device function. It is the purpose of this chapter to provide an overview of the arrhythmia detection and therapy capabilities and summarize diagnostic functions such as data logging and telemetry in ICDs (Table 1).

II. SENSING FUNCTIONS OF THE ICD

The ICD sensing circuit must be able to detect R waves that may vary from over 20 mV during the patient's native rhythm to as low as 0.2 mV during fine ventricular fibrillation. Conventionally, permanent pacemakers have employed sensing amplifiers with fixed gain. By contrast, ICDs, with a few exceptions, such as the Telectronics 4202, 4203, and 4210 devices, operate on the basis of an automatic gain control by adjusting the amplification factor (ratio of output voltage to the input voltage) or the threshold for signal detection based on the amplitude of the preceding signals (Figs. 1 and 2) [7]. Devices with fixed sensitivity have the potential to undersense ventricular fibrillation and oversense T waves during the patient's native rhythm (Figs. 3 and 4). Because of the need for defibrillators to sense these low-amplitude signals, as may be present in ventricular fibrillation, manufacturers have developed automatic gain control. With this, the gain function is determined by the preceding amplitude of the sensed ventricular signal. The automatic gain control filter has a variable gain in which each sensed electrogram signal causes adjustment in the threshold for detection. After a sensed event there is rapid decline in sensitivity to allow for detection of lower-amplitude electrograms which may occur if a patient suddenly develops ventricular fibrillation (Fig. 5). For example, the Metronics PCD has a programmable maximal sensitivity down to 0.3 mV. An electrogram signal exceeding this signal raises the sensitivity to 75% of the amplitude of the detected electrogram (or six times the programmed setting—whichever is less). The sensitivity then delays exponentially with time with a constant of 560 ms to the minimum programmed sensitivity. The Telectronics 4211 has similar automatic sensitivity tracking, which adjusts to 40% of the preceding sensed event with a half-time at 400 ms to a maximal sensitivity of 0.375 mV.

In all current devices, the primary determinant of the presence of a tachycardia is rate. With the initial CPI devices, an algorithm for the analysis of the morphology of the ventricular electrogram, known as probability density function (PDF), was used to define the presence of a ventricular arrhythmia. The PDF was determined by analysis of electrogram characteristics from the patch leads. During normal sinus rhythm, atrial fibrillation, or other narrow-complex

Table 1 Summary of the ICDs

Manufacturer: Model Number:	AngeMed Sentinel 2001	Biotronic Phylax 03	CPI Ventak 1500	CPI Ventak 1510	CPI Ventak 1520
Physical characteristics:					
Wt (g)	115	169	250	250	250
Dimensions (mm) $W \times H \times T$	$80 \times 50 \times 16$	$100 \times 79 \times 21$	$76 \times 108 \times 20$	$76 \times 108 \times 20$	$76 \times 108 \times 20$
Volume (cm^3)	60	121	148	148	148
Therapy:					
Bradycardia pacing	+	+	—	—	—
Cardioversion	+	+	—	—	—
Antitachycardia pacing	+	+	—	—	—
Noncommitted	+	+	—	—	—
Shock waveform-programmable	+	+	—	—	—
Tachycardia detection:					
Automatic gain control	+	+	+	+	+
Rate	+	+	+	+	+
Other detection algorithms	+	+	+	+	+
Telemetry:					
Event counters	+	+	+	+	+
Stored electrograms	+	—	—	—	—
Real-time electrograms	+	+	—	—	—
Marker channel	+	+	—	—	—
Noninvasive programmed stimulation:					
VOO, VTT	—	—	—	—	—
Slaved PES	—	—	—	—	—
NIPS	+	+	—	—	—

Table 1 Continued

Manufacturer: Model name:	CPI 1550 Ventak	CPI 1555 Ventak	CPI 1600 Ventak P	CPI 1620/1625 P2	CPI 1700 Ventak PRx
Physical characteristics:					
Wt (g)	235	235	240	235	220
Dimensions (mm) $W \times H \times T$	76 × 101 × 20	76 × 101 × 20	76 × 101 × 20	76 × 101 × 20	107 × 68 × 24
Volume (cm^3)	145	145	145	145	130
Therapy:					
Bardycardia pacing	−	−	−	+	+
Cardioversion	−	−	+	+	+
Antitachycardia pacing	−	−	−	−	+
Noncommitted	−	−	−	+	+
Shock waveform-programmable	−	−	−	+	−
Tachycardia detection:					
Automatic gain control	+	+	+	+	+
Rate	+	+	+	+	+
Other detection algorithms	+	+	+	+	+
Telemetry:					
Event counters	+	+	+	+	+
Stored electrograms	−	−	−	+	−
Real-time electrograms	−	−	−	+	+
Marker channel	+	+	+	+	+
Noninvasive programmed stimulation:					
VOO, VVT	−	−	−	−	−
Slaved PES	−	−	−	+	+
NIPS	−	−	−	+	−

Overview of the ICD

Physical characteristics:						
Wt (g)	220	220	220	240	197	197
Dimensions (mm) $W \times H \times T$	107 × 68 × 24	107 × 68 × 24	98 × 82 × 20	98 × 82 × 20	101 × 70 × 21	101 × 70 × 20
Volume (cm^3)	130	130	140	159	113	113
Therapy:						
Bradycardia pacing	+	+	+	+	+	+
Cardioversion	+	+	+	+	+	+
Antitachycardia pacing	+	+	+	+	−	+
Noncommitted	+	+	+	+	+	+
Shock waveform-programmable	−	+	+	+	−	−
Tachycardia detection:						
Automatic gain algorithm	+	+	+	+	+	+
Rate	+	+	+	+	+	+
Other detection algorithms	+	+	+	+	+	+
Telemetry:						
Event counters	+	+	+	+	+	+
Stored electrograms	−	+	−	−	−	−
Real-time electrograms	+	+	+	+	+	+
Marker channel	+	+	+	+	+	+
Noninvasive programmed stimulation:						
VOO, VVT	−	−	−	−	−	−
Slaved PES	+	+	−	−	−	−
NIPS	−	−	+	+	+	+

Table 1 Continued

Manufacturer: Model name:	Medtronic 7217 B/D PCD	Medtronic 7219 Jewel	Pacesetter 2120 Siecure	Telectronics 4202 Guardian	Telectronics 4203 Guardian
Physical characteristics:					
Wt (g)	197	136	220	270	270
Dimensions (mm) $H \times W \times T$	$101 \times 70 \times 20$	$89 \times 64 \times 18$	$110 \times 70 \times 22$	$120 \times 80 \times 20$	$120 \times 80 \times 20$
Volume (cc)	113	82		176	176
Therapy:					
Bradycardia pacing	+	+	+	+	+
Cardioversion	+	+	+	+	+
Antitachycardia pacing	+	+	+	−	+
Noncommitted	+	+	+	+	−
Shock waveform-programmable	−	+	−	−	−
Tachycardia detection:					
Automatic gain control	+	+	+	−	−
Rate	+	+	+	+	+
Other detection algorithms	+	+	+	−	−
Telemetry:					
Event counter	+	+	+	+	+
Stored electrograms	−	+	−	−	−
Real-time electrograms	+	+	+	+	+
Marker channel	+	+	+	+	+
Noninvasive programmed stimulation:					
VOO, VVT	−	−	−	−	−
Slaved PES	−	−	+	−	−
NIPS	+	+	−	−	−

Overview of the ICD

Physical characteristics:				
Wt (g)	272	272	270	240
Dimensions (mm) $W \times H \times T$	115 × 81 × 20	115 × 81 × 20	117 × 83 × 20	97 × 82 × 24
Volume (cm^3)	159	159	184	145
Therapy:				
Bradycardia pacing	+	+	+	+
Cardioversion	+	+	+	+
Antitachycardia pacing	−	+	+	+
Noncommitted	+	+	+	+
Shock waveform-programmable	−	−	+	+
Tachycardia detection:				
Automatic gain control	+	−	+	+
Rate	+	+	+	+
Other detections algorithms	+	+	+	+
Telemetry:				
Event counters	+	+	+	+
Stored electrograms	+	+	+	+
Real-time electrograms	+	+	+	+
Marker channel	+	+	+	+
Noninvasive programmed stimulation:				
VOO, VVT	+	+	+	−
Slaved PES	−	−	−	−
NIPS	−	−	−	+

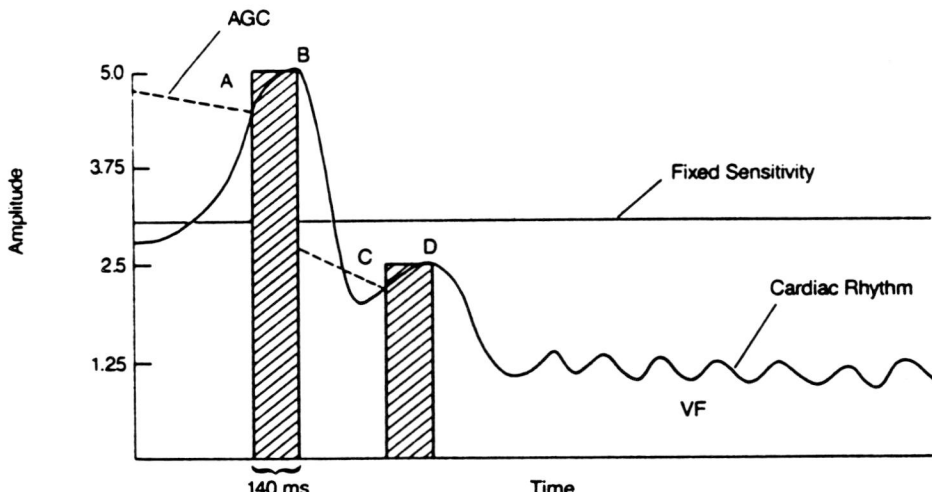

Figure 1 The principle of automatic gain control (AGC) is represented as an event is sensed (A), followed by a 140-ms refractory period (shaded portion). The cycle amplitude is measured at (B), the peak of the waveform. The sensing level for the next event (C) is determined by the peak amplitude of the last sensed event at (B). A device with fixed sensitivity as represented by the solid horizontal line would not sense the second event (C) or the subsequent low-amplitude ventricular fibrillation. By contrast, a device of AGC would sense the event C and establish the next sensitivity setting based on D.

rhythm, the majority of the electrical activity is at or near the isoelectric point, with abrupt deviations during ventricular depolarization. By contrast, with ventricular arrhythmias such as ventricular tachycardia, flutter, or fibrillation, there is relatively little activity around the isoelectric line. For satisfaction of PDF, the ratio of electrogram signal to cycle length had to be greater than 0.3 [4]. The limitations of this criterion in appropriately classifying VT and VF become apparent with the early-generation devices, resulting in the addition of an independent

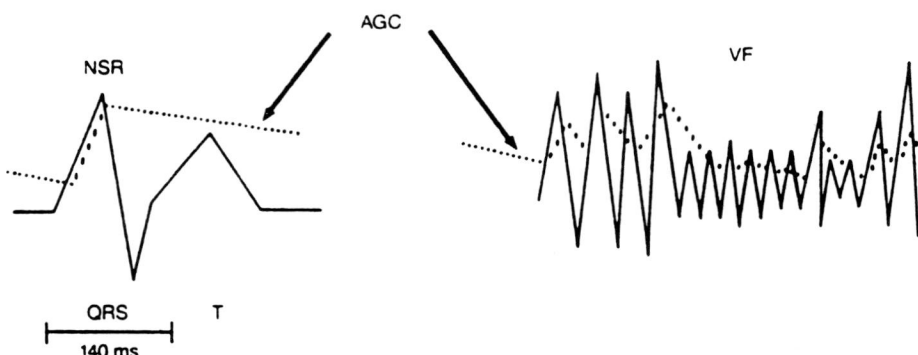

Figure 2 Automatic gain control (AGC) represented during normal sinus rhythm with a 140-ms refractory period. With the sensing level set by the R wave and an appropriate refractory period of 140 ms, the probability of double counting a QRS complex or oversensing the T wave is greatly reduced. When ventricular fibrillation develops, there is a decrease in the sensitivity down to as low as 0.2 mV to ensure appropriate detection of ventricular fibrillation.

Overview of the ICD

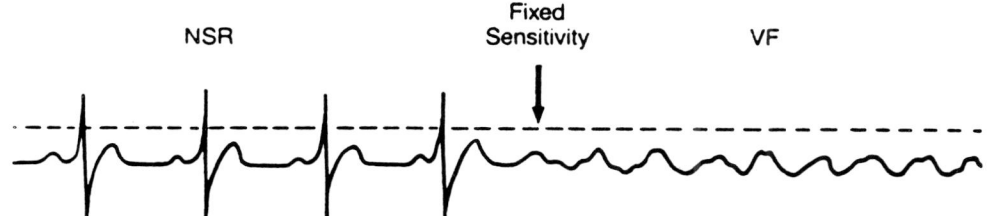

Figure 3 A fixed-sensitivity device in this instance would have normal sensing of R waves during normal sinus rhythm without oversensing the T waves. However, the sensitivity setting required to avoid oversensing of T waves during sinus rhythm may prevent sensing of VF and arrhythmia detection.

sensing channel for rate. When a tachycardia exceeds a predetermined rate limit by monitoring the R wave via the rate-sensing lead, the device delivers therapy. If PDF was programmed on, both rate and PDF had to be satisfied for the device to detect the arrhythmia and delivery therapy. One had the option of programming PDF off, using rate alone for arrhythmia classification. However, the use of PDF alone for detection was eliminated. With the early CPI AICD devices, a minimum of 8 beats at a rate faster than the programmed rate were required to satisfy the rate detection criterion. Current third-generation devices allow programming of duration of arrhythmia before therapy based on number of beats of tachycardia before therapy to allow for self-termination of slower, hemodynamically tolerated arrhythmia. With the Siemens Siecure device, for example, when this criterion is programmed on, a specific number of cycles (programmable from 4 to 150 cycles) at a rate greater than the detection limit must occur before

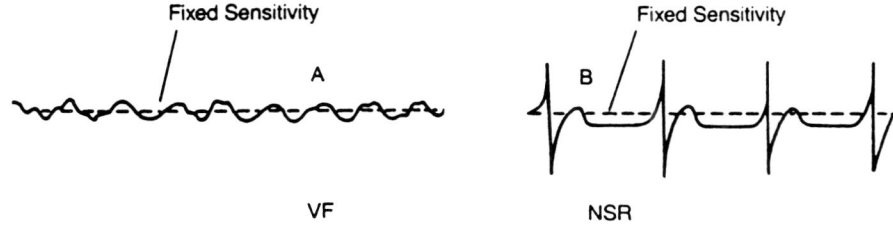

Figure 4 A device with fixed sensitivity could be programmed to a low sensitivity level to ensure detection of ventricular fibrillation (A). However, this sensitivity level would also increase the probability of oversensing T waves (B).

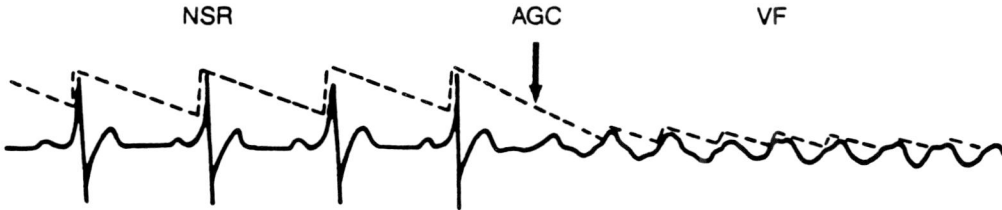

Figure 5 Automatic gain control is represented during normal sinus rhythm and ventricular fibrillation. Notice that the automatic increase in sensitivity with the onset of ventricular fibrillation ensures appropriate sensing of this rhythm without T-wave oversensing.

detection. However, when this criterion is programmed on, it must initially be met before other confirmatory criteria such as rate stability are initiated. This can potentially cause delays before final confirmation of the tachycardia and delivery of therapy.

To supplement the rate criteria and improve arrhythmia classification, some manufacturers allow programming of alternative criteria alone or in combinations. In an effort to distinguish between atrial fibrillation with a rapid ventricular response and ventricular tachycardia, rate stability has been developed as a feature of some devices. The rate or interval criterion for stability has been incorporated as a programmable option by most manufacturers. Based on the observations of R-R variability in a atrial fibrillation being greater than in ventricular tachycardia, arrhythmias that meet the rate criterion must also show R-R variability less than a programmed amount to be classified as ventricular tachycardia. For example, when rate stability is activated in the Siemens Siecure device, it requires that the difference between the measured interval and the three immediately preceding R-R intervals be equal to or less than the allowed amount of variability (programmable from 10 to 200 ms).

The Ventritex Cadence V-100 has two programmable, extended-high-rate (EHR) criteria— the detection time and the detection interval, which are programmable options to supplement rate and improve arrhythmia classification [28]. The EHR detection time is programmable from 10 s to 5 min and a nominal value of 20 s. The number of intervals required for arrhythmia detection can be programmed from 6 to 100. This can be changed separately for the slowest tachycardia detection interval and the fibrillation detection interval. Suddenness of onset or prematurity criteria can be useful in differentiating sinus tachycardia from ventricular tachycardias. Sinus tachycardia generally accelerates gradually without an abrupt change in cycle length. By contrast, ventricular tachycardia usually is initiated with an abrupt change in cycle length. When a sudden-onset criterion is programmed on, the initial beat of the tachycardia must show sufficient prematurity to satisfy the onset criterion. This "sudden onset delta" can be programmed from 50 to 500 ms with the Ventritex V-100 Cadence device. However, this algorithm has limited utility in distinguishing supraventricular tachycardia from ventricular tachycardia, both of which have a sudden onset. The rate stability, extended-high-rate, sudden onset, and other algorithms supplement the rate criterion for detection of tachycardia or fibrillation. Using additional characteristics of the rate in an effort to distinguish ventricular tachycardia from alternate arrhythmias may improve specificity of arrhythmia classification but may also decrease sensitivity. To program these options on in any individual patient, the ability of the patient's ventricular tachycardia to satisfy the detection algorithm must be confirmed with intraoperative or predischarge testing.

Despite considerable improvements in third-generation devices with regard to tachycardia detection and discrimination, inappropriate shocks continue to be a clinical problem. A number of approaches are being assessed, including electrogram analysis, template matching, and gradient pattern detection for electrogram potential to distinguish ventricular arrhythmias from other tachycardias [2,27]. An alternative approach that has been proposed is the use of a hemodynamic sensor such as right ventricular pressure to differentiate hemodynamically stable from unstable tachycardias [3]. This or alternative sensors may be incorporated into future-generation devices.

With future-generation devices, once an arrhythmia event was detected, the delivery of the shock was mandatory. Under these circumstances, the delivery of the shock was termed to be "committed." It became apparent that many spontaneously terminating tachycardias would be detected and therapy would be delivered into normal sinus rhythm. To obviate this problem, devices which reconfirmed the persistence of tachycardia before delivering any therapy were developed. Such devices are deemed "noncommitted" and divert the change into an internal resistor instead of into the defibrillation leads if the tachycardia has terminated spontaneously. Similarly, if the arrhythmia is classified as one appropriate for antitachycardia pacing but terminates spontaneously, therapy is withheld. The importance of arrhythmia confirmation is underscored by the fact that in one recent clinical investigation (Telectronics 4210), over 70% of 62,936 episodes of ventricular tachycardia were self-terminating.

III. BRADYCARDIA PACING

In approximately 15% of patients with first-generation devices, permanent pacemaker implantation for bradyarrhythmias was necessary. VVI pacing was incorporated into second-generation devices such as the Telectronics 4202 and 4203 in an effort to eliminate the need for a separately placed permanent pacemaker. Incorporating the pacemaker into the defibrillator itself eliminated potential interactions between separately implanted permanent pacemakers and ICDs [8–10]. When separately implanted permanent pacemakers undersense a ventricular arrhythmia, the pacemaker spike may be sensed by the ICD and inhibit arrhythmia detection and therapy. This is particularly true when permanent pacemakers are programmed to low sensitivity and when the pacemaker output is unipolar. Oversensing of the pacemaker spikes and the patient's native electrogram also can contribute to double sensing by the ICD rate-sensing lead, resulting in satisfaction of the rate detection criteria and delivery of therapy. In some of the patients in whom VVI pacing was performed by the ICD, it became necessary to implant a separate DDD pacemaker due to pacemaker syndrome. Future generations of ICDs are currently being designed with dual-chamber pacing capability both for treatment of bradyarrhythmias and for antitachycardia pacing.

IV. ANTITACHYCARDIA PACING

One of the major limitations of second-generation devices was the inability to treat sustained ventricular tachycardia with pacing techniques. Pacing therapy has been shown to be effective in over 90% of episodes of hemodynamically stable sustained ventricular tachycardia [23,29–40] (Fig. 6). The success of antitachycardia pacing is favored by slower rates of ventricular tachycardia, particularly when the cycle length is >350 ms. This painless therapy significantly reduces the frequency of shocks in the individual patient and the proportion of patients shocked overall. Refinement of antitachycardia pacing techniques has allowed for a greater overall success rate in termination of sustained ventricular tachycardias [3]. The strategies for antitachycardia pacing include single-capture termination methods such as a scanning extrastimuli or multiple-capture techniques including multiple extrastimuli, burst, ramp (autodecremental), shifting bursts, scanning bursts, scanning ramps, and incremental-decremental. The single-scanning extrastimulus technique may be appropriate for well-tolerated slow VT. Efficacy rates of 48% were reported by Fisher et al., with 139 of 290 episodes of VT terminated with only one arrhythmia acceleration [31–33]. With multiple-capture techniques there is an increase in both efficacy of termination and acceleration of ventricular tachycardia. Efficacy rates ranging from 21% to 92% have been reported with burst or ramp pacing techniques with acceleration rates ranging from 2% to 21% [29–40]. No mode of pacing has proven clearly superior with regard to either efficacy or risk of acceleration. Considerable flexibility exists with regard to the number of stimuli, cycle length, coupling interval, and repetition sequences. Comparative trials with randomization of the burst versus autodecremental ramp stimulation have shown comparable efficacy for sustained monomorphic ventricular tachycardia [23]. Frequently, ramp pacing with trains of 4 to 12 pulses are used with a rate-adaptive algorithm. The coupling interval

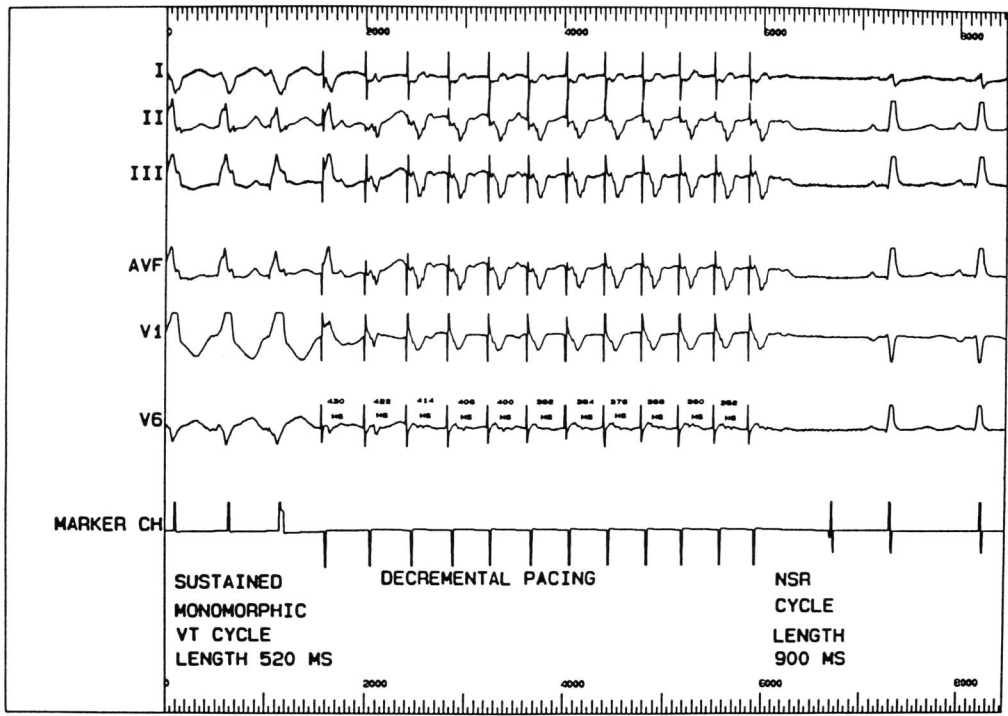

Figure 6 Surface leads I, II, III, AVF, VI, and V6 are shown with a marker channel for a third-generation, tiered-therapy device (CPI PRx). Sustained monomorphic ventricular tachycardia (VT) with a cycle length of 520 ms is sensed by the device. Decremental pacing with 8-ms decrements is successful in reestablishing normal sinus rhythm (NSR).

is specified a percentage of cycle length of the tachycardia ranging from approximately 90% to 65% of the VT cycle length. Using a rate-adaptive algorithm there is a decrement in the percentage of the tachycardia cycle length between trains. Some algorithms also allow for decrementing within each train. Generally, adaptive rate pacing has increased efficacy as the train cycle length is reduced as a percentage of the tachycardia cycle length. However as one paces more rapidly, particularly at cycle lengths less than 250 ms, a 1:1 relationship between the pacing stimulus and ventricular capture may not occur and acceleration of the tachycardia is more likely (Fig. 7). Generally, it is recommended that the lower limit of such pacing trains be 70% of the VT cycle length [3,23]. When acceleration does occur with antitachycardia pacing, cardioversion or defibrillation is then used to reestablish normal sinus rhythm (Fig. 8).

Tiered or hierarchical antitachycardia therapy is incorporated into all third-generation devices. The zones of therapy are defined by tachycardia rate, with the assumption that more rapid tachycardias are likely to be associated with hemodynamic compromise and should be treated more aggressively [4]. Generally, a lower rate and upper rate for each therapy zone is programmed. Typically, slower tachycardias will be treated with antitachycardia pacing. More rapid tachycardias can be treated with more aggressive burst pacing techniques or low-energy cardioversion. Tachycardias which are rapid or those accelerated by burst pacing are treated with high-energy cardioversion or defibrillation therapy. A zone for "monitoring" has also been

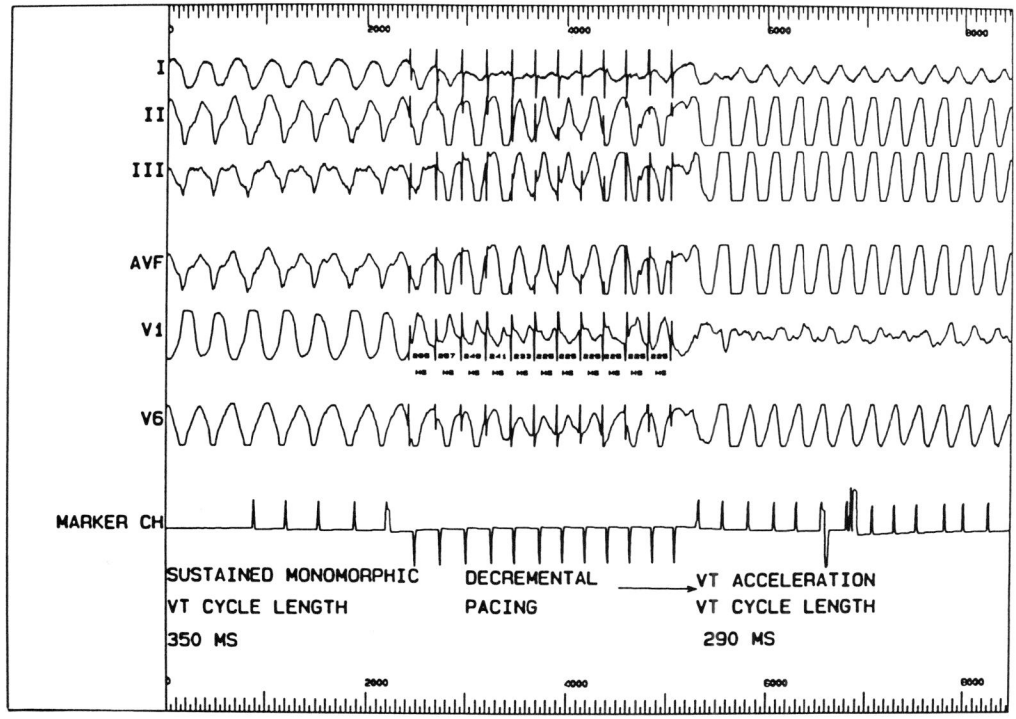

Figure 7 Sustained monomorphic ventricular tachycardia (VT) with a cycle length of 350 ms is sensed by the ICD, and ramp pacing with 8 ms decrements to a minimum burst cycle length of 225 ms results in VT acceleration to a cycle length of 290 ms.

incorporated in some devices, such as the CPI PRx ICD, which allows for storage of events in a data log within the ICD without therapy delivery.

V. SHOCK THERAPY

Most episodes of sustained monomorphic ventricular tachycardia are amenable to termination with low-energy shock or cardioversion therapy (Fig. 9). One prospective study demonstrated an 83% success rate in termination of ventricular tachycardia using shocks ranging from 0.5 to 2.7 J [23]. First-generation ICDs would treat such tachycardias with high-energy shocks, resulting in considerable patient discomfort and psychological stress. In the largest reported experience to date, the multicenter experience with the Medtronic PCD noted overall success for cardioversion (0.2–5 J) of 63% with an acceleration rate of 13% for tachycardia with cycle lengths <300 ms. For tachycardias with cycle length >300 ms, cardioversion was successful in 87% with acceleration in 4% [40]. Low-energy cardioversion have been compared to antitachycardia pacing using decremental fixed-rate burst [23,40]. It has been determined that with slow tachycardias (mean cycle length <391 ms), cardioversion had an 83% efficacy with an acceleration rate of 11%. By contrast, pacing was 80% effective, with a risk of acceleration of 6%. These investigators found a higher frequency of transient supraventricular arrhythmias after cardioversion (23%). As the tachycardia becomes more rapid, with cycle lengths <270 ms, the efficacy of pacing decreased to 77%. When pacing failed, cardioversion increased efficacy

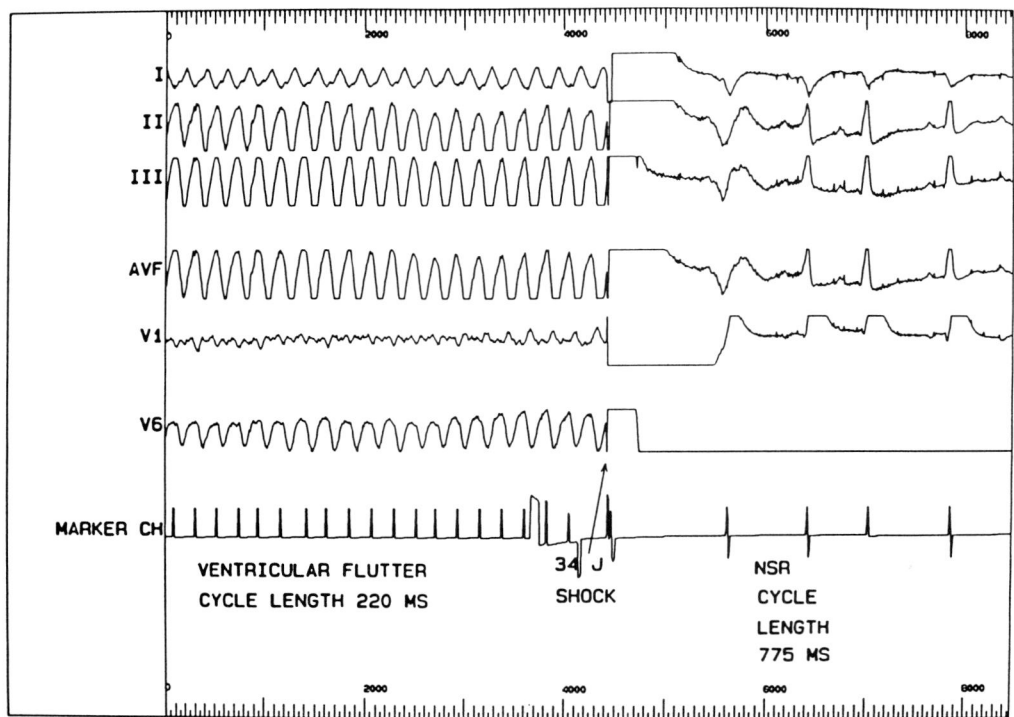

Figure 8 Ventricular flutter with a cycle length of 220 ms is sensed by the device. This rhythm had resulted from an acceleration of sustained monomorphic ventricular tachycardia with a cycle length of 350 ms, which was treated with antitachycardia pacing and resulted in acceleration to a VT cycle length of 290 ms (Fig. 6), which then deteriorated to ventricular flutter. The CPI PRx detected this and delivered a 34-shock to reestablish normal sinus rhythm with a cycle length of 775 ms.

by only 8%. These observations and those of others indicate that the gains made by low- to moderate-energy cardioversion are modest once pacing has failed [42].

The optimal waveform for lower cardioversion and defibrillation energy remains to be determined. The waveform used by early ICD devices was the monophasic truncated exponential wave form. When the voltage has declined to a certain value or after a predetermined time interval, the capacitors abruptly and automatically disconnect from the output circuitry to avoid the low-voltage trailing edge of a straight capacitor discharge, which can cause refibrillation. The truncated and exponential waveform is described in terms of its tilt [4]. The tilt is defined as a percentage tilt which is equal to $1-$ (trailing-edge voltage divided by leading-edge voltage).

While the truncated exponential monophasic waveform has a single polarity phase, biphasic waveforms have an initial phase followed by a second phase of reverse polarity. When the positive and negative phases are equal in emplitude, this is referred to as a symmetric biphasic. When they are unequal they are referred to as asymmetric biphasic. Multiple investigators have now determined that a biphasic waveform results in lower cardioversion and defibrillation energy and decreases the time to return to sinus rhythm [4,17,22]. Preliminary evidence suggests that biphasic waveforms with a longer first- and a shorter second-phase duration may have advantages in lowering cardioversion and defibrillation energy compared with monophasic wave-

Overview of the ICD

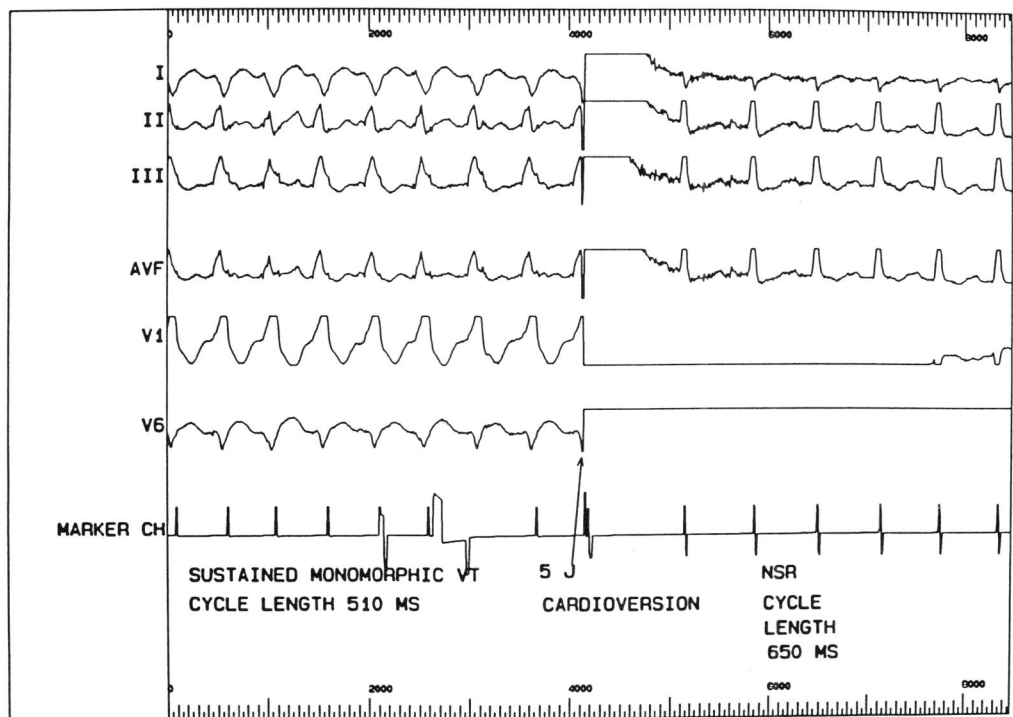

Figure 9 Sustained monomorphic ventricular tachycardia (VT) with a cycle length of 510 ms is treated with low-energy cardioversion (5 J) to reestablish normal sinus rhythm (NSR) with a cycle length of 650 ms.

forms. In addition to the simultaneous monophasic and simultaneous biphasic waveform, several alternative methods of cardioversion and defibrillation are being investigated, including sequential, dual, and simultaneous pulsing. With the simultaneous or single-pulse method, a single, unidirectional shock is delivered between two electrodes. Sequential pulses require three electrodes, one of which serves as a common cathode or a common anode and the other two as dual anodes or dual cathodes. The shock energy is temporarily interrupted and delivered across two different pathways. Preliminary data with triphasic waveforms show no significant benefits when compared to sequential biphasic waveforms.

Manufacturers currently are developing biphasic shock capability in third-generation ICDs with the option of programming it to monophasic. Some devices, such as the Telectronics 4211, will allow programming of the duration of the positive and negative portions of the asymmetric biphasic waveforms.

VI. NONINVASIVE PROGRAMMED STIMULATION

Virtually all third-generation ICDs and those in development allow noninvasive arrhythmia induction (Fig. 10). Some devices such as the Telectronics 4210 have VOO pacing at rapid rates to induce arrhythmias. This devices also allow for noninvasive arrhythmia induction with VVT pacing. Slaved programmed electrical stimulation is available in devices such as the CPI PRx 1705. Programmed stimulation can be performed by relaying the input from a conventional stimulator to the ICD through the device programmer. True noninvasive programmed stimu-

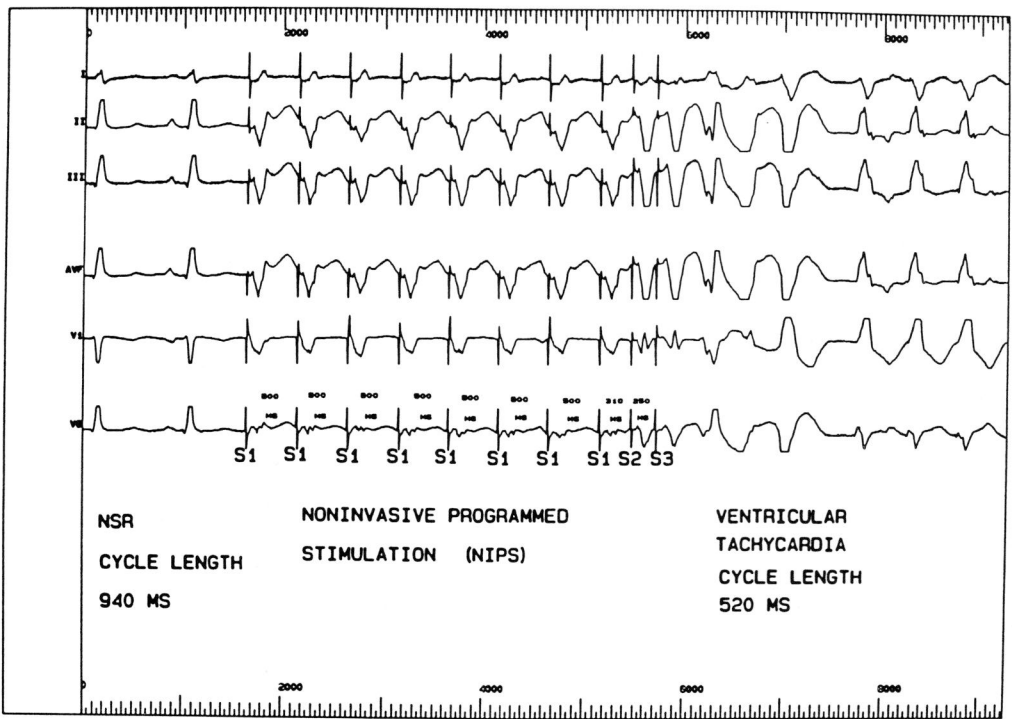

Figure 10 Noninvasive programmed stimulation (NIPS) is delivered through a CPI PRx device with an 8-beat drive with a cycle length of 500 ms and double extrastimuli coupled at 310 and 250 ms. This induces sustained monomorphic ventricular tachycardia with a cycle length of 520 ms.

lation (NIPS) can be performed with the device programmer without the need for a stimulator with devices such as the Medtronic PCD 7216. Premature stimuli or burst pacing are used via the pace/sense lead to induce either VT or VF. This ability to reinduce the tachycardia allows for noninvasive assessment of tachycardia rates, influence of antiarrhythmic drugs, effectiveness of antitachycardia pacing, shock therapy, and redetermination of defibrillation threshold.

VII. DIAGNOSTIC CAPABILITIES

First-generation devices provided only information regarding the number of shocks delivered to the patient or used to reform the capacitors. It became apparent that the lack of diagnostic capabilities severely limited the clinical interpretation of shock therapy. All third-generation devices incorporate some degree of data storage, including RR intervals, cycle length of detected arrhythmia, therapy delivered, impedance during the shock delivery, and the date and time of the event. Many third-generation ICDs also store electrograms at the time of arrhythmia detection and immediately after therapy (Telectronics 4210, 4211, Ventritex V100). Analysis of these electrograms can provide insights into the electrical events preceding ICD therapy [13–15]. Using bipolar rate-sensing leads, these electrograms can be stored or telemetered in real time to a physiological recorder. When intraoperative testing or postoperative evaluation is being performed, event markers can supplement the telemetered bipolar electrograms. The storage capability of third-generation ranges from an isolated "snapshot" of 1 s of the cardiac rhythm at the time of detection, confirmation, and after therapy to considerably more extensive electrogram storage. The Ventritex Cadence ICD provides programming options for electrogram storage include one 64-s event, three 32-s events, or seven 17-s events. With this device, if the total tachycardia duration from onset to termination is greater than programmed storage for an individual unit, the earliest portion of the tachycardia will not be stored. Because of the limits of memory of this device, if the number of spontaneous tachycardia episodes exceeds the number of stored electrogram events, only the most recent tachycardia will be stored. These are particularly valuable in diagnosing of rate-sensing lead fracture or lead connection, or electrical noise which may mimic arrhythmia detection and result in inappropriate therapy.

REFERENCES

1. Mirowski M, Reid PD, Mower MM, et al. Termination of malignant ventricular arrhythmias with an implanted defibrillator in human beings. N Engl J Med 1980; 303:322–324.
2. DiMarco JP. Nonpharmacological therapy of ventricular arrhythmias. PACE 1990; 13(II): 1527–1532.
3. Kolettis TM, Sakesena S. Implantable cardioverter-defibrillators for prevention of sudden death. Arrhythmia Management 1992:3–18.
4. Gessman L. Brief history of implanted cardioverter-defibrillator (ICD) product development. In: Morse DP, Parsonnet V, Gessman LJ, Droege TL, Shimmel JB, Bernstein AD, White M, eds, A Guide To Cardiac Pacemakers. Droege Computing Services, 1993.
5. Saksena S, Camm J. Implantable defibrillators for prevention of sudden death: technology at a medical and economic crossroad. Circulation 1992; 85:2316–2320.
6. Furman S, Kim S. The present status of implantable cardioverter defibrillator therapy. J Cardiovas Electrophysiol 1992; 3:602–625.
7. Troup PJ. Implantable cardioverters and defibrillators. Curr Probl Cardiol 1989; 679–815.
8. Calkins H, Brinkler J, Veltri EP, et al. Clinical interactions between pacemakers and automatic implantable cardioverter-defibrillations. J Am Coll Cardiol 1990; 16:666–673.
9. Cohen AI, Wish MH, Fletcher RD, et al. The use and interaction of permanent pacemakers and the automatic implantable cardioverter defibrillator. PACE 1988; 11:704–711.
10. Epstein AE, Kay GN, Plump VJ, et al. Combined automatic implantable cardioverter-defibrillator and pacemaker systems: implantation techniques and follow-up. J Am Coll Cardiol 1989; 13: 121–131.
11. Hammill S, Stanton M, Packer D. The effect of therapy type (autodecremental, burst, cardioversion) on subsequent ventricular tachycardia cycle length in patients with an implantable antitachycardia pacing-cardioversion-defibrillation device (abstr). PACE 1991; 14:623.
12. Klein LS, Miles WM, Zipes DP. Antitachycardia devices: realities and promises. J Am Coll Cardiol 1991; 18:1349–1362.
13. Callans DJ, Hook BG, Marchlinski FE. Paced beats following single nonsensed complexes in a "codependent" cardioverter defibrillator and bradycardia pacing systems: potential for ventricular tachycardia induction. PACE 1991; 14:1281–1287.
14. Hurwitz JL, Hook BG, Callans DJ, et al. Importance of abortive shock capability with electrogram storage in cardioverter-defibrillator devices. Circulation 1991; 84 (suppl II):427.
15. Wang PJ, Mandalakas N, Clyne C, et al. Accuracy of rhythm classification using a data log system. PACE 1991; 14:1911–1916.
16. Gurvich NL, Markarychev VA. Defibrillation of the heart with biphasic electrical impulses. Kardiologiia 1967;7:109–112.
17. Schuder JC, McDaniel WC, Stoeckle H. Defibrillation of 100-kg claves with asymmetrical, bidirectional, rectangular plueses. Cardiovasc Res 1984; 18:419–426.

18. Dixon EG, Tang ASL, Wolf JT, Meador MJ, Fine RV, Calfee, Ideker RE. Improved defibrillation thresholds with large contoured epicardial electrodes and biphasic waveforms. Circulation 1987; 76:1176–1184.
19. Chapman PD, Vetter JW, Souza JJ, Troup PJ, Wetherbee JN, Hoffman RG. Comparative efficacy of monophasic and biphasic truncated exponential shocks for nonthoracotomy internal defibrillation in dogs. J Am Coll Cardiol 1988; 12:739–745.
20. Chapman PD, Vetter JW, Souza JJ, Wetherbee JN, Troup PJ. Comparison of monophasic with single and dual capacitor biphasic waveforms for nonthoracotomy canine internal defibrillation. J Am Coll Cardiol 1989; 14:242–245.
21. Tang ASL, Yabe S, Wharton JM, Dolker M, Smith WM, Ideker RE. Ventricular fibrillation using biphasic waveforms: the importance of phasic duration. J Am Coll Cardiol 1989; 13:207–214.
22. Bardy GH, Ivey TD, Allen MD, Johnson G, Mehra R, Greene L. A prospective randomized evaluation of biphasic versus monophasic wave for pulses on defibrillation efficacy in humans. J Am Coll Cardiol 1989; 14:728–733.
23. Saksena S, Chandran P, Shah Y, Boccadamo R, Pantopoulos D, Rothbart ST. Comparative efficacy of transvenous cardioversion and pacing in patients with sustained ventricular tachycardia: a prospective, randomized, crossover study. Circulation 1985; 72:153–160.
24. Calvo RA, Saksensa S, Patopoulos D. Sequential transvenous pacing and shock therapy for termination of sustained ventricular tachycardia. Am Heart J 1988; 115:569–575.
25. Hook BG, Marchlinski FE. Value of ventricular electrogram recordings in the diagnosis of arrhythmias precipitating electrical device shock therapy. J Am Coll Cardiol 1991; 17:985–990.
26. Callans DJ, Hook BG, Marchlinski FE. Use of bipolar recordings from patch-patch and rate sensing leads to distinguish ventricular tachycardia from supraventricular rhythms in patients with implantable cardioverter defibrillators. PACE 1991; 14(II):1917–1922.
27. Callans DJ, Hook BG, Kleiman RB, Mitra RL, Flores BT, Marchlinski FE. Unique sensing errors in third generation implantable cardioverter-defibrillators. J Am Coll Cardiol 1993; 22:1135–40.
28. Fain ES, Winkle ES. Implantable cardioverter defibrillator. Ventritex Cadence. J Cardiovas Electrophysiol 1993; 4;211–223.
29. Gillis AM, Leitch JW, Wyse DG, Randomization comparative trial of methods of ventricular tachycardia pace termination (abstr). PACE 1992; 15:505.
30. Newman D, Dorian P, Hardy J. A randomized prospective comparison of ventricular antitachycardia pacing modalities. (abstr). PACE 1992; 15:506.
31. Fisher JD, Ostrow E, Kim SG, Matos JA. Ultrarapid single-capture train stimulation for termination of ventricualr tachycardia. Am J Cardiol 1983; 51:1334–1338.
32. Fisher JD, Kim SG, Matos JA, Ostrow E. Comparative effectiveness of pacing techniques for termination of well-tolerated sustained ventricular tachycardia. PACE 1983; 6:915–922.
33. Fisher JD, Mehra R, Furman S. Termination of ventricular tachycardia with bursts of rapid ventricular pacing. Am J Cardiol 1978; 41:94–102.
34. Naccarelli GV, Zipes DP, Rahilly GT, Heger JJ, Prystowsky EN. Influence of tachycardia cycle length and antiarrhythmic drugs on pacing termination and acceleration of ventricular tachycardia. Am Heart J 1983; 105:1–5.
35. Roy D, Waxman HL, Buxton AE, et al. Termination of ventricular tachycardia: role of tachycardia cycle length. Am J Cardiol 1982; 50:1346–1350.
36. Gardner MJ, Waxman HL, Buxton AE, Caine ME, Josephson ME. Termination of ventricular tachycardia. Evaluation of a new pacing method. Am J Cardiol 1982; 50:1338–1345.
37. Jentzer JH, Hoffman RM. Acceleration of ventricular tachycardia by rapid overdrive pacing combined with extrastimuli. PACE 1984; 72:922–924.
38. Charos GS, Haffajee CI, Gold RL, Bishop RL, Berkovits BV, Alpert JS. A theoretically and practically more effective method of interruption of ventricular tachycardia: self-adapting autodecremental overdrive pacing. Circulation 1986; 73:309–315.
39. Cook JR, Kirchhoffer JB, Fitzgerald TF, Lajzer DA. Comparison of decremental and burst overdrive pacing as treatment for ventricular tachycardia associated with coronary artery disease. Am J Cardiol 1992; 70:311–315.

40. Hammill S, Stanton M, Packer D. The effect of therapy type (autodecremental, burst, cardioversion) on subsequent ventricular tachycardia cycle length in patients with an implantable antitachycardia pacing-cardioversion-defibrillation device. (abstr). PACE 1991; 14:623.
41. Calvo RA, Saksena S, Pantopoulous D. Sequential transvenous pacing and shock therapy for termination of sustained ventricular tachycardia. Am Heart J 1988; 115:569–575.
42. Waspe LE, Kim SH, Matos JA, Fisher JD. Role of catheter lead system for transvenous countershocks and pacing during electrophysiologic tests: an assessment of the usefulness of catheter shocks for terminating ventricular tachyarrhythmias. Am J Cardiol 1983; 52:477–484.

37

Automatic Implantable Cardioverter-Defibrillators: The Ventak Devices

Antonis S. Manolis

*Tufts University School of Medicine
and New England Medical Center
Boston, Massachusetts*

The implantable cardioverter-defibrillator (ICD) devices approved by the U.S. FDA and presently available for implantation are the CPI Ventak P automatic implantable cardioverter-defibrillator (AICD) series, models 1550, 1555, and 1600. The B, BR, and C models are no longer available. The Ventak P2 (1625), PRX (1700/1705), and PRX II models are under clinical investigation. Various other newer-generation devices from other manufacturers (see respective chapters) are either under development or in the stage of clinical investigation or in the process of getting FDA approval. In this chapter the FDA-approved Ventak AICD series will be described.

I. HISTORICAL BACKGROUND

For more than a decade, the only available automatic implantable cardioverter-defibrillator devices were those of a single manufacturer, Cardiac Pacemakers Inc. (CPI, St. Paul, MN), being the pioneer in the field after buying the company that initially developed and manufactured the first clinical model of the automatic implantable defibrillator (Medrad, Inc./Intec Systems, Inc., Pittsburg, PA) under the trademark AID [1]. The first AID device, capable of detecting and treating ventricular fibrillation (VF) only, was implanted in a patient in 1980 [2], and it was monitoring the probability density function (PDF) of the heart by analyzing the QRS complex morphology and recognizing the time spent by the electrical signal (QRS) away from the isoelectric line. Sinusoidal rhythms that satisfied the PDF criterion would trigger the capacitor charge and defibrillation. The device utilized one pair of electrodes for both sensing and defibrillation. However, it soon became apparent that the inability of the AID device to recognize and cardiovert ventricular tachycardia was a major limitation of the device. In 1982 a subsequent model (AID-B), functioning both as a cardioverter as well as a defibrillator, incorporated the rate criterion by monitoring the heart rate. The AID-B device, which became the standard automatic implantable cardioverter-defibrillator (AICD), used both the PDF and heart rate criteria for arrhythmia detection, thereby allowing recognition and treatment of both ventricular tachycardia and ventricular fibrillation. This device and each subsequent model utilized separate sensing and defibrillation leads. Another model, the AID-BR, used only the heart rate criterion to detect the arrhythmia and trigger a device discharge when the heart rate exceeded a preset limit.

The AICD was approved for clinical use by the U.S. FDA in October 1985. The evolution in device technology led in 1986 to the development of the Ventak series, with a fully integrated circuit. The initial models, 1500, 1510, 1520, and 1530 (no longer available), where nonprogrammable, but the devices currently available and in clinical use (models 1550, 1555, and 1600) are programmable. Capability for telemetry was very limited with the nonprogrammable devices. An external analyzer (AIDCHECK) with a doughnut-shaped magnet and an electromagnetic transducer/probe placed over the pulse generator was used to communicate with the device and monitor the capacitor charge time and the number of discharges (''patient pulses'') already delivered to the patient (Fig. 1). Placing the magnet over the pulse generator for a brief period of time (> 2 s but < 25 s) triggered the charging of the capacitor and internal dumping of the discharge into a built-in resistor (''magnet test''). The magnet was also used to activate (QRS-synchronous tones emitted) and deactivate (continuous tone heard) the devices (by leaving the magnet in place for > 30 s) or divert a shock internally or temporarily blind the device by inhibiting the detection circuit (''EP mode'': standby status entered by not removing the magnet after initial activation of the device). All these nonprogrammable models were ''committed'' devices which, once charging had started, would proceed to deliver the shock even if the arrhythmia had meanwhile self-terminated, unless again a magnet was applied to internally divert the shock [3–5]. Two models (1500 and 1530) could deliver standard energy shocks (24 J), and two other models (1510 and 1520) were high-energy devices (28 J), with models 1500 and 1510 available with rate and morphology detection criteria, and models 1520 and 1530 with rate-only detection. Subsequent discussion in this chapter will concentrate on the presently available devices (models 1550, 1555, and 1600).

II. VENTAK 1550

The Ventak 1550 pulse generator weighs 235 g, is hermetically sealed in a titanium case, has a volume of 145 cm^3, dimensions of 10.1 cm H × 7.6 cm W × 2.0 cm D, is powered by two lithium-silver vanadium pentoxide cells connected in series, and accepts two 6.1-mm (morphology-sensing/defibrillating) and two 4.75-mm (rate-sensing) lead terminals (Fig. 2). It has four programmable parameters (mode, rate criterion, PDF criterion, and first-shock energy) (Table 1) and delivers monophasic truncated exponential, synchronized to the R-wave, shocks of 26–30 J with a pulse width of about 7 ms [6]. This and the other AICD models are constant-energy devices utilizing a constant energy waveform, also known as ''fixed tilt,'' and a self-adjusting pulse-width waveform, ensuring the delivery of the programmed energy, even in the presence of varying impedance [1].

A. Arrhythmia Detection

This system has two independent sensing channels for arrhythmia detection. One is for rate sensing and the other for morphology sensing [6]. The former determines when the rate exceeds the programmed rate cutoff by monitoring intrinsic R waves via the rate-sensing leads. A minimum of 8 beats at a rate faster than the programmed rate are required to satisfy this rate detection criterion. According to a rate-counting algorithm, the device tracks cardiac cycles (RR intervals) and the rate integrator advances by 1 (to a maximum of 15) for each RR interval

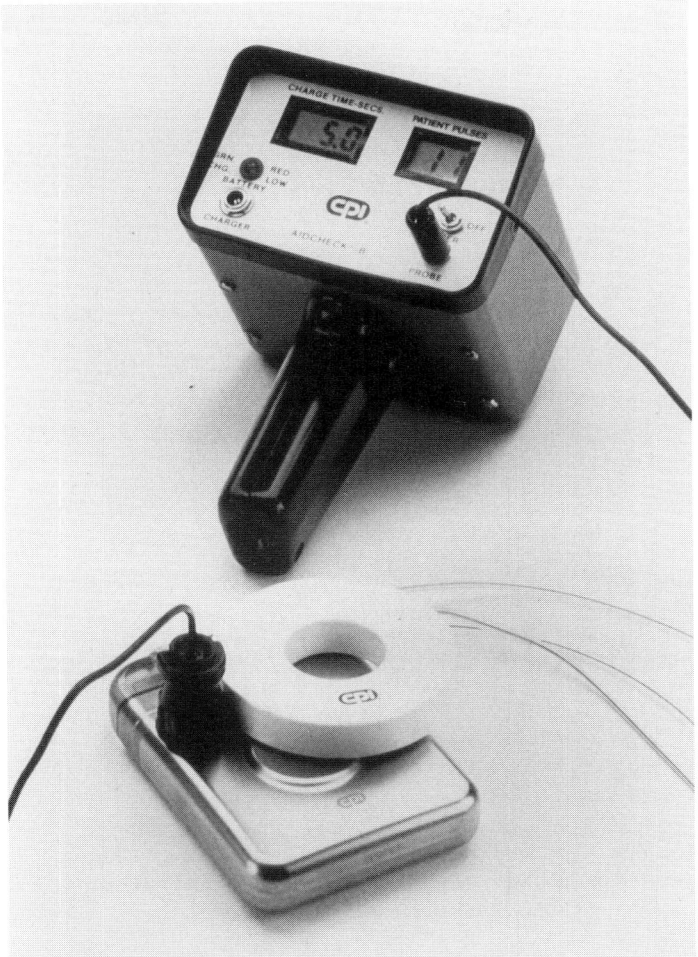

Figure 1 Early models of the AICD had very limited telemetry, obtained during a magnet test with the use of an external testing device (AIDCHECK, shown on top), a probe, and a doughnut-shaped magnet placed over the pulse generator (bottom). The telemetric parameters thus obtained included the charge time and the number of shocks delivered. (Courtesy of CPI.)

shorter than the programmed rate; when it reaches 8, arrhythmia detection has occurred. For RR intervals longer than the programmed rate criterion, the rate integrator decreases by 1 each 320 ms (to a minimum of 0) and has to reach 8 again before the first shock delay begins and has to remain at or above 8 for the duration of the first shock delay for the pulse generator to charge and deliver a shock. The rate criterion is programmable from 125 to 200 beats/min in 5-beats/min increments. The morphology detection criterion, also called PDF (probability density function), is determined by electrogram characteristics from the patch leads and is fulfilled when a significant absence of isoelectric time, characteristic of wide-QRS complex or sinusoidal rhythms, occurs. This criterion can be programmed on or off. Electrical noise may fulfill the PDF criterion. When it is programmed on, both the rate and the morphology criteria must

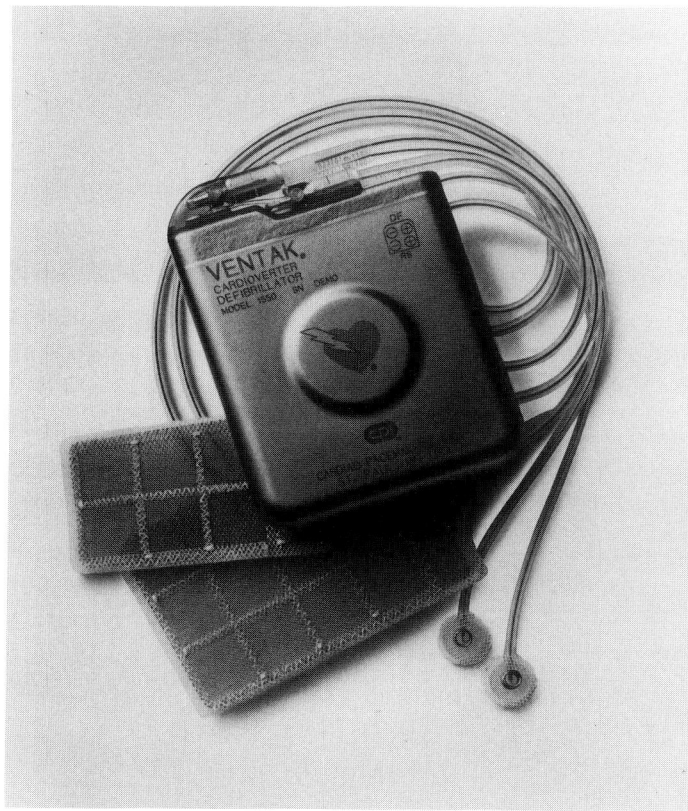

Figure 2 A Ventak AICD, model 1550, is shown connected to the standard leads (two defibrillating patch leads also used for morphology sensing and two epimyocardial rate-sensing leads). (Courtesy of CPI.)

be fulfilled and sustained for the shock delay period before the Ventak 1550 device proceeds with delivery of a shock. When the rate-only criterion is operative (PDF programmed off), the device will deliver therapy if the rate exceeds the programmed value and if it is sustained for a nonprogrammable shock-delay period of 2.5 s. The device has a refractory period of 140 ms after sensing an R wave, to prevent oversensing of the trailing edge of the R wave.

The morphology algorithm (PDF) was the initial method of arrhythmia detection used in the original AICD models, with the input signal for analysis obtained from the shocking leads. It was initially designed as a sensing algorithm used to discern ventricular fibrillation from asystole. However, it was not very sensitive or responsive to ventricular tachycardia and has since required design modifications in addition to the subsequent development of the rate-counting circuit. The morphology signal passes through an "operational" linear amplifier, which amplifies the voltage difference between inputs and performs various signal modifications [1]. The output signal has a voltage amplitude analogous to the slew rate of the input signal. During signal processing, the absolute-value signal represents the total of the positive and negative derivative voltages of the input signal, and this is sent to a comparator (another operational amplifier), which has a reference "window" voltage. When the voltage of the

Table 1 Features and Parameters of Ventak AICD devices[a]

	Ventak 1550	Ventak 1555	Ventak 1600	Ventak P2 1625
Programmable parameters				
Mode	Active/inactive	Active/inactive	Active/inactive	Active/inactive
Rate criterion	125–200 beats/min	125–200 beats/min	110–200 beats/min	110–200 beats/min[b]
PDF criterion	On/off	On/off	On/off	NA
First-shock delay	NA (2.5 s)	NA (2.5 s)	2.5–10 s	2.5–10 s
First-shock energy	26/30 J	NA (35 J)	0.1–30 J	0.1–34 J
Committed shock	NA	NA	NA	No/yes
VF protection	NA	NA	NA	On/off
Waveform	NA	NA	NA	Biphasic/monophasic
Polarity	NA	NA	NA	Initial/reverse
VVI pacing	NA	NA	NA	On/off
Postshock pacing	NA	NA	NA	On/off
EGM	NA	NA	NA	On/off
Nonprogrammable Parameters				
Second–fifth shock energy	30 J	35 J	30 J	34 J
Second–fifth shock delay	2.5 s	2.5 s	2.5 s	2.5 s
Refractory period	140 ms	140 ms	140 ms	140 ms

[a]AICD = automatic implantable cardioverter-defibrillator; EGM = (stored) electrograms; NA = not applicable/available; PDF = probability density function; VF = ventricular fibrillation.
[b]VF rate: 130–220 beats/min

absolute-value signal exceeds the voltage of the reference window, the comparator switches on a constant current source which charges a fibrillation-detecting capacitor. The voltage on this capacitor is proportional to the time the absolute-value signal spends above the window reference voltage level and is monitored by another comparator, which in the original AID device could then trigger the charge of the high-voltage capacitors. In the newer device models, however, the trigger from the PDF detection circuit (when PDF is on) is only one of the two inputs (the other being the rate-integrating circuit output) to the circuitry finally initiating charging of the high-voltage capacitors.

To provide a safety margin for detection of ventricular tachycardia (VT), it is recommended that the rate criterion be programmed at least 10 beats/min lower than the patient's VT rate if VT is monomorphic, or at least 30 beats/min lower if the VT is polymorphic, as R-wave variability of the latter may more frequently prevent sensing of all R waves. The rate cutoff should, of course, be higher than the patient's maximum normal heart rate. Use of a rate-only criterion for arrhythmia detection makes the device more sensitive but less specific, with risk of treating supraventricular tachyarrhythmias (SVTs), but such an approach may be preferred if PDF is not fulfilled during testing of spiky VTs. With certain characteristics of electrograms detected via the patches, such as those that are narrow, the VT may not satisfy the PDF criterion. This would result in failure of the device to detect and deliver therapy. During implantation of the leads, their signals are measured intraoperatively; ideally, for the rate-sensing leads, one should obtain an R-wave amplitude of at least 5 mV and a duration of less than 100 ms, and for the morphology-sensing leads the signal should be continuous with an R-wave amplitude of at least 1 mV and duration of >100 ms during native rhythm.

With regard to signal sensing and detection, the device operates on the basis of *automatic gain control* by adjusting its amplification factor (ratio of output voltage to input voltage) or the threshold for detection of a signal based on the amplitude of the preceding signals [1]. Thus, for detection of small-amplitude signals, such as those occurring during ventricular fibrillation, the device increases its sensitivity or lowers its detection threshold until the signals are detected. Although some VF signals of very low amplitude (<0.2 mV) may not be sensed (signal dropout), the majority of them are detected and therapy is delivered.

B. Delivery of Therapy

The Ventak 1550 device requires about 7 s to charge and deliver a 30-J shock at the beginning of life status. Over time, capacitor deformation occurs and the charge time increases. This is prevented by periodic capacitor reformation and battery testing. The shock is monophasic, it is delivered synchronously with the R wave, has a programmable energy of 26 or 30 J (only for the first shock), a typical pulse width of 7 ms, and a relatively constant energy output over the life of the device. Up to five shocks can be delivered in a given series if the first one is not successful. The energy is fixed at 30 J for the second to fifth shocks. Delivery of five sequential shocks may last more than 2 min, as the device takes about 10–25 s for each detection and charging. After the five shocks are delivered, the device will reset and deliver further shocks only if the heart rhythm has meanwhile changed and does not satisfy the detection criterion for at least 35 s. If the arrhythmia recurs within 35 s after the last delivered first to fourth shocks, the device will deliver the next shock in the five-shock sequence. To prevent inappropriate shocks from oversensing noise, the device has noise protection circuitry. If more than 38 signals per second are sensed in the rate-sensing channel, the device classifies this as noise and is inhibited and thus does not charge or shock; subsequently, the rate integrator count is reset to zero. Delivery of therapy can be affected by use of a programmer or a magnet. A shock can be diverted via a programmer, but also by placing a magnet for 2–3 s over the upper right-hand corner of the device after the pulse generator has begun charging. Inappropriate delivery of a shock may be precipitated by noninvasive testing of the device or pacemaker programming [4].

C. Programmable and Nonprogrammable Parameters

The Ventak 1550 model has four programmable parameters. The device can be programmed to active or inactive *mode* (Table 1). Therapy is delivered in the active mode only. In the inactive mode the device does not respond to an arrhythmia but retains all programmed parameters. In addition to the standard use of a programmer for activating or deactivating a device [7], a doughnut-shaped magnet can be used instead. The magnet should not be used during a programming session, as the programmer will not recognize the change unless the AICD is reinterrogated. Other programmable features, as mentioned earlier, are the *rate* criterion, which can be programmed from 125 to 200 beats/min in 5-beat/min increments, and the *PDF* criterion, which can be programmed on or off. Energy (26 or 30J) can be programmed for the *first shock* only. Nominal values include: inactive mode, rate criterion 155 beats/min, PDF off, first shock energy level 30 J. Nonprogrammable features of the device include a shock delay period set at 2.5 s, a factory preset energy level of 30 J for the second to fifth shocks, a refractory period of 140 ms, and a high-energy rescue shock of 30 J (STAT shock), which can be delivered to the patient with use of the programmer even when the device is inactive.

D. Other Device Functions

Data in the memory of the device that can be retrieved via the programmer and printed out include the model number and manufacturer, programmed parameters, total patient shock count with separate counters for the first and second through fifth shocks that have been delivered to the patient (when each counter reaches 255, it resets to 0), number of shocks dumped into the internal test load (this counter advances to 63 before resetting to 0), recent charge time, lead impedance, and battery status. Each device has an individual elective replacement indicator (ERI), which is printed on the pulse generator label. It represents $1.33 \times$ battery charge time at the beginning of life (BOL) and is used to determine the time when the pulse generator should be replaced. Functions provided via the programmer include stat (rescue) shock delivery, EP test data, event markers, capacitor reformation, charge time by performing battery test, shock diversion, extending the telemetry communication range, and obtaining a printed copy with all the above data.

When a doughnut magnet is placed over the device and within 2–8 in. (5–20 cm), the reed switch is actuated. For reliable use of the magnet, it should be positioned over the upper right-hand corner of the device and held firmly against the pulse generator. If the device is active and has been implanted, audible tones are emitted from the pulse generator which are synchronous to the R wave; if the device has not been implanted, no tones are heard. If the device is deactivated, a continuous tone is emitted. Holding the magnet in place for at least 30 s, if active the device will be deactivated and a synchronous tone will become continuous, or if inactive it will be activated and the continuous tone will become synchronous with each R wave. The magnet can also be used to divert a shock from the patient to the internal load, if it is held over the device for 2–3 s after the pulse generator has begun to charge. Tones are also emitted from the device in the presence of strong magnetic fields or during charging if the battery level is low.

III. VENTAK 1555

This device is a *high-energy* version of the previous model and functions in essentially the same way as described above for the VENTAK 1550 model, with a few differences which will be discussed here. The Ventak 1555 pulse generator delivers nonprogrammable shocks of 35 J. Thus only three instead of four parameters are programmable: mode, rate criterion, and PDF criterion; the energy level is preset at 35 J for all shocks [6]. Due to higher energy level, the charge time for this model is slightly higher (7.5 s) than for the 1550 model. The model 2825 module is used with the model 2035 programmer to program the Ventak 1555.

IV. VENTAK P 1600

This upgraded device has more (five) and a wider range of programmable features than the previous models, but its basic design encompasses the same principles of function [6]. The mode is programmable to active and inactive and the PDF criterion on or off as in the previous models. However, the rate criterion can be programmed to a lower rate of 110 beats/min; the range of rates is therefore 110 to 200 beats/min in 5-beat/min increments. In addition, the first shock delay is now programmable to 2.5, 5.0, 7.5, and 10 s. Also the first shock energy has a wider range of programmable values for *low-energy cardioversion*, with energy as low as 0.1 J (0.1, 0.5, 1-4, 6, 8, 10, 12, 14, 17, 20, 23, 26, 30 J) (Table 1). The output energy and the shock delay for the second to fifth shocks are nonprogrammable and remain fixed at 30 J and 2.5 s, respectively. The shock delay is applied before charging begins and ensures that a shock is not delivered for nonsustained arrhythmias that terminate spontaneously prior to the delay time. However, once the device starts charging, it is committed to deliver therapy. The charge time varies in a linear relationship with the programmed energy, from 0.08 s for a 0.1-J shock to 7 s for a 30-J shock. The Ventak P 1600 is programmed with use of the hand-held programmer (model 2035) and the model 2830 module (Fig. 3).

V. VENTAK P2

This new AICD model (1625) has, in addition to the features of the Ventak P, programmable monophasic or biphasic waveform output and bradycardia (VVI) pacing capability, and is designed to store electrograms and detailed therapy history (Table 1). It has already been implanted in Europe with the thoracotomy and nonthoracotomy (Endotak) lead systems, and clinical investigation is about to start in the United States as well. The device can be programmed with the CPI programmer (model 2035; software module 2835). Other diagnostic features of the device include noninvasive arrhythmia induction, impedance measurements, and stored electrograms of episode onset, and the periods immediately before and after therapy delivery. The stored electrograms are sensed via the shocking leads. The storage capacity is about 2.5 min. For noninvasive fibrillation induction, the device delivers rapid pulses via the shocking leads or continuous pace trains (bursts) at 50-, 75-, 100-, or 125-ms intervals through the pace/sense electrodes. In addition to VVI pacing, the device has separately programmable postshock pacing.

As of September 1992, 51 patients had received the Ventak P2 for malignant ventricular tachyarrhythmias, with 20% having concomitant bradyarrhythmia indications [6]. All patients were programmed to receive biphasic shock waveforms, and 88% were programmed to have noncommitted shocks. In eight patients tested, DFT was lower with a biphasic than with a monophasic waveform (9.8 versus 15.1 J). Using the stored electrograms, it was determined

The Ventak Devices

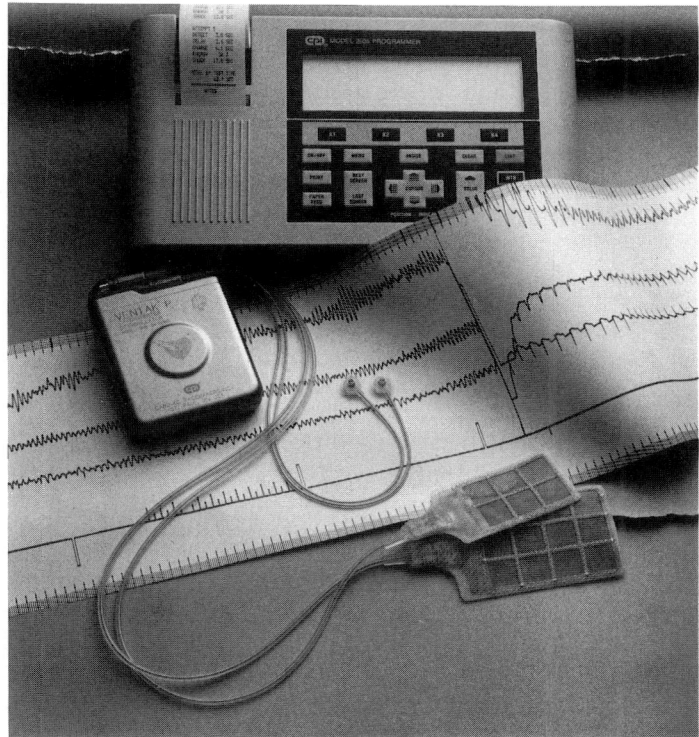

Figure 3 Shown are a Ventak P (1600) device with its leads, the hand-held programmer (model 2035), and arrhythmia recordings with the event markers providing information regarding detection and delivery of therapy. (Courtesy of CPI.)

that 43% of symptomatic shocks and 43% of asymptomatic shocks were appropriate. During the 9-month study period, three non-device-related deaths occurred (one cardiac and two noncardiac); two nonimplanted and two implanted devices were found to be malfunctioning. The results with the approved devices are discussed separately below.

VI. LEAD SYSTEM

The header of the Ventak devices is designed to accept defibrillation leads with 6.1-mm terminals (upper two ports) and rate-sensing leads with 4.75-mm terminals (lower two ports) (Figs. 2 and 3). Thus, if other than CPI leads are used, suitable adaptors will most likely be needed. For defibrillation leads, available options include the use of two patches or a combination of one patch and a transvenous superior vena cava lead (spring electrode) (see Chapter 35 for further details of lead design and positions). For rate sensing, a transvenous (bifurcated) bipolar endocardial lead or, alternatively, two sutureless epimyocardial leads can be used. [The nonthoracotomy lead system (Endotak) is described separately in Chapter 45]. After the lead signals are evaluated intraoperatively and cardioversion/defibrillation threshold testing is performed, as described below, the leads are tunneled to the implantation pocket, the lead signals are reevaluated, the pulse generator is tested, and finally the leads are connected to the pulse generator. Proper lead connection and set-screw tightening is important to ensure appropriate ICD function. To verify good connection, a magnet can be used to permit audible confirmation of R-wave synchronous sensing tones.

VII. IMPLANTATION AND INTRAOPERATIVE TESTING

Sterile accessories and equipment needed for the implantation procedure include the Ventak pulse generator, the rate-sensing and defibrillating leads, a bipolar cable, a high-voltage cable, bipolar and high-voltage monitoring cables, regular pacing cables, internal and external defibrillator paddles, a programmer wand (model 6577), a doughnut-shaped magnet, and duplicates of all these accessories. Nonsterile equipment comprise external defibrillator (R2) pads, the external cardioverter defibrillator (ECD) (model 2806), the programmer (2035) with the appropriate module, ECD monitoring cables, a multichannel strip-chart recorder, two external defibrillators, a fibrillator box, and preferably a pacing system analyzer (PSA) and a magnetic tape recorder [8].

A. External Cardioverter-Defibrillator (ECD)

The Ventak ECD (model 2806) is designed for use during implantation of the Ventak pulse generators [8] (Fig. 4). This external cardioverter defibrillator is a 25-lb portable, battery-powered device employed in the operating room for cardioversion and defibrillation threshold testing. It can operate in automatic or manual modes. It has five monitoring functions, which include the heart rate, amplitude of the electrogram, QRS, rate, and PDF arrhythmia detection. Measured parameters include energy, pulse width, impedance, and peak current. It connects to the defibrillation leads with the high-voltage cable, to the rate-sensing leads with the bipolar cable, and to the recorder with input/output cables. Selected output energy ranges from 0.1 to 35 J; a rescue shock of 40 J can also be delivered separately. Rate values can be selected from 110 to 200 beats/min. Detection criteria can include rate only or rate and PDF. The shock can be delivered synchronously or asynchronously with the QRS complex. An external stimulation source can be connected to the ECD for arrhythmia induction via the rate-sensing lead system. The device can be connected to a magnetic tape recorder. It has a rechargeable battery and incorporates a built-in printer.

B. Lead System Implantation and Testing

Various surgical and interventional techniques are employed for implantation of the ICD lead system [9] (Fig. 5) (see respective chapters). As mentioned above, with the previously conventional thoracotomy systems for rate sensing, either a bipolar transvenous lead or two sutureless epicardial leads can be implanted. For morphology sensing and defibrillation, either two patches or one patch and a superior vena cava lead can be used. The patches can be placed intra- or extrapericardially. Currently, however, the nonthoracotomy Endotak lead system with similar lead terminals is routinely employed. After the lead(s) are implanted, intraoperative electrical testing is performed. Initially the lead signals are evaluated with use of the CPI ECD system and a multichannel recorder. The two 4.75-mm rate-sensing lead terminals are therefore inserted into the two large ports of the bipolar cable, which is connected to the ECD. The R wave thus measured should be at least 5 mV in amplitude and less than 100 ms in duration during native rhythm. Similarly, the morphology-sensing/defibrillating leads (6.1-mm terminal pins) are connected to the ECD via the high-voltage cable and tested. The signal from these leads should be continuous and without artifact, with an R-wave amplitude of 1–10 mV (preferably >5 mV).

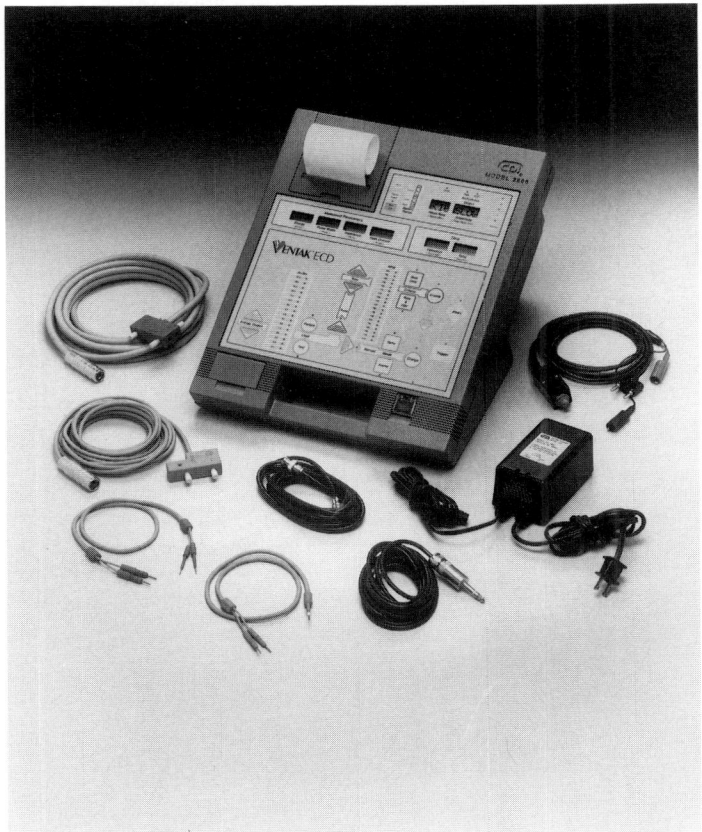

Figure 4 The external cardioverter defibrillator (ECD device, model 2806) used for intraoperative electrical testing. (Courtesy of CPI.)

Arrhythmia induction and cardioversion/defibrillation threshold (DFT) testing is subsequently performed to ensure adequate safety margins for available or programmable shock energy levels [10]. A minimum of three successful DFT tests are routinely performed. At least a 10-J "safety margin," or difference between the DFT and the maximum output of the device, is required. Ideally DFTs of ≤15 J are sought for all implants, but with a 30-J device a 20-J DFT would be acceptable. Arrhythmia induction can be accomplished through the ECD console and via the implanted rate-sensing or morphology-sensing leads or preferably through separate pacing wires attached to the heart if a thoracotomy technique is employed. At least ventricular fibrillation is induced and tested, but an attempt should also be made to induce and test the patient's clinical arrhythmia, especially if low-energy cardioversion is to be used with a Ventak 1600 device.

C. Pulse Generator Implantation and Testing

Following DFT testing, the implantation pocket is fashioned, usually in the left paraumbilical area, and the pulse generator is connected to the leads after it has been appropriately programmed. The ICD device is also connected to the ECD in a way that allows the parallel op-

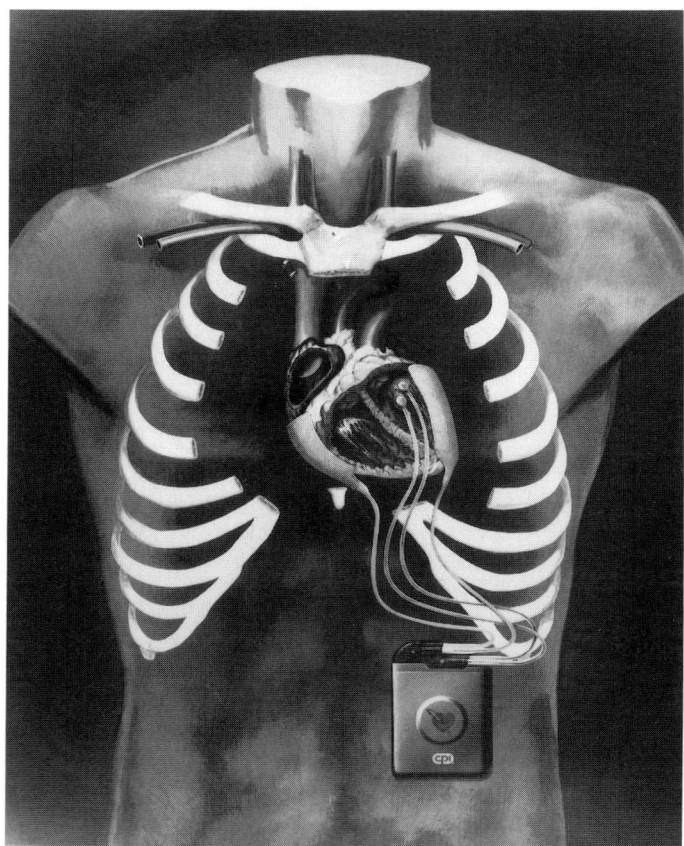

Figure 5 The figure demonstrates the old implantation technique of a full AICD system employing two patches and two rate-sensing leads implanted on the epicardium via thoracotomy and then tunneled down and connected to the pulse generator, which is implanted in a left paraumbilical pocket. (Courtesy of CPI.)

eration of the two defibrillators following precise instructions as outlined in the manufacturer's manual to avoid device damage. With use of a sterile wand and the programmer and with event marker monitoring in the EP test mode, as detailed below, the arrhythmia is induced and conversion is tested intraoperatively to ensure appropriate device function. Test results are printed out and records are kept for future reference. If it tests successfully, the device is inactivated and the leads are then properly connected to the pulse generator, which is subsequently implanted in the abdominal pocket (Fig. 5). Routinely, repeat device testing to verify efficacy with arrhythmia induction and conversion is scheduled in the electrophysiology laboratory prior to the patient's discharge from the hospital.

VIII. PROGRAMMING

Programming of the Ventak devices is performed through radiofrequency telemetry with use of the CPI hand-held, battery-powered programmer (model 2035), an external wand (model 6575 or 6577), and the appropriate software module (model 2820 or 2825 for the Ventak 1550, model 2825 for the Ventak 1555, model 2830 for the Ventak 1600, and model 2835 for the Ventak 1625) [7] (Fig. 3). The programming system also contains a printer and a built-in telemetry antenna. An electrogram cable is available for event marker detection and monitoring. Communication is established with use of the antenna (on the back of the programmer) or the external wand placed over the pulse generator, while proper positioning is indicated when performing interrogation with an illuminating light and a double beeping sound. Normal (5-cm) or extended (7.5-cm) telemetry range is available. After successful interrogation, the screen with the parameters is displayed and appropriate programming with selected new values can thus be performed (Fig. 6). Other data screens are also available via menu keystrokes and can be ac-

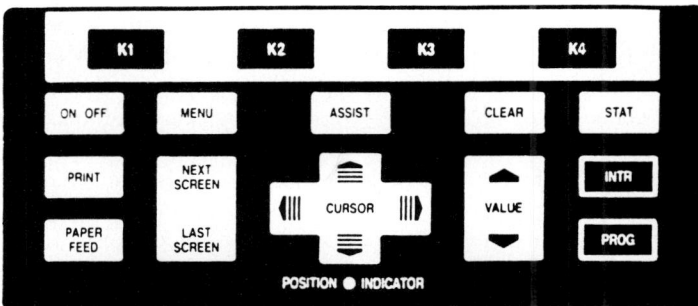

Figure 6 The keyboard of the universal hand-held CPI programmer (model 2035) is shown on top, the *parameters* screen accessed during initial interrogation of the AICD is shown in the middle, and the *menu* screen allowing access to other data screens is displayed at the bottom. (Courtesy of CPI.)

cessed with the use of a cursor and the next screen/last screen key. These include pulse generator data, electrophysiological (EP) test, form the capacitors screen, telemetry range, and new patient screen (Fig. 6). The pulse generator (PG) data screen provides current pulse generator data, such as the last recorded charge time, defibrillating lead impedance, number of delivered first shocks, total patient shocks, and test shocks, and allows one to perform a battery test, measure the charge time, and thus monitor the battery life. The pulse generator needs to be replaced when the battery test charge time reaches the ERI, which is listed on the pulse generator's label. Prior to battery test the capacitors are reformed with use of the form the capacitors screen.

The EP test screen allows one to perform arrhythmia induction and conversion with EP testing to confirm the ICD system's detection and conversion capability. Upon entering the EP test mode, the device is temporarily disabled and remains at standby. It therefore does not deliver therapy until it is enabled again by pressing the appropriate key. Monitoring of the produced event markers during the EP test procedure is accomplished with use of the model 6580 EGM cable, which connects the programmer with a multichannel recorder. After proper connections are made, the programmer transmits event markers (not real-time markers) to the recorder. By initially pressing the appropriate key, calibration pulses are transmitted to indicate the key events represented by the event markers, including generator charging, satisfaction of the rate-detection criterion and/or the PDF criterion, type of shock (test, first, stat, second, or third to fifth) delivered, and noise detection. Then the EP test mode with temporary device disabling is entered by pressing a key. The arrhythmia is induced with use of a separate induction source (e.g., endocardial wire and a programmed stimulator or fibrillator box) and at about 5 s the ICD device is enabled by pressing a key, detects and appropriately converts the arrhythmia (Fig. 7). During the EP test the telemetry link should be maintained throughout the procedure for accurate monitoring. A shock can be diverted to internal load by pressing the appropriate programmer key, or by using the magnet after the device has started charging; during pulse generator charging, the programmer emits a continuous tone and displays the divert screen. A continuous tone is also emitted by the programmer when telemetry communication is interrupted or a noisy environment is sensed. Other programmer functions available during programming and testing include the activation of a stat (rescue) high-energy shock delivery and report printing (Fig. 8).

Noninvasive Testing During Follow-up

Regular follow-up of patients with a Ventak device is conducted every 2 months in a facility with available means for cardiopulmonary resuscitation, including an external defibrillator. During noninvasive testing the device is initially interrogated, the number of shocks delivered is noted, and a full report is printed out (Fig. 8). Then the capacitors are reformed and a battery test is performed, during which the charge time is calculated and displayed. The charge time is compared to the ERI. The device is reprogrammed appropriately as needed and reinterrogated to confirm and verify that the desired values have been programmed. Finally, a full report is printed out at the end of the session, and a follow-up form is completed.

IX. ELECTROMAGNETIC INTERFERENCE/PACEMAKER INTERACTION

Electromagnetic interference (EMI) may inhibit or deactivate the Ventak devices or cause inappropriate shocks. Sources of potential EMI may include equipment for electrosurgical cau-

The Ventak Devices

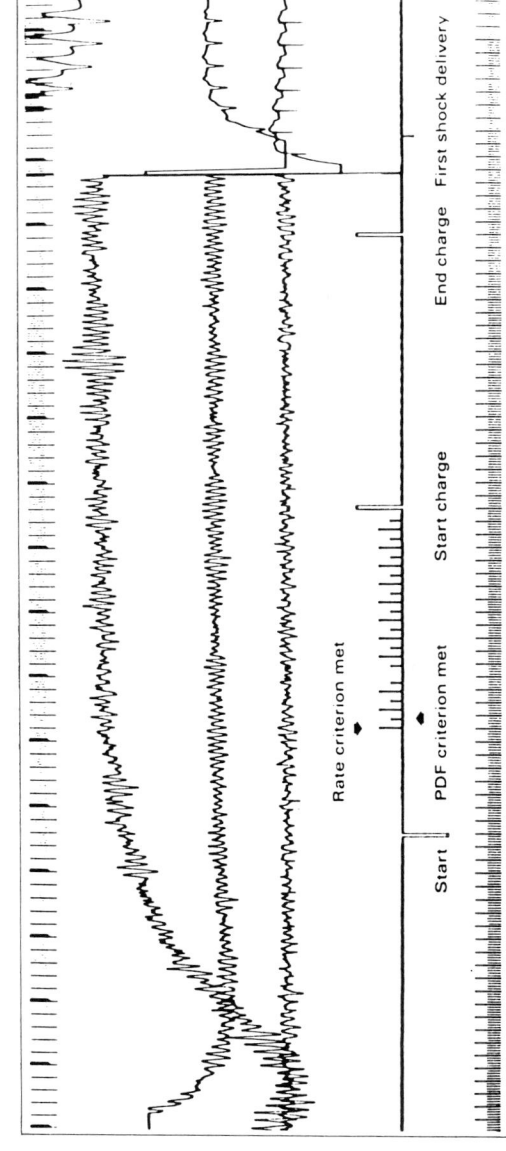

Figure 7 The rhythm strip shows ventricular fibrillation, which is induced either intraoperatively or before discharge in the electrophysiology laboratory for AICD testing. The programmer is used to transmit EP test event markers to the strip-chart recorder. These markers facilitate monitoring of proper device function. (Courtesy of CPI.)

```
         CONVERSION SUMMARY          PATIENT
ATTEMPT 1
DETECT       5.8 SEC                 PHYSICIAN
DELAY        2.5 SEC                 DATE
CHARGE       5.6 SEC
ENERGY       26 J
SHOCK        15.5 SEC                      VENTAK 1550
ATTEMPT 2                                PULSE GENERATOR
DETECT       5.9 SEC
DELAY        2.5 SEC                   PRESENT PARAMETERS
CHARGE       6.1 SEC
ENERGY       30 J
SHOCK        16.0 SEC                MODE         ACTIVE
ATTEMPT 3                            RATE         155 BPM
DETECT       5.9 SEC                 PDF          ON
DELAY        2.5 SEC                 DELAY        2.5 SEC
CHARGE       6.1 SEC                 SHOCK ENERGY
ENERGY       30 J                    1ST          26 JOULES
SHOCK        16.0 SEC                2-5          30 JOULES
ATTEMPT 4
DETECT       5.9 SEC                 CHARGE TIME
DELAY        2.5 SEC                              6.1 SEC
CHARGE       6.1 SEC                 LEAD IMPEDANCE
ENERGY       30 J                                 45 OHMS
SHOCK        16.0 SEC                PG BATTERY STATUS
ATTEMPT 5                                    EVALUATE ERI
DETECT       5.9 SEC                 CAPACITOR FORM
DELAY        2.5 SEC                              SEC
CHARGE       6.1 SEC                 COUNT
ENERGY       30 J                    1ST SHOCK        16
SHOCK        16.0 SEC                2-5 SHOCK         5
TOTAL TEST TIME                      TOTAL PATIENT    21
             79.5 SEC                TEST SHOCKS       3

             NOTES                             NOTES

       EP TEST PRINTOUT              PULSE GENERATOR
                                      DATA PRINTOUT
```

Figure 8 Printed reports are shown of a typical EP test conversion summary, displaying information about the delivery of the entire five-shock sequence (left), and a typical final report that includes the current parameters and memory information (right). (Courtesy of CPI.)

tery or diathermy, arc welding, robotic jacks, magnetic resonance imaging, running motors, transformers, radiofrequency transmitters, radar, radioactive cobalt, linear accelerators, betatrons, magnets, large stereo speakers, and lithotripsy equipment. Patients with an ICD should not be subjected to magnetic resonance imaging or diathermy, and before using electrocautery the ICD device should be deactivated; magnets should be kept away from the pulse generator; if lithotripsy is to be used, it should not be focused on the pulse generator site, while the device should be shielded during ionizing radiation therapy. The ICD should be checked if exposed to above EMI sources to verify proper device function. The Ventak devices have noise protection circuitry which helps to prevent false shocks caused by electrical noise. If the device senses through the rate-sensing lead more than 38 events per second (e.g., from a fibrillation induction source), it is inhibited and thus does not charge and deliver therapy; the detection algorithm is reset to zero. If noise is sensed by the morphology lead, the device will revert to a rate-only detection mode.

Possible interaction problems may be encountered in a patient with both an atrial and/or ventricular cardiac pacemaker, either temporary or permanent, and a Ventak ICD device [11,12]. Such problems may include inability of the pacemaker to sense the arrhythmia resulting in inappropriate pacing, which then may interfere with ICD sensing, especially if large pacemaker artifacts are seen by the ICD device, making the device adjust its automatic gain to a higher setting and thus leading to inhibition of arrhythmia detection, as the arrhythmia is interpreted as normal rhythm at the pacemaker rate. On the other hand, oversensing of the pacemaker artifacts by the ICD, due to various reasons, may result in inappropriate shocks. Use of bipolar pacemakers may minimize or avoid these problems. The ICD rate-sensing leads should be implanted as far from the pacing leads as possible, and the signals from the ICD rate-sensing leads should be examined intraoperatively to confirm that no pacing artifacts are sensed [12]. Also, arrhythmia induction and ICD device testing should be done with the pacemaker programmed to the asynchronous mode at maximum output, to provide the best opportunity to observe for possible ICD inhibition due to sensing of pacemaker artifacts. Eventually, programming the smallest pacing artifacts with the lowest allowable amplitude and pulse width may prevent such interactions. The ICD should be deactivated when a temporary pacemaker is being used or a permanent pacemaker is being tested or reprogrammed, as well as when the patient is taken to the operating room for noncardiac surgery. At such times an external defibrillator should be used if needed.

X. CLINICAL RESULTS AND AICD STATISTICS

As of August 1992, 32,474 CPI AICD devices had been implanted worldwide in 25,333 patients. Of these devices, 2069 were early models (AID B/BR), 6899 were old Ventak (1500, 1510, 1520, 1530) AICD models, 14,862 were Ventak 1550 and 1555 models, and 8644 were Ventak P (1600) models. The mean age of patients was 62 years, and the mean left ventricular ejection fraction was 33%. Coronary artery disease was present in the majority of patients (74%), while nonischemic cardiomyopathy was present in 10% and other underlying diagnoses (valvular, congenital, or primary electrical disorders or long QT syndrome) comprised about 16%. Sudden-death-free survival was 99.2% at 1 year, 98.8% at 2 years, 98.6% at 3 years, 98.3% at 4 years, and 98.1% at 5 years, according to the manufacturer. Nonsudden-cardiac-death-free survival was 98.5% at 1 year and 96.5% at 5 years. Total survival was 95.8% at 1 year and 90.1% at 5 years. Thus, by large numbers it has been clearly shown that these pioneer devices have been very effective in preventing sudden cardiac death [13–18], and the standard remains that the newer models must continue to be at least as effective as their predecessors, and hopefully become more convenient, flexible, and versatile. Whether overall survival is also improved will probably need to await the results of planned or ongoing prospective randomized trials [19]. With the newer models described herein, device longevity has been consistently improved compared with that of the older models, reaching 97–99% at 24 months (versus 77–92% of AICD models 1500, 1510, 1520) [20]. With regard to cost-effectiveness issues, recent studies from our institution and elsewhere have confirmed that use of these devices in patients with life-threatening arrhythmias is cost-effective [21–24]. Indeed, ICD implantation falls in the realm of use of other common cardiac and medical or surgical treatments, such as coronary bypass surgery, cardiac transplantation, hemodialysis, or medical therapy for hypertension or hypercholesterolemia, or electrophysiological testing-guided antiarrhythmia therapy.

XI. DEVICE LIMITATIONS

The Ventak 1550, 1555, and 1600 models, although improved versions of previous devices, still have limitations which may occasionally become important [25]. They are still partially committed devices, as they monitor the cardiac rhythm during the shock delay period (which is programmable only in the 1600 model) and no shock is delivered until the counter's value remains equal to or higher than the critical value at the end of the delay, but once capacitor charging has begun, these devices are committed to deliver a shock. The herein-described Ventak AICD models have no antibradycardia pacing capability (except for the Ventak P2 model, which is currently in clinical investigation); are still very costly, heavy, and bulky devices, and have only elementary programmability and capability for telemetry. Furthermore, there was a recent (5/1992) worrisome recall of these devices by the manufacturer as a result of a faulty production process that resulted in contamination of a diode in the charging circuit and led to replacement of all units which were not yet implanted, creating major problems for both patients and physicians due to shortage in device supply and potential risk to those who had already received such faulty devices. As a result of the diode failure, 8 devices were found to have a prolonged charge time that could have resulted in failure to deliver therapy, while 29 devices exhibited a premature ERI.

Among other limitations, albeit common to other similar ICD devices, one was, until recently, concerned about the need for thoracotomy to implant the patches for these devices, contributing to a 1.5–5.4% perioperative mortality. Such concern is now overcome with the recent FDA approval of nonthoracotomy lead systems. However, despite a notable reduction in perioperative mortality ($\leq 1\%$) with these systems, other device-related complications persist (2–10%), including infection, sensing problems, lead dislodgement or fracture, device malfunction, inappropriate shocks, lack of antibradycardia, and antitachycardia pacing capability, or finally, there is still concern about important quality-of-life or health-care cost issues and considerations [17].

REFERENCES

1. Troup PJ. Implantable cardioverters and defibrillators. Curr Probl Cardiol 1989:679–815.
2. Mirowski M, Reid PR, Mower MM, et al. Termination of malignant ventricular arrhythmias with an implanted defibrillator in human beings. N Engl J Med 1980; 303:322–324.
3. Cannom DS, Winkle RA. Implantation of the automatic implantable cardioverter defibrillator (AICD): practical aspects. PACE 1986; 9:793–809.
4. Manolis AS, Rastegar H, Estes NAM III. Automatic implantable cardioverter defibrillator: current status. JAMA 1989; 262:1362–1368.
5. Manolis AS. Nonpharmacologic management of malignant ventricular tachyarrhythmias: role of the automatic implantable cardioverter-defibrillator. Hellenic J Cardiol 1991; 32:14–24.
6. Cardiac Pacemakers, Inc. Physician's Manual: Ventak, model 1550 AICD, 1989; Ventak, model 1555 AICD, 1990; Ventak P AICD, model 1600, 1991; Ventak P2, Clinical Summary Report, 1992.
7. Cardiac Pacemakers, Inc. Physician's Manual: Ventak AICD, model 2820 software module, 1988; Ventak AICD, model 2825 software module, 1990; Ventak P AICD, model 2830 software module, 1991.
8. Cardiac Pacemakers, Inc. User's Manual: Ventak ECD 2805, 1991.
9. Frank G, Lowes D. Implantable cardioverter defibrillators: surgical considerations. PACE 1992; 15(III):631–635.
10. Singer I, Lang D. Defibrillation threshold: clinical utility and therapeutic implications. PACE 1992; 15:932–949.

11. Calkins H, Brinker J, Veltri EP, Guarnieri T, Levine JH. Clinical interactions between pacemakers and automatic implantable cardioverter-defibrillators. J Am Coll Cardiol 1990; 16:666–673.
12. Spotnitz HM, Ott GY, Bigger JT, Steinberg JS, Livelli F Jr. Methods of implantable-cardioverter defibrillator-pacemaker insertion to avoid interactions. Ann Thorac Surg 1992; 53:253–257.
13. Winkle RA, Mead RH, Ruder MA, et al. Long-term outcome with the automatic implantable cardioverter-defibrillator. J Am Coll Cardiol 1989; 13:1353–1361.
14. Manolis AS, Tan-DeGuzman W, Lee MA, et al. Clinical experience in seventy-seven patients with the automatic implantable cardioverter defibrillator. Am Heart J 1989; 118:445–450.
15. Horowitz LN. The automatic implantable cardioverter defibrillator: review of clinical results, 1980–1990. PACE 1992; 15(III):604–609.
16. Thomas AC, Moser SA, Smutka ML, et al. Implantable defibrillation: eight years clinical experience. PACE 1988; 11:2053–2058.
17. Lehman MH, Saksena S. NASPE Policy Statement. Implantable cardioverter defibrillators in cardiovascular practice: report of the policy conference of the North American Society of Pacing and Electrophysiology. PACE 1991; 14:969–979.
18. Newman D, Sauve J, Herre J, et al. Survival after implantation of the cardioverter defibrillator. Am J Cardiol 1992; 69:899–903.
19. Connolly SJ, Yusuf S. Evaluation of the implantable cardioverter defibrillator in survivors of cardiac arrest: the need for randomized trials. Am J Cardiol 1992; 69:959–962.
20. Song SL. The Bilitch Report. Performance of implantable cardiac rhythm management devices. PACE 1991; 14:1198–1200.
21. O'Donoghue S, Platia EV, Brooks-Robinson S, Mispireta L. Automatic implantable cardioverter-defibrillator: is early implantation cost-effective? J Am Coll Cardiol 1990; 16:1258–1263.
22. Kuppermann M, Luce BR, McGovern B, Podrid PJ, Bigger JT, Ruskin JN. An analysis of the cost effectiveness of the implantable defibrillator. Circulation 1990; 81:91–100.
23. Larsen GC, Manolis AS, Sonnenberg FA, Beshansky JR, Estes NAM, Pauker SG. Cost-effectiveness of the implantable cardioverter-defibrillator: effect of improved battery life and comparison with amiodarone therapy. J Am Coll Cardiol 1992; 19:1323–1334.
24. O'Brien B, Buxton M, Rushby J. Cost effectiveness of the implantable cardioverter defibrillator: a preliminary analysis. Br Heart J 1992; 68:241–245.
25. Farre J, Fraile J, Martinell J, Artiz V, Rabago G. The automatic implantable cardioverter defibrillator: limitations of the newest devices. PACE 1992; 15(III):659–664.

38

The Telectronics Guardian 4202/4203

Paul J. Wang

*Tufts University School of Medicine
and New England Medical Center
Boston, Massachusetts*

I. GENERAL CHARACTERISTICS

The Telectronics Guardian 4202/4203 is a multiprogrammable telemetric implantable defibrillator with bradycardia VVI pacing capability [1,2]. The device is rectangular in shape, with dimensions 120 × 80 × 20 mm. It weighs 270 gms and has a volume of 176 mL. Its radiographic code is TAJ(4202) or TPW(4203). The Guardian 4202 and 4203 both accept 3.2-mm in-line bipolar leads with a short terminal pin for rate sensing/pacing. The header has sealing rings. The Guardian 4202 accepts 6-mm patches. CPI patch (5.75 mm) terminals require an adapter to extend the terminal pin (e.g., Telectronics 040-045 adapter). An upsizing adaptor (e.g., Telectronics 040-054 adaptor may be used to adapt Telectronics patches to the Guardian 4202. The Guardian 4203 accepts 3.2-mm HV-1 patches. Telectronics patches or other HV-1 patches fit the Guardian 4203 without adapters. Six-millimeter (CPI) patches may be made to fit the Guardian 4203 by using Telectronics Adaptor #040-047.

II. ENGINEERING ASPECTS OF DESIGN

A. Battery Source

The defibrillator has a lithium/silver-vanadium pentoxide battery (WGL 8512, made by Wilson Greatbatch, Ltd., Clarence, NY) with a theoretical capacity of 5.6 A-h (ampere-hours). The bradycardia pacemaker component is lithium iodine (WGL 7905) with a theoretical capacity of 1.7 A-h. The lithium-iodine cell also powers the telemetry, pacer, and defib control integrated circuits.

The device has the capacity to delivery approximately 250 maximum energy defibrillation shocks to the patient at the time of implantation. The average generator life is estimated to be between 3 and 5 years.

B. Logic Circuitry

The defibrillation control integrated circuits which perform VT/VF detection and control therapy are interfaced with the telemetry and pacer integrated circuits. They also interface with the telemetry integrated circuit and the pacer integrated circuit.

III. PROGRAMMABLE FEATURES AND DEVICE FUNCTION
A. Sensitivity

Guardian 4202/4203 sensitivity values apply to both bradycardia pacing and tachycardia detection. They range from 0.7 ± 0.3 mV to 4.5 mV. The device does not have an "automatic gain" sensing function, and sensing does not change with arrhythmia confirmation.

B. Pulse amplitude

Pulse amplitude is available in only two voltages, 2.5 and 5.0 V. There is no increase in pacing voltage following defibrillation.

C. Pulse Width

There are only four programmable pulse widths. There is no pulse width above 1.0 ms. The maximum output, which is 1.0 ms at 5.0 V, may result in failure to capture if the thresholds become high, particularly with epicardial lead systems (see Section VII). When the end-of-life (EOL) indicator for the pacemaker cell has been exceeded, the pulse width will automatically increase to 1.5 ms, compensating for the reduced pulse amplitude.

D. Standby Rate

The maximum standby rate is 105 beats/min. However, standby rates are affected by the tachycardia detection interval which has been selected. Only by turning tachycardia detection off may one achieve, for example, pacing at 105 beats/min. The standby rate will be reduced by 20% when the pacemaker cell EOL has been reached.

E. Refractory Period

The refractory period is used only for bradycardia pacing and may be programmed to 250 or 312 ms.

F. Magnet Operation

The proper positioning of the magnet is in the lower right-hand corner. The maximum effective range of the doughnut magnet in this position is 8.0 cm above the device.
   When a magnet is applied, both bradycardia support and defibrillation are disabled as long as the magnet is held in place. Therefore, magnet application to temporarily disable the defibrillator function should not be used in the pacemaker-dependent patient unless an adequate escape rhythm is present. Application of the magnet immediately disables both of these functions. If a magnet is applied during charging and held in place for at least 30 s, the discharge will be diverted to an internal load or "dumped." If the magnet is applied during charging but removed prematurely, before the end of the charging sequence, a shock may still be delivered to the patient if the tachycardia is reconfirmed at the reconfirmation points in the charging sequence.

G. EMI Detection Criteria

The EMI detection window spans from 44 ms after a sensed event (the end of the absolute refractory period) to 76 ms after a sensed event. Sensed events during this window are considered to be the result of electromagnetic interference. When EMI has been detected, the Guardian will revert to VOO pacing at the programmed standby rate.

H. Detection and Recognition Algorithm

The Guardian 4202/4203 device uses a rate-only system. If the sensed events occur for the programmed number of intervals at a cycle length shorter than the tachycardia detection interval but longer than 76 ms (the end of the EMI detection window), the tachycardia detection criteria are met. Either 6 out of 7 or 12 out of 14 intervals may be required to meet this criteria. For the "12 out of 14" criterion to be met, two consecutive 6-out-of-7 intervals must be met. Other criteria, such as morphology, onset detection, or tachycardia stability, are not used in this device. Use of 12-out-of-14 criteria in some cases has been helpful to minimize the number of charges and shocks for rapid supraventricular arrhythmias such as atrial fibrillation.

Tachycardia detection may be programmed ON or OFF independently of turning the system ON or OFF in the Guardian 4202/4203.

I. Reconfirmation

Reconfirmation occurs at the programmed shock delay, either 6 or 20 s, from the time of detection, and again at full charge or 30 s whichever comes first.

If sensed events are present within the tachycardia detection window for 6 out of 7 intervals, reconfirmation criteria are met. If these criteria are met at both reconfirmation points, the shock will be delivered to the patient. After delivery of this shock, charging to the next higher sequence will begin automatically. If the criteria are not met at either reconfirmation point, an internal discharge or "charge dump" will occur after charging to the programmed voltage.

J. Antitachycardia Pacing Algorithms

Antitachycardia pacing algorithms are not applicable to this device.

K. Parameters of Shock Therapy

The device synchronizes the patient shock to within 50 ms following a sensed or paced event. There are 12 programmable initial energies, which are based on delivery into a 50-Ω load. Energy incrementation during a charging sequence occurs automatically after the initial energy has been delivered and the tachycardia is reconfirmed. Energies for shocks in the series are determined by the first shock energy, and subsequent shock energies are not programmable independently. The number of shocks that can be delivered in a series ranges from 4 to 7. If the last programmed shock in a series has been delivered and the tachycardia is reconfirmed 6 s after the last shock, the defibrillation function will be turned off automatically, without affecting bradycardia pacing. The indicator "Max shocks in series" will be seen upon interrogation with a programmer. The defibrillator function must be reactivated using a programmer to turn the system on. If the tachycardia is not confirmed at 6 s after the last shock in the series, the defibrillator function will remain on.

L. Emergency Shock

A MAX shock is a 30-J shock initiated by a command from the programmer. This command will result in shock delivery even if the system is turned off. After discharge of the MAX shock, the defibrillator returns to the standby condition, but the initial energy will be 30 J. Initiation of the MAX shock can be stopped only by holding a magnet over the device for at least 30 s.

M. Replacement Indicator for Pacing and Defibrillator Energy Sources

The pacer cell impedance measurement is obtained by selecting "Tests" using the 9600 or 4810 programmer. At the beginning of life, pacer cell impedance is less than 5 kΩ. When a pacer cell impedance of 21 kΩ has been reached, the end-of-life indicator is present. When the end-of-life indicator of the pacer cell has been exceeded, nominally at 35 kΩ, the standby rate will increase by 20% of the programmed rate and the pulse width will increase to 1.5 ms.

Defibrillator capacitor charge time is used to determine the end-of-life indicator. The charge time is performed by using a DEFIB test. This charges the capacitor to 650 V and dumps the energy internally. The first defib test is used to reform the capacitors. A second defib test may be performed immediately after the first defib test to determine the end-of-life indicator. When the second charge time is greater than or equal to 23.5 s, there are no more than 25 shocks and generator replacement should be scheduled. When three successive defib tests have charged time equal to 30 s, immediate generator replacement is recommended since the output of the device could be potentially significantly decreased.

N. Sensing System

This device uses a programmable sensitivity system. The sensitivity is independent of the magnitude of the sensed electrogram and does not change once initial detection criteria have been met. The maximum programmable sensitivity is 0.7 mV. Double sensing of the leading and trailing edge of the ventricular activation may occur, particularly at more sensitive settings. Undersensing of ventricular fibrillation with a low-amplitude ventricular electrogram signal may be possible. Clinical observations regarding sensing are discussed in Section VII.

O. Defibrillation Waveform

The defibrillator waveform used by the device is a monophasic truncated exponential. The leading edge in voltage and pulse width is altered with changes in the programmed shock energy. The measured energy delivered by the 30-J programmed energy will be listed on the test certificate accompanying each device. Sequential shocks and biphasic energy waveforms are not available with this device.

IV. IMPLANTATION AND INTRAOPERATIVE TESTING

A. Implantation

No new Guardian 4202/4203 defibrillators are currently being implanted. The procedure for implantation is as follows. Two defibrillation tests are performed. Typically, the first and second charge times are 18 and 12 s. Both the Guardian 4202 and 4203 have a 3.2-mm bipolar in-line connection for sensing and pacing leads. If two 5-mm unipolar myocardial leads are used, the adapter (for example, Telectronics 030-308) may be used to fit the 3.2-mm in-line connection. The set screws on the adapter and on the Guardian must be tightened. It should be noted that the 030-308 adapter does not have sealing rings, but sealing rings are present in the 4202 and 4203 headers. The Guardian 4202 header has 6-mm terminals for the patches. However, in order to accept standard 6-mm or 5.75-mm patches (e.g., CPI patches), an adapter (e.g., Telectronics 040-045) must be used to extend the pin length. The set screw on this adapter must be tightened securely. When looking down the barrel of the defibrillator facing the patch openings, the negative terminal is on the left and the positive terminal is on the right.

B. Intraoperative Testing

Using the 4510 implant support device (ISD), one can obtain marker channels using a standard EKG or a physiologic recorder. From the ISD one can continuously display the marker channel and the intracardiac electrogram as obtained from the pacing/sensing leads. With the 4510 implant support device one can obtain the pacing threshold and the sensed R-wave amplitude. By using the fibrillator cables, one can induce ventricular fibrillation and then deliver the appropriate energies for DFT testing. Using amplifiers that are similar to the implanted device, the marker channel can be used to determine whether sensing is appropriate at different programmed sensitivities.

Once the Guardian 4202 or 4203 has been attached to the pacing/sensing leads and the patches, the device may be tested. The simplest method of testing the device is first to turn the system off. Next, arrhythmia is induced either by rapid ventricular pacing or AC current. While the system is off during the induction period, the device is blinded. When the desired arrhythmia has been successfully induced, one turns the system back on, unblinding the device, Diversion of a shock may be accomplished by placing a magnet on the device for at least 30 s or by quickly turning the system off.

V. TELEMETRY, DATA STORAGE, AND NONINVASIVE TESTING

A. Telemetry

Real-time marker channels as well as the intracardiac electrogram may be telemetered using the 9600 or 4810 programmer. In addition, the pacer cell impedance may be measured and telemetered. The lead impedance may be measured and telemetered (see Section V. C). The patch impedance cannot be measured or telemetered in the Guardian 4202/4203. Data storage electrograms or R-R intervals are not stored by this device.

B. Event Counters

Three separate event counters are available in the Guardian 4202/4203:

1. Patient shock count is the number of shocks which have been delivered to the patient. This number includes shocks delivered through automatic device function and shocks delivered manually. The maximum counter value is 255, after which there will be no change to this counter.
2. Total shock count is the sum of the number of shocks which have been delivered to the patient, added to the number of dump discharges including the capacitor charge-time defib test. The dump discharge counter is not displayed directly using the programmer. There-

fore the total shock count may not be accurate if either the patient shock counter or the number of dump discharges has exceeded 255.
3. The defib activation count gives the number of charging sequences which have been initiated. These include automatic charge sequences, manual shocks, maximum shocks, and defib tests which have been initiated. When this counter reaches 255, the value will return to 0 until programming of any bradycardia parameter occurs. Thus, a defibrillation activation count of 0 indicates that the maximum count was reached. For example, when a tachycardia is detected resulting in device charging and is converted by the first shock delivered to the patient, the defib activation count will be advanced by 1 while the total shock count will be advanced by 2, since one shock will be delivered to the patient and the second charge will be dumped.

In the Guardian 4202/4203, the shock energy is not recorded, and the time of last shock is not recorded.

C. Noninvasive Testing

Several tests may be performed using the device programmer. Lead threshold testing results in 16 paced events at full amplitude at 85 to 100 pulses/min, depending on the pacer cell impedance, and then 16 paced events of decaying amplitude at 120 pulses/min. During this period the test can be stopped by using any key on the 4810 programmer and by using the "stop test" key on the 9600 programmer. The 9600 or 4810 programmer displays the amplitudes of each decaying pulse. The pacing threshold is determined by the amplitude of the last pacing pulse before loss of capture as seen on the surface ECG. During lead threshold testing, the system is automatically turned to OFF and will automatically be turned ON after completion of testing. Therefore, if the patient develops a tachycardia during threshold testing, the arrhythmia will not be sensed. The pacer cell test can also be used to determine the impedance of the pacer cell.

Programmed stimulation cannot be performed using this device, either directly through the device or using a VVT pacing mode.

VI. TROUBLESHOOTING

Undersensing may be detected by using the marker channel during intraoperative testing or device testing. Reprogramming the defibrillator to a more sensitive setting typically eliminates undersensing. However, occasionally a revision of the lead system may be necessary (see Section VII). In all cases, careful documentation of appropriate sensing is mandatory for accurate rhythm detection and patient safety.

Nonsustained arrhythmias are the most frequent cause of frequent dump discharges. Device interrogation at regular intervals and after patient shocks are important in detecting multiple dump discharges due to spontaneous tachycardia termination after detection and charging have occurred. As discussed in Section VII, these frequent dump discharges may use substantial amounts of generator energy and have even resulted in energy depletion. Documentation of the rhythm resulting in these spontaneous reversions is critical. Since the Guardian 4202/4203 does not have data log episode recording capability, ambulatory or loop monitoring or telemetry are the only methods for rhythm classification. Atrial fibrillation, for example, will be treated differently from nonsustained ventricular tachycardia. In addition, the programming of the 12-out-of-14 detection criterion may decrease the detection of many episodes of atrial fibrillation and short runs of nonsustained ventricular tachycardia.

Troubleshooting Failure to Capture

Threshold testing is the initial step in assessing failure to capture. Using the telemetered lead impedance, one may be able to identify problems of a lead fracture or insulation break. Because the maximal pacing output is 5 V at 1.0 ms, in some cases capture may not be attainable if the pacing threshold is elevated.

VII. CLINICAL STUDIES
A. Demographics

A total of 547 Guardian 4202/4203 implants were performed worldwide. [3]. These represented 322 Guardian 4202 and 255 Guardian 4203 implants. The primary indications for defibrillator implantation was ventricular tachycardia (44%), ventricular tachycardia/ventricular fibrillation (28%), ventricular fibrillation (22%), and cardiac arrest (6%). Coronary artery disease was present in 78% of patients. The mean left ventricular ejection fraction was 34%. The mean age was 62 years.

B. Tachyarrhythmia Detection and Therapy Delivery

In the 547 Guardian 4202/4203 implants, there have been a total of 16,473 device activations or charges. Therapy was delivered in only 12% of these episodes, with the remaining 88% of episodes representing spontaneous reversions without therapy delivery. These data suggest that reconfirmation in a noncommitted device may significantly decrease the frequency of shock delivery.

C. Sensing

In chronic follow-up electrophysiological studies, in seven patients undersensing of induced ventricular tachyarrhythmias resulted in delay or failure of therapy delivery. In three of these patients the devices were explanted. In two patients the devices were reprogrammed; one patient had an endocardial sensing lead implanted, and in the remaining patient subsequent testing demonstrated appropriate sensing. In chronic EPS, 5% of patients programmed to 0.7 mV sensitivity had undersensing noted [3].

Wilbur et al. [4] reported that undersensing at 1.0 mV or greater programmed sensitivity during induced sustained ventricular arrhythmias was identified in 20 of 205 (10%) of patients at implant. Reprogramming or lead repositioning resulted in normal sensing in all patients. None of these patients had undersensing resulting in failure of shock delivery. During prior-to-discharge testing in 159 patients, undersensing of induced sustained ventricular arrhythmias at programmed sensitivity values of 1.0 mV or greater was identified in 23 (14%) of patients. Two of the five patients with undersensing at 0.7 mV sensitivity had at least one episode of failure of shock therapy due to undersensing. A total of three patients required lead revision because of undersensing. At 4-month follow-up testing in 105 patients, undersensing at programmed sensitivity values of 1.0 mV or greater was seen in 11 (10%) patients. Of the seven patients with undersensing at 1.0 mV sensitivity, three had undersensing resulting in failure of shock delivery. All patients had resolution of undersensing with reprogramming. In three out of four patients with undersensing at 0.7 mV, failure to delivery shock therapy was observed, requiring lead revision in one patient and device explanation in two patients. All of the episodes of failure of shock delivery were due to failure to reconfirm rather than failure of initial detection. After the 4-month follow-up, 48 of 130 patients (37%) were programmed at 0.7 mV. No deaths attributed to sensing failure have been reported.

Oversensing resulting in an inappropriate shock has been observed in five patients.

D. Device Function and Complications

Lead-related observations were common. Twenty-seven patients displayed loss of capture. Lead or adaptor fracture was seen in seven patients. Undersensing and oversensing have been reported (see Section VII. C). Premature end of generator life was reported in four patients, and loss of telemetry occurred in two patients. Dump discharges due to nonsustained arrhythmias were also a cause of generator energy depletion [5].

Device explants have been performed in 82 patients. Reasons for explant included infection (18 patients), replacement with ATP device (8 patients), increased defibrillation threshold (8 patients), end of generator life (7 patients), increased counters/charge times (6 patients), lead problems (5 patients), adaptor failures (4 patients), heart transplants (2 patients), loss of telemetry function (2 patients), leak in header (1 patient), pocket erosion (1 patient), and other causes (17 patients). Three of these explants were due to undersensing (see Section VII. C).

E. Morbidity and Mortality

As of June 30, 1992, a total of 95 deaths had been reported in the 547 implants. These deaths were classified as sudden cardiac death (25 patients), nonsudden cardiac death (51 patients), and noncardiac death (19 patients). The actuarial survival using Kaplan-Meier analysis revealed a sudden-cardiac-death survival of 96.2%, 93.9%, and 93.9% at 1, 2, and 3 years, respectively. The total cardiac-death survival was 87.6%, 83.6%, and 82.5%, at 1, 2, and 3 years, respectively. The total overall survival was 85.0%, 79.7%, and 78.6% at 1, 2, and 3 years, respectively. The perioperative mortality was 3.6% (19 deaths).

VIII. SUMMARY

The Guardian 4202/4203 is an implantable defibrillator with bradycardia pacing capabilities. Arrhythmia reconfirmation combined with the 12-out-of-14 detection algorithm during nonsustained arrhythmias including atrial fibrillation may decrease patient shock frequency. Interrogation of counters after shocks is advisable to identify frequent device dump discharges. Clinically significant undersensing has been observed in clinical studies in a small percentage of patients. Careful documentation of appropriate sensing is critical for accurate rhythm detection and safety.

REFERENCES

1. Telectronics Pacing Systems, Inc. Guardian 4202 Implantable Cardioverter Defibrillator System. Physician Manual.
2. Telectronics Pacing Systems, Inc. Guardian 4203 Implantable Cardioverter Defibrillator System. Physician Manual.
3. Telectronics Pacing Systems, Inc. Guardian 4202/4203 implantable cardioverter defibrillator system. Clinical Study Annual Report, 1992.
4. Wilber D, Poczobutt-Johanos M, and Guardian Clinical Investigators. PACE 1991; 14:624.
5. Telectronics Pacing Systems, Inc. Guardian 4202/4203 PMA submission to FDA, 1991.

39

The Medtronic PCD Pacemaker Cardioverter-Defibrillator

Raymond Yee and George J. Klein

University of Western Ontario
and University Hospital
London, Ontario, Canada

Kevin Wolfe

University of Manitoba
and Health Sciences Centre
Winnepeg, Manitoba, Canada

I. INTRODUCTION

The pacemaker cardioverter defibrillator (PCD, Medtronic, Inc., Minneapolis, MN) is a fully programmable antitachycardia management device designed to deliver comprehensive, tiered therapy to patients with malignant ventricular arrhythmias. Following initial evaluation of a prototype (PCD model 7215) in a limited number of patients in 1985 [1], two models (PCD 7216A and 7217B) began large-scale clinical studies in 1989. Each successive model has differed slightly from its immediate predecessor in small ways while maintaining the same fundamental principles and features of operation (Table 1). This report outlines the hardware and software features of this device and presents data related to clinical experience with this device.

II. PACEMAKER CARDIOVERTER DEFIBRILLATOR (PCD) SYSTEM FEATURES

The PCD system consists of an implantable generator and lead system, the radiofrequency programmer and printer, and a separate external cardioverter defibrillator unit for intraoperative testing of the lead system prior to device implantation. The PCD device is designed to recognize two zones of tachycardia: a slower tachycardia zone designated as ventricular tachycardia (VT), and a rapid tachycardia or ventricular fibrillation (VF) zone (Table 2). The device is capable of delivering tiered therapy for ventricular tachycardia (antitachycardia pacing or cardioversion shocks), committed defibrillation shocks, and bradycardia pacing. Bidirectional telemetry permits flexible programming of the device parameters and retrieval of stored information. The marker channel is particularly helpful in evaluating the device's function and is operational while the radiofrequency programmer head is applied only. The present model does not store electrograms or marker channel information of spontaneous events. The device

Table 1 Models of the PCD

	7215	7216A	7217B
Available	1987	1989	1989
Mass (g)	180	281	197
Volume (mL)	112	209	113
Maximum shock energy (J)	15	34	34
Pace/sense configuration	Integrated bipolar	Integrated/true bipolar	Integrated/true bipolar
Leads	Epicardial	Epicardial and nonthoracotomy leads	

can also function as a programmable stimulator, delivering up to three ventricular extrastimuli or rapid autodecremental ventricular pacing to a minimum cycle length of 100 ms.

A. The PCD Generator

The PCD housing is constructed of titanium, and the device is powered by a twin-cell lithium silver vanadium oxide battery. The current PCD 7217B (Table 1) is roughly equivalent in mass and displacement volume to the prototype model (model 7215), even though the maximum energy output is more than double that of the prototype.

The development of the Medtronic model 7217 PCD implantable defibrillator presented numerous technical challenges. Although the device included pacemaker features which had previously been developed and miniaturized for bradycardia pacemakers, the designs of the implantable defibrillator circuitry and power source were highly influenced by the required flexibility of the tachyarrhythmia detection algorithms and the high-voltage aspects of the device.

The PCD circuitry uses a combination of various microelectronic technologies, including digital and linear CMOS (complementary metal oxide semiconductor) and linear bipolar inte-

Table 2 PCD Device Features

Full programmability
Two zones of tachycardia detection and therapy: VT and VF
Tiered antitachycardia therapy: up to 4 therapies per VT or VF episode
   VT: Antitachycardia pacing sequences: autodecremental "ramp" or burst modalities
      Up to 15 pacing sequences per therapy
      Cardioversion 0.2–34 J by single, simultaneous, or sequential methods
      Uncommitted
   VF: Programmable defibrillation energy 0.2–34 J
      Single-pathway, bidirectional simultaneous, or sequential methods
      Committed
Bradycardia Pacing   Demand pacing at 30–80 beats/min
                           Cannot be disabled
Diagnostic facilities
  Marker channel and ventricular electrogram: on-line transmission
  Memory storage: Battery voltage, charge circuit status, last charge time, all programmed settings
                  Last therapy data: RR intervals prior to and after therapy, result
                  Cumulative VT and VF episode and therapy result counters

grated circuits to optimize the performance of the device while maintaining a low battery drain during normal conditions. The circuitry uses a combination of multilayer co-fired ceramic and printed circuit board substrates.

The circuitry has been selected to provide the tachyarrhythmia functions associated with detection, therapy delivery, and data recording. The primary circuitry that controls these operations, which are generally more mathematically intensive than are typical for bradycardia pacemakers, is a custom microprocessor. This integrated circuit implements the features based on the embedded software (firmware), designed specifically for this device. The microprocessor responds to each sensed or paced cardiac event with an analysis of the present cardiac rhythm and then establishes the operation of the device until the time of the next sensed or paced event. The microprocessor, in essence, acts to change the operation of the device on a beat-to-beat basis, much the same as an external programmer might be envisioned to change the operation of a pacemaker if it could be accomplished during each cardiac cycle.

The high-voltage PCD circuitry consists of a charging circuit, high-voltage energy storage capacitors, and high-voltage semiconductor switches. The charging circuit is used to transfer the energy from the device battery onto the high-voltage output capacitors. This circuit uses a miniature "flyback" transformer that is switched at high frequency to convert the low voltage on the battery (approximately 5 V) to a potential greater than 750 V stored on the high-voltage energy storage capacitors.

The energy storage capacitors are constrained by the small volume of the device yet need to store a large amount of energy. The PCD capacitors use an aluminum electrolytic technology and have major advantages over other technologies in terms of volume (energy density) and mass. The primary disadvantage is the tendency for these capacitors to exhibit higher leakage current if the capacitor is not used for long periods (deformation). This tendency is the result of microscopic "cracks" in the dielectric material, which may occur when the capacitors have not been charged for long periods of time. This leakage current affects the charge time for a device, similar to trying to fill a leaky bucket with water. Fortunately, the dielectric is regrown (reformed) by applying a voltage for a short time, and the impact on the charge time for repeated charging cycles is minimal.

The high-voltage switches connect the energy storage capacitors to the defibrillation electrodes. Each switch consists of a number of power transistors to provide added protection from inappropriate electrical current, which may otherwise come from the device. The primary switching elements include both insulated gate bipolar transistors (IGBTs) and triacs.

The single battery used in the PCD provides both the low current for the control circuitry and the high current (power) for charging the high-voltage energy storage capacitors. The battery consists of two lithium/silver vanadium oxide cells (model 8830, manufactured by Wilson Greatbatch, Ltd.) with a stoichiometric capacity of 2.2 A-h. The chemistry was particularly suited to meeting both the low- and high-current requirements of the device because of (1) the relatively high energy density needed to meet the device size constraints, (2) the low self-discharge rate, and (3) the ability to respond quickly to charging after being under a low current condition for long periods of time. The chemical reactions of this battery result in a voltage discharge curve which exhibits plateaus at various voltages and a decline in the voltage through the device's life. This decline in the battery voltage provides an added benefit of allowing a gross assessment of the remaining capacity of the battery. At implantation battery voltage is 6.4 V and gradually declines as battery power is consumed. When the battery voltage reaches 5.11 V (model 7216A) or 4.97 V (model 7217B), elective replacement is indicated. Potential loss of function indicators include a battery voltage of $\leq$4.91 V (model 7216A) or $\leq$4.74 V (model 7217B). The time from elective replacement indicators to imminent device failure is estimated to be at least 4 months, based on: (1) 100% pacing at 65 beats/min, (2) 5.4-V pulse amplitude, (3) 0.49-ms pulse width, (4) 500 Ω pacing load, and (5) two 34-J capacitor charging periods per month.

Capacitor charge time to the maximum device output of 34 J requires approximately 6 s and increases gradually as battery voltage depletes, typically to less than 25 s by the time of elective generator replacement. If charging is not completed within 35 s, the device aborts the charge, reconfirms the VT and VF, and attempts to charge the capacitors again. After three consecutive unsuccessful charging attempts, the device automatically disables all VT and VF detections and therapies as well as any manually initiated shock therapies until they are manually reprogrammed.

B. Epicardial and Nonthoracotomy Lead System

Contact with the heart is provided by a set of epicardial or nonthoracotomy leads (Fig. 1). Epicardial defibrillation patch electrodes consist of helical coiled platinum alloy conductor wire in a spiral configuration embedded in a silicone insulation backing. To accommodate variations in heart size, epicardial electrodes are available in three sizes with total surface areas ranging from 54.7 to 67 cm^2. Sensing and pacing are provided by one or two screw-in intramyocardial electrodes. In early devices, an "integrated" bipolar pacing and sensing configuration was utilized. A single screw-in electrode and the cathodal defibrillation patch electrode was the electrode pair. The PCD 7217B incorporates "true" bipolar electrogram sensing between two screw-in electrodes, while pacing is still performed using the integrated bipolar configuration.

In 1989, a nonthoracotomy lead system was introduced to reduce the risks that accompany the implantation of epicardial leads [2]. Components of this nonthoracotomy lead system include transvenous leads for placement in the superior vena cava, right ventricular apex, or cor-

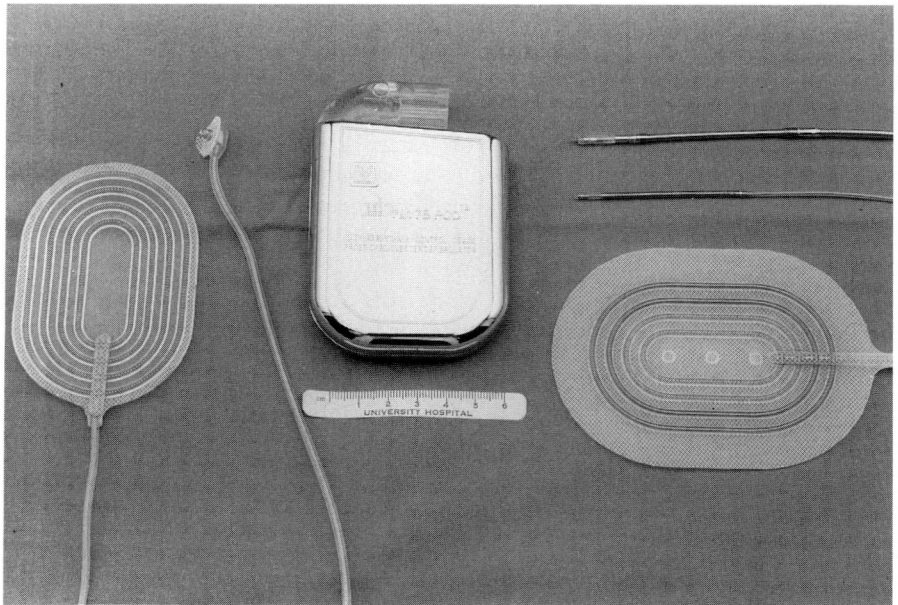

Figure 1 The PCD 7217 device system is shown with the generator (center) flanked by epicardial patch and screw-in leads (left) and nonthoracotomy leads (right).

onary sinus, and an alternative subcutaneous patch electrode for implantation in the left chest wall. The right ventricular lead is a 10.5-Fr tripolar electrode catheter with active fixation using a screw-in electrode and a 5-cm (surface area 4.48 cm^2) defibrillation coil. Initially, these two electrodes served as the integrated bipolar pacing and sensing pair. Subsequently, a separate distal ring electrode was inserted 5 mm from the screw-in electrode for true bipolar sensing. The 8-Fr unipolar defibrillation lead with a defibrillation coil electrode surface area of 3.61 cm^2 is positioned in the superior vena cava or coronary sinus.

C. Device Features

The PCD device provides automatic electrical therapy for bradycardias or tachycardias, with detection based on cycle length or rate-related criteria only. In addition to the bradycardia zone, there are two nonoverlapping tachycardia zones: a slower tachycardia or VT zone, and a rapid tachycardia or VF zone. Each of these zones is independently programmable and can be individually enabled or disabled.

The device utilizes a feature called an auto-adjusting sensitivity threshold system to detect the local ventricular electrogram while rejecting other low-amplitude signals. Otherwise, T-wave and far-field P-wave activity might be detected as a result of the high sensitivity settings used to ensure detection of potentially low-amplitude electrograms during ventricular fibrillation. Sensitivity threshold is programmable from 0.3 to 2.4 mV in increments of 0.3 mV (Table 3). An electrogram signal exceeding this threshold setting temporarily raises the sensing level to 75% of the electrogram's amplitude (or six times the program setting, whichever is less). This sensitivity level then decays exponentially with a time constant of 560 ms, approaching the programmed sensitivity threshold setting. The net effect is similar to the auto-adjusting gain mechanism employed by other ICDs.

Blanking periods are nonprogrammable and follow both paced and sensed events (Table 4). These prevent multiple sensing of a single electrical event or electrical noise, whether it be generated by the device during pacing or capacitor charging, external noise, or that related to lead fracture. Certain refractory periods are nonprogrammable, while others may be programmed to further reject inappropriate detection of electrical signals. Electrical events sensed within the blanking period are simply ignored by the device, whereas events detected within the various refractory period windows do reset the device event timer. Noise detected during bradycardia pacing does not revert the device to an asynchronous ventricular pacing mode (VOO).

1. TACHYCARDIA DETECTION ALGORITHM

Ventricular tachycardia detection is based on four available criteria, two of which are mandatory and the other two are optional (Table 3 and 5). The cycle length of the tachycardia must be less than the programmed tachycardia detection interval, or TDI, but greater than the interval for ventricular fibrillation detection (FDI). The number of consecutive intervals that are less than the TDI (number of intervals for detection or NID) must also be satisfied before a VT is detected. The TDI is programmable from 600 to 250 ms in increments of 10–20 ms, while the NID ranges from 6 to 30 consecutive beats in increments of 6 beats. To distinguish sinus tachycardia or other tachycardias characterized by gradual acceleration from VT, an onset criterion is available. If this is activated, a tachycardia must start abruptly with shortening of the cycle length by the programmed percentage of the averaged previous four intervals.

The interval stability criterion places further restrictions on fulfillment of VT detection and is intended to distinguish atrial fibrillation from ventricular tachycardia. When it is activated,

Table 3 Programmable Device Parameters

Functions	Capability	Increments
Pace/sense		
Mode	VVI	
Rate	30–90	2.0 beats/min
pulse width	0.03–1.59 ms	0.03 ms
Sensitivity	0.3–2.4 mV	0.3 mV
Amplitude	2.8/5.4 V	
Refractory period after pace	320–480 ms	40 ms
VT detection		
Enable	On/off	
Detection interval	280–600 ms	10 ms
No. of intervals to detect (NID)	4–52 (4–128, model 7216A)	4
Onset criteria	56–97%	3%
Interval stability	30–130 ms 10–150, 7216A	10 ms
VF detection		
Enable	On/off	
Detection interval	240–400	10 ms
NID	6–30	6
VT therapy (0–4)		
Enable	On/off	
Burst/ramp		
No. of S1 pulses	1–15	1
S1–S1 interval	50–97%	3%
No. of sequences	1–15	1
Decrement per:		
Sequence (burst)	0–40 ms	10 ms
Pulse (ramp)	0–40 ms (0–70, 7216A)	10 ms
Min. interval	150–300 ms (150–400, 7216A)	10 ms

it requires that the difference between the current interval and the average of the three immediately preceding RR intervals be equal to or less than the programmed allowed amount of variability. Any cycle length variability exceeding this programmed value resets the counter to zero, thus preventing detection.

Detection of ventricular fibrillation applies a probabilistic approach to detection, since the electrogram cycle length and amplitude may show considerable interbeat variability. A cycle

Table 4 Refractory Periods

	Blanking	Refractory
After sense	120 ms	200 ms
After pace	320 ms	320–480 ms
After charge or shock	300 ms	400 ms
VT/VF therapy	300 ms	520 ms

Table 5 Cardioversion and Defibrillation Therapy

Enable	On/off	
Current path	Single	
	Simultaneous	
	Sequential	
Pulse width	0.5–8.1 ms	0.5 ms
Energy stored	0.2–1.8 J	0.2 J
	2.0–15 J	1.0 J
	16–34 J	2.0 J

length interval called the fibrillation detection interval or FDI and the number of intervals to be counted in order to fulfill detection (NID) are programmed in a manner analogous to VT detection. The device then continuously scans a moving window encompassing 33% more intervals than are programmed for the NID. When the required number of intervals meeting the FDI criterion fall within that window, VF detection is fulfilled. For example, if the NID is programmed to 18 intervals, the device continuously evaluates a 24-beat window for 18 beats that are less than the programmed FDI. There are no other programmable criteria associated with VF detection.

In the event that a tachycardia is irregular and oscillates between the VT and VF detection zones, intervals falling within the VF detection zone do not increment the VT counter. In the uncommon event that VF detection occurs during VT detection, VF therapy intervenes. Tachycardia detection is disabled if the function is turned off, three consecutive 35-s charge intervals have failed to attain the programmed energy value, or if the PCD is used to deliver manual therapies. Detection is temporarily suspended during situations such as magnet application, delivery of therapy, capacitor charging, or if all programmed therapies are ineffective. In the latter case, detection does not resume until termination by any mechanism subsequently occurs or unless detection is actively reprogrammed on. Following a defibrillation shock, VT detection is temporarily suspended for the ensuing 64 cardiac cycles.

2. Therapies

For each detected VT or VF episode, up to four separate therapies may be programmed. Each therapy can be turned on or off, but turning a particular therapy off disables it and any following therapies (Table 5). When ventricular tachycardia has been detected, automatic therapy commences immediately after reconfirmation of the tachycardia. In the case of ventricular fibrillation, the device is committed to delivering defibrillation therapy without reconfirming that VF is ongoing. After each automatic therapy, the device evaluates the response to the therapy and considers an episode to have been successfully terminated when eight consecutive cardiac cycles after the therapy all have intervals greater than the TDI before tachycardia is redetected.

In the case of ventricular tachycardia, a single therapy may consist of one countershock attempt or up to 15 antitachycardia pacing sequences. Antitachycardia pacing is rate adaptive; that is, the cycle length of the pacing stimulus train is a function of the ventricular tachycardia cycle length. Following each delivered pacing train, the device determines whether it was effective or reconfirms the ongoing tachycardia before instituting a second rate-adaptive pacing sequence based on the newly measured tachycardia cycle length. The PCD device determines the tachycardia cycle length by averaging the last four intervals preceding VT detection, then delivers the burst sequence at the programmed percentage of the VT cycle length. The adaptive pacing percentage is programmable from 50% to 97%. The number of pulses for the first sequence, the number of sequences, and the amount of decrement between sequences and between pulses within a specific pacing train are programmable in 10-ms increments. The minimum antitachycardia pacing cycle length can be set from 150 to 300 ms.

Antitachycardia pacing is possible by adaptive burst pacing or adaptive ramp (autodecremental) pacing modalities. With a burst pacing train, the interpulse interval for any sequence is fixed. If a first pacing sequence is ineffective, one more pacing stimulus is added to each subsequent sequence and the pacing sequence cycle length is decremented by the programmed amount. For ramp pacing therapy, the interval between pacing stimuli is successively shortened by the programmed value. If the first ramp sequence is ineffective, then a pulse is added to each following pacing sequence and the entire pacing cycle length is decremented by the programmed amount.

If the ventricular tachycardia cycle length after an ineffective pacing therapy is accelerated by ≥ 60 ms compared to the cycle length of the initial VT, the device immediately advances to the next therapy. If the tachycardia cycle length is accelerated sufficiently to meet VF detection criteria, the VF detection algorithm is then invoked.

The device delivers shock of trapezoidal monophasic waveform, but the shock energy, pulse width, number of pathways, and timing of pulses is programmable. The simplest is a single-pathway shock between two defibrillation electrodes. Dual-pathway shocks are also possible using one common cathode and two anodes. The two pulses of these bidirectional shocks can be delivered simultaneously or sequentially. Actual delivered energy is dependent on pathway impedance. The percentage tilt of the pulse will be dependent on the programmed pulse width.

During capacitor charging, electrogram sensing and bradycardia pacing are suspended, marker channels and electrogram telemetry are not available, and programming is disabled. If the charging period exceeds 35 s without reaching the stored energy intended, charging is terminated. After capacitor charging, the device initiates a synchronization sequence which serves to reconfirm the presence of VT and to synchronize shock delivery. For defibrillation shocks, the device attempts to synchronize to a ventricular depolarization but is committed to delivering the shock with the first nonrefractory sensed cardiac cycle or at the end of the synchronization period (500 ms), whichever occurs first. After a VF therapy, VT detection is automatically suspended for 64 events, to avoid treatment of transient VT after a VF therapy.

There are no other special electromagnetic interference (EMI) detection criteria in either model of the Medtronic PCD. Integrated bipolar sensing in model 7216A and true bipolar sensing in model 7217B make either model relatively insensitive to the effects of electromagnetic interference. However, transthoracic and direct defibrillation, electrosurgical cautery, and strong magnetic fields all may damage circuitry, increase pacing threshold, trigger VT or VF detection, or inhibit VT and VF detection.

III. CLINICAL PERFORMANCE

A. Patient Characteristics

The PCD has been implanted in well over 1500 patients to date at over 52 centers worldwide and has been approved by regulatory agencies in several countries for clinical use. Comprehensive data concerning the clinical performance of these implanted devices have been made

Table 6 Demographic Profile of Patients Receiving a PCD

Lead system	Nonthoracotomy	Epicardial
Number of patients	317	434
Mean follow-up time	4.5 mo	11.0 mo
Number, % male	82.0%	86.2%
Mean age	58.5 yr	58.3 yr
Primary indication:		
SCD	37.9%	27.2%
VT	45.7%	53.7%
SCD + VT	16.4%	19.1%
Coronary artery disease	72.2%	74.7%
Mean ejection fraction	36.7%	34.6%
Defibrillation pathway:		
Sequential	77.4%	42.4%
Simultaneous	21.0%	1.6%
Single	1.6%	56.0%
Mean DFT	13.7 J ($N = 147$)	9.2 ($N = 264$)
Nonthoracotomy lead	DFT (J)	
RV-SVC-SQ	14.6 ($n = 84$)	
RV-CS-SQ	11.6 ($n = 48$)	
RV-CS-SVC	15.5 ($n = 15$)	

available to investigative centers for patients implanted prior to November 1991 [3]. At the time of the report, 751 patients had received PCD devices, 317 of whom were implanted with nonthoracotomy lead systems and 434 with epicardial patch electrodes (Table 6). The implantation of the devices with epicardial leads began in May 1989, while nonthoracotomy lead implantation with a PCD device began in October 1989. Despite this, the mean age of patients receiving either lead system was remarkably similar (58 years). As expected, the majority of patients were male and suffered from coronary artery disease. The mean left ventricular ejection fraction in the nonthoracotomy lead group was 37%, which is not significantly different from patients receiving the epicardial lead system.

Because the device system allows for two or three defibrillation electrodes to be connected, a variety of defibrillation lead configurations are possible. The specific choice was left to the discretion of each implanting center. More than half the patients received two epicardial patch electrodes. This was in distinct contrast to those patients receiving nonthoracotomy leads. Almost all patients in that group received a triple-electrode configuration, with the majority undergoing sequential pulse waveform defibrillation testing intraoperatively. At the time of the report was presented, results of intraoperative defibrillation testing were available for 289 patients, but defibrillation threshold was measured in only 147 patients (Table 6). Most patients had received a lead configuration consisting of RV, SVC, and subcutaneous pach electrodes. The remaining patients received a lead configuration which incorporated a coronary sinus electrode. In these 147 patients receiving nonthoracotomy leads, the mean defibrillation threshold was 13.7 J, as compared to 9.2 J in those patients receiving an epicardial lead system. These mean DFT values encompass patients who receive either two- or three-electrode configurations, and no comparative analysis of defibrillation threshold according to specific lead configuration is currently available.

In considering the results of device implantation, it is important to bear in mind the criteria governing implantation. Ventricular fibrillation must have been terminated by shocks of 18 J or less on three out of four VF episodes. However, the ultimate decision as to whether a patient received the device or not rested with the implanting physician. Ultimately, 60 patients in the nonthoracotomy lead group received a device even though the implant criteria were not met, while 44 patients of the epicardial lead population received a PCD. Reasons for failing to meet implantation criteria included failure to induce ventricular fibrillation, deteriorating hemodynamic condition of the patient, or failure to reach the defibrillation energy criteria.

B. Follow-Up Results

The mean follow-up time for the patient group receiving epicardial leads was more than twice that of the nonthoracotomy lead group, since implantation of PCD devices with epicardial lead systems started nearly 4 months before the nonthoracotomy leads were available (Table 7). In the epicardial implant group, there were 8672 spontaneous episodes of ventricular tachycardia (that is, episodes detected by the device as having met the criteria for VT detection) in 227 patients. Overall, 97.7% were treated successfully by programmed automatic VT therapy, with 91.1% being treated by antitachycardia pacing. Over 82% of patients experienced spontaneous VT episodes within the first 3 months following device implant. The choice of programmed therapy was left to the judgment of the individual physician, making comparison of relative efficacies of various VT therapies difficult. Nonetheless, autodecremental (ramp) antitachycardia pacing sequences were successful in almost 90% of episodes in which it was attempted (4814), and burst antitachycardia pacing sequences were successful on almost 84% of occasions. Of the 203 VT episodes registered by the device which failed to be terminated effectively, over half were documented to be due to inappropriate therapy for sinus tachycardia or atrial fibrillation with a rapid ventricular response. In the remaining 97 episodes involving 29 patients, reprogramming of VT therapies and/or modification of antiarrhythmic drug therapy resolved problems of device efficacy. There were no patient death resulting from ineffective VT therapy.

During this same time period, there were 1034 spontaneous episodes of tachycardia registered by the device as ventricular fibrillation in 177 patients. Sixty-nine percent of these occurred within the first 3 months following implantation. PCD successfully terminated 98.1% of these episodes, leaving 20 episodes in 11 patients in which the PCD was ineffective, despite delivering all four programmed VF therapies. Fourteen of these episodes (70%) were due to inappropriate therapy for atrial fibrillation, sinus tachycardia, or resensing of external noise as

Table 7 Resutls of Automatic Device Therapy for Spontaneous VT and VF Episodes

	Nonthoracotomy leads		Epicardial leads	
	Success/attempts	Percent efficacy	Success/attempts	Percent efficacy
VT therapy				
Ramp	1158/1245	93.0%	4329/4814	89.9%
Burst	388/426	90.9%	3392/4026	84.4%
Cardioversion	88/102	86.3%	748/884	84.6%
VF therapy	373/376	99.2%	1014/1034	98.1%
Sequential	317/320	99.1%	317/320	99.1%
Simultaneous	56/56	100.0%	56/56	100%

a result of failure to disable the device at the time of explantation of the PCD. This left six episodes (0.5%) in 4 patients wherein the PCD failed to terminate apparently true VF. In 2 patients, modification of drug therapy or reprogramming of the device resolved the problem. In the remaining 2 patients, cardiac rhythm was monitored at the time of death. In both cases, ventricular fibrillation occurred and were appropriately detected and treated by the device but were ineffective.

The experience in the nonthoracotomy lead population was similarly good. However, it is important to note that the results of therapy for spontaneous tachycardia events involve several assumptions. First, every episode is assumed to be a true episode of VT or VF. In addition, it is assumed that every VF episode is occurs de novo and is not the result of therapy for VT. The PCD counters cannot distinguish VF episodes that result from degeneration of VT secondary to antitachycardia pacing or cardioversion shocks.

The complication rate for patients receiving a PCD with an epicardial lead system has been low but involves a variety of expected problems. Pocket infection was observed in 2.5% of implants, while defibrillation patch lead fracture was observed in only 3 cases (0.7%). Fracture of a pace/sense lead was observed in only 1 patient, but loss of pacing capture occurred in 2% (8 patients). All these above-noted complications required surgical intervention to correct the problem.

In 14 patients, devices were explanted, 8 because of infection and 6 because of subsequent heart transplantation. During follow-up there were 64 patient deaths. Each death was reviewed by an independent clinical-event review committee. There were 46 cardiac-related deaths, 15 of which were sudden. Eighteen of the deaths were due to noncardiac causes. The 1-year actuarial survival for sudden cardiac death was 98.8% and for nonsudden cardiac death was 94.5% (Table 8). Perioperative mortality, defined as death within 30 days following device implantation, was 5.5%. This rate was slightly higher than previous published reports, and a contributing factor could include patient selection.

In the group of patients receiving nonthoracotomy leads, there were no sudden cardiac deaths. There were 4 nonsudden cardiac deaths, yielding a 1-year actuarial sinus survival rate of 97.9% for this patient group. The use of nonthoracotomy leads with a PCD resulted in a very low perioperative mortality rate of 0.3% as compared to 5.5% for the epicardial lead population. The device was explanted in 12 patients for reasons of infection or heart transplantation. Complications such as pocket infection and skin erosion were seen in a similar number of patients as in those receiving epicardial lead systems. However, nonthoracotomy or transvenous leads are attended by a series of unique risks. Transvenous lead dislodgment was observed in 25 patients (7.8%). In considering that many patients received more than one transvenous lead, the actual rate of lead dislodgment is considerably lower. Lead dislodgment was equally distributed among the three transvenous leads (RV, SVC, or coronary sinus). Many episodes of dislodgment were felt to be the result of tension and traction on a loosely anchored transvenous lead. Nonthoracotomy lead fracture was observed on only 2 occasions (0.6%).

Table 8 Actuarial Survival Rates in the PCD Population

	Nonthoracotomy leads	Epicardial leads
Sudden cardiac death	100%	98.8%
All cardiac death	97.9%	93.3%
Noncardiac death	99.3%	97.2%
Perioperative death rate	0.3%	5.5%

IV. CONCLUSIONS

These results involving the PCD support the fundamental principles that have driven development of this device system. First, incorporation of antitachycardia pacing into implantable cardioverter-defibrillators substantially reduces the number of shocks delivered to recipient patients while maintaining an efficacy rate comparable to the earlier AICD experience [4]. Second, the incorporation of newly developed nonthoracotomy lead systems substantially reduces the risks of PCD implantation, although defibrillation threshold is somewhat higher than is observed for epicardial electrodes. However, the efficacy of PCD therapy for spontaneous episodes of VT or VF remains high. The ultimate goal remains the implantation of a nonthoracotomy lead system with the PCD in all candidate patients so that the implant procedure becomes as simple as that for bradycardia pacemakers. No doubt, improvements in lead systems, alternative lead configuration, and defibrillation waveforms will contribute to the achievement of this goal.

REFERENCES

1. Yee R, Klein GJ, Guiraudon GM, Jones DL, Sharma AD, Norris C. Initial clinical experience with the pacemaker-cardioverter-defibrillator. Can J Cardiol 1990; 6(4):147–56.
2. Yee R, Klein GJ, Leitch JW, et al. A permanent transvenous lead system for an implantable pacemaker cardioverter-defibrillator. Nonthoracotomy approach to implantation. Circulation 1992; 85:196–204.
3. Medtronic Investigators' Interim Report. Model 7217B PCD Transvene Lead System Study Report (Draft), March 18, 1992.
4. Leitch JW, Gillis AM, Wyse G, et al. Reduction in defibrillator shocks with an implantable device combining antitachycardia pacing and shock therapy. JACC 1991; 18:145–151.

40

The VENTAK PRx Implantable Cardioverter-Defibrillator

N. A. Mark Estes III

*Tufts University School of Medicine
and New England Medical Center
Boston, Massachusetts*

I. INTRODUCTION

The CPI VENTAK PRx implantable cardioverter-defibrillators (model 1700 and 1705) are third-generation devices [1–4] with VVI bradycardia pacing capability designed to detect and terminate ventricular tachycardia and ventricular fibrillation. The devices are multimodal treatment systems, with antitachycardia pacing, low-energy cardioversion, and high-energy defibrillation shock therapy [5,6]. This chapter will provide a description of the device [6] and its features, as well as the results of its initial use in clinical investigation [5].

The nominal mechanical specifications of the model 1700 and 1705 are shown in Table 1. The VENTAK PRx device has an oval shape, weighing 220 to 230 g, with a volume of 130 to 140 cm^3. The model 1700 accepts CPI 3.2-mm morphology/defibrillating leads and 3.2-mm in-line bipolar sensing/pacing leads. By contrast, model 1705 accepts CPI 6.1-mm morphology/defibrillating leads and 4.75-mm sensing/pacing leads. The devices are otherwise functionally identical (Fig. 1). The pulse generators have an identifier that is visible on an X-ray (Fig. 2), which serves as a noninvasive confirmation of the manufacturer and model number. The serial number of the pulse generator must be determined from a patient identification card or from the programmer for the VENTAK PRx, the CPI model 2850 Prescriptor, which shows a "pulse generator status screen" when the pulse generator is initially interrogated using the model software application 2860 disk. Using the programmer and appropriate software, the VENTAK PRx pulse generator can have its detection and therapy parameters noninvasively reprogrammed. The programmer also provides access to diagnostic data stored in the memory of the device.

The VENTAK PRx is programmable to a number of detection and therapy options [5,6]. The tachyarrhythmia detection and therapy can be programmed to Off, Monitor Only, or Monitor and Therapy. When programmed Off, no tachyarrhythmia detection or therapy will occur. When programmed to Monitor Only, the device will detect and record tachyarrhythmia history in memory without therapy delivery. When programmed to Monitor and Therapy, the device

Table 1 Nominal Mechanical Specifications, PRX [6]

	Model 1700	Model 1705
Size	10.7 cm wide × 6.8 cm high × 2.4 cm deep	10.7 cm wide × 7.5 cm high × 2.4 cm deep
Volume	130 cm^3	140 cm^3
Weight	220 g	230 g
Case material	Hermetically sealed titanium	Hermetically sealed titanium
Header material	Implantation-grade polymer	Implantation-grade polymer
Power supply	Two lithium-silver vanadium pentoxide cells	Two lithium-silver vandium pentoxide cells
Morphology/defibrillating ports	Accepts CPI 3.2-mm defibrillating leads (defibrillating lead ports will not accept 3.2-mm in-line pace/sense leads)	Accepts CPI 6.1-mm defibrillating leads
Pace/sense lead port	Accepts CPI 3.2-mm in-line bipolar defibrillation sensing/pacing leads	Accepts CPI 4.75-mm sensing/pacing leads

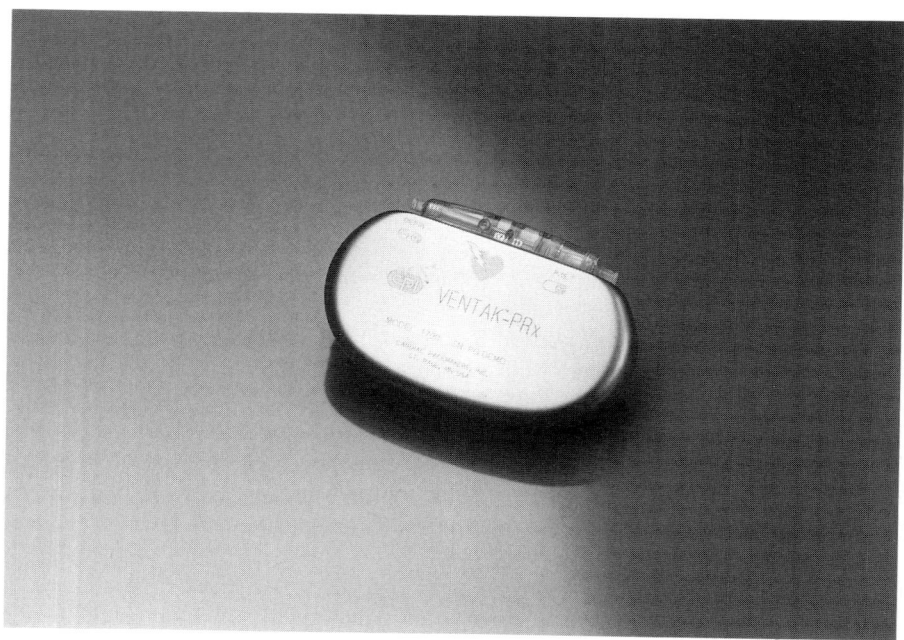

Figure 1 Photograph of the VENTAK PRx 1700 showing an oval-shaped, hermetically sealed titanium case with a polymer header. The model 1700 weighs 220 g and has a volume of 130 cm^3.

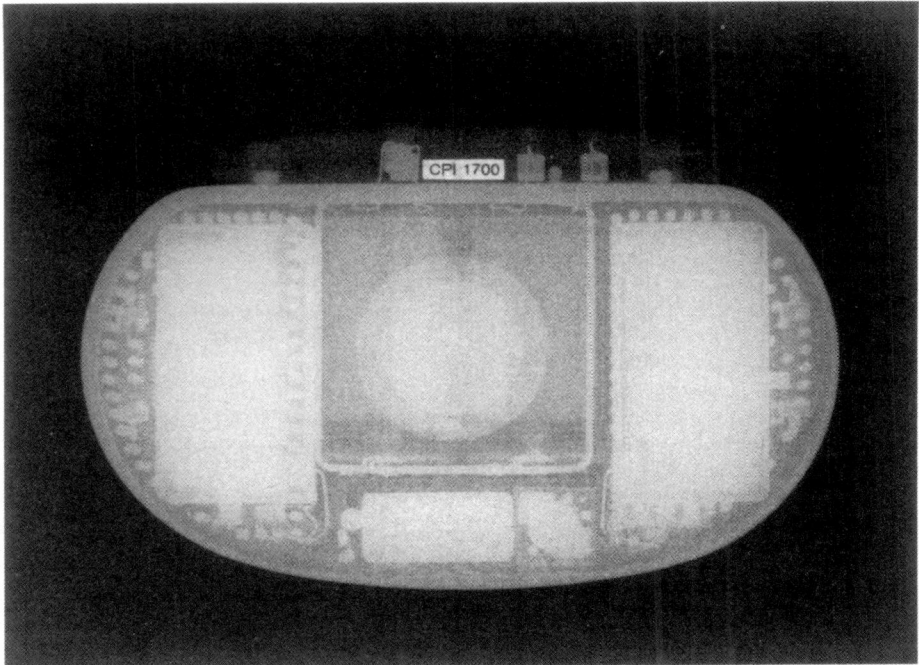

Figure 2 Radiographic appearance of the VENTAK PRx 1700 with identifier shown on the header.

will detect and respond to tachyarrhythmias. Bradycardia pacing can be programmed to Off or to VVI pacing. Postshock VVI pacing can be programmed to respond to bradyarrhythmias following shock therapy independently of the bradycardia pacing.

II. TACHYARRHYTHMIA ZONES

An essential design feature of the device includes "zone" therapy (Fig. 3). A tachyarrhythmia management zone is defined by a range of heart rates within which detection criteria and therapy have been programmed. Up to three separate tachyarrhythmia management zones can be defined. Each zone is defined by a rate threshold-independent detection criterion, and separately programmable therapy may be programmed. A representative configuration using three available tachyarrhythmia detection therapy zones, a normal rhythm zone, and a bradycardia pacing zone, is shown in Fig. 4. A minimum of one and a maximum of three zones can be set up for tachyarrhythmia detection and therapy.

III. TACHYARRHYTHMIA DETECTION

With a single zone or rate boundary, the pulse generator has only one tachyarrhythmia zone, and any sustained heart rate greater than the programmed rate criteria is treated as defined by tachyarrhythmia therapy programmed for that zone [5,6]. When two rate boundaries are programmed, the pulse generator has two zones. Any heart rate that falls between the two rate

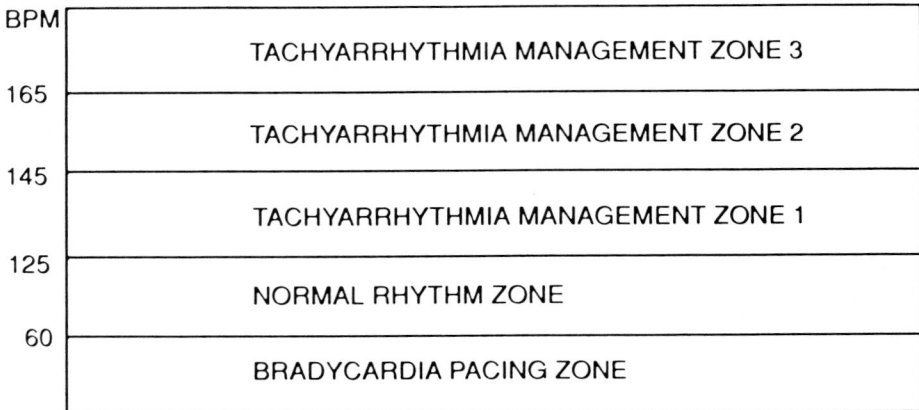

Figure 3 Tachyarrhythmia management zones are defined by the sensed heart rate. In this example, bradycardia pacing would occur for heart rates less than 60 beats/min. Heart rates of 125 to 144 beats/min would define tachyarrhythmia management zone 1; 145 to 164 beats/min zone 2; and greater than or equal to 165, zone 3. Separately programmable therapy is possible within each tachyarrhythmia management zone.

criteria is in zone 1, and if the heart rate accelerates above the higher rate criterion it enters zone 2. Similarly, when a three-zone device is configured, if the heart rate exceeds the upper limit of zone 2, tachyarrhythmia therapy is managed as defined in zone 3. In Fig. 3, zone 1 would be defined with heart rates from 125 to 144, zone 2, heart rates from 145 to 164, and zone 3, 165 beats/min or greater. The rate criteria can be programmed from 90 to 200 beats/min

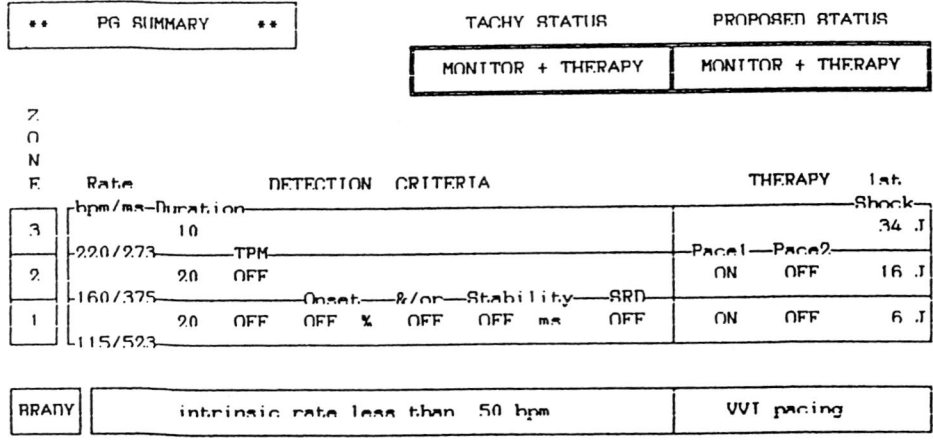

Figure 4 Pulse generator (PG) summary for a VENTAK PRx programmed for three-zone therapy. Bradycardia pacing (brady) occurs for intrinsic heart rates less than 50 beats/min in the VVI mode. Heart rates greater than 115 beats/min and less than 160 beats/min that persist for 20 cycles will be treated initially with antitachycardia pacing followed by 6-Joule shock. Tachycardias occuring at heart rate of 160 to 219 beats/min persisting for 20 cycles will be treated with antitachycardia pacing followed by a 16-Joule shock. Heart rates greater than 220 beats/min for 10 cycles will be treated with a 34-Joule shock.

by 5-beats/min increments, 210 beats/min, and 220 beats/min. The zones are contiguous and not overlapping with the minimum width of 10 beats/min. Most commonly, a rate zone is established for each tachyarrhythmia that can be treated by a separate therapy prescription. Generally, the lower rate value should be programmed at least 10 beats/min below and the upper rate value should be programmed to at least 10 beats/min above the rate of a monomorphic tachycardia to be treated in that zone.

Although rate is the primary detection criterion in defining the zones, one has the option of programming "detection enhancements" including turning-point morphology, onset, and rate stability [5,6]. When programmed On, the features apply only to the zone in which they are enabled. Additionally, sustained rate duration can be prescribed in zone 1 of a multizone configuration. When the turning-point morphology, "TPM," is programmed On, it continuously monitors the shocking lead electrogram real time and evaluates morphology by examining slew rate and evaluation of the electrogram's isoelectric time. During a 2-s segment, if the isoelectric time is less than a preset percentage of the total duration, TPM is partially satisfied. If two of three consecutive 2-s segments satisfy this percentage criterion, TPM is satisfied. TPM analysis begins only after three consecutive cardiac cycles with the rate falling above the lower limit for that zone. If a single interval occurs in the TPM zone before duration, TPM analysis will be reinitiated. TPM cannot, however, be used in zone 1 if the onset and stability are programmed On in this zone.

In an effort to separate physiological tachycardias such as sinus tachycardia, which typically accelerates slowly, from pathological tachycardias such as ventricular tachycardia, which more commonly begin abruptly, the onset feature measures the rate of transition from the normal monitored rhythm to the rapid rhythm [5,6]. The suddenness of onset of an arrhythmia is measured after the eighth fast cardiac cycle in a two-stage algorithm. Onset is programmed as a percentage of the cycle length with programmable values Off, 9 to 15%, 19 to 34%, and 38 to 50%, in 3% increments. Programming of Onset is limited to the lowest zone of a two-zone or three-zone configuration.

The stability detection feature is designed to distinguish treatable ventricular rhythms from such unstable rhythms as atrial fibrillation or frequent premature ventricular contractions, which may not be treatable by antitachycardia pacing. When the rate exceeds the lowest rate criterion for three consecutive intervals, the pulse generator classifies each interval as stable or unstable. The stability measurement is made by comparing the R–R interval with the four-interval running average. Any interval which differs from the four-beat running average by more than the programmed stability parameter is declared unstable by the algorithm. The maximum number of unstable intervals allowed before the rhythm is declared unstable is 20% of the programmed duration of the zone. Programming of stability is also limited to the lowest zone of a multizoned configuration, with programmable values of Off, 8, 16, 23, 31, 39, 47, or 55 ms.

The sustained rate duration (SRD) feature is included to allow therapy for a sustained tachycardia after a period of time beyond a preset duration when the programmed onset and/or stability criteria are not satisfied [5,6]. Thus, the SRD feature can only be programmed On when onset is programmed On, stability is programmed On, or when stability and onset are programmed On. Programmable sustained rate duration values range from 1 s to 60 min.

When rate is used as the only detection criterion, the tachyarrhythmia must be sustained for at least a programmed number of cardiac cycles or total duration before the pulse generator responds to the programmed therapy [5,6]. When the duration count is satisfied in a particular zone, if the last four intervals have occurred in that rate zone, the therapy programmed will be delivered. The average of those four intervals prior to therapy is used to determine the therapy zone and to compute the rate for adaptive antitachycardia pacing when used. Duration is programmed separately for each rate zone. Although intervals in a lower tachycardia rate zone are not counted in the higher zone, intervals in higher zones are counted in that zone and all lower zones. For example, with three programmed zones, a cycle length that falls into zone 3 increments the duration counts in zones 1, 2, and 3. Programmable values for duration are 8 to 30 cardiac cycles in 1-cycle increments, 30 to 50 cardiac cycles in 5-cycle increments, 50 to 100 cardiac cycles in 10-cycle increments, and 100 to 250 cardiac cycle in 50-cycle increments.

An acceleration measurement that is independent of zone boundaries is also included in the VENTAK PRx [5,6]. Rate acceleration is determined by comparing the four-interval average at the end of posttherapy monitoring to the 4-cycle interval average before the previous therapy. The acceleration percentage is programmable from 9 to 50%. If acceleration is met, the device will deliver 34 J next, independent of programmed therapy.

After antitachycardia pacing is attempted, rate analysis for redetection begins with the third R–R interval after termination of antitachycardia pacing and evaluates the next four consecutive R–R intervals to determine rate [5,6]. If the device detects four consecutive intervals within the same zone, it considers the therapy to have been unsuccessful and the next therapy is employed. Otherwise, posttherapy monitoring is extended one interval (up to a maximum of four intervals) and then reevaluation is done. At the end of the tenth interval, if three of four intervals fall below the lowest tachyarrhythmia rate zone boundary, the episode is considered to have been terminated successfully. If the tachyarrhythmia episode is not ended by the tenth interval, the average of these last four intervals is used to determine therapy progression. Following shock therapy, the postshock detection delay is programmable within each zone from 5 to 20 cardiac cycles in 1-cycle increments and 20 to 100 cardiac cycles in 10-cycle increments [5, 6]. Again, the device looks for four intervals in the same zone at the end of postshock detect delay. Postshock monitoring extends one interval (up to a maximum of four intervals) and then reevaluation is done. If necessary, at the end of the additional four intervals, if three of four intervals fall below the lowest tachyarrhythmia rate zone boundary, the episode is considered to have been terminated successfully. This is called a detection reset. However, if three of four intervals fall above the lowest tachyarrhythmia rate zone, the episode is considered to be persistent. As with redetection after antitachycardia pacing, the last four-interval average is used to determine whether the arrhythmia is terminated, and this average is used to decide which therapy to deliver next.

IV. TACHYARRHYTHMIA THERAPY

Within each detection zone there is independently programmable therapy that consists of antitachycardia pacing, low-energy cardioversion shocks, and high-energy defibrillating shocks [5,6]. Therapy regimens within a zone include up to two antitachycardia pacing schemes and five shocks. The antitachycardia pacing options are numerous. Burst pacing that is coupled at a percentage of the tachycardia cycle length, fixed burst, adaptive burst, scan, burst with ramp, increasing pulse count bursts, and a combination of the above are possible within each zone (Fig. 5). The shock therapy is delivered as a single truncated exponential pulse which is synchronized to detected electrical activity (Fig. 6). The maximum number of shocks per episode is five. The first two shocks are programmable, with delivered energy levels ranging from 0.10 to 34 J. The final three shocks of 34 J are nonprogrammable; only five shocks are available per one episode.

When in a single zone configuration, the device will also deliver five shocks. However, in a multizone configuration, each prescription, except in the highest zone, can be programmed

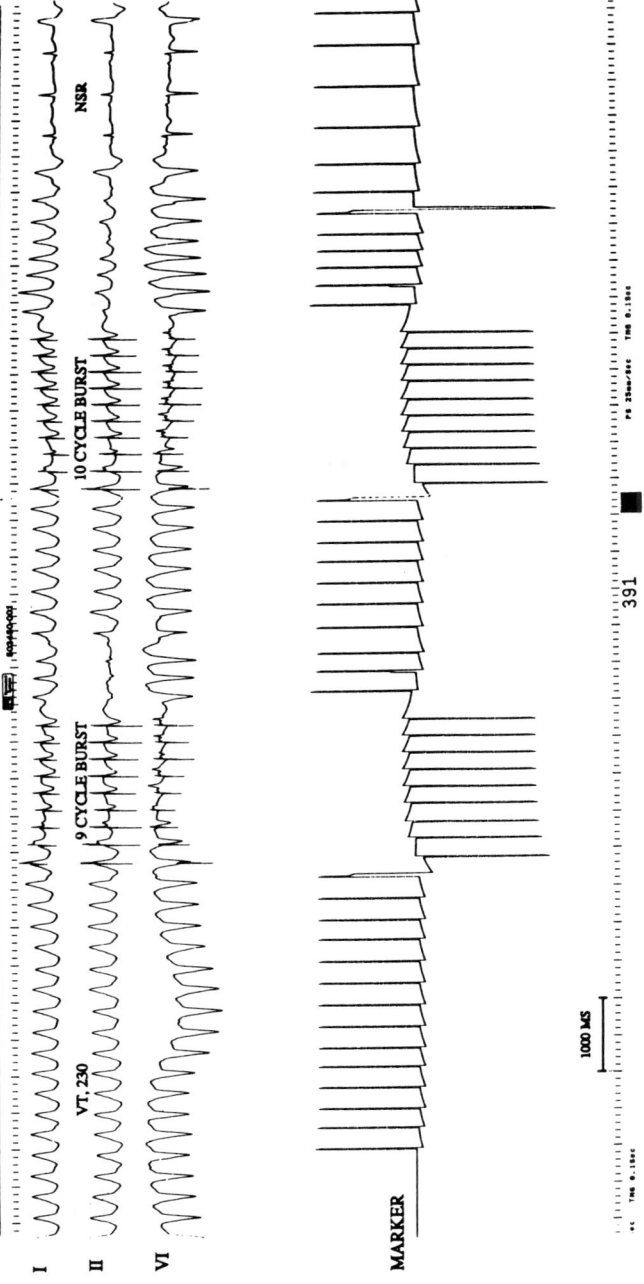

Figure 5 Tracing showing EKG leads I, II, and V1 with marker channel during sustained monomorphic left bundle ventricular tachycardia (V1) with a cycle length of 230 ms. The initial 9-cycle burst of antitachycardia pacing is not successful in terminating the VT. Immediate redetection of the tachycardia results in a 10-cycle burst followed by tachycardia termination.

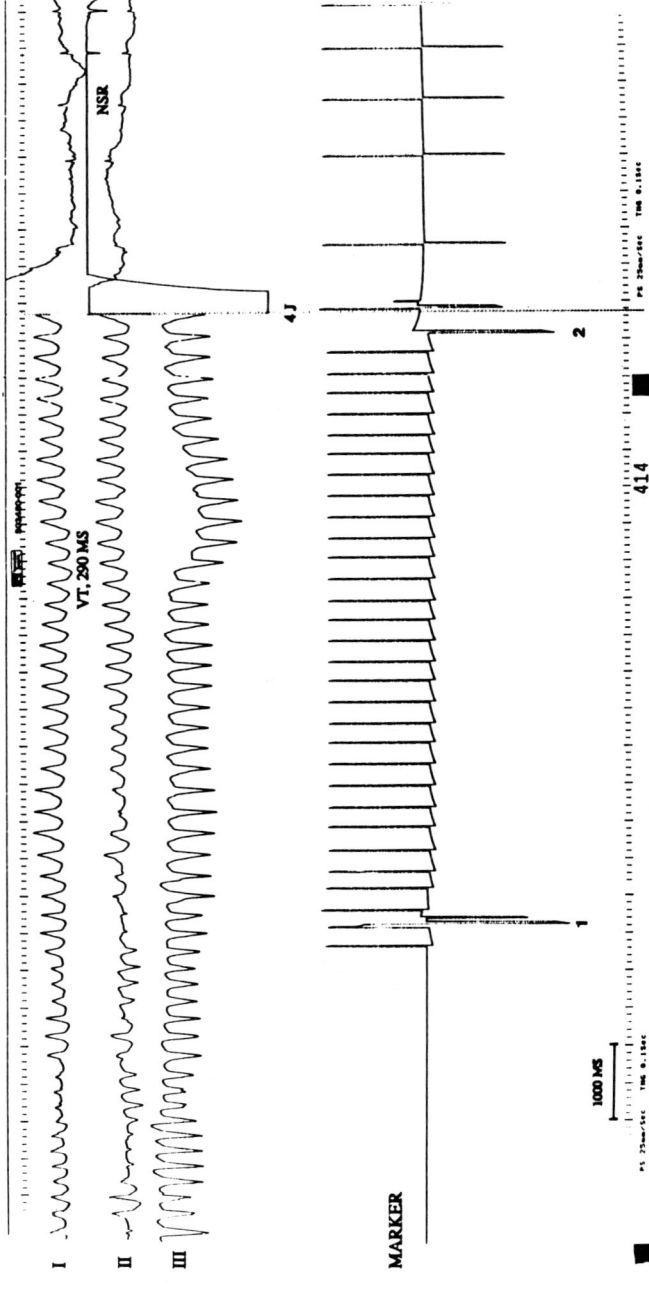

Figure 6 Tracing show VT with a cycle length of 290 ms. Event markers begin when the device is activated (1), detection of ventricular tachycardia occurs with charging of the capacitors to 4 J (2), and delivery of low-energy cardioversion (4 J) to reestablish normal sinus rhythm (NSR).

to include up to two antitachycardia schemes and five shocks. Zone 3 always contains five shocks. Zone 1 in a three-zone configuration can contain antitachycardia pacing, only antitachycardia pacing and five shocks, five shocks only, or be programmed to a "monitor only" status with no therapy. Additionally, in a multizone configuration, the antitachycardia pacing schemes and programmable shock energies can be programmed to one set of values in zone 1 and a different set in zone 2.

When detection criteria are met within a zone, the first therapy is initiated [5,6]. If redetection occurs, the therapies progress from pacing to shock, with shock energies always equal to or higher than the previous shock within the same zone. If redetection occurs of an arrhythmia that has crossed zone boundaries, the next most aggressive therapy in the new zone is delivered. If five shocks have delivered for an episode of tachycardia with subsequent redetection, no further shocks are available until the pulse generator has sensed all cardiac cycles below the tachycardia zone for four intervals. A limit can be set on the amount of time for attempts at termination of a tachycardia with antitachycardia pacing. When the antitachycardia pacing reaches the programmed time limit, it is discontinued and the programmed shock scheme appropriate for that tachycardia rate is initiated. The antitachycardia pacing time out ranges from Off to 5 s, to 5 min.

The VENTAK PRx device can be programmed to the committed or noncommitted mode for shock therapy. In the committed mode, the shock is delivered on the first sensed R wave following a 200-ms delay after the capacitors are charged. If there is no R wave detected within 2 s after the 200-ms wait, the pulse is delivered asynchronously at the end of the 2-s interval. In the noncommitted mode, detection is verified at the time that the capacitors are fully charged. If the tachycardia is terminated, the charge is diverted to an internal load at the end of the episode. Charge times vary from 0.2 s for a 0.5-J shock to 13 s for a 34-J shock.

V. BRADYCARDIA PACING

The VENTAK PRx pulse generator has a single-chamber VVI bipolar pacemaker which has programmable sensitivity ranging from 0.4 to 8.0 mV [6]. This fixed sensitivity for bradycardia pacing is not used for tachyarrhythmia detection. Automatic gain control tracks for tachyarrhythmias down to 0.2 mV in the ventricle. The VVI pacemaker has a programmable lower rate for 30 to 120 beats/min with or without hysteresis. The pulse amplitude is programmable to 2.5 to 7.5 V and is independently programmable for pacing after shock therapy. The pulse width is programmable from 0.03 to 2 ms. The duration of postshock pacing can be programmed from 30 s to 5 min. The postshock amplitude can be programmed to 2.5, 5, or 7.5 V, and the pulse width can be programmed from 0.03 to 2.0 ms in 1-ms increments. The postshock amplitude and pulse width cannot be programmed to less than regular bradycardia parameters.

VI. DIAGNOSTIC DATA

Using the model 2850 programmer, information on the pulse generator status can be retrieved noninvasively. This includes the model number, serial number, total number of charges, number of charges diverted, battery status, and the high-voltage lead impedance from the last shock delivered [5,6]. The programming system can transmit real-time event markers from the implanted pulse generator to a physiological recorder. Additionally, real-time electrograms can be transmitted from both the rate-sensing and the shocking leads of the VENTAK PRx. Analysis of the electrograms and event markers can be extremely useful at the time of pulse generator implantation, electrophysiological evaluation, or follow-up for detection of lead fractures, insulation breaks, dislodgement, or other troubleshooting maneuvers.

The programmer is used to re-form the capacitors. To optimize battery-capacitor performance during periods of inactivity with this device, the capacitors are re-formed with the programmer every 2 months at follow-up evaluation.

A therapy history for any detected tachycardia is also available for the last 128 therapy attempts. The information included in this therapy history includes the time of occurrence, zone of detection, and therapy delivered. A four-interval average of the rate pre- and post-therapy is given, as well as a determination as to whether the therapy was successful, accelerated the tachycardia, or aborted. For any episode in which shock therapy was delivered, the pulse generator stores 16 R–R intervals prior to initial therapy and 16 R–R intervals preceding the end of the episode. Electrograms are not stored with the current-generation device.

VII. SLAVED PROGRAMMED ELECTRICAL STIMULATION

Using the 2850 programmer with the 2860 programming disk, it is possible to perform programmed electrical stimulation through the VENTAK PRx in a slaved mode [5,6]. Thus, any standard stimulator used for programmed stimulation can be connected to the programming system. The pulse is sent from the stimulator to the programmer, translated to pace commands by the programmer, and communicated via telemetry to the pulse generator. Rates up to 800 beats/min can be achieved. There is a 30-ms delay from the stimulator output to the pulse generator output. With slaved programmed electrical stimulation it is possible to induce ventricular tachycardia (Fig. 7) and ventricular fibrillation (Fig. 8) noninvasively, and to assess the efficacy of programmed therapy (Fig. 9). The programmer also has two other models of induction, Manual Delivery and External Induction. Manual Delivery offers programmable commanded shock delivery from 0.1 J to 34 J. PES is also provided via Manual Pace with burst +1, ramp schemes available. External Induction provides a means for temporarily blinding the device if performing invasive testing intraoperatively or with an EP catheter.

Additional features [5,6] which are programmable in the device include the ability to have the device emit electronic tones at the time of elective replacement time, when there is a charge in progress, with valid telemetry, with tachycardia detection or for sensed events by the bradycardia pacing amplifier. The programmer also allows for enabling or disabling magnet use. When a magnet is applied to a device that has the magnet use enabled, it will terminate any therapy being delivered after 750 ms. Thus any charge on the capacitors will be diverted to the pulse generators' internal test load. No further therapy will be delivered while the magnet is in place. Leaving the magnet in place for 30 s, when the Ventak has been programmed to monitor therapy, will change the status to Monitor Only; while the magnet is in place in the Monitor Only mode, the device will emit a continuous electronic tone. When the magnet is applied for 30 s to a device which is in the Monitor Only mode, it will change its status to Monitor and Therapy and emit an electronic tone which is synchronous with each sensed R wave. When telephone monitoring with magnet application is enabled, battery status, system performance information, and indication that a shock has been delivered since the last magnet application can be determined with transtelephonic monitoring (Fig. 10). For transtelephonic monitoring, the pulse generator must be on Monitor Only or Monitor and Therapy status. With magnet application to the VENTAK PRx held for approximately 10 s, the pulse generator operates in VVT pacing mode with stimuli that are R-wave synchronous, and two sets of double pulses signal the initiation of the code. The third through seventh cycles provide the status code as indicated in Table 2. Cycle 3 gives therapy enabled status, cycles 4 through 5 provide battery

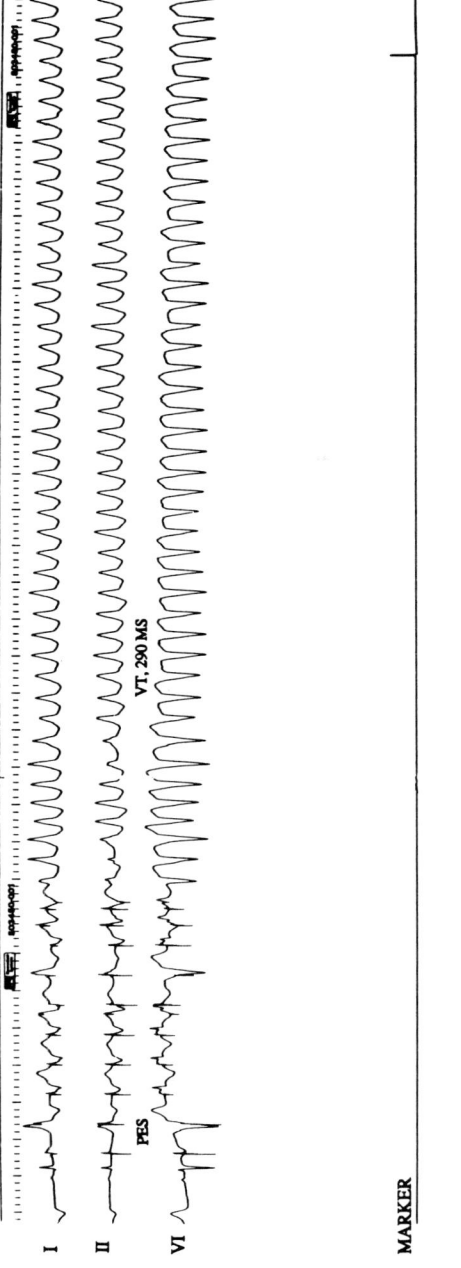

Figure 7 Tracing show noninvasive programmed electrical stimulation (PES) with induction of sustained monomorphic left bundle VT with cycle length of 290 ms.

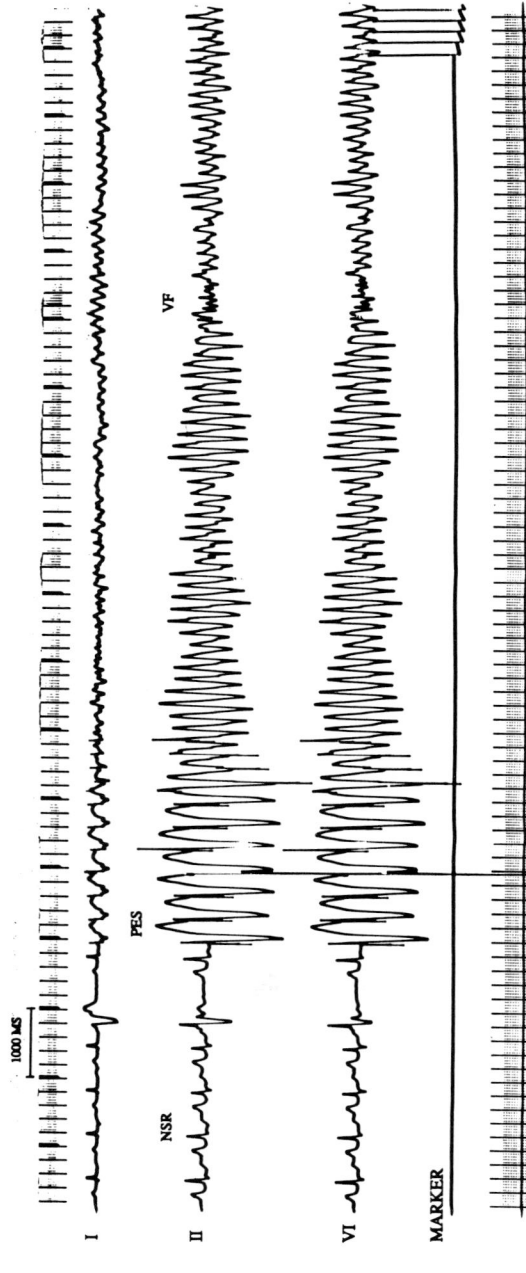

Figure 8 After normal sinus rhythm (NSR), programmed electrical stimulation (PES) is used noninvasively to induce ventricular fibrillation (VF). When the device is activated, the marker channel indicates immediate sensing of the VF.

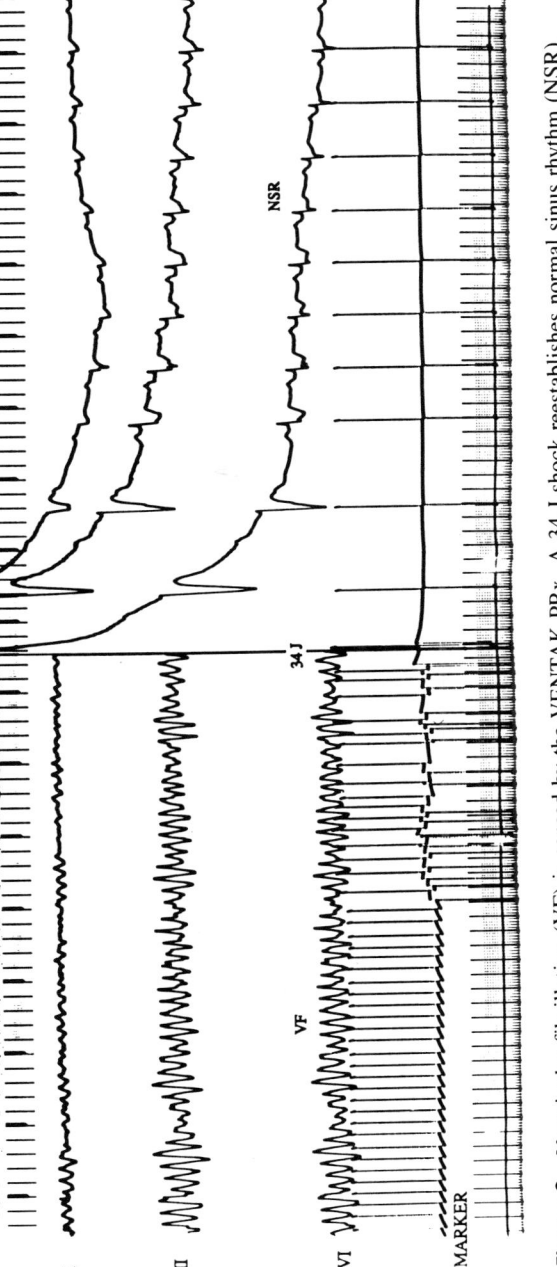

Figure 9 Ventricular fibrillation (VF) is sensed by the VENTAK PRx. A 34-J shock reestablishes normal sinus rhythm (NSR).

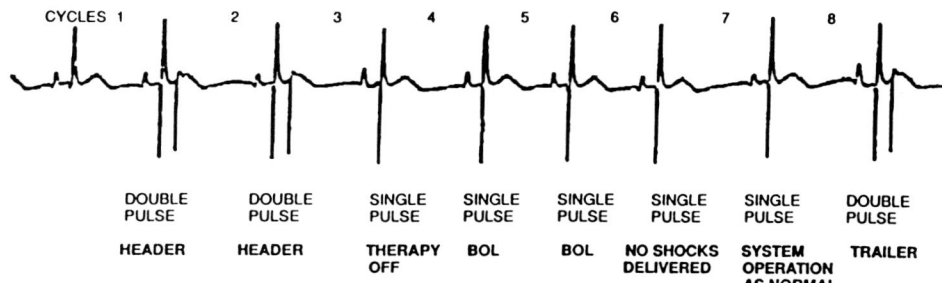

Figure 10 Transtelephonic monitoring of the VENTAK PRx. With magnet application held approximately 10 s (or at least 10 cardiac cycles), the pulse generator operates in a temporary VVT pacing mode. Eight cardiac cycles are required to complete the transmission. Two double pulses (the header) signal initiation of the code. The third through seventh cycles provide the status code. Pulse 3 gives the therapy enabled status, pulses 4 and 5 provides battery status information. Pulse 6 provides shock delivery information. Pulse 7 provides system status information. A double pulse at the eighth cardiac cycle (the trailer) signals termination of the transmission.

Table 2 Battery Status and Voltage [6]

Battery status level	Battery Status	Voltage	Condition
Beginning of life	BOL1	6.0 V	All therapy available.
	BOL 2	5.75 V	
	BOL 3	5.5 ± 0.1 V	
Middle of life	MOL1	5.25 V	All therapy available.
	MOL2	5.0 ± 0.1 V	
Elective replacement time	ER11	4.75 V	All therapy available. If Beep on ERI feature is programmed ON, pulse generator emits audible 16 beeps at 0.5-s, intervals every hour. Patient should contact contact physician immediately to schedule replacement. (Twenty 34-J shocks, or 4 months of monitoring, or 3 months of pacing (if pacing parameters are set at nominal values) remain at beginning of ERI.)
	ER12	4.4 V	
End of life	EOL		No outputs available. Antitachycardia Pacing and Bradycardia Pacing disabled.

status information, cycle 6 provides shock delivery information, and cycle 7 provides system status information. A double pulse of the termination indicates the end of the transmission. During routine clinic follow-ups every 2 months, therapy history is reviewed, the capacitors are re-formed, and battery status is reviewed (Table 2).

VIII. CLINICAL RESULTS

Between November 30, 1990, and June 1, 1992, 533 patients received the VENTAK PRx for treatment of life-threatening ventricular arrhythmias [5]. The mean age of the patient population was 63.3 ± 11.7 years. There were 445 (83.5%) males and 88 (16.5%) females. The mean left ventricular ejection fraction was 32.2 + 13%. Coronary artery disease was present in 436 of the 533 patients (81.8%). Nonischemic cardiomyopathy was present in 53 (9.9%) patients. Other cardiac diagnoses were present in 44 (8.3%) of patients.

The presenting clinical arrhythmia was sustained monomorphic ventricular tachycardia in 421 (79%) patients. Ventricular fibrillation was the diagnosis in 73 (13.7%), and monomorphic ventricular tachycardia and ventricular fibrillation in 39 (7.3%).

At the time of this writing, data regarding antiarrhythmic drug use are complete for the initial 372 patients enrolled in the protocol. Of these, 232 (62.4%) were receiving concomitant drug therapy. Amiodarone was used in 42.2% of the patient population. No antiarrhythmic medications were being used in 37.6% of the patient population. Similarly, complete data regarding configuration programming are available for the initial 372 patients. Of this patient population, single-zone therapy was employed in 126 (33.9%). Two-zone therapy was employed in 179 (48.1%), and three-zone therapy in 67 (18%). When programmed to the one-zone configuration, the median rate for delivery of therapy was 165 beats/min with a range of 135 to 220 beats/min. The median duration and cycles was 10 cycles with a range from 10 to 30. When programmed to the two-zone configuration, the median rate was 145 beats/min with a range from 90 to 195. The median duration was 8 cycles with a range of 8 to 100 cycles. In the three-zone configuration, the median rate was 200 beats/min with a range from 135 to 220 with a median duration of 10 cycles in a range of 8 to 20 cycles. The rate and duration in three-zone configuration is represented in Table 3. In this patient population, the use of onset, stability, sustained rate duration, and turning-point morphology as ''detection enhancements'' are represented in Table 4. When programmed to a one-zone configuration, the first shock energy was 0 .1 to 2 J in 7% of the patients, 3 to 30 J in 28% of the patients, and 34 J in 65% of the patients.

The cardioversion threshold, determined at the time of intraoperative placement of the device in 346 patients, was less than or equal to 1 J in 179 patients (50%), 2 to 5 J in 76 patients

Table 3 Rate and Duration Programming in Three-Zone Configuration [6]

Parameter		Median	Range
Zone 1	Rate (beats/min)	125	90–175
	Duration (cycles)	10	10–150
Zone 2	Rate (beats/min)	165	130–210
	Duration (cycles)	10	10–25
Zone 3	Rate (beats/min)	220	165–220
	Duration (cycles)	10	10–24

Table 4 Detection Enhancements Programmed [5]

Detection enhancement[a]	Range of programmed settings	Percent of patients using enhancement	Spontaneous episodes appropriate response[b]
Onset	9–31%	12.1%	95.8% (D)
Stability	8–39 ms	21%	98.6% (D)
SRD	0:02–6:00 min:s	26.3%	90.9% (I)
TPM	On	18.8%	96.2% (D)

[a]20 patients (5.4%) are programmed to use onset and/or stability.
[b]D indicates therapy delivery was initiated, I indicates therapy was inhibited [6].

(21.2%), and greater than 6 J in 91 patients (25.4%). The defibrillation threshold testing was tested in 533 patients and was less than 20 J in 462 (86.7%). The mean defibrillation threshold was 15.7 J ($\pm$5.6 J), with a range of 2 to 25 J.

In the 533 patients, there have been a total of 14,141 spontaneous episodes treated with therapy as represented in Table 5. Note that 79% of spontaneous episodes of ventricular tachycardia were terminated with antitachycardia pacing, and 10% with low-energy shocks. High-energy shocks were necessary in only 10% of patients.

In clinical investigation, the observations and complications included infection in 9 (1.6%) patients. High defibrillation thresholds were found in 2 patients (0.4%). Pulmonary edema was reported in 4 patients (0.7%), and other complications in 8 patients (1.5%).

For mortality analysis, deaths were classified as a tachyarrhythmic sudden death if there was an unwitnessed death, or death that occurred within 1 h of the onset of symptoms and was cardiac in nature [5]. By contrast, it was considered tachyarrhythmic and nonsudden if the death occurred more than 1 h after the onset of symptoms and was cardiac in nature. A death was classified as a nontachyarrhythmic cardiac death if it was due to cardiac process not related to a tachyarrhythmic event, such as a myocardial infarction or congestive heart failure. Finally, noncardiac deaths were those which were not cardiac in nature. Survival analysis yields a 1-year actuarial sudden cardiac death rate of 1.0%. Overall, 90.4% of patients were free of cardiac mortality, with the total mortality being 13.3% in follow-up.

IX. CONCLUSIONS

The CPI VENTAK PRx ICDs (models 1700 and 1705) are tiered-therapy third-generation devices which in clinical evaluation have been shown to reduce the frequency of sudden death in this high-risk population to a rate comparable to second-generation and other third-generation

Table 5 Distribution of Therapy Delivery [5]

Number of spontaneous episodes	14,141
ATP conversions	11,190 (79.1%)
Low-energy shocks	1,540 (10.9%)
High-energy shocks	1,411 (92.4%)
Episodes converted by initial therapy	13,073 (92.4%)
Total episodes converted	14,140 (99.99%)

devices [1–4]. The zone therapy for tachyarrhythmia management is a practical, logical, and effective format for detection and monitoring and therapy of tachycardias. The next-generation VENTAK PRx II will extend the memory capabilities with enhanced detection and therapy history and smaller device size.

REFERENCES

1. Saksena S, Mehta D, Krol RB, Tullo NG, Kavshik R, Neglia J. Experience with a third-generation implantable cardioverter-defibrillator. Am J Cardiol 1991; 67:1375–1384.
2. Fromer M, Schlapfer J, Fischeer A, Kappenberger L. Experience with a new implantable pacer-, cardioverter-, defibrillator for therapy of recurrent sustained ventricular tachyarrhythmias: a step toward a universal tachyarrhythmia control device. PACE 1991; 14:1288–1298.
3. Bardy G, Troutman C, Poole JE, et al. Clinical experience with a tiered-therapy multiprogrammable antiarrhythmic device. Circulation 1992; 85:1689–1698.
4. Fromer M, Brachman J, Block M, et al. Efficacy of automatic multimodal device therapy for ventricular tachyarrhythmias delivered by a new implantable pacing cardioverter-defibrillator: Results of a European Multicenter Study of 102 implants. Circulation 1991; 86:363–374.
5. VENTAK PRx Clinical Summary Report, Cardiac Pacemakers, Inc., March 1992.
6. VENTAK PRx 1700/1705 Automatic Implantable Cardioverter Defibrillator Physicians Manual, Cardiac Pacemakers, Inc., 1992.

41

The Telectronics Guardian 4210/4211

Paul J. Wang

*Tufts University School of Medicine
and New England Medical Center
Boston, Massachusetts*

I. GENERAL CHARACTERISTICS

The Telectronics Guardian 4210 and 4211 (Table 1) are multiprogrammable telemetric implantable defibrillators with VVI bradycardia pacing (Fig. 1), antitachycardia pacing, low-energy cardioversion, data logging, and telemetry capability [1,2]. The Guardian 4210 device is rectangular in shape, with its inferior aspect having a truncated oval appearance with dimensions 115 × 81 × 20 mm. It weighs 272 g and has a volume of 159 m L [1]. The Guardian 4211 device has dimensions of 117 × 83 × 20 mm, weighs 270 g, and has a volume of 184 mL [2]. Radiographs of the devices are shown in Chapter 31. The radiographic code for the Guardian 4210 is TWV. The radiographic code for the Guardian 4211 is TIZ. The Guardian 4210 and 4211 have VS-1B headers. They accept a 3.2-mm in-line bipolar lead with a short terminal pin for rate sensing/pacing and 3.2-mm HV-1 patches. The header has sealing rings. The Guardian 4210 and 4211 require use of a Telectronics 030-308 adaptor in order to use two unipolar myocardial rate-sensing and pacing leads. Telectronics patches or other HV-1 patches fit the Guardian 4210/4211 without adaptors. Use of 6-mm patches (e.g., CPI L67 or CPI A67) requires Telectronics adaptor 040-047.

II. ENGINEERING ASPECTS OF DESIGN

A. Battery Source

The Guardian 4210 and 4211 have a lithium/silver-vanadium pentoxide energy cell. This cell powers defibrillation, telemetry, pacer, and defib-control integrated circuits.

These devices have the capacity to deliver approximately 500 maximum-energy defibrillation shocks or provide 6 years of monitoring only. The average generator life is estimated to be between 3 and 5 years, depending on the number of patient shocks delivered.

Table 1 Comparison of Guardian 4210 and 4211

	4210	4211
Dimensions	115 × 81 × 20 mm	117 × 83 × 20 mm
Weight	272 g	270 g
Volume	159 mL	184 mL
Radiographic code	TWV	TIZ
Microprocessor-based	Yes	Yes
Sensing	Programmable	Automatic tracking
High rate detection	Fixed at 250 ms	160–600 ms
Tachycardia detection criteria	8/10 12/15 16/20	8/10 12/15 16/20, . . . 48/60
Tachycardia detection intervals	300–600 ms	180–600 ms
Number of maximum TCL for shock	1	2
Onset detection algorithm	Yes	Yes
Confirmation criteria	5/6 ATP, 8/10 shock	6/10 ATP and shock
Therapy reversion	Y − X + 1	Y − X + 1, ≥ 5 s
Confirmation modes	Noncommitted	Confirm—noncommitted Standby—11th undelivered shock committed Commit—all committed
Number of ATP zones	1	2
ATP time limit	No	Programmable
ATP Pasar-O	Yes	Yes
ATP autodecremental ramp	No	Yes
Recall of last successful ATP	Yes—single	Yes—multiple
Shock waveform	Monophasic	Programmable Monophasic or biphasic
Shock energy range	0.5–33 J (range 30–43 J)	50–680 V
Number of shock in series	4–9	4–9 for defibrillation 0–3 for cardioversion
Automatic capacitor reformation	60 days	60 days
Bradycardia pacing	Enabled/disabled	Enabled/disabled
Bradycardia amplitude	2.5 V, 5.0 V, 75 V	2.5 V, 5.0 V, 7.5 V
Bradycardia pulse width	Up to 1.0 ms	Up to 1.5 ms
Emergency VVI	7.5 V at 1.0 ms	7.5 V at 1.5 ms
Bradycardia pacing available during charging	No	Yes
Noninvasive VT/VF induction	VOO or VVT	VVT, PES, or burst pacing 1–240 intervals at 50–600 ms 0–4 extrastimuli
Electrogram snapshots	1 s	1 s in therapy 2 s after reversion
Data episode logs	Yes	Yes

```
Patient:                                                    08:47 Dec 31, 1992
Device:     Guardian ATP II 4211  V2.1 #:    ; SYSTEM ON

Brady Support      Enabled              Post Shock Delay    0 sec
   Standby Rate    50 ppm, 1200 ms      Post Shock Brady    Enabled
   Hysteresis      50 ppm,    0 ms         Standby Rate     55 ppm, 1100 ms
   Pulse Amplitude 5.0 V                    Duration        5 min
   Pulse Width     0.5 ms                   Energy          High

   | Sense/Pace Lead Impedance    700 ohms |
```

Figure 1 Printout from Telectronics 9600 programmer showing bradycardia parameters for the Guardian 4211. Postshock bradycardia pacing has independently programmable standby rate, duration, and energy (up to 7.5 V at 1.5 ms).

B. Current Leakage

The patient leakage currents are measured to be less than 100 nA into a 500-Ω load via the sensing leads and a maximum of 25 µA at 680 V into a 50-Ω load via the defibrillation leads.

C. Logic Circuitry

The Guardian 4210 and 4211 use microprocessor-based control circuits. The defibrillation-control integrated circuit performs VT/VF detection and interfaces with the telemetry integrated circuit and the pacer integrated circuit.

III. DEVICE FUNCTION

A. Sensing

The Guardian 4210 uses a programmable sensitivity system. The minimum initial sensitivity is 1.0 mV. In order to maximize the ability of the device to reconfirm ventricular fibrillation which may have electrograms of decreasing amplitude, during shock confirmation, the sensitivity increases to a programmable percentage of 25% to 71% of the initial programmed value, up to 0.5 mV. For example, if the initial programmed sensitivity is 1.4 mV and the percentage programmed is 71%, the resulting sensitivity will be 1.0 mV during shock confirmation. During ventricular fibrillation induction and device testing, it is extremely important that adequate sensing at the programmed sensitivity be carefully documented. Evidence of undersensing of ventricular fibrillation should be addressed by demonstrating appropriate sensing at more sensitive settings. Because of possible changes in sensing chronically, evaluation of sensing during ventricular fibrillation several months postimplant as well as predischarge may be important. In the Guardian 4210 clinical studies, a small number of patients exhibited undersensing, resulting in delay or failure of therapy during chronic testing at sensitivity settings which previously had demonstrated appropriate sensing. However, most commonly, reprogramming helped resolve these sensing problems (see Section VIII).

The Guardian 4211 has automatic sensitivity tracking, which adjusts the sensitivity based on the amplitude of the preceding sensed event. Using automatic sensitivity tracking, after a 96-ms window, the sensitivity is adjusted to 40% of the preceding sensed event. The sensitivity then decreases gradually over time, with a half-time of 400 ms. The minimal sensitivity is 3.1 mV, and the maximal sensitivity is 0.375 mV. After bradycardia pacing, the sensing system is blanked: double-sided for 160 ms and single-sided for 348 ms. This results in tracking to the maximal sensitivity of 0.375 mV postbradycardia pacing. If the feature called "Compensate" is programmed, the sensing threshold is set at 1.4 m V after each paced event with subsequent decay in order avoid sensing of a large pace-evoked response. In clinical studies to date, no undersensing or oversensing has been reported.

B. Recognition and Classification Algorithm

Both the Guardian 4210 and 4211 devices use rate as the primary determinant of the presence or absence of a tachycardia. In the Guardian 4210, if at least 8 out of 10 sensed intervals are less than or equal to 250 ms, nonprogrammable fibrillation detection interval criteria will be met. In the Guardian 4211, a high rate-detection interval of 160–600 ms is used to detect tachyarrhythmias which are converted by defibrillation only. Thus, cardioversion therapy may be used initially for tachycardias which fail to terminate with ATP, but defibrillation therapy may be delivered immediately for faster tachycardias. The tachycardia detection algorithm consists of an X-out-of-Y-interval detector. One may choose from 8 out of 10, 12 out of 15, or 16 out of 20 intervals. Guardian 4211 also has up to a 48/60 detector. If X number of intervals fall within the tachycardia detection window, then a tachycardia is detected. Programming to a greater X-out-of-Y criterion has been quite successful in preventing detection of many episodes of atrial fibrillation. This detection algorithm offers considerable flexibility, but does not prevent detection of long runs of ventricular tachycardia or detection of sinus tachycardia.

The tachycardia detection interval (TDI) may be programmed from 300 ms to 600 ms in the Guardian 4210 and from 180 ms to 600 ms in the Guardian 4211 (Fig. 3). Slow tachycardias with cycle lengths greater than 600 ms cannot be treated by the 4210/4211 and should be identified prior to implant when possible. In the Guardian 4210, an independently programmable Maximum Tachycardia Cycle Length (TCL) for shock is used to define the slowest tachycardia for which shock therapy may be initially given. For most patients the Max TCL for shock should be programmed to be equal to the TDI. If the Max TCL for shock is programmed to be less than the TDI (to a minimum of 260 ms), a tachycardia may result in ATP therapy without shock therapy unless acceleration to a cycle length faster than the Max TCL for shock occurs. Such programmed settings should be used only in the unusual patient with hemodynamically stable ventricular tachycardia for which one does not want to deliver shock therapy. In the Guardian 4211, there are two separate TCLs for shock which may be programmed.

By adjusting another parameter, the Min TCL for ATP, one defines the most rapid tachycardia for which ATP therapy may be given, allowing one to deliver ATP therapy only for slower tachycardias. In the Guardian 4211 there is a separate Min TCL for ATP for ATP1 and ATP2 in order to increase the ability to treat different tachycardias with distinct ATP algorithms. A separate Max TCL for ATP2 permits ATP2 to be used only for faster tachycardias (Fig. 4).

The onset detection algorithm enables the device to detect tachycardias which have a sudden onset from sinus rhythm. For the onset detection criterion to be met, all of the intervals must be less than the average sinus interval minus the programmed onset delta interval, and the X-out-of-Y intervals must be less than the tachycardia detection interval. For example, if the average sinus interval is 1000 ms or 60 beats/min and the onset delta is programmed to 200 ms, the cycle length must decrease to 800 ms or 75 beats/min or faster. For the Guardian 4211, the intervals must be less than the onset detection interval within 2 beats. Onset delta is programmable from 150 ms to 250 ms in the Guardian 4210 and from 50 ms to 250 ms in the Guardian 4211. Onset detection may potentially be useful in distinguishing sinus tachycardia from ventricular tachycardia, but careful programming must be performed in order to make certain that

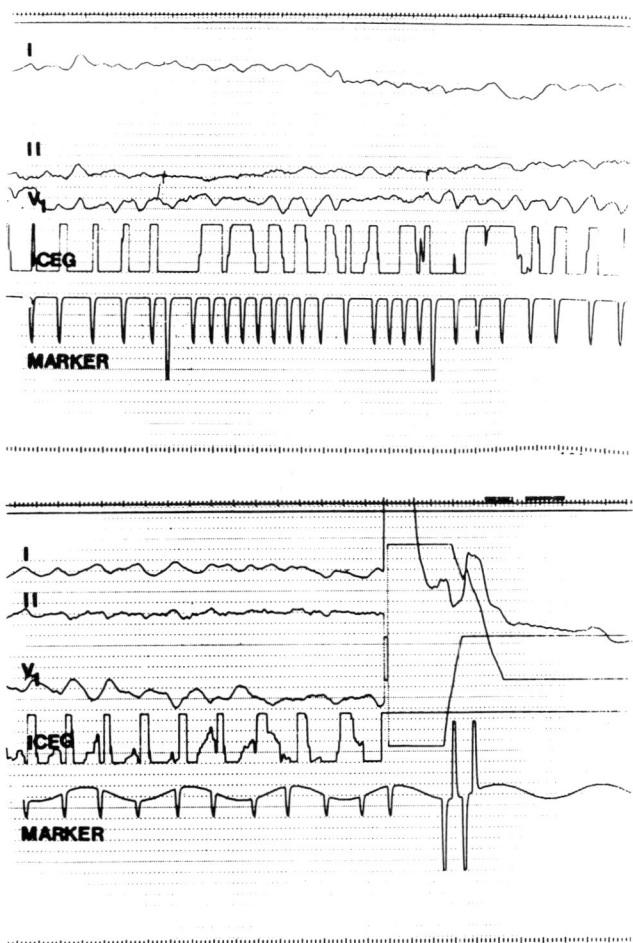

Figure 2 ECG recording of noise detection resulting in delay in detection of ventricular fibrillation. Surface ECG leads (I, II, V1), intracardiac electrogram (IECG), and marker channels revealing main timing events (MTE) are present from top to bottom. Ventricular fibrillation was oversensed, resulting in delay in detection and misclassification of VF as noise. Noise detection results in VOO pacing, despite VF as underlying rhythm (top). In the bottom tracing, ventricular fibrillation is no longer oversensed, probably because of a decrease in electrogram amplitude. Ventricular fibrillation is then detected, resulting in appropriate shock therapy.

ventricular tachycardia occurring during sinus tachycardia will be detected. In addition, the Guardian 4210 and 4211 do not have programmable time limits, which would minimize this risk by overriding the onset detection criterion if a sustained high rate occurred.

C. Tachyarrhythmia Confirmation

In order to make certain that the tachycardia is still present, tachyarrhythmia confirmation occurs at several points: (1) after detection has occurred; (2) before each ATP train is delivered; (3) after leaving ATP therapy mode; (4) after charging has occurred and the minimum shock

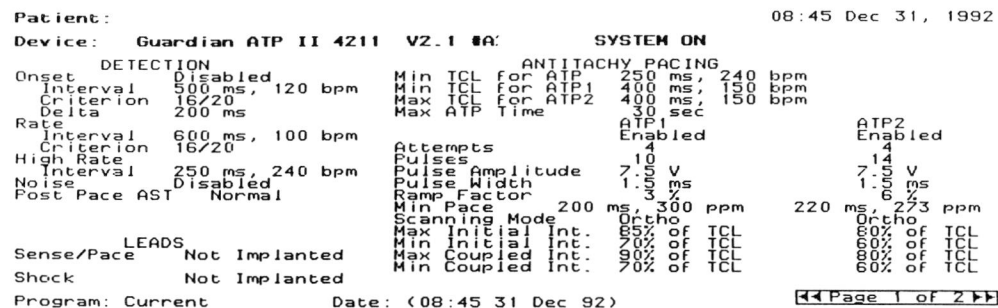

Figure 3 Printout from Telectronics 9600 programmer showing detection parameter, lead description and antitachycardia pacing parameters for the Guardian 4211. Onset detection, tachycardia detector, and high rate intervals are independently programmable. Noise may be programmed enabled or disabled. Postpacing automatic sensitivity tracking (AST) may be "normal" or "compensate," during which sensing threshold is set at 1.4 mV after each paced event with subsequent decay in order to avoid sensing of a large pace-evoked response. The two antitachycardia protocols, ATP1 and ATP2, are independently programmable.

delay has been met; and (5) after each shock has been delivered. Tachycardia is confirmed if its cycle length is less than or equal to the slowest tachycardia detection interval, either the tachycardia detection interval or halfway between the rate and the onset detection interval if it is programmed On. In the Guardian 4211, confirmation is not performed prior to charging if detected by the high rate detection interval in order to deliver therapy quickly.

For the Guardian 4210, if 5 out of 6 intervals fall within the tachycardia confirmation interval, reconfirmation criteria for ATP therapy are met. For shock therapy, 8 out of 10 intervals must meet the detection criteria. For the Guardian 4211, 6/10 confirmation is used for either ATP or shock therapy. If the confirmation criteria are not met, ATP therapy or shock therapy will not be delivered. In the Guardian 4210, if the X-out-of-Y criterion is used for detection, reversion from ATP or shock therapy requires $Y - X + 1$ long intervals. This rule also applies in the Guardian 4211, but for shock reversion a 5-s period must also elapse, during which reconfirmation results in progression to the next shock in the series. For the Guardian 4211 but not the 4210, confirmation prior to shock therapy is programmable. In the nominal "standby" mode,

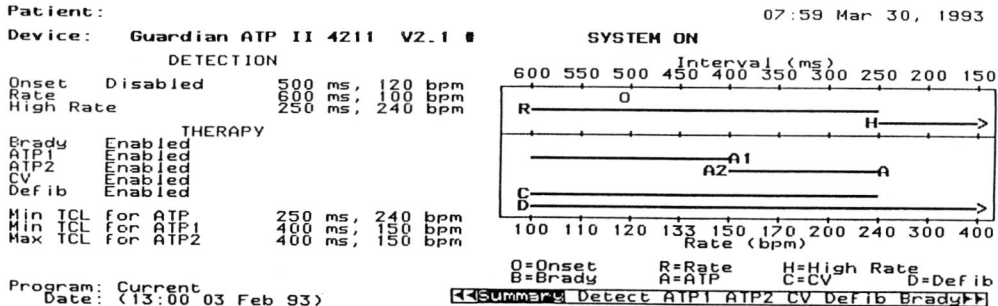

Figure 4 Printout from Telectronics 9600 programmer showing therapy and detection windows for the Guardian 4211 on the right. O = onset, B = bradycardia, R = tachycardia detection rate, A = ATP, H = high rate detection, C = cardioversion, D = defibrillation, A1 = ATP1, A2 = ATP2.

after 10 undelivered charges occur, the subsequent charge will be committed. Interrogation of the device after delivery of a shock to the patient might alert the patient and the physician that frequent nonsustained tachyarrhythmias leading to charging had occurred. This feature may decrease the likelihood that undelivered charges might result in significant generator depletion. In the "confirm" mode, all arrhythmias are confirmed prior to shock delivery. In the "commit" mode, shock therapy is delivered without reconfirming the presence of the arrhythmia.

It has been difficult to obtain clinical data about the accuracy and efficacy of confirmation of spontaneous arrhythmias, since only a limited number of such arrhythmias have been documented using electrocardiography. However, confirmation appears to be accurate for spontaneous arrhythmias which have been documented, as well as for induced arrhythmias. Use of confirmation in the Guardian 4210 and 4211 seems to have significantly reduced the frequency of therapy deliver for nonsustained arrhythmias, as demonstrated by the large number of spontaneously reverting arrhythmias on data logs. In recent clinical studies in 401 Guardian 4210 patients, there were 64,590 episodes which met detection criteria but did not fulfill confirmation criteria because of spontaneous termination.

D. Detection and Therapy Zones for Tiered-Therapy Devices

The Guardian 4210 may provide one zone of bradycardia therapy, while the 4211 provides two zones. Both devices provide up to three zones of tachycardia therapy. As discussed in Section III. C, the three zones of tachycardia therapy include a zone of ATP-only therapy, a zone of ATP followed by shock, and a zone of shock-only therapy. These zones are defined by adjusting the tachycardia detection interval (TDI), Max TCL for shock, and Min TCL for ATP (Fig. 4).

Acceleration may result in a shift from the ATP zone to the shock zone. However, the ATP therapy zone cannot be entered after shock therapy has been delivered, despite an increase in tachycardia cycle length. As described in Section III.C, in the ATP and shock therapy zones, if the tachyarrhythmia is not converted by ATP and cycle length is less than the Max TCL for shock, shock therapy will be delivered.

E. Antitachycardia Pacing Algorithms

Two pacing algorithms are available in the Guardian 4210 and 4211: PASAR (Programmable Automatic Scanning Arrhythmia Reversion) and PASAR-O (orthorhythmic PASAR). PASAR is never used, since the same pacing drive cycle is used in all trains and only the initial interval between the last sensed beat and the first beat of the ATP train decreases from one train to the next train. PASAR-O, in contrast, is widely used and is effective in treating many tachycardias. In PASAR-O, both the initial interval preceding the first beat of the train and subsequent intervals of the train are expressed as a percentage of the average tachycardia cycle length of 4 sensed beats. The percentage decreases from one train to the next train. The minimum pace interval may be adjusted in order to provide a "floor" for the shortest intervals which may be delivered in a train. In PASAR-O the first and the last trains are identical, and the remaining trains are delivered in proportionate steps determined by the minimum and maximum initial interval and the maximum coupled interval. In the Guardian 4210, the coupled interval, the interval between pacing stimuli in the train, decreases by the same percentage as the initial interval. However, in the Guardian 4211, the coupled interval is determined independent of the initial interval and is set by the maximum and minimum coupled interval. The Guardian 4211 also combines the capability of PASAR-O with an autodecremental ramp. Within each train, the coupled intervals may be decreased by a percentage, and the initial and coupled in-

```
Patient:                                                       08:01 Mar 30, 1993
Device:     Guardian ATP II 4211    V2.1           SYSTEM ON
                         Saved ATP Scan Lists
TCL(ms) ATP1 ATP2   TCL(ms) ATP1 ATP2   TCL(ms) ATP1 ATP2   TCL(ms) ATP1 ATP2
 94-108   -    -    297-311   -    -    500-515   -    -    703-718   -    -
109-124   -    -    312-327   -    -    516-530   -    -    719-733   -    -
125-140   -    -    328-343   -    0    531-546   -    -    734-249   -    -
141-155   -    -    344-358   -    -    547-561   -    -    250-265   -    -
156-171   -    -    359-374   -    -    562-577   -    -    266-280   -    -
172-186   -    -    375-390   -    -    578-593   -    -    281-796   -    -
187-202   -    -    391-405   -    -    594-608   0    -    797-811   -    -
203-218   -    -    406-421   -    -    609-624   -    -    812-827   -    -
219-233   -    -    422-436   -    -    625-640   -    -    828-843   -    -
234-249   -    -    437-452   -    -    641-655   -    -    844-858   -    -
250-265   -    -    453-468   -    -    656-671   -    -    859-874   -    -
266-280   -    -    469-483   -    -    672-686   -    -    875-890   -    -
281-296   -    -    484-499   -    -    687-702   -    -    891-905   -    -
```

Figure 5 Guardian 4211 scan list providing a record of previous tachycardias for which ATP therapy was delivered and successful. In each column is a memory or "mem" value corresponding to train in ATP sequence. 0 = first train, 1 = second train, 2 = third train, etc. When a new tachycardia occurs in the future, the previous tachycardia with the closest tachycardia cycle length will be used by the device to select which train of ATP to begin therapy.

tervals of each train may be decreased as in PASAR-O. The Guardian 4211 has an additional feature that stores in memory a scan listing the trains which resulted in successful tachycardia reversions (Fig. 5). When a new tachycardia occurs in the future, the previous tachycardia with most similar characteristics will be recalled and the first ATP train will have the same percentage of tachycardia cycle length as was used previously. While the superiority of this function has not yet been demonstrated in clinical studies, it may be helpful in many clinical circumstances. While the Guardian 4210 may have only one ATP therapy programmed, the Guardian 4211 permits two ATP therapies to be programmed independently: ATP1 and ATP2 (Fig. 4). Programming both therapies permits tachycardias which are more rapid to be treated by ATP2 only. Alternatively, ATP1 and ATP2 may be programmed so that the memory scan selects the most successful previous therapy and, if the first therapy is not successful, the second therapy will be delivered. Since the Guardian 4210 does not have a separately programmable maximum time for ATP, it is important to estimate the time for ATP therapy which is felt to be acceptable for the individual patient. Using the 9600 programmer and an estimated tachycardia cycle length, one may calculate the duration of ATP therapy if all trains are used. For the Guardian 4211, a time limit of 5 to 180 s may be selected for ATP therapy.

F. Parameters of Shock Therapy

The device synchronizes the patient shock to within 100 ms following a sensed or paced event. The Guardian 4210 programmed energy ranges from 0.5 J to maximal energy, which is 680 V and 11.5 ms, nominally 33 J with a range of 30–43 J. The voltage range of the Guardian 4211 is 50 to 680 V. Energy incrementation during a charging sequence occurs automatically after the initial energy has been delivered and the tachycardia is reconfirmed. The number of shocks that can be delivered in a series ranges from 4 to 7 in the Guardian 4210 and from 4 to 9 in the Guardian 4211 for defibrillation (Fig. 6). In Guardian 4211 up to 3 cardioversion shocks may be delivered. The minimum shock delay is programmable from 5 s to 40 s and applies only to the first shock in a series. The tachyarrhythmia must be reconfirmed during this period for shock therapy to be delivered. If the last programmed shock in a series has been delivered, as long as the tachycardia is reconfirmed, no further shock therapy will be delivered while bradycardia pacing will continue. The indicator "max shocks in series" will be seen upon first interrogation with a programmer. If the X out of Y intervals fail to be met at any time, detection criteria will no longer be met and the device will return to the monitoring state. If the detection criteria are then again met, the device may delivery tachyarrhythmia therapy.

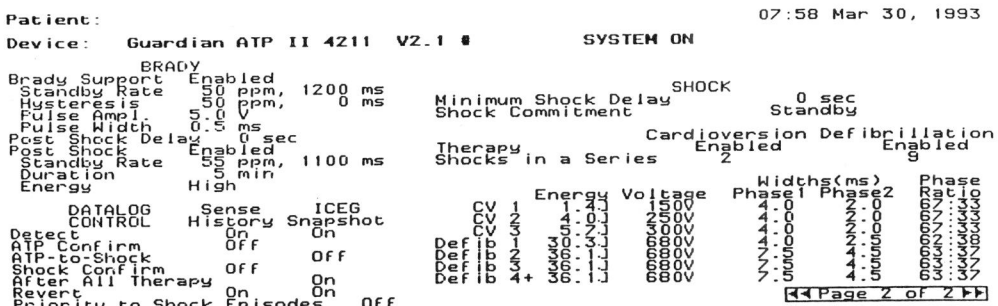

Figure 6 Guardian 4211 bradycardia parameters and data log parameters. The cardioversion energies and defibrillation energies are independently programmable. Defibrillation shocks 4 to maximum are at the same energy voltage. The phase widths and ratios for biphasic waveforms are programmable.

G. Defibrillation Waveform

The defibrillation waveform used by the Guardian 4210 is a monophasic truncated exponential. The Guardian 4211 is programmable to monophasic truncated exponential or biphasic truncated exponential. The initial voltage and phase ratios of the biphasic shocks are programmable, with a nonprogrammable interphase delay (0.5 ms). Most commonly a phase ratio of 60:40 is employed. The phases may ranges from 0.5 to 11.5 ms (Fig. 6).

Sequential shocks are not available with either the Guardian 4210 or 4211 device.

H. Capacitor Reformation and Replacement Indicator

For both the Guardian 4210 and 4211, defibrillator capacitor formation is automatically performed by the device once every 60 days if a maximum shock is not delivered. The elective replacement indicator is reached when 5% of generator energy remains, as determined by interrogation by the 9600 programmer. At this point only about 25 maximum shocks (up to 3 per day) or 3 months of monitoring is available.

I. Bradycardia Therapy

Bradycardia pacing is programmable as Enabled or Disabled in both the Guardian 4210 and the 4211. The pulse amplitude is available in three voltages, 2.5, 5.0, and 7.5 V. In the Guardian 4210, there is a programmable increase in pacing voltage following defibrillation to 7.5 V and 1.0 ms, which continues for 5 min after shock. In the Guardian 4211, high-output postshock pacing is programmable and may be set to 7.5 V at 1.5 ms for 0.25 to 30 min. A separate standby rate may be programmed postshock in the 4211. The Guardian 4210 has four programmable pulse widths with a maximum of 1.0 ms, while in the Guardian 4211 the pulse width may be increased up to 1.5 ms (Fig. 1). The standby rate ranges from 30 ppm to 120 ppm. Hysteresis intervals of 0 to 500 ms may be programmed On or Off.

J. Telemetry

Telemetry range is 0.5 to 7 cm and can be extended to 10 cm using the 9600 programmer. Programmed parameters are telemetered using the 9600 programmer. Real-time marker channels and intracardiac electrograms may be telemetered simultaneously from the device. The lead impedance may be measured and telemetered. The patch impedance from the most recent shock delivery may also be telemetered.

K. Magnet Operation

The range is 0.5 to 7 cm using the recommended magnet, a Telectronics Donut Magnet 840-370 with a field strength of 90 gauss at 4 cm. The field sensitivity of the device is 24 gauss.

The proper positioning of the magnet is in the lower mid portion of the generator. When a magnet is applied, the ATP and defibrillation therapies are disabled as long as the magnet is held in place and for an additional 5 s after magnet removal if the system if programmed On. Programming may be performed after magnet removal but not during magnet application. Magnet application does not affect bradycardia function and cannot be used to initiate bradycardia pacing. Postshock bradycardia pacing is halted by magnet application in the Guardian 4210 but not in the Guardian 4211.

If a magnet is applied during charging and held in place for at least 15 s, the discharge will be diverted and not delivered to the patient.

L. Noise Detection

Noise detection is a programmable feature available using the 9600 Telectronics programmer. If 7 out of 10 intervals are less than 100 ms (Guardian 4210) or 120 ms (Guardian 4211) with noise detection programmed On and bradycardia pacing enabled, tachyarrhythmia detection is disabled and VOO pacing will occur. Once the noise-detection algorithm is no longer satisfied, VOO pacing will continue for one additional second. Noise detection is automatically suspended if tachycardia detection has occurred. When noise detection is programmed On, it is possible that oversensing during ventricular fibrillation will result in a delay in detection (Fig. 2). While this phenomenon has been observed in the Guardian 4210, it has not been observed in the Guardian 4211 Nominally, noise detection is programmed Off in the Guardian 4211 and only if the patient is likely to experience oversensing due to EMI should the feature be programmed On.

M. Refractory Period

In the Guardian 4210, the refractory periods used for detection and shock confirmation are not programmable. The detection channel has a refractory period of 70 ms after sensed events in the monitoring state with noise detection enabled and 100 ms with noise detection disabled. These relatively short refractory periods may result in double counting of ventricular electrograms, depending on the sensitivity programmed. The refractory period is 120 ms after a paced event in the monitoring state or in the ATP therapy state. The shock confirmation channel has a refractory period of 120 ms after all sensed or paced events. The refractory period may be extended by up to 50 ms. A postshock refractory period of 1 s occurs following a shock delivered by the ICD. In the Guardian 4211, the absolute refractory period is 100 ms after a sensed event and 160 ms after a paced event.

IV. SYSTEM STATES AND EMERGENCY FUNCTION

A. System States

"System Off" may be programmed and prevents all tachyarrhythmia therapy, noise detection, and capacitor reformation. In the Guardian 4211, bradycardia therapy, emergency shocks, real-time data, and programming are available when the device is programmed to System Off. In the Guardian 4210 programming and emergency shocks are available when the system is programmed Off.

B. Fault Recovery and Self-Tests

Because the Guardian 4211 is a microprocessor-based device, every hour it initiates a self-test, which does not interfere with any function. If an internal fault is detected, automatic correction is attempted. During this fault-recovery period (less than 30 s), all tachycardia detections and tests are suspended, while bradycardia pacing is available. Recoverable faults may include transient memory errors caused by external defibrillation or single-bit soft memory errors caused by natural ionizing radiation. If a high-energy system fault is identified while the system is programmed On, a Back Up System On mode is entered, resulting in all shock therapy being set to maximum energy with ATP disabled. If an irrecoverable fault occurs, the system will enter a Shutdown Mode and all tachyarrhythmia detection and therapy will be suspended while bradycardia pacing will be available. In the Guardian 4210, no Backup System On mode is available, and detection of a fault by the self-check will automatically result in a Shutdown Mode.

C. Emergency Values

A Max Shock command initiated by the programmer stops any therapy or programmer-initiated actions and results in charging and delivery of maximum energy shock.

Emergency VVI pacing at high output, 7.5 V and 1.0 ms (Guardian 4210) or 1.5 ms (Guardian 4211) and a rate of 67 ppm may be also initiated by the programmer. Use of the emergency VVI program results in turning the System On in the Guardian 4210 but not in the Guardian 4211.

V. IMPLANTATION AND DEVICE TESTING

A. Implantation

Prior to implantation, the device should be interrogated and generator energy noted. The device should have the system turned Off prior to implantation. The Guardian 4210 and 4211 have 3.2-mm bipolar in-line connections for sensing and pacing leads. If two 5-mm unipolar myocardial leads are used, an adaptor (for example, the Telectronics 030-308) may be used to fit the 3.2-mm in-line connection. The set screws on the adaptor and on the Guardian must be tightened. It should be noted that the 030-308 adaptor does not have sealing rings, but sealing rings are present in the 4210 and 4211 headers. The Guardian 4210 has 3.2 mm terminals for the patches. However, in order to accept standard 6-mm or 5.75-mm patches (e.g., CPI patches), an adaptor (e.g., the Telectronics 040-047) must be used. When looking down the barrel of the defibrillator header, the negative terminal is on the left and the positive terminal is on the right.

B. Intraoperative Testing

Using the 4510 implant support device (ISD), one can obtain marker channels via an EKG machine or physiological recorder. From the ISD one can display the marker channel and the intracardiac electrogram as obtained from the pacing/sensing leads continuously and simultaneously. Using the 4510 implant support device, one can obtain the pacing threshold, the sensed R-wave amplitude, and the patch impedance. The ISD can be used to induce ventricular fibrillation and to deliver the appropriate shock energies for DFT testing. Using amplifiers that are similar to the implanted device, the marker channel can be used to determine whether sensing is appropriate at different programmed sensitivities if the Guardian 4210 is to be implanted.

Once the Guardian 4210 or 4211 has been attached to the pacing/sensing leads and the patches, the device may be tested. Arrhythmia induction may be performed by first blinding the device in the Therapy Assessment mode. Diversion of a shock may be accomplished by placing a magnet on the device for at least 15 s or quickly turning the system off or shock therapy off. In the 4211 the charge from undelivered shocks is kept on the capacitors, (and thus subsequent shocks (within 10 min) can deliver higher than programmed energy. Thus, it is essential that programmed and delivered energies be checked carefully.

C. Noninvasive Testing

Using both the Guardian 4210 and 4211 and the 9600 programmer, several tests may be performed:

1. Pacing threshold using alternating pulses of constant and decreasing amplitude.
2. Rate-sensing lead impedance.
3. VT or VF induction using VOO pacing or VVT pacing. Programmed stimulation or burst pacing using 1–240 intervals at 50–600 ms and 0–4 extrastimuli may be used for noninvasive induction via the Guardian 4211.

VI. DATA STORAGE

A. Event Counters

The Guardian 4210 and 4211 have event counters which indicate the total number of patient shocks delivered, the number of tachycardia detections, the number of onset detections, the number of episodes of fibrillation detection, the number of episodes requiring shock therapy, the number of episodes reverted by ATP therapy, the number of reversions after one, two, three, or more shocks, the number of spontaneous reverting episodes, and the number of delayed reversions (Fig. 7). Delayed reversions refer to reversions occurring during charging or without therapy being given since the previous confirmation.

B. Episode Logs

The episode logs provide detailed information about detected tachyarrhythmias, therapy delivered, and resultant rhythm. The episode summary provides a quick guide to all the episodes which have been recorded (Fig. 8). The number of episodes which may be recorded varies according to the length of the data episodes, but frequently about 25 episodes may be recorded. For each episode, a log is available which describes the tachycardia cycle length at time of detection and multiple R–R intervals prior to therapy delivery. In addition, the cycle length of tachycardia and R–R intervals are given before and after each ATP or shock therapy. These data permit one to detect acceleration and other responses to therapy delivered. This extensive data is extremely helpful in classifying the arrhythmia and selecting proper therapy. In a study of the data-logging function, two independent blinded investigators were able to classify ECG-documented arrhythmias based on data logs alone with a predictive accuracy of 96%. The sensitivity, specificity, and predicting accuracy using data logs were greater than using symptoms alone [4].

Only tachyarrhythmias which meet the tachycardia detection interval will be recorded on the data log. Thus, the device will not help determine if tachycardias slower than the TDI are occurring.

C. Electrogram

Intracardiac electrogram "snapshots" may be stored at several points: postdetection, reversion, and advancing from ATP to shock therapy, in the Guardian 4210. In the Guardian 4210, all

Patient: 08:01 Mar 30, 1993

Device: Guardian ATP II 4211 V2.1 SYSTEM ON

DETECTIONS	
Total Tachy	0
Onset	0
Rate	0
High Rate	0
Noise	0
Magnet	0

BRADY THERAPY	
Percent Pacing	80 %

LONGEVITY	
Life Remaining	> 40 %
Last Max Charge	16 sec

ATP THERAPY COUNTERS	ATP1	ATP2	ATP 1or2
Reversions			
By Therapy	0	0	
Spontaneous			0
Acceleration from ATP	0	0	
Used Maximum Attempts	0	0	
ATP Timed Out			0
Telemetry or Magnet Interrupt			0
Acceleration to ATP2	0		
Deceleration to ATP1		0	
Acceleration of TCL by >50ms	0	0	
Total Delivered Trains	0	0	

Data from 12:57 03 Feb 93 to 08:00 30 Mar 93 ◄◄Page 1 of 3►►

Patient: 08:01 Mar 30, 1993

Device: Guardian ATP II 4211 V2.1 #A SYSTEM ON

SHOCK THERAPY

	CV or Defib
Total Delivered Shocks	11
Undelivered Charges	0
Committed Shocks	0
Used Max. Number of Shocks	0
Telemetry or Magnet Interrupt	0

	CV
Acceleration of TCL by >50ms	0
Acceleration from CV to Defib	0

Reversions	CV	Defib
By 1st Shock	0	0
By 2nd Shock	0	0
By 3rd Shock	0	0
By 4th+ Shock		0
Delay/Spont	0	0

Last Capacitor Reform at 09:02 01 Mar 93

Equiv BOL Max Charges 11.3

Last Shock at	Nominal Energy	Nominal Voltage	Nominal Widths(ms)		Nominal Ratio	Delivered Energy	Delivered Impedance	Delivered Charge Time
09:56 31 Dec 92	1.4J	150V	4.0	2.0	67:33	1.7J	34 ohms	1 sec

Data from 12:57 03 Feb 93 to 08:00 30 Mar 93 ◄◄Page 2 of 3►►

Figure 7 Guardian 4211 detection, bradycardia, and ATP therapy counters (top) and shock counters (bottom). The energy, voltage, and pulse width of the last shock with its measured energy and impedance are given.

snapshots which are selected are 1 s in duration; in the Guardian 4211, 1-s snapshots occur in therapy and 2-s snapshots occur after reversion. The morphology of electrograms has been shown to be potentially helpful in arrhythmia classification for another ICD device [6], but a study of the usefulness of electrogram "snapshots" for the Guardian 4210 or 4211 has not been performed. Changes in morphology along with appropriate R–R intervals may suggest whether the tachyarrhythmias is likely to be of ventricular origin (Fig. 9).

Patient: 18:14 Dec 30, 1992

Device: Guardian ATP II 4211 V2.1 SYSTEM ON

Episode Date	Detect	TCL ms (bpm)	Trains ATP1	Trains ATP2	Shocks CV	Shocks Defib	Reversion	Time to Reversion
08 30 Dec 92	Rate	328 (183)	4	1	2	-	CV	00:00:57
03 30 Dec 92	Rate	359 (167)	4	1	-	-	ATP2	00:00:34
59 30 Dec 92	Rate	316 (190)	4	2	-	1	Defib	00:00:59

Datalog Read at 18:14 30 Dec 92

Figure 8 Guardian 4211 episode summary. In this example, three episodes had met detection. For the three episodes, cardioversion, ATP2, or defibrillation were successful. In the first episode, ATP1 and ATP2 were unsuccessful and cardioversion was required. In the second episode, ATPI was unsuccessful but ATP2 was successful. In the third episode, ATP1 and ATP2 were unsuccessful, resulting in acceleration, and requiring defibrillation for conversion.

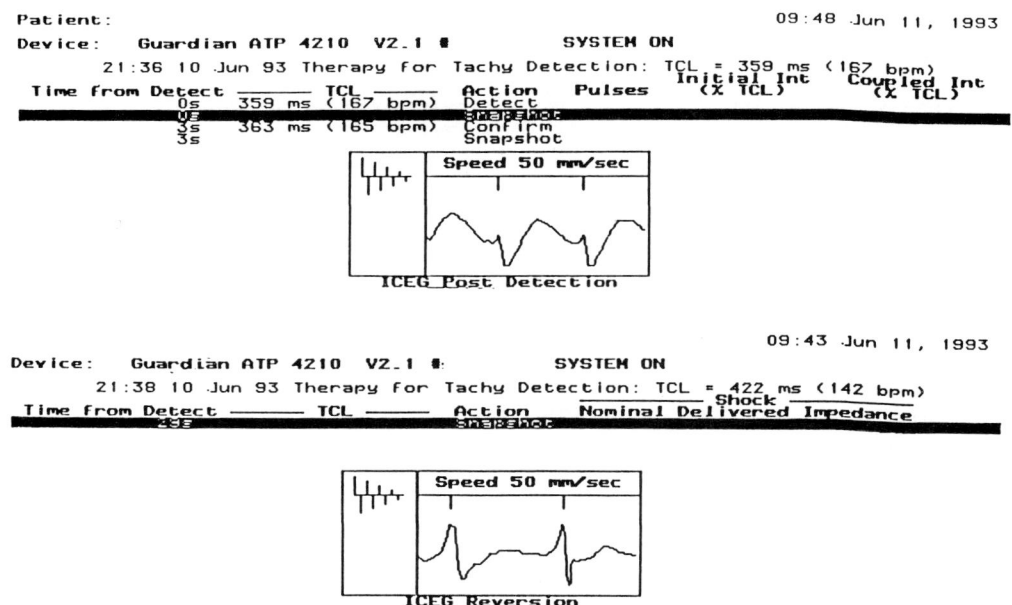

Figure 9 Intracardiac electrogram (ICEG) and log episode data for sustained monomorphic ventricular tachycardia in a patient with a Guardian 4210. The top ICEG was obtained during ventricular tachycardia and the bottom ICEG was obtained during sinus rhythm.

VII. TROUBLESHOOTING

A. Frequent Shocks and Rhythm Classification

The data logs provide an outstanding method for initial evaluation of frequent shocks not preceded by warning symptoms. Monomorphic ventricular tachycardia may be distinguished from sinus tachycardia by its sudden onset and fast regular rate (Fig. 10). Alternatively, rapid irregular R–R intervals may indicate atrial fibrillation but do not rule out polymorphic ventricular tachycardia. In contrast, extremely short intervals which are erratic suggest a lead abnormality and/or electromagnetic interference (Fig. 11), and other tests such as lead impedance may be performed noninvasively.

Detection of undersensing in the Guardian 4210 is important in the thorough evaluation of its performance. Adjusting programmed sensitivity and examining marker channels to demonstrate appropriate sensing are valuable steps in troubleshooting (Fig. 12). Most often, intermittent oversensing of tachyarrhythmias does not result in clinically significant problems. However, as discussed in Section III.L, appearance of oversensing at short intervals raises particular concern about misclassification of ventricular fibrillation as noise if noise detection is programmed on. Oversensing rarely causes misclassification of sinus rhythm as a tachyarrhythmia, and usually programming resolves this problem. The data log usually allows accurate classification of frequent spontaneous reversions, since it records R–R intervals whether therapy is delivered or not. This allows one to distinguish between frequent nonsustained ventricular tachycardia and sinus tachycardia (Fig. 13).

Telectronics Guardian 4210/4211

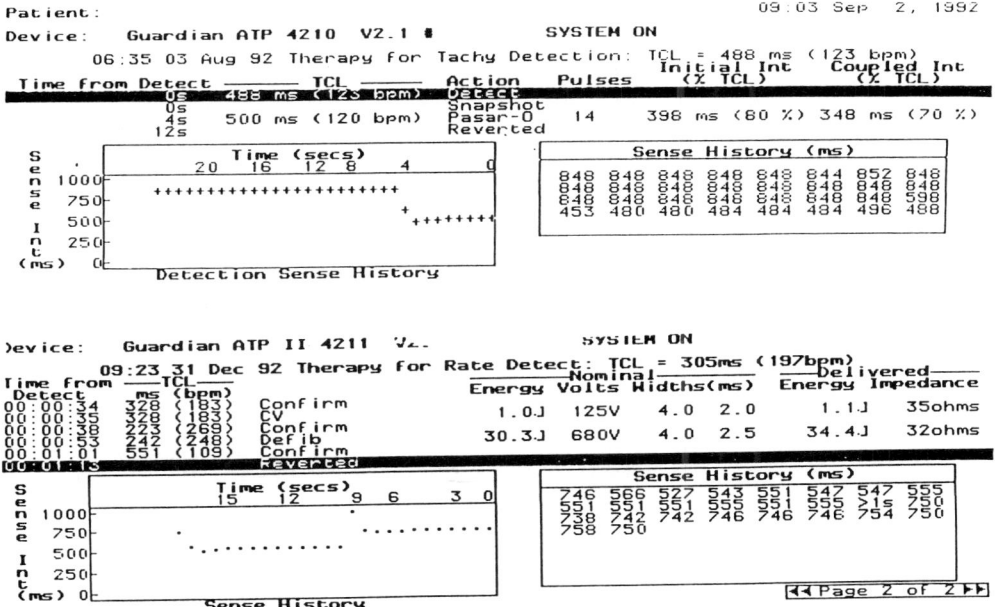

Figure 10 Guardian 4210 data log episode revealing detection of monomorphic ventricular tachycardia (top). The sinus cycle length is 848 ms, and ventricular tachycardia cycle length is 480–488 ms. This sudden onset and regularity is characteristic of a sustained tachyarrhythmia rather than sinus tachycardia or atrial fibrillation. In the bottom panel, the Guardian 4211 data log reveals tachycardia reversion from ventricular tachycardia at 543–555 ms cycle length to sinus rhythm at 742–758 ms cycle length.

B. Ventricular Tachycardia Close to the Tachycardia Detection Interval

Ventricular tachycardias may occur at a cycle length equal to greater than the tachycardia detection interval, particularly with drug therapy. If one sees on the data log that the tachycardia is detected but only slightly slowed by ATP shock therapy and the tachycardia recurs almost immediately, the likely diagnoses are sinus tachycardia or monomorphic ventricular tachycardia close to TDI. Occasionally, ATP therapy may result in transient slowing of a tachycardia to greater than the TDI without termination, followed by recognition as new tachycardia.

VIII. CLINICAL STUDIES

A. Demographics

A total of 527 Guardian 4210 implantations were performed worldwide between December 4, 1989, and March 1, 1993, with 364 implants in the United States alone [3]. The mean left ventricular ejection fraction was 33%. The mean age was 61.2 years. Coronary artery disease was present in 78% patients, and cardiomyopathy was present in 12%. Primary indications include VT (71.5%), VT/VF (9.9%), VF (13.4%), and cardiac arrest with no arrhythmia type

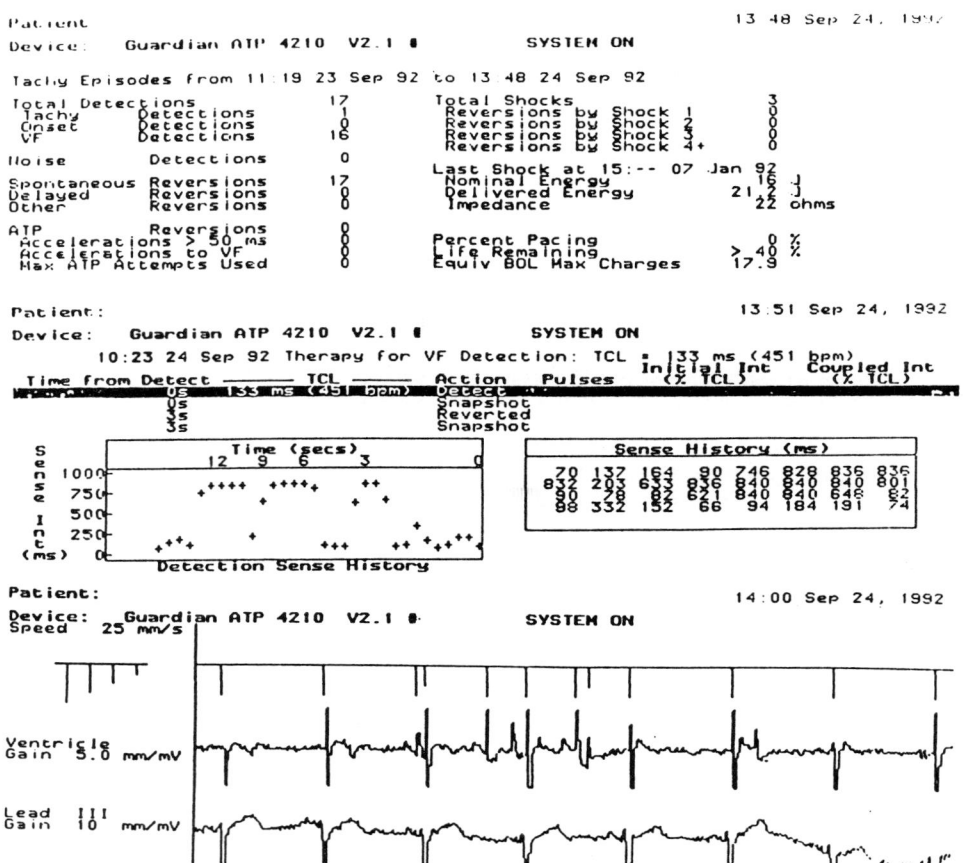

Figure 11 Guardian 4210 event counters (top), data log episode (middle), and telemetry (bottom) in patients with multiple spontaneous reversions of episodes recorded by the device as VF detections (top). Such an observation should immediately raise the possibility of oversensing due to lead/adaptor abnormality. The data log episode (middle) reveals marked fluctuation of R–R intervals, with some very short (<100 ms) intervals. The telemetry of the marker channel, ventricular electrogram, and lead III during manipulation of the generator in this patient revealed oversensing, demonstrated by ventricular electrograms and events of marker channel without corresponding QRS on surface ECG.

reported (5.2%). The mean implant duration was 14.5 months as of March 1, 1993. A total of 146 Guardian 4211 implantations were performed in the United States as of December 1, 1993. The mean ejection fraction was 32%. The mean age was 65 years. Coronary artery disease was present in 79% of patients. Primary indications included ventricular tachycardia in 99 patients, ventricular fibrillation in 24 patients, ventricular tachycardia/ventricular fibrillation in 19 patients, and nonspecified in 4 patients.

B. Tachyarrhythmia Episodes and Therapy Delivery

In the 527 Guardian 4210 implants, 401 patients had 90,484 spontaneous episodes recorded [3]. These episodes included 82,117 by VT detection algorithm, 6,154 by VF detection algorithm, and 2,213 by onset detection. While 62,169 episodes (68.7%) reverted spontaneously at

Telectronics Guardian 4210/4211

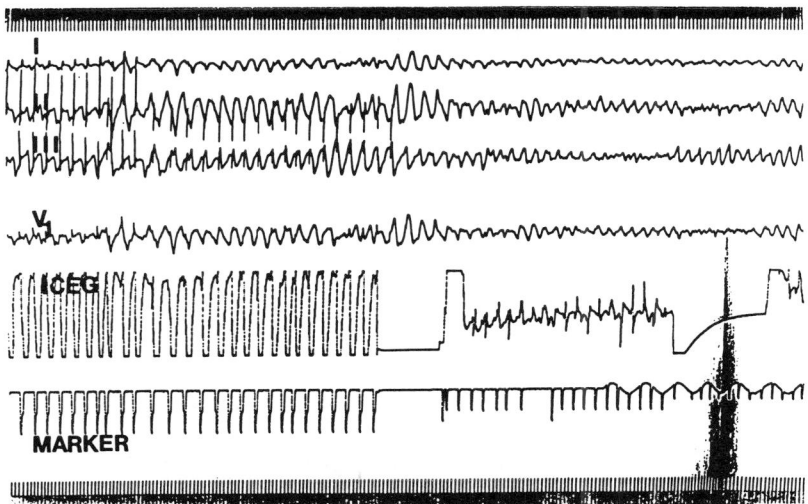

Figure 12 Induction of VF during defibrillation testing. The ventricular electrogram (second from bottom tracing) is shown during induction and VF (right). The bottom tracing shows the marker channel, with each downward deflection corresponding to a sensed event. Onset of the wavy line in the market channel indicates tachycardia detection. This example shows transient undersensing of VF but without delay in tachyarrhythmia detection. In this patient, this degree of undersensing was not felt to be clinically significant.

first confirmation and 2,421 episodes (2.7%) reverted spontaneously prior to shock delivery, 25,797 episodes (28.5) resulted in therapy delivery. The great majority of these episodes (92%) reverted after ATP therapy, while the remaining 1,945 episodes reverted after shock therapy. The PASAR-O algorithm was used in all of the ATP reversions, and in only 2.0% of episodes did the rate accelerate from VT by detection algorithm to VF by detection criteria. All accelerations to VF were converted successfully by shock therapy.

In the 146 Guardian 4211 implants, 606 spontaneous tachyarrhythmias were detected in 35 patients. Of these 606 episodes, 546 were detected by the rate detection algorithm, 52 by the

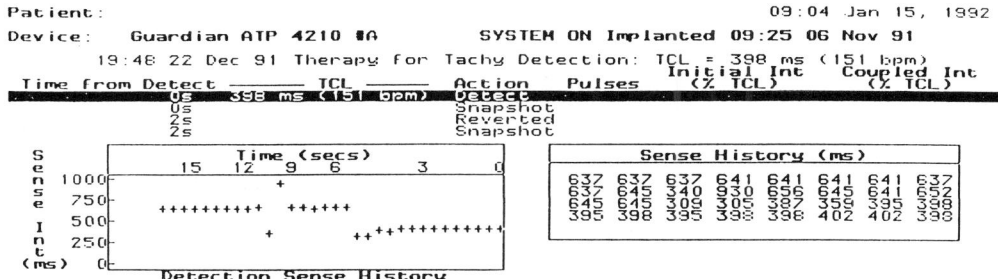

Figure 13 Guardian 4210 log episode revealing a spontaneously terminating tachyarrhythmia. The sudden onset of the tachycardia during detection suggests ventricular tachycardia or atrial flutter rather than sinus tachycardia or atrial fibrillation.

high rate detection algorithm, and 8 by the onset detection algorithm [5]. The spontaneous arrythmic episodes were terminated by ATP (132 episodes), cardioversion (18 episodes), defibrillation (42 episodes), and spontaneous or delayed ATP acceleration (407 episodes) occured in 2.0% of episodes.

C. Sensing

As of June 1, 1992, in 401 Guardian 4210 patients, sensing at implant was appropriate in 99.5% of patients [7]. At prior-to-discharge EPS, undersensing resulting in delay or failure of therapy which could not be resolved with reprogramming was reported in 5 patients. In one patient the device was explanted "due to high DFTs," and in one patient the device was explanted due to undersensing. Two patients had lead revision, with subsequent appropriate sensing and detection documented. One patient had a loose set screw, which was corrected. One additional patient had sensing of noise with resultant VOO pacing and failure of therapy, which was felt to be due to a lead connector/header problem.

At chronic EPS 2 to 6 months postimplant, 3 Guardian 4210 patients had undersensing resulting in failure of therapy. In 1 patient, the device was explanted and the remaining 2 patients had appropriate sensing after reprogramming. One additional patient had undersensing with delay in therapy, which resolved after reprogramming. Oversensing resulting in VOO pacing, and failure of therapy was seen in 2 patients and was resolved by programming the noise mode Off [7].

Thus, while sensing in the Guardian 4210 is usually appropriate, delay or failure of therapy may occur due to undersensing, and careful testing of sensing at implant and subsequent follow-up visits is important. In addition, noise detection should be programmed Off to prevent delay or failure of therapy because of misclassification of VT or VF as noise. Oversensing due to double counting of complexes has been noted, but has not been reported to cause a clinical problem.

The Guardian 4211, which uses automatic sensitivity tracking rather than programmable sensitivity, has demonstrated appropriate sensing.

D. Morbidity and Mortality

Analysis of deaths in the clinical trial of the Guardian 4210 was performed by an independent group of physicians who were not investigators in this clinical trial. Based on clinical data forms, final device interrogations, and physician notes, the board completed CAST trial mortality forms. CAST definitions were used to determine sudden death, cardiac death, and noncardiac death rates. Sudden death was defined as cardiac death occurring unexpectedly within 1 h of the onset of new symptoms or a death that was unwitnessed.

As of March 1, 1993, in the Guardian 4210 clinical study, 11 sudden cardiac and 34 non-sudden cardiac deaths were reported, representing a sudden-cardiac-death survival rate of 97.8% at 1 and 2 years and a total cardiac survival rate of 92.9% at 1 year and 88.6% at 2 years [3]. The total cumulative survival was 90.0% at 1 year and 84.3% at 2 years. These survival rates include perioperative deaths within 30 days of implant or prior to discharge, which occurred in 1.8% of patients.

Seventy explants in the Guardian 4210 clinical study have been reported. Infection resulted in 23 of these explants, while device failure resulted in 16 explants [3]. In addition, 5 devices were explanted due to high defibrillation thresholds. Six patients underwent heart transplantation. Two devices were explanted due to inappropriate sensing, and four devices were explanted due to lead header problems. One device was explanted due to surgical complications and one device was explanted due to physician error. Twelve devices were electively explanted.

In the Guardian 4211 clinical study, there have been three deaths. One death was noncardiac and one death was nonsudden cardiac in origin. The remaining death was determined to be nonsudden cardiac by the investigator but has not yet been reviewed by the medical review board. The actuarial survival analysis revealed a 98.6% total survival rate at 11 months.

E. Device Function and Complications

Device failure has been reported in the Guardian 4210 clinical studies [3,6]. As of March, 1993, 16 Guardian 4210 devices out of a total of 527 implants had been explanted due to device failure. Because of changes in the design and manufacture of the Guardian 4210, a second population of devices began to be implemented in May 1991. In addition, error-correcting software was programmed into the initial population of device. Causes of shutdown have included random soft errors in memory, random component and random manufacturing faults, solder joint failures, transient anomaly, and external factors (defibrillation, electrocautery) [3].

No shutdown cases have been reported for the Guardian 4211 [5]. In one Guardian 4211 device, outside the U.S., telemetered data logs showed intermittent noise, which was found to be due to an intermittent connection between the indifferent terminal and the internal electronic module. Five Guardian 4211 devices have been explanted due to infection, and in four of these cases the devices were reimplanted [5].

A significant number of adaptor and lead complications have been reported in the Guardian 4210 clinical study. Fifty-one lead complications and 35 adaptor complications have been reported as of March 1, 1993. Eleven of the 51 lead complications were due to lead insulation breaks, and 17 were due to lead dislodgements. Of 35 adaptor complications, 22 were adaptor connection problems. Some investigators have advised securing the rate/pacing lead at several points using multiple anchoring sleeves to minimize stress on the lead at several points using multiple anchoring sleeves to minimize stress on the lead and reduce dislodgement. Physical exertion, often consisting of repetitive motions of the torso, may contribute to lead and adaptor complications. In some cases, repetitive movement of the lead and adaptor next to the generator casing has been implicated, but substantiation has not been possible. Selecting a rate-sensing lead that does not require adaptors may minimize the risk of lead-related complications.

IX. SUMMARY

The Guardian 4210 and 4211 are tiered-therapy devices with antitachycardia pacing, bradycardia pacing, and shock capabilities. Clinical studies of the Guardian 4210 have shown an excellent sudden-death survival. Based on data log events, both shock and ATP therapy have also demonstrated successful treatment of spontaneous tachyarrhythmias. The recognition and therapy algorithms of both the Guardian 4210 and 4211 permit significant flexibility in programming the devices to treat multiple different tachyarrhythmias in the individual patient. Guardian 4211 provides the additional capability of two separate ATP therapy protocols and biphasic waveform for cardioversion or defibrillation. Reconfirmation is used extensively in these devices, reducing the risk of inappropriate therapy delivery. In addition, the Guardian 4211 has a "standby" confirmation mode, resulting in delivery of a committed shock after 10 undelivered charges. This feature may minimize the risk of significant battery depletion from repetitive, spontaneously terminating arrhythmia resulting in charging but not therapy delivery.

Because of the potential for clinically significant undersensing in the Guardian 4210 because of its programmable sensitivity system [3,7,8], careful testing to confirm appropriate sensing is essential at the time of implantation and follow-up. Also, the addition of programmable noise-detection mode may decrease risks of oversensing and increase safety. The Guardian 4211 employs automatic sensitivity tracking rather than programmable sensitivity. This system will likely eliminate significant problems in sensing, and no sensing abnormalities have been observed in clinical studies to date.

In the initial clinical studies of the Guardian 4210, device shutdown occurred due to a variety of component and software abnormalities. Some of these were due to external factors such as defibrillation, but others were due to factors such as manufacturing faults. As a result of changes in device manufacture/design and software capable of recovering software abnormalities, the problem of device shutdown has been significantly decreased. The Guardian 4211 has several fault-recovery modes, with an internal automatic recovery system for software abnormalities.

The data logging capabilities of both the Guardian 4210 and 4211 are outstanding. Extensive R–R interval logs are given before and after each ATP train or shock, permitting one to analyze the efficacy of each therapy. R–R intervals during and prior to detection with or without therapy delivery are particularly valuable in arrhythmia classification, even in spontaneously terminating arrhythmias.

Overall, many advances have occurred in these third-generation tiered-therapy devices. Improved ATP algorithms, biphasic shock waveforms, reconfirmation and fault-recovery modes, automatic sensitivity tracking, and outstanding data logging capabilities represent particular strengths of the Guardian 4211 device.

REFERENCES

1. Telectronics Pacing Systems, Inc. Guardian ATP 4210 implantable cardioverter/defibrillator. Physicians manual.
2. Telectronics Pacing Systems, Inc. Guardian ATPII 4211 implantable cardioverter/defibrillator. Training protocol. 1992.
3. Telectronics Pacing Systems, Inc. Guardian ATP 4210 implantable cardioverter/defibrillator. Clinical report. April 1993.
4. Wang, PJ, Mandalakas N, Clyne C, et al. Accuracy of rhythm classification using a data log systems in implantable cardioverter defibrillators. PACE 1991; 14:1911–1916.
5. Telectronics Pacing Systems, Inc. Guardian ATPII 4211 implantable cardioverter/defibrillator. Phase I clinical report. April 1993.
6. Marchlinski FE, Gottlieb CD, Sarter B, et al. ICD data storage: value in arrhythmia management. PACE 1993; 16:527–534.
7. Telectronics Pacing Systems, Inc. Guardian ATP 4210 implantable cardioverter/defibrillator. Clinical report. November 24, 1992.
8. Sperry RE, Ellenbogen KA, Wood MA, Stamber BS, DiMarco JP, Haines DE. Failure of a second and third generation implantable cardioverter defibrillator to sense ventricular tachycardia: implications for fixed gain sensing devices. PACE 1992; 15:749–755.

42

Siecure: Tiered Antitachycardia Therapy with Bradycardia Support Pacing and Extensive Diagnostics

Asa Hedin and Martin Obel

Siemens Elema AB
Solna, Sweden

Paul A. Levine

Siemens Pacesetter, Inc.
Sylmar
and Loma Linda University Medical Center
Loma Linda, California

Siecure is a fully implantable ventricular antitachycardia device capable of providing tiered therapy comprised of antitachycardia pacing, low-energy shocks for ventricular tachycardia (cardioversion), and high-energy shocks for ventricular fibrillation (defibrillation). This is combined with single-chamber backup bradycardia (VVI) support pacing therapy and extensive diagnostic and monitoring features. As such, its NBG identification code would be VVICD. This chapter describes the features of the Siecure model 2120 along with the defibrillation system analyzer and programmer which comprise the full system.

I. GENERAL CHARACTERISTICS

Siecure is presently configured to weigh 200 g and measures 22 × 70 × 110 mm. It has a conservative projected longevity of 3 years, with the capability of delivering 200 shocks at an average of 30 J per shock. This includes the energy for reforming the capacitors. There are versions available which will be compatible with the CPI defibrillation patch terminal pins as well as the new HV-1 terminal pin configuration. The sensing and pacing lead connector are bipolar and IS-1 compatible (Fig. 1).

II. BRADYCARDIA SUPPORT FUNCTION

Upwards of 20% of patients have been reported as having asystolic pauses following successful termination of either ventricular tachycardia or fibrillation. Siecure provides backup VVI bradycardia pacing. This is also available should the patient require bradycardia support inde-

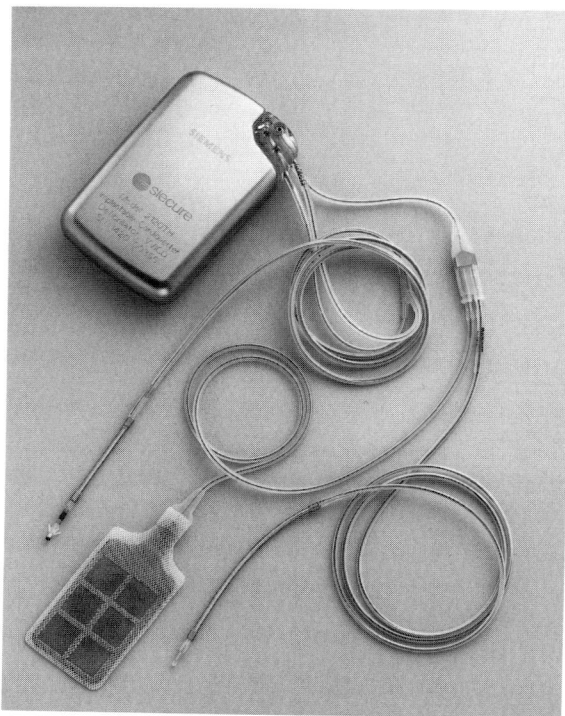

Figure 1 Illustration of the Siecure pulse generator and endocardial lead system.

pendent of posttachycardia asystolic episodes. As the posttachycardia capture threshold may be higher than that assessed during a hemodynamically stable bradycardia, two outputs will be able to be programmed. One is for standard bradycardia support pacing. The second, a high-output option up to a maximum output of 11 V at 0.5-ms pulse duration, is able to be programmed to follow delivery of antitachycardia therapy. The duration of the high-output option, the postshock pacing energy, is programmable based on the number of output pulses, varying from a low of 100 to a high of 2000. This function can also be programmed Off.

The programmable options of bradycardia support pacing include mode (VVI, VVT, and OVO), rate including hysteresis, sensitivity, refractory period, pulse amplitude, and pulse duration. The available options are detailed in Table 1.

Application of a magnet to the Siecure has no effect on its bradycardia pacing support function. VOO function can be programmed in a temporary mode only for diagnostic purposes under careful medical supervision. It will not be induced by magnet application, as this mode was deemed to be too dangerous in a population of patients who have been identified as being electrically unstable prior to receiving this system.

An OVO mode is achievable by programming the output to a subthreshold setting. The system is effectively in an OVO mode as shipped from the manufacturer in that the output is set to 0 V and 0.05-ms pulse width. The OVO mode can be used as a diagnostic monitoring mode in conjunction with the real-time event marker telemetry function when one wishes to monitor the native rhythm while withholding stimulation therapy.

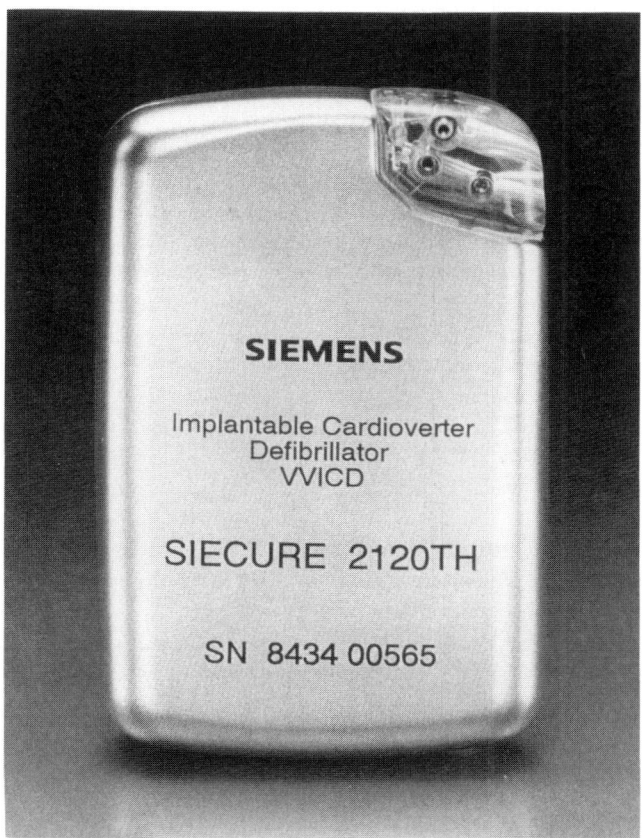

Table 1

Modes:	VVI, VVT, VOO (temporary)
Rates:	30–110 ppm in steps of 5 ppm
Hysteresis:	Off, 30 to programmed base rate in steps of 5 ppm
Sensitivity:	0.4–5.7 mV in 0.4-mV steps
Refractory period	
After sensing:	120–250 ms in 10-ms steps
After pacing:	250–500 ms in 25-ms steps
Pulse amplitude:	2.7, 5.4, 8.3, and 11.0 V
Pulse width:	0.05–1.0 ms in 0.05-ms steps
Postshock pulse width also:	1.25 and 1.5 ms

III. ARRHYTHMIA IDENTIFICATION

Siecure incorporates tiered logic for both the detection and response to ventricular tachyarrhythmias. Three levels of tachycardia can be identified and will be simplistically labeled as a low-rate ventricular tachycardia (VT low), a high-rate ventricular tachycardia (VT high), and ventricular fibrillation (VF).

The primary criteria for each of these tachycardias is rate (Fig. 2). Both VT low and VT high are allowed to begin at any rate between 100 to 250 beats/min. These two rhythms, however, cannot be programmed to start at the same rate nor at discrepant rates, with VT high beginning at a rate lower than VT low. For example, if a VT low initial rate of 150 beats/min is chosen, VT high cannot begin at a rate which is below this. The rate range for VT low is defined by the minimum rate for VT low which is programmed by the physician, and 1 beat/min below the minimum rate for VT high. By the same token, the VT high rate range extends from the minimum VT high rate, which is programmed, to the VF rate which is programmed into the device. Ventricular fibrillation can be defined as starting at any rate between 175 to 300 beats/min, but the lowest rate at which VF is diagnosed cannot be slower than the VT high rate. One does not need to set criteria for all three tachycardia ranges—one can choose to program VT high and VF or only VF.

Patients who require ICD therapy tend to have at least occasional premature beats, both atrial as well as ventricular. These premature beats often are tightly coupled to the preceding native conducted beat, such that the rate for this one cycle is relatively rapid and could be expected to fall into either the VT high or possibly the VF rate zones. To reduce the likelihood of the device responding to abrupt variations in rate based on isolated ectopic beats, the sam-

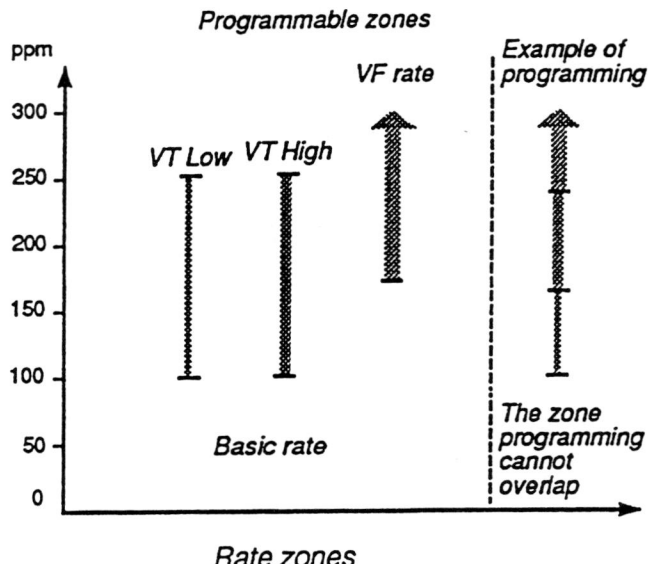

Figure 2 Schematic diagram of the rate ranges for VT low, VT high, and ventricular fibrillation. Once the base rate for each rate zone has been programmed, the progression and interaction are shown to the right.

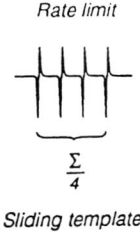

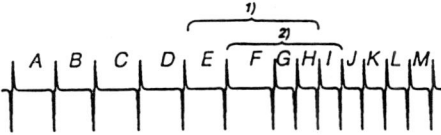

Rate Limit Criterion = RLC

Rate limit criterion is compared to the mean of the last four intervals.

1) $\dfrac{\Sigma \text{ Intervals } E+F+G+H}{4}$ > RLC means that Rate limit is not crossed

2) $\dfrac{\Sigma \text{ Intervals } F+G+H+I}{4}$ < RLC means that Rate limit is crossed

Rate limit can be within 4 zones: Sinus, VT Low, VT High and VF rate.

Figure 3 Schematic diagram of the rate limit criterion. This is determined by a running average of the last four consecutive intervals. In this way, a single isolated premature beat cannot inappropriately trigger the rate detection criteria.

pled heart rate for the tachycardia rate zone analysis is determined by a continuously running average of four consecutive sensed ventricular cycles. This is illustrated in Fig. 3.

While the identification of ventricular fibrillation is based solely on rate, additional criteria can be programmed into the Siecure to enhance the specificity with which the device identifies VT low and VT high. When these additional criteria are employed, they too must be fulfilled before the device will make a diagnosis and initiate therapy. These include rate of onset, duration, and stability.

Pathological tachycardias, particularly those amenable to antitachycardia pacing, often begin abruptly, having been initiated by a premature beat. The rate of onset criterion will help the device differentiate between the progressive acceleration of a physiological tachycardia, particularly in the VT low rate ranges, from a pathological tachycardia. To fulfill this criterion, the average cycle length of the ventricular rhythm must decrease by a programmable minimum interval based on two consecutive four-cycle groups. This is shown in Fig. 4 and is termed *sudden cycle length decrease*.

A second supporting criterion is duration of the tachycardia. This is achieved by counting a programmable number of cycles after a tachycardia is "diagnosed" by rate criteria before

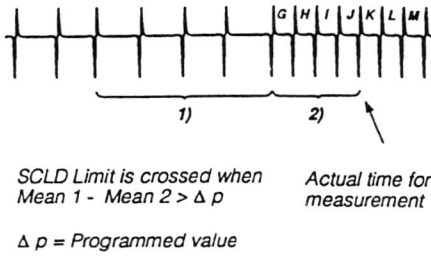

Figure 4 Schematic diagram of the sudden cycle length decrease or rate-change criterion. This criterion compares the average rate determined by the last four cycles prior to the rate change to the first four cycles at the faster rate.

other confirmation criteria are initiated such as stability (Fig. 5). This will delay the final confirmation of the tachycardia and the time before antitachycardia therapy or a low-energy shock (cardioversion) can be initiated. The intent of this criterion is to make the system as noncommitted as possible. If a tachycardia, i.e., ventricular tachycardia, is diagnosed but is nonsustained, the device will not automatically deliver therapy when it is no longer needed. It will also not begin to charge when it is programmed to deliver a shock until there is reasonable certainty that the tachycardia is persisting. This minimizes the frequency of charging and having to dump the charge internally when, upon reconfirmation, the rhythm has resolved so that the shock is no longer required. The length of the delay before delivery of therapy is a programmable option varying between 4 and 150 cycles. A long delay is a reasonable choice only when the physician knows that the ventricular tachycardia is either frequently nonsustained and/or hemodynamically stable.

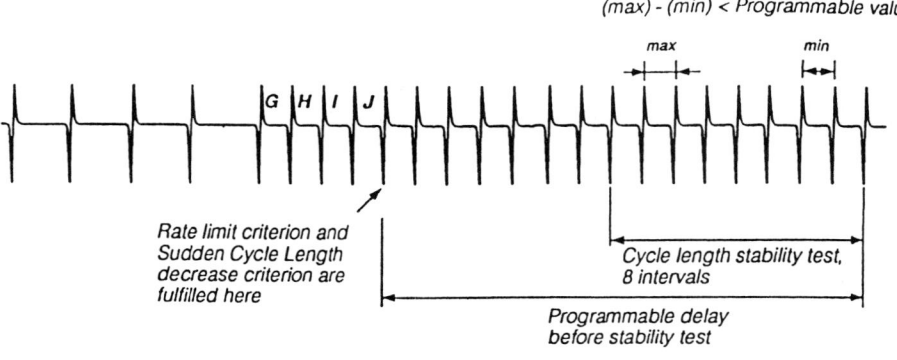

Figure 5 Schematic diagram of the delay before stability test or sustained tachycardia rate criterion. After the sudden cycle length criteria have been met, there is a programmable number of cycles which must occur at the faster rate before the system will initiate the cycle length stability test. This minimizes the chance of responding to a nonsustained tachycardia that is greater than four cycles (hence fulfilling the sudden cycle length criteria) but ends spontaneously.

The third supplementary criterion is rate stability. The goal of this criterion is to differentiate monomorphic ventricular tachycardia, which tends to be very stable, from paroxysmal atrial fibrillation, which will fulfill the rate and sudden-onset criteria but not the rate stability criterion. The majority of patients who require ICD therapy have poor ventricular function, based on either coronary artery disease or a cardiomyopathy. Thus they also have an increased incidence of atrial fibrillation. In patients who have known episodes of paroxysmal atrial fibrillation or who develop it sometime after the ICD unit is implanted, rate stability criteria can be programmed into the tachycardia diagnostic criteria to minimize false positive responses. However, if one knows that the primary rhythm which is being treated is polymorphic ventricular tachycardia or ventricular fibrillation, both of which tend to be very fast as well as irregular, then the rate stability criteria need not be utilized. To determine whether cycle length variability is present in a rhythm, the rate template continuously analyzes the last eight cardiac cycles and determines the cycle length for each. It then compares the shortest (minimum) detected cycle length with the longest (maximum) detected cycle length. If the difference between the cycle lengths is less than the programmed value, the stability criterion is fulfilled. The programmable options are Off, or 10 to 200 ms in steps in 5 ms each.

Thus, in addition to the essential rate criteria, one also has the option of utilizing rate of onset, rate stability and duration of tachycardia criteria to enhance the specificity of the device's response to the tachycardias of an individual patient. There is extensive programmability within each of these options. If one provides the system with very wide latitude with respect to tachycardia identification, there is an increased risk of responding to nonpathological tachycardias or supraventricular tachycardias. On the other hand, extremely stringent criteria, while increasing the specificity of the system, will also decrease the sensitivity and may fail to identify rhythms for which the device is intended. The physician has a significant responsibility for programming the system appropriately for each patient.

IV. REQUIRED RATE SAMPLES

The ventricular fibrillation detection criteria include both rate as well as a parameter called *required rate samples*. This feature is designed to allow the physician to determine if the device should respond to early rapid detection of fibrillation or to avoid detection of short, non-sustained runs of polymorphic ventricular tachycardia (Fig. 6). Each rate average at or above

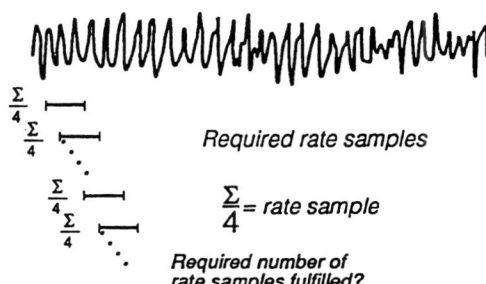

Figure 6 Schematic diagram of ventricular fibrillation detection using an average of four consecutive sensed cycles a programmable number of times before a diagnosis of ventricular fibrillation will be made.

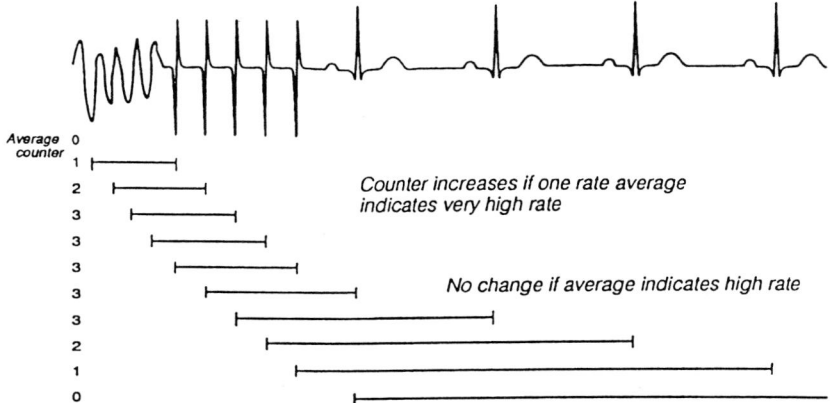

Figure 7 Demonstration of counter function for monitoring ventricular activity. When the counter resets to zero, having detected repeated cycles at a nontachycardia rate, the rhythm is diagnosed as having ended.

the programmed VF rate will increase the average counter by 1. Should one rate sample indicated either a VT low or a VT high rate, the required rate samples counter will hold stable; it will neither increase nor decrease. However, should one rate sample indicate sinus rhythm or asystole, the counter will be decremented by one toward zero. If asystole, backup pacing support will also be initiated. The number of rate samples required for identification of ventricular fibrillation include 15 to 25 in steps of 1, 30 to 50 in steps of 5, and 60 to 100 in steps of 10 (Fig. 7).

V. TACHYCARDIA RECONFIRMATION

The reconfirmation procedure continuously monitors the heart activity to confirm if the status of the arrhythmia has changed to another arrhythmia or terminated. Should a detection of an accelerated or decelerated arrhythmia occur, the device immediately selects appropriate treatment. Reconfirmation is done using rate only, but only after ignoring a programmable number of intervals prior to the onset of the reconfirmation procedure. This is designed to minimize recognition of nonsustained tachyarrhythmias. The number of intervals to be ignored are programmable separately for antitachycardia pacing and shock therapy (Fig. 8).

Reconfirmation is made as follows. When the rate belongs to the zone for the arrhythmia presently being treated, the arrhythmia is declared as being unchanged and the defined treatment continues. When, six times in a row, the running average of the rate corresponds to some other tachycardia zone other than the initial tachycardia which was diagnosed, treatment for the new zone is initiated, but only if that therapy is more vigorous than the original therapy. Thus, the system will not switch from VT high with shock delivery to VT low with antitachycardia pacing. It will continue with shocks as long as a tachycardia is still diagnosed. However, when a nonarrhythmia zone is diagnosed, the arrhythmia is considered to be terminated and the therapy ceases.

Reconfirmation continues continuously while the capacitors are being charged, so that shock is delivered *only* if the criteria for the arrhythmia continue to be met (Fig. 9).

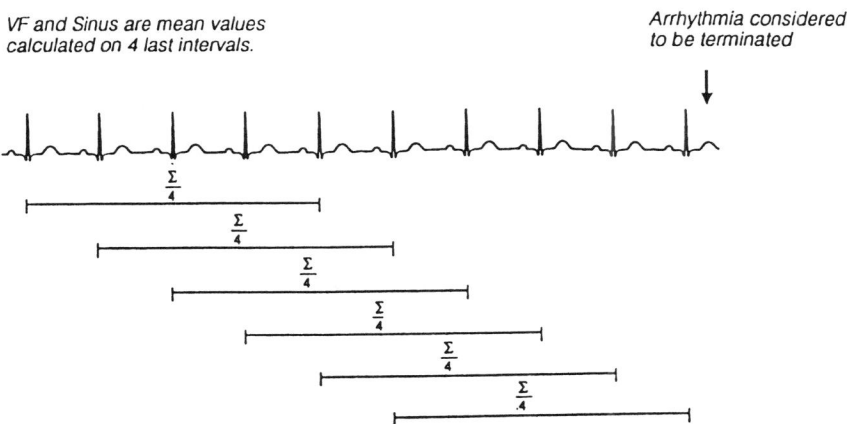

Figure 8 Six successive mean rate of four consecutive cycles is required to define a tachycardia as having ended.

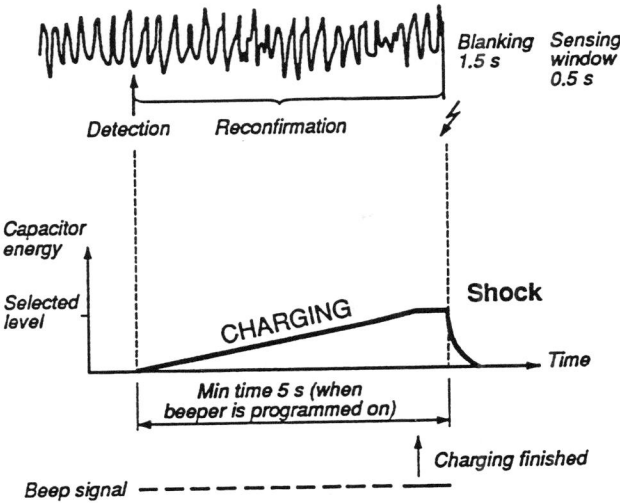

Figure 9 The system continues to reconfirm the presence of the tachycardia during charging of the output capacitor to deliver a shock. Once it is fully charged, there is a final reconfirmation before the shock is delivered. Once it is delivered, the system is incapable of sensing for 1500 ms, and this is followed by a 500-ms alert window. If nothing is sensed during this time period, bradycardia support pacing is initiated at the programmed base rate.

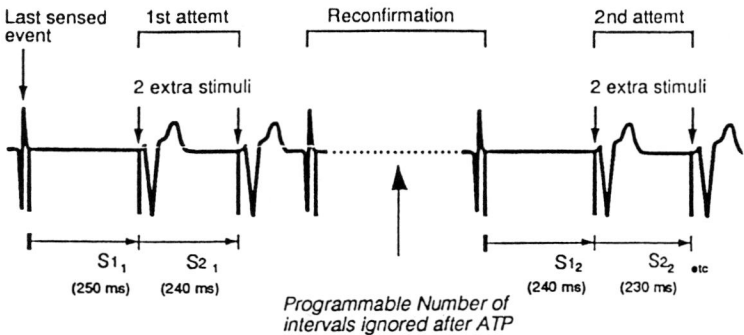

Figure 10 After delivery of an antitachycardia pacing attempt, there is a programmable number of sensed intervals where the system makes no attempt to confirm the success of the therapeutic intervention. Once this number of cycles ends, reconfirmation is resumed based only on rate criteria to determine if the next therapy in the sequence needs to be delivered.

With respect to antitachycardia pacing, there is a period of reconfirmation after each delivery of therapy. This is preceded by a programmable number of intervals which are ignored for purposes of diagnosing persistence of the tachycardia before reconfirmation is initiated (Fig. 10).

VI. THERAPEUTIC OPTIONS

With respect to tiered therapy, VT low or VT high can be treated by antitachycardia pacing followed by one or more series of shocks, by ATP only, or by shocks only. Ventricular fibrillation must be treated by shock therapy. If the ATP or low-energy shocks convert one of the ventricular tachycardias to ventricular fibrillation, VF therapy will go into effect immediately.

Antitachycardia pacing is defined as a sequence of stimuli coupled to a sensed event during a detected tachyarrhythmia in an effort to terminate that rhythm. Each extra stimulus or burst of pacing pulses is referred to as an *attempt*. The VT low and VT high tachycardias each have a separately programmable maximum number of attempts at ATP. ATP would utilize standard pacing pulses delivering energy in the microjoule energy range. This is virtually undetectable by the patient and, if successful, markedly reduces the battery current drain associated with each therapeutic intervention. Anywhere from 1 to 31 pulses can be provided during each antitachycardia attempt.

If more than five stimuli are programmed for a burst attempt, the programmer allows the timing of the first two (S1, S2) and the last two stimuli (S4, S5) of the attempt to be programmed individually if the physician desires. All the intervening cycles are at an S3 coupling interval. The minimum cycle length that can be programmed is 100 ms, and the maximum is 595 ms. Further, the bursts can be scanned with progressive decrements in intervals on successive bursts. The scanning step size is programmable from 2 to 40 ms (Fig. 11).

One can also alternate bursts between a primary burst set to one set of intervals and an alternate programmed to a second set of intervals (Fig. 12). The primary search will be followed by the alternate search, which will then return to the primary search if the ATP attempt was unsuccessful, until either the tachycardia is terminated or the programmed number of

Siecure

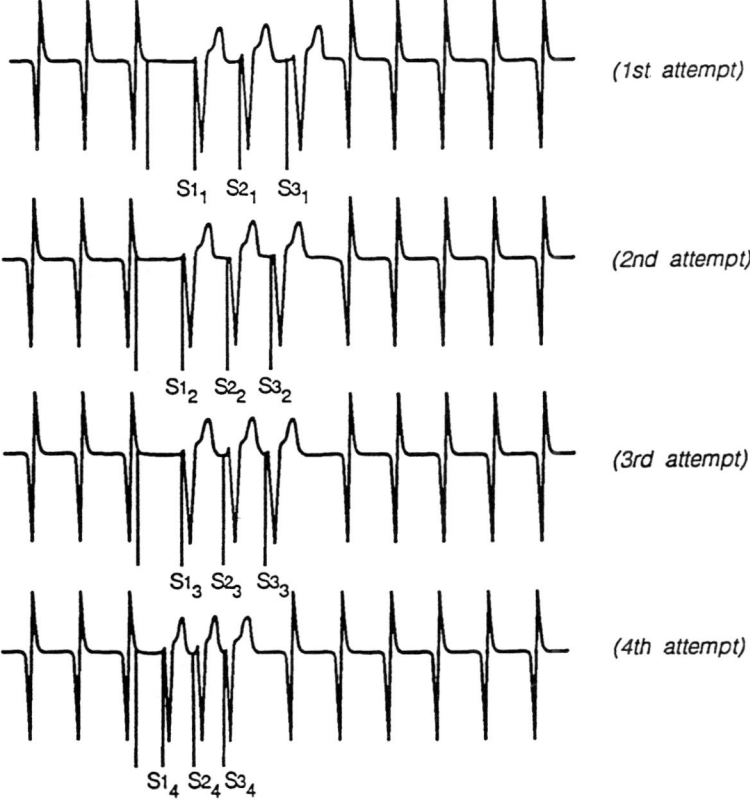

Programmed values: S1, S2 and S3 with *4 attempts*

Figure 11 A series of attempts at antitachycardia pacing demonstrating the scanning function by which each burst starts at a successively shorter coupling interval.

attempts have been completed, at which time the system will automatically move on to the next level of therapy (shock).

One of the concerns is that the programmable intervals for the burst may be longer than the tachycardia which develops. Thus, in the diagnosis phase, if the tachycardia cycle length is shorter than the initial S1 coupling interval, the system will automatically proceed to the first programmed coupling interval which is shorter than the tachycardia cycle length (Fig. 13).

With respect to ventricular fibrillation, only shock therapy is allowed. In choosing the number of shocks, one can program the device from 0.5 to 40 J. All shocks are synchronized to a sensed R wave delivered 30 ms after the R wave is sensed. Up to seven shocks can be programmed with respect to cardioversion (VT low and VT high). Only five shocks can be delivered when the diagnosed rhythm is ventricular fibrillation. These too are programmable, but for fibrillation the starting shock can be no lower than 10 J. It can then proceed up to 40 J. The shock is a monophasic, truncated exponential waveform with a pulse duration of 7.75 ms.

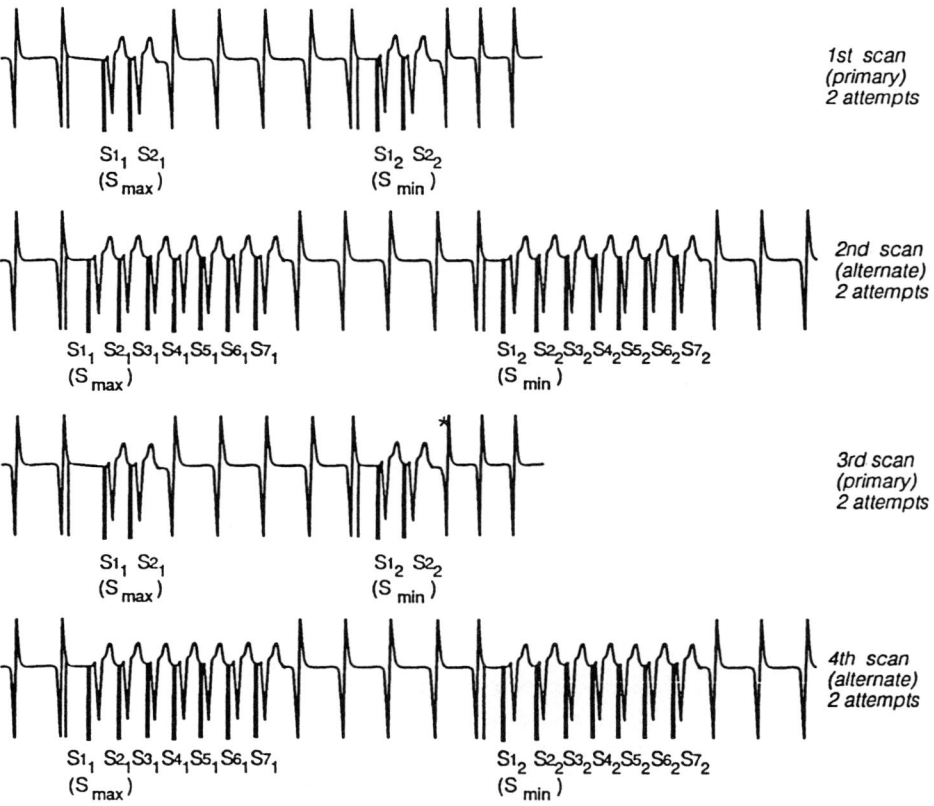

Figure 12 A diagrammatic representation of the alternation between primary and alternate antitachycardia therapy.

VII. SENSING OF VENTRICULAR TACHYCARDIA AND FIBRILLATION

At the time of implantation, capture and sensing thresholds are assessed routinely. However, the sensing threshold refers to the amplitude of the intrinsic deflection of the sinus or native ventricular depolarization. The amplitude of the intrinsic deflection associated with either ventricular tachycardia or ventricular fibrillation may be significantly smaller than that associated with sinus rhythm. The literature has reported fibrillation signals as being anywhere from 25% to only 10% of the intrinsic deflection of the sinus QRS complex. Recognition of the ventricular intrinsic deflection associated with both VT and VF is essential if the system is going to deliver the desired therapy. There are a number of ways by which optimal sensing is assured in the Siecure.

The first is the utilization of different refractory periods after a sensed and paced complex. Both VT high and VF are characterized by relatively rapid rates, commonly above 200 ppm, which means that the refractory period needs to be significantly shorter than 300 ms. In fact, the standard refractory period following a sensed complex is 140 ms, with a programmable range between 120 to 250 ms. T-wave oversensing, which is most commonly associated with

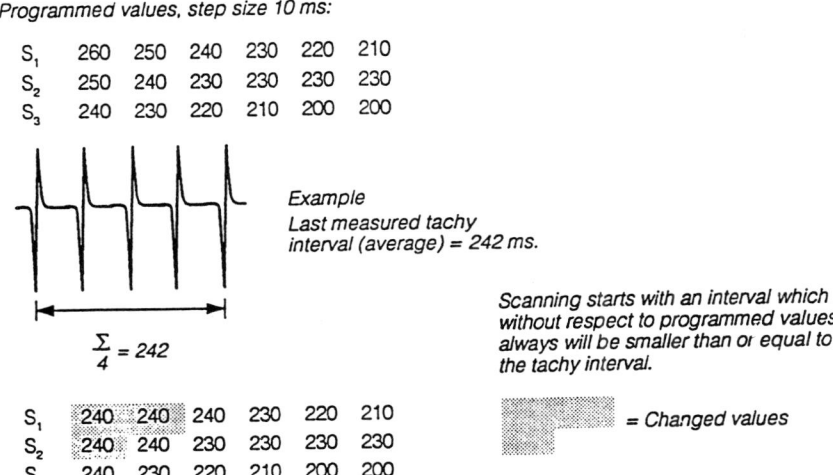

Figure 13 Schematic representation of the behavior of a Siecure should a tachycardia develop which has a shorter cycle length than the first and even second burst intervals. The pacemaker will start at the longest interval which is still shorter than the tachycardia cycle length and stay there for the requisite number of attempts until that stage in the sequence of attempts is reached.

paced beats, is prevented not only with the bandpass filter of the sense amplifier but by having a longer refractory period following release of an output pulse which is programmable from 250 to 500 ms.

The second method is a programmable feature termed *automatic sensitivity control* (ASC). It can be enabled or disabled. While one could simply program the pacemaker to its most sensitive setting, this would predispose to oversensing of T waves and other signals despite the bipolar sensing configuration, at which point there might be double and even triple counting with delivery of ATP or shock therapy when the rhythm was otherwise normal. ASC automatically adapts the sensitivity of the system, within limits, to the amplitude of the intracardiac signal during normal sinus rhythm, anticipating that the fibrillation signal will be a percentage of the sinus electrogram.

The automatic sensitivity control operates within a programmable range of parameters identified as minimum and maximum sensitivity. The minimum sensitivity is the least sensitive setting to which the device can automatically adjust itself, no matter how large the intracardiac signal. The maximum sensitivity is the most sensitive setting to which the system can automatically adjust itself. Sensitivity is identified by the amplitude of the signal which can be sensed, a high or maximum sensitivity being the ability to recognize a very small signal. Siecure is able to be programmed between a high sensitivity of 0.4 mV and a low of 5.7 mV. If a bradycardia pacing pulse is released, the ASC automatically programs the system to its most sensitive setting looking for low-amplitude ventricular fibrillation signals (Fig. 14).

VIII. EMI DETECTION CRITERIA AND RESPONSE

All ICDs are generally more sensitive to electromagnetic interference (EMI), despite the bipolar sensing configuration. The sense amplifier passed the European EMI draft requirements as defined in EN50061 from SENELEC. Each refractory period is divided into two

SIECURE:

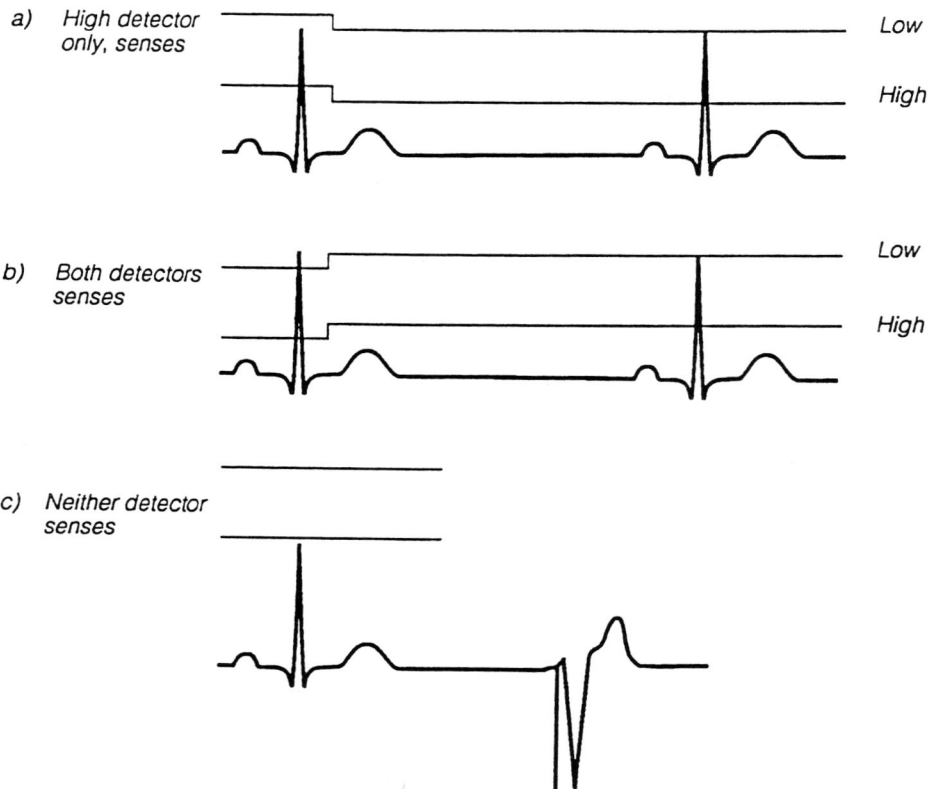

Figure 14 Schematic diagram of the automatic sensitivity control. If only the high detector senses (a), the sensitivity of the detectors is automatically adjusted to become more sensitive until the low sensor also detects the QRS. If both detectors (b) sense the QRS, the system becomes less sensitive until the low detector loses sensing. The system continues to modulate itself within the programmable range. If neither detector senses, bradycardia pacing is initiated and the system proceeds to its most sensitive setting to look for low-amplitude ventricular fibrillation.

subintervals—an absolute and a relative refractory period. This latter is also called a noise sampling period and is a fixed 30 ms in duration. If an event is sensed during the noise sampling period, a second, shorter refractory period is reset. It too is comprised of an absolute and a relative refractory period (Fig. 15). If there is continuous electrical noise, the refractory periods are repeatedly reset until the ventricular escape interval times out and ventricular output pulse is released at the programmed base rate. This is termed the noise reversion mode.

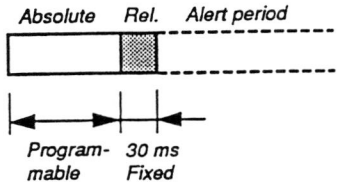

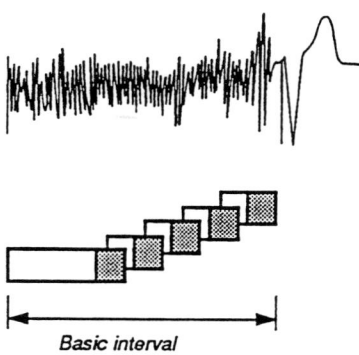

Figure 15 Schematic diagram of the absolute and relative refractory period and the behavior of the system in response to electrical noise.

The refractory period behaves differently after a paced event, after a sensed event, and after delivery of a shock. The refractory period after a sensed event is shorter than after a paced event. This facilitates the sensing of the rapid signals associated with ventricular tachycardia and fibrillation. It is lengthened after a paced event to minimize oversensing of the paced T wave. After a cardioversion or defibrillation shock has been delivered, no detection is feasible for 1500 ms. The terminal 30 ms of this 1500 ms is also a relative refractory period. This is then followed by a 500-ms alert period, giving a total escape interval of 2000 ms. If a cardiac depolarization is not sensed during the alert period, bradycardia pacing at the programmed rate is then initiated.

IX. DIAGNOSTIC TELEMETRY

As with most modern pacemakers, the ability to program the various parameters in the Siecure is based on a radiofrequency link from the programmer, P3060. Communication is at a speed of 2 kilobaud and has a block-oriented transmission with block check bytes with frequent checks to detect transmission faults. Active communication between the ICD and the programmer can continue even during device charging. Thus, one can continue to obtain telemetered intracardiac electrograms or event marker information during testing procedures such as predischarge DFT testing.

There are extensive diagnostic features in the Siecure. These include utilization of the implanted device for noninvasive EP testing, obtaining a multiplicity of measured data, real-time telemetered intracardiac electrograms, and even markers. In addition, implant data including lead model, position, and measurements can be entered into the random access memory of the Siecure for retrieval at the time of routine follow-up.

Noninvasive electrophysiological studies (NIEPS) can be obtained when the Siecure is used in combination with the programmer. In the model 2121, an external programmable stimulator can be slaved to the implanted device via the programmer, allowing the physician to do the NIEPS using the equipment that he is most familiar with. Premature stimuli as well as bursts can be used to induce either ventricular tachycardia or ventricular fibrillation via the pacing/sensing lead. If one wishes, the system can be used as a slave to the external device to also do antitachycardia pacing rather than relying on the algorithms programmed into the device. One also has the ability to deliver an emergency shock at any time during the study, even before the device is fully interrogated.

Extensive measured data is provided with regard to the battery current, battery voltage, and history of battery function. The system can display the relationship between the remaining voltage, RRT, and EOL. The Siecure automatically measures its battery voltage on a daily basis and can be set to initiate a regular beeping sound when the battery voltage reaches RRT. If it is determined that this would induce too much anxiety in the patient, the beeping function can be disabled, with the battery status reported at each routine follow-up when the system is interrogated.

The frequency with which the patient must be seen in the office for follow-up can be determined by the physician based on the clinical status of the patient. The prior requirement associated with the first generation of ICDs, mandating frequent office visits to reform the capacitors, is no longer necessary. While reforming the capacitors is still required to assure proper function, this has been incorporated in the Siecure as an automatic function that is done on a monthly basis.

X. ELECTROGRAM AND EVENT MARKER TELEMETRY

Real-time endocardial electrograms from the sense/pacing lead can be telemetered to the programmer by being displayed on the LCD screen as well as by being printed. They may also be sent to the external input of a standard ECG machine and recorded in this manner as well. Electrograms can continue to be telemetered during a pathological tachycardia, even while the system is charging to deliver a shock.

In addition, there are event markers that can be obtained from the implanted system. The markers are variable-amplitude pulses that will be displayed and recorded simultaneously with a surface ECG (Fig. 16). Markers identify paced and sensed complexes, end of the refractory period, VF and VT detection (a large marker is released when the diagnostic criteria are met), and upon confirmation of tachycardia termination.

XI. TEMPORARY MODE

One can also program the Siecure to a set of temporary parameters for performing capture and sensing threshold tests. At either the end of the test sequence or if telemetry contact is interrupted during the testing sequence, the unit promptly returns to its initially programmed pa-

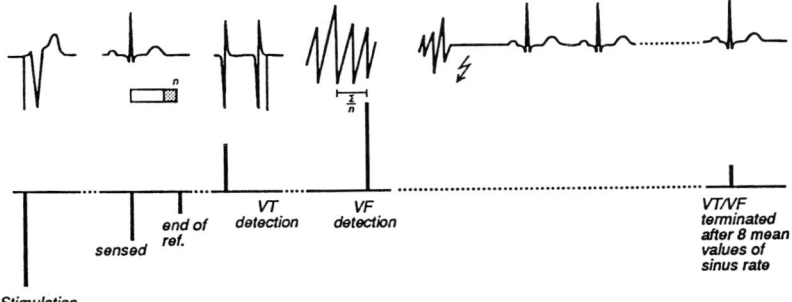

1. Stimulus and start of total refractory period. (-0.75V)
2. Detection outside total refractory period and start of total refractory period. (-0.5V)
3. End of total refractory period.(-0.25V)
4. VT detected all criteria fulfilled (+0.5V)
5. VF detected all criteria fulfilled (+0.75V)
6. VT/VF terminated (+0.25V)

Figure 16 Diagrammatic representation of the various event markers utilized in the Siecure. The downward pulses refer to bradycardia pacing events and the upright pulses identify tachyarrhythmias.

rameters to minimize the chances of asystole, under- or oversensing that might occur during the evaluation sequence.

All of the telemetered data can be either printed via the P3060 programmer/printer or dumped directly into a PC database such as the Patientlog database system, which was originally developed as a PC-based system for data collection with respect to bradycardia pacing systems.

XII. EVENT COUNTERS AND OTHER DATA STORAGE

The Siecure has the capability of storing a variety of data, which is obtainable at the time of routine office follow-up utilizing the P3060 programmer. This includes administrative data and extensive event counters.

XIII. ADMINISTRATIVE DATA

Utilizing the programmer, basic data can be stored in the device. This includes the models and serial numbers not only of the ICD but of the various lead systems, their locations and dates of implantation, patient and physician identifying information, as well as a cryptic patient history (Fig. 17). All of this can be printed at the beginning at each follow-up visit.

XIV. EVENT COUNTER TELEMETRY

The event counter in the Siecure collects the number of paced and sensed events, the numbers and types of tachycardias recognized, the therapeutic trials, and results of these interventions, all with respect to real time, as there is a real-time clock in the Siecure. Examples of the data

```
SIEMENS                        Siecure®
Software version: 3061f
10 Apr 1992 14:22

Model: P63                     Serial: 1400-63298
Patient ID:                    Implant date: 19 Mar 1992
Hospital:
```

INITIAL ADMINISTRATIVE DATA

```
Last Program. .. 19 Mar 1992 13:36    Implant Date ......... 19 Mar 1992
Name ....................              Physician .............
Patient ID ....................        Hospital ..............
```

Doctors Notes

Lead Data

```
Pace/Sense:
 1 ID ..........................
        Position .............. UNSPEC.
 2 ID ..........................
        Position .............. UNSPEC.
Shocking:
 1 ID ..........................
        Position .............. UNSPEC.
 2 ID ..........................
        Position .............. UNSPEC.
```

Device Data

```
Connectors:
Pace/Sense 1 ................... T
Pace/Sense 2 ................... K
Shocking 1 ................... DEF
Shocking 2 ................... DEF

Program Version ............ 07.e3
Battery ID ................ WG8615
```

INITIAL BASIC PARAMETERS

```
Mode ............. VVI          Pulse Amplitude ... 5.4 V
Basic Rate ........ 80 ppm      Pulse Width ...... 0.50 ms
Hysteresis Rate .... 40 bpm     Refractory Sensed . 140 ms
ASC ............... ON          Refractory Paced .. 350 ms
Min. Sensitivity .. 4.5 mV
Max. Sensitivity .. 0.7 mV
```

Figure 17 Administrative data which can be stored in the random-access memory of the Siecure for retrieval at any follow-up visit.

which will be stored and reported for a VT episode (are shown in Fig. 18.) From within this database, specific episodes can be examined in greater detail. If a therapy is unsuccessful, this too will be shown (Fig. 19a), and one can examine the next level of intervention (Fig. 19b). Data are retained for documentation purposes if any antitachycardia therapy is initiated, even it is unsuccessful. By referring to the date and time, since there is a real-time clock in the Siecure, one can reconstruct the sequence of events. In addition, data with respect to the 32

Diagnostic Data/VT High Episodes 1(2)							
Date	Time	Rate	Term.	Date	Time	Rate	Term.
89-Mar-30	10:07	190	Yes	89-Feb-17	06:38	187	Yes
89-Mar-27	22:13	182	Yes	89-Jan-31	14:30	197	Yes
89-Mar-21	06:44	130	Yes	89-Jan-29	10:01	210	Yes
89-Mar-16	16:07	192	No	89-Jan-25	03:25	216	Yes
89-Mar-03	15:18	193	Yes				NEXT
				Clear	Read	Initial	RETURN

Diagnostic Data/VT High Episodes 1(2)		
89-Jan-29 10:01	Therapy Successful	
Detection Rate .... 210 bpm	Term. Coupling Int: S1 .... 250 ms	
	S2 .... 230 ms	
Preceded by VT Low .... 130 bpm	S3-S5 .... 220 ms	
	S6 .... 210 ms	
No of Extra Stimuli Attempts 15	S7 .... 210 ms	
No of Stimuli in Last Attempt 7	RETURN	

Figure 18 Representative data which is stored for a series of VT episodes, and the data available for each individual episode.

intervals preceding and following delivery of the last three therapies in each rate zone are retained and are retrievable at the time of follow-up.

The event-counter data can be displayed as tables (Fig. 18) as well as histograms (Fig. 20). Sixteen arrhythmic episodes in each rate zone can be stored with respect to the exact time and date of each, the therapy which was initiated, and whether or not it was successful in terminating the arrhythmia. Histograms showing the extrastimuli attempts to treat VT low, to treat VT high, cardioversion energies for VT low and VT high, defibrillation energies, and tachyarrhythmia rates are all stored and retrievable as desired by the physician.

XV. CLINICAL EXPERIENCE

As of November 1992, there have been 35 ICD implants in Europe, the last five of which were nonthoracotomy lead systems utilizing a transvenous lead and subcutaneous patch. The results have been excellent. The experience with the first six implants at Guy's Hospital in London has been published [1] demonstrating the effectiveness of the antitachycardia pacing algorithms as well as the shocks. There have been no patient deaths attributable to failure to sense ventricular fibrillation or to terminate a tachycardia, but the experience is still small and the patients have been carefully selected at a limited number of centers.

XVI. FUTURE DEVELOPMENTS

Actively under development is a a dual-chamber, rate-modulated bradycardia support system with full antitachycardia pacing and defibrillation capability. It would be identified by the NBG code as DDDRD. The rationale behind this very complex system is that the majority of patients who require ICD therapy have marked ventricular dysfunction. If they require pacing

VT High Episodes

1991 Jul 16 04:48   *Therapy not successful*

Detection rate .... 179 bpm
Predetection rate .... 113 bpm
Cycle length stability .... 44 ms

No of extra stimuli attempts...3
No of stimuli in last attempt...5

Figure 19A   Representative data for an episode of ventricular tachycardia which did not convert with ATP therapy. In fact, it accelerated the rhythm to ventricular fibrillation.

support, they will benefit from maintenance of AV synchrony, assuming that the atrial function is intact. In addition, there has been recent work suggesting that dual-chamber pacing with a short AV delay may be beneficial as a primary therapy for dilated myopathic ventricles [2,3], in which case the primary mode of exit becomes sudden death rather than progressive congestive heart failure. It is further proposed that a hemodynamic sensor can be utilized to help determine which tachyarrhythmias are hemodynamically stable versus unstable as a further guide to therapy, ATP versus proceeding directly to delivery of a shock even if the rate criteria indicate the rhythm is ventricular tachycardia for which ATP therapy was prescribed as the first tier of treatment.

This new system will have programmable shock pulse morphology (monophasic, biphasic), as well as extensive diagnostics including stored electrograms combined historical data as to arrhythmia diagnosis and intervention as presently incorporated in the Siecure and bradycardia pacing system behavior as implemented in the Synchrony series of pacemakers [4].

VF Episodes

1991 Jul 16 04:48

Detection rate.............. 219 bpm   Preceded by VT High....179 bpm
No of shock in sequence...3   VT to VF time ....16.0 sec
Energy in last shock........40 J   No of extra stim attempts 3
Charge time for   No of stim in last attempt 5
last shock....................11.5 sec

Figure 19B   The continuation of the data from Fig. 19a but now showing the response including time since the initial diagnosis of VT until the rhythm was successfully terminated with a shock.

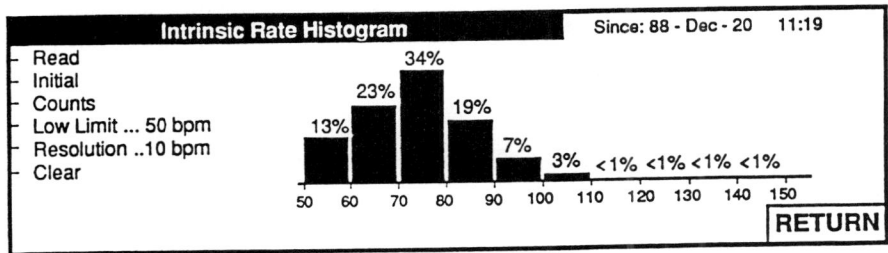
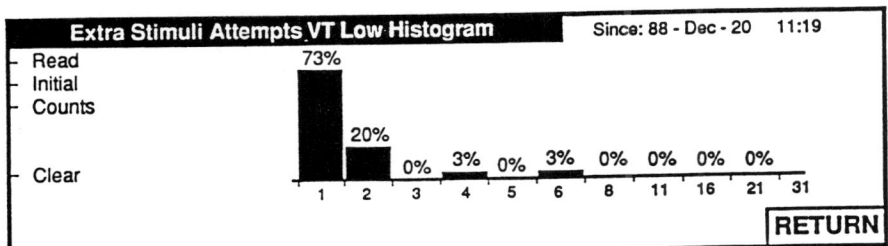
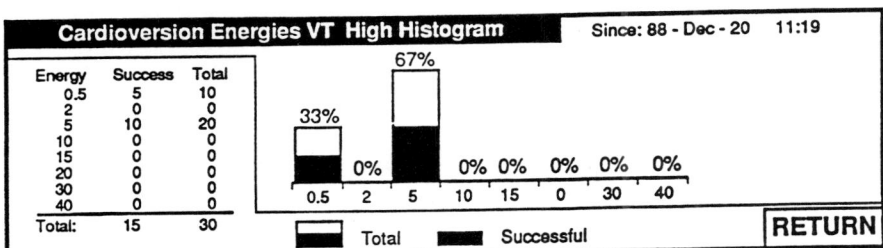
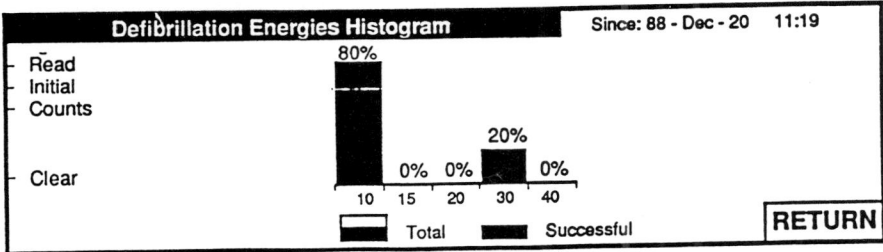

Figure 20 Representative histograms showing intrinsic rates, the number of extrastimuli attempts for VT low, the cardioversion energies used to treat VT high, and the defibrillation energies utilized since the last time each of these histograms was cleared.

REFERENCES

1. Sowton E, Sulke N. Clinical experience with the Siemens Pacesetter Siecure. J Cardiovasc Electrophysiol 1992; 3:515–522.
2. Hochleitner M, Hortnagl H, Hortnagl H, et al. Long-term efficacy of physiologic dual-chamber pacing in the treatment of end-stage idiopathic dilated cardiomyopathy. Am J Cardiol 1992; 70:1320–1325.
3. Brecker SJD, Xiao HB, Sparrow J, Gibson DG. Effects of dual-chamber pacing with short atrioventricular delay in dilated cardiomyopathy. Lancet 1992; 340:1308–1312.
4. Levine PA. Utility and clinical benefit of extensive event counter telemetry in the follow-up and management of the rate modulated pacemaker patient. Siemens Pacesetter Inc. Sylmar, Calif., Feb 1992.

43

The AngeMed Sentinel Implantable Antitachycardia Pacer Cardioverter-Defibrillator

Patrick J. Tchou

*University of Pittsburgh
and University of Pittsburgh Medical Center
Pittsburgh, Pennsylvania*

Mark W. Kroll

*AngeMed, Division of Angeion Corporation
Plymouth, Minnesota*

I. INTRODUCTION

The future of implantable antitachycardia device therapy lies in the direction of smaller devices, nonthoracotomy transvenous lead systems, and more energy-efficient defibrillation pathways and waveforms. These devices will incorporate antitachycardia pacing, low-energy cardioversion, as well as high-energy defibrillation shock therapy. They will also have the capability of low rate pacing to prevent excessive bradycardia, especially following delivery of antitachycardia therapy. There has been considerable progress in this field within the last decade. The initial human implants involved devices which delivered an unsynchronized shock having a monophasic, truncated exponential waveform during ventricular tachycardia/fibrillation. Recently approved "third-generation" devices can deliver biphasic shocks, perform antitachycardia pacing therapy using sophisticated algorithms, apply low-energy synchronized shocks for cardioverting ventricular tachycardia, use nonthoracotomy lead systems, and offer bradycardia pacing, all in a single device. However, there is still much to be improved. The current devices are relatively large and are not suitable for subpectoral implantation. They require implantation subcutaneously over the abdomen. Subpectoral implantation would offer several advantages. The length of a transvenous lead system can be shortened considerably, thus improving handling during implantation and reducing potential sources of malfunction. The surgical procedure can be simplified to be similar to a pacemaker implant. Subpectoral implant of the device can also offer an alternative subcutaneous electrode that is defined by the container of the device itself.

The optimal defibrillator waveform, pulse amplitude, and pulse duration combination has yet to be clearly defined. Clearly, devices that can take advantage of developing knowledge in this field and improve defibrillation thresholds would facilitate the development of generators which are small enough for subpectoral implantation. The Angemed Sentinel is a device that is aimed at taking advantage of the developing knowledge in the field of cardiac defibrillation and recent technological developments in the electronics field to achieve some of the above desired goals. The device will have two models, a full-featured model (2002) with complex diagnostic and therapeutic pacing modalities which will be described in this chapter, and a model 2000 prophylactic device for those patients who may need all the features of the model 2002.

II. PHYSICAL PARAMETERS OF THE DEVICE

A model of the device with its lead system is shown in Fig. 1. The physical dimensions are 3.18 in. length, 2.46 in. width, and 0.65 in. thickness. The device will have a weight of 115 g and a volume of 60 cm^3. The header of the device will have four sockets that will allow insertion of a transvenous lead, a subcutaneous patch electrode, and a sense/pace lead. In addition, the container of the generator itself can serve as one of the shocking electrodes. All lead connections to the device will be via standard DF1 connectors. While the device can be used with conventional epicardial patch electrode systems, its size and weight make it most suitable for subpectoral implantation with a subcutaneous and transvenous lead system.

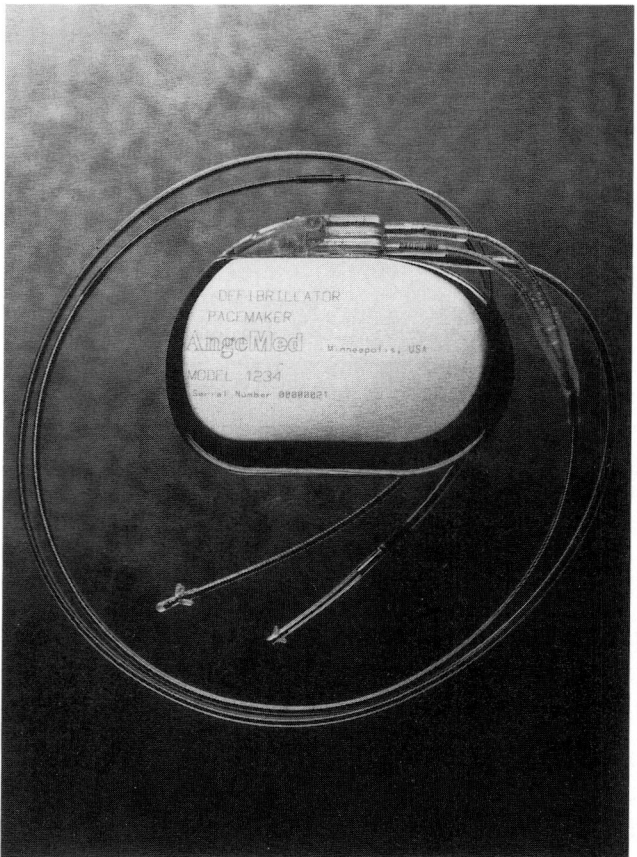

Figure 1 Photograph of the AngeMed defibrillator and transvenous lead system. Note the comparable size of the shocking electrode to the pacing and sensing electrode. Dimensions and other specifications are listed in the text.

III. ENERGY SOURCE AND EXPECTED LONGEVITY

In order to take advantage of the available battery technology for optimizing the longevity of such devices, the Sentinel will utilize a dual power source. Lithium Iodide batteries with lower voltage and current outputs, but higher energy density, are used to power the monitoring circuits and operate the initial detection circuitry in the device. A lithium silver vanadium pentoxide battery, which has a higher voltage and current output, is used to power pacing and shock delivery. This dual-power-source approach could improve longevity of the device by matching the voltage and current outputs of the batteries to the demands of its function. The design of the system would also allow use of the vanadium pentoxide battery to power the monitoring circuits once the lithium iodide batteries start to lose power. The switching of the power source for the monitoring portion of the device from the lithium iodide batteries to the vanadium pentoxide batteries can extend the life of the device considerably, depending on prior energy depletion with shocks or pacing. Figure 2 is an illustration of the projected device longevity based on reception of one shock per month and no pacing. The faster drop in the remaining shock counts after 60 months is due to switching of the power source for monitoring from the lithium iodide cell to the vanadium pentoxide battery. Based on this scenario, one can expect a longevity of approximately 6 years in a typical patient.

IV. LEAD SYSTEM

While the Sentinel is capable of utilizing standard epicardial patch systems, it is designed primarily for use with a transvenous electrode together with a subcutaneous patch electrode. The electrode systems are also illustrated in Fig. 1. The transvenous lead has a diameter of 6.5 Fr. The length of the distal shocking coil electrode is 8 cm, with a surface area of 4.14 cm^2. This

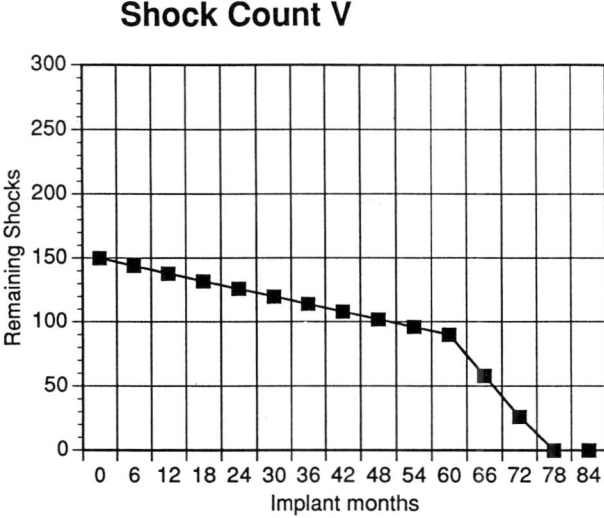

Figure 2 Projected longevity of the AngeMed device based on no pacing and one shock per month. The device has a dual power supply, one for monitoring and a second one for pacing and shock delivery (see text for details). However, once the monitoring circuit power supply becomes depleted, the device then switches entirely to operating from the pacing and shocking power source. The graph shows this switch occurring at approximately 60 months thus prolonging useful device life for another 12 months.

somewhat-longer-than-usual electrode has been demonstrated to yield lower defibrillation thresholds in animal studies [1]. The proximal electrode is designed to be located in the high right atrium or superior vena cava. It is located at various distances from the tip of the catheter. It is 5.2 cm in length and has a surface area of 2.70 cm^2. A subcutaneous patch electrode could also be used with this system to enhance defibrillation efficacy. A unique feature of this device is the ability to use the device container as one of the electrodes. For cardioversion or defibrillation, shocks can be delivered from the distal shocking electrode to the proximal electrode, to the subcutaneous patch, or to the device canister. Alternatively, a combination of these pairs can be used. The specific combination will be programmable. A unique feature of this device is the ability to deliver a QRS synchronized shock from the proximal lead electrode to the subcutaneous patch. This pathway of delivered current would be suitable for cardioverting atrial fibrillation or flutter.

V. ARRHYTHMIA DETECTION AND THERAPY ZONES

The device will have five detection zones for cardiac rhythm. The bradycardia pacing zone will have a programmable upper limit of 40 to 120 beats/min. Between a detected heart rate of zero and the upper programmed rate of this zone, the device would deliver bradycardia pacing through the tip electrode and the defibrillation cathode. The next higher rate zone is the "no therapy" zone. The upper limit of this zone is programmable from 120 to 250 beats/min. Within this zone, no therapy would be delivered. This zone is typically used to define the expected range of normal rhythm for a patient that does not overlap with tachyarrhythmia rates. Above the "no therapy" zone, there will be three tachycardia detection zones. The upper rate limits of these zones are programmable from 120 to 250 beats/min. The lowest of these tachyarrhythmia zones is designed primarily for response to slower ventricular tachyarrhythmia, which would typically be readily treatable with antitachycardia pacing or lower-energy cardioversion. All forms of therapy will be available in this zone, including antitachycardia pacing, lower-energy cardioversion, and high-energy defibrillation. A maximum of five sequential forms of therapy would be available for each episode of tachyarrhythmia. The next higher zone of tachycardia detection essentially allows the same type of therapeutic programming as the lowest zone. That is, antitachycardia pacing and low-energy cardioversion as well as high-energy defibrillation are all available. However, the last three of the five treatment forms are mandated to be maximum-energy shocks. In the highest tachyarrhythmia zone, all therapies are mandated to be at the highest defibrillation shock output. Presumably, this zone would be used to treat extremely rapid (>250 beats/min) monomorphic or polymorphic ventricular tachycardia as well as ventricular fibrillation. This arrhythmia therapy scheme is illustrated in Fig. 3.

Besides heart rate, several other parameters can be used to enhance the accuracy of tachycardia detection. These include sudden onset, rate stability, and a "rate modal change index." The latter is a rate distribution comparison of beats before and after the rate cutoff criterion is met. This parameter has been successful in discriminating exercise-induced high sinus rates from ventricular tachycardia is preliminary studies (unpublished observations from AngeMed, Inc.) These detection enhancements can be programmed only in the first and second tachyarrhythmia detection zones.

VI. ANTITACHYCARDIA PACING THERAPY

Antitachycardia pacing will consist of a series of overdrive pacing impulses delivered through the pacing lead of the system. There are multiple parameters of antitachycardia pacing which can be altered with telemetry programming. The cycle length of the burst of pacing impulses

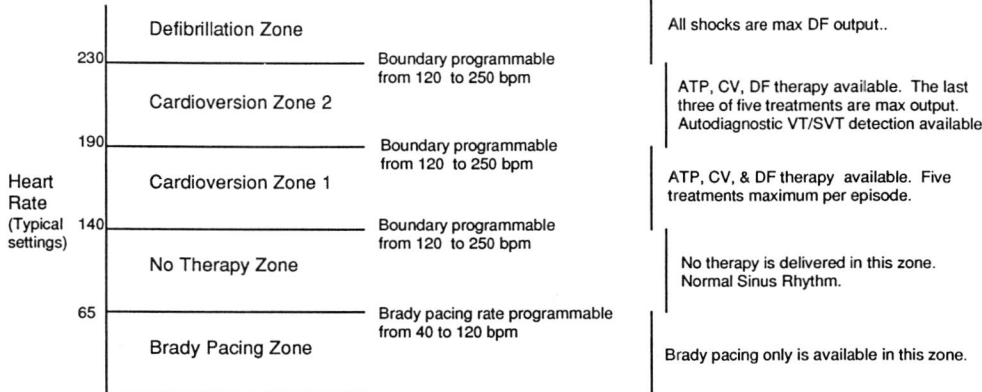

Figure 3 Therapy zones of the AngeMed defibrillator. The figure illustrates the programmable therapy zones and the type of therapy available in each zone. See text for details.

is programmable as a percentage of the detected tachycardia cycle length from 60% to 90%. The coupling interval of the first paced impulse to the last sensed electrogram will be equal to the burst cycle length. The number of pulses in the burst will be programmable from 1 to 250 beats. The maximum number of pacing bursts in an antitachycardia pacing sequence will be programmable from 1 to 50. Within a sequence, the number of impulses in sequential bursts can be incremented using a feature labeled "burst pulse increment." When activated, one pulse is added to each subsequent burst until the pulse increment limit is reached. This limit will be programmable.

Each subsequent burst can also be programmed to have a shorter cycle length. This feature, labeled "scan decrement," will allow shortening of a burst cycle length from the preceding burst by a fixed decrement (5, 10, 15, 20, or 25 ms) or by a percentage from the preceding burst cycle length (5, 10, or 15%).

Within a burst, each sequential pulse can have a decremented interval as programmed by a feature called "ramp decrement." When activated, each pulse within a burst following the first one can be decremented by a fixed value (5, 10, 15, 20, or 25 ms) or a percentage of the preceding interval (5, 10, or 15%). A minimum cycle length will be programmable (200 to 400 ms), which will apply to burst pulses. When the minimum cycle length is reached, subsequent bursts of pulses within a burst will have the minimum cycle length. When the maximum number of bursts has been delivered in a particular antitachycardia protocol, it can be repeated from 0 to 10 times as programmed. If a tachycardia persists beyond the repeated protocols, the next programmed therapy is activated. As a safety feature, there will be an antitachycardia pacing therapy time-out. This will be programmable from 10 s to 30 min. If the time-out is reached during antitachycardia pacing, therapy progresses to the first shock in the programmed regimen, skipping any intervening antitachycardia pacing.

Antitachycardia pacing pulse amplitude will not be programmable. The pacing amplitude will be at the voltage output of the lithium silver vanadium pentoxide battery, which will be approximately 6 V at beginning of life (two 3-V cells in series). Antitachycardia pacing therapy is available in the lowest and the middle zones of antitachycardia therapy. In the lowest zone, all therapies can be defined as antitachycardia therapy. In the middle zone, only the first two therapies can be defined as antitachycardia pacing therapies. The remaining three therapies must be a defibrillation shock at maximum energy. In the highest tachycardia therapy zone, all therapy must be at the maximum shock output, and antitachycardia pacing is not available.

VII. LOW-VOLTAGE CARDIOVERSION AND HIGH-VOLTAGE DEFIBRILLATION

Recent studies have suggested that a smaller capacitor may optimize the defibrillation energy requirement [2,3]. While the use of smaller capacitors may require somewhat higher voltages for defibrillation, energy requirements may be lower than the standard capacitors used in currently available implantable devices, which use a 140- or 150-μF capacitor. The savings in energy translates into longer battery life. More important, however, the use of smaller capacitors allows a reduction of device size to the extent that subpectoral implantation is feasible. The Sentinel will have defibrillation output that is biphasic. It will utilize a truncated exponential waveform. After a 44% tilt, the waveform is extended by 1.6 ms. At this point, the waveform is inverted to produce a second phase. The second phase will have a pulse width of 2.5 ms. Given a typical 50-Ω resistance across defibrillation electrodes, the first phase will have approximately a 60% tilt and a pulse width of 4.1 ms. The rationale for using such waveforms is based on the idea that defibrillation, like pacing, has a representative chronaxie and a rheobase [4,5]. The capacitor size, pulse duration, and waveform of the Sentinel are based on values that would be closer to the defibrillation chronaxie time than values used in currently approved defibrillation devices. The above-quoted experimental studies [2,3] suggest that such waveforms may indeed be more efficient.

Another unique feature of this device is the ability to proportionally deliver the energy of a shock to various electrode combinations, independent of the impedance between the electrodes. This is accomplished by initiating the shock in one direction, for example, between the right ventricular apex electrode (cathode) and a subcutaneous patch (anode). At a programmable delay after initiation of the shock, an additional electrode, for example, the superior vena cava electrode, can be connected as one of the anodes. The latter portion of the shock can be directed from the right ventricular apex electrodes toward both the subcutaneous patch and the superior vena cava electrode. This approach permits the rationing of total energy delivered in the two different directions in a manner that could not be accomplished if the shock was delivered in both directions simultaneously. In the latter case, the rationing would be predetermined by the respective impedances. However, by allowing the programmable delay before incorporation of a second electrode direction, there is more control over the amount of energy directed at the second electrode. This concept of "energy steering" may be useful in optimizing defibrillation thresholds. The maximum leading edge voltage of the device is 750 V, and the maximum stored energy is 27 J. However, the output of a shock can be programmed to have a leading-edge voltage of 50 to 750 V.

Lower-voltage shocks are frequently adequate for converting monomorphic ventricular tachycardias that do not respond to overdrive pacing. Another unique feature of the Sentinel is the shorter pulse width of a low-energy shock, meant to cardiovert monomorphic ventricular tachycardia. These shocks are delivered using a 2-ms pulse width and are monophasic and thus will not have low trailing-edge voltages associated with conventional cardioverting shocks constrained to have the same pulse width as a defibrillating shock. Such a shock with shorter pulse width may provide the advantage of being less proarrhythmic.

VIII. DIAGNOSTIC CAPABILITIES

In the full-featured model (2002), the device will have a range of transtelephonic diagnostic capabilities. This includes a patient interrogator module which the patient can place over the device to interrogate it. The patient can do this on schedule, on request, or when concerned. The interrogator will then display a code or sequence of codes which the patient can relay over the telephone to the physician's office. These codes will alert the physician to any potential problems with the device. For example, a code could state that the patient had a brief high sinus rate or received an appropriate shock. The patient interrogator can also be set into a transtelephonic fax machine. The fax machine can then transmit a full interrogation report to the physician's office. This would include not only the programmed therapeutic modalities but also arrhythmic events, therapeutic interventions, and a stored electrogram associated with these events with up to 240 s of recording. Such a report would also include battery status and any battery end-of-life indices.

IX. EXTERNAL SYSTEM PROGRAMMER AND EXTERNAL DEFIBRILLATOR

The system programmer will be a standard PC with appropriate off-the-shelf hardware and dedicated software to communicate and control the various components. It will communicate with the various components via standardized communication ports. One of these components will be the programming wand used to program the implantable defibrillator generator. The device can also be used to perform noninvasive programmed electrical stimulation as guided by the external programmer. A second component is the external defibrillator. The system programmer will be used to control the external defibrillator to be used during intraoperative testing of the pacing and defibrillating lead system. The external defibrillator will have a cable system that will attach to the patient's leads during implantation.

X. CONCLUSIONS

Certainly, implantable cardioverter-defibrillator therapy has advanced considerably since its initiation in the early 1980s. The ability to implant a subpectoral unit with nonthoracotomy leads will represent a significant advance in reducing the morbidity and mortality associated with implantation of these devices. The Sentinel will offer this ability. It is hoped that implantation of these devices in the future can become technically similar to pacemaker implantation.

REFERENCES

1. Leonelli FM, Kuo CS, Kroll MW, Koch C, Anderson KM. Increased right ventricular coil length lowers defibrillation thresholds despite reduction in catheter diameter and total electrode surface. PACE 1993; 16(4, part II):887.
2. Leonelli FM, Kuo CS, Fujimura O, Kroll MW, Koch C. Defibrillation thresholds are lower with small output capacitor values. PACE 1993; 16(4, part II):888.
3. Rist K, Kroll M, Mowrey K, et al. Comparison of epicardial defibrillation energy requirement using 140 and 85 microfarad capacitors. PACE 1993; 16(4, part II):914.
4. Kroll M, Lehman, Tchou P. Defining a defibrillation dosage. In: Kroll M, Lehmann LH, eds. Implantable Cardioverter Defibrillator Therapy. Boston: Kluwer, 1993.
5. Kroll MW. A minimal model of the monophasic defibrillation pulse. PACE 1993; 16(4, part I):769.

44

The Ventritex Cadence Tiered-Therapy Defibrillator: Device Description and Clinical Experience

Michael J. Reiter

*University of Colorado Health Sciences Center
and University Hospital
Denver, Colorado*

I. GENERAL DESCRIPTION

The introduction of implantable devices capable of antitachycardia pacing and defibrillation has expanded the population of patients with ventricular arrhythmias who can be effectively treated with device therapy. The Ventritex Cadence model V-100 tiered-therapy defibrillator is a multiprogrammable antitachycardia device, capable of antitachycardia pacing, cardioversion, and defibrillation, with backup ventricular pacing. The device has recently completed clinical trials in the United States.

In addition to ventricular fibrillation, tachycardia detection options allow for identification of up to two separate tachycardias (tachycardias A and B), with different termination strategies for each. A programmable monophasic/biphasic cardioversion/defibrillation waveform can be utilized. Persistence of tachycardia is reassessed during and after capacitor charging and before shock delivery. The Cadence model V-100 pulse generator has extensive tachyarrhythmia diagnostic capabilities. A valuable feature is the capability of recording and storing continuous bipolar ventricular electrograms of arrhythmias that trigger antitachycardia therapy.

Noninvasive programmed stimulation for induction of both ventricular tachycardia and ventricular fibrillation is possible, simplifying postoperative evaluation and troubleshooting.

II. DESCRIPTION OF PROGRAMMED DEVICE PARAMETERS

Available implantable antitachycardia devices require extensive programmability to provide the flexibility necessary to manage changing clinical situations (e.g., changing antiarrhythmic therapy) in patients with ventricular arrhythmias. Initial experience with the Cadence model V-100 suggests that reprogramming of device parameters is frequent after hospital discharge and is often based on review of telemetered diagnostic data and stored intracardiac electrograms [1]. An outline of the specific programmable features of the device is provided in Table 1.

Table 1 Programmable Features Available in the Ventritex Cadence Model V-100 Tiered-Therapy Defibrillator

Function	Options
Configuration	All functions off; bradycardia pacing only; defibrillator; defibrillator with one or two tachycardias
Fibrillation detection	
Detection rate (or interval)	140–222 beats/min (430–270 ms)[a]
Detection time	Nominal; fast; slow
Ventricular tachycardia detection	
Detection rate	102–200 beats/min (590–300 ms)
Duration[b]	6–100 beats
Sudden-onset criterion	On; off
Sudden-onset change	50–500 ms
Extended high rate (EHR) detection	On; off
EHR time	10 s–5 min
EHR rate[c]	Tachycardia CL–fibrillation CL
Cardioversion/defibrillation	
Capacitor voltage	50–750 V[d]
Waveform	Biphasic; monophasic
Pulse duration[e]	3.0–12.0 ms
Number of attempts	2–6
Antitachycardia therapy	
Burst pacing	On; off
Burst pacing rate	Fixed (200–550 ms); adaptive (50–100% average tachycardia CL)
Burst duration	2–20 stimuli
Burst pacing attempts	1–15
Autodecremental burst	On; off
Intraburst step size	5–25 ms
Scanning burst	Decremental; decrem/increm; off
Scanning step size	5–25 ms
Minimum burst CL	150–600 ms
Pulse amplitude[f]	1–10 V
Pulse width[f]	0.5–2.0 ms
Ventricular Demand Pacing	On; off
Demand rate	25–90 beats/min
Pulse amplitude[f]	1–10 V
Pulse width[f]	0.1–2.0 ms
Refractory period	350–500 ms
Posttherapy pause	0–15 sensed or suppressed paced events
Electrogram memory	On; off
Number of events	1; 3; 7[g]
Events stored	Fibrillation; tachycardia; EHR; all
Trigger	Therapy delivery; return to sinus rhythm
Pretrigger duration	1–60 s[h]
Noninvasive stimulation	
Programmed stimulation	On; off
Number of drive beats	1–20 beats
CL of drive train	140–960 ms
Number of ES	1–3
Coupling interval of ES	140–960 ms

Table 1 Continued

Function	Options
Pulse amplitude[f]	1–10 V
Pulse width[f]	0.5–2.0 ms
Fibrillation induction[i]	On; off
Number of stimuli	25–250
CL of drive train	20–50 ms
Pulse amplitude[f]	1–10 V
Pulse width[f]	0.5–2.0 ms

Abbreviations: CL = cycle length; ES = extrastimulus
[a]Fibrillation detection rate options differ slightly depending on programmed configuration.
[b]Minimum number of intervals satisfying rate criteria.
[c]Nominally equal to the tachycardia cycle length, but can be programmed separately.
[d]Energy (in joules) for selected voltage, waveform, pulse width, and impedance is displayed by the programmer.
[e]For biphasic waveforms, the pulse width of the positive and negative phases may be programmed independently.
[f]Independently programmable for antitachycardia pacing, bradycardia pacing, and noninvasive stimulation.
[g]Number of events selected for storage determines the duration of each stored event.
[h]Number of events selected for storage determines pretrigger duration options.
[i]Fibrillation induction requires a two-step programmer function as a safety precaution.

The Cadence model V-100 pulse generator can be programmed to one of three different antitachycardia configurations (in addition to an inactive mode or as a bradycardia pacemaker only): as a defibrillator with zero, one, or two additional tachycardia discriminations, with each having distinct rate recognition ranges and antitachycardia responses.

Fibrillation detection is based on rate. The time necessary to detect fibrillation can be adjusted and is generally under 3 s (nominal setting). Tachycardia recognition depends on rate and duration parameters. Fulfillment of sudden rate-change criteria may also be added to the tachycardia recognition algorithm.

Antitachycardia therapy consists of either burst pacing or cardioversion as the initial therapy, followed by up to four synchronous cardioversion shocks at programmable voltages.

After detection of fibrillation, a maximum of six synchronous defibrillation shocks can be delivered. For cardioversion and defibrillation, capacitor voltage, waveform, pulse duration, and number of attempts are programmable. Ventricular demand bradycardia pacing may be programmed to a rate between 25 or 90 beats/min, or turned off.

The Cadence model V-100 pulse generator may be interrogated and programmed with the Cadence programmer, a modified Compaq II portable computer with custom hardware and software. The programmer communicates with the pulse generator through a programming wand positioned over the device. A light pen is used to select parameters displayed on the screen of the programmer. The programmer is menu-driven, and the software contains safeguards designed to prevent selection of conflicting or inappropriate parameters.

III. SENSING SYSTEM

The sensing algorithm is an important parameter of device function. Use of a fixed sensitivity at a level that avoids oversensing during sinus rhythm may result in inability to sense small-amplitude signals that can occur during ventricular tachycardia or ventricular fibrillation. This could result in the inappropriate interpretation of a potentially lethal ventricular arrhythmia as a bradycardia or asystole. The device uses an automatic gain control circuit in order to compensate for changing electrogram amplitude.

Ventricular bipolar signals from the sensing leads are utilized. The high-voltage leads are not used for sensing. The gain control in the model V-100 is performed by a microprocessor which automatically selects sensitivity from one of eight settings based on the amplitudes of prior electrograms. By evaluating a number of previous electrogram amplitudes, the automatic gain control determines the sensitivity setting appropriate to detect the next cardiac event. The automatic gain control will respond more rapidly during a fast rhythm than during a slow rhythm. If the electrogram amplitude changes significantly and suddenly, undersensing or oversensing can occur for a brief period while the gain control adjusts the sensitivity. More gradual amplitude changes are tracked by the automatic gain microprocessor, usually without any sensing abnormalities. The setting of the gain control at any time (e.g., during induced ventricular fibrillation) can be viewed on the status screen or obtained by real-time measurement.

In the presence of large-amplitude signals of 50 Hz or faster (interpreted as noise) for longer than 300 ms, tachyarrhythmia therapy (and bradycardia pacing) will be inhibited (noise-detection mode). This mode reverts once noise is no longer sensed.

IV. RECOGNITION ALGORITHM

The model V-100 constantly monitors the ventricular electrogram recorded via the sensing lead and utilizes both the current interval and a running interval average to define the underlying rhythm. The programmed number of tachycardia intervals is the minimum number of intervals required for initial detection of a tachycardia, but frequently, more than the minimum number of intervals will be necessary for detection if there are large variations in signal amplitude or rate. If a tachycardia is detected, the rate-specific programmed therapy sequence will be delivered until the rate drops below the tachycardia detection rate or until all therapies are delivered. After each therapy is delivered, a minimum of six intervals is required to determine tachycardia continuance and initiate the next therapy.

A sudden-onset criterion can be enabled, in an attempt to prevent therapy delivery if there is a gradual increase in rate (as may occur with sinus tachycardia) while delivering therapy for the usually more abrupt onset of ventricular tachycardia. If this is enabled, therapy cannot be delivered unless the sudden-onset criterion is satisfied. Once tachycardia intervals have been detected, the average interval is compared to previous interval averages to determine if the difference between averages satisfies the sudden-onset change criterion. Since average intervals are used for the comparison, a single long interval during a gradual increase in rate will probably not result in satisfaction of the sudden-rate criterion.

The model V-100 incorporates an additional parameter that prevents prolonged attempts at pace termination of tachycardias in patients who may only tolerate their arrhythmias for a limited amount of time. This extended high-rate (EHR) parameter is used to deliver fibrillation therapy to a sustained tachycardia in the event that the therapies delivered within a (programmable) time limit have not been successful. If the tachycardia accelerates to rates exceeding fibrillation at any time, fibrillation therapy will be delivered without requiring the EHR timer to expire. If all tachycardia therapies have been delivered and the arrhythmia is still present and has not accelerated, no further therapy will be delivered until the EHR timer expires. In the event that no tachycardia therapies are delivered as a result of the sudden-onset criterion not being satisfied, fibrillation therapy will be delivered when the EHR timer expires.

V. ANTITACHYCARDIA ALGORITHMS

The initial antitachycardia therapy for ventricular tachycardia may be either antitachycardia pacing or a cardioversion shock. The availability of antitachycardia pacing is important to avoid uncomfortable, and sometimes psychologically intolerable [2], shocks for well-tolerated arrhythmias. Burst pacing rate, duration, and number of attempts (before progressing to a second antitachycardia therapy) are programmable within a wide range. Burst pacing rate may be specified at either a fixed interval or as an "adaptive" interval (i.e., at a given percentage of the average sensed tachycardia cycle length). The cycle length of antitachycardia pacing is also variable within a given burst and from burst to burst. When autodecremental antitachycardia pacing is turned on, each interval after the first in each burst will be decreased by the intraburst step size. When the scanning function is enabled, the pacing intervals of each subsequent burst will be decremented (or alternatively decremented and incremented) by the scanning step size. When autodecremental pacing and scanning are both turned off, the programmed burst cycle length is the interval between all pulses in all bursts. The first antitachycardia pacing stimulus in a burst is delivered synchronously with a sensed event. Antitachycardia pacing will never be performed at an interval shorter than the programmed minimum burst cycle length.

After each burst, the arrhythmia is reassessed to determine its rate. If the tachycardia remains within the same recognition range, then the next programmed antitachycardia pacing burst will be delivered. If, however, the tachycardia has accelerated into another tachycardia rate range, then cardioversion of defibrillation therapy will be delivered. When all programmed bursts have been delivered, the next programmed therapy (cardioversion at the first programmed voltage) will be delivered (Fig. 1). If the tachycardia persists for longer than the EHR time, then defibrillation therapy is delivered.

VI. PARAMETERS OF SHOCK THERAPY

Several features of cardioversion and fibrillation high-voltage therapies are programmable: voltage, waveform, pulse width, and number of times therapy is to be delivered. Successive therapy voltages must be greater than or equal to previous therapy voltages. All high-voltage therapies are delivered synchronously with sensed ventricular electrograms.

Cardioversion and defibrillation may be performed with either a biphasic or monophasic truncated exponential waveform. For the biphasic waveform, which is generally associated with lower defibrillation thresholds than the monophasic waveform [3], the leading-edge voltage of the second phase is one-half the residual voltage of the first phase. Pulse widths are programmable, and the programmer suggests a recommended pulse duration to maintain a relatively constant 60% waveform tilt based on high-voltage lead impedance. Delivered energy is dependent on the impedance of the high-voltage lead system. The device is capable of a maximum output of approximately 38 J (750 V into a typical impedance of 35 Ω). An estimate of the energy that will be delivered is calculated and displayed by the programmer based on the selected waveform, voltage, pulse width, and estimated (or measured) high-voltage lead impedance.

Once a tachyarrhythmia requiring cardioversion or defibrillation is detected, the high-voltage capacitors begin charging. Persistence of the tachyarrhythmia is checked continuously during charging. When the capacitors are completely charged, the presence of a tachyarrhythmia is reconfirmed before therapy is delivered. If sinus rhythm is detected prior to therapy delivery, charging is terminated and no therapy is delivered (i.e., the device is noncommitted to therapy delivery). This avoids painful (and potentially arrhythmogenic) shock delivery in

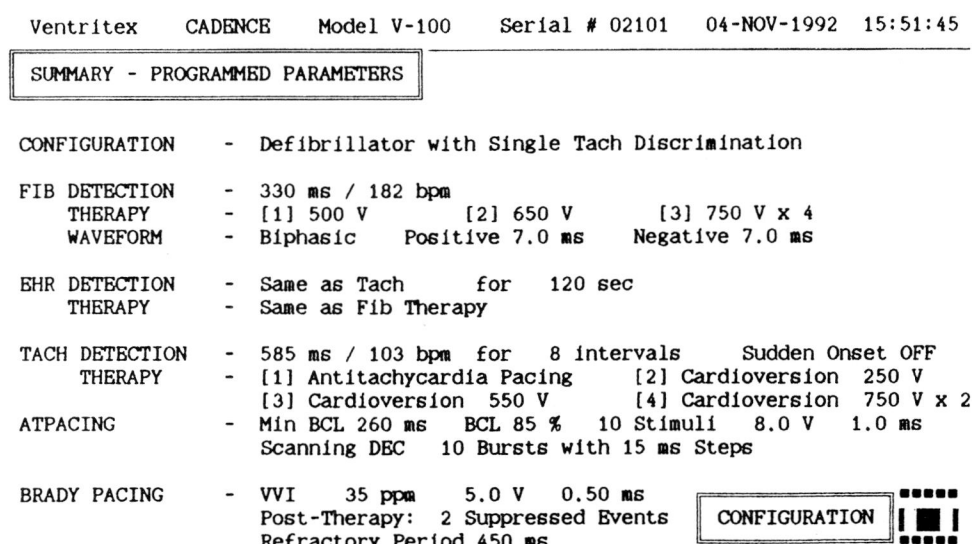

Figure 1 Programmed parameters for a device configured to recognize one ventricular tachycardia (VT), defined by a cycle length ≤ 585 ms. Fibrillation is defined by a cycle length ≤ 330 ms. Initial antitachycardia therapy consists of rapid (85% of the VT cycle length) ventricular pacing for 10 beats. If this is unsuccessful, pacing will be repeated up to nine times, with the cycle length of each burst decreased 15 ms each time (burst cycle length will not be decremented below 260 ms). If antitachycardia pacing is ineffective (or if termination takes longer than 120 s), then cardioversion (at 250 V with a biphasic waveform) will be delivered. An additional 550-V, and two 750-V shocks, will be delivered if necessary. Fibrillation therapy consists of an initial 500-V biphasic shock. Subsequent shocks are 650 V (×1) and 4 × 750 V shocks. Demand ventricular pacing at 35 beats/min will occur during bradycardia.

sinus rhythm in patients with nonsustained or self-terminating tachycardia [4]. Therapy will be delivered even if the arrhythmia rate slows but remains within any programmed tachyarrhythmia detection range.

The voltage on the capacitors is not "dumped" when charging is terminated but instead decreases gradually with time. Within 10 min, very little voltage is left on the capacitors. The residual voltage on the high-voltage capacitors can be measured and displayed. If another tachycardia is detected shortly after an aborted shock, capacitor charging time will be abbreviated due to the residual capacitor charge.

Deformation of the dielectric material within the high-voltage capacitors between charges may result in a prolonged initial charge time following a period of prolonged disuse. In order to minimize this possibility, the model V-100 automatically charges and "reforms" the high-voltage capacitors if 6 months pass without charging for therapy.

VII. DATA STORAGE AND TELEMETRY

Extensive diagnostic information is stored between programming episodes and can be retrieved (Table 2). The numbers of detected and treated tachyarrhythmias (in each category) and the number of delivered and aborted shocks are tracked by diagnostic counters. The maximum number that can be displayed for any detection category is 255. Diagnostic counters are cleared each time the model V-100 is programmed. Minimum and maximum average cycle lengths of

Table 2 Diagnostic and Telemetered Information Available in the Ventritex Cadence Model V-100 Tiered-Therapy Defibrillator

Stored information
Device charging history[a]
  Number of times device has charged to:
    50–200 V
    250–400 V
    450–600 V
    650–750 V
Diagnostic summary information[b]
  Number of detected and treated episodes of:
    Fibrillation
    EHR[c]
    Tachycardia A[c]
    Tachycardia B[c]
  Number of shocks
  Number of aborted shocks
  Minimum and maximum average cycle lengths of VT
Therapy sequencing information[b]
  For the last 11 arrhythmias:
    Detected arrhythmia
    Delivered therapy
    Outcome of therapy
    Duration of therapy
Stored electrograms[b]

Real-time information
Status
  Current setting of automatic gain control
  Progression of tachycardia detection
  Progression of fibrillation detection
  Current status of EHR timer
  Current sensed cycle length
Real-time measurements
  Battery voltage
  Residual HV capacitor voltage
  Pacing lead impedance
  Automatic gain-control setting (R-wave amplitude)
Real-time electrogram

[a]Counters not cleared by programming. Device charging history reflects charging for the life of the device.
[b]Counters cleared by programming.
[c]If applicable.

tachycardia are also displayed. Tachycardias shorter than the programmed tachycardia detection duration are not logged.

For the last 11 arrhythmia episodes for which therapy was delivered, the detected tachycardia is shown, along with the delivered therapy, the outcome of therapy (e.g., acceleration to fibrillation, sinus rhythm, etc.), and therapy duration (time from first therapy delivery to redetection of sinus rhythm). In addition, delivered energy, high-voltage lead impedance, charge time, and battery voltage for the last delivered shock are also available. The device also keeps a history of the number of times the device was charged to various voltages. Aborted shocks and capacitor maintenance charges are included in this history, and this information is not cleared by reprogramming but is kept for the life of the device.

During an induced or spontaneous tachycardia, the current status of the automatic gain control, cycle length of the sensed arrhythmia, and tachycardia, fibrillation, and EHR detection counters can be monitored in real time. These data are useful during implantation (or troubleshooting) to evaluate the suitability of programmed settings and the adequacy of the sensed electrograms.

Additional information about device function is provided by real-time measurement of battery voltage, residual capacitor voltage, pacing lead impedance, high-voltage lead impedance, and sensing amplifier automatic gain setting. An estimate of the input R-wave amplitude is also displayed.

A valuable feature of the Cadence model V-100 pulse generator is its ability to record and store bipolar ventricular electrograms. The type of events to be stored, criteria for storage (therapy delivered or redetection of sinus rhythm), and the number and duration of the events to be stored are programmable functions.

The pulse generator can be programmed to store the last one, three, or seven arrhythmic episodes, with storage times of 64, 32 or 16 s, respectively. Each additional event will overwrite the oldest stored event. The trigger for storage can be either therapy delivery or detection of sinus rhythm after therapy is initiated. The available storage time can be divided, with different pre- and posttrigger durations. Most implanted devices have been left at the nominal settings: storage of three 32-s events with return to sinus rhythm being the trigger for electrogram storage, and a pretrigger duration of 30 s (Fig. 2).

Electrogram review available in the model V-100 pulse generator has proven to be of significant value in determining the character of recurrent arrhythmias. Lack of ability to confirm the specific cause for shock delivery is an important limitation of other devices. Appropriate discharges have, historically, been defined as those occurring in association with syncope or presyncope. Since ventricular arrhythmias may occur in the absence of symptoms before discharge [5,6], shocks for ventricular arrhythmias (especially if better tolerated) can be erroneously labeled "inappropriate." Moreover, supraventricular arrhythmias associated with a rapid ventricular rate can be accompanied by hypotensive symptoms and device discharge, and can be classified as "appropriate." Availability of bipolar electrograms allows more accurate categorization of tachyarrhythmias leading to device activation. Episodes can be determined to be supraventricular on the basis of a comparison of the electrogram obtained during tachycardia with electrograms obtained during sinus rhythm (Fig. 3). In a majority of patients who receive a Cadence model V-100 pulse generator, stored electrograms are available to confirm the nature of recurrent arrhythmias. At least one episode of recurrent ventricular arrhythmia was confirmed by examination of stored electrograms in all but 1 of 205 patients with recurrent ventricular arrhythmias [7]. Overall, 17% of episodes were documented by stored electrograms. In 337 patients, 29 patients (9%) had device activation exclusively for supraventricular arrhythmias. Of 205 patients who had documented recurrent ventricular arrhythmias, 42 (20%) also had one or more supraventricular arrhythmias. In these 42 patients, 81% of device activations were for ventricular arrhythmias.

Use of the electrogram to define the nature of a tachyarrhythmia is not infallible. There is a change in electrogram morphology when supraventricular arrhythmias are associated with aberrant conduction. Additionally, local electrogram morphology during ventricular tachycardia may be identical to that during sinus rhythm [6]. However, composite criteria using rate,

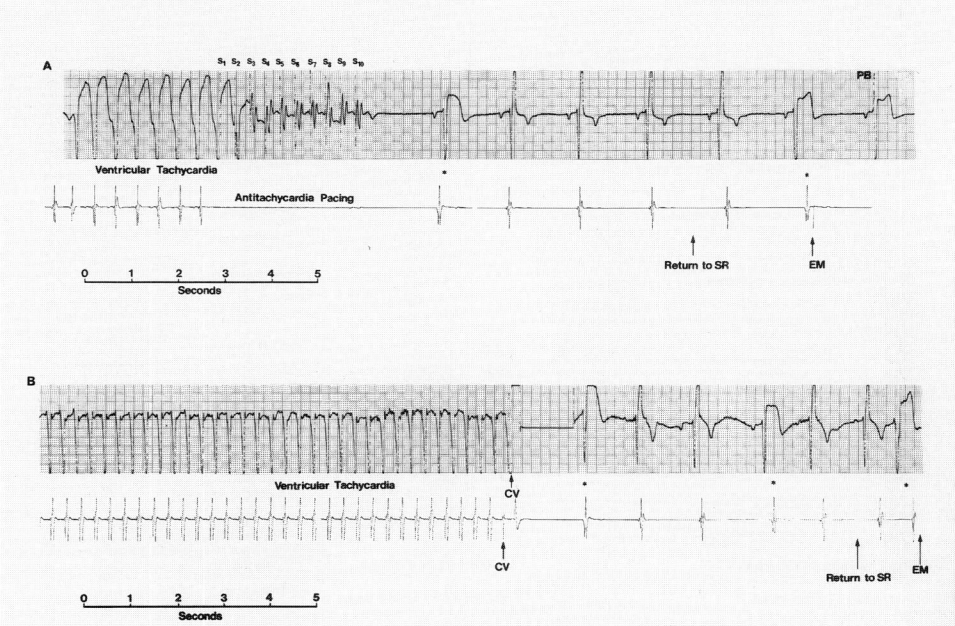

Figure 2 Simultaneous surface electrocardiogram (top) and stored ventricular electrogram (bottom) are shown for two episodes of ventricular tachycardia. Pulse generator programmed parameters are as illustrated in Fig. 1. The last 20 s of the stored electrogram are shown. Slight differences in recorder speed account for the lack of exact correspondence. (A) Monomorphic ventricular tachycardia (cycle length 420 ms), satisfying criteria for tachycardia A detection ($\leq$585 ms). Antitachycardia pacing, initially at a cycle length of 360 ms (85% of ventricular tachycardia cycle length) and at 345 ms (360−15 ms), failed to terminate tachycardia. The tachycardia immediately after the second episode of burst pacing is shown at the beginning of the record. After 7 beats of ventricular tachycardia, antitachycardia pacing (cycle length 330 ms) for 10 beats is delivered. The first stimulus (S_1) is synchronous with the sensed beat. The second stimulus (S_2) is a fusion beat. Capture with termination of ventricular tachycardia is accomplished by S_3–S_{10}. The first and sixth beats after termination are nonsinus beats (*). The approximate time the device recognizes return to sinus rhythm (return to SR) is shown. The end of memory (EM) for the event (approximately 2 s after the return to sinus rhythm trigger) is also shown. The last beat illustrated on the surface ECG is a fusion of a ventricular beat and ventricular pacing (PB), initiated at rates $\leq$ 35 beats/min. (B) Ventricular tachycardia (cycle length 320 ms) satisfying "fibrillation" criteria (cycle length $\leq$ 330 ms). One 500-V biphasic shock (CV) terminates the arrhythmia. Nonsinus beats (*), the return to sinus rhythm trigger (return to SR), and end of memory (EM) are shown.

interval variability, abruptness of onset and termination (after therapy), and electrogram morphology [8] allow accurate diagnosis of the vast majority of arrhythmias.

In addition to stored electrogram review, the model V-100 pulse generator permits review of real-time electrograms from the implanted ventricular sensing lead. This optimizes assessment of sensing parameters of the implanted device and facilitates troubleshooting. For example, suspected lead fracture causing inappropriate device discharge during arm movement can be evaluated by transmitting and displaying the sensed electrogram during movement.

All diagnostic data stored between programmings are telemetered to the programmer during interrogation. The initial step is to interrogate the implanted device. This results in the display of a summary screen (Fig. 1) indicating the currently programmed parameter values.

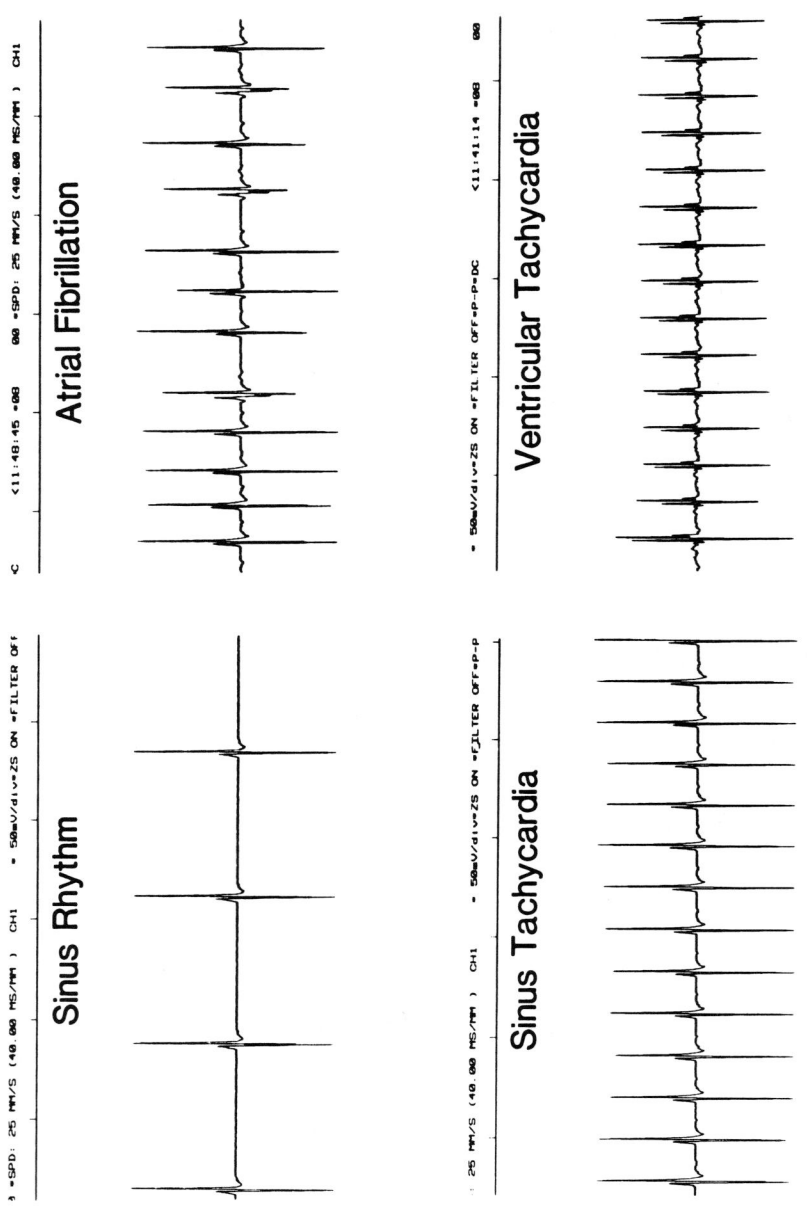

Figure 3 Enlargement of electrogram morphology during sinus rhythm, sinus tachycardia, atrial fibrillation, and ventricular tachycardia. Electrogram morphology is seen to be essentially identical in sinus rhythm, sinus tachycardia, and atrial fibrillation, although in the latter case there is significant variation in electrogram amplitude and intervals. Electrogram morphology is distinctly different during ventricular tachycardia.

Transfer of telemetered information is indicated by an audible tone. A chart recorder may be used to record stored or real-time electrograms.

VIII. BACKUP PACING CAPABILITIES

Ventricular demand pacing (VVI) may be enabled with any antitachycardia configuration and is also available when all antitachycardia modes are off. Bradycardia pacing amplitude and pulse width can be programmed independently of pacing for antitachycardia termination or during noninvasive programmed stimulation. Thus, bradycardia pacing parameters can be programmed for maximum device longevity while allowing antitachycardia pacing parameters to be sufficient in amplitude to assure capture during ventricular tachycardia. Because bradycardia pacing immediately after termination of a tachycardia may be arrhythmogenic in some patients [9], demand pacing may be delayed after delivery of antitachycardia therapy.

IX. NONINVASIVE EECTROPHYSIOLOGICAL FUNCTIONS

Tachyarrhythmias and fibrillation can be induced by the model V-100 pulse generator. Programmed stimulation allows ventricular pacing with one, two, or three ventricular extrastimuli. In addition, a fibrillation induction mode allows for trains (up to 250 beats) at short cycle lengths for induction of ventricular fibrillation. Programming of the noninvasive stimulation function is performed with the programming wand positioned over the implanted device. As soon as the device has completed stimulation, normal detection and tachyarrhythmia therapy capabilities are restored.

X. TECHNICAL DESCRIPTION

The Cadence model V-100 pulse generator is a 240-g device (9.7 × 8.2 × 2.4 cm; approximately 145 cm^3 displacement volume), sealed in a titanium case. The microelectronics consists of a hybrid circuit made up of four integrated circuits (including one RAM integrated circuit), additional discrete components, and a telemetry coil. There are two high-voltage aluminum electrolytic 300-uF capacitors. Power is provided by two lithium silver vanadium oxide cells in series (initial capacity 1.33 A-h).

The implantation life of the pulse generator is dependent on the frequency of high-voltage charging. It has been estimated that with 100% bradycardia pacing (60 beats/min, pulse amplitude of 5.0 V, and a pulse width of 0.5 ms) and approximately one high-voltage charge per month, the life of the device is approximately 4 years.

The voltage of the battery is used as an elective replacement indicator. The unloaded voltage of a new device is >6.0 V. Replacement is indicated when the unloaded battery voltage decreases to ≤5.1 V. Approximately 6 months of device life (at conditions described above) are available when the elective replacement battery voltage has been reached. The unloaded battery voltage should be checked at each follow-up visit. Battery voltage measured within 1 day of a high-voltage charge may be inappropriately low and should not be used as an indicator for device replacement.

Two high-voltage (female) lead connectors on the header of the model V-100 accept the 5-mm lead tips of the Ventritex contoured defibrillation patches (investigational; available with either 19 or 38 cm^2 surface area). The sensing/pacing connector is a single in-line VS-1. Bifurcated bipolar endocardial leads or two unipolar epicardial leads can be adapted to the in-line connector with an adapter. The pulse generator is also available with two additional header configurations, allowing use of commercially available high-voltage leads (Cardiac Pacemakers, Inc., 6.4-mm proximal connector) and/or two epicardial screw-in leads (5-mm connectors) without adapters.

Magnet application (over either end of the device) will inhibit delivery of tachyarrhythmia therapy as long as the magnet is in place. No audible tones result from magnet application. Bradycardia pacing and noninvasive stimulation are unaffected by magnet application. The device cannot be permanently programmed Off by magnet application.

XI. CLINICAL DATA ON DEVICE PERFORMANCE

Clinical evaluation of the Ventritex Cadence started July 11, 1989. As of September 30, 1992, 1185 implants had been done in 45 participating centers in the United States and Europe. FDA (Circulatory System Devices Panel) approval was recommended in February 1992, and commercial release was expected by the end of 1992.

Analysis of the first 337 patients after at least 6 months of follow-up [7] revealed that at least one recurrent ventricular arrhythmia occurred in 61% of patients, with a mean of 37 ± 5 (range 1–441 per patient) recurrent ventricular arrhythmias per patient (mean follow-up = 360 ± 10 days). Analysis of predictors of recurrent ventricular arrhythmias suggested that patients presenting with monomorphic ventricular tachycardia were more likely to experience recurrent ventricular arrhythmias (and had more frequent and earlier recurrences) than patients presenting with ventricular fibrillation. This is important, since previously published studies [2,10] with patients presenting with sudden death have probably underestimated the benefits of device therapy.

Therapy for ventricular fibrillation accounts for approximately 5% of spontaneous recurrent ventricular arrhythmias [11]. In 569 instances in which therapy was delivered for ventricular fibrillation, the first shock was successful in 91%. Subsequent shocks were required (and were successful) in 9% of episodes. Antitachycardia pacing was the initial therapy in 96% of 14,005 episodes of ventricular tachycardia. Antitachycardia pacing was successful in 93% of instances, was unsuccessful in 5%, and accelerated tachycardia in 2% (subsequent cardioversion was successful in all cases in which antitachycardia pacing was unsuccessful or accelerated the rhythm).

In a recent series [7], 33 patients died during follow-up (mean follow-up 360 ± 10 days). There were 7 perioperative deaths, 3 sudden deaths, and 16 nonsudden cardiac deaths. Thus, the 1-year sudden-death-free survival was 99% and the cardiac death-free survival was 94%. In 5 patients, the device was explanted because of infection (3 patients) or in association with cardiac transplantation (2 patients) after initial implantation.

XII. INTRAOPERATIVE TESTING AND FOLLOW-UP EVALUATION: DEVICE-SPECIFIC FEATURES

Cardioversion or defibrillation is accompanied via two defibrillation leads. Of the first 951 implants, nearly all patients (896) received two epicardial high-voltage patches. Limited experience is available using a superior vena caval spring electrode and either a single epicardial patch (41 patients) or an intracardiac lead and an apical subcutaneous patch (3 patients). Nine patients received CPI Endotak leads only (in Europe). For ventricular sensing and pacing, either a bipolar endocardial lead or two epicardial screw-in electrodes can be utilized. Epicardial leads should be positioned within 3 cm of each other. In the first 942 patients, ventricular bi-

Ventritex Cadence

Table 3 Implant and Follow-up Procedures for the Ventritex Cadence Model V-100 Tiered-Therapy Defibrillator

Implant procedures
1. Position sensing/pacing lead and determine threshold, R-wave amplitude, and impedance.[a]
2. Position high-voltage defibrillation leads and determine lead impedance.[b]
3. Determine defibrillation threshold using the HVS-02 Diagnostic Electrophysiology Device with the appropriate waveform. High-voltage lead revision is required if the threshold is ≥ 650 V.
4. Implant V-100.
5. Examine real-time electrograms to assess sensing lead integrity and interrogate the device.
6. Program device to appropriate configuration and settings.
7. Induce ventricular fibrillation[c] and assess adequacy of recognition[d] and termination.
8. Induce ventricular tachycardia and assess adequacy of recognition and termination, if applicable.
9. Assess bradycardia pacing and sensing, if applicable.
10. Retrieve stored electrograms and reprogram to clear diagnostic counters.

Predischarge and first follow-up (4–6 weeks postimplant)
1. Interrogate and retrieve diagnostic data and stored electrograms.
2. Induce clinical arrhythmias and assess adequacy of recognition and termination.
3. Retrieve diagnostic data and stored electrograms.
4. Measure battery voltage, pacing lead impedance, and gain control setting.
5. Reprogram to clear diagnostic counters.

Subsequent follow-up
1. Interrogate device and retrieve relevant diagnostic information. Retrieve and play back stored electrograms, if applicable.
2. Measure real-time values, including unloaded battery voltage (for EOL determination).
3. Examine real-time electrogram.
4. Program device to clear diagnostics.

[a]Acute pacing threshold should be ≤ 2 V (chronic ≤ 5 V); acute R-wave amplitude should be ≥ 5 mv (chronic ≥ 2 mv); acute lead impedance should be ≥ 25 Ω (chronic ≥ 20 Ω).
[b]High-voltage lead impedance can be determined by delivering a synchronous shock in sinus rhythm. Acute high-voltage lead impedance should be >25 Ω (chronic >20 Ω). Damage to the pulse generator can occur with delivery of the maximum capacitor voltage to a load of <20 Ω.
[c]Ventricular fibrillation should be induced, whether or not it is the clinical arrhythmia, since antitachycardia pacing of a well-tolerated ventricular tachycardia may accelerate the arrhythmia. Fibrillation can be induced with the implanted device, noninvasively.
[d]Progress of fibrillation recognition can be assessed in real time using the status screen.

polar endocardial leads were endocardial in 499 patients, and epicardial leads were used in 443 patients. More recently, endocardial bipolar leads have been preferred because of a perception of lower long-term pacing thresholds.

Equipment required for intraoperative implantation and testing includes, in addition to the Ventritex Cadence model V-100 pulse generator, (1) two defibrillation leads; (2) two unipolar or one bipolar ventricular sensing/pacing electrodes; (3) the Ventritex Cadence programmer, model PR-1000 or 1001; and (4) a Ventritex HVS-02 diagnostic electrophysiology device for intraoperative testing of the lead system. Intraoperative implant and evaluation procedures are summarized in Table 3. Adequate sensing and pacing parameters must be confirmed after lead implantation. Low-amplitude sensed signals during tachycardia or fibrillation can result in prolonged arrhythmia detection time or inability to detect an arrhythmia. High pacing thresholds may result in difficulty in pace terminating ventricular tachycardia.

In the clinical evaluation of the Cadence model V-100 pulse generator, patients have undergone a predischarge induction of ventricular fibrillation to confirm effective defibrillation and returned routinely 4–6 weeks after discharge from the hospital following implantation for a similar evaluation. In nearly all cases, adequate intraoperative defibrillation thresholds were reaffirmed by comparable thresholds postoperatively. In at least 6 instances, significantly higher defibrillation thresholds were obtained at postimplant testing; and in 3 of these cases, higher thresholds were correlated with lead migration or displacement.

Routine follow-up is recommended every 2–3 months after implantation. Follow-up evaluations (Table 3) should include assessment of diagnostic data (including retrieval of stored electrograms) and measurement of real-time parameters.

XIII. NONINVASIVE TESTING AND TROUBLESHOOTING

The design philosophy of the Cadence model V-100 pulse generator, extensive programmability, and availability of both real-time and stored electrograms of arrhythmias greatly assists in the management of postimplantation problems. The status screen provides a window that is useful in assessing the device's arrhythmia detection process and the function of the automatic gain-control circuit during induced arrhythmias. Real-time measurements provide information about R-wave amplitude, and the real-time electrogram displays the filtered signal used by the device to sense the heart rate. Lead problems may manifest as a noisy, abnormal, or absent real-time signal. Extensive diagnostic data and electrograms of tachycardia therapy allow assessment of how effectively antitachycardia therapy is functioning.

Avoidance of frequent, painful shocks in patients with nonsustained ventricular tachycardias is an advantage of the the noncommitted nature of the device. However, frequent capacitor charging may lead to early battery depletion. In this case, the time necessary for tachycardia recognition can be prolonged.

The Extended High Rate feature prevents continued delivery of ineffective therapy (or nondelivery of therapy due to inability to satisfy the sudden-onset criterion). A potential problem is the delivery of painful defibrillation shocks for well-tolerated ventricular arrhythmias. In this case, the EHR detection interval (nominally equal to the detection rate of the slowest tachycardia) can be reprogrammed independently should a patient's tachycardia be well tolerated.

REFERENCES

1. Winkle RA, Fain ES, Hardage ML, Senelly KM, and the CADENCE Investigators. The value and usage of programmability in a tiered therapy defibrillator (abstr). J Am Coll Cardiol 1992; 19:365A.
2. Echt DS, Armstrong K, Schmidt P, Oyer PE, Stinson EB, Winkle RA. Clinical experience, complications, and survival in 70 patients with the automatic implantable cardioverter/defibrillator. Circulation 1985; 71:289–296.
3. Bardy GH, Ivey TD, Allen MD, Johnson G, Mehra R, Greene HL. A prospective randomized evaluation of biphasic versus monophasic waveform pulses on defibrillation efficacy in humans. J Am Coll Cardiol 1989; 14:728–733.
4. Hurwitz JL, Hook BG, Callans DJ, et al. Importance of aborted shock capability with electrogram storage in cardioverter/defibrillator devices (abstr). Circulation 1991; 84 (suppl II): 427.
5. Tchou PJ, Kadri N, Anderson J, Caceres JA, Jazayeri M, Akhtar M. Automatic implantable cardioverter defibrillators and survival of patients with left ventricular dysfunction and malignant ventricular arrhythmias. Ann Intern Med 1988; 109:529–534.
6. Hook BG, Marchlinski FE. Value of ventricular electrogram recordings in the diagnosis of arrhythmias precipitating electrical device shock therapy. J Am Coll Cardiol 1991; 17:985–990.

7. Reiter MJ, Fain ES, Senelly KM, and the Cadence Investigators. Determinants of recurrent ventricular arrhythmias in patients with implantable pacemaker/defibrillators (abstr). Circulation 1991; 84:II-426.
8. Callans DJ, Hook BG, Marchlinski FE. Use of bipolar recordings from patch-patch and rate sensing leads to distinguish ventricular tachycardia from supraventricular rhythms in patients with implantable cardioverter defibrillators. PACE 1991; 14(II):1917–1922.
9. Callans DJ, Hook BG, Marchlinski FE. Paced beats following single nonsensed complexes in a "co-dependent" cardioverter defibrillator and bradycardia pacing system: potential for ventricular tachycardia induction. PACE 1991; 14:1281–1287.
10. Kelly PA, Cannom DS, Garan H, et al. Predictors of automatic implantable cardioverter defibrillator discharge for life-threatening ventricular arrhythmias. Am J Cardiol 1988; 62:83–87.
11. Winkle RA, Fain ES, Sweeney MB, Senelly KM, and the Cadence Investigators. Survival in patients with ventricular tachyarrhythmias treated with programmable tiered therapy implantable defibrillators (abstr). J Am Coll Cardiol 1992; 19:209A.

45

The CPI Endotak Nonthoracotomy Lead System

Ferdinand J. Venditti, Jr., David T. Martin, David Shahian

Harvard Medical School
Boston
and Lahey Clinic Medical Center
Burlington, Massachusetts

I. INTRODUCTION

The efficacy of the implantable cardioverter-defibrillator (ICD) in preventing sudden cardiac death has been well established [1–5]. However, there remains resistance from patients and physicians to this life-saving therapy because of the cost, discomfort, and risk associated with standard implant techniques. Either a lateral thoracotomy or a median sternotomy, both with the attendant risks of major surgery, have been the approaches used in the vast majority of implants [5]. Both have associated discomfort as well as significant perioperative risks [5].

Several manufacturers have recently developed transvenous or nonthoracotomy lead systems to reduce risks and discomfort associated with implantation of an ICD system. The Endotak lead system (Cardiac Pacemakers, Inc.) was the first lead to move from animal testing to implantation in patients [6].

II. PREVIOUS REPORTS

Lead systems for ICDs have evolved strikingly since the early design and animal work in the 1970s. The earliest prototype ICD utilized two transvenous leads: a distal right ventricular lead, and a proximal spring coil in the superior vena cava. There was a pressure transducer at the tip of the ventricular lead for arrhythmia detection, using changes in the "mechanogram" to determine rhythm [7]. This design was rapidly abandoned when lead dislodgement in canine experiments severely limited longevity of the system.

The initial clinical ICD was a simple shocking device that utilized a spring electrode in the superior vena cava combined with a cup electrode over the cardiac apex for energy delivery. This transvenous lead was also used for arrhythmia detection, using morphology alterations in the cardiac electrogram for diagnosis of ventricular fibrillation [8]. Early transvenous leads still required an epicardial patch and were supplanted by completely epicardial systems in which more reliable defibrillation thresholds (DFT) were demonstrated [9,10].

A subsequent transvenous lead system manufactured by CPI, used in conjunction with a subcutaneous or submuscular patch, was reported to be efficacious in short-term use [6]. A report of a single patient appeared in 1988 in whom thoracic surgery was contraindicated and implantation of the early Endotak lead system achieved a satisfactory DFT. The most successful shock configuration in this case utilized the right ventricular spring electrode as the common cathode and delivered bidirectional shocks to both the proximal spring and submuscular epicostal patch anodes. This configuration (the "configuration 2" of the ultimate clinical trial) gave reliable defibrillation with less than 10 J.

Early trials showed this lead lacked chronic durability due to conductor fracture, often at the site of subclavian venous entry. After a complete redesign, including altering the materials used for conduction and insulation, clinical trials resumed in 1990 with the Endotak C. Two recent reports from the Cleveland Clinic describe short-term experience with this system [11,12]. These reports describe a total of 14 patients in whom implantation was attempted. Five of the 14 patients did not receive the transvenous system because their DFT was too high; they went on to receive a thoracotomy or subxiphoid implant. Of the patients who were successfully implanted with the redesigned system, all were tested with configuration 2, and in most instances, this was the implanted configuration. The authors readily acknowledge their bias in favor of this electrode configuration based on animal data [13,14], but the nonrandomized nature of the clinical testing, and their a priori preference for configuration 2 make definitive conclusions about the truly optimal human implant electrode configuration and current pathway impossible.

Mean follow-up in this study was only 15 months (range 7–26), which prevents definitive conclusions about the longevity of these leads. At the 8- to 12-week postimplant system evaluation, all induced arrhythmias in 9 patients were sensed and terminated. During the short follow-up period there were significant complications in this small patient group. At least 1, and probably 2 patients received inappropriate shocks because of patch conductor fracture leading to oversensing. This problem led to a redesign of the patch lead, and no further fractures have been reported. In addition, 2 patients complained of pain at the patch site, requiring instillation of local anesthesia in one case.

III. DESCRIPTION OF THE DEVICE

The Endotak lead system is composed of a tripolar, tined, transvenous lead (Endotak C), a Y connector, and a subcutaneous patch (Fig. 1). The 100-cm transvenous lead is capable of bipolar sensing (distal tip cathode versus distal spring anode) and defibrillation (distal spring cathode versus proximal spring anode) in a single lead. The subcutaneous patch and Y connector allow for the versatility of multiple pathways to enhance the likelihood of successful defibrillation with the system.

The lead has two drawn brazed strand cable conductors coated with Teflon connecting the titanium spring electrodes used for defibrillation to 6.1-mm titanium pins. The third electrode, used for sensing, is a porous electrode tip with a diameter of 2.72 mm connected by a MP35N nickel-cobalt alloy conductor to a 4.75-mm titanium pin. All three conductors are enclosed in silicone rubber, with a maximum lead body diameter of 3.95 mm (12 F).

The distal and proximal defibrillation electrodes are 295 mm^2 and 617 mm^2, respectively, with a coil diameter of 3.56 mm. The distal-to-proximal electrode distance is available in three sizes (10 cm, 13 cm, and 16 cm). Variable interelectrode spacing allows for optimal electrode separation in small as well as large hearts. The distal sensing-to-distal defibrillating electrode distance is 0.6 cm.

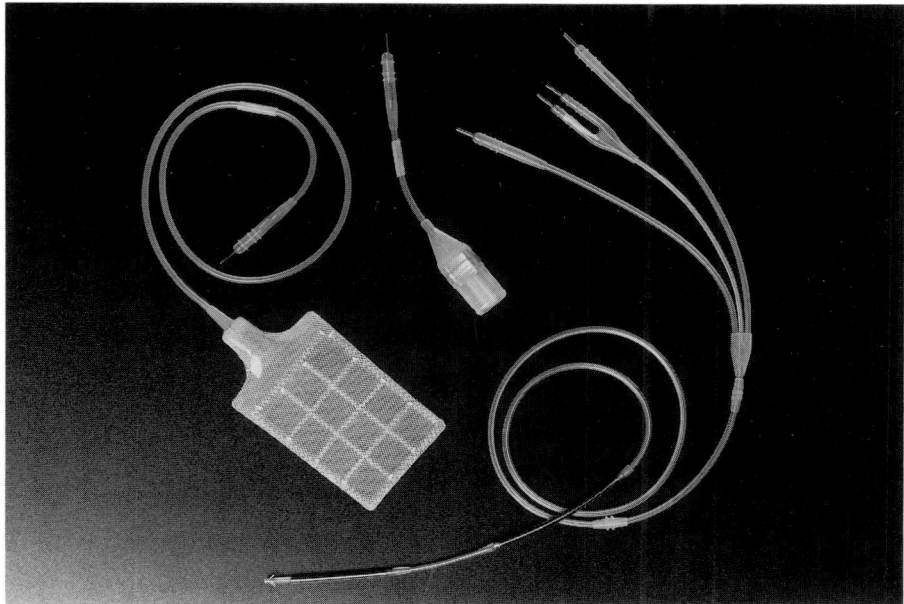

Figure 1 The Endotak nonthoracotomy lead system, which includes a subcutaneous patch, a tripolar Endotak C lead, and a Y connector.

The subcutaneous or submuscular patch lead is a 63-cm lead with a titanium mesh patch, which has silicone rubber reinforced with Dacron as its backing. The conductor to a titanium pin is also drawn brazed strand cable with silicone rubber insulation. The surface area of the 12-mesh windows is 28 cm^2. The Y connector, which is used when bidirectional shocks are given, consists of two 6.1-mm ports connected to a 6.1-mm titanium pin.

IV. LEAD CONFIGURATIONS

Three defibrillation electrodes permit multiple configurations for the delivery of energy (Fig. 2). Using only two electrodes, unidirectional shocks can be given in two configurations (configuration 3 and 4). With two electrodes made electrically common (anode) by using the Y connector, bidirectional shocks may be delivered in two additional configurations (configuration 1 and 2).

Multiple configurations can be tested in an individual patient in an effort to minimize the defibrillation threshold. In addition, reverse polarity has been demonstrated to be helpful in some patients with epicardial patches [15], and can be used to expand the number of possible transvenous configurations.

If the standard configurations are unsuccessful, repositioning of either lead can be tried, as can nonprotocol configurations.

The experience with the new system, Endotak C, is growing. We will describe our experience in a large series of patients implanted in a single center and briefly summarize pooled data from the initial 536 patients who have undergone implantation in a large, multicenter clinical trial begun in September 1990.

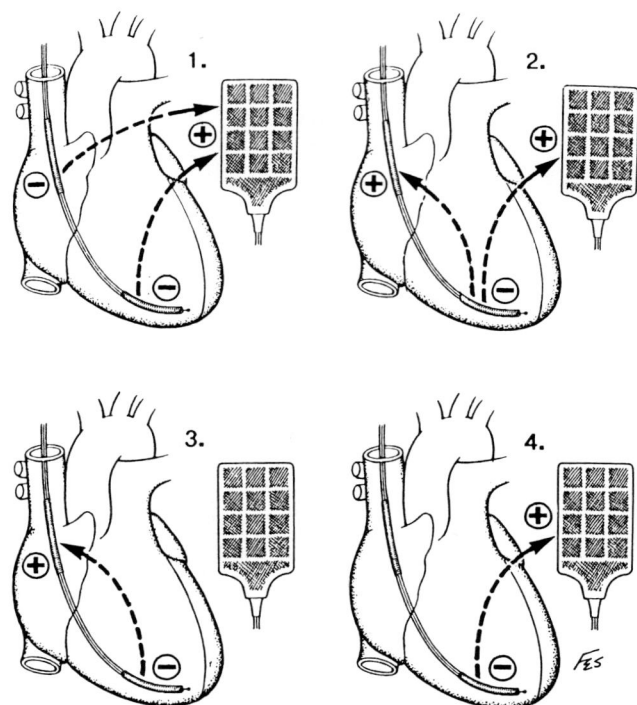

Figure 2 The four configurations evaluated in the clinical trial of the Endotak nonthoracotomy lead system. There are two unidirectional configurations (3 and 4) and two bidirectional configurations (1 and 2). Common electrodes were made anodal.

V. PATIENT POPULATION

A total of 75 patients requiring ICD implantation were entered into this protocol at our institution from May 1991 to December 1992 after giving written informed consent. This protocol was approved by the Human Studies Committee of the research division of the Lahey Clinic.

Evaluation included cardiac catheterization and electrophysiological testing in all patients. Holter monitoring, 2-D echocardiogram, and exercise testing were performed as indicated.

There were 62 men and 13 women in the group, with a median age of 68 (range 23–78). The predominant disease process was coronary artery disease, with 61 (82%) having previous myocardial infarctions; valvular heart disease and nonischemic cardiomyopathy were present in 4 patients each, hypertrophic cardiomyopathy and primary electrical disease were present in 2 patients each, and arrhythmogenic RV dysplasia was present in 1 individual. The mean ejection fraction was $35.2 \pm 16.6\%$ (range 10–76%). The presenting clinical problem was sustained hypotensive monomorphic ventricular tachycardia in 40 patients (53%), ventricular fibrillation or out-of-hospital cardiac arrest in 23 (31%), and syncope in the presence of structural heart disease with provokable sustained monomorphic ventricular tachycardia at the time of electrophysiological testing in 12 (16%). All patients were ruled out for acute myocardial infarction at the time of their initial presentation. All reversible causes were also excluded (i.e., hypokalemia, ischemia, etc.).

All patients with provokable arrhythmias (72 patients) underwent serial drug testing prior to ICD implantation. A mean of 2.4 antiarrhythmic drugs failed prior to ICD implantation.

Clinical variables in the group undergoing transvenous ICD implantation were similar to patients who underwent thoracotomy implantation previously in our institution [7].

VI. IMPLANTATION TECHNIQUE

All aspects of the implantation were performed during the same procedure in the surgical theater. This includes transvenous lead placement as well as subcutaneous patch placement, lead tunneling, and generator implant.

All patients were monitored intraoperatively with a pulmonary artery catheter capable of monitoring mixed venous oxygen saturation. Continuous mixed venous oxygen saturation monitoring allows for the prompt identification of cardiovascular problems during the procedure [16]. In addition, patients with profound left ventricular dysfunction or unrevascularized coronary disease were frequently supported with an intraaortic balloon pump perioperatively.

Patients were prepared to undergo a thoracotomy immediately if the transvenous approach failed. To facilitate this, the patients were placed with their upper torso elevated 30–40° from the table, with the left arm at the side. A large field was draped in both the abdomen and chest. This allowed us to proceed immediately to thoracotomy if necessary without repositioning or redraping the patient.

The left or right cephalic vein was exposed via a 4- to 5-cm incision over the deltopectoral groove. The cephalic vein was exposed with sharp and then blunt dissection. A venotomy was then made in the exposed vein, and a 0.025-gauge guide wire was inserted into the cephalic vein. The vein was then dilated or sheared away with the introduction of a 14F peelaway introducer, a modification of the Ong-Barold technique for pacemaker lead insertion [17]. Through this sheath the Endotak lead was inserted. This technique was used in all but 3 implants, where subclavian puncture was necessary because of the lack of an appropriate cephalic vein.

The Endotak was positioned in the apex of the right ventricle under fluoroscopic guidance. Care was taken to advance the tip of the lead into the apex of the ventricle to ensure close proximity to the interventricular septum. Stability of the lead was tested, as was measured R-wave and pacing thresholds prior to anchoring the lead with a redundant loop using two anchoring sleeves (to ensure no stress on the intracardiac portion of the lead).

The subcutaneous patch was then placed in a small pocket in the inframammary crease, centered at the expected level of the left ventricular apex. The patch can be moved as necessary in this region to improve the defibrillation threshold. Also, this incision was placed so that it could be expanded in either direction to an anterolateral thoracotomy. The subcutaneous patch was secured with stitches, to be certain that the edges did not curl or fold.

The leads were tunneled from the infraclavicular and inframammary areas to the generator pocket with a long clamp and chest tube or with a special tunneling tool available from the manufacturer. All testing was performed after tunneling to ensure that any damage done to the leads during tunneling would be promptly detected.

VII. DEFIBRILLATION THRESHOLD MEASUREMENTS

Defibrillation threshold is a misnomer. The likelihood of successful defibrillation at a given energy is a probability function [18]. A sigmoid curve with energy on the x axis and percent success on the y axis more accurately describes the likelihood of success at a given energy level (Fig. 3).

Despite the difficulty inherent in using a DFT measurement, clinical practice limits our ability to define exactly the relationship between energy and efficacy. However, if step-down

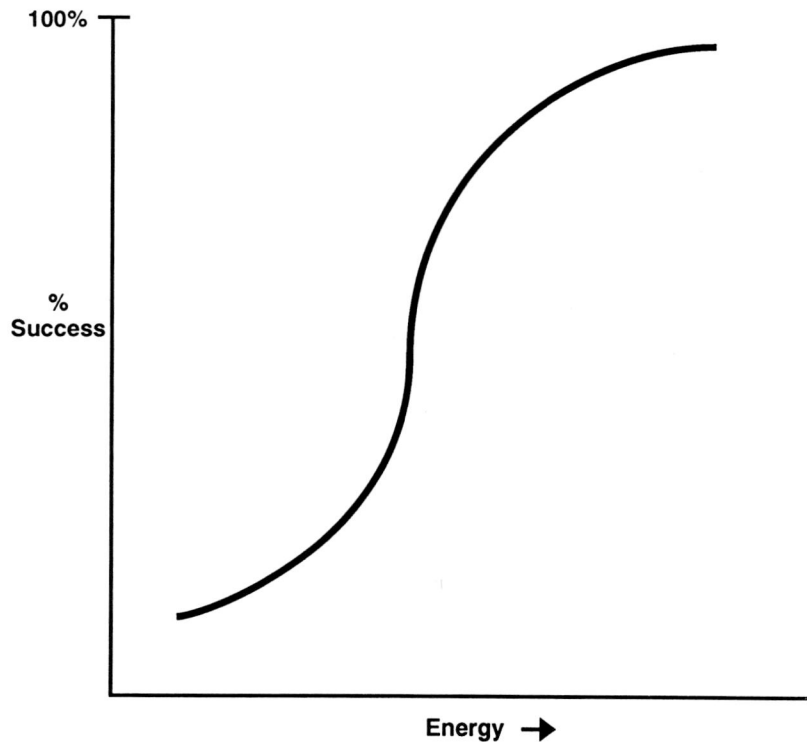

Figure 3 The efficacy of defibrillation is related to the energy in a sigmoid fashion, as demonstrated by this curve. The percent success approaches 100% at higher energies. The E_{75} point is the point at which 75% of attempts at a given energy level are successful.

testing to determine a DFT is begun above the expected threshold, the value will likely represent the E_{75} point on the sigmoid curve (the energy at which 75% of defibrillation attempts are successful). Three consecutive successful conversions at a measured DFT also strongly suggests that the measured DFT is at E_{75} or higher on the curve. If the DFT is high ($\geq$20 J), repeat attempts at that same energy level will more accurately define the relationship between energy and efficacy of conversion, enhancing the clinical utility of the DFT determination [19]. This is important when the DFT is near the maximum energy delivered by the device.

The standard protocol employed in determining DFTs in our series is outlined in Fig. 4. All testing during implantation was performed with an external cardioverter-defibrillator using monophasic shocks. DFT was defined as the minimum energy that successfully resulted in defibrillation with a step-down protocol that began with an energy level likely to be higher than the DFT. If the measured DFT was 20 or 25 J, two additional attempts at defibrillation were made at that energy level. If both were successful, the likelihood was that the measured DFT was high on the success curve, and system implantation was performed. Patients with a DFT of 25 J who received a high-energy device were considered to have "inadequate" thresholds. These patients were implanted without the required 10-J safety margin because of their clinical circumstances.

Most patients had a minimum of two electrode configurations tested. The configuration with the lowest DFT was used as the final implanted configuration. In those patients with

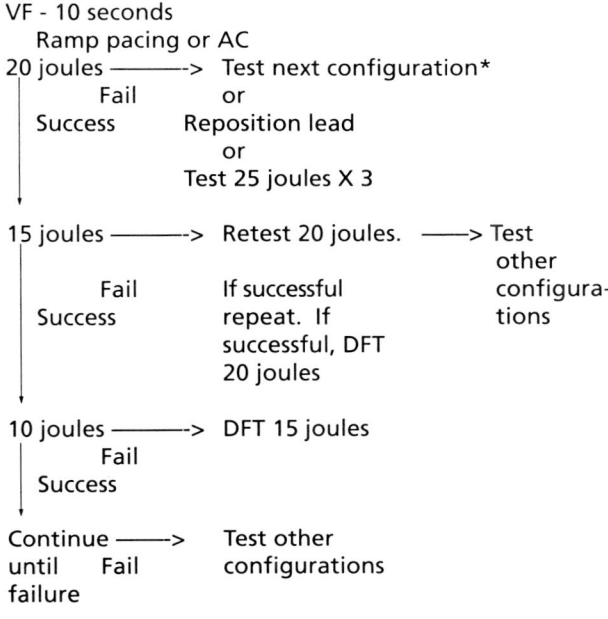

Figure 4 This is the testing protocol used in the operating room as well as at the time of the 2-month and 6-month follow-up EP studies. All protocol configurations as well as reverse-polarity configurations were tested using this scheme. Testing was started at 20 J and stepwise decreased until a shock was unsuccessful. The lowest successful shock was defined as the DFT. If 20 J was unsuccessful, a new configuration was tried.

an unacceptably high DFT with the transvenous system (less than a 10-J margin of safety), thoracotomy implantation of a standard ICD was performed in all but 1 patient during the same operation.

VIII. POSTOPERATIVE TESTING

All patients underwent predischarge, 2-month, and 6-month conversion testing of their system and two-view chest radiography. All postoperative invasive testing was done with IV anesthesia, using propofol 0.5–3 mg/kg given continuously [20]. The predischarge test was used to demonstrate appropriate system function. One to three conversion tests of ventricular fibrillation were performed at maximum energy of the device.

The 2- and 6-month tests were more detailed. Repeat defibrillation threshold testing was performed when possible with the use of a programmable ICD (Ventak P, CPI). Testing was performed in an identical fashion to the protocol in the operating theater (Fig. 4). If there was a significant rise in the DFT, repeat testing was performed after several weeks, antiarrhythmic drug therapy was altered, or the system was revised (1 patient each).

Sensing was tested with a magnet over the generator activating audible tones with each sensed event. Arm and shoulder motion was then used to determine if conductor or insulation defects were present at the insertion site. In addition, all patients were subjected to at least one redetection after a failed low-energy discharge, to assess the effect of defibrillation on R-wave sensing.

IX. RESULTS: IMPLANTATION

At the time of DFT testing in the operating theater, 66 of 75 (88%) patients had acceptable thresholds and underwent implantation of a full system. In the 9 patients with high thresholds, 7 patients underwent a full thoracotomy system implant during the same procedure. The transvenous lead was used as a rate-sensing lead in 1 patient with epicardial patches after threshold testing with the Endotak and a single epicardial patch revealed persistently high thresholds. One patient had high epicardial patch thresholds. This was a patient with Ebstein's anomaly, who became unstable during the first procedure and was ultimately implanted during a second operation with a measured epicardial patch defibrillation threshold of 23 J.

During DFT testing, a mean of three configurations were tested in each patient (range 1–13). The possible configurations tested include the four standard configurations as well as their reverse-polarity versions and retesting of a configuration after repositioning of either lead. The majority of patients received a "lead only" system (configuration 3), without the need for the subcutaneous patch (Fig. 5). In most patients ($n = 54$), other configurations were tested and configuration 3 was used only if it resulted in the lowest DFT. The other unidirectional configuration (configuration 4) was seldom used due to high thresholds.

The reverse-polarity configuration of a standard configuration was used in 8 patients (12% of implanted patients). Reverse polarity was utilized only after testing with standard polarity failed to demonstrate adequate thresholds. This nonrandomized use of reverse polarity obscures its utility, though we have found individual cases where it allowed for successful implantation of the system because of a seemingly marked reduction in DFT.

A mean of 10 episodes of ventricular fibrillation were provoked during DFT testing (range 3–18) with AC current or ramp pacing. The mean impedance of the implanted configuration was $45 \pm 7 \, \Omega$ (range 33–57 Ω). The median threshold measured at implant was 15 J (Fig. 6).

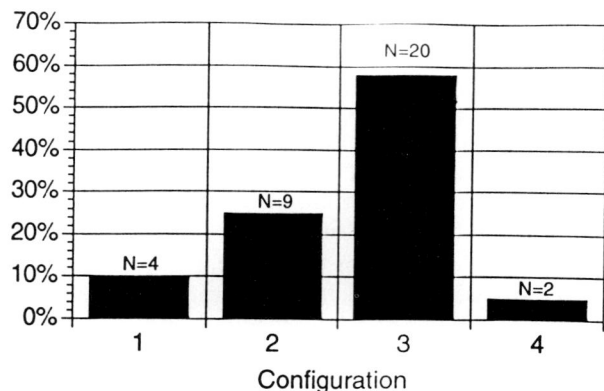

Figure 5 The majority of implanted configurations were configuration 3, which represents a transvenous-lead-only system without a subcutaneous patch. This is a unidirectional configuration. Configuration 4, though frequently tested, was rarely useful due to high DFTs.

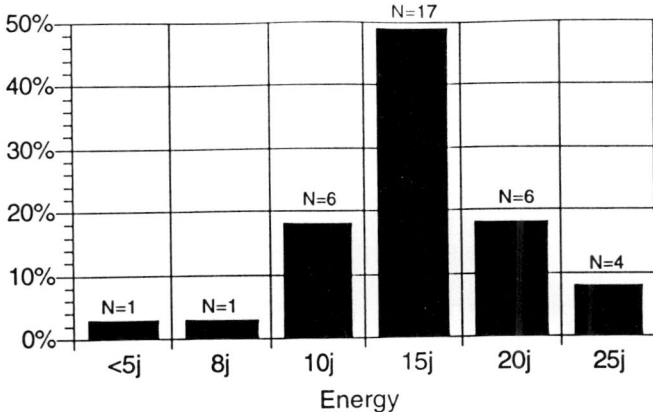

Figure 6 The median defibrillation threshold was 15 J with a mean of 13.5 J. All patients with DFTs of 20 or 25 J had three consecutive conversions at that energy level before implantation was undertaken.

X. PREDICTORS OF ADEQUATE THRESHOLDS

In the initial series of 44 consecutive patients, 31 (70%) had "adequate thresholds," defined as a DFT of 20 J or less. Multiple clinical variables (Table 1) were evaluated to determine if we could predict the likelihood of adequate thresholds [21]. Included in the variables were two X-ray parameters felt likely to be related to outcome. The standard cardiothoracic ratio was evaluated as was a lateral/AP chest cavity ratio felt likely to semiquantify the degree of lung insulation present between the subcutaneous patch and the heart. This measurement was a simple ratio of the sternum-to-spine measurement on a lateral chest X-ray divided by the largest left-to-right chest wall measurements on the PA film.

Those patients with adequate DFT had higher left ventricular ejection fractions and smaller right ventricular size (Table 2). We speculate that the latter relationship occurred because in a small right ventricular chamber it is more likely that the Endotak will be in close proximity to the interventricular septum. Adequate voltage gradients in this area of the heart are felt to be important for successful defibrillation [22].

Table 1 Clinical Variables Evaluated for Prediction of Successful Implantation

Age	Lowest impedence
Sex	Interelectrode spacing size
Ejection fraction	Right ventricular size
Type of heart disease	Dilated right ventricular
Presenting arrhythmia.	Extent of coronary artery disease
CT ratio	Myocardial infarction location
Lat/PA dimension	Configurations tested
Number of drugs failed	

Table 2 Univariate Analysis of Predictors

	DFTs ≤ 20 J	DFTs > 20 J	p value
Age	62 ± 14	65 ± 7	NS
M/F	64%/90%	36%/10%	0.13
EF	38.8 ± 15.3	26.6 ± 16.7	0.03
CT ratio	0.61 ± 0.08	0.61 ± 0.05	NS
LAT/PA	0.78 ± 0.09	0.75 ± 0.07	NS
RV size	37.6 ± 5.5	43.9 ± 10.5	0.03
Dilated RV	8%	54%	0.003

*Mean ± SD.
Type of heart disease, myocardial infarction location, extent of coronary artery disease, presenting arrhythmia, lead size, number of failed antiarrythmic drugs, and configurations tested were unrelated to DFTs.
NS = not significant.

In addition, the experience of the operator correlated with the adequacy of the defibrillation threshold, suggesting a "learning curve" for this procedure. As we have implanted more systems, the likelihood of adequate thresholds has risen (Fig. 7).

XI. COMPLICATIONS

There was no operative or 30-day mortality. There were 4 patients with perioperative myocardial infarctions. All 4 had creatinine phosphokinase elevations with positive myocardial fractions, but without ECG evolution (persistent T-wave abnormalities or new Q waves).

Significant postoperative bleeding (requiring transfusion) occurred in 2 patients, who were anticoagulated with heparin postoperatively because of prosthetic heart valves. One required surgical exploration during which diffuse oozing was noted along the course of the leads and in the generator pocket; however, no point source of bleeding was identified.

One patient developed ICD system infection with *Staphylococcus aureus* 6 weeks postimplantation. This patient had had two previous *Staphylococcus aureus* infections in the year prior to his implantation. Despite preoperative antibiotic coverage, he developed systemic infection requiring complete ICD system removal and 4 weeks of IV antibiotics. He subsequently refused reimplantation and is now receiving amiodarone.

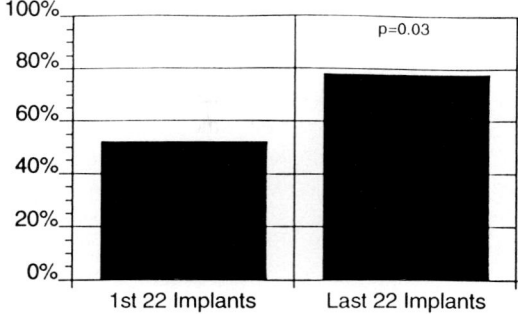

Figure 7 A "learning curve" effect was noted in our series. The percentage of patients with adequate DFTs increased as the operators became more experienced. This was statistically significant ($p = 0.03$).

XII. RESULTS: FOLLOW-UP

The 66 patients implanted with the full system have been followed for a mean of 9 months (range 1–20). There have been 120 spontaneous defibrillator discharges in 18 patients followed for >3 months. These discharges were accompanied by symptoms or documented ventricular arrhythmias in 40% of patients.

There has been 1 sudden cardiac death, 1 nonsudden cardiac death, and 1 patient who underwent cardiac transplantation. The latter patient developed worsening heart failure during follow-up, but was not on the transplant list prior to ICD implantation. He underwent transplantation 5 months postimplant after receiving 25 appropriate shocks, many documented on telemetry.

The only sudden cardiac death was witnessed, and the first recorded rhythm was asystole. The patient was resuscitated but died 24 hours later in hospital. The terminal rhythm was complete heart block and asystole. During the prolonged resuscitation efforts, ventricular tachycardia and fibrillation were documented to be appropriately detected and terminated by the ICD. We speculate that the patient initially suffered a primary bradycardia event without antecedent ventricular tachyarrhythmias.

XIII. SENSING PROBLEMS

Sensing difficulties have been reported with the Endotak C lead (23–25). These problems stem from a reported reduction in the magnitude of the recorded R wave from the rate-sensing leads after an unsuccessful shock has been delivered. Initial detection of arrhythmias is not influenced by this transient undersensing, which is noted only during redetection after an unsuccessful shock. Altered electrophysiological properties in close proximity to the rate-sensing electrodes after defibrillation may explain the phenomenon.

In one report [23], 5 patients with an Endotak system were carefully evaluated for sensing problems. A significant decline in R-wave amplitude was noted by these investigators. In addition, 2 patients demonstrated failure to redetect VF after an unsuccessful shock during the predischarge test. They state that their initial experience with the next generation of this lead system, where the electrode spacing is larger (Endotak Plus) is more favorable without sensing problems in the first 3 patients implanted in their institution.

We reviewed 410 episodes of ventricular fibrillation during DFT testing in the operating room, measuring R-wave amplitude of normal sinus rhythm at 30–35 s after successful shocks. This time was selected to determine if there was a significant reduction in R-wave amplitude at the critical point beyond which this ICD would recognize the ongoing arrhythmia as a "new" event. If this were to occur, a potentially lethal ineffective loop could occur, with the device delivering nonefficacious shocks if programmed to less than the maximum output.

The mean R-wave amplitude decreased from 9.26 ± 0.67 mV to 8.52 ± 0.53 mV ($p < 0.001$). Though statistically significant, the magnitude of the decline seems to be clinically irrelevant in the majority of patients. We did, however, identify 4 patients with prolonged detection times at the time of their 2- or 6-month DFT test. During this testing, patients receive at least one unsuccessful shock and therefore redetection is required. In 3 of 35 patients the redetection times were prolonged by 12–25 s. In 1 patient, one redetection time was greater than 25 s. A 30-J stat shock was required to terminate the arrhythmia (Fig. 8).

There have been no instances of failure to redetect arrhythmias clinically, but the lack of significant diagnostic data from the implanted generators precludes a definitive statement in this regard.

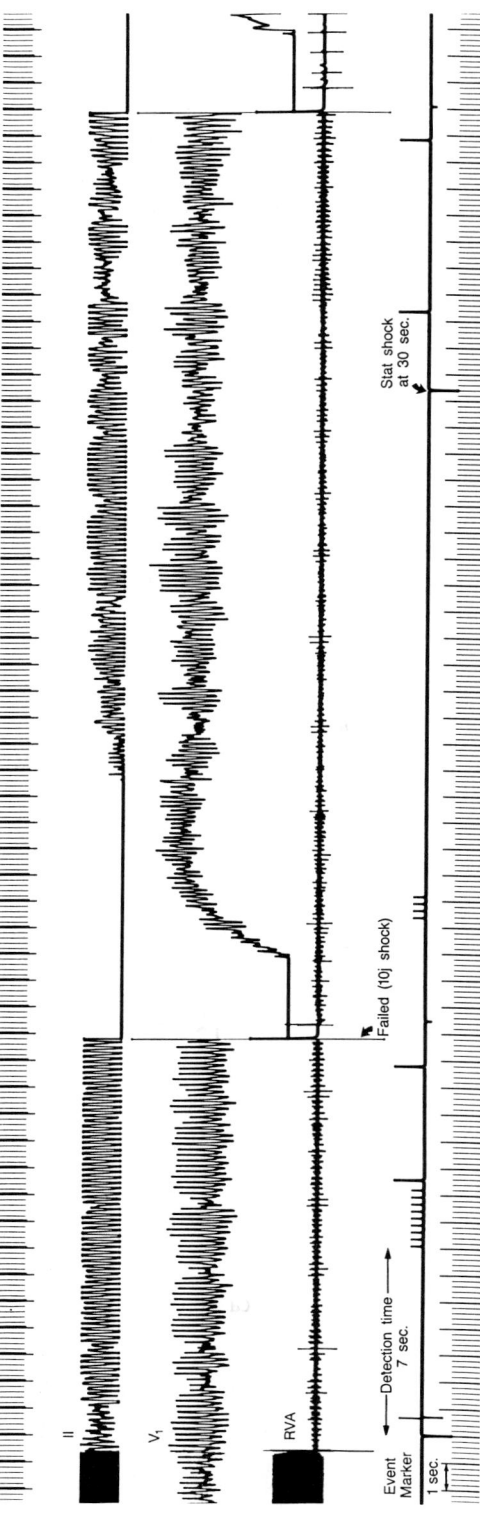

Figure 8 This figure demonstrates initially adequate sensing with the first shock (10 J) delivered without conversion. The redetection time is markedly delayed, with no detection at 25 s, requiring a "stat shock" for the termination of the arrhythmia. Such an event spontaneously might result in an "ineffective loop," occurring without the delivery of the maximum shock energy.

XIV. LONG-TERM DEFIBRILLATION THRESHOLD STABILITY

Thirty-five patients have returned for 2-month conversion testing, and 20 patients have had 6-month tests. In those patients with programmable ICDs, repeated DFTs were measured at both follow-up tests ($n = 20$). The latter retesting was added after the first 5 patients tested demonstrated a trend upward in DFTs at 2 months.

There appears to be a trend upward in the measured DFTs over time, with the mean DFT at implant of 13.5 ± 8 J rising at 2 months to 15.8 ± 4.7 J and at 6 months to 18.0 ± 5 J ($p < 0.05$ and $p < 0.02$, respectively). Though the number of patients tested thus far is small, this is a disturbing trend that merits further observation.

XV. COST

Since the Endotak C system requires a less invasive approach with less morbidity, hospital costs could be expected to be less for each patient. To test this hypothesis, we compared 25 patients who underwent an Endotak C system implant to 15 patients who received a standard thoracotomy implant to determine if costs were reduced by this new approach [26]. The Endotak C patients were all successful implants. The thoracotomy patients were all implanted either prior to the availability of the Endotak C or during periods when the device was not available.

Hospital *and* physician fees were examined at the Lahey Clinic, where all charges are billed by a central computerized system. Bills were divided into implant, convalescent, and total charges. As expected, there was no difference in the implant charges; however, there was a significant reduction in convalescent charges. The Endotak C system resulted in a $11,446 mean savings per patient in convalescent charges ($p < 0.005$) and a mean decrease in length of convalescence of 8 days ($p < 0.001$). Though these decreases were significant, total charges and length of stay were not statistically different, though a trend was present, with declines similar to the convalescent declines noted. This analysis was not performed on an "intention to treat" basis.

XVI. MULTICENTER STUDY OF SAFETY AND EFFICACY

Thirty-five centers have participated in a multicenter study organized by the manufacturer to prove for licensing purposes in the United States that the Endotak system is safe and efficacious [27]. A total of 536 patients with out-of-hospital cardiac arrest or recurrent sustained ventricular tachycardia underwent attempted implantation of the system between September 1990 and February 1992. The implantation protocol and configurations used were the same as outlined above.

There were 403 (75%) successful protocol implants during the initial study period. In the remaining 133 patients, 110 were not implanted because of high DFTs, 17 patients were implanted in a nonstandard configuration, 4 were not tested because of difficulty placing the transvenous lead, and 2 patients had inadequate sensing thresholds.

The mean age was 62.4 ± 12.3 years in the 299 males and 104 females successfully implanted. The mean ejection fraction reported was 33%, with the majority of patients having coronary artery disease [77%]. The primary arrhythmia was monomorphic ventricular tachycardia in 51%, ventricular fibrillation in 34%, both in 12%, and polymorphic ventricular tachycardia in 3%.

The phase II protocol required investigators to attempt at least two different configurations at the time of implantation. Patients were randomly assigned on the day of surgery to be tested

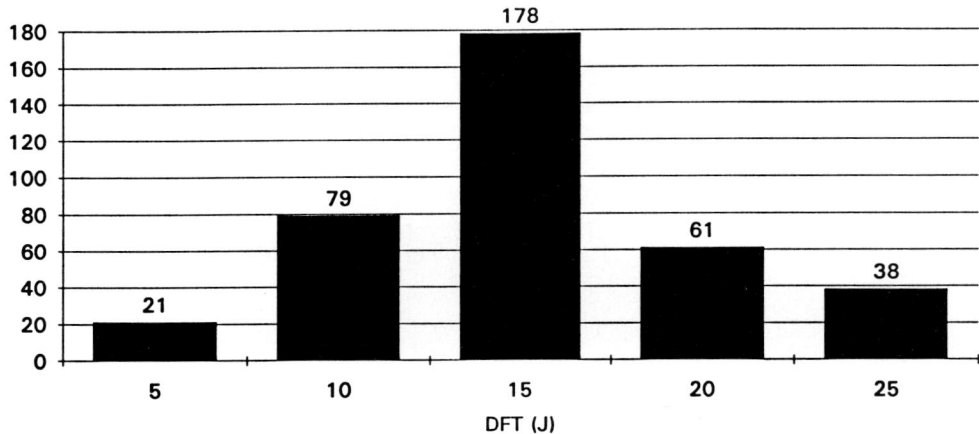

Figure 9 The lowest defibrillating energy during intraoperative testing in the multicenter study of efficacy ($n = 377$). True DFTs were not measured in all patients. Twenty-five patients were not included in this figure, because DFT testing was indeterminant.

in configuration 3 and one of the other configurations. A DFT of 20 J or less was required unless a high-energy device was implanted, in which case a DFT of 25 J was accepted. The testing scheme was as outlined previously (Fig. 4).

The mean R-wave for sensing was 11.0 ± 5.3 mV (range 3.0–30.0 mV). The mean pacing threshold was 0.86 ± 0.78 V (range 0.1–6.0 V). The mean impedance for the shocking electrodes was 43.5 ± 8.9 Ω (range 29–90 Ω). The mean DFT was 15.2 J. Figure 9 demonstrates the range of values.

The configuration most commonly implanted was configuration 2, used in 60% of patients ($n = 241$), with configuration 3 used in only 31%. A high-energy device was used in 20% of patients. Twenty-one patients had concomitant permanent pacemakers implanted before or at the time of Endotak C implantation. One patient developed intermittent sensing secondary to pacemaker-ICD interaction, requiring explanation of the Endotak C.

Lead dislodgement was noted in 1.2% of implants. Implant difficulty such as stylet handling problems and lead perforation were seen in less than 1%. Intermittent sensing problems also occurred in less than 1%.

A total of 169 patients have reported 1275 spontaneous shocks during a mean follow-up of 6 months. Associated symptoms occurred in 566 episodes (44%). The sudden cardiac death rate at 1 year for this group was reported by the manufacturer to be 2.8%. This compares favorably with the mortality reported with epicardial systems.

The reliability over time for this system is demonstrated by the 384 successful shocks > 90 days postimplant occurring in 80 patients. This finding suggests that the system remains reliable at least until the postoperative healing phase is over. However, the trial is ongoing, and complete data are not yet available.

XVII. CONCLUSION

ICD therapy has had a significant impact on sudden cardiac death. Current systems rely on an epicardial lead system which requires the risk and discomfort of a thoracotomy. The transvenous lead system developed by CPI in our initial experience has proven reliable in the short term and is cost-saving compared to conventional systems. Sensing problems have been reported, but will likely be addressed in a modified lead system. As this and other nonthoracotomy lead systems are proven chronically reliable, epicardial systems will likely be used only if concomitant cardiac surgery is required.

REFERENCES

1. Winkle RA, Thomas A. The automatic implantable cardioverter defibrillator: the US experience. In: Brugada P, Wellens HJJ, eds. Cardiac Arrhythmias: Where Do We Go from Here? Mount Kisco, NY: Futura, 1987:663–680.
2. Kelly PA, Cannom DS, Garan H, et al. The automatic implantable cardioverter-defibrillator: efficacy, complications, and survival in patients with malignant ventricular arrhythmias. J Am Coll Cardiol 1988; 11:1278–1286.
3. Mirowski M, Reid PR, Winkle RA, et al. Mortality in patients with implanted automatic defibrillator. Ann Intern Med 1983; 98 (part 1):585–588.
4. Gaby MD, Brodman R, Johnston D, et al. Automatic implantable cardioverter-defibrillator: patient survival, battery longevity and shock delivery analysis. J Am Coll Cardiol 1987; 9:1349–1356.
5. Winkle RA, Mead RH, Ruder MA, et al. Longterm outcome with the automatic implantable cardioverter-defibrillator. J Am Coll Cardiol 1989; 13:1353–1361.
6. Saksena S, Parsonnet V. Implantation of a cardioverter-defibrillator without thoracotomy using a triple electrode system. JAMA 1988; 259:69–72.
7. Troup PJ. Implantable cardioverters and defibrillators. Curr Prob Cardiol 1989; 14:675–843.
8. Mirowski M, Mower MM, Langer A, Heilman MS, Schreibman J. A chronically implanted system for automatic defibrillation in active conscious dogs. Experimental model for treatment of sudden death from ventricular fibrillation. Circulation 1978; 58:90–94.
9. Reid PR, Griffith LS, Mower MM, et al. Implantable cardioverter-defibrillator: patient selection and implantation protocol. PACE 1984; 7:1338–1344.
10. Winkle RA, Stinson EB, Bach SM, Jr., Echt DS, Oyer P, Armstrong K. Measurement of cardioversion/defibrillation thresholds in man by a truncated exponential waveform and an apical patch-superior vena caval spring electrode configuration. Circulation 1984; 69:766–771.
11. McCowan R, Maloney J, Wilkoff B, et al. Automatic implantable cardioverter-defibrillator implantation without thoracotomy using an endocardial and submuscular patch system. J Am Coll Cardiol 1991; 17:415–421.
12. Moore SL, Maloney JD, Edel TB, et al. Implantable cardioverter defibrillator implanted by nonthoracotomy approach: initial clinical experience with the redesigned transvenous lead system. PACE 1991; 14:1865–1869.
13. Chang MS, Inoue H, Kallok MJ, Zipes DP. Double and triple sequential shocks reduce ventricular defibrillation threshold in dogs with and without myocardial infarction. J Am Coll Cardiol 1986; 8:1393–1405.
14. Wetherbee JN, Chapman PD, Klopfenstein HS, Bach SM Jr, Troup PJ. Nonthoracotomy internal defibrillation in dogs: threshold reduction using a subcutaneous chest wall electrode with a transvenous catheter electrode. J Am Coll Cardiol 1987; 10:406–411.
15. O'Neill PG, Boahene KA, Lawrie GM, Harvill LF, Pacifico A. The automatic implantable cardioverter-defibrillator: effect of the patch polarity on defibrillation threshold. J Am Coll Cardiol 1991; 17(3):707–711.
16. Venditti FJ, Qiang ZZ, Grubelich F, Martin D. Hemodynamic stability of tachyarrhythmias determined by use of pulmonary artery O_2 saturation monitoring (abstr). PACE 1991; 14:708.
17. Ong LS, Barold SS, Lederman M, Falkoff MD, Heinle RA. Cephalic vein guide wire technique for implantation of permanent pacemakers. Am Heart J 1987; 114:753–756.
18. Singer I, Lange D. Defibrillation threshold: clinical utility and therapeutic implications. PACE 1992; 15:932–949.

19. Lange DJ, Cato EL, Echt DS. Protocol for evaluation of internal defibrillation safety margins (abstr). J Am Coll Cardiol 1989; 13:(2):111A.
20. Mendoza IG, Kleiman RB, Marchlinski FE. Electrophysiologic effect of the anesthetic propofol at post-operative defibrillation testing (abstr). J Am Coll Cardiol 1992; 19:221A.
21. Venditti FJ, Vassolas G, Bowen S, Shahian D. Predictors of successful implantations of a transvenous defibrillator system (abstr). PACE 1992; 15:541.
22. Ideker RE, Hillsley RE, Wharton JM. Shock strength for the implantable defibrillator: can you have too much of a good thing? (edit). PACE 1992; 15:841–844.
23. Jung W, Manz M, Moosdorf R, Luderitz B. Failure of an implantable cardioverter-defibrillator to redetect ventricular fibrillation in patients with a nonthoracotomy lead system. Circulation 1992; 86:1217–1222.
24. Jung W, Manz M, Tebbenjohans J, Moosdorf R, Schneider C, Luderitz B. Failure of an implantable cardioverter/defibrillator to redetect ventricular fibrillation using a nonthoracotomy lead system (abstr). PACE 1992; 15:531.
25. Isbruch F, Block M, Wietholt D, et al. Reduction of the endocardial sensing signal of an integrated sense/pace/defibrillation lead after application of defibrillation shocks (abstr). PACE 1992; 15:562.
26. O'Connell M, Venditti FJ. Implantable cardioverter defibrillator implantation: effect of a transvenous lead system on length of hospitalization and cost (abstr). PACE 1992; 15:565.
27. Cardiac Pacemaker Incorporated. Endotak lead system clinical report. July 1, 1992.

46

The DF Endocardial Defibrillation and Pacing Nonthoracotomy Lead System

N. A. Mark Estes III

*Tufts University School of Medicine
and New England Medical Center
Boston, Massachusetts*

I. INTRODUCTION

The feasibility of using a nonthoracotomy lead system in conjunction with an implantable cardioverter defibrillator to sense, cardiovert, or defibrillate ventricular arrhythmias was supported by early animal laboratory research [1,8]. Subsequent, testing of lead systems in humans has demonstrated the ability to obtain adequate defibrillation thresholds without placement of epicardial or pericardial patches in the majority of patients who have been appropriately selected [2–7]. Currently, several manufacturers have nonthoracotomy lead systems at various stages of clinical investigation [2–7]. This chapter summarizes the design, animal studies, and results of both acute and chronic human testing in clinical investigation of a nonthoracotomy lead system: the Telectronics endocardial defibrillation lead system (DF system) (Telectronics Pacing Systems, Denver, Colo.).

DF Endocardial Defibrillation Lead System

The DF endocardial defibrillation lead system consists of the atrial DF lead (model 040-112) and the Accufix DF lead (model 040-113) [8]. In addition, a subcutaneous patch electrode (models 040-105, -106, and -107) and a bifurcated adaptor (model 040-051) can be used to achieve several different configurations for energy delivery. Both atrial and ventricular electrodes have sensing, pacing, and defibrillation capabilities.

The atrial DF lead, model 040-112, is a bifurcated, bipolar VS1/unipolar, 3.2-mm HV tined atrial "J" pacing/defibrillation lead (Fig. 1). It is 90 cm in length and is designed such that when the sensing electrode at the distal tip is placed in the atrial appendage, the defibrillation electrode will rest in the superior vena cava and right atrium. The Accufix DF lead, model 040-113, is a 100-cm, bifurcated, bipolar VS-1/unipolar, 3.2-mm HV, ventricular active-fixation pacing/defibrillation lead designed to be placed near the right ventricular apex (Fig. 2).

MODEL 040-112 GENERAL SPECIFICATIONS

ELECTRODE DESCRIPTION	BIFURCATED TERMINAL CONNECTOR	LEAD LENGTH (cm)	LEAD BODY DIAMETER (mm)	CONDUCTORS	CONDUCTOR RESISTANCE AT 25 °C (ohms)	ELECTRODE SEPARATION (cm)	ELECTRODE SURFACE AREA (mm²)
ATRIAL DF	Pace/sense: bipolar VS·1; High voltage: unipolar 3.2 mm (HV)	90	2.5	Inner: Quadrafilar MP35N Helical Coil Outer: Braided Titanium	Braid 5 (max) Inner 95 (max)	8.5	Distal 8.8 Braid 600

NOMINAL DIMENSIONS

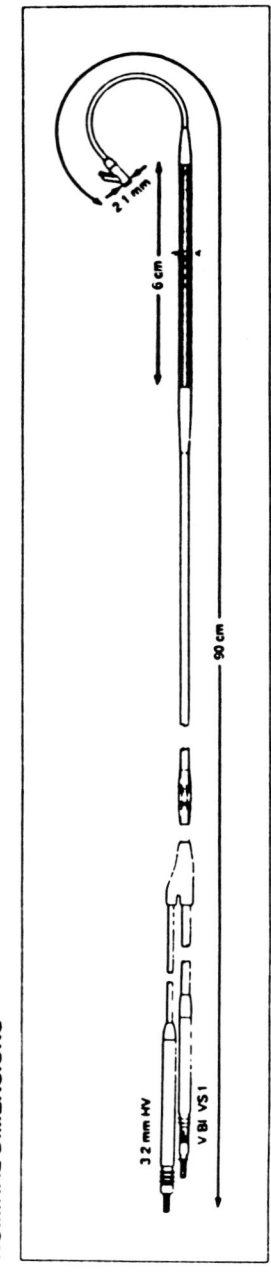

Figure 1 Atrial DF lead with electrode description and specifications [8].

MODEL 040-113 GENERAL SPECIFICATIONS

ELECTRODE DESCRIPTION	BIFURCATED TERMINAL CONNECTOR	LEAD LENGTH (cm)	LEAD BODY DIAMETER (mm)	CONDUCTORS	CONDUCTOR RESISTANCE AT 25 °C (ohms)	ELECTRODE SEPARATION (mm)	ELECTRODE SURFACE AREA (mm²)	MAX HELIX PENETRATION (mm)
ACCUFIX DF	Pace/sense: bipolar VS-1; High voltage: unipolar 3.2 mm (HV)	100	2.5	Inner: Quadrafilar MP35N Helical Coil Outer: Braided Titanium	Braid 5 (max) Inner 95 (max)	18	Distal 10.2 Braid 600	2.1

NOMINAL DIMENSIONS

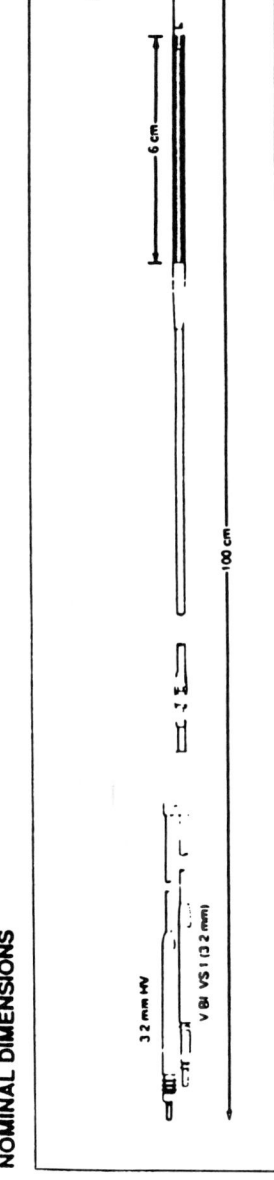

Figure 2 Accufix DF lead with electrode description and specifications [8].

In the absence of an atrial appendage, this lead could also be left free-floating in the junction of the superior vena cave and the right atrium.

The lead body of both the atrial DF and the Accufix DF lead consists of a quadrafilar cobalt-nickel conductor coil insulated by polyurethane. A braided titanium HV conductor surrounds this inner coil and is also insulated by polyurethane. The cathodal electrode used for pacing and sensing is platinum/iridium with a porous surface. The 3.2-mm HV terminal connector is made of titanium with silicone elastomer insulation, while the VS-1 terminal connector is made of stainless steel with silicone elastomer insulation.

The atrial DF lead has a tined tip for fixation in the atrial appendage, while the ventricular lead has a retractable platinum/iridium active-fixation helix which serves to fix the lead in position by penetrating the endocardial tissue. The helix is electrically isolated from the electrode. It is exposed with the use of a fixation stylet which is used to extend or retract the helix by rotating the fixation stylet clockwise or counterclockwise, respectively.

The patch lead used with this system comes in three sizes: small (model 040-105), standard (model 040-106), and large (model 040-107) [8]. The patches are composed of titanium mesh embedded in a Dacron-reinforced silicone sheet which forms a flexible conductive patch electrode. The titanium mesh is welded to a low-resistance conductor which is insulated by three layers, including a Teflon coating, a polyurethane sleeve, and a silicone sleeve. Each patch has a 3.2-mm/HV 1 unipolar connector. The exposed surface area is 15 cm^2 for the small, 28 cm^2 for the standard, and 40 cm^2 for the large patch. The DC resistance is <2 Ω with a voltage rating at 2 kV for all sizes.

The DF lead system allows the delivery of a cardioversion or defibrillation shock in a unidirectional or bidirectional pathway in a variety of waveforms [8]. Testing at the time of implantation of various configuration allows the physician to choose the most appropriate lead configuration (Fig. 3). During the course of the clinical study, the DF lead system was initially implanted with the Telectronics Guardian II 4204 and Guardian ATP 4210 implantable cardioverter-defibrillators.

II. ANIMAL STUDIES OF THE DF LEAD SYSTEM

Prior to acute testing in humans, investigations were undertaken in dogs to determine both the acute and chronic thresholds with this system [1]. In 15 dogs, a subcutaneous patch was implanted with atrial and ventricular electrodes. Implantable cardioverter-defibrillators were not used in this study, so the lead terminals were capped and required exposure at each follow-up, with subsequent capping and reimplantation. Defibrillation thresholds, pacing thresholds, and impedance were determined acutely at implant, at 6 weeks, and at 12 weeks. At each follow-up study the lead and patch integrity and positions were checked with fluoroscopy. Atrial and ventricular pacing and sensing thresholds were collected in a bipolar fashion prior to, and following, the determination of defibrillation thresholds at implant and at each follow-up.

Defibrillation thresholds were obtained at implant and at each follow-up in three configurations. These included monophasic, unidirectional (M/U); asymmetric biphasic, unidirectional (AB/U); and asymmetric biphasic, bidirectional (AB/B2). The implant, 6-week, and 12-week defibrillation thresholds data are summarized in Table 1 [1]. There were no statistically significant differences for any of the configurations in the mean voltage required for defibrillation when comparing the implant, 6-week, and 12-week values. The decrease in resistance did reach statistical significance.

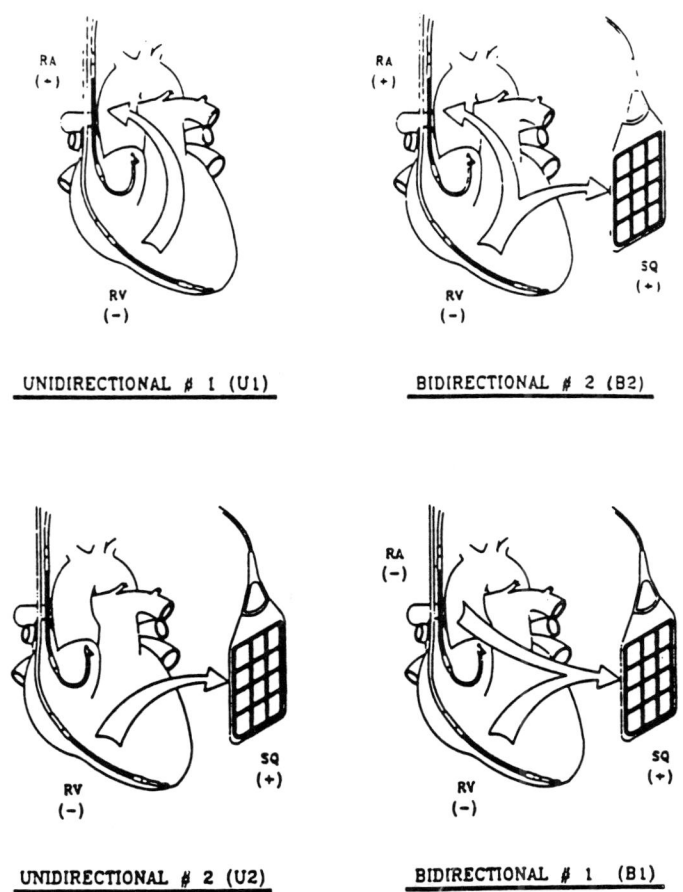

Figure 3 Electrode configurations for the Accufix DF nonthoracotomy lead system. With the U1 configuration, current flows from the right ventricular (RV) cathode (−) to the right atrial (RA) anode (+). With the B2 configuration, current flows from the RV cathode bidirectionally to the common anode of the RA and subcutaneous (SQ) patch. With the U2 configuration, and RV electrode is the cathode (−), with the SQ patch as the anode (+). With the B1 configuration, the RA and RV electrodes are used as a common cathode, with the SQ patch as anode [8].

Bipolar atrial and ventricular pacing thresholds were measured at implant and in follow-up. Threshold and impedance data are summarized in Table 2 [1]. The mean atrial postshock constant-voltage bipolar threshold was 0.5 V at 0.5-ms pulse width. This had increased at 6 and 12 weeks to 1.3 V. The mean ventricular pacing threshold was 0.7 V at implant and doubled to 1.4 V at 6 and 12 weeks.

Pathological studies were done after 12 weeks on the atrial and ventricular leads. A smooth fibrotic sheath encased both leads and was generally thicker around the ventricular lead [1]. Evidence of localized tissue irritation where the leads contacted the endocardium were present in several dogs. Evidence of fibroses at the sites was present. Dislodgment of the ventricular lead into the outflow tract was observed in 2 dogs, reportedly without any evident clinical

Table 1 Defibrillation Thresholds and Resistance [1]

		Implant	Week 6	Week 12
M/U	Mean	8.5 J (346 V)	13.5 J (410 V)	15.0 J (418 V)
	S.D.	4.0 J (69 V)	7.5 J (116 V)	6.0 J (97 V)
	Resistance	63Ω	53Ω	47Ω
AB/U	Mean	5.4 J (313 V)	6.9 J (330 V)	8.4 J (360 V)
	S.D.	1.3 J (69 V)	2.2 J (110 V)	2.3 J (96 V)
	Resistance	63Ω	53Ω	48Ω
AB/B2	Mean	7.9 J (333 V)	10.6 J (371 V)	11.8 J (390 V)
	S.D.	1.5 J (84 V)	3.0 J (110 V)	3.2 J (99 V)
	Resistance	46Ω	38Ω	36Ω

effect. Additionally, 1 dog had right ventricular perforation without any clinical signs, symptoms, or effects on resistance threshold or defibrillation thresholds [1,8].

III. ACUTE HUMAN STUDIES: DF LEAD SYSTEM

A multicenter acute study was performed using the DF atrial and ventricular leads with a cutaneous patch (R2 pad, R2 Corporation) or fast patch (Physio-Control) [25]. Once the atrial and ventricular leads had been placed at the time of electrophysiology study being done for clinical purposes, bipolar thresholds and impedance as well as R-wave amplitude were determined. When ventricular tachycardia or ventricular fibrillation was induced, R-wave amplitude was determined during the rhythm, and the Telectronics Pacing Systems Clinical Research System (CRS) was used to deliver cardioversion or defibrillation shocks.

During the study, a total of 23 patients were studied, including 21 males and 2 females [25]. The mean age was 65.5 years, ranging from 27 to 87 years. The mean left ventricular ejection fraction was 36.4% (range 11–59%). Coronary artery disease was present in 18 pa-

Table 2 Bipolar Atrial and Ventricular Pacing Thresholds and Impedances obtained Before and After Defibrillation Threshold Determination [1]

	Pre	Post	Pre	Post	Pre	Post
Atrial thresholds						
Pacing (V)						
Mean	0.5	0.5	1.4	1.3	1.4	1.3
S.D.	0.14	0.08	0.56	0.41	0.42	0.49
Impedance (Ω)						
Mean	855	740	764	693	770	694
S.D.	117	151	205	173	174	161
Ventricular thresholds						
Pacing (V)						
Mean	0.5	0.7	1.5	1.4	1.7	1.4
S.D.	0.14	0.18	0.59	0.61	0.91	0.55
Impedance (Ω)						
Mean	690	510	472	409	481	401
S.D.	257	76	106	77	116	81

Table 3 Prestudy and Poststudy Bipolar Pacing Analysis

	Mean	S.D.	Range
Prestudy Analysis			
0.5-ms pulse width	0.7 V	0.5 V	(0.3–2.0 V)
1.0-ms pulse width	0.7 V	0.5 V	(0.2–2.2 V)
Pacing impedance	375 Ω	75 Ω	(250–550 Ω)
R-wave amplitude	8.2 mV	3.6 mV	(1.8–15.4 mV)
Poststudy analysis			
0.5-ms pulse width	1.1 V	0.7 V	(0.3–2.9 V)
1.0-ms pulse width	0.9 V	0.5 V	(0.3–2.0 V)
Pacing impedance	368 Ω	57 Ω	(270–500 Ω)
R-wave amplitude	7.6 mV	3.9 mV	(1.7–15.4 mV)

tients, with 17 having had a prior myocardial infarction. Congestive heart failure was present in 8 patients, and coronary bypass grafting had been performed in 6. Cardiomyopathy was diagnosed in 5 patients, and hypertensive heart disease in 3 patients. The presenting clinical arrhythmia was ventricular tachycardia in 17 patients, ventricular fibrillation in 3 patients, nonsustained ventricular tachycardia in 2 patients, and one patient was labeled as having had a cardiac arrest.

The mean threshold for ventricular capture at 0.5-ms pulse width was 0.7 ± 0.5 V (range 0.3–2.0 V). At the conclusion of the study, the threshold at the same pulse width was 1.1 ± 0.7 V (range 0.3–2.9 V) (Table 3). The pacing impedance remained unchanged at 375 ± 75 Ω (range 250–550 Ω) at the beginning of the study and was 368 ± 57 Ω (range 270–500 Ω) at the end of the study. The R-wave amplitude in normal sinus rhythm average 8.2 ± 3.6 mV (range 1.8–15.4 mV) at initiation and 7.6 ± 3.9 mV (range 1.7–15.4 mV) at the conclusion of the study. No statistically significant changes were noted in threshold, impedance, or R-wave amplitude when values at the beginning and end of the study were compared.

When an arrhythmia was induced, the atrial electrode, ventricular electrode, and cutaneous patch were used in several different combinations as anode or cathode. In this investigation a total of 19 episodes of ventricular fibrillation were induced in 9 patients (Table 4). The mean successful energy necessary to defibrillate was 23 J (549 V). Four shocks were delivered at maximum voltage of the currently 14 available ICDs (35–40 J). Only 1 shock failed to defibrillate at maximum voltage. It should be noted that the intent of this study was not to establish the defibrillation threshold in the patient population. Preselected energy values were delivered regardless of the arrhythmia induced.

Twenty-three of 26 episodes of slow ventricular tachycardia were successfully cardioverted with a mean of 365 ± 97 (range 172–511 V). Seventeen of 20 episodes (85%) of slow ventricular tachycardia were successfully cardioverted with 400 V or less, while 6 of 6 (100%) were converted successfully with 101–550 V. Of the 33 episodes of fast ventricular tachycardia (cycle length <250 ms), 26 were successfully converted. Seven of 11 episodes (64%) were successfully converted with less than 400 V, 16 of 19 (84%) with 401–550 V, and 3 out of 3 (100%) with 551 through 700 V. The mean voltage for successful conversion of rapid ventricular tachycardia was 491 ± 95 V (271–684 V). All of the above measurements were made with monophasic, bidirectional shocks. In addition, most patients were tested with biphasic shocks. A cumulative logistic regression analysis showed significant improvement with biphasic shocks [24]. Based on these data showing the feasibility of detection, cardioversion, and defibrillation

Table 4

	Percent success of monophasic bidirectional shocks		
	Voltage range		
Arrhythmia	<400 V	401–500 V	551–700 V
Slow VT	85% (17/20)	100% (6/6)	No data
Fast VT	64%(7/11)	84% (16/19)	100% (3/3)
VF	No data	53% (8/15)	75% (3/4)

Mean of successful energy for monophasic bidirectional shocks			
Arrhythmia	Mean	S.D.	Range
Slow VT	9.9 J	4.9 J	(2.1–20.5 J)
Fast VT	17.7 J	6.2 J	(5.1–33.0 J)
VF	23.1 J	5.6 J	(17.4–32.8 J)

Mean successful voltage for monophasic bidirectional shocks			
Arrhythmia	Mean	S.D.	Range
Slow VT	365 V	97 V	(172–544 V)
Fast VT	391 V	95 V	(271–684 V)
VF	549 V	72 V	(497–692 V)

in acute human studies, the decision was made to proceed with clinical investigation and implantation of the DF lead system with implantable cardioverter-defibrillators [8].

IV. DF ENDOCARDIAL DEFIBRILLATION LEAD SYSTEMS: CLINICAL STUDY

The initial phase of the clinical investigation of the DF lead system was designed to further evaluate the efficacy and safety of the lead system in conjunction with an implantable cardioverter-defibrillator [8]. Patients who were considered candidates for this protocol were those who had had episodes of prior out-of-hospital ventricular fibrillation, who had sustained ventricular tachycardia, or who had syncope with induced sustained ventricular tachycardia.

Table 5

	Pacing thresholds @ 0.5 ms			Pacing thresholds @ 1.0 ms		
	AVG (STD)	Range	n	AVG (STD)	Range	n
Implant	0.71 (0.57)	0.10–4.00	64	0.54 (0.47)	0.10–3.30	63
Post tunnel	1.89 (0.96)	0.20–3.90	62	1.54 (1.07)	0.10–7.50	60
PTD	2.90 (1.43)	1.20–7.50	28	4.20 (2.31)	0.90–7.50	43
1 month	2.90 (1.58)	1.10–7.50	17	4.20 (2.42)	1.40–7.50	20
2 months	3.00 (1.45)	1.10–7.50	26	2.90 (1.46)	1.40–7.50	26
4 months	2.80 (1.37)	1.00–7.10	25	2.90 (1.67)	1.10–7.50	32
6 months	2.80 (1.23)	1.30–7.00	15	3.16 (1.67)	1.20–7.50	19

Patients with excluded if they had artificial valves in the tricuspid position or if they had ventricular and/or atrial pacemaker leads implanted. In addition, patients whose physical condition or recent illness would put them at additional risk of complications or death after implant could not be included in the study. During the initial phase, patients who were not candidates for standard thoracotomy implantation of an implantable defibrillator system were also excluded. The preimplant evaluation included a detailed cardiovascular history and, where possible, documentation of the clinical ventricular arrhythmia with 12-lead EKG or rhythm strip. Cardiac catheterization with determination of coronary anatomy and left ventricular ejection fraction as well as baseline comprehensive electrophysiological evaluation were also requested; however, no patients were excluded from the study because of low ejection fraction.

At the time of implantation, the protocol recommended that the implant be done in a one-step procedure. The site of venous access was left to the discretion of the implanting physician. The option of leaving a bifurcated active fixation lead at the junction of the superior vena cava and right atrium in place of the atrial J lead for patients who had no atrial appendage was present in the protocol. Prior to a subcutaneous patch implant, the physician had the option of using a cutaneous patch to determine the defibrillation efficacy of the bidirectional configuration. The bidirectional configuration in which the ventricular electrode was the cathode and the atrial electrode and cutaneous or subcutaneous patch were combined with an adaptor as a common anode (the B2 configuration) was the configuration most tested at implant.

At the time of implantation, pacing thresholds were determined at pulse widths of 0.5 and 1.0 ms. Additionally, the R-wave, P-wave, and lead impedance were determined. These values were repeated after the leads had been tunneled into the abdomen. In order for the DF lead system to be implanted, the patient's ventricular fibrillation had to be induced and reverted three times at an energy level which represented at least a 10-J safety margin. A minimum of 10 s had to occur after arrhythmia induction before shock delivery, and a minimum of 2 min was required between arrhythmia inductions to allow for stabilization.

The defibrillation threshold for the purpose of this protocol was defined as the lowest successful energy. Defibrillation was attempted at progressively lower discrete energy levels until there was a failure. Per protocol, effective sensing and defibrillation in the final electrode configuration after the DF system had been connected to the implantable defibrillator had to be demonstrated prior to the conclusion of the implant procedure. The follow-up required for patients enrolled in the clinical study included prior-to-discharge and 4-month postimplant EP studies, and routine follow-up visits at 2 and 6 months postimplant to evaluate the system noninvasively.

At all follow-up visits, documentation of any change in the patient's cardiovascular status was obtained, as well as noninvasive measurement of pacing threshold and lead impedance and reading of all event counters and data logs [8]. Additionally, sensing of the patient's intrinsic rhythm was analyzed to optimize the sensitivity of the implantable cardioverter-defibrillator. At the prior-to-discharge EP study, the function of the system was verified by inducing the patient's arrhythmia and allowing the implantable defibrillator to adequately sense the arrhythmia and deliver the programmed therapy. Therapy with antitachycardia pacing and low-energy cardioversion could also be refined at this time.

Induction of ventricular fibrillation was required at the 4-month electrophysiology study. During that study, the defibrillation threshold energy established at implant was to be tested first. If this energy was successful in converting the patient's ventricular fibrillation, the physician was requested to test successive lower discrete energy levels until there was a failure. If the defibrillation energy established at implant was not successful in reverting the patient's VF, successive higher discrete energy levels should be tested. Once an energy level was successful,

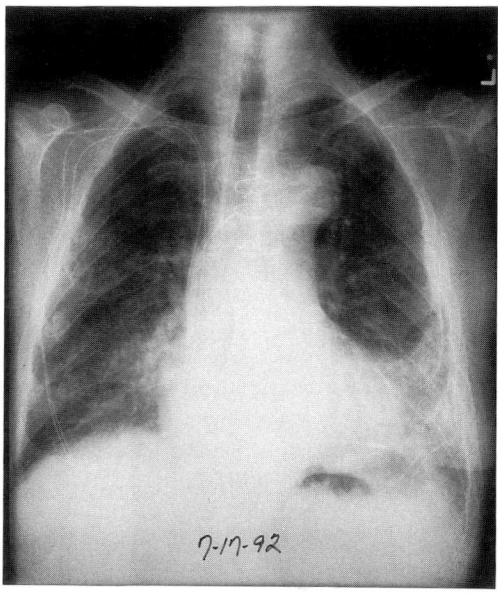

(a)

Figure 4 Chest X-ray including (a) AP and (b) lateral, showing atrial J electrode in the right atrial appendage, ventricular electrode in the right ventricular apex, and subcutaneous patch. These are tunneled to the implantable cardioverter defibrillator in the left upper quadrant of the abdomen. The 4210 ATP ICD, atrial and ventricular leads are seen in the abdominal film (c).

if the energy level was 20 J or below, two successful reversions at that energy level were necessary. If the new successful energy level was above 20 J, three successful reversions at that energy were necessary. Additionally, sensing of the patient's intrinsic rhythm and ventricular fibrillation was evaluated, and the lead positions were verified fluoroscopically.

Per protocol, all patients who received shock therapy were evaluated immediately for lead performance via telemetered pacing thresholds and lead impedance measurements. All data log and even counters were also checked. Verification of the position of the DF lead system via fluoroscopy or X-ray was left to physician discretion. Additional testing such as Holter monitoring or event monitors could be used at the discretion of the physician.

As of December 1992, 59 implants of the DF lead system had occurred in 58 patients [10]. The patient population consists of 51 males and 7 females with a mean age of 57 years. The presenting clinical arrhythmia and indication for implant was listed as sustained ventricular tachycardia in 36 patients, ventricular fibrillation in 21 patients, and cardiac arrest in 16 patients. In some patients, more than one indication was noted on the clinical report form. Four patients received their device as replacement devices, whereas 54 had new implants.

In 39 patients, the lead system was introduced using a retained guidewire technique through the subclavian vein (Fig. 4). In 17 patients, the leads were introduced through the cephalic vein. In 6 patients, a combined approach was used with the cephalic and subclavian veins. The axillary vein was used in 1 patient. Patch placement was subcutaneous in 43 patients, submuscular in 13, and in 5 patients, the implant configuration did not require a patch. In 1 patient a defibrillation lead was implanted in the coronary sinus position to serve as a common anode

DF Nonthoracotomy Lead System

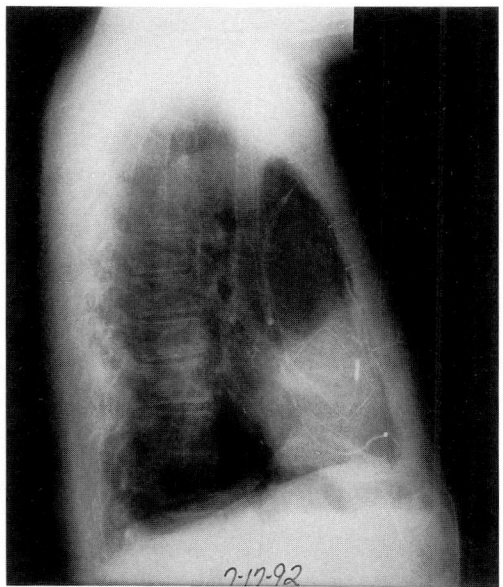

(b)

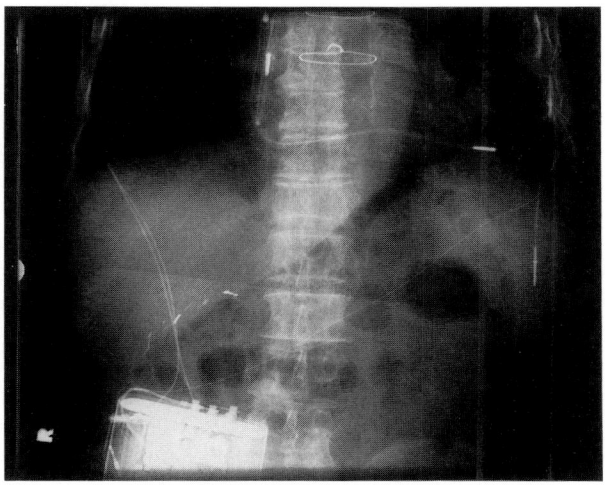

(c)

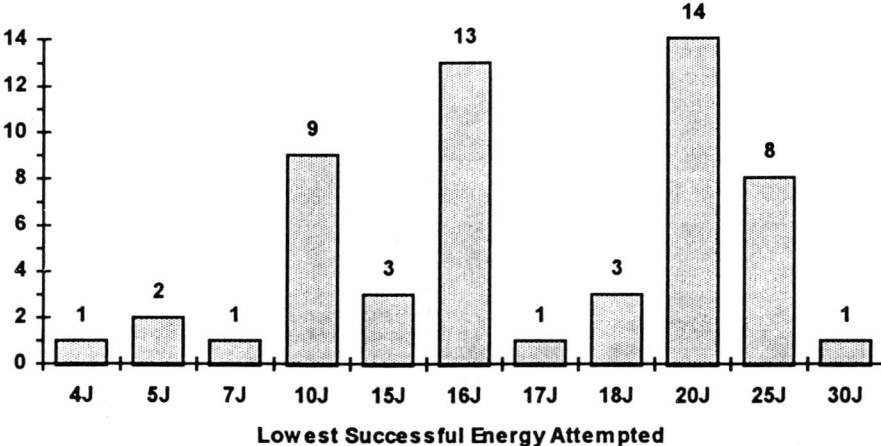

Figure 5 Distribution of the lowest successful energy attempted at the time of implantation with the B2 configuration for the DF lead system [10].

for a bidirectional configuration. In 54 patients the Guardian ATP 4210 was implanted, and 4 patients received a Guardian II 4204. Two patients implanted with the Guardian ATP 4210 were later upgraded to Guardian ATP II 4211 devices. At the time of implant, the B2 configuration, in which the ventricular lead is the cathode and the atrial lead and subcutaneous patch are combined as the anode, was tested in 58 patients; the U1 configuration, in which the ventricular lead is the cathode and the atrial lead is the anode, was tested in 22 patients; the U2 configuration, in which the ventricular lead is the cathode and the subcutaneous patch is the anode, was tested in 2 patients; and the B1 configuration, in which the atrial and ventricular leads are combined as the cathode and the subcutaneous patch is the anode, was tested in 3 patients. In 5 patients, other configurations were tested, including the following: unidirectional-atrial lead cathode, patch anode; bidirectional-atrial lead anode, ventricular lead and subcutaneous patch common cathode; bidirectional-ventricular lead cathode, atrial lead in coronary sinus and patch common anode; bidirectional-ventricular lead and patch anode, atrial lead cathode; and bidirectional-ventricular lead anode, atrial and patch common cathode.

There were a total of 377 inductions of ventricular fibrillation tested with B2 configuration, 93 with the U1, 4 with the B1, 7 with the U2, and 13 with the other configurations listed above. The mean number of inductions per implant was 7.7 ± 3.1. The final implant configuration was the B2 configuration in 54 patients, the U1 configuration in 4 patients, and the U2 configuration in one patient. In 3 patients, alternative configurations were implanted. These included the atrial and coronary sinus leads as the common anode with a ventricular lead as the cathode, the ventricular and subcutaneous patch as the common anode with the atrial lead as the cathode, and the atrial and subcutaneous patch as the common cathode with a ventricular lead as the anode.

The defibrillation energies tested at implant ranged from 4 J to 30 J in the B2 configuration (Fig. 5) [10]. The lowest successful energy for the U1 configuration ranged from 10 J to 25 J.

Defibrillation thresholds or lowest successful energy for defibrillation were reported on 37 patients who had undergone EPS testing. The protocol asked that defibrillation thresholds established at implant be tested. This, however, was not always done. In some cases, only the programmed energy was tested. The lowest successful energies attempted are represented in Fig. 6.

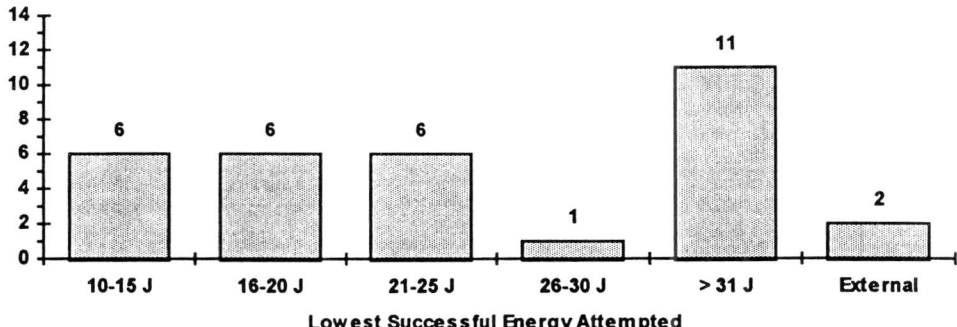

Figure 6 Distribution of the lowest successful energy attempted at 4-month follow-up study for the DF lead system [10]. Note that the programmed energy was the only energy delivered in many patients, with no attempt to determine the defibrillation threshold.

During the implant procedure, ventricular pacing thresholds were obtained at initial placement of the lead, after the lead was tunneled to the abdominal implant pocket after defibrillation testing, and after the lead was connected to the implantable defibrillator. A rise from an average value of 0.71 ± 0.57 to 1.89 ± 9.6 V was seen from the measurement taken at the time of initial lead placement to the measurement taken after defibrillation testing and tunneling of the leads. At the EPS follow-up (1–27 days postimplant), the thresholds had risen to an average of 4.2 V (± 2.3 V) at 1.0 ms. The data indicate the thresholds start declining at the 2-month follow-up and remain stable through the 6-month follow-up. Although the number of patients observed past 6 months remain small, pacing threshold average 3.2 ± 1.7 V at 1.0 V.

This rise in threshold was sometimes accompanied by a decrease in R-wave amplitude, which has been previously described with nonthoracotomy lead systems and may result in delayed detections or failure to detect ventricular arrhythmias [9,12]. Additionally, it has been noted that there is a reduction of the sensing signal with the combined use of endocardial sensing and defibrillation electrodes [13,26], particularly after application of defibrillation shocks [14–16]. Although the mechanism of this observation is not totally evaluated [17–22], low R-wave amplitudes with ventricular tachycardia or fibrillation can present a particular risk of failure to detect with fixed-sensitivity implantable cardioverter-defibrillators [22].

A total of 325 detections of spontaneous episodes of ventricular tachycardia or fibrillation have been reported in clinical investigation with the DF lead system. Of these, 306 were by the ventricular tachycardia detection algorithm (tachycardia cycle length >250 ms) and 19 by the VF detection algorithm (tachycardia cycle length <250 ms). Of the 325 total detections, 186 (57%) reverted at first confirmation, and 29 (9%) spontaneously reverted at confirmation prior to shock. The remaining 110 episodes (34%) required device intervention, including 84 episodes of ventricular tachycardia that were terminated by antitachycardia pacing therapy, and 26 by shock therapy.

During the course of the clinical study there have been a total of 5 deaths, including 4 which were classified by the investigators as congestive heart failure deaths and 1 in which the clinical data available are insufficient to determine the cause of death. Analysis of the explanted defibrillator and lead system revealed both to be within specifications.

The complications reported in the patient population implanted with the DF lead system reflect those reported with other endocardial lead systems, such as dislodgment, infection, telemetry corruption, sensing anomalies, and increased DFTs. However, there was a greater-than-anticipated incidence of elevated pacing thresholds and conductor fractures.

Based on the clinical data, in-vitro test methods were developed which better approximate the forces placed on endocardial lead systems in the body. The results of those tests, as well as extensive in-vivo animal testing, resulted in a modified lead system design based on standard bipolar bradycardia lead design with known historical implant reliability.

Long-term adequacy of pacing thresholds, R-wave amplitude, detection of ventricular fibrillation, and defibrillation thresholds will continue to be evaluated [8]. All are requisites for this nonthoracotomy and alternative nonthoracotomy systems for continued effectiveness of the implantable cardioverter-defibrillator in the prevention of sudden cardiac death [22,23].

REFERENCES

1. Saksena S, Scott S, Accorti P, Boveja B, Callaghan F, Abels D. Improved pacing and internal defibrillation using a porous electrode catheter with biphasic unidirectional and bidirectional shocks. PACE 1989; 12(4):663.
2. McCowan R, Malloney J, Wilcoff B, et al. Automatic implantable cardioverter defibrillator: implantation without thoracotomy using an endocardial and submuscular patch system. J Am Coll Cardiol 1991; 17:415–421.
3. Winkle RA, Bach SM, Mead H, et al. Comparison of defibrillation efficacy in humans using a new catheter and superior vena cava spring-left ventricular patch electrodes. J Am Coll Cardiol 1988; 11:365–370.
4. Jung W, Manz M, Moosdorf R, Luderitz B. Failure of an implantable cardioverter defibrillator to redetect ventricular fibrillation in patients with a nonthoracotomy lead system. Circulation 1992; 86:1217–1222.
5. CPI Endotak Clinical Summary Report. Phase II. Cardiac Pacemakers, Inc. September 1992: 1–8.
6. Medtronic Investigator's Interim Report Model 7217B PCD Transvene Lead System Study Report. Medtronic, Inc. March 8, 1992.
7. Yee R, Klein GJ, Leitch JW, Guiraudon GM, Jones DL, Norris C. A permanent transvenous lead system for an implantable pacemaker, cardioverter-defibrillation: nonthoracotomy approach to implantation. Circulation 1192; 85:196–204.
8. Telectronics Pacing Systems, Inc. Evaluation of the Accufix DF endocardial defibrillation/pace electrode system, protocol notebook. Telectronics Pacing Systems. Document 190-8031, Rev. 4. 1991.
9. Yee R, Jones DL, Klein GJ. Patch threshold changes after transvenous catheter countershock. Am J Cardiol 1984; 503–507.
10. Telectronics Pacing Systems, Inc. Clinical study report, EnGuard defibrillation lead system. Telectronics Pacing Systems. December 11, 1992.
11. Isbruch F, Block M, Hammel D, et al. Influence of defibrillation shocks on the endocardial sensing signals of an integrated sense/pace/defibrillation lead (abstr). Eur Heart J 1991; 12:1976.
12. Bardy GH, Ivey TD, Stewart R, Graham EL, Green HL. Failure of the automatic implantable defibrillator to detect ventricular fibrillation. Am J Cardiol 1986; 58:1107–1108.
13. Kuhlkamp V, Michael J, Hoffmeister HE, Seipel L. Reduction of the sensing signal with the use of combined endocardial sensing and defibrillation electrodes. Eur Heart J 1991; 12:363.
14. Isbruch F, Block M, Wiethold D, et al. Reduction of the endocardial sensing signal of an integrated sense/pace/defibrillation lead after application of defibrillation shocks. PACE 1992; 15:562.
15. Yee R, Jones DL, Jarvis E, Donner AP, Klein GJ. Changes in pacing threshold and R wave amplitude after transvenous catheter countershock. J Am Coll Cardiol 1984; 4:543–549.
16. Bardy GH, Olson WH. Does unsuccessful defibrillation adversely effect subsequent AICD sensing of ventricular fibrillation? PACE 1988; 11:485.
17. Crowley JM. Electrical breakdown of bimolecular lipid membranes as an electromechanical instability. Biophys J 1973; 13:711–724.
18. Jones JL, Lepershkin E, Jones RE, Rush S. Response to cultured myocardial cells to countershock-type electric field stimulation. Am J Physiol 1978; 235:H214–H222.

19. Jones JL, Proskauer CC, Paull WK, Lepeschkin E, Jones RE. Ultrastructural injury to chick myocardial cells in vitro following "electric countershock." Circ Res 1980; 46:387–394.
20. John JL, Jones RE, Balasky G. Microlesion formation in myocardial cells by high-intensity electric field breakdown in viable frog skin. Am J Physiol 1987; 253:H480–H486.
21. Powell KT, Morgenthaler AW, Weaver JC. Tissue electroporation: observation of reversible electrical breakdown in viable frog skin. Biophys J 1989; 56:1163–1171.
22. Sperry RE, Ellenbogen KA, Wood MA, Stambler BS, DiMarco JP, Haines DE. Failure of a second and third generation implantable cardioverter defibrillator to sense ventricular tachycardia: implications for fixed-gained sensing devices. PACE 1992; 15:749–755.
23. Bardy GH. Ensuring automatic detection of ventricular fibrillation. Circulation 1992; 1134–1135.
24. Saksena S, Scott SSE, Accorti PR, Boveja BK, Abel D, Callaghan F. Efficacy and safety of monophasic and biphasic waveform shocks using a braided endocardial defibrillation lead system. Am Heart J 1990; 120(6):1342–1347.
25. Saksena S, Luceri R, Tullo NG, et al. Clinical efficacy and safety of a braided endocardial pacing and defibrillation lead system for ventricular tachycardia and ventricular fibrillation using monophasic and biphasic shocks. Circulation 1990; 82 (suppl III) (4):III–166.
26. Accorti P, Brewer G, Livingston A, et al. Post shock R-wave attenuation as a result of electrogram spectral shifts in nonthoracotomy defibrillation lead systems. Eur J C P E 1992; 2(2):A–106.

47

The Implantable Cardioverter-Defibrillators: European Clinical Experience

Werner Jung, Matthias Manz, and Berndt Lüderitz

*Friedrick-Wilhelm University
and University Hospital Bonn
Bonn, Germany*

I. INTRODUCTION

After more than 10 years of research and development, Mirowski and colleagues performed the first human implantation of an automatic defibrillator (AID) in the United States at the Johns Hopkins University Medical Center on February 4, 1980 [1]. For the first year, defibrillator implantation was performed only at the Johns Hopkins Hospital, with expansion to Stanford University Medical Center in March 1981. Between 1980 and 1982, with the introduction of the automatic implantable cardioverter-defibrillator (AICD), expansion continued to several centers in the United States as well as in Canada and Europe [2,3].

II. ICD DEVELOPMENT AND USE IN EUROPE

The first European AICD implantation was performed at the Hôpital Lariboisière in Paris in December 1982 [4]. Up to September 1986, 127 systems were implanted in Europe. However, with the introduction of the first hybridized AICD (Ventak 1500 series, CPI, Inc., St. Paul, MN) in 1986, patients with frequent recurrences of hemodynamically well tolerated ventricular tachycardia (VT) had still to be excluded from implantation of an AICD capable of delivering only shocks but no antitachycardia pacing modalities. For these patients, the multiple defibrillator shock discharges would have been caused discomfort and a low acceptance rate. In order to include also patients with recurrent monomorphic VT, our group proposed the combined use of an antitachycardia pacemaker with an AICD for patients with multiple recurrences of hemodynamically well tolerated VT [5–7] (see Table 1). In the automatic mode, the antitachycardia pacemaker, Tachylog (Siemens-Elema, Solva, Sweden) functioned as a bipolar ventricular inhibited (VVI) device with antitachycardia burst stimulation. During follow-up of 47 ± 24 months, the Tachylog terminated VT 50 to 505 times per patient. In 5 patients, acceleration of VT occurred during burst stimulation and could also be reliably terminated by shock discharge thereafter (see Fig. 1). However, the occurrence of device interactions between

Table 1 Combined Use of Automatic Implantable Cardioverter-Defibrillator (AICD) and Antitachycardia Pacemaker (Tachylog) in Ventricular Tachyarrhythmias

Pt.	Age (yr) and sex	Diagnosis	Rate of VT (min^{-1})	Pacing mode; no. of stimuli; interval	Follow-up (shocks)		
					Tachylog (n)	AICD (n)	Months
1	66 M	CAD	171	Burst; 5; 260 ms[a] (stimulation no longer effective)	50	57	46[a,b]
2	53 M	CMP	160	Burst; 2; 270 ms	444	91	47[b]
3	70 M	CAD	162	Burst; 4; 300 ms	286	22	28[a]
4	59 M	CAD	188	Burst; 5; 4 × 300 ms 1 × 280 ms	505	19	29[c]
5	63 M	CAD	182	Burst; 3; 300 ms	346	30	41[a]
6	50 M	CAD	200	Burst; 4; 300 ms	0	8	1¼[a]

[a]Deceased.
[b]AICD replacement 2 times.
[c]AICD replacement 1 time.
CAD = coronary artery disease; CMP = congestive cardiomyopathy; n = number of interventions.

the antitachycardia pacemakers and the defibrillator and the anticipated arrival of a modern universal pacemaker utilizing antitachycardia pacing with backup defibrillation in one unit prevented the widespread use of the proposed combined use of an antitachycardia pacemaker as a separate unit besides implantation of an implantable cardioverter-defibrillator (ICD). In contrast to the United States, the nonthoracotomy ICD approach became increasingly widespread in Europe and the first choice of ICD management [8–14].

A comprehensive, independent ICD registry does not yet exist in Europe, and data tracking remains difficult, because there are several device manufacturers at the present time. In addition, as for any new therapy, there is a broad spectrum of opinions regarding the indications for implantation, the most appropriate implantation technique, measurements of device efficacy, and acceptable complication rates. It is therefore difficult to present a single report reflecting "the European experience" with an ICD. This chapter, therefore, represents the authors' best judgments concerning many areas where no objective data exist. In the following chapter, the European clinical experience with ICD devices already released or still under clinical investigation will be discussed.

III. EUROPEAN GUIDELINES FOR THE USE OF IMPLANTABLE CARDIOVERTER-DEFIBRILLATORS

ICD use in Europe is different from that in the United States, where most of the clinical data regarding these devices originate. Some high-level arrhythmology centers in Europe have implantation rates matching those in the United States, while in other, equally prestigious units, few if any devices have been used. U.S. guidelines for ICD use, which are widely publicized, may not meet European needs and may not accord with European opinions. Under the auspices of the European Society of Cardiology, a task force on the use of ICDs was established. It comprised designated individuals from the European Society of Cardiology's Working Groups on Cardiac Arrhythmias and Cardiac Pacing [15].

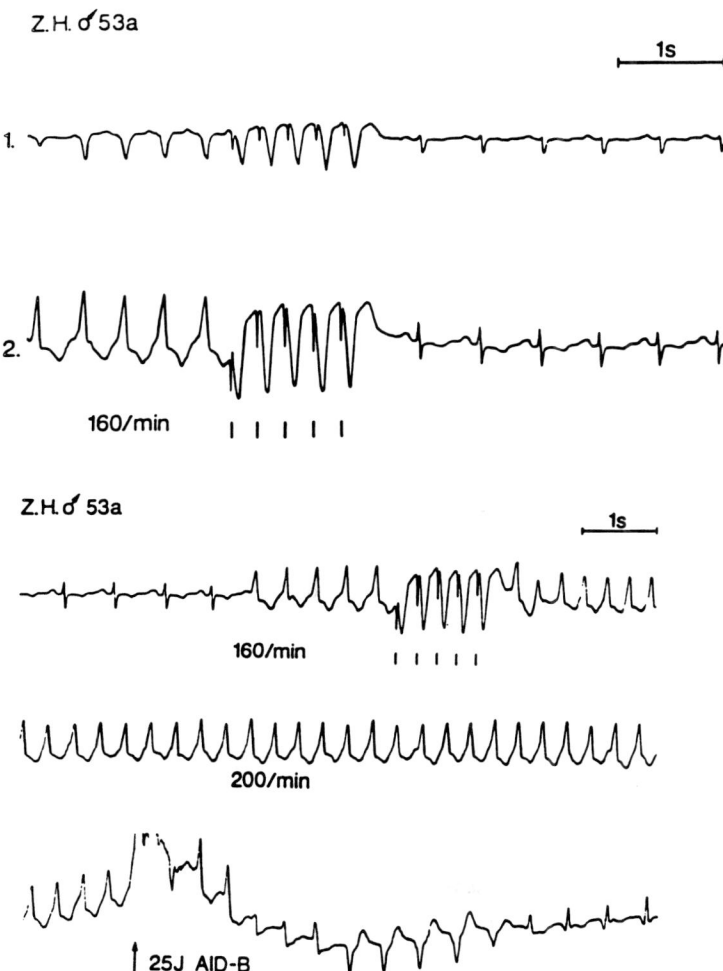

Figure 1 A 53-year-old male patient with persistent VT. *Upper panel*: Successful termination of a VT at a rate of 160 beats/min by burst stimulation with five pulses from implanted antitachycardia pacemaker (Tachylog). This ECG is a two-channel Holter recording. *Lower panel*: ECG of the same patient. After the first intervention by the Tachylog system with a burst stimulation, the VT was accelerated from 160 to 200 beats/min. The higher rate activated the ICD system, which terminated the VT with a high-energy shock of 25 J.

A. Implantation Indications for an ICD

Implantation indications depend on an ability to define patients at high risk of ventricular tachyarrhythmias. ICDs would have the most cost-effective utilization in patients with no or minimal heart disease or in whom the disease is of a nature that predisposes to repetitive VT or ventricular fibrillation (VF). ICDs would have their least cost-effective utilization in patients whose prognosis is poor, based on irrecoverable and progressive myocardial damage. We therefore believe that clinical guidelines for ICD use must address many dimensions, including the nature and extent of underlying disease and the current and predicted mechanical and electrical performance of the heart. Four groups of patients who have survived a cardiac arrest are discussed: (1) patients with no structural heart disease; (2) patients with severe irrecoverable cardiac damage whose prognosis is poor, and who are not candidates for cardiac transplantation; (3) a similar group of patients, but who are transplant candidates; (4) and an intermediate group of patients in whom prognosis is dictated both by the nature and extent of underlying disease and the propensity to electrical instability. Table 2 shows the elements which are relevant for determining that the prognosis is dictated more by electrical versus mechanical factors and lists some modulating influences which may be related to the risk of arrhythmia recurrence.

1. Cardiac Arrest Survivors: No Structural Heart Disease

Contrary to long-held beliefs, cardiac arrest survivors with no structural heart disease are now known to have a high rate of recurrent cardiac arrest. All patients should undergo a complete electrophysiological study using accredited protocols to exclude accessory pathways or atrial ventricular conduction abnormalities. In patients in whom sustained monomorphic VT can be reliably induced, suppressive antiarrhythmic therapy should be sought. If no effective drug is identified, or drugs are not tolerated, an ICD should be implanted. If, at the time of electrophysiological study, no ventricular arrhythmia is induced or only VF is provoked, an ICD should be considered; as yet there is no proven evidence that the ICD would be beneficial, but strong circumstantial evidence supports the intervention.

2. Patients with VT/VF and Severe Irremediable Cardiac Disease

At the other end of the disease spectrum, recurrence of VT and VF is common in some patients with severe irremediable cardiac disease but the prognosis is much more dependent on the un-

Table 2 Clinical Factors and Therapy Options Relevant to ICD Consideration [15][a]

Clinical presentation	Etiological diagnosis	Risk modifiers for recurrence	Therapy options
Ventricular tachycardia (VT)	Circumscribed completed event—MI stable EPS	Progression of primary disease	Nothing
Ventricular fibrillation	MI + EP inducible VT	Established arrhythmia substrate	Therapy directed at primary disease
Unspecified cardiac arrest	Subendocardial MI	Late potentials	Antiarrhythmic drugs including beta blockers
High risk of sudden death	CAD no MI	Autonomic status	Antiarrhythmic surgery
	Hypertrophic cardiomyopathy	Left ventricular function	Catheter ablation
	Long QT syndrome	Age	Implantable cardioverter defibrillator (ICD)
	Dilated cardiomyopathy		
	Other heart disease		
	No heart disease		

[a]For each individual patient considered for ICD implantation, several clinical factors must be taken into account to weigh the risk-benefit of the ICD versus other treatment options. The nature of the clinical presentation, the etiological, diagnosis, and some of the risk factors for arrhythmia recurrence are listed.

derlying disease than on the arrhythmia. In this population there is no convincing evidence of total mortality benefit from the ICD, although sudden cardiac death rates seem to be reduced. In the past, this group of patients has been regarded as appropriate for ICD therapy; this opinion may need to be reconsidered, as the cost-benefit ratio seems poor. Some patients with severe cardiac disease may be candidates for transplantation. Currently, studies are examining the role of the ICD as a bridge to transplantation [16,17]. Until additional data become available, this use of the ICD should be regarded as investigational. For individual patients, however, the ICD may offer improved quality of life. Our group evaluated the patient's acceptance of the ICD, the psychological profile of 57 consecutive patients using a specifically designed questionnaire and the state trait anxiety inventory (STAI test). The results of the questionnaire are listed in Tables 3–5. Figure 2 shows the state of anxiety in a subgroup of patients with respect to the experienced shocks of the ICD system. Our results demonstrated an improvement in quality of life in the majority of patients studied [18].

3. Patients with Structural Heart Disease and the Risk of Recurrent VT/VF

The majority of survivors of cardiac arrest have cardiovascular disease. Amelioration management must address that underlying disease; its amelioration may reduce the propensity to further arrhythmias. Unfortunately, this strategy has only a modest impact. Optimal use of the ICD mandates that the risk of death from progression of the underlying disease be assessed and weighed against the risk of ventricular tachyarrhythmia recurrence. This assessment procedure is complicated. It involves consideration of the presentation, the hemodynamic toleration of the arrhythmia, the nature and severity of the underlying disease, and the presence of modifying features (Table 2).

B. ICD Use Guidelines Regardless of Etiology of Primary Disease

If electrophysiological study reproducibly induces VT or VF, suppressive drug therapy should be sought. If spontaneous episodes recur or sustained VT or VF remain inducible on drugs, or if drugs are not tolerated and antiarrhythmic surgery is inappropriate, an ICD should be implanted. If electrophysiological stimulation is unreliable for drug assessment, an ICD may be used based on the individual patient. Implantation guidelines are not clear for this group. If electrophysiological stimulation does not provoke a sustained ventricular arrhythmia and the presenting arrhythmia has been judged as being secondary to a self-limiting event now resolved, no further antiarrhythmic action may be necessary. Similarly, if the arrhythmia can be proven to be based on ischemia, then revascularization may be the preferred option. If electrophysiological stimulation provokes VT or VF, and drug therapy is either ineffective or not tolerated, treatment options include not only ICD implantation but also less easily testable antiarrhythmic drugs (beta blockers, amiodarone), antiarrhythmic surgery, ablation, and treatment directed against the primary disease process.

C. ICD Use Guidelines Dependent on Etiology of Primary Disease

Few if any randomized control studies of the optimal management of cardiac arrest, VT, and VF survivors have been conducted. The following statements are offered as a present-day guidance when considering ICD use: Patients with sustained VT postmyocardial infarction (> 48 h after onset of symptoms) are candidates for consideration of nonpharmacological management if no effective drug can be identified or if there is a problem with intolerance or noncompliance. The nonpharmacological treatment consists of ICD, ablation technique, map-

Table 3 Answers to the Questionnaire (57 patients)

Do you feel more comfortable with the ICD?			
yes: 47		no:	10
Are you constantly aware of the device?	or just at particular times?		
yes: 32		yes:	25
How long did it take you to get used to the ICD?			
<2 months: 24		>2 months:	33
Battery replacement - EPS requested?			
yes: 27		no:	30
What is your greatest concern?			
—Fear of the ICD discharge			20
—Physical discomfort due to the device			12
—Limited quality of life (job, sport, social activity)			8
—None			17
Was it worth having an ICD device implanted?			
yes: 55		no:	2
Has the ICD allowed you to return to active life?			
yes: 30		no:	27
Would you advise another patient to undergo ICD implantation if necessary?			
yes: 56		no:	1

EPS = electrophysiological study

Table 4 Questionnaire: Anxiety and Social Impact ($n = 57$)

	Yes	No
Anxiety		
Pain during ICD discharge	27	30
Limited physical activity	40	17
Fear of ICD shock	20	37
Fear of device failure	16	41
Decreased sexual activity	15	42
Social Impact		
Return to active lifestyle	35	22
Return to work	7	50
Hobby (sports)	39	18
Unemployment	32	25

Table 5 State of Anxiety in 57 ICD Recipients

		Number of patients (n)	Before ICD Implantation (percentile scores)		After ICD Implantaton (follow-up: 12 ± 2 months) (percentile scores)	
Total patient population:			39.4	n.s.	37.5	
ICD indication:	VT	27	39.5	n.s.	39.7	n.s.
	VF	30	39.8		41.7	
Cardiac disease:	CAD	40	39.3	n.s.	39.8	n.s.
	IDC	11	39.7		39.6	
	Other	6				
Age:	<50 years	17	38.7	$p < 0.05$	44.6	$p < 0.05$
	≥50 years	40	38.6	n.s.	38.8	
Ejection fraction:	<35%	25	38.5	n.s.	38.4	n.s.
	≥35%	32	39.2		39.9	
Gender:	Male	47	40.2	n.s.	39.0	n.s.
	Female	10	42.1		43.8	
Number of experienced shocks:	<5	33	38.2	n.s.	36.3	$p < 0.001$
	≥5	24	38.4	$p < 0.001$	46.4	

CAD = coronary artery disease; ICD = implantable cardioverter/defibrillator; IDC = idiopathic dilated cardiomyopathy; n.s. = not significant; VF = ventricular fibrillation; VT = ventricular tachycardia.

directed surgery and, for those patients with severely impaired left ventricular function, heart transplantation. ICDs are not indicated in those patients presenting VF complicating acute myocardial infarction (< 48 h after the onset of symptoms). In patients surviving an out-of-hospital cardiac arrest with subsequent diagnosis of non-Q-wave myocardial infarction, or surviving cardiac arrest without evidence of infarction but of coronary artery disease, ICDs are rarely indicated. Theoretically, nothing more than revascularization is necessary for the majority of those patients. In patients with hypertrophic cardiomyopathy, therapies for this condition are controversial. Controlled but nonrandomized data suggest that empirical amiodarone therapy can improve prognosis; currently, this is widely considered the best option. Among patients with dilated cardiomyopathy, the ICD is indicated for those patients with sustained VT or a history of cardiac arrest in whom these arrhythmias are not inducible, and who do not respond to antiarrhythmic drug therapy during electrophysiological testing. In those patients with severe left ventricular dysfunction, the risk-benefit of ICD implantation may be suboptimal unless it is used as a bridge to transplantation [16,17]. In patients with a congenital long QT syndrome, current evidence suggests that the administration of beta blockers, with or without left cardiac sympathetic denervation, is the best management option. A minority of treated individuals continue with serious and life-threatening arrhythmias. Within this group, antibradycardia pacing may be of value in selected patients, but in others, ICD implantation should be considered. In patients with mitral valve prolapse presenting arrhythmias, empirical beta-blocking therapy has been suggested as useful, but there is little controlled scientific evidence in support. The ICD may be indicated in individual patients with life-threatening ventricular tachyarrhythmias. In patients with WPW syndrome and atrial fibrillation, there is a risk of VF that is related directly to the anterograde conduction capability of the accessory pathway. In this

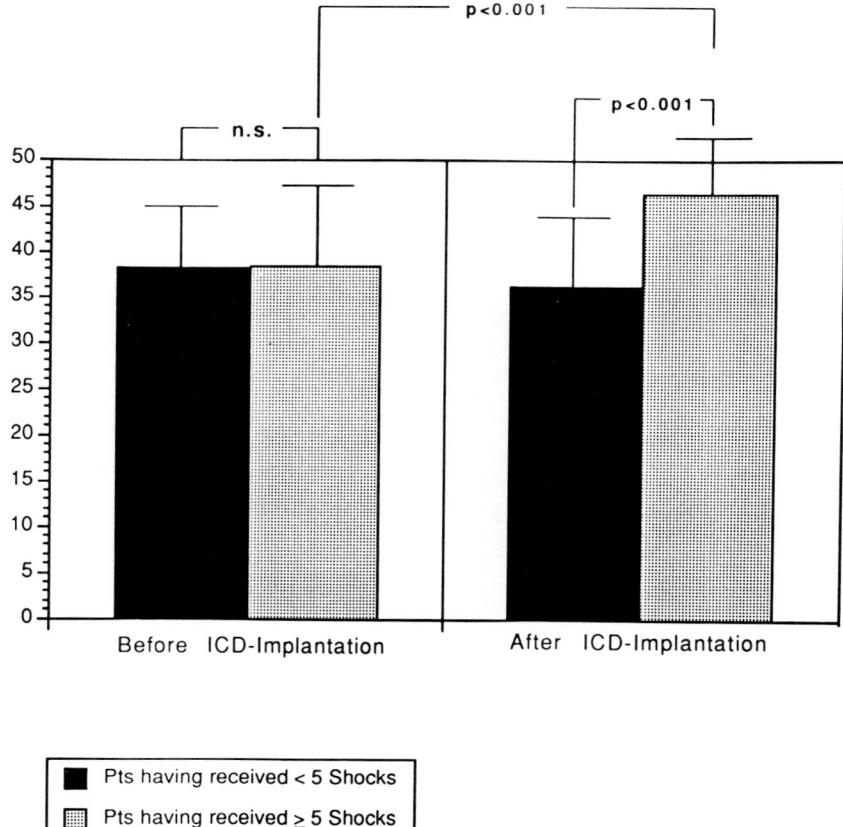

Figure 2 This figure illustrates the difference in the level of anxiety before and after implantation of an ICD in two patient subgroups, the group that had received ≥ 5 shocks, and the group that had received <5 shocks. This clearly demonstrates that the score of anxiety increased significantly in patients who have experienced multiple shocks ($p < 0.001$).

group of patients, ICD implantation is not indicated, but catheter ablation is the treatment of choice.

IV. ONGOING EUROPEAN MULTICENTER STUDIES

Table 6 provides information about the most important ongoing multicenter studies. Objectives, endpoints, and inclusion criteria are listed.

A. Cardiac Arrest Study Hamburg (CASH)

In 1987, the Cardiac Arrest Study Hamburg (CASH) was started in several centers in Germany [19]. CASH is a randomized controlled study of survivors of sudden cardiac death due to documented VT and/or VF, unrelated to myocardial infarction. The aim of the study is to compare the incidence of recurrence of cardiac arrest, sudden cardiac death, cardiac mortality, and total

Table 6 Ongoing European Multicenter Studies

	CASH	CAT	Cost/efficacy	Optimal	UCARE	SAMI	ICD/d-Sotalol versus placebo
Study design	Open, prospective, randomized	Prophylactic, open, prospective, randomized	Open, prospective, randomized	Prospective, consecutive	Retro-/prospective, consecutive	Open, prospective, randomized	Double-blind, prospective, randomized
Number of participating centres	Hospitals in Hamburg, Germany	11	Dutch study	Belgium study	Open to all	22	11 in Europe
Principal investigators	K.-H. Kuck	K.-H. Kuck	R. Hauer	P. Brugada	P. Schwartz	K.-H. Kuck, A. J. Camm	H. Klein, J. Brachmann
Projected number of patients	400	720	60	?	Unlimited	568	360
Inclusion criteria	Sudden cardiac death survivors	Idiopathic dilated cardiomyopathy (IDC), ejection fraction <30%, no symptomatic VT/VF, IDC known <9 months, age 18–70 years	Coronary artery disease, postinfarction (>4 weeks), sudden-cardiac-death survivors	Risk stratification based on: syncope during VT/VF, history of multiple myocardial infarction, dyspnoe with NYHA class III	Survivors of sudden cardiac death without structural heart disease	Coronary artery disease, documented VT, ejection fraction ≤40%, age 18–76 years. NYHA II–III	Spontaneous or inducible VT or VF, ejection fraction ≤40%, ICD with documentation capability, defibrillation threshold ≤20 J
Objective of the study	ICD versus antiarrhythmic drugs (amiodarone, metoprolol, propafenone)	ICD versus no antiarrhythmic drugs	Early ICD implantation versus conventional therapy	ICD (high-risk patients) versus conventional therapy (low-risk patients)	Outcome based on individual treatment	ICD versus antiarrhythmic drugs (sotalol, amiodarone)	d-Sotalol versus placebo in ICD patients

Table 6 continued

	CASH	CAT	Cost/efficacy	Optimal	UCARE	SAMI	ICD/d-Sotalol versus placebo
Primary endpoint	Total mortality, cardiac arrest	Total mortality	Cost per year of life saved (cost-effectiveness ratio)	Total mortality, cardiac arrest	Total mortality, cardiac arrest	Total mortality	Recurrence of sustained VT or VF during a 1 year follow-up, time to spontaneous recurrence, frequency of ICD discharge Time to arrhythmic death
Secondary endpoint	Unstable VT, heart transplantation, drug withdrawal, change in antiarrhythmic drug treatment	Heart transplantation, survival of cardiac arrest, sustained VT, symptomatic VT requiring antiarrhythmic drugs	Medical, economic, and quality-of-life issues	?	Unstable VT	Major complications, cardiac arrest, heart transplantation	
Projected duration of the study	5 years	3 years	3 years	?	Unlimited	3 years	1 year, thereafter extended follow-up

CASH = cardiac arrest study Hamburg; CAT = cardiomyopathy trial; SAMI = Sotalol or *Amiodarone* versus ICD; ICD = implantable cardioverter *defibrillator*; VF = ventricular fibrillation, VT = ventricular tachycardia, NYHA = New York Heart Association.

mortality among patients treated with antiarrhythmic drugs besides having an ICD. The projected enrollment includes 400 patients, whose admission has to occur within 3 months of the cardiac arrest event. After electrophysiological testing, all patients are randomized regardless of clinical findings or testing results to receive either amiodarone, metoprolol, propafenone, or primary implantation of ICD with no concomitant antiarrhythmic treatment. The primary endpoint of the study are total mortality and recurrence of cardiac arrest in the patients receiving antiarrhythmic drugs, and total mortality in the ICD patients. Through December 1991, 230 patients were included in the study. This time period represented an average follow-up of 11 months for all patients studied. To date, analysis of the primary endpoint showed no significant differences among the three populations treated with amiodarone, metoprolol, and the ICD. Conversely, a significantly higher evidence of total mortality and cardiac arrest recurrence was found in the propafenone group when compared to the ICD group. Due to the high incidence of sudden cardiac arrest under propafenone therapy, this drug treatment was eventually discontinued. However, the study is still ongoing with the ICD, amiodarone, and metoprolol arms [19].

B. Cardiomyopathy Trial (CAT)

The German dilated cardiomyopathy study was designed to (1) assess the natural history of patients with dilated cardiomyopathy and no documentation of sustained ventricular arrhythmias and (2) investigate the influence of the prophylactic implantation of an ICD based on the prognoses for these patients [20]. This investigation is a multicenter study currently including 11 centers in Germany. Patients that are between 18 and 70 years of age, and who have dilated cardiomyopathy proven by left ventricular catherization, are enrolled in the study. The patients must have no coronary artery disease, no symptomatic ventricular arrhythmias, and a left ventricular ejection fraction $< 30\%$. Idiopathic dilated cardiomyopathy should not have been diagnosed for more than 9 months before enrollment in the study. Patients with either documented cardiac arrest or documented sustained VT are excluded from the study. The primary endpoint of this study is the assessment of the total mortality in this group of patients, while secondary endpoints are to assess the incidence of (1) heart transplantation; (2) survival of cardiac arrest; (3) sustained VT; and (4) symptomatic ventricular arrhythmias requiring antiarrhythmic drug treatment. The calculated number of patients enrolled in this study will be 360 in each group for a total of 720 patients. After the basic clinical assessment, the patients are randomized to either no antiarrhythmic treatment or to the implantation of an ICD. This prospective, randomized, and prophylactically designed multicenter study started on July 1, 1991. Up to now, more than 40 patients are enrolled in this study.

C. The Dutch Prospective Study of the ICD as First-Choice Therapy: Cost-Effectiveness Considerations

A randomized prospective cost-effectiveness analysis in successfully resuscitated postinfarction patients was started in 1989 [21]. In one group, an ICD was implanted as a first-choice therapy (early defibrillator implantation), whereas the other group was subject to conventional therapy strategy. Items to be considered for comparison were medical, economic, and those related to assessment of quality of life. In both groups, cost-effectiveness was expressed as cost per year of lives saved (cost-effectiveness ratio). A category of patients in the chronic stage of myocardial infarction (at least 4 weeks of the acute infarction) was selected, because this group was large and relatively homogenous. Candidates for the study had to have at least one cardiac arrest episode due to VF or rapid VT. As of June 1992, 46 patients had entered the study. A total of 60 patients will be included. Results are expected in late 1993 and will be expressed as cost-effectiveness ratio in both study arms. Another model to assess cost-efficiency of the ICD has been published recently by an investigator group from the United Kingdom [22].

D. Optimal Study

In the Optimal study, high-risk patients were consecutively assigned to ICD treatment, whereas low-risk patients received conventional therapy. The risk stratification was based on the following variables: syncope during ventricular tachyarrhythmia, history of multiple myocardial infarction, dyspnoe with NYHA functional class III. To date, 230 patients have been enrolled in this study. At a mean follow-up of 13 months, the ICD improved the sudden cardiac death and total mortality in patients at high risk of recurrent ventricular tachyarrhythmias [23].

E. UCARE Registry

The UCARE, unexplained cardiac arrest registry of Europe was started to enroll patients with idiopathic VF, and it is expected to provide a definite answer to the prognosis and management of patients with idiopathic VF [24]. The project started out as a retrospective analysis. A total of 120 cases were evaluated; 60% of the episodes occurred in the age group of 20 to 45 years, about 70% in men. Electrophysiological evaluation showed inducible VF in 12%, VT in 35%, and no inducibility in 53%. Therapy was given to 95% of patients and included antiarrhythmic drugs, beta blockers, and the ICD. During follow-up, 12 patients died suddenly or had a successful defibrillation by the ICD. The overall recurrence of major arrhythmic events was 21%. This registry is open to any center willing to participate. A prospective analysis of patients presenting idiopathic VF has recently been started.

F. SAMI Study

A new multicenter study is planned including patients randomized to either an ICD or a class III antiarrhythmic drug (amiodarone, sotalol). This multicenter trial is called the SAMI study: *s*otalol, *ami*odarone versus *I*CD. The goal of the study is to assess the influence of an ICD on the prognosis of patients with coronary artery disease, impaired left ventricular ejection fraction (EF < 40%, NYHA functional class II–III), and documented symptomatic, hemodynamically unstable, ventricular tachycardia. As scheduled, the study will be completed within 3 years.

G. d-Sotalol Versus Placebo/ICD Study

The aim of the *d*-sotalol versus placebo/ICD multicenter study is to assess the efficacy and safety of oral *d*-sotalol in patients with malignant VT or VF and ICDs. The trial will be conducted in 360 patients in Europe and North America and will utilize a double-blind, randomized, parallel-group design. *d*-Sotalol will be tested at a dose of 200 mg administered twice daily. Placebo will also be administered twice a day. The primary data analysis will be based on patient outcome at 1 year, or for patients who discontinue randomized medication prior to 1 year, at the time of discontinuation of blinded therapy. Inclusion criteria are as follows: spontaneous or inducible sustained VT or VF, left ventricular ejection fraction below 40% (VF patients only), ICD with arrhythmia documentation capabilities, and DFT < 20 J. After a 1-year-follow-up, a phase II with extended long-term follow-up is planned.

V. IMPLANTABLE CARDIOVERTER-DEFIBRILLATORS

Several third-generation ICDs have been introduced by different manufacturers for clinical evaluation in Europe.

A. Ventak Defibrillators (CPI)

The Ventak P, recently approved by the U.S. Food and Drug Administration (FDA) for use in the United States and already market-released in Europe, allows programming of the first shock energy down to 0.1 J, the cutoff rate, the first shock delay, and the probability density function. In the majority of European patients, the Ventak P was combined with epicardial patch electrodes.

1. Ventak P with Epicardial Leads

In a prospective and parallel, randomized study, our group evaluated the long-term stability of epicardial defibrillation threshold (DFT) in 22 patients using a patch-patch lead configuration at the time of implantation and generator replacement [25,26]. The concomitant antiarrhythmic drug treatment consisted of either mexiletine (720 mg/day) or amiodarone (400 mg/day) and was administered to patients in a randomized and parallel manner. During a mean follow-up of 24 ± 6 months, the DFT increased significantly from 14.3 ± 2.8 to 17.9 ± 5.3 J ($p < 0.05$) for the entire patient group. The increase in the chronic DFT was due to a marked increase in defibrillation energy needs in the subgroup of patients receiving amiodarone. Whereas no significant changes in DFT were documented in the subgroup of patients receiving mexiletine, the mean DFT increased from 14.1 ± 3.0 J to 20.9 ± 5.4 J ($p < 0.001$) in those receiving amiodarone (Fig. 3). The only variable associated with an increase in the chronic DFT was amiodarone treatment [25,26].

2. PRx Device with Endotak C Lead

a. Study Population. The PRx is currently undergoing investigation in the United States in accordance with FDA guidelines. European market release of the PRx-I system took place in May 1991. In the majority of patients in Europe, the Ventak PRx pulse generator was combined with a transvenous defibrillation lead, the Endotak C lead model 0062. This lead is a tripolar, tined transvenous catheter that combines rate sensing, pacing, and defibrillation in a single lead. Another investigational nonthoracotomy lead system, the 50-series model, was implanted in a small group of patients in the United States during 1987 [27,28]. However, early lead fractures terminated the use of that lead system in a clinical trial. The 50-series lead models were never implanted in Europe. During the European Endotak study, 170 patients were evaluated [29]. The first Endotak implant took place in Hanover, Germany, in early 1990. DFT testing was performed according to the investigators' individual protocol. In general, defibrillation was performed using the right ventricular electrode as a cathode and the proximal coil plus the subcutaneous patch as the anodes. Of the 170 patients tested, 159 (89%) underwent Endotak lead implantation; 74% were implants using an additional subcutaneous patch electrode and 25% with the lead alone.

b. Complications and Observations. The perioperative mortality rate for the implanted patients was 2%; three postoperative deaths were due to coagulopathy, pulmonary embolism, and acute hydrocephalus internus. Two patients died during the late follow-up period (average, 4.7 months; longest, 14 months); one patient died suddenly due to an incessant arrhythmia, while the other patient's death was due to congestive heart failure. Twenty-three patients received clinically appropriate shocks, and two received inappropriate shocks that were related to

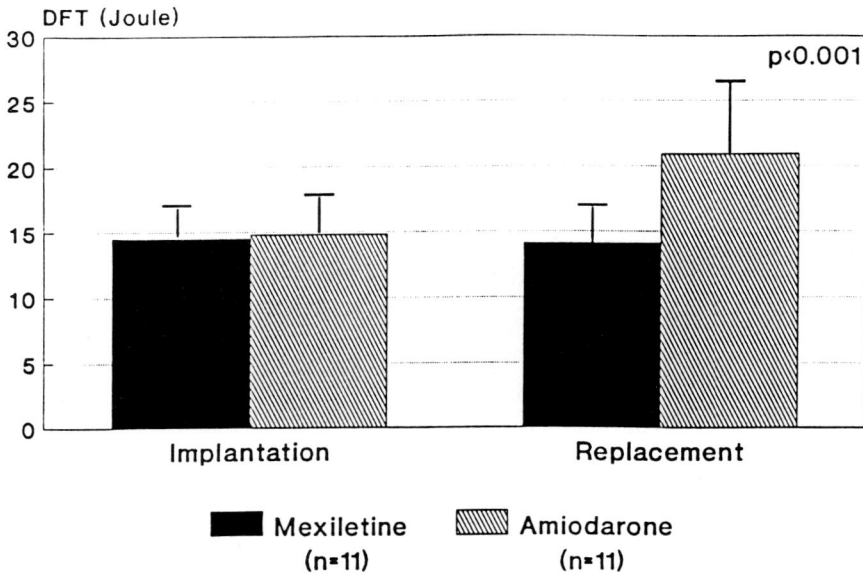

Figure 3 Comparison of defibrillation threshold (DFT) at the times of implantation and generator replacement. Patients were separated into two groups receiving either mexiletine ($n = 11$) or amiodarone ($n = 11$). At replacement, DFT increased significantly ($p < 0.001$) in patients receiving amiodarone compared to those receiving mexiletine.

atrial fibrillation during the postoperative period. As expected, antiachycardia pacing was successful in terminating the majority of monomorphic VTs induced prior to discharge and during follow-up [30]. In the European trial, two lead-related complications occurred after implantation. One lead dislodged 3 days postoperatively due to the absence of adequate strain relief at the venous entry site. One lead had a high DFT 4 weeks postimplant due to displacement within the right ventricle.

c. *Endotak C leads, Models 0062 and 0072.* Aside from these problems, we recently reported on a failure of a third-generation defibrillator to redetect VF after an unsuccessful attempt in patients using the Endotak C lead system, model 0062 [31] (Fig. 4). In that study, we observed a significant decrease in endocardial electrogram amplitudes following shock delivery. The decrease in intracardiac electrogram amplitudes following a high-energy defibrillation shock is probably a temporary tissue effect caused by the high current density in the tissue surrounding the high-voltage electrode during the shock. Accordingly, the transvenous Endotak C lead, model 0062, was redesigned and introduced as model 0072 for clinical evaluation in Europe. The redesigned lead version, the model 0072, differs from the model 0062 with respect to the distance between the distal tip and the distal coil, which was extended to 12 mm in the modified electrode system. Comparing the effects of defibrillator shocks on the amplitude of endocardial electrograms, the redesigned version 0072 demonstrated a substantial improvement in the postshock endocardial electrogram amplitudes [32].

d. *Array Electrode.* As the PRx-I device provides only the capability of delivering monophasic shock waveforms, some patients did not meet the implant criteria despite using a transvenous subcutaneous electrode configuration. To further improve DFT and to minimize discomfort due to the subcutaneous patch electrode, a new lead, the array electrode, was de-

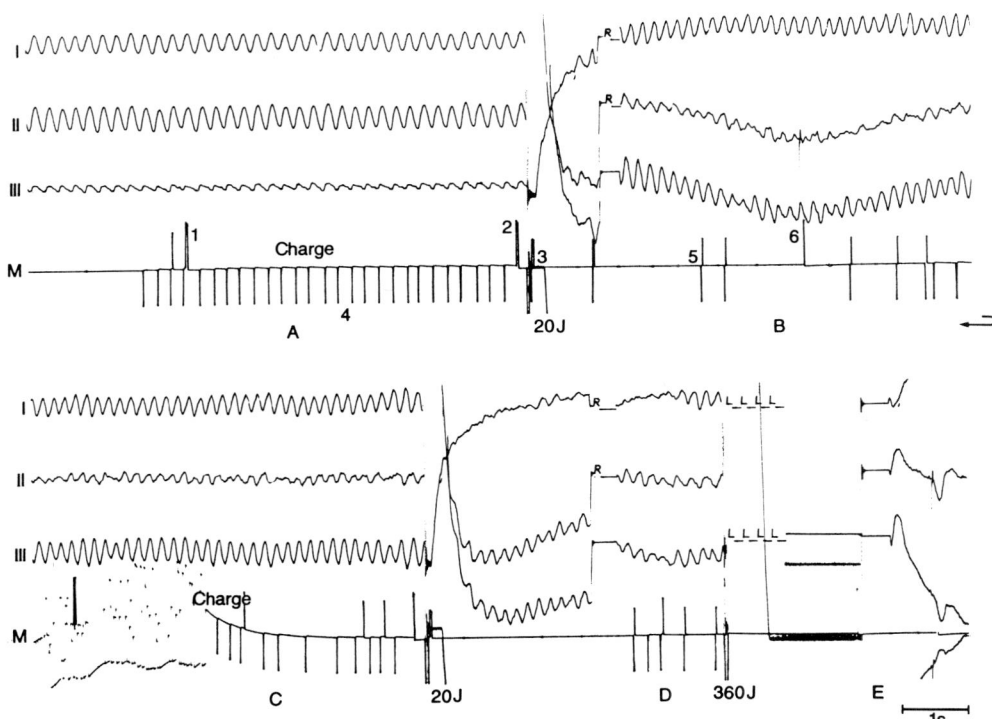

Figure 4 Failure of redetection of ventricular fibrillation (VF) after delivery of unsuccessful shock. VF was noninvasively induced by manual rapid ramp pacing. After detection of VF, the device (PRx-I) charged for delivery of a first therapy (20 J), which failed to terminate VF (A). Thereafter, sensing was inappropriate. Only a few intraventricular depolarizations (slow beats) were recognized during persistent VF (B). After a period of 12 s, the device started to charge for delivery of first therapy again (20 J) (C). According to the printout ("first therapy"), it is obvious that the device considered the previous VF episode as effectively terminated. After delivery of the second shock (20 J), undersensing occurred again (D). Sinus rhythm had to be restored by external defibrillation (360 J) (E). Event marker (M): 1, start charge; 2, stop charge; 3, shock delivery; 4, tachy sense; 5, slow beat (sensed intervals occur below the detection rate); 6, paced beat (after a programmed escape interval of 4 sec); 7, noise caused by activation of an external defibrillator. Surface leads I, II, and III are shown.

veloped and introduced for clinical evaluation in Europe in 1992 (Fig. 5). Preliminary data with the use of this electrode demonstrated that the DFT could be lowered by approximately 5 J compared to the subcutaneous patch electrode. In particular, the patient's discomfort due to the location of the electrode, and problems associated with the subcutaneous patch electrode such as hematoma, were reduced [33].

3. Ventak P2

a. Study Population. The Ventak P2, capable of providing stored electrograms (see Figs. 6 and 7) underwent clinical evaluation in Europe and was implanted in 162 patients between September 27, 1991, and July 20, 1992, by 39 centers in 11 countries in Europe [34]. The patient population consisted of 81.5% males and 17.5% females. The mean age was 55.5 years, with a range of 16 to 78 years. Implant duration ranged from 6.5 to 16 months, with a mean

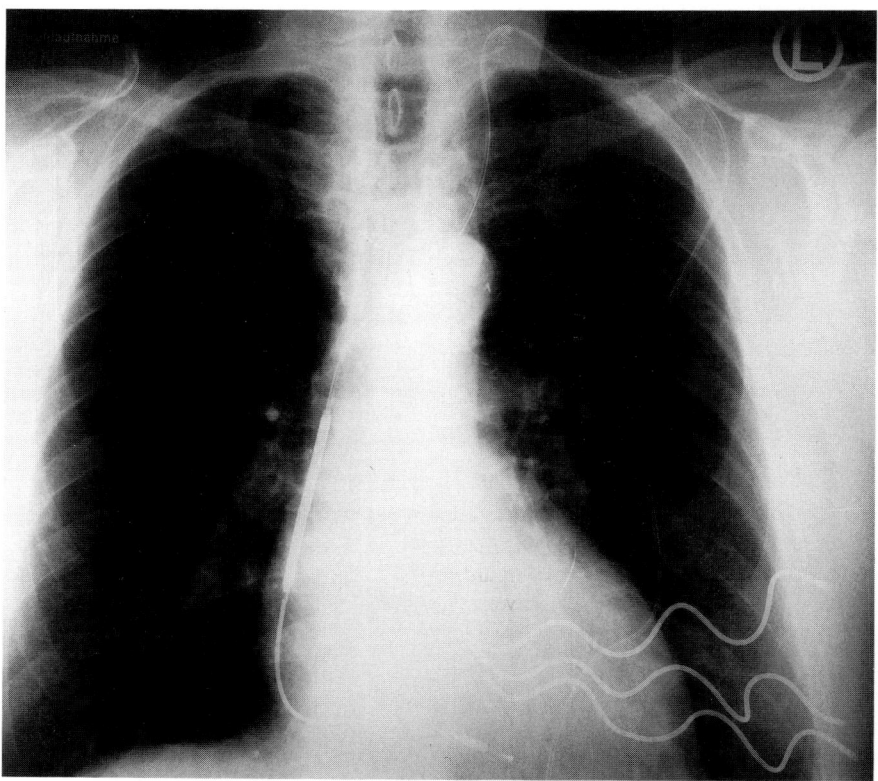

Figure 5 This figure illustrates a chest X-ray with an implanted transvenous Endotak C lead system in combination with a subcutaneous array electrode. The array electrode consists of three 20.5 cm-long coils which cover a larger area (approximately 150 cm^2) and allow a more homogenous field during defibrillation.

implant duration of 10.75 months, providing 1010.9 months of cumulative device experience. The mean left ventricular ejection fraction was 36%, with a range of 13% to 83%. The primary cardiac disease was coronary artery disease in 91 patients (56.2%), nonischemic cardiomyopathy in 36 patients (22.2%), and others including congenital heart disease, arrhythmogenic right ventricular dysplasia, primary electrical disease, valvular disease, myocarditis, idiopathic VF, hypertrophic cardiomyopathy, and long QT syndrome in 24 patients (14.8%). The underlying heart disease was not reported in 11 patients (5.3%). The primary rhythm disturbance was reported for 157 of the 162 patients. 78 patients (48.1%) had VF, 30 patients (18.5%) had VT, and 46 patients (28.4%) had both VT and VF. The Ventak P2 was implanted prophylactically in 3 patients (1.9%). No indication was reported in 5 patients (3.1%). At implant, 81 patients (50%) were receiving concomitant drug therapy. For 45 patients, the drug therapy was continued after implant. Seventy-two patients received no drugs, 43 patients were administered amiodarone, and 80 patients received sotalol. Most patients ($n = 150$; 92.6%) had never had a previous ICD device prior to implant of a Ventak P2. Twelve patients (7.4%) underwent replacement of a pulse generator and were connected with epicardial lead systems. Of the 150

European Clinical Experience

M.H., f., 25 a.

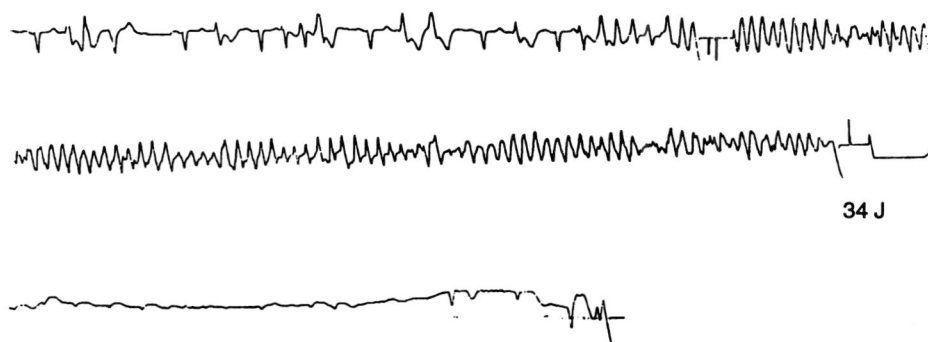

Figure 6 Continuous stored electrograms (25 mm/s) recorded from the shocking leads, demonstrating successful conversion of spontaneous occurrence of ventricular fibrillation in a 24-year-old female patient. Ventricular fibrillation was preceded by premature ventricular contractions. After the detection criterion was met (short and long vertical downward markers), the programmed delay was initiated and the Ventak P2 device started to charge for delivery of a 34-J shock (long vertical upright marker), which successfully terminated the arrhythmia.

A.L., m., 50 a.

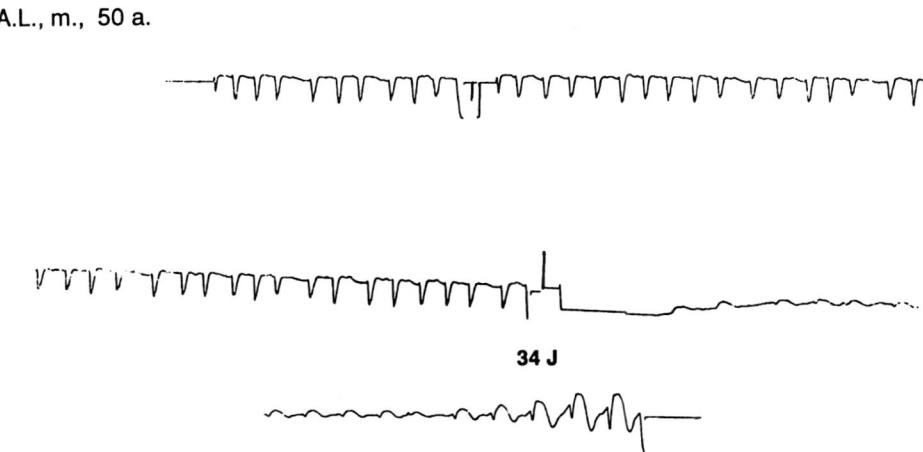

Figure 7 Continuous stored electrograms (25 mm/s) documenting inappropriate shock delivery due to atrial tachyarrhythmias with rapid ventricular response in a 50-year-old male patient. After the detection criterion was satisfied (short and long vertical downward markers), a 34-J shock was delivered (long vertical upright marker) during persistent supraventricular tachyarrhythmia.

patients who received the Ventak P2 as their first ICD device, the majority ($n = 136$, 90.7%) were implanted with a transvenous Endotak lead system. Most of these patients ($n = 92$; 67.6%) were implanted with the Endotak C lead only. A transvenous/subcutaneous approach was chosen in 44 patients (32.4%).

b. Lead Signals and DFT. The sensing signal amplitude obtained in 136 patients with transvenous leads was 13.1 mV (6–28 mV), the shocking amplitude was 12.1 mV (3–55 mV), and the pacing threshold obtained at 0.5-ms pulse duration was 0.56 V (0.1–2.1 V). Once the lead system was implanted and signal amplitudes and pacing thresholds were obtained, the patients were randomized to receive either biphasic or monophasic shocks to determine the DFT. A true DFT was obtained in 33 patients using monophasic shocks, and in 108 patients using biphasic shock waveforms. A paired-waveform test was performed in 61 patients. Biphasic conversion energies were lower than monophasic energies in 55 (90.2%) patients, although 4 patients had lower DFTs with a monophasic waveform, where the difference was less than 5 J. The mean monophasic DFT was 17.4 J, and the mean biphasic DFT was 10.2 J for those patients with paired comparison testing. Using 15 J or less, the cumulative success rate was still 70% in patients with only the Endotak C lead and 89% success rate in patients using a transvenous/subcutaneous lead configuration.

c. Complications and Observations. By the end of January 1993, 338 appropriate and 6 inappropriate shocks were reported in 49 patients (ranging from 1 to 51 shocks per patient). All these episodes were documented with the capability of stored electrograms derived via shocking leads (Figs. 6 and 7). During the study period, the clinical observations included lead dislodgement in 3 patients, insulation damage in 2 patients, tamponade of the right ventricle in 1 patient, seroma in 2 patients, and hematoma in 1 patient. Five Ventak P2 devices were out of service for reasons other than patient mortality: 1 device produced an error during an induction of a tachyarrythmia by means of using the burst-pacing induction scheme. The reason was that the patient's Endotak C lead was dislodged in such a way that the proximal spring touched the distal spring. This caused a short circuit that initiated the error code 35. A second device probably detected the induced tachyarrhythmia at implant, but after charging diverted all five shocks. In the programmer, the error code 35 was reasonable. The exact cause was not identified, but probably the shocking lead resistance was too low. Another device was explanted 7 months postimplant, because the patient underwent heart transplantation. The fourth device was explanted 5 weeks postimplant. The patient's Endotak C lead was dislocated, and then the patient was informed about a revision, but he refused to receive a new system. The fifth device was explanted 10 months after implantation. The patient was seen by the hospital for normal follow-up examination. Attempts to interrogate the device failed. Applying a magnet over the device did not change the device mode. Test results are still pending. Up to January 27, 1993, 6 deaths were reported in this clinical investigation. Two patients died in the perioperative period (< 30 days). The first patient died 3 weeks postimplant due to reentrant tachycardia complicated by severe heart failure. The second patient's death was attributed to myocardial infarction complicated by refractory VF 4 weeks postimplant. The third patient died 5 months postimplant secondary to end-stage cancer. The fourth patient died 6 months postimplant by unknown cause. The patient's general physician informed the implanting physician after the patient's death. The device was not explanted. The fifth patient, who received a Ventak P2 pulse generator as a replacement for a competitive device due to extremely high DFT, died suddenly 7 months postimplant due to a ventricular storm.

In summary, 90.7% of the patients received a transvenous/subcutaneous Endotak C lead system. In the total group, the DFT was < 20 J in 95.6% of the patients using monophasic shock waveforms and < 15 J in 68.2% of the patients using biphasic shock waveforms. In paired conversion tests, this resulted in energy saving of about 40%. During a mean follow-up of 10.7 months, the actuarial survival rate of total mortality was 96.4%, and the actuarial survival rate of sudden cardiac death was 99.4% [34].

d. Comparison of Mono- and Biphasic Waveforms. In our institution, we determined the defibrillation efficacy of simultaneous monophasic and biphasic waveforms in 43 patients using either a unidirectional or a bidirectional transvenous lead configuration. The bidirectional lead configuration consisted of a cathodal right ventricular lead with an anodal subcutaneous patch coupled to the superior vena cava lead. The unidirectional lead configuration consisted of a cathodal right ventricular lead with an anodal superior vena cava lead. DFT was determined using monophasic and biphasic single-capacitor 63% tilt pulses. The leading-edge voltage of the second phase was equal to the trailing-edge voltage of the first phase. In the total patient group, the stored-energy DFT decreased from 22.5 ± 5.5 J using monophasic shock waveforms to 15.0 ± 4.9 J using biphasic shock waveforms ($p < 0.001$). The mean defibrillation energy saved was in the range of 30%. The bidirectional lead system seemed to have no advantage over the unidirectional defibrillation efficacy [35]. Figure 8 illustrates the comparison of monophasic and biphasic shock waveforms in the 43 patients studied.

4. Ventak PRx-II

In late 1992, the Ventak PRx-II was introduced for phase I clinical evaluation in Europe. The new device is similar in weight and volume to the Ventak PRx-I, but it is capable of delivering biphasic shock waveforms and provides extensified Holter features including stored electrograms which can be retrieved by a new programmer system, model 2950. To date, 67 Ventak PRx-II pulse generators have been implanted in 10 centers throughout Europe. The device was

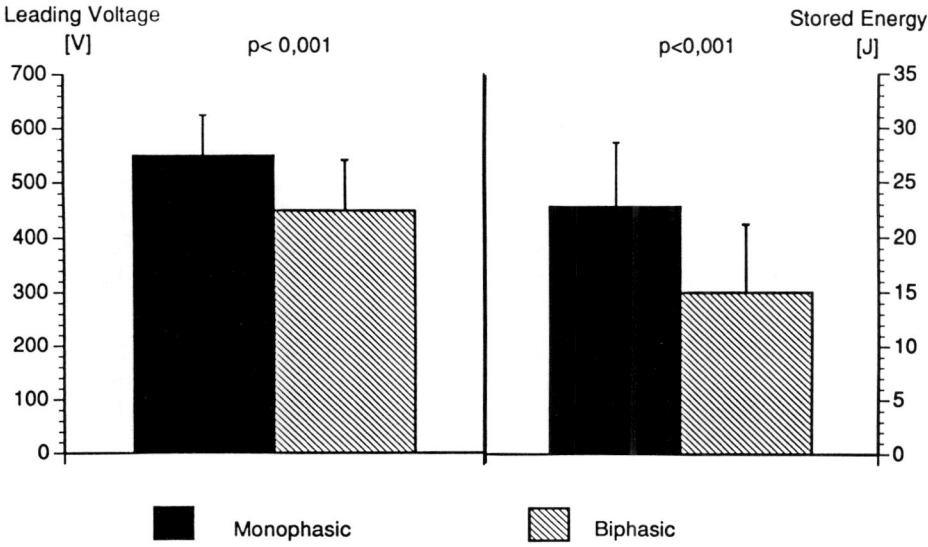

Figure 8 Comparison of defibrillation threshold data (leading-edge voltage and stored energy) in 43 patients using monophasic and biphasic shock waveforms. The leading-edge voltage decreased significantly from 580 V using monophasic shock waveforms to 470 V using biphasic pulses. Correspondingly, the stored energy decreased from 22.5 J with monophasic to 15 J using biphasic waveforms ($p < 0.001$).

implanted with 100% success rate using a transvenous approach. During the follow-up period (range 7 days to 22 weeks), a total of 217 spontaneous episodes occurred in 13 patients. Fifty-nine shock episodes occurred in 4 patients and were all successfully converted, 1 patient needing the fifth shock on two occasions. All therapy was appropriate with 100% conversion rate based on stored data.

B. Pacer Cardioverter-Defibrillator (PCD) (Medtronic)

The Medtronic model 7210 multiprogrammable tachyarrhythmia control device, capable of both antitachycardia pacing and low-energy (max. 2 J) shocks, was the first chronically implanted device employing a totally endocardial catheter electrode, the model 6682, for shock delivery. A few of these devices have been implanted in Europe.

1. PCD Model 7215

The PCD 7215 was first implanted in May 1988 in London, Ontario, Canada [36]. This device weighed 180 g, and was capable of delivering bradycardia pacing support as well as antitachycardia pacing and high-voltage energy shocks up to 15 J. Tachycardia detection was composed of rate, sudden onset, rate stability, and duration. This device was never implanted in Europe.

2. PCD Models 7216 and 7217

Later, the PCD models 7216A and 7217B were introduced in Europe for clinical evaluation. Apart from size and weight, the two models differ only in configuration. The model 7216A features integrated bipolar sensing, whereas the model 7217B has conventional bipolar sensing. The PCD is a committed device for VF but not for VT. Shocks can be delivered over two or three patches, and bidirectional sequential shocks may be delivered through the device. However, it cannot deliver biphasic shocks. A nonthoracotomy lead system is available consisting of a tripolar, endocardial screw-in ventricular lead, model 6966, a unipolar subcutaneous oval patch lead, model 6999, and a unipolar, endocardial coronary sinus or superior vena cava lead, model 6963. The ventricular lead is a true bipolar sensing lead. The first model 7216A PCD implant in Europe with an epicardial patch electrode took place in Lausanne, Switzerland, on May 19, 1989 [37]. The first model 7217B was implanted in February 1990. From May 1989 to November 1991, more than 450 PCD devices were implanted in Europe. The European clinical evaluation study using epicardial patch electrodes was completed in March 1991, when safety and efficacy of the system had been demonstrated. Market approval for the epicardial patch systems was recommended by the FDA advisory panel on February 3, 1992.

a. PCD with Epicardial Leads

1. Study Population. The European clinical evaluation report of the first 109 of 170 patients using epicardial patch electrodes is available [38]. The mean age of this study population was 55.4 years, the mean ejection fraction was 34.8%, the underlying heart disease was coronary heart disease in 70 patients, dilated cardiomyopathy in 19 patients, and other diseases in 14 patients. In 6 patients, the underlying heart disease was not available. The primary indication for ICD implantation was aborted sudden cardiac death in 38 patients, recurrences of monomorphic VT in 42 patients, and both VT and VF in 29 patients. Thirty patients were not receiving antiarrhythmic drugs at the time of implantation. The majority of the patients received a class III drug, which was either amiodarone in 35 patients, or sotalol in 14 patients. The surgical approach was a median sternotomy in 89 patients (82%). PCD implantation was the only surgical procedure in 83% of the patients ($n = 91$). A subxiphoidal approach was performed in 9 patients, a subcostal approach in 7 patients, and a lateral thoracotomy in 4 patients. Concomitant heart surgery was performed in 18 patients. The epicardial sensing and pacing thresholds were as follows (mean ± S.D.): electrogram amplitude 13.7 ± 5.9 mV, pacing threshold at 0.5 ms 0.96 ± 0.50 mV, pacing resistance 467 ± 137 Ω, slew rate 1.45 ± 0.98 V/s. A true DFT could be determined at implantation in 54 patients, with a mean value of 10.0 J ± 5.0 (range 2–18 J).

2. Complications and Observations. Nine perioperative deaths occurred. Causes of death were end-stage heart failure in 5 patients, acute myocardial infarction in 1 patient, pneumonia in 1 patient, and septicemia in 2 patients. Follow-up results are available for the first 100 patients, with a mean follow-up period of 5.6 months. A total of 1829 spontaneous episodes of VT was detected in 49 patients, an average of 37 and a medium of 15 per patient. Overall, 98.3% of the detected episodes of VT were terminated successfully. The PCD device interpreted 330 spontaneous arrhythmias in 39 patients as VF. Probably in two of the patients with more than 50 episodes, the circumstances suggested that most of these therapies were provoked by atrial fibrillation with rapid ventricular response. The overall efficacy in terminating episodes of VT has been 97%. Apart from the 9 patients who died in the hospital, 6 patients died after hospital discharge. All of these deaths were cardiac; two were classified as sudden, and four as nonsudden. Complications and observations were as follows: Seven patients received inappropriate therapies due to atrial fibrillation; pocket infection occurred in 6 patients, requiring explantation of the device in 5; five patients lost capture on the myocardial screw-in electrodes; but the problem was solved by placement of an intravenous lead; patch repositioning was required in 3 patients; in 2 of them, crumbling of patches occurred, and in 1, rubbing of the patch edge against the aorta ascendens caused arterial bleeding. At 1 year after implant, the actuarial survival rate for sudden cardiac death and total mortality was 98.5% and 86.3%, respectively. These results were confirmed by a large European multicenter study including 102 implants from 11 European centers. Patients were enrolled in this study between May 1989 and February 1991 [39].

b. PCD with Transvene Lead System. The first European implantation of a model 7216A with a nonthoracotomy lead system occurred on November 10, 1989, in Münster, Germany. From November 1989 to July 1992, 139 patients were enrolled in the European PCD clinical investigation using the nonthoracotomy lead system, the Transvene leads [40]. As of November 1991, over 290 PCD devices with Transvene leads had been implanted by 38 European centers.

1. Study Population. 139 patients received their devices in 14 European centers, with an average of 7.4 (range 1–39 implants per investigator). The mean age was 55.3 years, the mean ejection fraction was 40.4%. The underlying heart disease was coronary heart disease in 66% of the patients, dilated cardiomyopathy in 26% of the patients, and other diseases in 8% of the patients. The primary indication for the PCD implantation was aborted sudden cardiac death in 37% of the patients, recurrent VT in 41%, and both VT and VF in 22%. At the time of implantation, 30 patients were off any antiarrhythmic drugs, and 32 patients were taking either amiodarone ($n = 15$) or sotalol ($n = 17$). The sensing and pacing thresholds at implantation were as follows: electrogram amplitude 12.6 ± 5.5 mV, pacing threshold at 0.5 ms 0.9 ± 0.5 V, resistance 531 ± 134 Ω, slew rate 1.5 ± 1.0 V/s. The mean DFT was 15.5 ± 3.7 J from 5 to 24 J. There was no significant difference in DFT between patients receiving a right ventricular superior vena cava-subcutaneous patch electrode configuration (DFT: 15.3 ± 3.8; range 5–25 J) or those receiving a right ventricular coronary sinus-subcutaneous patch electrode configuration (DFT: 17.3 ± 1.5; range 15–18 J). Sequential current pathway was used in 76% of patients, simultaneous current pathway in 22%, and single-current pathway in 2%.

2. Efficacy. A total of 437 spontaneous episodes of VT as defined by the programmed detection parameters in the PCD was treated in 30 patients, an average of 14.6 and a median of 3 per patient. Antitachycardia pacing as a first therapy had a termination rate of 85.3%. There was no significant difference in termination success rates between ramp pacing (85.7%) and burst pacing (81%). The effectiveness of the second antitachycardia pacing therapy was much lower than the first, with 16% success rate. Success rates for burst and ramp as second VT therapy were also very similar: 15.3% and 16.7%, respectively. The success rate for cardioversion as first VT therapy was 80%, and as second VT therapy 77% (Fig. 9). Regarding all four available VT therapies, the success rate increased gradually from 85% after delivery of VT therapy 1 to 98.8% after therapy 4. A total of 212 spontaneous arrhythmias in 21 patients occurred during follow-up and were interpreted by the device as VF. There was a 98.6% therapy effectiveness for defibrillation via the Transvene lead system.

3. Complications and Observations. The most frequently reported complication in this European study has been lead dislodgement of the lead model 6963 (Fig. 10). In 5 patients, the lead retracted from the superior vena cava or moved deeper into the right atrium. In another 3 patients, the lead dislodged from its coronary sinus position. Two lead dislodgements occurred with the lead model 6996 from the right ventricle. Two lead fractures of the subcutaneous patch electrode were observed. Two patients experienced pocket infection, and all implanted materials were removed. Hematoma in the pulse generator pocket or in the pocket of the subcutaneous electrode was reported in 2 and 1 patient, respectively. Seroma occurred in 5 patients. Substantial fibrosis around the subcutaneous patch electrode was observed in 1 patient. Loss of

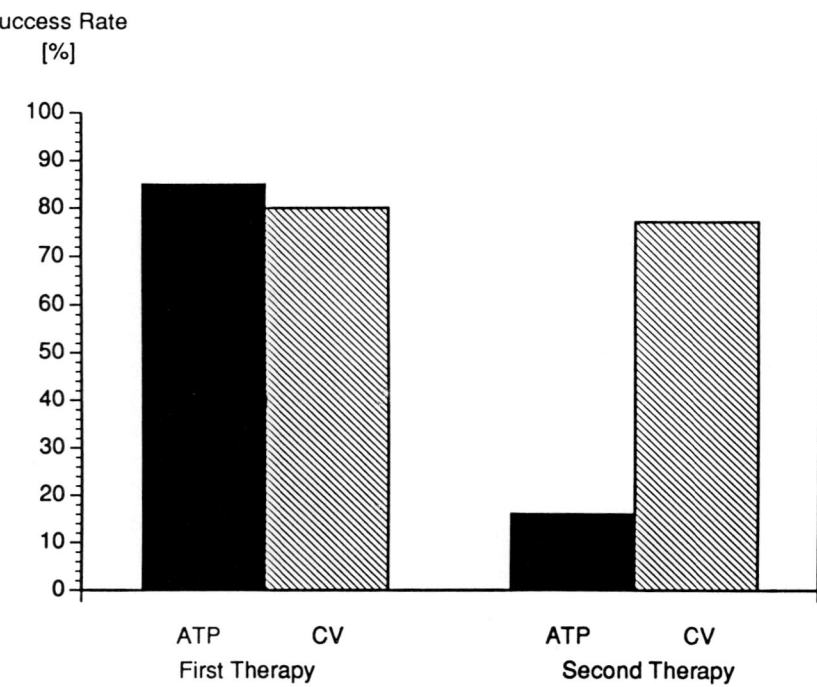

Figure 9 Success rates of antitachycardia pacing (ATP) and cardioversion (CV) therapies. In the first therapy, the efficacy rate in terminating VT is similar for ATP and CV therapies. In contrast to these findings, the success rate for termination of VT using ATP decreased to 16% during the second therapy as compared to 77% using cardioversion therapy.

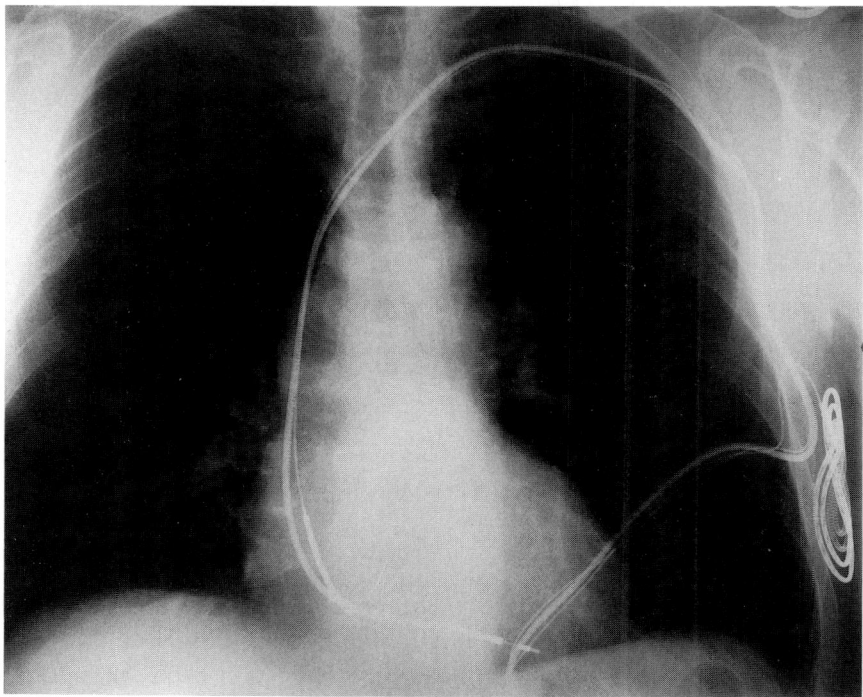

Figure 10 Chest X-ray of a patient with a dislodged vena cava superior electrode into the deep right atrium. The defibrillating lead system consists of a screw-in lead in the right ventricular apex, a free-floating vena cava superior lead at the junction of the right atrium, and a left lateral subcutaneous patch electrode.

ventricular capture was observed postimplant in two patients, and was resolved by fixing one of the set screws for the right ventricular lead in the first and by replacing a fractured right ventricular lead in the second patient. One patient experienced thrombosis of the left subclavian vene, which was treated with anticoagulants. One patient developed a sero-pneumothorax requiring drainage. Two patients received cardiac transplant. One of the 103 patients died within 1 month after implantation, in contrast to 9 in-hospital deaths from the series of 109 epicardial implants. Between November 1989 and November 1991, 3 deaths occurred in the Transvene patient group. One patient died suddenly; there was 1 patient death due to progressive heart failure, and 1 noncardiac death. The true survivor curve for sudden cardiac death was 99.1%, and for total mortality was 97.1%.

3. PCD Model 7219

A new PCD defibrillator, the Jewel, model 7219LD, capable of delivering biphasic pulses, extensified Holter storage, and reduced in size to approximately 130 g has been recently introduced in Europe for clinical evaluation. The first implant was performed in March 1993 in Munich, Germany. To date, approximately 30 of these defibrillators have been implanted in Europe. Due to the reduced size and weight, this defibrillator can be implanted pectorally in selected patients (Fg. 11). Details of the introduced third-generation ICDs are provided in Table 7.

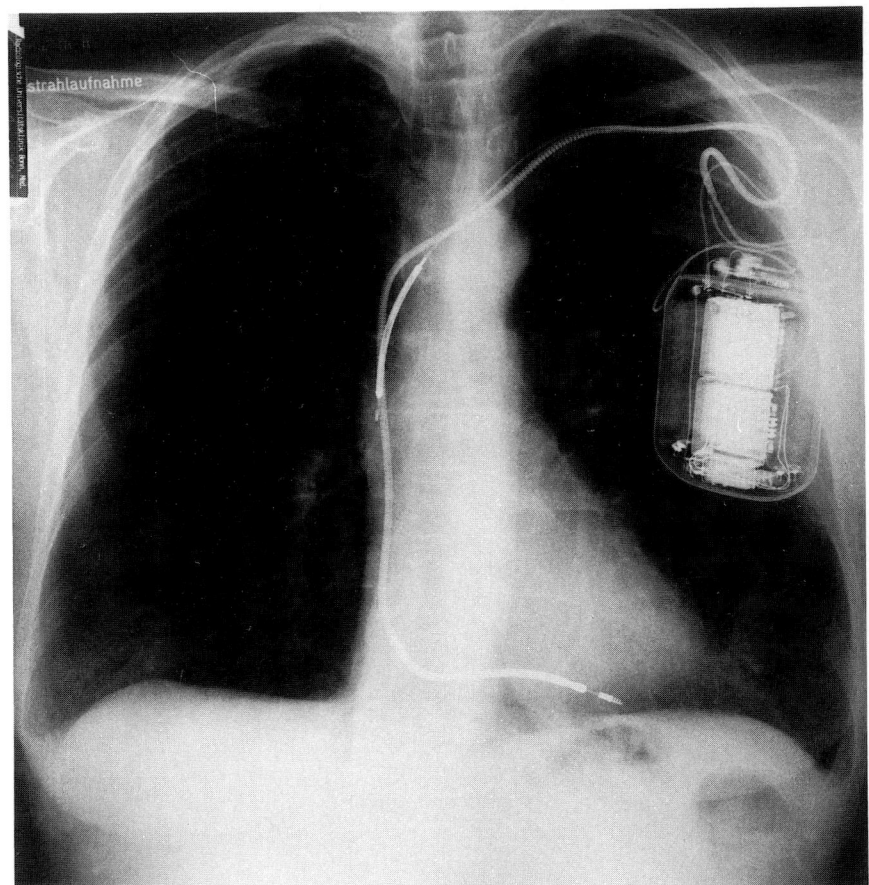

Figure 11 Chest X-ray of a 50-year-old female patient with a subpectoral implantation of a PCD. The defibrillator is connected with a free-floating lead in the vena cava superior and a right ventricular screw-in lead.

C. Guardian (Telectronics)

The Guardian 4201/3 provides two major advantages over the Ventak P: bradycardia support as well as reconfirmation that VT is still present, and it has the ability to dump the charge internally if the arrhythmia terminates before shock delivery. A major drawback of this device is the fixed gain sensitivity sensing, which has been demonstrated to cause undersensing of VF during follow-up [41]. In Europe, these devices have rarely been implanted because of the possibility of undersensing due to the fixed gain setting. A new third-generation, multi-programmable pulse generator, the ATP 4210 has been introduced for clinical evaluation. For arrhythmia detection, an automatic sensitivity adjustment is used in the Guardian ATP 4210 and the Guardian 4204. The user programs the sensitivity of the low- and high-gain detection channels. Once an arrhythmia is detected and shock therapy might be required, the defibrillator automatically switches to a higher (more sensitive) gain channel depending on the RR interval.

Table 7 ATP-ICD Pulse Generators: Third Generation

	CPI Ventak P2	CPI PRx I	CPI PRx II	Intermedics Res-Q	Siemens Siecure	Telectronics Guardian 4211	Ventritex Cadence	Medtronic 7217	Medtronic Jewel, 7219
Antitachycardia pacing	−	+	+	+	+	+	+	+	+
Bradycardia pacing	+	+	+	+	+	+	+	+	+
Programmable rate/energy	+	+	+	+	+	+	+	+	
Waveforms	M,B	M	M,B	B	M	M,B	M,B	M,S	M,B
Tiered therapy	−	+	+	+	+	+	+	+	+
Noninvasive EPS	+	+	+	+	+	+	+	+	+
Weight (g)	240	220	220	220	200	270	237	200	132

M = monophasic; B = biphasic; S = sequential; EPS = electrophysiological programmed stimulation.

1. Guardian ATP 4210

   a. Study Population. As of May 1, 1992, 131 Guardian ATP 4210 implants had been performed by 29 centers in Europe. The patient population was predominantly male (85%). The mean age was 61 years, the mean ejection fraction 34%. The underlying heart disease was coronary heart disease in 78% of the patients, and dilated cardiomyopathy in 12%. The indication for implantation of the ICD was VT in 20%, VF in 14%, and both arrhythmias in 12%. The mean implant duration was 10 months as of June 1, 1992. The actuarial analysis for patient survival showed a 98.4% sudden cardiac death survival rate at 2 years, a total cardiac survival rate of 93.7% at 1 year, and an 89.6% overall patient survival rate at 1 year. Perioperative deaths amounted to 1.7% overall. In 6 cases, the device program was inactivated or had never been activated prior to death. Forty explants were reported: 17 were due to infection and 9 were a result of device failure; 1 device was explanted due to inappropriate sensing of an induced arrhythmia, and 2 devices were electively replaced at the time of lead revision. There were 6 explants as a result of high DFTs, and 5 devices were explanted during heart transplantation. During follow-up, spontaneous episodes of VT were reverted by antitachycardia pacing in 93%. The acceleration rate was only 1.3%. Clinical data indicates that 74.5% of the spontaneous clinical events reverted spontaneously at the first confirmation prior to therapy delivery.

2. Guardian ATP-II 4210 and 4211

The Guardian ATP 4210 device, as previously designed, performs a number of safety checks every hour. These include checks of the integrity of the microprocessor memory and checks of the validity of all programmable parameters. If either of the two safety checks fail, the device shuts down. In this mode, the device cannot deliver the required therapy for ventricular tachyarrhythmias, but continues to provide antibradycardia pacing support. As of January 1991, six shutdowns had been documented in Europe in 55 implants [42]. The cause of the shutdowns may be due to random component failure or may be software-related. As an interim measure, an external device (Guardimate) has been provided by the manufacturer so that the patient can monitor the state of the implanted device. Initial experience with the shutdown feature of the Guardian ATP 4210 led to a revision of design and manufacturing during the trial. In May 1991, the new population of ATP-II 4210 devices were introduced with modified shutdown features. As of April 24, 1992, the shutdown rate due to random component failure was significantly lower using the new population of 4210 devices. In late 1992, the Guardian ATP 4211 was introduced for clinical evaluation. This device differs from the 4210 in the following features: The sensing circuit has been changed from automatic sensitivity adjustment using two gain channels to an automatic sensitivity tracking mode, i.e., the sensitivity automatically tracks beat to beat; the device is capable of delivering biphasic shock waveforms. In the new device model 4211, a new current-shunting protection circuitry has been implemented to prevent current leakage back through the lead to the patient, resulting in elevated pacing thresholds. Up to March 1993, 22 patients received the Guardian ATP 4211 in 7 centers in Europe. To date, no deaths or complications have been reported.

3. Transvenous Lead Systems

The first transvenous lead system, the Accufix DF, was introduced in 1990. However, several lead fractures occurred, resulting in the suspension of the transvenous electrode system [43].

   a. Enguard I Lead System. A new electrode system, the Enguard I lead, consisting of atrial and ventricular braided endocardial electrodes, was introduced in November 1991 and continued in use until March 1992, when the study was suspended due to both the occurrence of several lead fractures and elevated pacing thresholds resulting in exit block. Of the 60 attempted implants, 58 patients received the Enguard I system. The clinical update presents data as of December 11, 1992. In one patient the lead system was not implanted because of failure to meet the implant criteria; a second system was not implanted due to variability of the patient's electrogram amplitude postshock, which was observed during testing. There are currently 7 centers in Europe participating in the clinical study. The mean age of the patient population is 57 ± 15 years, the mean ejection fraction 33 ± 16%. A bidirectional lead configuration was utilized in 86% of the patients, and the unidirectional configuration was used in the remainder. The successful defibrillation energies tested at implant ranged from 4 J to 30 J in the bidirectional configuration, and from 10 to 25 J in the unidirectional configuration. The system detected 325 episodes of clinical, spontaneous arrhythmias in 25 patients. Of these episodes, 110 were terminated by either antitachycardia pacing or defibrillation therapy from the device. The remainder reverted spontaneously. Relevant medical events were reported in 21 patients. There were 5 patient deaths and 16 explants that resulted in the termination of the study. Lead conductor fractures were reported in 11 patients. The fractures were all within either the clavical/first rib area or in the tunnel/pocket area. An analysis of all leads indicated that the conductor fractures were associated with constraint of the lead. Early in the clinical study it was found that there was a higher number of patients with elevated pacing thresholds than anticipated. Eleven patients presented with exit block at a mean time of 8 days after implant. The actuarial survival rate at 1 year after implant was 98.3% for cardiac death and 91.8% for overall mortality. Due to the elevated pacing thresholds and high incidence of lead fractures, a newly redesigned lead system, the Enguard PFx, was introduced for clinical evaluation in the beginning of 1993. The new right ventricular lead is a passive-fixation lead and, additionally, the conductor material has been changed.

b. Enguard PFx Lead System. As of February 26, 1993, there had been 15 implants with the Enguard PFx endocardial defibrillation lead system in Europe, among 7 different centers. The mean implant duration was 17 days, ranging from 1 to 48 days. The mean age of the patients enrolled was 60.4 ± 7.3 years. All of the patients were male. The mean ejection fraction reported was 34.3 ± 11.9% (range from 19 to 57%). Primary indication to implant the device was sudden cardiac death in 10%, aborted sudden cardiac death as well as recurrent VT in 20%, and recurrent episodes of VT in 70%. The underlying heart disease was coronary heart disease in 80% of the patients, dilated cardiomyopathy in 10%, and other diseases in 10%. The DFT voltage ranged between 350 and 550 V. Forty percent of the patients received a transvenous lead system only; the other 60% required an additional subcutaneous patch electrode. Pacing threshold at implant at a pulse duration of 0.5 ms was 0.43 ± 0.13 V (range 0.3–0.6 V). No deaths or explants of the Enguard PFx system and no severe complications have been observed to date.

D. Cadence (Ventritex)

The Cadence is a 240-g device with the capability of performing antitachycardia pacing, bradycardia pacing, and defibrillation with a maximum energy of 34 J. Biphasic shocks are available to be delivered via two patches. At present, no transvenous lead system is available. Noninvasive electrophysiological testing can be performed with the Cadence, and ventricular electrograms can be recorded via the sensing leads. In Europe, only limited experience has been gained with the Cadence defibrillator because of two reasons: One, the system used to be available to only two investigational centers in Europe; second, the device had to be implanted using epicardial patch electrodes. This is a major drawback, particularly in Europe, where transvenous leads from other manufacturers are already market-released. Thus, some Cadence pulse generators have been connected to an Endotak transvenous lead system from the CPI manufacturer. The Endotak C lead had to be connected with an adaptor provided by a third supplier to fit into the header of the Cadence defibrillator. At least 2 patients experienced inappropriate shock discharges due to a connector defect in the sensing lead circuit. Widespread use of this defibrillator will not be expected in Europe until the manufacturer is able to provide its own transvenous lead system. The device was studied extensively using epicardial patch electrodes in the United States and showed reliable detection and termination functions [44]. A recent report described the value of ventricular sensing electrograms in the diagnosis of arrhythmias causing electrical devices to administer shock therapy [45].

E. Res-Q (Intermedics)

The Res-Q defibrillator was introduced into phase I clinical evaluation in Europe in 1989.

1. Res-Q with Epicardial Leads

Initially, the Res-Q device consisted only of contoured epicardial patches. The Res-Q is a committed pulse generator capable of delivering biphasic shock waveforms. In Europe, the Res-Q has been implanted with contoured patches in only three centers, in London (England), Bonn (Germany), and Marseille (France). About 15 units were implanted with large-surface-area, asymmetrically contoured patches placed epicardially. DFTs achieved were in the range of 3 to 7 J [46–48]. However, further implantations had to be discontinued because of frequent inappropriate shocks due to oversensing during normal sinus rhythm.

2. Res-Q with Transvenous Leads

In the spring of 1992, a nonthoracotomy lead system was introduced for phase I clinical evaluation consisting of a subcutaneous patch electrode and a screw-in right ventricular lead with a 10-cm coil. Sensing was accomplished between the distal tip and the right ventricular coil. To date, the Res-Q pulse generator has been implanted with a transvenous/subcutaneous lead configuration in 17 patients in only one center in Europe (Bonn, Germany).

a. Study Population. The mean age of the study population was 53 ± 12 years; the mean ejection fraction was 45 ± 17%. The underlying heart disease was coronary artery disease in 10 patients, nonischemic dilated cardiomyopathy in 5 patients, and other cardiac diseases in 2 patients. The primary indication for ICD implantation was VF in 10 patients, recurrent VT in 5 patients, and both VT and VF in 2 patients. At implant, 7 patients were off any antiarrhythmic drug treatment. The mean DFT utilizing biphasic pulse waveforms was 21.1 ± 7.4 J at the time of implantation and decreased to 16.3 ± 6.1 J prior to hospital discharge (Fig. 12). The Res-Q can also be programmed to triphasic shock waveforms. There was no significant difference in required energies between bi- and triphasic shock waveforms in the patients studied. The mean DFT for biphasic shock waveform was 21 ± 7 J and for triphasic shock pulses was 20 ± 6 J (Fig. 13). The endocardial electrogram amplitudes and pacing thresholds were as follows: electrogram amplitude 8.1 ± 3.5 mV, pacing threshold at 0.5 ms 0.8 ± 0.4 V.

b. Efficacy. During the follow-up of 2.4 ± 2.3 months, a total of 23 spontaneous episodes of ventricular tachyarrhythmias was detected in 4 patients. Due to the committed function of the Res-Q pulse generator, inappropriate shock delivery occurred in 3 patients due to sinus tachycardia or atrial fibrillation with rapid ventricular response. During follow-up, no rise in pacing threshold was observed. Besides infection of the ICD system in 1 patient, no further complications were noted. In this patient, the complete ICD system had to be explanted

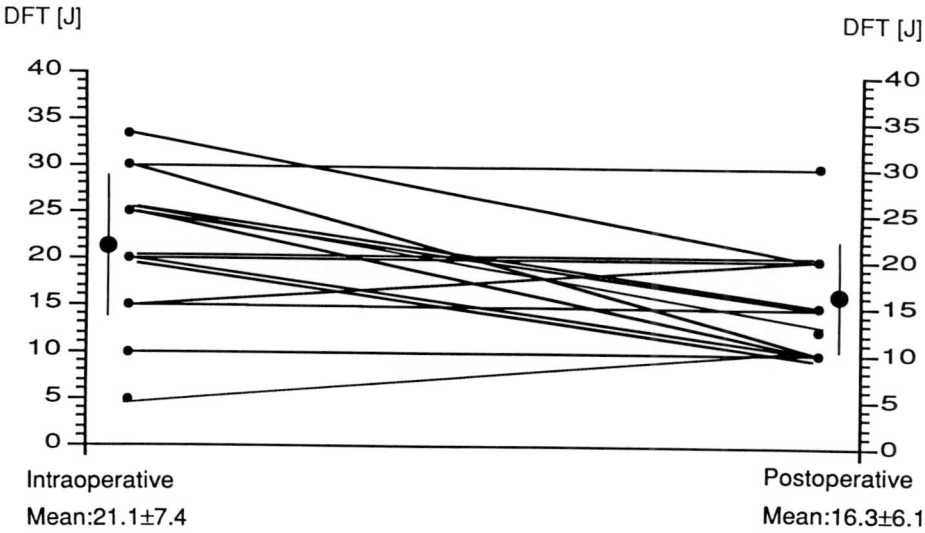

Figure 12 The relation of intraoperative to postoperative defibrillation threshold (DFT). This figure demonstrates the change in DFT in 17 patients using biphasic shock waveforms with a pulse duration of 10 ms and a unidirectional lead configuration consisting of a cathodal right ventricular screw-in lead and an anodal subcutaneous patch electrode. There was a significant decrease in DFT from 21.1 ± 7.4 J at the time of implantation to 16.3 ± 6.1 J prior to hospital discharge.

1 week after implantation due to *Staphylococcus aureus* infection. The overall actuarial survival rate of this patient population is 100%. Further implantations in other European centers are expected in the near future.

F. Siecure (Siemens Pacesetter)

Because of the lack of a transvenous lead system, the Siecure ICD device has been implanted in Europe in only a few centers.

1. Siecure with Epicardial Leads

In one report from London, United Kingdom, the device was implanted transthoracically with no peri- or postoperative complications in 6 patients with a mean age of 49 years. All patients had malignant arrhythmias induced perioperatively and noninvasively 6 weeks postoperation, confirming appropriate device response and tachycardia sensing functions [49]. One patient has required reintroduction of amiodarone due to increasing frequency of VT, but the remainder of the patients were free of antiarrhythmic drug therapy up to 1 year postimplantation. The antitachycardia pacing function was used successfully six times to terminate arrhythmias in these patients. The implant DFT was < 10 J in all 6 patients.

2. Siecure with Transvenous Leads

In midsummer 1992, a transvenous lead system consisting of a right ventricular electrode, a superior vena cava electrode, and an additional subcutaneous patch electrode became available. Despite introduction of a transvenous system, the Siecure pulse generator was not used increas-

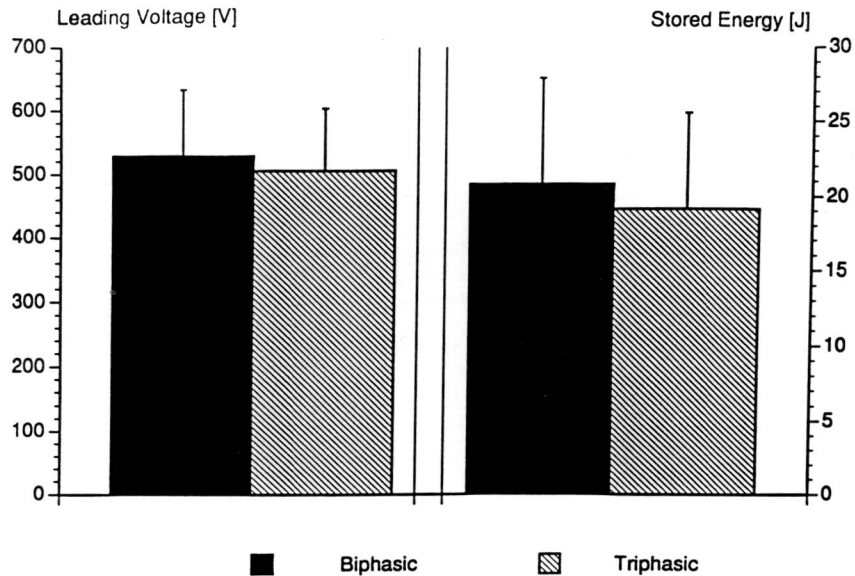

Figure 13 Defibrillation efficacy of biphasic and triphasic shock waveforms in 17 patients. Comparing the defibrillation efficacy of the biphasic and triphasic shock waveforms, there was no significant difference in leading-edge voltage and stored energy between shock waveforms tested.

ingly because the device was only capable of delivering monophasic shock waveforms. In a recent report, the device was implanted in 18 patients (mean age 56 ± 9 years, mean ejection fraction 46 ± 14%). The underlying heart disease was coronary artery disease in 16 patients, and dilated cardiomyopathy in 2 patients. An epicardial patch-patch lead system was employed in 13 patients, and the transvenous lead configuration in 5 patients. The mean intraoperative DFT was 17.3 ± 8.1 J in those patients using epicardial leads and 25.0 ± 10.0 J in those patients using transvenous lead systems. An additional subcutaneous patch electrode was necessary in only 2 of the 5 patients with transvenous lead systems [50].

VI. FUTURE ASPECTS OF ICD DEVELOPMENT

With the increasingly widespread use of the transvenous ICD approach, some technological advances will be expected in the near future (Table 8). Progress will occur in the development of improved sensing function of the ICD. More accurate automatic arrhythmia diagnoses need to be guaranteed. This will occur in association with atrial sensing leads and template recognition formats. Hemodynamic monitoring will allow for the optimum utilization of tiered therapy. Dual-chamber bradycardia pacing will be routine in the near future. The size of the devices will be reduced so that a transvenous pectoral approach will be the first choice of implantation. To reduce the size of the devices, new capacitor technology will be implemented. In addition, besides the optimal shock waveform, new transvenous leads with smaller diameters will be developed, possibly including new electrode materials. Furthermore, the Holter functions of the ICD system will be extended to allow analysis of the mechanism of the onset of ventricular tachyarrhythmias. Improved battery technology will ensure increased longevity. Finally, preventive pacing techniques will be developed and incorporated into the device to preclude the

Table 8 Future Aspects of ICD Development

- Sensing function
  New detection algorithms, atrial sensing leads, hemodynamic sensors
- Tiered therapy
  DDD/VVI-R pacing capability, preventive pacing techniques, optimal shock waveforms
- Surgical approach
  Pectoral implantation, new lead technology (smaller diameters)
- Size of the device
  New capacitor technology, low-energy units (20 J)
- Battery longevity
- Holter functions
  Extended ECG documentation, telephone monitoring

development of symptoms which may be associated with the onset of frequent recurrent ventricular tachyarrhythmias.

REFERENCES

1. Mirowski M, Reid PR, Mower MM, et al. Termination of malignant ventricular arrhythmias with an implanted automatic defibrillator in human beings. N Engl J Med 1980; 303:322–324.
2. Lüderitz B. Historical aspects of device therapy for cardiac arrhythmias. In: Lüderitz B, Saksena S, eds. Interventional Electrophysiology. Mount Kisco, NY: Futura, 1991: 333–352.
3. Coumel P. Historical milestones of implanted defibrillation. PACE 1992; 15:598–603.
4. Kulbertus HE, Nisam S. The implantable defibrillator AICD: European clinical experience. In: Brugada P, Wellens HJJ, eds. Cardiac Arrhythmias: Where to Go from Here? Mount Kisco, NY: Futura, 1987; 681–686.
5. Manz M, Gerckens U, Funke HD, Kirchhoff PG, Lüderitz B. Combination of antitachycardia pacemaker and automatic implantable cardioverter/defibrillator for ventricular tachycardia. PACE 1986; 9:676–684.
6. Lüderitz B, Gerckens U, Manz M. Automatic implantable cardioverter/defibrillator (AICD) and antitachycardia pacemaker (Tachylog): combined use in ventricular tachyarrhythmias. PACE 1986; 9:1356–1360.
7. Lüderitz B. The impact of antitachycardia pacing with defibrillation. PACE 1992; 14:312–316.
8. Block M, Hammel D, Isbruch F, et al. Results and realistic expectations with transvenous lead systems. PACE 1992; 15:665–670.
9. Hief CH, Podczeck A, Veit F, et al. Transvenous-subcutaneous lead system for implantable cardioverter-defibrillator. Wien Klin Wochenschr 1993; 105:12–16.
10. Trappe HJ, Klein H, Fieguth HG, Kielblock B, Wenzlaff P, Lichtlen PR. Initial experience with a new transvenous defibrillation system. PACE 1993; 16:134–140.
11. Block M, Hammel D, Borggrefe M, et al. Transvenous-subcutaneous implantation of leads for implantable defibrillators. Z Kardiol 1991; 80:657–664.
12. Schmitt C, Brachmann J, Saggau W, et al. Integrated antibradycardiac/antitachycardiac pacemaker-cardioverter-defibrillator systems in patients with recurrent ventricular tachyarrhythmias. Z Kardiol 1991; 80:665–672.
13. Neuzner J, Huth Ch, Friedl A, Reinisch P, Pitschner HF, Schlepper M. Cardioverter-defibrillator implantation without thoracotomy: clinical experience with various defibrillation lead configura-

tions and defibrillation waveforms of a nonthoracotomy defibrillator system. Z Kardiol 1993; 82:99–107.
14. Jordaens L, Trouerbach JW, Vertongen P, Herregods L, Poelaert J, Van Nooten G. Experience of cardioverter-defibrillators inserted without thoracotomy: evaluation of transvenously inserted intracardiac leads alone or with subcutaneous axillary patch. Br Heart J 1993; 69:14–19.
15. A Task Force of the Working Group on Cardiac Arrhythmias and Cardiac Pacing of the European Society of Cardiology. Guidelines for the use of implantable cardioverter defibrillators. Eur Heart J 1992; 13:1304–1310.
16. Haverich A, Tröster J, Wahlers T, Fieguth HG, Klein H. The automatic implantable cardioverter defibrillator (AICD) as a bridge to heart transplantation. PACE 1992; 15:701–707.
17. Defibrillat Study Group. Actuarial risk of sudden death while awaiting cardiac transplantation in patients with atherosclerotic heart disease. Am J Cardiol 1991; 68:545–546.
18. Lüderitz B, Jung W, Deister A, Marneros A, Manz M. Patient acceptance of the implantable cardioverter-defibrillator (ICD) in ventricular tachyarrhythmias. PACE 1993; 16:1815–1821.
19. Siebels J, Cappato R, Rüppel R, Schneider MAE, Kuck KH, and the CASH investigators. ICD versus drugs in cardiac arrest survivors: preliminary results of the Cardiac Arrest Study, Hamburg. PACE 1993; 16:552–558.
20. The Cardiomyopathy Trial Investigators. Cardiomyopathy Trial. PACE 1993; 16:576–581.
21. Hauer RNW, Wever EFD, Crijns HJGM. Automatic implantable cardioverter defibrillator: cost effectiveness. PACE 1993; 16:559–563.
22. Anderson MH, Camm AJ. Implications for present and future applications of the implantable cardioverter-defibrillator resulting from the use of a simple-model of cost efficacy. Br Heart J 1993; 69:83–92.
23. Brugada B, Andries E. The rationale for prophylactic implantation of a defibrillator in "high risk" patients. PACE 1993; 16:547–551.
24. Priori SG, Borggrefe M, Camm AJ, et al. Idiopathic ventricular fibrillation: a clinical dilemma (abstr.). J Am Coll Cardiol 1993; 21:24A.
25. Jung W, Manz M, Pfeiffer D, Tebbenjohanns J, Pizzulli L, Lüderitz B. Effects of antiarrhythmic drugs on epicardial defibrillation energy requirements and the rate of defibrillator discharges. PACE 1993; 16:198–201.
26. Jung W, Manz M, Pizzulli L, Pfeiffer D, Lüderitz B. Effects of chronic amiodarone therapy on defibrillation threshold. Am J Cardiol 1992; 70:1023–1027.
27. McCowan R, Maloney J, Wilkoff B, et al. Automatic implantable cardioverter-defibrillator implantation without thoracotomy using an endocardial and submuscular patch system. J Am Coll Cardiol 1991; 17:415–421.
28. Saksena S, Tullo NG, Krol RB, Mauro AM. Initial clinical experience with endocardial defibrillation using an implantable cardioverter/defibrillator with a triple-electrode system. Arch Intern Med 1989; 149:2333–2339.
29. Hauser RG, Mower MM, Mitchell M, Nisam S. Current status of the Ventak PRx pulse generator and Endotak nonthoracotomy lead system. PACE 1992; 15:671–677.
30. Wietholt D, Block M, Isbruch F, et al. Clinical experience with antitachycardia pacing and improved detection algorithms in a new implantable cardioverter-defibrillator. J Am Coll Cardiol 1993; 21:885–894.
31. Jung W, Manz M, Moosdorf R, Lüderitz B. Failure of an implantable cardioverter-defibrillator to redetect ventricular fibrillation in patients with a nonthoracotomy lead system. Circulation 1992; 86:1217–1222.
32. Jung W, Manz M, Pfeiffer D, et al. Substantial improvement in redetection of ventricular fibrillation with a new nonthoracotomy lead system (abstr.). Circulation 1992; 86:I–791.
33. Block M, Hammel D, Böcker D, Isbruch F, Wietholt D, Breithardt G. Subcutaneous array lead for internal defibrillation—a new lead configuration (abstr.). PACE 1993; 16:896.
34. Jung W. Clinical experience with the Ventak P2 defibrillator system: results of a European multicenter study (abstr.). Z Kardiol 1993; 82:190.

35. Jung W, Pfeiffer D, Moosdorf R, et al. Effects of transvenous electrode configuration and shock waveforms on defibrillation threshold in man (abstr.). Circulation 1992; 86:I-792.
36. Yee R, Klein GJ, Guiraudon GM, Jones DL, Sharma AD, Norris C. Initial clinical experience with the pacemaker-cardioverter-defibrillator. Can J Cardiol 1990; 6:147-156.
37. Fromer M, Schläpfer J, Fischer A, Kappenberger L. Experience with a new implantable pacer-, cardioverter-defibrillator for the therapy of recurrent sustained ventricular tachyarrhythmias: a step toward a universal ventricular tachyarrhythmia control device. PACE 1991; 14:1288-1298.
38. Lindemans FW, van Berlo AMW. European PCD Study, First Report. Clinical Report, Medtronic Bakken Research Center, Maastricht, The Netherlands, February, 1991.
39. Fromer M, Brachmann J, Block M, et al. Efficacy of automatic multimodal device therapy for ventricular tachyarrhythmias as delivered by a new implantable pacing cardioverter-defibrillator. Circulation 1992; 86:363-374.
40. Lindemans FW, van Binsbergen EJ, Roberts D, Bourgeois E. Technical aspects and clinical results of transvenous defibrillation. In: Adornato E, Galassi A, eds. The '92 Scenario on Cardiac Pacing. Roma, Italy: Edizioni: Luigi Pozzi, 1992:104-115.
41. Saksena S, Poczobutt-Johanos M, Castle LW, et al. Long-term multicenter experience with a second-generation implantable pacemaker-defibrillator in patients with malignant ventricular tachyarrhythmias. J Am Coll Cardiol 1992; 19:490-499.
42. Singer I, Austin E, Nash W, Gilbo J, Kupersmith J. The initial clinical experience with an implantable cardioverter defibrillator/antitachycardia pacemaker. PACE 1991; 14:1119-1128.
43. Paul VE, Anderson M, Jones S, Shekan DJ, Camm AJ, Ward DE. Cardiologist implanted cardioverter/defibrillators: early experience of three systems. Eur J CPE 1991; 1:21-26.
44. Winkle RA. The implantable defibrillator: progression from first to third generation devices. In: Zipes DP, Jalife J, eds. Cardiac Electrophysiology—From Cell to Bedside. Philadelphia: Saunders, 1990: 963-969.
45. Hurwitz JL, Hook BG, Flores BT, Marchlinski FE. Importance of abortive shock capability with electrogram storage in cardioverter-defibrillator devices. J Am Coll Cardiol 1993; 21:895-900.
46. Wong C, Davies DW, Rees GM, Edmondson SJ, Nathan AW. Early experience with a combined antitachycardia pacemaker and implantable defibrillator (abstr.). PACE 1990; 13:1215.
47. Jung W, Mletzko R, Manz M, Mohr F, Lüderitz B. Clinical experiences with a new antibradycardia/antitachycardia pacemaker and implantable defibrillator (abstr.). PACE 1990; 13:1199.
48. Manz M, Jung W, Lüderitz B. Selection of the individual therapeutic program with new implantable defibrillators. In: Lüderitz B, Saksena S, eds. Interventional Electrophysiology. Mount Kisco, NY: Futura, 1991:437-446.
49. Sowton E, Sulke N. Clinical experience with the Siemens Pacesetter Siecure. J Cardiovasc Electrophys 1992; 3:515-522.
50. Weismüller P, Hemmer W, Wiecha J, et al. Initial clinical experiences with the new ICD Siecure (abst.). PACE 1993; 16:874.

48

The Implantable Cardioverter-Defibrillator: Future Directions

Sanjeev Saksena*

Eastern Heart Institute
Passaic
and UMD-NJ Medical School
Newark, New Jersey

I. INTRODUCTION

The specialty of implantable defibrillator therapy has spanned a mere 25 years, with most of this period being devoted to prototype device development or clinical investigation. In less than one decade, however, a series of successor devices and investigations has produced a knowledge base large enough to warrant consideration as a specialty. The presentations preceding this chapter have established that there is already a definite role for implantable cardioverter-defibrillator (ICD) devices in the treatment of patients with malignant ventricular tachyarrhythmias. The future evolution of this approach in the treatment of tachyarrhythmias will be considered in this chapter. Due to the diversity and depth of investigation, this commentary can serve only as an overview. The reader is referred to the references for more detailed treatment of each area.

The concept of implantable device therapy for tachyarrhythmias is neither novel nor restricted to devices that revert such rhythms. Earliest clinical efforts used implanted pacemakers to suppress ventricular and atrial ectopy [1,2]. This effort was directed at least in part at tachyarrhythmia prevention. This goal still remains elusive but is a focus for future investigative effort. Implantable antitachycardia pacemakers, cardioverters, and defibrillators demonstrated the feasibility of tachyarrhythmia reversion in clinical practice and have been combined in the current generation of ICDs [3,4]. It appears reasonable to project the basic elements of such devices and identify persisting technological needs. Technological improvizations are likely as an interim measure. Application to new patient populations is under study. Issues relative to each target group can be assessed to a certain degree. Tangential, but on occasion critical, to such development are economic implications of such therapy. Finally, use of such devices as adjunctive therapy in other clinical arenas can be considered.

---

*Present affiliation: Private practice, Milburn, New Jersey.

II. ELEMENTS OF FUTURE ICD GENERATORS

The ICD is, certainly for the foreseeable future, likely to remain a hybrid device. It is reasonable to examine this proposition more critically. It is often suggested that an implantable defibrillator with a limited shock capacity alone may be adequate in many patient populations. The evolution of the current third-generation ICD has been derived from experience with demand pacemakers, antitachycardia pacemakers, implantable cardioverters, and implantable defibrillators [1–4]. The need for each component in ICD devices should be scrutinized.

Sudden death due to bradyarrhythmias has been demonstrated in cardiac arrest victims, patients with severe heart failure, and recipients of ICD devices for ventricular tachycardia (VT)/ventricular fibrillation (VF) [5–9]. In patients who are deemed at risk or who have had a cardiac arrest, it is presently difficult to differentiate prospectively those at risk for primary bradyarrhythmic arrest as opposed to those likely to have a tachyarrhythmic event. Furthermore, tachyarrhythmic events often culminate in bradycardic agonal phase [5,9]. In other instances, bradycardia may predispose to VT/VF. It is highly desirable and probable that demand pacing be retained in implantable devices used for the primary prevention of sudden death.

Antitachycardia pacing has been shown to offer patients benefits with respect to reduced shock exposure [10]. These benefits are, in general, restricted largely to patients experiencing monomorphic VT episodes with rates <220 beats/min. Prediction of future events of this nature is usually indirect. Most commonly, individuals who have previously demonstrated such a predilection, i.e., presented clinically with recurrent sustained VT, are primary candidates for this electrical intervention. Another method utilizes prediction of such events based on the results of invasive electrophysiological testing. Data derived from such studies indicate that spontaneous tachycardia recurrence rates are often at variance with induced tachyarrhythmias [11,12]. This difference nearly invariably takes the form of slower spontaneous events. The basis for this observation can be elucidated by prior reports on the reproducibility of programmed stimulation used in the electrophysiological study. Table 1 shows the patient population for a group of patients with recurrent sustained VT in whom the spontaneous event was recorded electrocardiographically in the absence of antiarrhythmic drugs. These patients subsequently underwent electrophysiological testing. Figure 1 shows the comparison of cycle lengths of spontaneous VT with induced VT stratified by induction mode. While single and

Table 1

24 patients with recurrent sustained VT and organic heart disease:
  20 men, 4 women
  Mean age 65 (range 32–80) years
Clinical presentation:
  5–25 episodes of spontaneous sustained VT requiring pharmacological electrical termination
  No recent myocardial infarction
  1–10 episodes of spontaneous VT recorded on ECG in the absence of antiarrhythmic drugs; >2 episodes in 18 patients
Methods:
  Programmed stimulation performed with 1, 2, 3, and 4 extrastimuli during sinus rhythm and ventricular pacing and burst of rapid ventricular pacing. Base drive cycle lengths were 600 and 400 ms.
  Stimulation sites included right ventricular apex, right ventricular outflow tract and left ventricle.
  VT cycle length and morphology analyzed for 10 consecutive complexes during sustained rhythm (spontaneous or induced) without antiarrhythmic drugs.

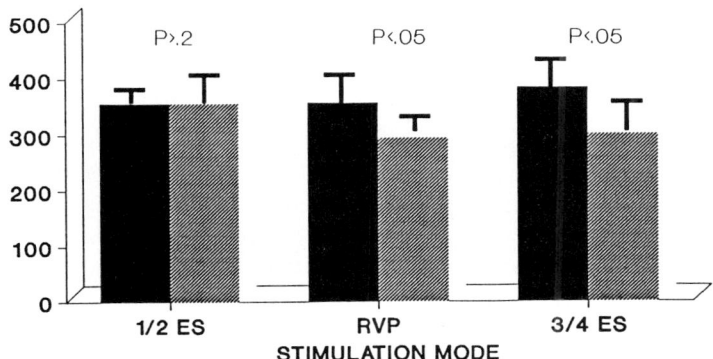

Figure 1 Comparison of cycle length of spontaneous VT determined on electrocardiographic recordings with induced VT in the electrophysiology laboratory in 24 patients with recurrent sustained VT. The mean cycle length is shown on the Y axis in milliseconds, and the induction mode is shown on the X axis. Abbreviations: ES = extrastimuli; RVP = rapid ventricular pacing; (■) spontaneous; (▨) induced. Note that there is a significant reduction in induced tachycardia cycle length with use of rapid ventricular pacing or triple or quadruple extrastimuli for tachycardia induction.

double extrastimuli faithfully reproduced the spontaneous rhythm rate, triple extrastimuli and burst pacing shortened the induced VT cycle length (Fig. 1). This is best explained by reduction in tissue refractoriness induced by the stimulation modes, thus abbreviating revolution time. The importance of this observation lies in the knowledge that the efficacy of pacing is influenced by the event rate. Thus, inefficacy of a pacing therapy for an induced tachycardia may not predict a similar interaction with a spontaneous event in the same patient. Empirical activation of antitachycardia pacing may have significant success. Nominal algorithms have been tested [13]. Different pacing modes often have comparable success. Furthermore, such success is not confined to patients with VT but is also seen in cardiac arrest of VF survivors receiving third-generation ICDs. In patients with declared risk undergoing secondary prevention with the ICD, activation of antitachycardia pacing appears to be highly likely. This feature will therefore be retained, especially for this population.

Utilization of antitachycardia pacing in primary prevention applications is more controversial. Electrophysiological prediction of the high-risk patient is being undertaken in populations with nonsustained VT and myocardial infarction. While noninvasive methods such as ambulatory ECG recording, signal averaging, or heart rate variability are often employed to predict risk of sudden death, none of these is being utilized in such patients to suggest the nature of the tachyarrhythmic event, i.e., VT or VF. The predictive value of electrophysiological testing specifically to predict risk for VT or VF or bradyarrhythmic death in these populations requires further study. Thus, the role of antitachycardia pacing in devices used for this application remains a less certain one than the need for bradycardia pacing. The latter is more likely to be retained. The availability of the former may depend simply on device complexity and cost introduced by its institution. Alternatively, the feature may be simply locked out in the generic ICD. Elimination of all pacing functions from the ICD, particularly in patients at high risk for VT/VF with depressed ventricular function, appears premature in view of the demonstrated propensity for bradyarrhythmic arrest [6].

Programmable shocks and cardioversion capabilities have established their value in current and past clinical trials of the ICD. Reduced exposure to high-energy shocks can be anticipated, but this patient benefit declines with programmed energies over 2 J [14,15]. Thus, this feature is of value only to a small, select group of patients with VT that is unresponsive to antitachycardia pacing. Biphasic low-energy shocks have greater efficacy and could enlarge this role to include more fast-VT patients [16]. Reprogramming of this feature is most often to higher energies [14]. Thus, limited programmability may have a role. Reducing the range of current programmable shock energies may still be appropriate. In contrast, elimination of programmed shock energies from devices used for primary prevention can be clinically acceptable. High-energy cardioversion/defibrillation shocks remain the mainstay of sudden-death prevention in such devices. This essential feature of all ICD devices will, however, be redefined as more effective defibrillation shock modes and lead systems are developed. Recent data suggest that use of biphasic simultaneous shocks and an axillary or pectoral anode can achieve nearly universal defibrillation at 15 J [17,18]. Maximum shock outputs of 20 to 25 J can now be considered.

Programmable tachycardia detection has contributed to reduced shock exposure by establishing zones for antitachycardia pacing therapies to be delivered [19]. A reconfirmation feature has eliminated committed therapies for nonsustained arrhythmias. Differentiation of sinus tachycardia or other supraventricular arrhythmias is also feasible. Reprogramming of tachycardia detection rates is likely during follow-up with changes in drug regimens, etc. Extensive programmability of this feature is likely in devices used for secondary prevention of sudden death. A more limited programmability is likely in primary prevention applications if advantages in device complexity and cost can be realized.

Tachycardia event data storage is invaluable in follow-up of ICD recipients, particularly when frequent device activation is observed. Differentiation of supraventricular rhythms and the nature of VT/VF events and their clinical impact is an essential component of patient management [20]. In contrast, devices used in primary prevention have low event rates and may accept significantly lesser capabilities in this area. Hybrid devices using pacemaker-cardioverter-defibrillator technology and extensive programmability and memory will become standard in secondary prevention. A more limited version of this hybrid device, i.e., a pacemaker-defibrillator, may be more applicable to primary prevention.

III. EVOLUTION OF ICD LEAD SYSTEMS

The lead systems used in ICD devices have now crystallized with respect to implant technique but await further refinements. The nonthoracotomy implant technique is now clearly the method of first choice [21–23]. The technique has low implant risk, with a perioperative mortality of 1% or less. Figure 2 shows implant risk as compared to epicardial lead implantation in one study [23]. Figure 3 shows that this benefit exists across different clinical subgroups in this study despite highly variable implant risk in each group. The major limitation of the nonthoracotomy approach, namely, high defibrillation energy requirements with monophasic shock waveforms, has been largely overcome with the use of biphasic shocks. A variety of devices are now either commercially available or under investigation with the feature, e.g., the Medtronic 7219, CPI Ventak-P2 and PRX-II, Ventitrex Cadence, Intermedics Res-Q, Angeion Sentinel and Telectronics model 4215. The lead configuration most frequently employed utilizes two catheter electrodes combined usually with a left thoracic patch electrode. Catheter electrodes utilize a right ventricular location of pacing, sensing, and defibrillation and a superior venacaval or right atrial site for defibrillation. With the likely advent of dual-chamber pacing and sensing in these devices, the atrial lead would assume importance to fulfill these functions. The left thoracic patch electrode is most valuable to reduce defibrillation energy requirements and improve reliability. In some patients with low thresholds, this may be avoided. The atrial elec-

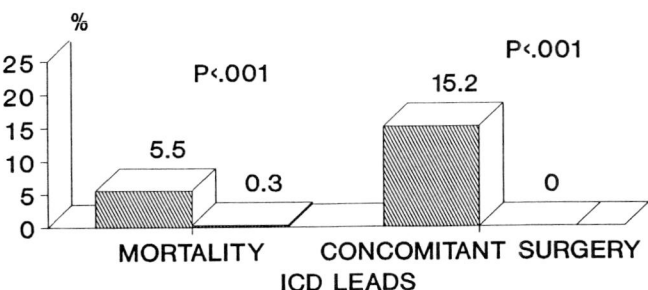

Figure 2 Perioperative 30-day mortality and the incidence of concomitant cardiac surgery in patients receiving the Medtronic model 7216A/7217 implantable defibrillator with epicardial or endocardial leads. Note the significant reduction in perioperative mortality and the absence of concomitant surgery with endocardial-lead nonthoracotomy implantation. (▨) epicardial; (▧) endocardial. Medtronic PCD study 1989–1991.

trode may occasionally be replaced by an alternate location such as the coronary sinus [24]. However, recent data suggest that axillary and pectoral electrode locations offer reduced defibrillation thresholds [17]. A simplified configuration using one catheter electrode and the pectoral electrode has been suggested. Use of a patch lead or the pulse generator casing as the anode has been evaluated. Figure 4 is a prototype generator casing used in testing this concept. This is feasible for biphasic shock devices with lower defibrillation energy requirements. Due to significant dislodgement rates reported for coronary sinus lead locations and complexity of implant, it is likely that thoracic electrodes will be preferred. While a variety of other concepts such as intrapericardial electrodes inserted percutaneously or other lead locations such as the right ventricular outflow tract have been offered to refine the system [25,26], it is more likely that innovation in existing electrodes will be tested. One such approach is the use of intercostal electrodes such as electrode catheters or an array of spring electrodes placed along the intercostal spaces [27–29]. Initially tested as single-wire intercostal electrodes by Obel and colleagues in experimental studies, subsequent variations included subcutaneous placement of a

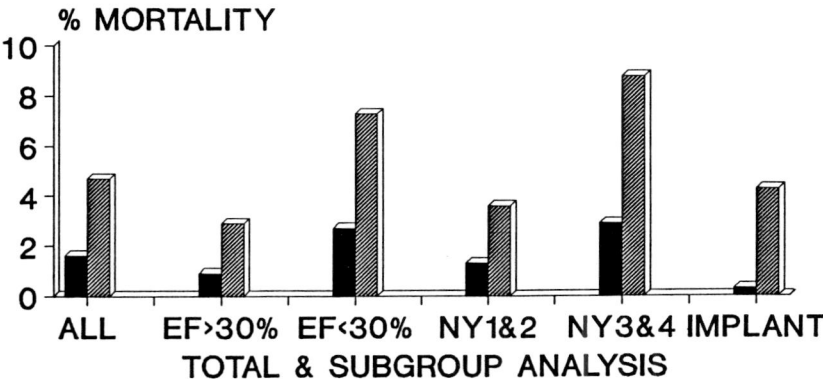

Figure 3 Stratification of perioperative mortality based on an intention-to-treat and actual implant basis and by left ventricular ejection fraction and New York Heart Association class. Note that the endocardial nonthoracotomy implant has lower risk of perioperative mortality in all subgroups. Abbreviations: EF = ejection fraction; NY = New York Heart Association class. (■) endocardial; (▨) epicardial.

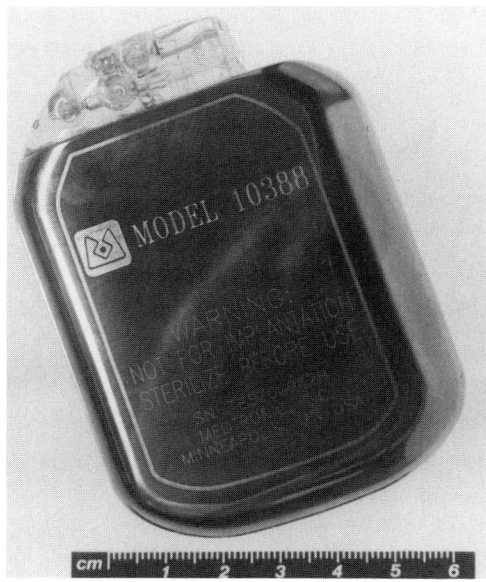

Figure 4 Shell electrode for use as a thoracic electrode in a nonthoracotomy lead configuration. This electrode can be used in conjunction with one or two endocardial leads.

single or multiple catheter leads along the left thorax and a subcutaneous array. Experimental modeling of energy fields with different lead systems has been increasingly employed to develop new leads or optimize existing systems [30].

IV. THE IMPLANT TECHNIQUE

Implantation of ICD devices by the nonthoracotomy technique is now the primary method of choice. This technique, first performed with a triple-electrode system in a human in 1986, has been refined and standardized [21]. The current technique is described in detail elsewhere and in this volume [21]. Many limitations imposed by device technology in the early reports were overcome by clinical innovation. Most frequent was the high endocardial defibrillation threshold seen with monophasic shock generators [22–24]. Mean defibrillation threshold in the early clinical series varied from 13.7 to 18 J in successful implants [22,23]. While implant success rates were reported as up to 86% in multicenter reports, the higher-end success rates were achieved by use of patch or catheter electrode relocations and exhaustive testing procedures [22,23,31]. The availability of biphasic waveforms provides lower defibrillation thresholds and near-universal nonthoracotomy implant [16,32–34].

Future developments will focus initially on refinement and simplification of the nonthoracotomy technique. Suggestions include subpectoral, prepectoral, or submammary generator implantation [35–38]. Significant down-sizing in the fourth-generation ICD pulse generator to approximately 135 g and 60 cm^3 volume will permit these approaches (Fig. 4). Further decline in size with lower-output generators may be feasible as defibrillation thresholds decline. Simplification of lead systems will be dependent on the latter development [37,38]. With high-output ICD generators, i.e., > 30 J, two-electrode systems may permit adequate safety margins. Configurations currently tested include the two catheters alone or a catheter-patch/generator [34]. Preliminary data suggest lower defibrillation thresholds with the latter using a pectoral or axillary location for the thoracic electrode [17,37,38]. As a general principle, improvement of shock vectors to provide an optimal field can be achieved by electrode location and addition. Use of an appropriately located third or fourth electrode can be anticipated to reduce cardioversion and defibrillation thresholds [17]. This would be important as low-output generators are evolved [17].

V. CLINICAL APPLICATIONS

Several new directions in clinical development of ICD therapy can be expected. These include:
1. Improving total outcome when ICD devices are used for secondary prevention of sudden death
2. Evaluation of ICD devices for the primary prevention of sudden death in high-risk populations
3. Reducing cardiovascular morbidity and mortality associated with atrial tachyarrhythmias, particularly atrial flutter-fibrillation, with devices
4. As an adjunctive therapy to antiarrhythmic drugs for patients at risk for arrhythmic relapses
5. A role as secondary therapy for patient safety during the evaluation of an alternative primary therapy

More distant new horizons will include offshoot devices for implantable cardiac monitoring and drug delivery and prevention of tachyarrhythmia recurrences or emergence. While very limited substantive analysis of these applications can be done at the present time, more definitive comment is possible for the former five scenarios.

A. Improving Total Survival of ICD Recipients

It has been widely suggested that continued nonarrhythmic mortality in ICD recipients dilutes survival benefits anticipated from sudden-death prevention. Methods for limiting this dilution have not been hitherto widely contemplated. Progressive myocardial dysfunction and other cardiovascular events such as cerebrovascular accidents are the predominant cause for this attrition. Available therapies for established myocardial dysfunction have limited impact on survival [39]. The use of vasodilators in such patients is well established. Any beneficial effects of such therapy on cardiac mortality may already be factored in current ICD trial data. The general lesson from existing heart-failure therapy trials suggests that only a modest impact can be achieved once class IV or advanced class III symptoms are established [40,41]. The use of an ICD as a bridge to cardiac transplant is an attractive option in advanced heart failure patients who are candidates for transplant therapy and are likely to receive it. Widespread ICD use in all screened transplant patients is not likely to be cost-effective or have an overall impact on patient survival. Alternatives such as best available drug therapy should be evaluated in such patients.

Prevention of heart failure development has more impact on improving survival. Preventing progressive myocardial dysfunction and other cardiovascular events has been achieved by some drug therapies. Prophylactic use of ACE inhibitors has been recommended for the former [40]. Antiplatelet therapy or anticoagulation with warfarin has reduced cerebrovascular accidents in patients with atrial fibrillation [42,43]. One electrical therapy that has affected both areas is dual-chamber atrioventricular or single-chamber atrial pacing [44–46]. Atrial fibrillation is an independent marker of mortality in patients with advanced heart failure [47]. The use of atrial pacing after development of heart failure has been shown to improve long-term outcome. It has also been shown to reduce recurrent atrial flutter-fibrillation in patients with these

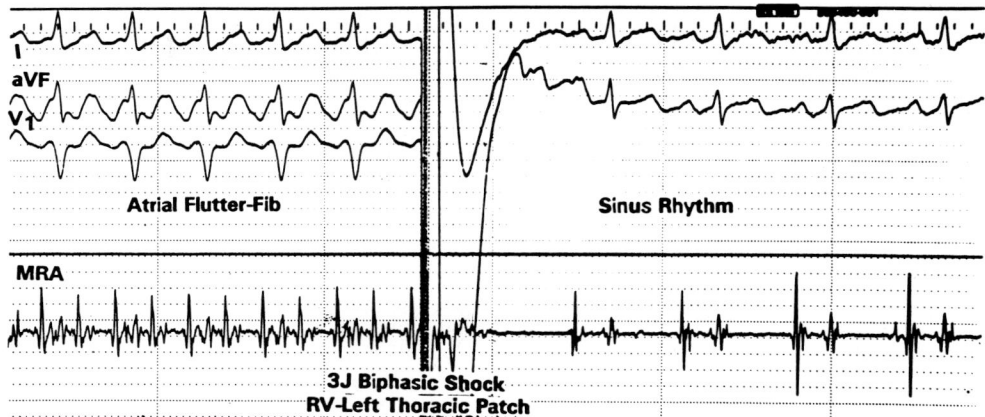

Figure 5 Endocardial defibrillation of atrial flutter/fibrillation with a 3-J biphasic unidirectional shock using a right ventricular and left thoracic electrode pair. Note that the endocardial electrogram in the mid right atrium (MRA) shows variable electrical signals differentiating it from atrial flutter.

disorders or bradyarrhythmias [44,45]. Furthermore, early reversion of atrial fibrillation to sinus rhythm has been shown to improve atrial transport function and result in progressive improvement in atrial mechanical function over several weeks [49]. Continuation of atrial fibrillation in patients with paroxysmal atrial fibrillation has had the reverse effect and promoted development of atrial dilatation and chronic atrial fibrillation with its attendant hemodynamic and thromboembolic consequences. Availability of atrial pacing and atrial defibrillation will permit testing of this potential benefit. Early clinical studies from our and other laboratories suggest that lead configurations and waveforms used for ventricular defibrillation may be useful for atrial cardioversion/defibrillation (Fig. 5). New endocardial pacing and defibrillation leads are already available to allow for these applications (Fig. 6).

Comparative benefits of ICD therapy vis-à-vis antiarrhythmic drug therapy in VT/VF patients will be an important focus of future study. One multicenter trial (Antiarrhythmics Versus Implantable Defibrillator or AVID trial) has been initiated in pilot form in 1993. Total mortality is the primary endpoint, though secondary endpoints include sudden death and quality-of-life indicators. Drugs used are empiric amiodarone or guided sotalol therapy. Another trial (the Canadian Implantable Defibrillator Study or CIDS) compares the ICD to oral amiodarone therapy. Over 200 patients have been enrolled in this study. Similar endpoints are used. These will be pivotal studies for ICD benefit in VT/VF.

B. Primary Prevention of Sudden Death in High-Risk Populations

In earlier chapters of this volume, detailed treatment of ICD clinical trials relating to this subject has been presented. Three major studies are evaluating the role of ICD intervention in high-risk coronary artery disease populations, and at least one trial is directed at dilated cardiomyopathy patients. In coronary artery disease patients, the rationale for such therapy is clearly defined, and an extensive clinical database supports it. The risk of sudden death has been linked to coronary risk factors, but interventions directed at such factors may produce only gradual long-term results, and their final impact is unknown [49]. Long-term sudden death rates remain unacceptably high in patients with prior myocardial infarction despite major ad-

Future Directions

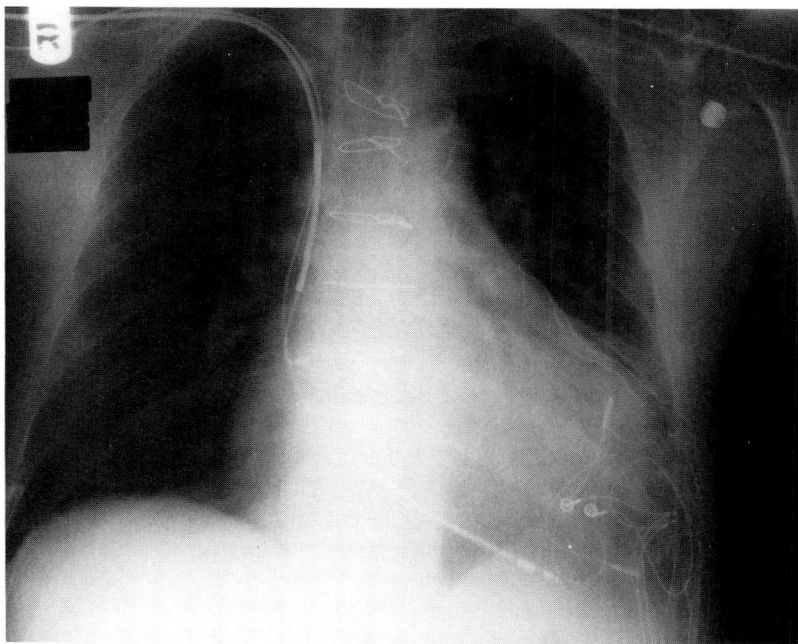

Figure 6 Endocardial lead system used for atrial defibrillation in conjunction with a left thoracic patch in the axillary region. Unidirectional and bidirectional shocks can be delivered using this configuration. Bipolar atrial sensing and pacing and bipolar ventricular sensing and pacing is feasible. In this patient, a previously implanted epicardial lead system for an ICD is also seen.

vances in treatment of acute myocardial infarction, with thrombolysis and anticoagulation improving short- and intermediate-term mortality [50]. High event rates in patients after myocardial infarction have been defined by risk factors such as ventricular dysfunction, ectopy, late potentials, loss of heart rate variability, and inducibility of sustained monomorphic VT [51–54]. A combination of noninvasive indices or combined noninvasive/invasive data have been used to predict high event rates for these studies. These indices have been extended to the postsurgical coronary bypass patient in whom high-risk subgroups have been defined [55]. Different studies test the ICD in different roles. In the CABG patch study, the ICD is compared with standard antiischemic therapy [55]. In the MADIT study, benefit vis-à-vis conventional antiarrhythmic drug therapy is analyzed [56]. There is no direct evidence for quantitative benefit of either therapy in the absence of a placebo arm. In the MUSTT trial, the ICD is used in drug-refractory patients and a placebo limb is present to assess actual benefit, if any accrues [57]. In the latter study, benefits of guided antiarrhythmic drug therapy will also be analyzable.

Critical to all of these studies is the need to document adequate arrhythmic event rates to justify intervention and, thus, validate the predictive accuracy of the risk stratification schema used. The pilot CABG patch study has done so for the coronary bypass surgery patient [55]. The other studies will evaluate the nonsustained VT population in this light. Another crucial factor will be the contribution of nonarrhythmic cardiac death to total mortality. Dilution of the benefit of sudden-death prevention may occur if this component is substantial and will limit the role of ICD therapy. Third, a definitive benefit for the ICD with respect to alternative therapy in patient survival, safety, or quality of life will need to be demonstrated.

For patients with dilated cardiomyopathy, the challenge is greater. Risk stratification is still rudimentary, with few prospective studies evaluating predictive indices [58]. Ventricular dysfunction and nonsustained VT are clearly risk factors for sudden death. The value of invasive electrophysiological testing is tenuous. The contribution of nonarrhythmic mortality can be substantial. The definition of a high-risk sudden-death subgroup appears more diffuse at the present time. The use of transplantation as long-term therapy is limited by its logistic issues. Diverse etiologies for this disorder with variable prognoses, e.g., myocarditis, right ventricular dysplasia, hypertrophic cardiomyopathy, etc., further complicate subgroup definition. It is likely that the next decade will be devoted to clinical studies extending our knowledge in many of these areas. Prophylactic new applications for ICD devices are initially most likely in coronary artery disease patients, but empirical application to other substrates may be instituted pending formal study.

C. Atrial Defibrillation

This application has been partially discussed in Section V.A. However, a stand alone application of ICDs for this purpose can be discussed briefly. While demonstration of successful atrial cardioversion and defibrillation by intracavitary shocks is not novel, more detailed experimental and clinical studies are now in progress. The rationale for this use is also now apparent. Over 500,000 individuals suffer from this rhythm disorder annually. The morbidity associated with this arrhythmia is now well documented and is a major contributor to impairing function and quality of life, and reducing survival in middle-aged and geriatric individuals [43–46]. Stroke is a major public health problem for the elderly and is linked directly to atrial fibrillation. While anticoagulation has affected this result, the risk still remains substantial. Prompt reversion of paroxysmal atrial arrhythmias can delay the onset of chronic fibrillation and preserve atrial hemodynamic function.

Recent experimental studies have followed similar paths as prior evaluations for ventricular defibrillation. A transvenous catheter or catheter patch method is under study. Popular configurations used are similar to the ventricular application. Right ventricular or atrial leads, coronary sinus or superior venacaval sites, and left thoracic patch leads are currently under study [57]. Monophasic and biphasic shocks are being tested. Biphasic shocks show advantages with respect to lower atrial defibrillation thresholds. In general, dual- and triple-electrode configurations are being studied. Early clinical studies in our laboratory suggest that defibrillation thresholds below 10 J are attainable (Fig. 7). In one preliminary clinical study, mean defibrillation threshold was 6.7 J in 8 patients with chronic atrial fibrillation [58]. Critical to the whole issue for this application is patient pain perception during shock delivery. Since the arrhythmia rarely impairs consciousness and cardioversion shocks > 2 J are often perceived as painful, patient acceptance of this therapy is an issue. The absence of imminent risk of death with atrial fibrillation is another important factor. ICD intervention has to be balanced with the alternatives of drug therapy or external cardioversion in a hospital environment in these patients. Clinical studies will be needed to assess this issue, which may be pivotal to this ICD application.

D. Adjunctive or Alternative Therapy

The use of ICD devices in conjunction with antiarrhythmic drugs is not new. Early clinical studies documented high frequency of this combination therapy. Antiarrhythmic drugs were most frequently introduced for frequent VT and VF recurrences, management of additional arrhythmias such as atrial fibrillation, or slowing of tachycardia rate to limit its hemodynamic effects. In most early reports, over 50% of patients used such combination therapy. Nonprogrammability was often a major factor in such decisions. More recently, third-generation ICDs

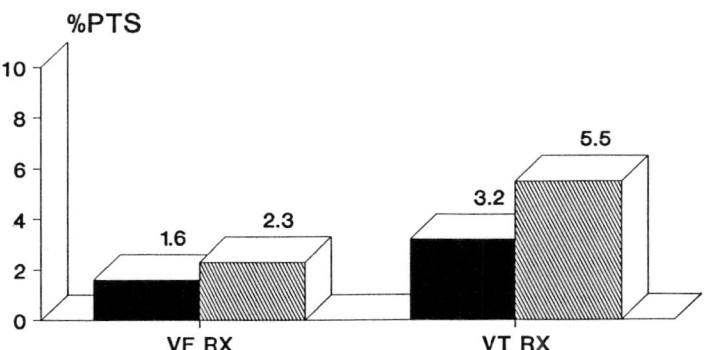

Figure 7 Incidence of antitachycardia therapies for atrial fibrillation in patients with the Medtronic 7216A/7217 ICD. The incidence of delivery of this therapy for arrhythmias characterized by the device in the ventricular fibrillation zone (VF RX) and in the ventricular tachycardia detection zone (VT RX) are shown. Note that there is a significantly higher incidence of activation of antitachycardia therapy in the VT zone. Differences in incidence may be related to variable length of follow-up. (■) endocardial; (▨) epicardial. Medtronic PCD study 1989–1991.

were widely expected to decrease antiarrhythmic drug usage. While some centers have reported a decline in concomitant antiarrhythmic drug use to 30% of patients or less, multicenter reports indicate that concomitant antiarrhythmic drugs are still used in approximately 50% of patients receiving a third-generation ICD [61]. Major reasons for continued use remain frequent tachycardia recurrences or need for tachycardia slowing to make it more amenable to pacing therapies. In contrast, the use of ICD devices as adjuncts to antiarrhythmic drug therapy is likely to face resurgence for a variety of other reasons. Recent clinical studies examining antiarrhythmic drug efficacy in this patient population have indicated high tachyarrhythmia recurrences during intermediate-term follow-up. In the ESVEM study, type I antiarrhythmic drugs associated with arrhythmia recurrence rates in excess of 50% at 3 years and one type III drug had recurrence rates of 20% in that period [62,63]. The rationale for concomitant device use in these patients at continued risk for highly symptomatic or life-threatening recurrences is established from these data. It can be expected that the hypothesis that combined therapy affords superior patient protection and quality of life will be tested in the immediate future.

The relationship between drug and device therapy is a complex one and has been reviewed in earlier chapters. Specific antiarrhythmic drugs have been shown to affect the efficacy of electrical therapies. Elevation of defibrillation thresholds is most frequently cited. Uncontrolled studies and one recent controlled clinical trial have demonstrated this phenomenon conclusively for amiodarone [64]. Individual patients may be affected by other agents such as mexiletine. Alternatively, beneficial effects on defibrillation thresholds of drugs such as sotalol have been suggested [65]. True decreases in defibrillation energy requirements have been observed in experimental studies with clofilium [66]. Clinical trials to address this question and other benefits, e.g., reduced ICD activation, are now being formulated or initiated. Further information from such trials will delineate this application.

E. Secondary Therapy with ICDs in Other Clinical Trials

As a further extension to the remarks in the previous section, ICD therapy is now being considered as a second line of therapy when patients enter clinical trials with a significant risk of sudden death. In the past, such clinical trials were precluded in patient populations with sustained VT and VF, for obvious ethical and clinical reasons. Availability of ICD devices has radically changed this perception. Clinical trials in which a significant sudden-death risk can be anticipated, e.g., clinical evaluation of a new antiarrhythmic agent with unknown proarrhythmic potential or a controlled study design with a placebo limb may now be considered [67,68] and are feasible in patients with previously implanted ICD devices. With the experience of the CAST study emphasizing the need for a placebo arm in evaluation of antiarrhythmic drugs, the possibility of such trials assumes enormous importance. Careful analysis of quantitative benefits as well as proarrhythmia potential of such drugs can be undertaken. This concept can be extended to drugs outside the antiarrhythmic arena, e.g., agents being evaluated for the treatment of heart failure. Significant increases in sudden-death risk have been reported with drugs such as milrinone and manoplax [67]. The availability of small, pectorally implanted ICD generators with endocardial lead systems and low implant risk will clearly make such efforts feasible.

VI. FUTURE TECHNOLOGICAL DEVELOPMENTS FOR ICDS

Technological innovation in these devices can be expected to continue, with a variety of different goals. It is obvious that the very nature of this technology will spawn a series of offshoot medical devices with further specific clinical applications. In the short term, technological effort will be devoted to refinement of the ICD generator and lead technology. Focus on device down-sizing will lead inevitably to a search for still lower defibrillation energy levels and newer modes of energy storage and delivery. The goal of pacemakerlike device of similar size and implantation technique will be pursued with vigor in the next few years. This is quite realizable, at least in part, even with existing technology.

Intermediate-term efforts will focus on improving tachycardia management and could take three different directions.

A. Improved Tachycardia Detection and Monitoring

Nonprogrammable ICDs encountered significant clinical problems differentiating supraventricular and ventricular tachyarrhythmias with overlapping rates or nonsustained and sustained arrhythmias. Use of programmable tachycardia detection rates, stratification of arrhythmic events by zones, and reconfirmation of tachycardia maintenance has greatly reduced the incidence of these problems. Figure 7 shows the incidence of misdiagnosis of atrial fibrillation in one large multicenter study [61]. Figure 8 shows the incidence of aborted therapies in a multicenter third-generation ICD study using a relatively abbreviated detection algorithm [68]. A significant number of spontaneous reversions and late reversions after institution of staged therapy are noted. Thus, the focus of improvements in tachycardia detection will need to address the following:

1. Eliminate the overlap detection of sinus tachycardia, atrial flutter/fibrillation, or paroxysmal supraventricular tachycardia with slow VT.
2. Establish the hemodynamic impact of the arrhythmia.
3. Refine monitoring of spontaneous events. This application can be extended to patients suspected to be at risk for such events but not documented or otherwise defined.
4. Refine algorithms for tachycardia detection toward high specificity and establish nominal values.

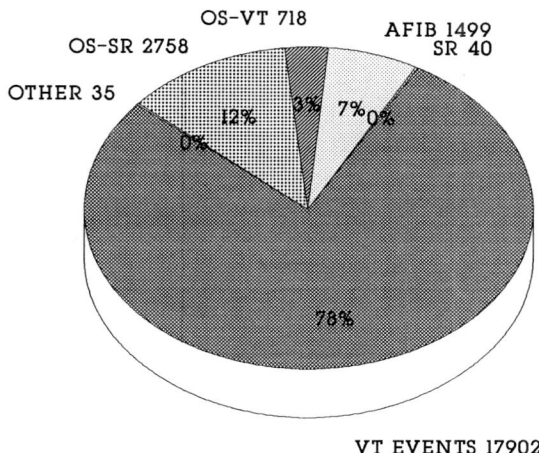

Figure 8 Incidence of different types of tachyarrhythmia events in the initial Guardian 4210 multicenter ICD study (1990–1991). Oversensing (OS) during sinus rhythm (SR) and VT as well as atrial fibrillation (AFIB) and sinus tachycardia account for up to 22% of all events.

A variety of approaches has been envisaged. Testing of dual-chamber sensing appears imminent. This permits analysis of atrial and ventricular rates and their relationship. Atrial sensing should resolve the misdiagnosis of atrial flutter and, with adequate sensitivity, atrial fibrillation. While one-to-one AV relationships are observed in some VTs, absence of this concordance will clearly delineate many VT episodes from supraventricular tachycardia or sinus tachycardia. The atrial activation sequence may have value in differentiating the latter arrhythmia. In an early report, we noted change in frequency content of antegrade and retrograde atrial activation by fast Fourier analysis [68,69]. Amikam and Furman found slew rates to be faster during antegrade activation than during retrograde activation [70]. This would explain the shift to lower frequency content observed during Fouier analysis (71). This has also been observed in our laboratory in Fourier analysis of the ventricular electrogram (Figs. 9A and 9B).

Hemodynamic impact of ventricular arrhythmias has been evaluated in several pilot studies. A variety of parameters has been suggested, but technology for the measurements on a chronic basis has been difficult to develop. An early concept was measurement of right ventricular pressure or impedance, suggested by Bouvrain and Zacuoto and tested experimentally by Mirowski and Mower [1,68]. However, lead technology to measure right ventricular pressure was slower to develop. Impedance changes to evaluate right ventricular volumes including stroke volume were easier to incorporate in such catheter systems. Recently, left ventricular hemodynamics in sinus rhythm and VT have been studied [71–75]. In an early study, we examined the hemodynamic changes associated with ventricular ectopy as well as slow and fast VT in patients with recurrent sustained VT/VF. While the details of the physiological changes seen in VT are beyond the scope of this discussion, decreases in systolic and diastolic ventricular function were apparent, as were alterations of preload [73]. Baseline ventricular function, filling pressure, and volumes influence the overall impact of these alterations. Right and left ventricular impact from these changes may not be identical (Fig. 10). Data obtained recently in our laboratory indicate a significant variability in the impairment of systolic and diastolic performance in the two chambers [75]. Thus, prediction of systemic pressure during VT or VF to select or accelerate electrical intervention remains a more distant goal. These complex interrelationships need further definition prior to implementation in implanted sensors for tachycardia detection.

Analysis of electrogram characteristics has been implemented in early and current ICD systems. Rate detection has been uniformly present. Morphology analysis in the original form used the duration of electrogram absence from an isoelectric baseline. This was referred to as the probability density function. Thus, wide electrogram tachycardias with multiphasic components and fragmentation were presumed to be ventricular in origin. More recently, in similar fashion to pacemaker telemetered electrograms, ventricular electrograms from sensing leads or

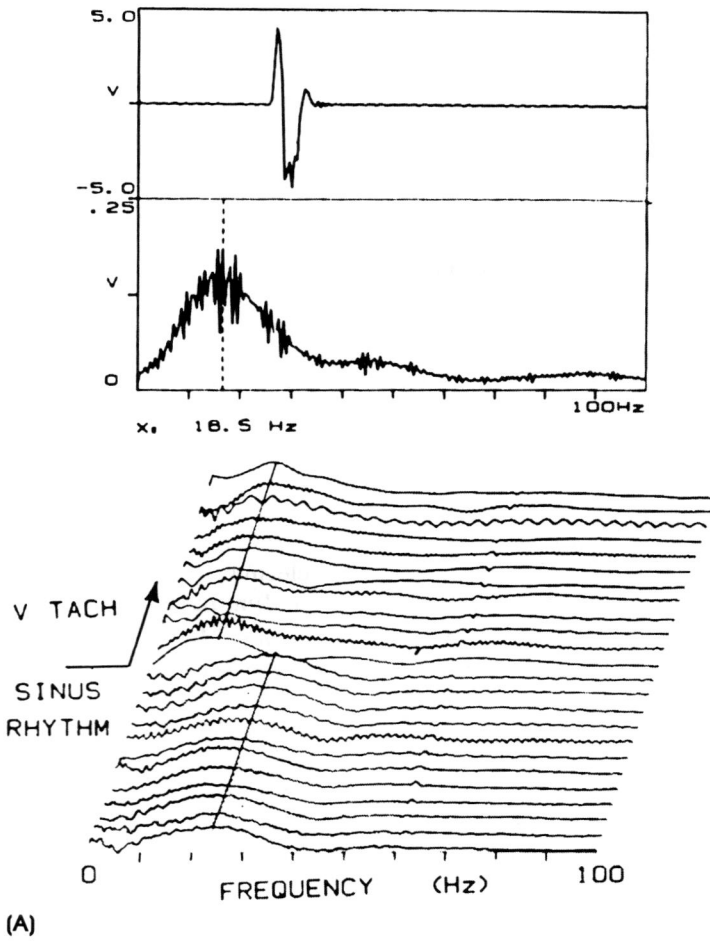

(A)

Figure 9 Spectral analysis of ventricular potentials during VT. Panel A (upper portion) shows ventricular potential recorded during VT. Lower portion of Panel A shows averaged spectrum of eight potentials as shown above. Panel B shows spectra obtained on filtered potentials in sinus rhythm from another patient (lower portion). Spectra obtained during VT begin at the arrow. Note the regularity of peaks at 22.5 Hz obtained during sinus rhythm and the shift to 13 Hz during VT. (Reproduced with permission from Saksena S, Craelius W, Hussain SM, et al. Intraoperative spectral analysis of ventricular electrograms during sinus rhythm, and ventricular tachycardia. In: Steinkopff D, ed. Cardiac Pacing. Darmstadt, Federal Republic of Germany: GmbH & C. Verlag, 1983:680.)

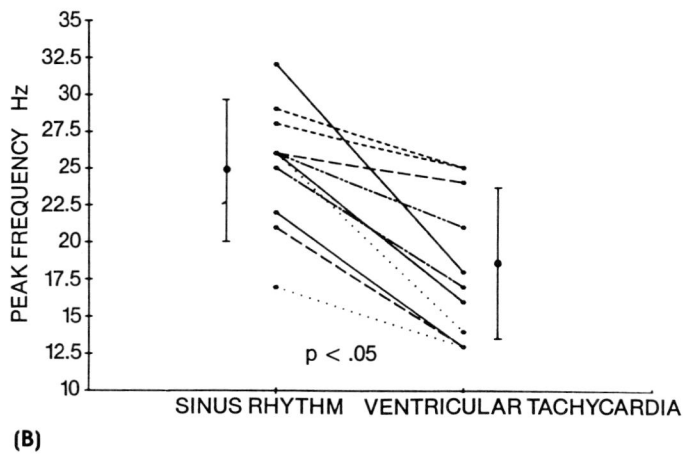

(B)

defibrillation electrodes have been stored or made available on line by telemetry [76]. Storage of these electrograms is possible from spontaneous detected tachycardia events for later analysis and classification of the tachyarrhythmia [19]. This could help in differentiating supraventricular and ventricular tachycardias based on the premise that the ventricular activation sequence is modified in the two rhythms and thus the activation wavefront inscribes a different potential. Figure 11 shows electrograms stored by a Telectronics model 4210 ICD during sinus rhythm and VT. Note the change in the electrogram configuration. This feature has also been used to correlate symptoms with supraventricular and ventricular tachycardias in ICD recipients experiencing both arrhythmias. The concomitant existence of bundle branch aberrancy or accessory pathway conduction is an important limitation.

More complex waveform analysis can be performed and is alluded to only in principle here. Template matching of the spontaneous-event electrogram with sinus rhythm or development of an index to analyze electrograms such as gradient pattern detection can be more sophisticated tools [77,78]. The former involves digitization of the analog signal and comparison with a sinus rhythm template, akin to computerized Holter analysis [77]. In contrast, gradient pattern detection evaluates timing and amplitude but analyzes a first derivative of the electrogram after analog-to-digital conversion [78]. The electrogram turning points are specific for each tachycardia morphology. This has been validated clinically. Autocorrelation analysis of sequential electrograms has also been suggested. A phase angle is calculated for the sinus and tachycardia electrogram [76]. Normally conducted supraventricular beats may have a low phase angle. This would be greater for ventricular arrhythmias. A high degree of specificity is claimed for each of these methods. The impact of aberrant conduction and pathological tachycardias is as yet unknown. These concepts may be more distant in their implementation in ICD devices.

Another technique that is being studied is the use of the coherence spectrum to differentiate fibrillatory and nonfibrillatory rhythms [77]. This method is successful in distinguishing organized and disorganized rhythms but has yet to be tested in implanted devices. Furthermore, the clinical problem is more in the overlap between regular tachycardias. We and others performed fast Fourier analysis of ventricular electrograms during sinus rhythm and VT. In our study, a shift to lower frequencies was instantaneous during VT. Pannizzo reported an 85% success in discrimination of VT on this basis [78]. Aubert accurately differentiated VT from

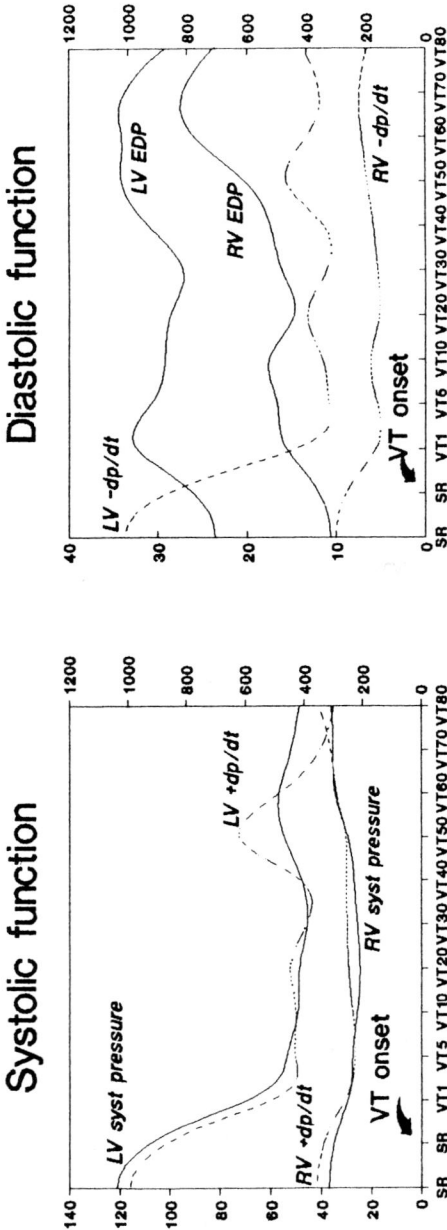

Figure 10 Behavior of right and left ventricular pressures and pressure indices at the onset of VT in patients with sustained VT. Pressure recordings are obtained with high-fidelity micromanometer recordings (after Kolettis et al. [75]). Abbreviations: dp/dt = first derivative of pressure; EDP = end diastolic pressure; SR = sinus rhythm; syst pressure = systolic pressure; + = positive; − = negative. Numbers indicate individual beats of tachycardia from onset.

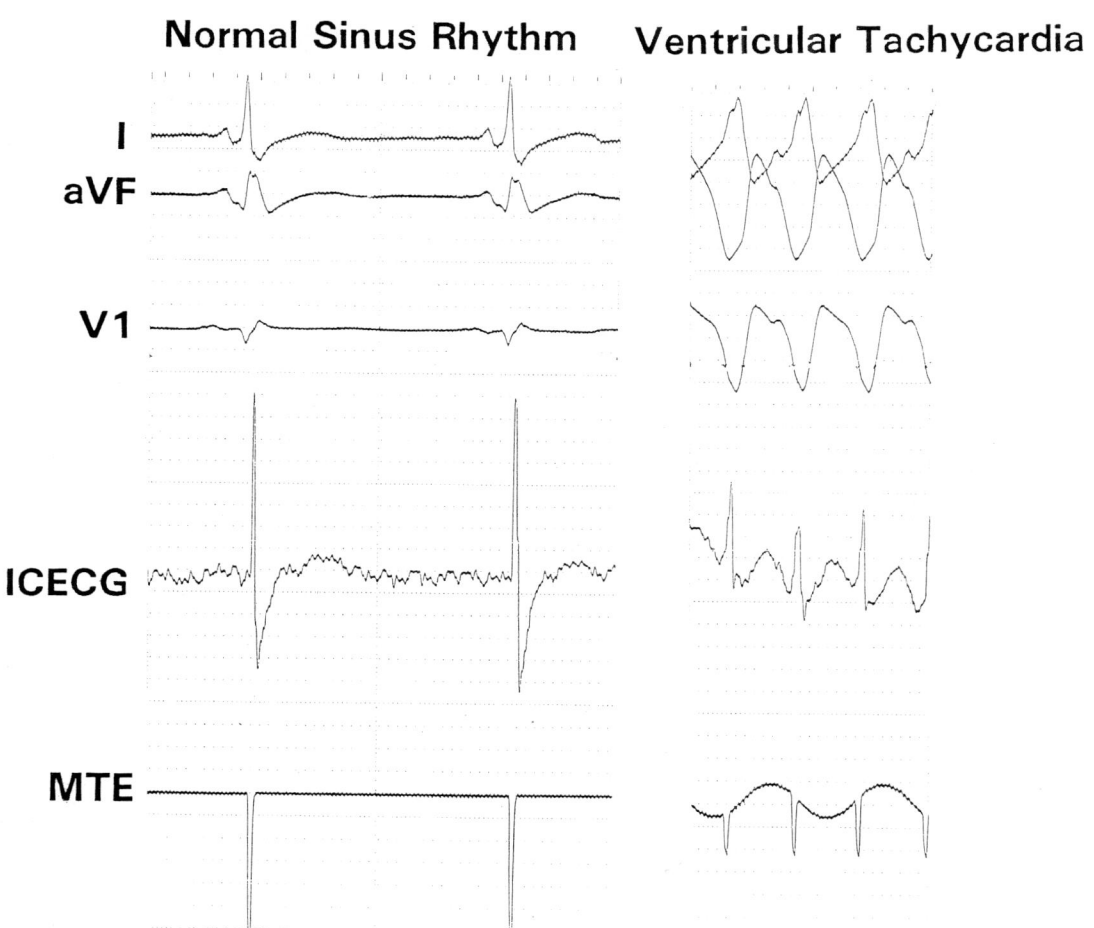

Figure 11 Intracardiac electrogram recording during sinus rhythm and VT in a patient with a Telectronics model 4210 ICD. Note the difference in intracardiac electrogram configuration during the two rhythms. Abbreviations: ICECG = intracardiac electrogram; MTE = mean timing events. Downward deflections on the MTE channel reflects individual sensed events, and the wavy line indicates satisfaction of tachycardia detection parameters.

other rhythms. Different acquisition electrodes have been used, and a standardized method is awaited. Monophasic action potentials have shown abbreviation in duration during VT and VF [79]. This method is presently unavailable for implanted systems.

Implantable devices for the purpose of cardiac event monitoring are a natural offshoot of pacemaker and defibrillator devices with these functions. In recent years the concept of a device with this sole function for diagnostic and therapeutic use along with drug or other device therapy has been considered [80]. Leitch and colleagues used a prototype device temporarily in patients undergoing pacemaker implantation. Bipolar recordings in which atrial and ventricular activity could be discussed could be obtained in all patients. Pectoral muscle contraction was an interfering factor and could be addressed by lead configuration. Further refinements clearly will follow.

B. Tachycardia Prevention

The optimal goal of ICD devices is arrhythmia prevention by electrical interventions rather than reversion after initiation. The objective has been pursued for many years using cardiac pacing systems, and a variety of concepts have been presented. Tachycardia initiation is a poorly understood concept, with many areas in need of further study. Trigger mechanisms may depend on autonomic tone, prior electrical events, and spontaneous triggers such as ectopic beats or intercurrent disturbances such as hypoxia, ischemia, heart failure, or mechanical distension or irritation. Thus, it is not surprising that single or multiple factors may be operative in any patient. Individual examples have stressed the importance of any one factor with this potential. These provide fundamental impetus for further study.

Several different approaches have been categorized by Mehra:

1. Prevention of heart rate-dependent ventricular tachyarrhythmias
2. Prevention of pause-dependent tachycardia
3. Prevention of ventricular arrhythmias by modulation of autonomic tone
4. Preexcitation of "ischemic" tissues
5. Prevention of ventricular tachyarrhythmias by stimulation in the protective zone
6. Subthreshold stimulation at critical sites for reentry

Each of these mechanisms has an extensive array of theoretical considerations and some clinical data. These are too extensive for detailed review in this overview. However, the general principles of some of these approaches can be outlined here.

Pacing interventions can alter the electrical milieu and impair the ability to sustain reentry or modify automaticity. Sudden changes in ventricular refractoriness occur with pacing trains and extrastimuli. Bradycardia or heart rate-dependent tachycardias have been well described. Rate support to prevent bradycardias or the electrical conditions necessary for tachycardia initiation has been reported to be effective in case reports. Overdrive pacing has been used to prevent emergence of these arrhythmias by modifying repolarization properties of the arrhythmogenic substrate. This is often used in drug-toxic polymorphic VT to homogenize dispersion

Figure 12 (A) Induction of sustained VT with a single ventricular extrastimulus (S_2). Monomorphic VT with a cycle length of 380 ms is induced. Simultaneous atrial and His bundle recordings as well as right heart pressures and aortic pressure are shown. Abbreviations: Ao = aortic pressure; c.l. = cycle length; HRA = high right atrium; HBE = His bundle electrogram; MRA = mid right atrium; RVP = right ventricular pressure; S_1 = basic ventricular pacing cycle; S_2 = extrastimulus. (B) Delivery of a 40-V endocardial shock in an attempt to prevent induction of VT by intracavitary shocks. This is unsuccessful, as can be seen by the induction of more rapid sustained VT, cycle length of 300 ms. Abbreviations: as in Panel A; ECVD = external cardioverter-defibrillator. Note that this tachycardia is hemodynamically more unstable. Delivery of the shock appears to have modified the tachycardia circuit and abbreviated revolution time.

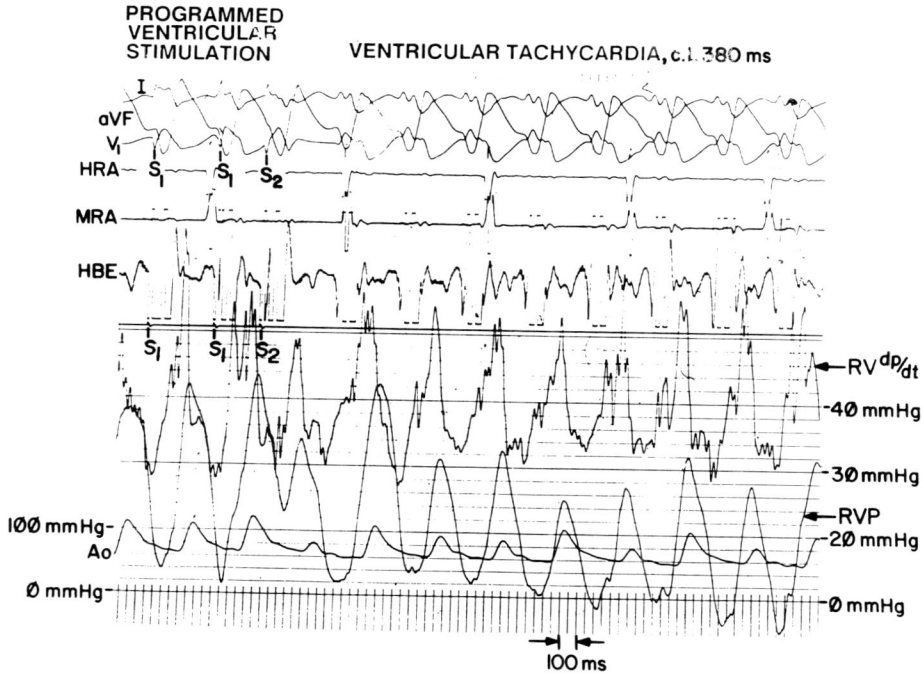

(A)

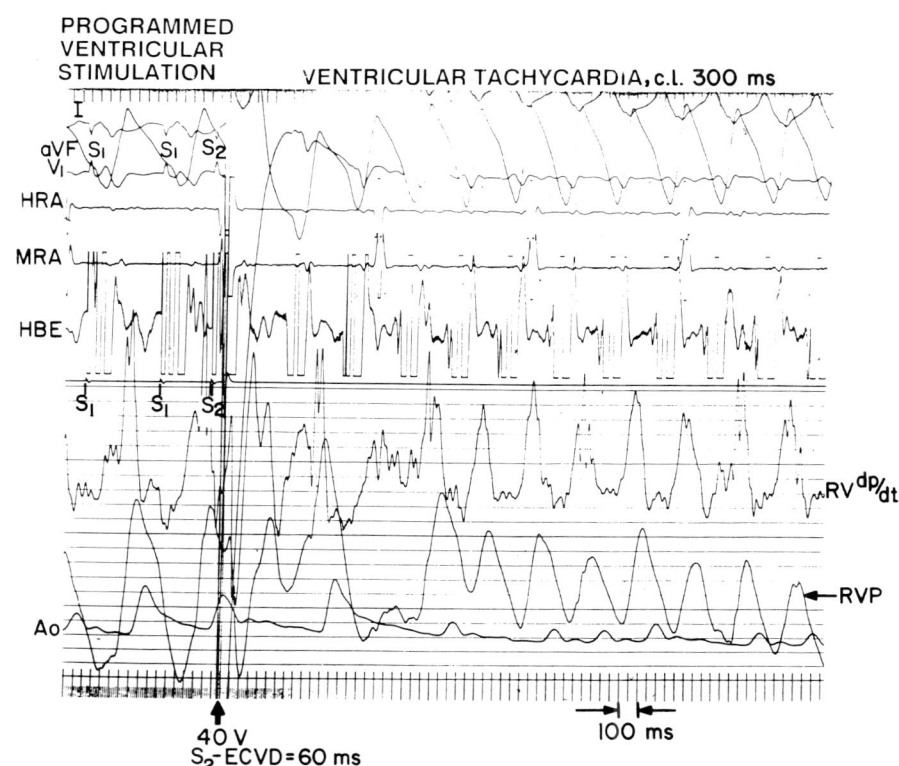

(B)

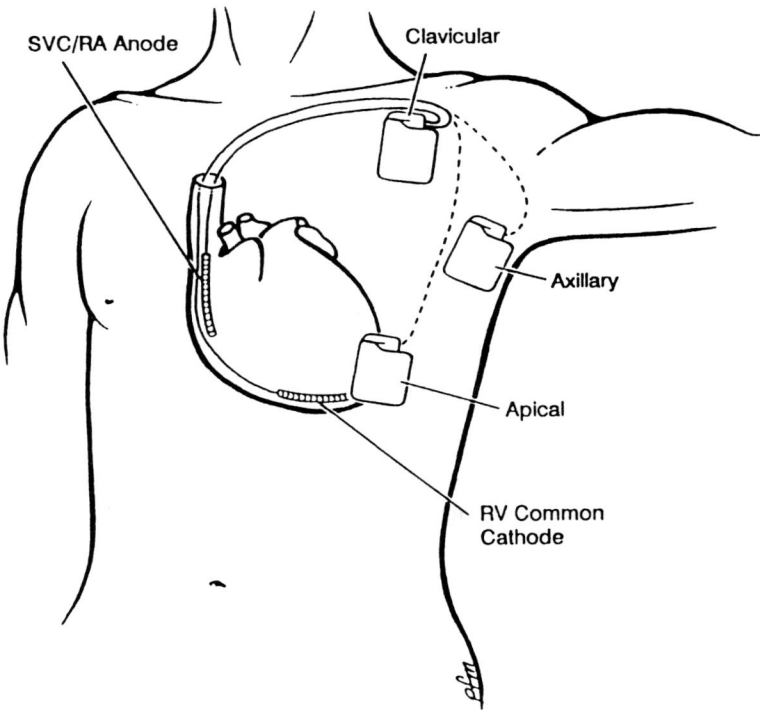

Figure 13 Potential thoracic locations of shell electrode in an implantable defibrillator system. In a prospective randomized study, axillary and clavicular locations were associated with lower defibrillation thresholds.

of refractoriness and repolarization [2]. These approaches are also valuable in the long-QT syndrome. Rapid atrial pacing and dual-chamber demand pacing are effective in supraventricular tachycardia prevention, particularly when due to AV reentry [84,85]. In contrast, dual demand pacing in the ventricle has had more modest success, probably due to the limited range of electrical modification achieved in the large ventricular substrate for VT/VF [86]. High-energy pacing has also been used for this purpose [87]. In an attempt to achieve more widespread effect, low-energy shocks have been used to prevent tachycardia induction at electrophysiological study [88]. Unfortunately, as shown in the example in Fig. 12, these have usually not been successful. Accepting the more limited effects of the electrical interventions, another approach is to apply them at critical sites for reentry. Subthreshold pacing stimuli have been effective and are painless [89]. Single and multiple critically timed stimuli or stimulation at suprathreshold values has been considered [89–91]. These modes have been effective in individual patients with recurrent sustained VT, but their general applicability remains unknown [88]. At best, these are important early steps forward toward this elusive goal.

Alternative approaches that can be used alone or in combination with ICD insertion include autonomic blockade with surgical, medical, or device techniques. These are generally in their infancy. Stellate ganglionectomy has shown promise in reducing the incidence of sudden arrhythmic death in infarcted animals and patients after acute myocardial infarction. Beta-blocking drugs have similar value [92]. Devices with neurocardiologic application are being suggested for achieving a favorable effect on sudden-death risk. Catheter ablation methods are also being used to modify the arrhythmogenic substrate for tachycardia prevention. This technique can be combined with device insertion. Preliminary studies indicate that substrate modification can have favorable effect on the frequency of ICD use in patients with frequent VT/VF. These avenues are being actively investigated at the present time.

C. ICD Therapy as an Empirical Approach to Treatment of VT/VF

It is reasonable at this time to consider that the place of ICD devices in the treatment of VT/VF may undergo significant and rapid change. Currently used as second-line therapy in most patients, it is likely that this will be modified in the immediate future. It can be projected that these devices, when implanted pectorally and transvenously, will be the first line of therapy for these patients (Fig. 13). Electrophysiological assessment and drug therapy may be adjunctive to device implant and may not necessarily precede its insertion. Significant health-care cost savings may be realized [93,94]. More important, other therapies influencing total survival of these patients will be implemented concomitantly, e.g., revascularization in patients with advanced coronary artery disease or vasodilator therapy in patients with heart failure. Integration with monitoring and drug delivery systems is feasible and, with demonstrated benefit for tachycardia prevention, can be implemented [95]. Further long-term development of ICD technology appears promising and likely.

REFERENCES

1. Sowton E, Leatham A, Carson P. The suppression of arrhythmias by artificial pacing. Lancet 1964; 2:1098.
2. Friedberg CK, Lyon LJ, Donoso E. Suppression of refractory recurrent VT by transvenous rapid pacing and antiarrhythmic drugs. Am Heart J 1970; 79:44.
3. Mirowski M, Mower MM, Staewen WS, et al. Standby automatic defibrillator—an approach to prevention of sudden death. Arch Intern Med 1970; 126:158.
4. Zipes DP, Heger JJ, Miles WM, et al. Early experience with an implantable cardioverter. N Engl J Med 1984; 311:485–490.
5. Myerburg RJ, Castellanos A. Cardiac arrest and sudden cardiac death. In: Braunwald E, ed. Heart Disease. A Textbook of Cardiovascular Medicine. 3d ed. New York: Saunders, 1987:742–777.
6. Luu M, Stevenson WG, Stevenson LW, Baron K, Walden J. Diverse mechanisms of unexpected cardiac arrest in advanced heart failure. Circulation 1989; 80:1675–1680.
7. Luceri RM, Habal SM, Castellanos A. Mechanisms of death in patients with the automatic implantable cardioverter-defibrillator. PACE 1988; 11:2015–2022.
8. Mehta D, Saksena S, Krol RB. Survival of implantable cardioverter-defibrillator recipients: role of left ventricular function and its relationship to device use. Am Heart J 1992; 124:1608–1614.
9. Bayes de Luna A, Coumel P. Leclercq JF. Ambulatory sudden cardiac death: mechanisms of production of fatal arrhythmia on the basis of data from 157 cases. Am Heart J 1989; 117:151–156.
10. Mehta D, Saksena S, Krol RB, et al. Device use patterns and clinical outcome of implantable cardioverter defibrillator patients with moderate and severe impairment of left ventricular function. PACE 1993; 16:179–185.
11. Vandepol CJ, Farshidi A, Spielman SR, Greenspan AM, Horowitz LN, Josephson ME. Incidence and clinical significance of induced ventricular tachycardia. Am J Cardiol 1980; 45:725–733.
12. Krol RB, Saksena S, Tullo NG, et al. Clinical efficacy of antitachycardia pacing in patients with ventricular tachyarrhythmias with implanted third-generation cardioverter-defibrillators (abst). J Am Coll Cardiol 1991; 17:86A.

13. Saksena S. Implantable antitachycardia devices—the next generation. In: Saksena S, Goldschlager N, eds. Electrical Therapy for Cardiac Arrhythmias. Philadelphia: Saunders, 1990:554–573.
14. Saksena S, Poczobutt-Johanos M, Castle LW, et al., for the Guardian Multicenter Investigators Group. Long-term multicenter experience with a second-generation implantable pacemaker-defibrillator in patients with malignant ventricular tacharrhythmias. J Am Coll Cardiol 1992; 19:490–499.
15. McVeigh K, Mower MM, Nisam S, Voshage L. Clinical efficacy of low energy cardioversion in automatic implantable cardioverter defibrillator patients. PACE 1991; 14:1846–1848.
16. Saksena S, Luceri R, Krol RB, et al. Endocardial pacing, cardioversion and defibrillation using a braided endocardial lead system. Am J Cardiol 1993; 71:834–841.
17. Saksena S, DeGroot P, Krol RB, Raju R, Mathew P, Mehra R. Low energy endocardial defibrillation using an axillary or pectoral thoracic anode location. Circulation, 1993.
18. Bardy GH, Johnson G, Poole JE, et al. A simplified single lead unipolar transvenous cardioverter-defibrillator (abstr). Circulation 1992; 86:I-792.
19. Mehta D, Saksena S, Krol RB, John T, Duque L. Antitachycardia pacing & programmable tachycardia detection independently contribute to reduced shock exposure in patients with programmable pacemaker-defibrillators (abstr). PACE 1992; 15(II):569.
20. Grimm W, Flores BF, Marchlinski FE. Symptoms and electrocardiographically documented rhythm preceding spontaneous shocks in patients with implantable cardioverter-defibrillators. Am J Cardiol 1993; 71:1415–1418.
21. Saksena S, Parsonnet V. Implantation of an implantable cardioverter-defibrillator without thoracotomy using a triple electrode system. JAMA 1988; 259:69–72.
22. Saksena S, Tullo NG, Krol RB, Mauro AM. Initial clinical experience with endocardial defibrillation using an implantable cardioverter-defibrillator with a triple electrode system. Arch Int Med 1989; 149:2333–2339.
23. Saksena S and The PCD Investigators and Participating Institutions. Defibrillation thresholds and perioperative mortality associated with endocardial and epicardial defibrillation lead systems. PACE 1993; 16:202–207.
24. Bardy GH, Troutman C, Poole JE, et al. Clinical experience with a tiered-therapy, multiprogrammable antiarrhythmia device. Circulation 1992; 85:1689–1698.
25. An H, Saksena S, Mehra R, Tullo N, Krol R, Smits K. Effect of right ventricular cathode configuration on endocardial cardioversion and defibrillation with dual electrode systems and monophasic shocks (abstr). PACE 1990; 13:511.
26. Kavanagh KM, Tang AS, Rollins DL, Smith WM, Ideker R. Comparison of internal defibrillation thresholds for monophasic and single capacitor biphasic waveforms. J Am Coll Cardiol 1990; 14:1343–1349.
27. Obel IWP, Poluta M, Jardine R, Smits K, Bourgeois I. Electrode system for closed chest ventricular defibrillation. In: Belhassen B, Feldman S, Copperman Y, eds. Cardiac Pacing And Electrophysiology. Tel Aviv, Israel: R & L Creative Communications, 1987:465–472.
28. Scott S, Accorti P, Callaghan F, Abels D, Boveja B. Ventricular and atrial defibrillation using new transvenous tripolar and bipolar leads with 5 French electrodes and 8 French subcutaneous catheters. PACE 1991; 14:1893–1898.
29. Jordaens L, Van Belleghein Y, Vertongen P. Defibrillation threshold testing using a subcutaneous wire array. PACE 1993; 16:895.
30. Mehra R, DeGroot PJ, Norenberg MS. Energy waveforms and lead systems for implantable defibrillators. In: Luderitz B, Saksena S, eds. Interventional Electrophysiology. Futura, Mount Kisco, NY: 1991:377–394.
31. McCowan R, Maloney J, Wilkoff B, et al. Automatic implantable cardioverter-defibrillator implantation without thoracotomy using an endocardial and submuscular patch system. J Am Coll Cardiol 1991; 17:415–421.
32. Saksena S, An H, Mehra R, et al. Prospective comparison of biphasic and monophasic shocks for implantable cardioverter-defibrillators using endocardial leads. Am J Cardiol 1992; 70:304–310.

33. Trappe HJ, Conrad-Weber O, Fieguth HG, et al. First experience with a new biphasic cardioverter-defibrillator system (abstr). J Am Coll Cardiol 1993; 21:308A.
34. Winter J, Vester EG, Kuhls S, et al. Defibrillation energy requirements with single endocardial lead. PACE 1993; 16:540–546.
35. Hammel D, Block M, Borggrefe M, Konertz W, Breithardt G, Scheld HH. Implantation of a cardioverter/defibrillator in the subpectoral region combined with a nonthoracotomy lead system. PACE 1992; 15:367–368.
36. Kolettis TM, Saxena A, Krol RB, Saksena S. Submammary implantation of a cardioverter-defibrillator using a nonthoracotomy lead system. Am Heart J 1993.
37. Bardy GH, Johnson G, Poole JE, et al. Simplicity & efficacy of a single incision pectoral implant unipolar defibrillation system (abstr). J Am Coll Cardiol 1993; 21:66A.
38. Adler SW, Remole SC, Lurie KG, et al. Prepectoral anode electrode position optimizes defibrillation efficacy for an unipolar transvenous implantable defibrillator (abstr). PACE 1993; 16:853.
39. The CONSENSUS Trial Study Group. Effects of enalapril on mortality in severe congestive heart failure. Results of the Cooperative North Scandinavian Enalapril Survival Study (CONSENSUS). N Engl J Med 1987; 316:1429.
40. Packer M, Rouleau JL, Moye LA, et al. Effect of captopril on ventricular arrhythmias and sudden death in patients with left ventricular dysfunction after myocardial infarction: SAVE trial (abstr). J Am Coll Cardiol 1993; 21:130A.
41. Rogers WJ for the SOLVD Investigators. Functional status and quality of life of 2569 patients with symptomatic CHF randomized between enalapril and placebo in the studies of left ventricular dysfunction (SOLVD) treatment trial (abstr). Circulation 1991; 84:II–311.
42. Petersen P, Boysen G, Godtfredsen J, Andersen B. Placebo controlled randomized trial of waveform and aspirin for prevention of thromboembolic complications in chronic atrial fibrillation. Lancet 1989; 1:175–179.
43. Stroke Prevention in Atrial Fibrillation Study Group Investigators. Preliminary report of the stroke prevention in atrial fibrillation study. N Engl J Med 1990; 322:863–868.
44. Rosenqvist M, Brandt J, Schulle HJ: Atrial versus ventricular pacing in sinus node disease: a treatment comparison study. Am Heart J 1986; 111:292.
45. Ebagosti A, Gueunoun M, Saadjian A, et al. Long-term follow-up of patients treated with VVI pacing and sequential pacing with special reference to VA retrograde conduction. PACE 1988; 11:1929.
46. Boccadamo R, Toscano S. Prevention and interruption of supraventricular tachycardia by antitachycardia pacing. In: Luderitz B, Saksena S, eds. Interventional Electrophysiology. Futura, Mount Kisco, NY: 1991:213–223.
47. MiddleKauf H, Stevenson WG, Stevenson LW. Prognostic significance of atrial fibrillation in advanced heart failure. Circulation 1991; 84:40–48.
48. Shapiro EP, Effron MB, Lima S, Ouyang P, Siu CO, Bush D. Transient atrial dysfunction after conversion of chronic atrial fibrillation to sinus rhythm. Am J Cardiol 1988; 62:1202–1207.
49. Cupples LA, Gagnon DR, Kannel WB. Long- and short-term risk of sudden coronary death. Circulation 1992; 85(suppl I):I-11–I-18.
50. ISIS-2 (Second International Study of Infarct Survival) Collaborative Group. Randomised trial of intravenous streptokinase, oral aspirin, both, or neither among 17,187 cases of suspected acute myocardial infarction: ISIS-2. Lancet 1988; 2:349–360.
51. Moss AJ, Davies HT, Decamilla J: Ventricular ectopic beats and their relation to sudden and non-sudden cardiac death after myocardial infarction. Circulation 1979; 60:998–1003.
52. Bigger JT, Fleiss JL, Kleiger R, et al., and the Multicenter Post-Infarction Research Group. The relationships among ventricular arrhythmias, left ventricular dysfunction and mortality in the two years after myocardial infarction. Circulation 1984; 69:250.
53. Schwartz PJ. The rationale and the role of left stellectomy for the prevention of malignant arrhythmias. Ann NY Acad Sci 1984; 427:199.

54. Iesaka Y, Nogami A, Aonuma K, et al. Prognostic significance of sustained monomorphic ventricular tachycardia induced by programmed ventricular stimulation using upto triple extrastimuli in survivors of acute myocardial infarction. Am J Cardiol 1990; 65:1057–1063.
55. Bigger JT Jr. Future studies with the implantable cardioverter-defibrillator. PACE 1991; 14:883–889.
56. MADIT Executive Committee. Multicenter Automatic Defibrillator Implantation Trial (MADIT): design and clinical protocol. PACE 1991; 14:920–927.
57. Kolettis TM, Saksena S. Prophylactic implantable cardioverter-defibrillator therapy in high risk patients with coronary artery disease. Am Heart J 1994; in press.
58. Goldschlager N. Myocardial dysfunction in patients with ventricular tachycardia: a prospective. In: Luderitz B, Saksena S, eds. Interventional Electrophysiology. Futura, Mount Kisco, NY: 1991: 471–487.
59. Alferness CA, Ilina MI, Wagner DO, Kreyenhagen PE, Griffin JC, Ayers GM. Comparison of a dual to a single lead system for transvenous atrial defibrillation (abstr). PACE 1993; 16(II):854.
60. Keane D, Salke N, Cooke R, Jackson G, Sowton E. Endocardial cardioversion of atrial flutter and fibrillation. PACE 1993; 16:928.
61. The PCD Investigator Group. Long-term clinical outcome of patients with malignant ventricular tachyarrhythmias implanted with a multiprogrammable cardioverter-defibrillator with or without thoracotomy: a prospective international multicenter study. J. Am. Coll. Cardiol, 1994 (in press).
62. Mason JW, for the ESVEM Investigators. A comparison of electrophysiologic testing with Holter monitoring to predict antiarrhythmic-drug efficacy for ventricular tachyarrhythmias. N Engl J Med 1993; 329:445–451.
63. Mason JW, for the ESVEM Investigators. A comparison of seven antiarrhythmic drugs in patients with ventricular tachyarrhythmias. N Engl J Med 1993; 329:452–458.
64. Jung W, Manz M, Pizzulli L, Pfeiffer D, Luderitz B. Effects of chronic amiodarone therapy on defibrillation threshold in man. Am J Cardiol 1993.
65. Wong M, Dorian P. D-L and D-sotalol decrease defibrillation energy requirements. PACE 1989; 12:1522–1529.
66. Dorian P, Wong M, David I, Feinedell C. Oral clofilium produces sustained lowering of defibrillation energy requirements in a canine model. Circulation 1991; 83:614–621.
67. Packer M, Carver JR, Rodeheffer R, et al. Effect of oral milrinone on mortality in severe chronic heart failure. N Engl J Med 1991; 325:1468–1473.
68. Domanski M, Saksena S. Evaluation of treatment strategies of malignant ventricular tachyarrhythmias in the era of the implantable defibrillator (editorial). Am J Cardiol 1993.
69. Craelius W, Saksena S, Pantopoulos D, Hussain SM, Parsonnet V, Gielchinsky I. Frequency analysis of cardiac potentials: a new technique for ventricular tachycardia detection (abstr). J Am Coll Cardiol 1984; 3:581.
70. Amikam S, Furman S. A comparison of anterograde and retrograde atrial depolarization in the electrogram. PACE 1983; 6:A-111.
71. Saksena S, Craelius W, Pantopoulos D, Rothbart ST. Influence of ventriculo-atrial conduction patterns on frequency spectra of retrograde atrial potentials (abstr). PACE 1984; 7:477.
72. Bouvrain Y, Zacuoto F. Lentrainment electrophysiologic du coeur. Presse Med 1961; 69:525–528.
73. Saksena S, Ciccone J, Craelius W, Pantopoulos D, Rothbart ST, Werres R. Studies on left ventricular function during sustained ventricular tachycardia. J Am Coll Cardiol 1984; 4:501–508.
74. Krol RB, Saksena S. Hemodynamic effects of tachycardias. B. Ventricular tachycardia. In Saksena S, Goldschlager N, eds. Electrical Therapy for Cardiac Arrhythmias. Philadelphia: Saunders, 1990:478–488.
75. Kolettis T, Saksena S, Mathew P, et al. Simultaneous left and right ventricular systolic and diastolic performance during induced ventricular tachycardia (abstr). PACE 1993; 16(II):933.
76. Hook BG, Marchlinski FE. Value of ventricular electrogram recordings in the diagnosis of arrhythmias precipitating electrical device shock therapy. J Am Coll Cardio 1991; 17:985–990.

77. Griffin JC, Nielsen AP, Finke WL, et al. A new method of rhythm identification: endocardial electrogram morphology. Circulation 1984; (suppl II):201.
78. Davies DW, Wainwright RJ, Tooley MA, et al. Detection of pathological tachycardia by analysis of electrogram morphology. PACE 1986; 9:200.
79. Tronstad A, Hoff PI, Ohm OJ. A new method for the detection of ventricular tachyarrhythmias. PACE 1987; 10:754.
80. Ropella KM, Sahakian AV, Baerman JM, et al. Discrimination of fibrillatory from nonfibrillatory rhythm: coherence spectra. PACE 1988; 11:485.
81. Panizzo MS, Furman S. Optimal tachycardia sensing for cardiac pacemakers. PACE 1985; 8:298.
82. Brachmann J, Stroobandt R, Aidonidis I, et al. Analysis of monophasic action potentials facilitates differentiation of ventricular tachyarrhythmias. PACE 1986; 9:308.
83. Leitch J, Klein G, Yee R, et al. Feasibility of an implantable arrhythmia monitor. PACE 1992; 15:2232–2234.
84. Akhtar M, Gilbert CJ, Al-Nouri M, Schmidt DH. Electrophysiologic mechanisms for modification and abolition of atrioventricular junction tachycardia with simultaneous and sequential atrial and ventricular pacing. Circulation 1979; 60:1443.
85. Haft JI. Treatment of arrhythmia by intracardiac electrical stimulation. Prog Cardiovasc Dis 1974; 16:539–567.
86. Mehra R, Gough WB, Zeiler R, et al. A Dual ventricular stimulation for prevention of reentrant ventricular arrhythmias (abstr). J Am Coll Cardiol 1984; 3:472.
87. Marchlinski FE, Buxton AD, Miller JM, et al. Prevention of ventricular tachycardia induction during right ventricular programmed stimulation by high current strength pacing at the site of origin. Circulation 1987; 76:332.
88. Mehra R, Santel D. Can a high voltage shock delivered immediately after premature beats prevent subsequent ventricular arrhythmias? In Belhessen B, Feldman S, Cooperman Y, eds. Cardiac Pacing and Electrophysiology. Tel Aviv, Israel: R & L Creative Communications, 1987:425–432.
89. Ruffy R, Friday KJ, Southworth WF. Termination of VT by single extrastimulation during a ventricular effective refractory period. Circulation 1983; 67:457.
90. Podczeck A, Borggrefe M, Martinez-Rubio A, et al. Termination of reentrant ventricular tachycardia by subthreshold stimulus applied to the zone of slow conduction. Eur Heart J 1988; 9:1146.
91. Waldo AL, Henthorn RW. Use of transient entrainment during ventricular tachycardia to localize a critical area in the reentry circuit for ablation. PACE 1989; 12:231.
92. Beta Blocker Heart Attack Trial Research Group. A randomized trial of propranolol in patients with acute myocardial infarction. I. Mortality results. JAMA 1982; 247:1707–1714.
93. Saksena S, Camm AJ. Implantable defibrillators for prevention of sudden death: technology at a medical and economic crossroads (editorial). Circulation 1992; 85:2316–2321.
94. Saksena S. The impact of the ICD on health care delivery systems. Am Heart J, 1994; in press.
95. Camilli L. Automatic implantable pharmacologic defibrillator. Proceedings, 9th International Congress on the New Frontiers of Arrhythmias, Marilleva, Italy, 1990.

ICD Devices Index

Antonis S. Manolis

*Tufts University School of Medicine
and New England Medical Center
Boston, Massachusetts*

ANGEMED (ANGEION CO.)
Sentinel 2001*

Functions	ATC, shock Rx, brady support
Modes	Tachy detection off/tachy detection on + tachy Rx off (monitor mode)/tachy detection on + tachy Rx on (Rx mode)/brady pacing on or off/postshock brady pacing on or off
Detection/Rx zones	3 (VT1/VT2/VF)
VT detection	2 zones
Rate	90–250 beats/min (separate for each zone)
Interval	240–(10)–670 ms
No. of cycles	6–(1)–25, 30–(5)–250 (separate for each zone)
Onset	On/off
Stability	On/off, 5–(5)–50% cycle length decrease
Prolongation	On/off, 1–(1)–30 min
VT/SVT discriminator	On/off
VT therapy	2 zones/5 therapies per zone
Rx 1,2	ATP/CV/DF
Rx 3,4, &5	Max. energy DF shock
ATP	
Burst CL	Adaptive, 90–(5%)–60%
Pulses per burst	1–(1)–100
No. of attempts	1–(1)–50
Burst pulse increments	1–(1)–50
Scanning	On/off; adaptive, 5–(5)–50% or fixed 4–(4)–250 ms
Ramping	On/off; adaptive, 5–(5)–50% or fixed 4–(4)–250 ms
Min. cycle length	200–(10)–400 ms
ATP time-out	30–(30)–1800 s

---

*Investigational devices are indicated by asterisk. Index sections were also edited by the respective manufacturers except where indicated otherwise.

Cardioversion
   No. of shocks   0,1,2
   Amplitude   50–(50)–750 V
   Waveform   Monophasic fixed width/monophasic custom tilt/biphasic

VF detection
   Rate   90–250 beats/min
   Interval   240–(10)–670 ms
   No. of cycles   6–(1)–25, 30–(5)–250

VF Therapy
   Shock voltage   100–(50)–750 V
   No. of shocks in series   6
   Shock form   Biphasic/monophasic custom tilt

Bradycardia pacing
   Mode   OFF/VVI
   Rate   30–(5)–135 ppm
   PA   6 V (fixed)
   PW   0.05–(0.05)–2 ms
   Sensitivity   Autothreshold control

Lead system
   Ports   1 pace/sense (IS-1)
           3 shock (DF-1; "PG can" may be used as a shock electrode)

NIPS
  VT induction
    No. of S1   1–(1)–20
    S1S1   100–(10)–1000 ms
    S2, S3, S4 coupling intervals   Off; 100–(10)–1000 ms
    PW   2 ms (fixed)
  VF induction
    Rate   5–(5)–50 pulses per second
    No. of pulses   10–(10)–250
    PW   2 ms (fixed)

Telemetry
  Interrogation/programming
  Real-time event markers, EGM
  Diagnostic data

Nonprogrammable functions
   Pacer PA   6 V
   NIPS PW   2 ms

Mechanical features
   Size   8 × 6 × 1.6 cm
   Weight   115 g
   Volume   60 cm^3
   Housing material   Titanium
   Battery   Lithium iodine for monitoring; lithium silver vanadium for shocks & pacing
   X-ray ID   AM37-2

Magnet functions
  ATP/shock Rx are temporarily suspended

Programmer
  AngeMed Programmer

ICD Devices Index

External device for intraoperative testing
  Angemed Defibrillation System Analyzer
Manual therapy
  Stat max. shock/stat Rx (selectable energy)
Routine follow-up
  At physician's discretion
  Capacitor reformation is automatic every 4 months
  Percent remaining battery life is telemetered
  Projected battery longevity: ? years

BIOTRONIK

Phylax 03*

Device functions	ATP, brady support, shock
VT detection	
Tachycardia detection	On/off
Interval	325–(25)–600 ms
No. of cycles	5–(1)–32
Onset criterion	On/off
Onset delta	Absolute: 100–(5)–500 ms; adaptive: 1.6%–(1.6%)–50%
VT Therapy	
Burst form	Equidistant, ramp, triangular ramp, equidistant + PES
Pulses per burst	1–32 (+PES)
Burst pulse start interval	Absolute: 100–(5)–650 ms
	Adaptive: 40.6–(1.6)–98.4%
PES interval	Adaptive: 40.6–(1.6)–98.4%
VF Detection	
VF detection	On/off
Interval	275–(25)–400 ms
No. of cycles, total (Y)	8–(4)–32
No. of fibrillation cycles (X from Y)	5–(1)–32
VF Therapy	
Shock voltage	100–(25)–700 V
Switch voltage for biphasic shock	75–(25)–650 V
No. of shocks in series	0–(1)–10
Energy (max)	30 J
Shock form	Biphasic/monophasic
Shock configuration	Polarity of shock leads (1, 2, 3) independently programmable for shock phases 1 & 2
Postshock pause	0.5, 1–(1)–10 s
Bradycardia pacing	
Mode	VVI, VOO
Rate	30 ppm, 40 ppm, 50–(5)–90 ppm, 100 ppm, 110 ppm
Hysteresis	None, 40 ppm, 50 ppm, 60 ppm
PA	2.4, 3.1, 3.6, 4.8, 6.2, 7.2, 9.6 V
PW	0.25, 0.5, 0.75, 1.0 ms
Sensitivity	0.2, 0.4, 0.6, 0.8, 1.2, 1.4 mV; automatic gain control

Lead system
  Ports   1 pace/sense (IS-1, bipolar)
                                         3 shock (DF-1, unipolar)
NIPS
  Burst   Adaptive: 40.6–(1.6)–98.4%
Mechanical features
  Size $100 \times 79 \times 21$ mm
  Weight   169 g
  Volume   121 cm^3
  Housing material   Titanium
  Battery   Lithium silver vanadiumoxide
  Capacity (nominal)   2.2 Ah
  X-ray ID   Biotronic logo PE
Magnet functions
  VOO, no ATP, no shock
Programmer
  Biotronik Programmer PMS 1000
External device for intraoperative testing
  Biotronik Defibrillation System Analyzer
Manual therapy
  Stat shock
Routine follow-up
  Every 2 months   ERI: charging time   Capacitor reformation: automatic
  Battery longevity: 100 shocks

CPI DEVICES

Ventak AICD 1550

Function   Shock therapy
Mode   Active/inactive
VT/VF detection
  Rate   125–(5)–200 bpm
  PDF   On/off
  Sensing   Fully automatic gain control
VT/VF therapy
  No. of shocks in a series   5
  First shock energy   26, 30 J (delivered)
  Second–fifth shock energy   30 J (delivered)
  First shock delay   2.5 s
Bradycardia pacing   NA
Lead system
  Ports   Sense (4.75 mm); defib (6.1 mm)
                                       Sense (4.75 mm); defib (6.1 mm)
NIPS   NA
Telemetry
  Programming and interrogation
  EP test (standby mode)
  Event markers
  STAT shock delivery
  During arrhythmia conversion
    Detection time
    Delay time

ICD Devices Index

    Charge time
    Shock delivery time & energy level
    Noise on the rate-sensing channel
    Noise detected by programmer
    Rate integrator count
  Diagnostic PG data
    No. of total patient shocks/patient
      first shocks/test shocks
    Last charge time & lead impedance
      of last shock
    PG battery status/evaluate ERI
      ERI = BOL battery charge time × 1.33
        (recorded on the PG's shipping container
        for each device)
  Reform capacitors/battery test
  Delivery of stat high-energy (30-J) rescue shock
  Divert shock

Telemetry range	Normal/extended
Nonprogrammable functions	
Second–fifth shock energy	30 J
Second–fifth shock delay	2.5 s
Refractory period	140 ms
Mechanical features	
Size	10.1 × 7.6 × 2 cm
Volume	145 cm^3
Weight	235 g
Case material	Titanium
Header material	Implantation-grade polymer
Power supply	2 lithium-silver vanadium pentoxide batteries in series
X-ray identifier	CPI 1550 AICD

Magnet functions
  Activate/deactivate/verify sensing; activation/
    deactivation time 30 s
  Divert shock
Programmer
  CPI model 2035 Handheld Programmer
  CPI model 2820 or 2825 Software Module
External device for intraoperative testing
  CPI model 2806 External Cardioverter Defibrillator (ECD)
Manual therapy delivery
  Stat high-energy (30-J) rescue shock
Routine follow-up
  Every 2 months
  Reform capacitors
  Perform battery test
  Check charge time and compare against ERI
    (on device packing label)

Ventak 1555

Function	Shock therapy
Mode	Active/inactive
VT/VF detection	
Rate	125–(5)–200 beats/min

PDF	On/off
Sensing	Fully automatic gain control
VT/VF therapy	
No. of shocks in a series	5
First–fifth shock energy	35 J
Shock delay	2.5 s
Bradycardia pacing	NA
Lead system	
Ports	Sense (4.75 mm); defib (6.1 mm)
	Sense (4.75 mm); defib (6.1 mm)
NIPS	NA

Telemetry
  EP test (standby mode)
  Event markers
  During arrhythmia conversion
    Detection time
    Delay time
    Charge time
    Shock delivery time & energy level
    Noise on the rate-sensing channel
    Noise detected by programmer
    Rate integrator count
  Diagnostic PG data
    No. of total patient shocks/patient first shocks/test shocks
    Last charge time & lead impedance of last shock
    PG battery status/evaluate ERI
      ERI = BOL battery charge time × 1.33
        (recorded on the PG's shipping container
        for each device)
  Reform capacitors
  Battery test
  Delivery of stat high-energy (35-J) rescue shock
  Divert shock

Telemetry range	Normal/extended

Nonprogrammable Functions

First–fifth shock energy	35 J
First–fifth shock delay	2.5 s
Refractory period	140 ms

Mechanical features

Size	10.1 × 7.6 × 2 cm
Volume	145 cm^3
Weight	235 g
Case material	Titanium
Header material	Implantation-grade polymer
Power supply	2 lithium-silver vanadium pentoxide batteries in series
X-ray identifier	CPI 1555 AICD

Magnet functions
  Activate/deactivate/verify sensing; magnet
    activation/deactivation time 30 s
  Divert shock
Programmer
  CPI model 2035 Handheld Programmer
  CPI model 2825 Software Module

External device for intraoperative testing
  CPI model 2806 External Cardioverter Defibrillator (ECD)
Manual therapy delivery
  Stat high-energy (35-J) rescue shock
Routine follow-up
  Every 2 months
  Reform capacitors
  Perform battery test
  Check charge time and compare against ERI
    (on the device packing label)

Ventak P 1600

Function	Shock therapy
Mode	Active/inactive
VT/VF detection	
Rate	110–(5)–200 beats/min
Rate integrator value (cardiac cycles)	8
PDF	on/off
Sensing	Fully automatic gain control
VT/VF therapy	
No. of shocks in a series	5
First-shock energy	0.1, 0.5, 1, 2, 3, 4–(2)–14–(3)–26, 30 J
Second–fifth shock energy	30 J
First shock delay	2.5, 5, 7.5, 10 s
Second–fifth shock delay	2.5 s
Bradycardia pacing	NA
Lead System	
Ports	Sense (4.75 mm); defib (6.1 mm)
	Sense (4.75 mm); defib (6.1 mm)
NIPS	NA

Telemetry
  EP test (standby mode)
  Event markers
  Programming and interrogation
  STAT shock delivery
  During arrhythmia conversion
    Detection time
    Delay time
    Charge time
    Shock delivery time & energy level
    Noise on the rate-sensing channel
    Beats above the rate criterion
  Diagnostic PG data
    No. of total patient shocks/patient first shocks/
      2–5 (rescue) shocks/test shocks
    Last charge time & lead impedance of last shock
    PG battery status/evaluate ERI
      ERI = BOL battery charge time × 1.33 (recorded on
        the PG's shipping container for each device)
  Reform capacitors/battery test
  Delivery of stat high-energy (30-J) rescue shock

Divert shock
　　Telemetry range　　　　　　　　Normal/extended
Nonprogrammable functions
　　Second–fifth shock energy　　　30 J
　　Second–fifth shock delay　　　　2.5 s
　　Refractory period　　　　　　　140 ms
Mechanical features
　　Size　　　　　　　　　　　　　$10.1 \times 7.6 \times 2$ cm
　　Volume　　　　　　　　　　　　145 cm^3
　　Weight　　　　　　　　　　　　235 g
　　Case material　　　　　　　　　Titanium
　　Header material　　　　　　　　Implantation-grade polymer
　　Power supply　　　　　　　　　2 lithium-silver vanadium pentoxide batteries in series
　　X-ray identifier　　　　　　　　CPI 1600 AICD
Magnet functions
　　Activate/deactivate/verify sensing; magnet activation/
　　　　deactivation time 30 s
　　Divert shock
Programmer
　　CPI model 2035 Handheld Programmer
　　CPI model 2830 Software Module
External device for intraoperative testing
　　CPI model 2806 External Cardioverter Defibrillator (ECD)
Manual therapy delivery
　　Stat high-energy (30-J) rescue shock
Routine follow-up
　　Every 2 months
　　Reform capacitors
　　Perform battery test
　　Check charge time and compare against ERI
　　　　(on device packaging label)

Ventak P2 1620/1625*

　　Functions　　　　　　　　　　　Brady pacing/shock Rx
　　　　　　　　　　　　　　　　　　1 (VT) or 2-zone (VT/VF) detection/therapy configuration
　　Mode　　　　　　　　　　　　　Active/inactive/Monitor only
　　VT Detection
　　　　Rate　　　　　　　　　　　110–(5)–210, 220 beats/min
　　　　　Rate integrator value　　　8
　　　　　　(cardiac cycles)
　　　　PDF　　　　　　　　　　　　NA
　　VF Detection
　　　　Rate　　　　　　　　　　　130–(5)–210, 220 beats/min, off
　　　　PDF　　　　　　　　　　　　NA
　　Sensing　　　　　　　　　　　　Fully automatic gain control
　　VT/VF therapy
　　　　VF protection　　　　　　　On/off
　　　　No. of shocks in a series　　5
　　　　First shock energy　VT zone　0.1, 0.3, 0.5, 0.8, 1, 1.5, 2, 3, 4, 5, 6–(2)–12, 15–(5)–30, 34 J
　　　　　　　　　　　　　VF zone　34 J
　　　　Second–fifth shock energy　　34 J
　　　　First shock delay　VT zone　2.5, 5, 7.5, 10 s

ICD Devices Index

VF zone	2.5 s
Second–fifth shock delay	2.5 s
Shock waveform	Biphasic/monophasic
Polarity	Initial/reverse
Committed shock	No/yes
Bradycardia pacing	Off, VVI
Rate	30–120 ppm
Hysteresis	NA
PA	2–10 V
PW	0.05–2 ms
Refractory period	250–400 ms
Sensitivity	Automatic gain control
Noise response	VOO/inhibit
Postshock pacing	Off, VVI
Delay	1.5–10s
PA	5–10 V
PW	0.05–2 ms
Pacing period	0.5–60 min
Lead system	
Ports 1625	2 sense/pace (4.75 mm, unipolar); 2 defib (6.1 mm)
1620	1 sense/pace (3.2 mm, in-line bipolar); 2 defib (3.2 mm DF-1)
NIPS	
VF induction (rapid pulses via shock leads)	Fib high, Fib low
Burst cycle length (via pace/sense leads)	50–(25)–125, 170, 240, 300, 350, 400, 500, 600 ms
Telemetry	
Programming and interrogation	
EP test (standby mode)	
Event markers	
EGM	On/off
STAT shock delivery	
During arrhythmia conversion	
Detection time	
Delay time	
Charge time	
Shock delivery time & energy level	
Noise on the rate-sensing channel	
Beats above the rate criterion	
Diagnostic PG data	
Episode counters, shocked & divert data, first attempt success rate, elapsed time, number of therapy attempts, shock energy level, detected heart rate, presence of EGMs, reconfirmation data	
Last charge time & lead impedance of last shock	
PG battery status/evaluate ERI	
ERI = BOL battery charge time × 1.33 (recorded on the PG's shipping container for each device)	
Stored EGM	2.5 min
Reform capacitors/battery test automatically	
Delivery of stat high-energy (34-J) rescue shock	
Divert shock	
Telemetry range	7.5 cm
Nonprogrammable functions	

Second–fifth shock energy	34 J
Second–fifth shock delay	2.5 sec
Refractory period	135 ms

Mechanical features
- Size: 10.7 × 7.2 × 2.4 cm (1620); 10.7 × 7.5 × 2.4 cm (1625)
- Volume: 143/144 cm^3
- Weight: 230/233 g
- Case material: Titanium
- Header material: Implantation-grade polymer
- Power supply: 2 lithium-silver vanadium pentoxide batteries in series
- X-ray identifier: CPI 1620/1625 AICD

Magnet functions
- Activate/deactivate/verify sensing; magnet activation/deactivation time 30 s
- Divert shock

Programmer
- CPI model 2035 Handheld Programmer
- CPI model 2835 Software Module

External device for intraoperative testing
- CPI model 2806 External Cardioverter Defibrillator (ECD)

Manual therapy delivery
- Stat high-energy (34-J) rescue shock

Routine follow-up
- Every 2 months
- Review battery status
- Perform pacing threshold test
- Check charge time and compare against ERI

Ventak PRX 1700/1705*

Functions	ATP/shock Rx/brady pacing
Therapy options	Off, monitor only, monitory & therapy, bradycardia pacing, postshock VVI pacing, 1-, 2-, or 3-zone tachyarrhythmia configuration
VT/VF detection	
Rate	90–(5)–200 ppm, 210 ppm, 220 ppm
	Zone 2 minimum = zone 1 rate + 10 beats/min
	Zone 3 minimum = zone 2 rate + 10 beats/min
Duration (cardiac cycles)	8–(1)–30, 30–(5)–50, 50–(10)–100, 100–(50)–250
Sustained rate duration	Off, 1–(1)–5 s, 5–(5)–45 s, 60–(10)–120 s, 2–(0.5)–5 min, 5–(1)–10 min, 15, 20, 25, 30, 45, 60 min
TPM	On/off
Onset	Off, 9–(3%)–15%, 19–(3%)–34%, 38–(3%)–50%
Stability	Off, 8, 16, 23, 31, 39, 47, 55 ms
Sensing	Fully automatic gain control
VT therapy	Burst/ramp/scan/burst + 1
ATP time-out	Off, 5–(5)–45 s, 45–(15)–120 s, 2.5 min, 3 min, 5 min
PW	0.03, 0.06, 0.1–(0.1)–2.0 ms
PA	2.5, 5, 7.5 V
No. of attempts	Off, 1–(1)–30
No. of pulses	1–(1)–30
Max. no. of pulses per attempt	1–(1)–30

ICD Devices Index

Coupling interval	SYNC, 50–(25)–300 ms, 300–(50)–650 ms, or 41%–(3%)–62%, 66%–(3%)–81%, 85%–(3%)–97%
Min. coupling interval	SYNC, 50–(25)–300 ms, 300–(50)–650 ms
Coupling interval decrement	0–(8)–16, 23–(8)–63, 70–(8)–94 ms
Burst cycle length (CL)	41–(3%)–97% or 50–(25)–300 ms, 300–(50)–650 ms
Min. burst cycle length	50–(25)–300 ms, 300–(50)–650 ms
Decrement burst CL between bursts & CL within bursts	0–(8)–16, 23–(8)–63, 70–(8)–94 ms
Shock therapy	
No. of shocks	Off, or 5 shocks
First shock energy	0.1 J, 0.25 J, 0.5 J, 0.75 J, 1–(1)–10 J, 10–(2)–20 J, 25 J, 30 J, 34 J
Second shock energy	0.1 J, 0.25 J, 0.5 J, 0.75 J, 1–(1)–10 J, 10–(2)–20 J, 25 J, 30 J, 34 J
Third–fifth shock energy	34 J
Postshock detect delay (cardiac cycles)	5–(1)–20, 20–(10)–100
Committed shock	Yes/no
Acceleration percentage	Off, 9–(3%)–15%, 19%–(3%)–34%, 38%–(3%)–50%
Manual shock energy	0.1, 0.25, 0.5, 0.75 J, 1–(1)–10, 10–(2)–20 J, 25, 30, 34 J
Lowest rate criterion	90–(5)–200, 210, 220 beats/min
Bradycardia pacing	
Mode	Off, VVI
Rate	30, 35, 40, 50–(1)–90 ppm, 95–(5)–120 ppm
PA	2.5, 5, 7.5 V
PW	0.03, 0.06, 0.1–(0.1)–2 ms
Sensitivity	0.4, 0.5, 0.7, 1.3, 2, 2.7, 4, 8 mV
Refractory period	100–(25)–300, 300–(10)–350, 375, 400, 450, 500 ms
Hysteresis rate	Off, 30, 35, 40, 45, 50–(1)–90, 95–(5)–120
Postshock VVI pacing	On/off
Postshock escape interval	1–(1)–10 s
Postshock pacing period	30, 60, 90, 100 s, 2–(0.5)–5 min
Postshock PA	2.5, 5, 7.5 V
Postshock PW	0.03, 0.06, 0.1–(0.1)–2 ms
Lead system	
Ports	
Model 1700	1 sense/pace (3.2 mm, bipolar); 2 defib (3.2 mm)
Model 1705	2 sense/pace (4.75 mm); 2 defib (6.1 mm)
NIPS	
Slaved PES	
Lowest rate criterion	90–(5)–200 beats/min, 210 beats/min, 220 beats/min
PW	0.03, 0.06, 0.1–(0.1)–2 ms
PA	2.5, 5, 7.5 V
Telemetry	
Programming	
Capacitor reformation	
Event markers	
Electrograms	
Transtelephonic monitoring	
Data	
Pulse generator status	Model number, serial number, no. of total charges, no. of charges diverted, battery status, high-voltage lead impedance from last shock delivered, last charge time

Battery status & voltage	BOL 1/6 V; BOL 2/5.75 V; BOL 3/5.5 V MOL 1/5.25 V, MOL 2/5.0 V ERI 1/4.75 V, ERI 2/4.4 V EOL 1
Therapy history	Last 128 therapy attempts are stored; information includes episode, zone, and therapy; time of occurrence; detection criteria satisfied; 4-interval average of rate; Rx successful/aborted, acceleration % exceeded. For last 15 episodes of shock Rx: 16 RR intervals prior to initial Rx and 16 RRs just before end of episode

Nonprogrammable functions
  Refractory period   140 ms
Mechanical features
  Size $10.7 \times 6.8 \times 2.4$ cm (1700); $10.7 \times 7.5 \times 2.4$ cm (1705)
  Volume   130 cm^3 (1700); 140 cm^3 (1705)
  Weight   220 g (1700); 230 g (1705)
  Case material   Titanium
  Header material   Implantation-grade polymer
  Power supply   2 lithium-silver vanadium pentoxide cells
  X-ray ID   CPI 1700/1705 AICD
Magnet functions   Enable/disable, inhibit/abort, no effect
  Activate/deactivate/suspend function/divert shock/cause tones to be emitted
Programmer
  CPI model 2850 Prescriptor system with model 2860 program disk; 6575 wand
External device for intraoperative testing
  CPI model 2806 External Cardioverter Defibrillator (ECD)
Manual therapy delivery
  Burst pacing
  Manual shock
  Stat shock   34 J
  Stat pace   65 ppm
  Therapy abort
Other programmable functions
  Tone generation
    ERT   On/off
    Charge in process   On/off
    Valid telemetry   On/off
    Rate amplifier sense   On/off
    Bradycardia pacing amplifier sense   On/off
Routine follow-up
  1 month after implant and every 2 months thereafter
  Review therapy history/battery status
  Reform the capacitors

Ventak PRX II 1710/1715*

Functions	ATP/shock Rx/brady pacing
Therapy options	Off, monitory only, monitory & therapy, bradycardia pacing, postshock VVI pacing, 1-, 2-, or 3-zone tachyarrhythmia configuration

ICD Devices Index

VT/VF detection	
Rate	90–(5)–200 ppm, 210 ppm, 220, 250 ppm
	Zone 2 minimum = zone 1 rate + 10 beats/min
	Zone 3 minimum = zone 2 rate + 10 beats/min
Duration	1–60 s
Sustained rate duration	Off, 10–(5)–45 s, 60–(10)–120 s, 2–(0.5)–5 min, 5–(1)–10 min, 15, 20, 25, 30, 45, 60 min
Onset	Off, 3–(3%)–15%, 19–(3%)–34%, 38–(3%)–50%, or 10–250 ms
Stability (inhibit if unstable)	Off, 6–120 ms
Stability (shock if unstable)	Off, 6–120 ms
Sensing	Fully automatic gain control (max sensitivity 0.2 mV)
VT therapy	2 schemes per zone (VT/VT-1)
ATP time-out (rescue timer)	Off, 10 s–60 min
PW	0.5–(0.1)–2.0 ms
PA	5, 7.5, 10 V
No. of bursts	Off, 1–(1)–30 (per scheme)
No. of pulses	1–(1)–30
Pulse count increment	0–(1)–5
Max. no. of pulses per attempt	1–(1)–30
Coupling interval	120–(25)–300 ms, 300–(50)–750 ms, or 50%–(3%)–97%
Coupling interval decrement	0–30 ms
Burst cycle length (CL)	50–(3%)–97% or 120–(25)–300 ms, 300–(50)–750 ms
Ramp decrement	0–30 ms
Scan decrement	0–30 ms
Min. interval	120–750 ms
Shock (CV/defib)therapy	
No. of shocks	Off, or 5 shocks
First shock (delivered) energy	0.1 J, 0.25 J, 0.5 J, 0.75 J, 1–(1)–10 J, 10–(2)–20 J, 25 J, 30 J, 34 J
Second shock (delivered) energy	0.1 J, 0.25 J, 0.5 J, 0.75 J, 1–(1)–10 J, 10–(2)–20 J, 25 J, 30 J, 34 J
Third-fifth shock energy	34 J
Postshock detect delay (cardiac cycles)	5–(1)–20, 20–(10)–100
Shock waveform	Biphasic/monophasic
Polarity	Initial/reverse
Committed shock	Yes/no
Manual shock energy	0.1, 0.25, 0.5, 0.75 J, 1–(1)–10, 10–(2)–20 J, 25, 30, 34 J
Lowest rate criterion	90–(5)–200, 210, 220 beats/min
Bradycardia pacing	
Mode	Off, VVI
Rate	30, 40, 50–(1)–90 ppm, 95–(5)–100 ppm, 110, 120 ppm
PA	2, 5, 7.5, 10 V
PW	0.03, 0.06, 0.1–(0.1)–2 ms
Sensitivity	0.4, 0.5, 0.7, 1.3, 2, 2.7 4, 8 mV
Refractory period	250–(25)–300, 300–(10)–350, 375, 400 ms
Hysteresis	NA
Postshock VVI pacing	On/off
Postshock pacing delay	1.5–10 s
Postshock pacing rate	30–120 ppm
Postshock pacing period	15 s–60 min
Postshock PA	5, 7.5, 10 V

Postshock PW	0.5–(0.1)–2 ms
Noise response	VOO or inhibit
Lead System	
Ports Model 1710	1 sense/pace (3.2 mm, bipolar); 2 defib (3.2 mm)
Model 1715	2 sense/pace (4.75 mm); 2 defib (6.1 mm)
NIPS	
Slaved PES	
Lowest rate criterion	90–(5)–200 beats/min, 210 beats/min, 220 beats/min
PW	0.5–(0.1)–2 ms
PA	2.5, 5, 7.5, 10 V
VF induction (rapid pulses via shock leads)	
Burst cycle length (via pace/sense leads)	50–(25)–125 ms
Telemetry	
Programming	
Capacitor reformation (manual or automatic every 60 days)	
Event markers	
Electrograms	On/off
Transtelephonic monitoring	
Data	
Pulse generator status	Model number, serial number, no. of total charges, no. of charges diverted, battery status, pacing/shocking lead impedances
Battery status & voltage	BOL/6-5.5 V
	MOL 1, MOL 2/5.25 V
	ERI/4.75
	EOL
Therapy history	Episode number, date and time; detection criteria satisfied; onset and stability measured; 4-interval average rate (pre- and post-attempt); detailed counter data; zone, Rx type; Rx success/aborted; post-Rx redetection; up to 512 annotated RR intervals stored; up to 2.5 min of stored EGMs from shocking electrodes
Nonprogrammable functions	
Refractory period	140 ms
Mechanical features	
Size	10.7 × 7.2 × 2.4 cm (1710); 10.7 × 7.5 × 2.4 cm (1715)
Volume	143/144 cm^3
Weight	230/233 g
Case material	Titanium
Header material	Implantation-grade polymer
Power supply	2 lithium-silver vanadium pentoxide cells
X-ray ID	CPI 1710/1715 AICD
Magnet functions	
Activate/deactivate/suspend function/divert shock	
Programmer	
CPI model 2950 PRM (Programmer/Recorder/Monitor) system; model 2870 software application	
External device for intraoperative testing	
CPI model 2806 External Cardioverter Defibrillator (ECD)	
Manual therapy delivery	
Burst pacing	
Stat shock	34 J

Stat pace	65 ppm
Therapy abort	
Other programmable functions	
Tone generation	
ERI	On/off
Charging	On/off
Sensing	On/off

Routine follow-up
 1 month after implant and every 2 months thereafter
 Review therapy history/battery status. Autothreshold/impedance test
 Reform the capacitors (manually or automatically every 60 days)

INTERMEDICS
RES-Q 101-01 and 101-01R*

Functions	ATP/shock Rx/brady support
VT detection	
No. of VT classes	2 (TACH-1, TACH-2) or 3 (TACH-1, TACH-2, TACH-3)
SR to TACH-1 boundary	90–(5)–220 beats/min
TACH-1 to TACH-2 boundary	105–(5)–220 beats/min
TACH-2 to TACH-3 boundary	150–(5)–220 beats/min
TACH-3 to FIB boundary	200–(5)–300 beats/min
Rate criterion	
No. of intervals	4–(1)–250
Sudden onset	
Delta	50–(5)–500 ms
Rate stability	
Delta	1–(1)–100 ms
No. of intervals	3–(1)–249
Sustained high rate	
No. of intervals	50–(10)–20,000
Automatic gain control	
Automatic gain control	On/off
Sensitivity	Automatic/manual: 0.15–15.65 mV
Max sensitivity	0.15–2 mV
T-wave window	
Start	225–(5)–400 ms
End	310–(5)–600 ms
Sensing margin	1.8, 2.1, 2.7, 3.5, 5.3
Dither	1/256–(1/256)–255/256
Jump	1/256–(1/256)–255/256
VF Detection	
TACH-3 to FIB boundary	200–(5)–300 beats/min
No. of intervals	4–(1)–30
No. of FIB intervals (x/y)	5/5–(1/1)–31/31
Sinus detection	
No. of SR intervals (x/y)	3/3–(1/1)–31/31
Tachycardia redetection	
Rate	
No. of intervals	4–(1)–250
Rate stability	
Delta	1–(1)–100 ms
No. of intervals	3–(1)–249

VT therapy (ATP)
  No. of S1   1–(1)–100
  No. of S2 & S3   0–(1)–100
  S1 delay   50–(3.125%)–97% or 148–(2.56)–653 ms
  Burst CL (S1, S2 or S3)   50–(3.125%)–97% or 148–(2.56)–653 ms
  No. of attempts   1–(1)–100
  Add S1 pulse/attempt   On/off
  Autodecremental step   3–(3.125%)–25% or 3–(2.56)–100 ms
  Min CL   50–(3.125%)–97% or 148–(2.56)–571 ms
  Scanning   On/off
    Sequence   Decrement, increment/decrement
    Step size (delay or S1, S2,   3–(3.125%)–25% or 3–(2.56)–100 ms
      & S3)
    Bursts per attempt   1–(1)–100
Shock therapy
  No. of attempts   1–(1)–10
  Waveform   Biphasic
  Amplitude   50–(10)–700 V
  Energy   0.2–38.5 J (into a 50-Ω impedance)
  Coupling interval   3–(2.56)–653 ms
Therapy control
  Therapies available   4(A, B, C, D)
    A, B, C: either pacing or
      shock Rx
    D: only shock Rx
  Rachet   On/off
  Memory   Off/retry last successful Rx/retry last successful burst/retry both
  Repeat/no repeat
Bradycardia pacing
  Mode   VVI, VOO, OOO
  Rate   30–(1)–120 ppm
  Escape interval   500–2,000 ms
  PA   2.2, 4.4, 6.6 V
  Sense refractory period   135–(5)–185 ms
  Pace refractory period   375–(5)–665 ms
  Noise reversion mode   VOO, OOO
  Runaway protection   185 ppm
  Postshock PA   2.2, 4.4, 6.6 V
  Duration of postshock PA   2–(2)–100 min
Lead system   Pace/sense (3.2 mm)
                                                    Defib (4 mm)
                                                    Defib (4 mm)

NIPS
  No. of pulses   1–(1)–100
  S1 delay   10–(10)–650 ms
  Cycle length (S1, S2, S3, S4)   20–(10)–650 ms
  PW   0.03–(0.01)–1.5 ms
  Voltage   2.2, 4.4, 6.6 V
Telemetry
  Programmed values/ERI status
  Diagnostic data
    Bradycardia diagnostics

ICD Devices Index

      No. of paced/sensed events
      No. of noise-induced events/inhibitions
   Arrhythmia therapy history
      No. of times TACH-1/2/3 and FIB were first episodes/broken by therapies A, B, C, D or self-terminated/accelerated/decelerated
      No. of shocks with details of last shock delivered
      Last tachycardia treatment/details of last successful therapy
   Battery status
   Intracardiac EGM telemetry
Nonprogrammable functions
   Shock waveform (biphasic)
Mechanical features

Size	9.83 × 8.22 × 2.03 cm (101-01)
	11.43 × 8.22 × 2.03 cm (101-01R)
Volume	140 cm^3 (101-01)
	159 cm^3 (101-01R)
Weight	220 g (101-01)
	240 g (101-01R)
Case	Titanium
Header	Biologically compatible epoxy
Screw cap	Acetal polymer
X-ray ID code	IFC

Magnet functions
   Inhibits arrhythmia detection
   Invokes battery/capture test
Programmer
   Intermedics Rx2000, model 522-06 Graphics Programmer with model 531-30 Graphics program module
External device for intraoperative testing
   Intermedics model 370-04 Arrhythmia Control Device (ACD) Test Box
Manual therapy

Amplitude	50–(10)–700 V
Energy	0.2–38.5 J (into 50-Ω load)

Routine follow-up
   Every 2 months. Reform capacitors. Perform battery/charge-time test
   ERI: Postcharge battery voltage ≤ 4.7 V
      Battery voltage < 8.15 V (± 0.5 V) 8-1/2 h following a shock
   EOS: charge time 30 s at 2nd battery/charge-time test

MEDTRONIC

PCD 7217B/D

Functions	ATP/shock Rx (2 zones—VT, VF; 4 slots per zone)/brady support
VT detection	
Enable	On/off
Interval	280–(10)–600 ms
No. of intervals	4–(4)–52
Onset criterion	On/off
RR%	56%–(3%)–62%, 66%–(3%)–87%, 91%–(3%)–97%
Onset counter	On/off

Interval stability	Off, 30–(10)–130 ms
VT therapy	0–(1)–4
Burst (VVI)	
Enable	On/off
No. of S1	1–(1)–15
S1-S1	50%–(3%)–62%, 66%–(3%)–87%, 91%–(3%)–97%
No. of sequences	1–(1)–15
Decrement per sequence	0–(10)–40 ms
Min. pulse interval	150–(10)–300 ms
Ramp (VVI)	
Enable	On/off
Initial no. of S1	1–(1)–15
First R-S interval	50%–(3%)–62%, 66%–(3%)–87%, 91–(3%)–97%
Decrement per pulse	0–(10)–40 ms
No. of sequences	1–(1)–15
Min. pulse interval	150–(10)–300 ms
Cardioversion (noncommitted)	
Enable	On/off
Current path	Single, simultaneous, or sequential
Shock form	Monophasic
PW	0.5–(0.5)–2, 2.4–(0.5)–5.9, 6.3–(0.5)–7.8 ms & 8.1 ms
Energy	0.2–(0.2)–1.8 J, 2–(1)–15 J, 16–(2)–34 J
VF detection	
Enable	On/off
Interval	240–(10)–400 ms
No. of intervals	6–(6)–30
VF therapy	0–(1)–4
Defibrillation (committed)	
Enable	On/off
Current path	Single, simultaneous, or sequential
Shock form	Monophasic
PW	2 & 2.4–(0.5)–5.9 ms, 6.3–(0.5)–7.8 ms & 8.1 ms
Energy	0.2–(0.2)–1.8 J, 2–(1)–15 J, 16–(2)–34 J
Bradycardia pacing	
Mode	VVI
Rate	30–(2)–64, 65, 66–(2)–82, 85, 86, 88, 90 ppm
Hysteresis	NA
PA	2.8 & 5.4 V
PW	0.03–(0.03)–1.59 ms
Sensitivity	0.3–(0.3)–2.4 mV (autoadjusting)
Refractory period	320–(40)–480 ms
Lead system	
Ports	Pace/sense, sense 2 (3.2 mm, bipolar or IS-1, bipolar)
	Pulse 1 (6.5 mm, unipolar)/(ISO DF-1 draft standard)
	Common (6.5 mm, unipolar)/(ISO DF-1 draft standard)
	Pulse 2 (6.5 mm, unipolar)/(ISO DF-1 draft standard)
NIPS	
S1-S1	300–(10)–2000 ms
S1-S2	150–(10)–600 ms
S2-S3	150–(10)–600 ms
S3-S4	150–(10)–600 ms
No. of S1	1–(1)–20, 20–(5)–95

ICD Devices Index

High-rate pacing	
Manual—interval	100–(10)–400 ms
Automatic interval limit	100–(10)–200 ms, 210–(20)–250 ms, 300–(50)–400 ms
Telemetry	
Permanent	Off, 1–(1)–63 h, continuous
Type	Marker Channel (coded & annotated), EGM near field, EGM far field
Stored episode data	1 episode (20 intervals before detection & 10 intervals after therapy delivery)
Data	
PCD status	
Memory retention	OK, reset
Charge circuit	OK, timeout, inactive
Last charge time	10 ms–34.95 s
Battery voltage	Measured voltage
VT onset counter	0–65,535
VT episode and therapy data	
Episode count	0–255
VT Rx success count	0–255 (reports for each 4 therapies)
No. of VTs PCD ineffective	0–255
PCD efficacious on last VT	Yes/no
Last therapy used	0–4
No. of sequences in last Rx	1–15
RR average for last pace Rx	None, 150–600 ms
VT episode and therapy data	
Episode count	0–255
VF Rx success count	0–255 (reports for each 4 therapies)
No. of VFs PCD ineffective	0–255
PCD efficacious on last VF	Yes/no
Last therapy used	0–4
Last episode sequence	20 intervals
Cycle length intervals	100–2000 ms
Last therapy sequence	10 intervals
Manual capacitor charging	0.2–(0.2)–1.8 J, 2–(1)–15 J, 16–(2)–34 J
Nonprogrammable functions	
Blanking	120 ms (after sensed event)
	320 ms (after paced event)
	300 ms (after charging period)
	300 ms (after VT/VF therapy)
Refractory	200 ms (after sense)
	400 ms (after charging period)
	520 ms (after VT/VF therapy or failure to synchronize)
VF synch period	500 ms
Escape interval after a Rx delivery	1000 ms
Max. allowable charging period	34.95 s
Time between sequential pulses	244 μs
Disabling of VT detection	64 events
Rate limit (protective feature)	120 ppm
Input impedance (min)	50 kΩ

Mechanical features
  Size
    Height   101 mm/93 mm
    Length   70 mm
    Width   20 mm
  Weight   197 g/191 g
  Volume   113cm^3/108cm^3
  External shield   Titanium
  Battrey   Lithium silver vanadium oxide (6.4-V nominal at BOL)
  X-ray ID   Medtronic logo ZB2
Programmer
  Model 9710E + appropriate MemoryMod software cartridge
External device for intraoperative testing
  Medtronic model 5355 External Tachyarrhythmia Control Device (ETCD)
Magnet function
  VT/VF detection & therapy are temporarily suspended
  Bradycardia support function is not affected
Routine follow-up
  Every 3 months after implant and every 1 month after the battery voltage drops below 5.25 V
  Check battery status. Note last charge time, condition capacitors
  Evaluate episode data/pacing threshold. Test for oversensing

PCD 7219 (Jewel) (Information for this model was not edited by Medtronic. 7219C is the "active can" model.)

Functions   ATP/shock Rx (3 zones—VT, fast VT, VF; 4 slots per zone)/brady support
VT detection
  Enable   On/off
  Interval   280–(10)–600 ms
  No. of intervals   4–(4)–52
  Onset criterion   On/off
    RR %   56%–(3%)–97%
  Onset counter   On/off
  Interval stability   Off, 30–(10)–130 ms
VT therapy & fast VT therapy   0–(1)–4
  Burst (VOO)
    Enable   On/off
    No. of S1   1–(1)–15
    S1-S1   50%–(3%)–97%
    No. of sequences   1–(1)–15
    Decrement per sequence 0–(10)–40 ms
    Min. pulse interval   150–(10)–300 ms
  Ramp (VVI)/ramp+ (VOO)
    Enable   On/off
    Initial No. of S1   1–(1)–15
    First R-S interval   50%–(3%)–97%
    Decrement per pulse   0–(10)–40 ms
    No. of sequences   1–(1)–15
    Min. pulse interval   150–(10)–300 ms
  Cardioversion (noncommitted)
    Enable   On/off

ICD Devices Index

Current path	Single, or simultaneous
Shock form	Monophasic/biphasic (65% tilt)
PW	0.5–(0.5)–2, 2.4–(0.5)–5.9, 6.3–(0.5)–7.8 ms & 8.1 ms
Energy	0.2–(0.2)–1.8 J, 2–(1)–15 J, 16–(2)–34 J
VF detection	
Enable	On/off
Interval	240–(10)–400 ms
No. of intervals	6–(6)–30
VF therapy	
Defibrillation (noncommitted for VF Rx#1)	
Enable	On/off
Current path	Single, or simultaneous
Shock form	Monophasic/biphasic (65% tilt)
PW	2 & 2.4–(0.5)–5.9 ms, 6.3–(0.5)–7.8 ms & 8.1 ms
Energy	0.2–(0.2)–1.8 J, 2–(1)–15 J, 16–(2)–34 J
Bradycardia pacing	
Mode	VVI/OVO
Rate	30–(2)–64, 65, 66–(2)–82, 85, 86, 88, 90 ppm
Hysteresis	None
PA	2.8, 5.4 & 8.4 V
PW	0.03–(0.03)–1.59 ms
Sensitivity	0.15–(0.15)–0.6 mV, 0.9–(0.3)–1.5 mV, 2.1 mV
Refractory period	320–(40)–480 ms
Lead system	
Ports	Pace/sense, sense 2 (3.2 mm, bipolar or IS-1, bipolar)
	Pulse 1 (3.2 mm, DF-1, unipolar)
	Common (3.2 mm, DF-1, unipolar)
	Pulse 2 (3.2 mm, DF-1, unipolar)
NIPS	
S1-S1	300–(10)–2000 ms
S1-S2	150–(10)–600 ms
S2-S3	150–(10)–600 ms
S3-S4	150–(10)–600 ms
No. of S1	1–(1)–20, 20–(5)–95
High-rate pacing	
Manual—interval	100–(10)–400 ms
Automatic interval limit	100–(10)–200 ms, 210–(20)–250 ms, 300–(50)–400 ms
Telemetry	
Permanent	Off, 1–(1)–63 h, continuous
Type	Marker Channel, EGM near field, EGM far field (markers & EGM: available simultaneously)
Stored episode data	5 episodes (30 intervals before detection & 20 intervals after therapy delivery)
Data	
PG status	
Memory retention	OK, reset
Charge circuit	OK, timeout, inactive
Last charge time	10 ms–34.95 s
Battery voltage	Measured voltage
VT onset counter	0–65,535
Pacing lead/defibrillation lead impedance	Measured values

VT episode and therapy data	
Episode count	0–255
VT Rx success count	0–255
No. of VTs PCD ineffective	0–255
PCD efficacious on last VT	Yes/no
Last therapy used	0–4
No. of sequences in last Rx	1–15
RR average for last pace Rx	None, 150–600 ms
VF episode and therapy data	
Episode count	0–255
VF Rx success count	0–255
No. of VFs PCD ineffective	0–255
PCD efficacious on last VF	Yes/no
Last therapy used	0–4
Last episode sequence	20 intervals
Cycle length intervals	100–2000 ms
Last therapy sequence	10 intervals
Manual capacitor charging	0.2–(0.2)–1.8 J, 2–(1)–15 J, 16–(2)–34 J
Nonprogrammable functions	
Blanking	120 ms (after sensed event)
	320 ms (after paced event)
	300 ms (after charging period)
	300 ms (after VT/VF therapy)
Refractory	200 ms (after sense)
	400 ms (after charging period)
	520 ms (after VT/VF therapy or failure to synchronize)
VF synch period	500 ms
Escape interval after Rx delivery	1000 ms
Max. allowable charging period	34.95 s
Time between sequential pulses	244 μs
Disabling of VT detection	64 events
Rate limit	120 ppm
Input impedance (min)	50 kΩ
Mechanical features	
Size	8.9 × 6.4 × 1.8 cm
Weight	136 g
Volume	83 cm^3
External shield	Titanium
Battery	Lithium silver vanadium oxide (6.4 V nominal at BOL)
X-ray ID	Medtronic logo PAE 1 (7219D); TBL2 (7219C)

Programmer
  Medtronic model 9760 + model 9861 E MemoryMod software cartridge
External device for intraoperative testing
  Medtronic model 5358 Defibrillation System Analyzer (DSA)
Magnet function
  VT/VF detection & therapy are temporarily suspended
  Bradycardia support function is not affected

ICD Devices Index

Routine follow-up
  Every 3 months after implant and every 1 month after the battery voltage drops below 5.25 V
  Check battery status. Note last charge time. Capacitor reformation is automatic.
  Evaluate episode data/pacing threshold. Test for oversensing

PCD 7201 (Information for this model was not edited by Medtronic. 7202D model with biphasic shocks has also entered the phase of clinical investigation.)

Functions	Shock Rx/brady support ("shock only" version of PCD)
VT/VF detection	
Enable	On/off
Interval	240–(10)–400 ms
No. of intervals	6–(6)–30
VT/VF therapy	
Cardioversion	0–(1)–4
Enable	On/off
Current path	Single, simultaneous, or sequential
Shock form	Monophasic
PW	2, 2.4–(0.5)–5.9, 6.3–(0.5)–7.8 ms & 8.1 ms
Energy	0.2–(0.2)–1.8 J, 2–(1)–15 J, 16–(2)–34 J
Defibrillation	0–(1)–4
Enable	On/off
Current path	Single, simultaneous, or sequential
Shock form	Monophasic (biphasic shocks available with 7202 model)
PW	2 & 2.4–(0.5)–5.9 ms, 6.3–(0.5)–7.8 ms & 8.1 ms
Energy	0.2–(0.2)–1.8 J, 2–(1)–15 J, 16–(2)–34 J
Bradycardia pacing	
Mode	VVI
Rate	30–(2)–64, 65, 66–(2)–82, 85, 86, 88, 90 ppm
Hysteresis	NA
PA	2.8 & 5.4 V
PW	0.03–(0.03)–1.59 ms
Sensitivity	0.3–(0.3)–2.4 mV (autoadjusting)
Refractory period	320–(40)–480 ms
Lead system	
Ports	Pace/sense, sense 2 (3.2 mm, bipolar or IS-1, bipolar)
	Pulse 1 (6.5 mm, unipolar)/(ISO DF-1 draft standard)
	Common (6.5 mm, unipolar)/(ISO DF-1 draft standard)
	Pulse 2 (6.5 mm, unipolar)/(ISO DF-1 draft standard)
NIPS	
S_1–S_1	300–(10)–2000 ms
S_1–S_2/S_2–S_3/S_3–S_4	150–(10)–600 ms
Number of S_1	1–(1)–20, 20–(5)–95
High-rate pacing	
Manual—interval	100–(10)–400 ms
Automatic interval limit	100–(10)–200 ms, 210–(20)–250 ms, 300–(50)–400 ms

Telemetry	
Permanent	Off, 1–(1)–63 h, continuous
Type	Marker Channel (coded & annotated), EGM near field, EGM far field
Stored episode data	1 episode (20 intervals before detection & 10 intervals after therapy delivery)
Data	
PCD status	
Memory retention	OK, reset
Charge circuit	OK, timeout, inactive
Last charge time	10 ms–34.95 s
Battery voltage	Measured voltage
VT onset counter	0–65,535
VT/VF episode and therapy data	
Episode count	0–255
VT/VF Rx success count	0–255
No. of VT/VFs PCD ineffective	0–255
PCD efficacious on last VT/VF	Yes/no
Manual capacitor charging	0.2–(0.2)–1.8 J, 2–(1)–15 J, 16–(2)–34 J
Nonprogrammable functions	
Blanking	120 ms (after sensed event); 300 ms (after charging period)
	320 ms (after paced event); 300 ms (after VT/VF therapy)
Refractory	200 ms (after sense)
	400 ms (after charging period)
	520 ms (after VT/VF therapy or failure to synchronize)
VF synch period	500 ms
Escape interval after a Rx delivery	1000 ms
Max. allowable charging period	34.95 s
Time between sequential pulses	244 µs
Disabling of VT/VF detection	64 events
Rate limit (protective feature)	120 ppm
Input impedance (min)	50 kΩ
Mechanical features	
Size	
Height	101 mm/93 mm
Length	70 mm
Width	20 mm
Weight	197 g/191 g
Volume	113 cm^3/108 cm^3
External shield	Titanium
Battery	Lithium silver vanadium oxide (6.4 V nominal at BOL)
X-ray ID	Medtronic Logo 9J1 (7201); TBP 2 (7202D)
Programmer	
Model 9710E + appropriate MemoryMod software cartridge	
External device for intraoperative testing	
Medtronic model 5355 External Tachyarrhythmia Control Device (ETCD)	

ICD Devices Index

Magnet function
    VT/VF detection & therapy are temporarily suspended
    Bradycardia support function is not affected
Routine follow-up
    Every 3 months after implant and every 1 month after the battery voltage drops below 5.25 V
    Check battery status. Note last charge time, condition capacitors
    Evaluate episode data/pacing threshold. Test for oversensing

PACESETTER

Siecure 2120*

Functions	ATP/shock Rx/brady support
Available VT levels	3 (VT low, VT high, VF)
VT detection	
Rate	100–250 beats/min (VT low)
	100–250 beats/min (VT high) (> VT low)
No. of cycles	4
Sudden cycle length decrease	On/off
Delay before Rx delivery	4–150 cycles
Rate stability	Off, 10–(5)–200 ms
Reconfirmation (intervals to be ignored)	Programmable
Refractory period	
After sensed event	120–250 ms
After paced event	250–500
Postshock	1500 ms
Automatic sensitivity control	Enabled/disabled
Max. sensitivity	0.4 mV
Min. sensitivity	5.7 mV
VT therapy	
ATP	
Form	Burst
Pulses per burst	1–31
S1 timing	Programmable
S2 timing	Programmable
Sn timing	Programmable
Sn-1 timing	Programmable
S3 coupling interval (all intervening pulses)	100–595 ms
Scanning step size	2–40 ms
Cardioversion	
No. of shocks	1–7
Energy	0.5–40 J
Shock form	Monophasic
PW	7.75 ms
VF detection	
Rate	175–300 beats/min
No. of cycles, total	4
Required rate samples	15–(1)–25, 30–(5)–50, 60–(10)–100
Reconfirmation (intervals to be ignored)	Programmable

VF therapy
  No. of shocks in series   1–5
  Energy   10–40 J
  Shock form   Monophasic
  Shock PW   7.75 ms
  Postshock pause   1.5 s
Bradycardia pacing
  Mode   VVI/VVT/VOO
  Rate   30–(5)–110 ppm
  Hysteresis   Off, 30–(5)–110 ppm
  PA   2.7, 5.4, 8.3, 11 V
  PW   0.05–(0.05)–1 ms
  Sensitivity   0.4–(0.4)–5.7 mV
  Automatic sensitivity control   On/off
  Post shock PW   1.25, 1.5 ms
  Refractory period
    After sensing   120–(10)–250 ms
    After pacing   250–(25)–500 ms
Lead system
  Ports   2 pace/sense (IS-1, bipolar), 2 shock (6 mm/HV-1 version)
NIPS
  Slaved EPS
Telemetry
  Interrogation/programming
  Real-time event markers/ICEGM
  Perform capture and sensing threshold tests
  Data
    Battery current/voltage/function
    Administrative data
    Event counter telemetry displayed as tables or histograms
      (no. of paced/sensed events, types of VT, Rx trials & results)
      (real-time clock)
    Retrieval of 32 intervals preceding and following delivery of Rx
    Storage/retrieval of 16 arrhythmic episodes
Nonprogrammable functions
  Noise sampling period   30 ms
Mechanical features
  Size   11 × 7 × 2.2 cm
  Weight   220 g
  Volume   ?
  Housing material   ?
  Battery   Lithium silver vanadium oxide
  X-ray ID   S220
Magnet functions
  No effect on brady support
Programmer
  Siemens-Pacesetter P3060 Programmer/Printer
  Telemetered data can also be fed directly to a PC database
External device for intraoperative testing
  Pacesetter Defibrillation System Analyzer
Manual therapy
  Emergency shock

Routine follow-up
  At physician's discretion
  Capacitor reformation is automatic

TELECTRONICS

Guardian 4202/4203*

Functions	VT/VF detection, shock therapy, bradycardia support, telemetry
System	On/off
VT/VF detection	
Tachycardia detection	On/off
Interval	256, 288, 320, 352, 384, 416 ms
No. of cycles	6/7, 12/14
VT/VF therapy	
No. of shocks in series	4–(1)–7
Energy	3, 4, 7, 9, 10, 13, 16, 18, 21, 25, 28, 30 J
Shock form	Monophasic
Min. shock delay	6, 20 s
Bradycardia pacing	
Mode	VVI (nonprogrammable VOO with EMI, during programming, when doing impedance measurements, or during threshold testing)
Rate	30–(5)–105 ppm
Hysteresis	0, 125, 250, 375 ms
PA	2.5, 5 V
PW	0.25–(0.25)–1 ms
Sensitivity	0.7, 1, 1.4, 1.8, 2.5, 3.3, 4.5 mV
Refractory period	250, 312 ms
Lead system	
Ports	
Model 4202	Pace/sense (VS-1), 2 shock (6 mm)
Model 4203	Pace/sense (VS-1), 2 shock (HV-1)
NIPS	
Telemetry	
Interrogation/programming	
Real-time measurements (lead/pacer cell impedance & pacing threshold measurement)	
Real-time MTEs and ICEGs	
Performs defib tests	
Data	
Patient shock count/total shock count/defib activation count	
Nonprogrammable functions	
Absolute refractory period	44 ms
EMI detection window	76 ms
Mechanical features	
Size	12 × 8 × 2 cm
Weight	270 g
Volume	176 mL
Housing material	Titanium

Battery　　　　　　　　　　　Lithium silver vanadium pentoxide (defibrillator)
　　　　　　　　　　　　　　　Lithium iodine (pacemaker)
X-ray ID　　　　　　　　　　　TAJ (4202)
　　　　　　　　　　　　　　　TPW (4203)
Magnet functions
　Temporarily disables function (both bradycardia support and defibrillation)
Programmer
　Telectronics 4802 and 4810 Programmers, 5702 Universal Printer; 9600 Network Programmer
External device for intraoperative testing
　Telectronics Implant Support Device
Manual therapy
　Max. (30-J) shock
Routine follow-up
　Every 2 months
　Measure lead/pacer cell impedance (<2000 Ω/<5–21 kΩ) & pacing threshold
　Perform defib test (twice) to reform and charge the capacitors
　EOL indicator: 3 consecutive defib tests yield charge times of 30 s
　Battery longevity: 250 defib shocks

Guardian II 4204*

Functions	VT/VF detection/shock Rx/brady support
Operating modes	
System	On/off
ATP	NA
VT/VF detection	
Tachycardia detection	
Interval	250–(10)–600 ms
No. of cycles	8/10, 12/15, 16/20
Onset detection	On/off
Onset delta	150–(50)–250 ms
VT confirm	8/10
Sensitivity	1, 1.4, 2, 2.8, 4, 5.7 mV
Noise detection	On/off
Noise detection interval	100 ms
Noise detection criterion	7/10
VT/VF therapy	
Shock Rx	Enabled/disabled
No. of shocks in series	4–7
Shock voltage	100–680 V
Shock PW	4–11.5 ms
Energy	0.5 J, 1 J, 2–(2)–20 J, 25 J, max J
Energy (max)	≥33 J
Shock form	Monophasic
Min shock delay	5–(5)–40 s
Shock therapy confirm	25%, 50% or 71% of programmed sensitivity
Bradycardia pacing	
Mode	Off/VVI
Rate	30–120 ppm
Hysteresis	0–500 ms
PA	2.5, 5, 7, 5V

ICD Devices Index

PW	0.25, 0.5, 0.75, 1 ms
Sensitivity	1, 1.4, 2, 2.8, 4, 5.7 mV
Runaway interval	365 ms (164 beats/min)
Postshock brady support (× 5 min)	Normal/high (7.5 V, 1 ms)

Lead system
    Ports   Pace/sense (VS-1, bipolar)
                                 Shock (3.2-mm HV-1)
                                 Shock (3.2-mm HV-1)

NIPS

VT/VF induction	VOO, VVT
VOO train	5–250 pulses
Pulse interval	50–340 ms
PA	5, 7.5 V
PW	1 ms

Telemetry
  Programming/interrogation
  Impedance/pacing threshold/DFT
  Real-time MTEs/ICEG
  Emergency operations (max. energy shock/turn ICD off; emergency VVI)
  Telemetry range: up to 10 cm

Data
  Data logging

Sense history logging	None/detect only/all
ICEG snapshot	None/post-detect only/post-detect & revert/all

  Event counters
    No. of VT/VF/noise
      detections
    No. of successful spont./
      shock reversions
    Total no. of shocks
    Percentage brady support
      pacing

Last shock information	Date/time/energy/patch impedance

  Episode log
    Date/time/TCL
    Type of Rx
    Sense history (up to
      32 intervals) for detect, confirm and revert, as selected
    Snapshot (1 s) for detect, confirm & revert, as selected
    Information is stored for typically the most recent 25 episodes

Nonprogrammable functions
  Absolute refractory periods
    Detection channel

After sensed events	70 ms (with noise detection enabled)
	100 ms (with noise detection disabled)
After paced events	120 ms

    Shock confirmation
      channel

After sensed/paced events	120 + 50 ms
After shock	1 s

Mechanical features
  Size $11.5 \times 8.1 \times 2$ cm
  Weight   272 g
  Volume   159 cm^3
  Housing material   Titanium
  Top cap material   Silicone elastomer
  Battery   Lithium silver vanadium pentoxide
  X-ray ID code   TQW
Magnet functions
  Suspends detection/therapy
  Brady support is not affected
  Magnet detection range: 0.5–7 cm
Programmer
  Telectronics Programmer/Printer & 5302 wand; 9600 Network Programmer
External device for intraoperative testing
  Telectronics Implant Support Device
Manual therapy
  Shocks   3 (0.5–max J)
Routine follow-up
  At physician's discretion
  Capacitor reformation is automatic every 60 days or with each max. shock charge
  BOL: > 40% estimated longevity
  ERI: ≤ 5% estimated longevity
  Special condition: "shut down" after EOL or device malfunction
  Device longevity: 6 years of monitoring only, or 500 max. energy charge cycles

Guardian ATP 4210*

Functions   ATP/shock Rx/brady support
Operating modes
  System   On/off
  ATP   Enabled/disabled
VT detection
  Interval   300–(10)–600 ms
  No. of cycles   8/10, 12/15, 16/20
  Onset detection   On/off
  Onset delta   150–(50)–250 ms
  VT confirm   5/6 ATP; 8/10 shock
  Sensitivity   1, 1.4, 2, 2.8, 4, 5.7 mV
VT therapy
  ATP   Enabled/disabled
  Min. TCL   250–(10)–550 ms
  ATP algorithm   PASAR/PASAR O
  Min. pacing interval   160–(10)–260 ms
    (PASAR-O)
  Max. initial interval   60–(5%)–90%/200–(20)–460 ms
    (PASAR-O/PASAR)
  Min. initial interval   60–(5%)–90%/200–(20)–460 ms
    (PASAR-O/PASAR)
  Max. coupled interval   60–(5%)–90%/200–(20)–460 ms
    (PASAR-O/PASAR)
  Pulses per burst   1–(1)–20

ICD Devices Index

No. of attempts	1–(1)–10
PA	5, 7.5 V
PW	0.5–(0.5)–1.5 ms
VF detection	
VF detection	
Interval	250 ms (240 beats/min) (fixed)
No. of cycles, total (Y)	10
No. of fibrillation cycles (X from Y)	8/10
Noise detection	On/off
Noise detection interval	100 ms
Noise detection criterion	7/10
VF therapy	
Shock Rx	Enabled/disabled
No. of shocks in series	4–7
Max. TCL for defib	260–(10)–600 ms
Shock voltage	100–680 V
Shock PW	4–11.5 ms
Energy	0.5 J, 1 J, 2–(2)–20 J, 25 J, max J
Energy (max)	33 J
Shock form	Monophasic
Min. shock delay	5–(5)–40 s
Shock Rx confirm	25%, 50%, or 71% of programmed sensitivity
Bradycardia pacing	
Mode	Off/VVI
Rate	30–120 ppm
Hysteresis	0–500 ms
PA	2.5, 5, 7.5 V
PW	0.25, 0.5, 0.75, 1 ms
Sensitivity	1, 1.4, 2, 2.8, 4, 5.7 mV
Runaway interval	365 ms (164 beats/min)
Post shock brady support ($\times$ 5 min)	Normal/high (7.5 V, 1 ms)
Lead system	
Ports	Pace/sense (VS-1, bipolar)
	Shock (3.2-mm HV-1)
	Shock (3.2-mm HV-1)
NIPS	
VT/VF induction	VOO, VVT
VOO train	5–250 pulses
Pulse interval	50–340 ms
PA	5, 7.5 V
PW	1 ms
Telemetry	
Programming/interrogation	
Impedance/pacing threshold/DFT	
Real time MTEs/ICEG	
Emergency operations (max. energy shock/turn ICD off; emergency VVI)	
Data	
Data logging	
Sense history logging	None/detect only/all
ICEG snapshot	None/post-detect only/post-detect & revert/all

Event counters
    No. of VT/VF/noise detections
    No. of successful spont./ATP/shock reversions
    No. of accelerations
    Total no. of shocks
    Percentage brady support pacing
    Last shock information   Date/time/energy/patch impedance
Episode log
    Date/time/TCL
    Type of Rx
    Sense history (up to 32 intervals) for detect, confirm & revert, as selected
    Snapshot (1 s) for detect, confirm & revert, as selected
    Information is stored for typically the most recent 25 episodes
Nonprogrammable functions
    Absolute refractory periods
        Detection channel
            After sensed events   70 ms (with noise detection disabled); 100 ms (noise detection enabled)
            After paced events   120 ms
        Shock confirmation channel
            After sensed/paced events   120 ms
            After shock   1 s
Mechanical features
    Size   11.5 × 8.1 × 2 cm
    Weight   272 g
    Volume   159 cm^3
    Housing material   Titanium
    Top cap material   Silicone elastomer
    Battery   Lithium silver vanadium pentoxide
    X-ray ID code   TWV
Magnet functions
    Suspends detection/therapy
    Brady support is not affected
Programmer
    Telectronics Programmer/Printer & 5302 wand
External device for intraoperative testing
    Telectronics Implant Support Device
Manual therapy
    Shocks   3 (0.5–max J)
Routine follow-up
    At physician's discretion
    Capacitor reformation is automatic every 60 days or with each max. shock charge
    BOL: >40% estimated longevity
    ERI: ≤5% estimated longevity
    Special condition: "shut down" after EOL or device malfunction
    Longevity: 6 years of monitoring only, or 500 max. energy charge cycles

Guardian ATP II 4211*

Functions	ATP/Shock Rx/Brady support
VT detection	
Rate detect interval (RDI)	180–(10)–600 ms
Rate detect criterion	8/10–(4/5)–48/60
Onset detection	Disabled/Enabled
Onset detect interval (ODI)	180–(10)–600 ms
Onset detect criterion	8/10–(4/5)–48/60
Onset delta	50–(10)–250 ms
Automatic sensitivity tracking (AST)	(0.375–3.1 mV)
Confirmation criterion	6/10 (fixed)
Reversion criterion	4 long intervals plus 5 sec timeout
Postpace AST	Normal/compensate
VT therapy	
Orthorhythmic/nonorthorhythmic $ATP_{1/2}$	
ATP-1/ATP-2	Enabled/disabled
Scanning mode	Orthorhythmic/nonorthorhythmic
No. of pulses in train	1–(1)–20
No. of attempts	1–(1)–20
Max. initial interval	60–95%/160–580 ms
Min. initial interval	60–95%/160–580 ms
Max. coupled interval	60–95%/160–580 ms
Min. coupled interval	60–95%/160–580 ms
Ramp factor	0–20%
Min. pace interval	160–300 ms
ATP PW	0.25–1.5 ms
ATP PA	2.5–7.5 V
Max. ATP time	5–180 s
Min. TCL for ATP	180–(10)–600 ms
Min. TCL for ATP 1	180–(10)–600 ms
Max. TCL for ATP 2	180–(10)–600 ms
Cardioversion	
CV therapy	Disabled/enabled
CV shocks in series	1, 2, 3
CV phase 1 width	Biphasic: 0.5–(0.5)–7.5 ms
	Monophasic: 4–(0.5)–11.5 ms
CV phase 2 width	0–(0.5)–7.5 ms
CV voltage	50–(10)–100 V, 125 V, 150–(50)–650 V, 680 V
VF detection	
High-rate detect interval (HRDI)	160–(10)–600 ms
High-rate detect criterion	8/10 (fixed)
Noise detection	Disabled/enabled (7/10 intervals <120 ms)
VF therapy	
Defibrillation therapy	Enabled/disabled
Shocks in a series	4–9
Defib phase 1 width	Biphasic: 0.5–(0.5)–7.5 ms
	Monophasic: 4–(0.5)–11.5 ms

Defib phase 2 width	0–(0.5 ms)–7.5 ms (independently programmable for shocks 1–3)
Defib voltage	50–(10)–100 V, 125 V, 150–(50)–650 V, 680 V
Max. TCL for shock 1	180–(10)–600 ms
Max. TCL for shock 2+	180–(10)–600 ms
Min. shock delay	0–(1)–40 sec
Shock commitment	Commit, standby, confirm
Bradycardia pacing	
Brady support	Enabled/disabled
Rate	30,38,43,50,55,60,63,67,71,75,80,86,92,100,109,120 ppm
Hysteresis	0–(125)–500 ms
PA	2.5–(2.5)–7.5 V
PW	0.25–(0.25)–1.5 ms
Postshock brady delay	0–(1)–10 s
Postshock brady energy	High/normal
Lead system	
Ports	1 pace/sense (VS-1B, bipolar); 2 shock (HV-1)
NIPS	
Induction method	VOO, VVT, External
Induction PA	2.5–(2.5)–7.5 V
Induction PW	0.25–(0.25)–1.5 ms
VOO drive train interval	50–(10)–600 ms
VOO drive train length	1, 2, 4, 6, 8, 10–(5)–240 pulses
VOO extrastimulus (1st–4th)	Disabled, 50–(10)–600 ms
Telemetry	
Interrogation/programming	
Impedance/pacing threshold/DFT	
Real time MTEs/ICEG	
Emergency operations (max energy shock/turn ICD off; emergency VVI)	
Data	
Sense history ATP confirm	On/off
Sense history detect	On/off
Sense history revert	On/off
Sense history shock confirm	On/off
ICEG snapshot all therapy used	On/off
ICEG snapshot ATP to shock	On/off
ICEG snapshot detect	On/off
Episode Log	
Date/time/TCL	
Type of therapy	
Sense history (up to 64 intervals) for detect, confirm & revert, as selected	
Snapshot (1 or 2 sec) for detect, confirm & revert, as selected	
Information is stored for typically the most recent 25 episodes	
Nonprogrammable functions	
Automatic sensitivity tracking	0.375–3.1 mV
Absolute refractory period	100 ms (after sense)
	160 ms (after pace)
Mechanical features	
Size	11.7 × 8.3 × 2.0 cm

ICD Devices Index

Weight	270 g
Volume	184 mL
Case material	Titanium
Header	Silastic
X-Ray ID	TIZ

Magnet function
   Tachyarrhythmia detection and therapy suspended
   Bradycardia therapy is not affected
Programmer
   Telectronics, 9600 Network Programmer
External device for intraoperative testing
   Telectronics 4510 Implant Support Device
Manual therapy
   Stat max. shock/system off/emergency VVI
Routine follow-up
   At the physician's discretion
   Capacitor reformation is automatic every 2 months or with any max.
      shock charge
   Remaining cell capacity is displayed as percent life remaining (0–40%)
   ERT at 5%. EOL at 0%. Additional indicator of ERT: 30-s max. charge time
   Longevity: 5 years of monitoring only, or 500 max. energy charge cycles

Guardian ATP III 4215*

Functions	ATP/shock Rx/brady support
VT detection	
Rate detect interval (RDI)	180–(10)–600 ms
Rate detect criterion	8/10–(4/5)–48/60
Onset detection	Disabled/enabled
Onset detect interval (ODI)	180–(10)–600 ms
Onset detect criterion	8/10–(4/5)–48/60
Onset delta	50–(10)–250 ms
Automatic sensitivity tracking (AST)	(0.375–3.1 mV)
Confirmation criterion	6/10 (fixed)
Reversion criterion	6/10 (fixed)
Postpace AST	Normal/compensate
VT Therapy	
Orthorhythmic/nonorthorhythmic ATP$_{1/2}$	
ATP-1/ATP-2	Enabled/disabled
Scanning mode	Orthorhythmic/nonorthorhythmic
No. of pulses in train	1–(1)–20
No. of attempts	1–(1)–20
Max. initial interval	60–(5%)–95%/160–(10)–580 ms
Min. initial interval	60–(5%)–95%/160–(10)–580 ms
Max. coupled interval	60–(5%)–95%/160–(10)–580 ms
Min. coupled interval	60–(5%)–95%/160–(10)–580 ms
Ramp factor	0–20%
Min. pace interval	160–(10)–300 ms
ATP PW	0.25–(0.25)–1.5 ms
ATP PA	2.5–(2.5)–7.5 V
Max. ATP time	5–(5)–180 s

Min. TCL for ATP	180–(10)–600 ms
Min. TCL for ATP 1	180–(10)–600 ms
Max. TCL for ATP 2	180–(10)–600 ms
Cardioversion	
CV therapy	Disabled/enabled
CV shocks in series	1, 2, 3
CV phase 1 width	Biphasic/monophasic: 2–(0.5)–11.5 ms
CV phase 2 width	0–(0.5)–6 ms
CV 1–3 voltage	50–(10)–100 V, 125 V, 150–(50)–700 V
VF detection	
High-rate detect interval (HRDI)	180–(10)–600 ms
High-rate detect criterion	8/10 (fixed)
Noise detection	Disabled/enabled
VF therapy	
Defibrillation therapy	Enabled/disabled
Shocks in a series	4–7
Defib. phase 1 width	Biphasic/monophasic: 2–(0.5)–11.5 ms
Defib. phase 2 width	0–(0.5 ms)–6 ms (independently programmable for shocks 1–3)
Defib. 1–3 voltage	50–(10)–100 V, 125 V, 150–(50)–700 V
Defib 4+ voltage	700 V
Min. shock delay	0–(1)–40 s
Shock commitment	Commit, standby, confirm
Bradycardia pacing	
Brady support	Enabled/disabled
Rate	30,38,43,50,55,60,63,67,71,75,80,86,92,100,109,120 ppm
Hysteresis	0–(125)–500 ms
PA	2.5–(2.5)–7.5 V
PW	0.25–(0.25)–1.5 ms
Postshock brady	Enabled/disabled
Postshock brady delay	0–(1)–10 s
Postshock brady duration	0.25–(0.25)–1 min, 2–(1)–30 min
Postshock brady energy	High/normal
Lead system	
Ports	2 pace/sense (VS-1B, bipolar or unipolar), 3 shock (HV-1, 3.2 mm)
NIPS	
Induction method	VOO, VVT, external
Induction PA	2.5–(2.5)–7.5 V
Induction PW	0.25–(0.25)–1.5 ms
VOO drive train interval	50–(10)–600 ms
VOO drive train length	1, 2, 4, 6, 8, 10–(5)–240 pulses
VOO extrastimulus	Disabled, 50–(10)–600 ms
Telemetry	
Interrogation/programming	
Measurements	
Pacing lead impedance	
Pacing threshold	
Defibrillation threshold	
Real-time event markers/ICEGs	
Arrhythmia induction	
Manual delivery of Rx	

ICD Devices Index

Data logging
  Sense history
    ATP confirm   On/off
    Detect   On/off
    Revert   On/off
    Confirm   On/off
  ICEG snapshot
    All therapy used   On/off
    ATP to shock   On/off
    Detect   On/off
    Revert   On/off
  Prior to shock episodes   On/off
Episode Log
  Date/time/TCL
  Type of therapy
  Sense history (up to 64 intervals) for detect, confirm & revert, as selected
  Snapshot (1 or 2 sec) for detect, confirm & revert, as selected
  Information is stored for typically the most recent 25 episodes
Nonprogrammable functions
  Automatic sensitivity tracking   0.375–3.1 mV
  Absolute refractory period   100 ms (after sense)
                                   160 ms (after pace)
Mechanical Features
  Dimensions   9.2 × 6.4 × 1.9 cm
  Weight   175 g
  Volume   102 mL
  Case material   Titanium
  Header   Silastic
  X-Ray ID   tWW
  Cell type   WG8830-lithium silver vanadium oxide
Magnet function
  Tachyarrhythmia detection and therapy suspended
  Bradycardia therapy is not affected
Programmer
  Telectronics 9600 Network Programmer
External device for intraoperative testing
  Telectronics 4510 Implant Support Device
Manual therapy
  Stat max. shock/system off/emergency VVI
Routine follow-up
  At the physician's discretion
  Capacitor reformation is automatic every 100 days or with any max. shock charge
  Remaining cell capacity is displayed as percent life remaining (0–40%)
  ERT at 5%. EOL at 0%. Additional indicator of ERT: 30-s max. charge time
  Longevity: ≥4 years of monitoring only, or 200 max. energy charge cycles

Guardian ATP IV 4310*

Functions   ATP/shock Rx/brady support
VT detection
  Rate detect interval (RDI)   180–(10)–600 ms
  Rate detect criterion   8/10–(4/5)–48/60

High-rate detect interval	180–(10)–600 ms
Onset detection	Disabled/enabled
Onset detect interval (ODI)	180–(10)–600 ms
Onset detect criterion	8/10–(4/5)–48/60
Onset delta	50–(10)–250 ms
Automatic sensitivity tracking (AST)	(0.375–3.1 mV)
Confirmation criterion	6/10 (fixed)
Reversion criterion	6/10 (fixed)
Postpace AST	Normal/compensate
VT therapy	
Orthorhythmic/nonorthorhythmic ATP$_{1/2}$	
ATP-1/ATP-2	Enabled/disabled
Scanning mode	Orthorhythmic/nonorthorhythmic
No. of pulses in train	1–(1)–20
No. of attempts	1–(1)–20
Max. initial interval	60–(5%)–95%/160–(10)–580 ms
Min. initial interval	60–(5%)–95%/160–(10)–580 ms
Max. coupled interval	60–(5%)–95%/160–(10)–580 ms
Min. coupled interval	60–(5%)–95%/160–(10)–580 ms
Ramp factor	0–20%
Min. pace interval	160–(10)–300 ms
ATP PW	0.25 (0.25)–1.5 ms
ATP PA	2.5–(2.5)–7.5 V
Max. ATP time	5–(5)–180 s
Min. TCL for ATP	180–(10)–600 ms
Min. TCL for ATP 1	180–(10)–600 ms
Max. TCL for ATP 2	180–(10)–600 ms
Cardioversion	
CV therapy	Disabled/enabled
CV shocks in series	1, 2, 3
CV phase 1 width	Biphasic/monphasic: 2–(0.5)–11.5 ms
CV phase 2 width	0–(0.5)–6 ms
CV 1–3 voltage	50–(10)–100 V, 125 V, 150–(50)–700 V
VF detection	
High-rate detect interval (HRDI)	180–(10)–600 ms
High-rate detect criterion	8/10 (fixed)
Noise detection	Disabled/enabled
VF therapy	
Defibrillation therapy	Enabled/disabled
Shocks in a series	4–7
Defib. phase 1 width	Biphasic/monophasic: 2–(0.5)–11.5 ms
Defib. phase 2 width	0–(0.5 ms)–6 ms (independently programmable for shocks 1–3)
Defib. 1–3 voltage	50–(10)–100 V, 125 V, 150–(50)–700 V
Defib 4+ voltage	700 V
Min. shock delay	0–(1)–40 s
Shock commitment	Commit, standby, confirm
Bradycardia pacing	
Brady support	Enabled/disabled
Rate	30,38,43,50,55,60,63,67,71,75,80,86,92,100,109,120 ppm

ICD Devices Index

Hysteresis	0–(125)–500 ms
PA	2.5–(2.5)–7.5 V
PW	0.25–(0.25)–1.5 ms
Postshock brady	Enabled/disabled
Postshock brady delay	0–(1)–10 s
Postshock brady duration	0.25–(0.25)–1 min, 2–(1)–30 min
Postshock brady energy	High/normal
Lead system	
Ports	1 pace/sense (VS-1/IS-1, accepts all 3.2-mm bipolar leads), 3 shock (DF-1, 3.2 mm)
NIPS	
Induction method	VOO, VVT, external
Induction PA	2.5–(2.5)–7.5 V
Induction PW	0.25–(0.25)–1.5 ms
VOO drive train interval	50–(10)–600 ms
VOO drive train length	1, 2, 4, 6, 8, 10–(5)–240 pulses
VOO extrastimulus (1st-4th)	Disabled, 50–(10)–600 ms
Telemetry	
Interrogation/programming	
Measurements	
Pacing lead impedance	
Pacing threshold	
Defibrillation threshold	
Real-time event markers/ICEGs	
Arrhythmia induction	
Manual delivery of Rx	
Data logging	
Sense history	
ATP confirm	On/off
Shock confirm	On/off
Detect	On/off
Revert	On/off
ICEG snapshot	
All therapy used	On/off
ATP to shock	On/off
Detect	On/off
Revert	On/off
Priority to shock episodes	On/off
Episode Log	
Date/time/TCL	
Type of therapy	
Sense history (up to 64 intervals) for detect, confirm & revert, as selected	
Snapshot (1 or 2 sec) for detect, confirm & revert, as selected	
Information is stored for typically the most recent 25 episodes	

Nonprogrammable functions
   Automatic sensing tracking   0.375–3.1 mV
   Absolute refractory period   100 ms (after sense)
                                       160 ms (after pace)

Mechanical Features
   Dimensions   8.3 × 5.7 × 1.8 cm
   Weight   140 g
   Volume   80 mL
   Case material   Titanium
   X-Ray ID   tCL
   Cell type   Lithium silver vanadium oxide

Magnet function
   Tachyarrhythmia detection and therapy suspended
   Bradycardia therapy is unaffected

Programmer
   Telectronics 9600 Network Programmer

External device for intraoperative testing
   Telectronics 4510 Implant Support Device

Manual therapy
   Stat max. shock/system off/emergency VVI

Routine follow-up
   At the physician's discretion
   Capacitor reformation is automatic every 100 days or with any max. shock charge
   Remaining cell capacity is displayed as percent life remaining (0–40%)
   ERT at 5%. EOL at 0%. Additional indicator of ERT: 30-s max. charge time
   Longevity: ≥ 4 years of monitoring only, or 200 max. energy charge cycles

VENTRITEX^R

Cadence V-100, V-100B, V-100C

Available therapies	Off/defib/defib + tach A/defib + tach A & B/brady pacing only
VT detection	
Detection interval	300–(5)–590 ms (102–200 beats/min) ("1 tach system")
Tach A detection	330–(10)–590 ms (102–182 beats/min)
Tach B detection	300–(10)–550 ms (109–200 beats/min)
No. of intervals	6–(1)–25, 30–(5)–100
Sudden-onset delta	50–(50)–500 ms
Time for extended high-rate detection	10–(5)–30 s, 30–(10)–120 sec, 2.5–(0.5)–5 min
Continuous sensing	Yes
Noncommitted shock	Yes
VF detection	
VF detect CL	290–(10)–430 ms (140–207 beats/min) ("defib only" configuration)
	270–(10)–400 ms (150–222 beats/min) ("1 tach system" & "2 tach system")
VF detection time	Nominal/fast/slow
Sinus redetection time	Nominal/fast/slow
Postshock VF detection interval	From VF detect interval–(10 ms)–VT detect interval
Continuous sensing	Yes
Noncommitted shock	Yes

ICD Devices Index

VT therapy	
No. of therapies	4
Rx-1	ATP or 1 CV shock [50–(50)–750 V]
Rx-2	0 or 1 CV shock [50–(50)–750 V]
Rx-3	0 or 1 CV shock [50–(50)–750 V]
Rx-4	0, 1 or 2 CV shocks [550–(50)–750 V]
ATP	
Min. burst CL	150–(5)–600 ms
Burst CL	Adaptive: 50–(1%)–100%
	Fixed: 200–(5)–550 ms
No. of stimuli	2–(1)–20
No. of bursts	1–(1)–15
Autodecremental	On/off
Autodecremental intraburst step size	5–(5)–25 ms
Scanning	On/off
Sequence	Dec. or dec./inc. if autodec off; dec. only if autodec on
Step size	5–(5)–25 ms
PA	1–(1)–10 V
PW	0.5–(0.5)–2 ms
Shock waveform	Biphasic/monophasic
Shock PW	Biphasic, +ve phase: 3–(1)–10 ms
	Biphasic, -ve phase: 1–(1)–10 ms ($\leq$ +ve phase)
	Monophasic: 3–(1)–12 ms
Estimated CV lead impedance (for calculating delivered energy)	10–(5)–100 Ω, 100–(10)–150 Ω (measurement, not programmable)
VF therapy	
No. of shocks	6
Shock amplitude	
1st & 2nd	100–(50)–750 V
3rd–6th	750 V
Shock waveform	Biphasic/monophasic
PW	Biphasic, +ve phase: 3–(1)–10 ms
	Biphasic, −ve phase: 1–(1)–10 ms ($\leq$ +ve phase)
	Monophasic: 3–(1)–12 ms
Bradycardia pacing	
Mode	Off, VVI
Rate	25–(5)–90 ppm
PA	1–(1)–10 V
PW	0.02, 0.1–(0.1)–2 ms
Refractory period	350–(25)–500 ms
Lead system	
Ports	
Model V-100	1 sense/pace (VS-1 in-line bipolar), 2 defib (5 mm; with 1.4-mm pin)
Model V-100B	2 sense/pace (5 mm), 2 defib (5 mm; with 1.4-mm pin)
Model V-100C	2 sense/pace (5 mm), 2 defib (6.1 mm)
NIPS	
S1	1–(1)–20
S1 CL	140–(10)–960 ms
S2, S3, S4 coupling intervals	OFF, 140–(10)–960 ms

PA	1–(1)–10 V
PW	0.5–(0.5)–2 ms
VF induction	On/off
S1	25–(25)–250
S1 CL	20–(10)–50 ms
PA	1–(1)–10 V, 5.5 V
PW	0.5–(0.5)–2 ms

Telemetry
  Interrogation/programming
  Measurements
    Lead (sense/pace + high-voltage) impedance
    R-wave amplitude
  Data
    Autogain level
    No. of detected events/delivered shocks/shocks aborted
    Therapies delivered in last 11 episodes
    Detection counters (via status screen)
    Battery voltage

EGM storage	On/off
Type of EGM	Fib./tach/extended high rate/combination
No. of EGM events stored/ duration	Last event/64 s
	3 most recent events/each 32 s
	7 most recent events, each 16 s
Trigger for EGM storage	Rx or redetection of SR

Nonprogrammable functions
  Refractory periods

After CV/defib	1000 ms
After ATP	350 ms
After sensed events	145 ms (min. 135 ms)
Noise detection rate	≥50 sensed events/s

Mechanical features

Size	9.72 × 8.21 × 2.36 cm
Weight	240 g
Volume	145 cm^3
Case	Titanium
Header	Epoxy resin
Cap screw	Acetal resin
Power source	2 lithium/silver vanadium oxide cells
X-ray ID	V-100
Magnet functions	Normal/ignore

  Normal
    Closes reed switch that prevents delivery of tachyarrhythmia therapy
    Bradycardia pacing/NIPS are unaffected
    (When magnet is removed, previous programming is restored)
Programmer
  Ventritex Cadence programmer, models PR-1000 (110 V)/PR-1001 (220 V;)
    model AC-1010 light pen
External device for intraoperative testing
  Ventritex HVS-02 cardiac EP device (stimulator/defibrillator/pacing analyzer)
Manual therapy
  No stat shock available on programmer

ICD Devices Index

Routine follow-up
  Per physician's recommendation
  Fully automatic capacitor
    maintenance is programmable: 3, 6, 9, 12 months
  Longevity: about 4 years with 1 max. shock per month and 100% VVI pacing
  Battery voltage (BOL) > 6 V
  Elective replacement voltage 5.1 V
  End-of-service voltage 5 V

ABBREVIATIONS
    ATP = antitachycardia pacing
    BOL = beginning of life
     CL = cycle length
     CV = cardioversion
     DF = defibrillation
    DFT = defibrillation threshold
    EGM = electrograms
    EOL = end of life
    EOS = end of service
     EP = electrophysiology
    ERI = elective replacement indicator
    ERT = elective replacement time
    ICD = implantable cardioverter defibrillator
   ICEG = intracardiac electrogram
  ICEGM = intracardiac electrograms
    MOL = middle of life
   MTEs = main timing events
     NA = not available
   NIPS = noninvasive programmed stimulation
     PA = pulse amplitude
    PDF = probability density function
    PES = programmed electrical stimulation
     PG = pulse generator
    PW = pulse width
     Rx = therapy
    TCL = tachycardia cycle length
   TPM = turning-point morphology
     VF = ventricular fibrillation
     VT = ventricular tachycardia

Index

Abortive shock capability, stored ventricular electrogram and, 107
N-Acetylprocainamide (NAPA), effect on DFT of, 375, 376
Acoustic radiation, 141
Adjustment disorder, 409
  with depressed mood, 416
Adolescents. *See* Children and adolescents
Adult respiratory distress syndrome (ARDS), 354
  postoperative, 342, 348
Adverse PM-ICD interactions, prevention of, 485–493
  ICDs in patients with previously implanted PMs, 485–489
  PMs in patients with previously implanted ICDs, 489–491
  postoperative testing, 491–493
Airway management following ICD implantation, 330–331
Albuterol, 326
Alfentanil, 323
American College of Cardiology (ACC), 189
  development of database registry for ICD therapy by, 202
Amiodarone, 188, 192, 199, 229, 230, 237–238, 243–244, 372, 588
  cardiovascular risks associated with, 260–261
  effect on DFT of, 375, 377, 378, 380–381

[Amiodarone]
  interaction between antitachyardia pacing and, 81
  postoperative pulmonary complications due to, 348
  for prophylaxis of ventricular arrhythmias, 573–574
Anemia, 259
Anesthesia, 319–340
  anesthetic technique, 321–325
    induction agents, 322–323
    maintenance agents, 324–325
  intraoperative problems, 326–330
    defibrillation, 329–330
    hypertension and tachycardia, 328–329
    hypotension, 327–328
    hypoxemia, 326–327
    myocardial ischemia, 328
  one-lung anesthesia, 325–326
  patients having ICD and cardiac surgery, 325
  postoperative concerns, 330–336
    airway management, 330–331
    intensive care and monitoring, 331–332
    pain management, 332–336
  preoperative evaluation, 319, 320–321
  preparation for, 321
Anesthesia team, 295
Aneurysmectomy, 267–268

AngeMed Sentinel (ICD device), 755–761
  antitachycardia pacing therapy, 758–760
  arrhythmia detection and therapy zones, 758
  diagnostic capabilities, 761
  energy source and expected longevity, 757
  external system programmer and external defibrillator, 761
  lead system, 757–758
  low-voltage cardioversion and high-voltage defibrillation, 760
  physical parameters, 756
AngeMed Sentinel model 2001, 637, 871–873
Anger, 410
Anterolateral thoracotomy, 283–285
  technique, 284–285
Antiarrhythmic drug use, 371–386
  combined with ATP, 80–81
  effects on ATP, 464–465
  ESVEM for selection of, 229, 236
  influence of drugs and ICD discharge on pacing threshold, 382–383
  interactions between ICD and, 371–382
    class I agents, 374–380
    class II agents, 380
    class III agents, 380–382
    DFT, 373–374, 375, 376–378
    types of drug effects, 372, 373, 374
  medication summary sheet for ICD patients, 396, 398
  SCD death rate due to, 188
  See also names of drugs
Antibiotic prophylaxis for prevention of ICD device infection, 501–502
Antitachycardia pacing (ATP), 242, 645–647
  clinical performance of, 73–81
    adverse interactions, 76–80
    antiarrhythmic medication in combination with pacing, 80–81
    combined use of pacing and defibrillation systems, 76
    pacing without defibrillation backup, 73–76
  comparison with low-energy cardioversion, 95, 96
  failure mechanism of, 66–67
  hemodynamic stabilization technique, 63
  mechanisms of tachycardia interruptions, 63–64
    entrainment, 64–66
    resetting, 63–64
  prevention of tachycardia, 61–62
  strategies for, 67–73

[Antitachycardia pacing (ATP)]
  Telectronics Guardian 4210/4211 pacing algorithm, 719–720
  troubleshooting, 450–465
Anxiety, 259, 270–271, 411, 414–415
Aortic stenosis, 207–208
Aspirin therapy, 259
Asymptomatic ICD therapy:
  troubleshooting ICD shocks, 441–442, 443
  value of stored ventricular electrograms in, 105–106
Atelectasis, 354
Atracurium, 324
Atrial defibrillation, future directions in, 854
Atrial fibrillation:
  diagnosis using stored electrogram analysis, 103
  postoperative, 342, 344–346
Atropine, 326
Automatic gain control (AGC) sensing circuitry, 120
Automatic sensitivity tracking, 308
Autonomic nervous system (ANS):
  role in SCD of, 406–407
  tests to predict high risk of SCD after abnormal functions of, 567–572
Aviation environment, electromagnetic interference from, 147

Barbiturates, 323
Baroreflex sensitivity (BRS), 570–572
Batteries, 124–132
  for the cardioverter-defibrillators, 125–131
    battery chemistry, 125–126
    battery qualification and electrical testing, 130–131
    battery requirements, 125
    cell construction and configuration, 126
    cell discharge performance, 126–130
    the future, 131
  technology of, 124–125
Benzodiazepines, 322, 323
Beta-blockers, 328, 329, 372, 587
  interaction between ATP and, 81
Beta-2 agonists, 326
Bidisomide, effect on DFT of, 375, 379
Bilateral anterior thoracotomy, 288–289
Binary number system (data storage method), 155
Biotronik Phylax 03 (ICD device), 637, 873–874
Biphasic waveforms, 18–19, 296

Bipolar endocardial leads, 624–625
Blocking agents, neuromuscular, 324
Bradycardia, 61
Bradycardia pacing, 645
  inappropriate inhibition of pacing due to T-wave oversensing, 109–110
  pacing zone of Ventak PRx, 703
Bretylium, 230
  effect on DFT of, 378
Bretylium tosylate, effect on DFT of, 375, 381
Bronchial blockers to provide one-lung anesthesia, 325
"Buddy" system for ICD patients, 401
Bupivacaine, 335, 336

Calcium channel blockers, 328, 372
Calcium deficiency, 259
Canadian Implantable Defibrillator Study (CIDS), 199, 217, 244, 575
Canadian Myocardial Infarction Amiodarone Trial (CAMIAT), 574
Candida species causing ICD device infection, 498, 499
Capacitors, 132–137
  for cardioverter-defibrillators, 133–137
    discharge/charge performance, 136
    electrical and qualification testing, 136
    requirements, 133
    types, 133–136
  technology of, 132–133
Cardiac Arrest in Seattle—Conventional versus Amiodarone Drug Evaluation (CASCADE), 237
Cardiac Arrest Study of Hamburg (CASH), 192, 199, 237, 575, 818–821
Cardiac Arrhythmia Suppression Trial (CAST), 232
  ventricular premature complex (VPC) hypothesis and, 558
Cardiac complications following ICD placement, 354, 355–357
  cardiac laceration and trauma, 357
  congestive heart failure, 354, 355
  myocardial infarction, 354, 355–356
  pericarditis, 354, 356–357
Cardiac Pacemakers, Inc. (CPI), 99, 299, 607, 655
  follow-up procedure for, 429–430
  See also Endotak non-thoracotomy lead system; Ventak (AICD devices)
Cardiac perfusion imaging, 231

Cardiomyopathies in children and adolescents, 210–213
  hypertrophic cardiomyopathies, 211–213
  idiopathic dilated cardiomyopathies, 210–211
Cardiomyopathy Trial (CAT) of Germany, 819–820, 821
Cardiopulmonary resuscitation (CPR), importance of instructions in, 400–401
Cardiovascular risks in the ICD patient, 260–261
Cardiovascular surgeon, 295
Catheter ablation, 241
  interference of ICDs and PMs due to, 144
Catheterization for ICD candidates, 263–264
Catheter mapping, 268–269
Ceramic capacitors, 135–136
Children and adolescents, 205–227
  cardiovascular diseases and SCD in, 206–215
    cardiomyopathies, 210–213
    congenital heart disease, 207–209
    primary electrical diseases, 213–215
  considerations in use of ICDs in, 216–222
    anatomy, 216
    electrophysiology, 217–222
    future considerations, 222
  SCD in, 205–206
2-Chloroprocaine, 335
Chronic respiratory disease, 259
Clinical utility of data logging facility, 163–165
Clinic for ICD patient follow-up. *See* Patient follow-up
Clofilium, effect on DFT of, 378
Clofilium phosphate, effect on DFT of, 375, 381
Closed-circuit voltage (CCV) of a battery cell, 124–125
Cocaine, 335
Colonic perforation, 354
Complementary metal oxide semiconductor (CMOS) circuitry, 121, 155
Computed tomography (CT), 263, 513–517
Computer simulation of DFT, 35–39
Congenital heart disease in childhood, 207–209
  aortic stenosis, 207–208
  tetralogy of Fallot, 207
  transposition of the great arteries, 208
Congestive heart failure (CHF):
  following ICD placement, 354, 355
  SCD and, 587
  use of AICD for, 184
Contraindications for ICD implantation, 191

Cooperative North Scandanavian Enalapril Survival Study (CONSENSUS), 586, 587–588
Coronary artery bypass graft (CABG), postoperative care of, 341
Coronary Artery Bypass Graft Patch Trial (CABG Patch Trial), 192, 244, 577
Coronary artery bypass grafting (CABG), 239–241
Corynebacterium species causing ICD device infection, 498, 499
Costs and cost effectiveness of the ICD, 595–605
  benefits, 598–599
    choice of benefits, 598
    quality of life, 598–599
  cost-effectiveness analyses, 596
  expenses, 596–598
  literature review of, 600–604
  method of analysis, 599–600
  payment-benefit perspective, 595–596
  valuing future costs, 597–598
Critical mass hypothesis for defibrillation, 13–16

Database registry of ICD therapy (via ACC), 202
Data logging, 160–161, 636, 637–641
  detailed record of tachycardia episodes, 161
  intracardiac electrogram, 161
  long-term log, 160
Data storage, 153–171
  data logging of events, 160–161
  device comparison-data logging, 166, 167
  future development, 166–170
  presentation of stored data to users, 159–160
  storage methods, 154–159
    binary number system, 155
    memory, 155–159
    microprocessor system, 154
  utilities of data logging, 163–166
    clinical utility, 163–165
    engineering utility, 165–166
    research utility, 166
DC magnetic fields, 141
Deep vein thrombosis, 358
Deep venous thrombophlebitis, 342, 350
Defibrillation:
  adverse interactions between antitachycardia pacing and, 76–80
  antitachycardia pacing without backup of, 73–76
  combined use of pacing and, 76

[Defibrillation]
  definition of, 1
  during ICD implantation, 329–330
  interference on ICDs and PMs due to, 143
  mechanisms of, 10–21
  waveforms of, 18–19
Defibrillation leads, 607–622
  combined defibrillation-sense/pace leads, 625
  complications of, 616–617
  nonthoracotomy lead systems, 617–622
Defibrillation (DF) nonthoracotomy lead system (Telectronics), 795–809
  acute human studies, 800–802
  animal studies, 798–800
  endocardial defibrillation lead system, 795–798, 802–808
Defibrillation shock, 49–51
Defibrillation threshold (DFT), 29–54
  assessment of, 33–35
    alternative methods, 43–44
  clinical testing for, 40
  computer simulations of, 35–39
  concepts of, 30–31
  definition of, 19, 56–57
  effects of antiarrhythmic drugs on, 373–374, 375, 376–378
  efficacy predication from threshold determinations, 41–43
  elevated, 303–307
  estimated defibrillation efficacy, 45–46
  influence of patient size on, 31–33
  lead signal evaluation and DFT testing, 626–628
  mathematical models of, 35–39
  setting level of first shock therapy, 50–51
  timing test shock delivery, 49–50
  upper limit of vulnerability of, 46–48
Defibrillation threshold testing, 40, 48–49, 56–57, 296–298
  equipment for, 298–301
  practical aspects of, 301–303
Defibrillation Implant as a Bridge to Later Transplant (DEFIBRILAT) Trial, 245, 598, 591
Delirium, 417–418
Depression, 409, 416–417
  major depressive disorders, 410, 416
  myocardial, 81
Desflurane, 324
Diagnostic capabilities of ICDs, 650–651
  data logging, 160–161, 636, 637–641
  telemetry, 636, 637–641

Index

Digoxin, 372
    effect on DFT of, 375
Discharge teaching plans for ICD patients, 396, 397
Disopyramide, 230, 372
Doxacurium, 324
Dutch prospective study of ICD (as first-choice therapy), 819–820, 821–822
Dynamic RAM (DRAM), 115
Dysthymia, 417

Echocardiography, 231, 262, 517–518
Edrophonium, 324
Electrical stimulus, VF induced by, 4–8
Electrocardiogram (ECG):
    during intraoperative ICD testing, 296
    signal-averaged, 231, 261
    surface, 261
Electrochemical capacitors, 136
Electrolyte imbalance, 259
Electrolytic capacitors, 133–134, 135
Electromagnetic interference (EMI):
    detection criteria and response of Siecure devices, 745–747
    effects on ICDs and PMS, 140
    interaction of Ventak devices with, 668–671
    power frequency (50–60 Hz), 146–147
    protection against, 120–121
Electrophysiological study versus electrocardiographic monitoring (ESVEM) for selection of drug therapy, 229, 236
Electrophysiological (EP) testing for ICD candidates, 264–266, 408–410
Electrophysiologist (EP), 295, 387–388
EP nurse (as member of ICD patient team), 387–388
Electrosurgery, interference on ICDs and PMs due to, 143–144
Elevated defibrillation thresholds, 303–307
Encainide, 372
    effect on DFT of, 375, 376, 379
Endocardial leads, 624–625
Endocarditis, 354
Endotak nonthoracotomy lead system (CPI), 306, 617, 618, 779–799
    complications of, 788
    cost of, 791
    defibrillation threshold measurements, 783–785
    description of, 780–781
    follow-up results, 789
    implantation results, 786

[Endotak nonthoracotomy lead system (CPI)]
    implantation technique, 783, 786
    lead configuration, 781
    long-term defibrillation threshold stability, 791
    multicenter study of safety and efficacy, 791–792
    patient population, 782–783
    postoperative testing, 785–786
    prediction of adequate thresholds, 787–788
    sensing problems, 789–790
Energy storage and delivery, 123–137
    batteries, 124–132
        for the cardioverter-defibrillators, 125–131
        technology of, 124–125
    capacitors, 132–137
        for the cardioverter-defibrillators, 133–137
        technology of, 132–133
    requirements and operating environment for energy system, 123
Enflurane, 324
Engineering considerations in ICD systems design, 113–122
    functional characteristics, 114–116
        isolation/protection circuits, 116
        memory, 115
        microprocessor, 114–115
        pacing and high-voltage output sections, 115–116
    implementation considerations, 116–119
        hybridization, 118
        integration, 117–118
        power, 116–117
        size/shape/weight, 118–119
    other design considerations, 119–121
        ionizing radiation, 121
        protection against component failure, 119–120
        protection against interference, 120–121
        protection against memory errors, 119–120
Engineering utility of data logging facility, 165–166
Entrainment, 64–66
Environmental interferences effecting ICDS and PMs, 146–147
    aviation environments, 147
    power frequency (50–60 Hz), 146–147
    Scuba diving, 147
    security systems, 147
    stun guns, 147
Epicardial leads, 622–624
    for Medtronic PCD, 686–687

Epidocaine, 335
Esmolol, 329
Etomidate, 322–323
European clinical experience with ICDs, 811–843
　European guidelines for ICD use, 811–818
　future aspects of ICD development, 840–841
　ICD development and use, 811–812
　ongoing European multicenter studies, 819–821
　　Cardiac Arrest Study Hamburg (CASH), 818–821
　　cardiomyopathy trial (CAT), 819–820, 821
　　Dutch prospective study of ICD, 819–820, 821–822
　　Optimal study, 819–820, 822
　　SAMI study, 819–820, 822
　　d-sotalol versus placebo/ICD study, 819–820, 822
　　U-care registry, 819–820, 822
　third-generation ICDs, 832–840
European Dilated Cardiomyopathy Trial, 245
European Myocardial Infarction Amiodarone Trial (EMIAT), 574
European Society of Cardiology, 812
Exercise radionuclide scans, 262
External cardioverter-defibrillator (ECD) of Ventak devices, 664
External interferences effecting ICDs and PMs, 139–151
　differences between ICDs and PMs, 142–143
　environmental interferences, 146–147
　interference from medical devices and instruments, 143–146
　　cardiac defibrillation, 143
　　electrosurgery, 143–144
　　hyperbaric chambers, 146
　　ionizing radiation, 145
　　lithotripsy, 144–145
　　magnetic resonance imaging, 144
　　medical diathermy, 145
　　radiofrequency catheter ablation, 144
　　TENS and other stimulators, 145–146
　interference in specific occupations and activities, 147–148
　standards for interference testing, 148
　types of interference, timing, and spatial factors, 140–142
　　acoustic radiation, 141
　　DC magnetic fields, 141
　　directly conducted galvanic currents, 140–141

[External interferences effecting ICDs and PMs]
　　external pressure, 141
　　geometric factors, 142
　　ionizing radiation dose, 141
　　mechanical trauma and twiddling, 141
　　radiated electromagnetic fields, 140
　　temporal factors, 142
　　thermal heating, 141
Extracorporeal shock-wave lithotripsy, interference of ICDs and PMs due to, 144–145

Family education. See Patient and family teaching
Fear, 270–271
Fentanyl, 323
　transdermal, 334
Fibrillation. See Atrial fibrillation; Ventricular fibrillation (VF)
First-generation ICDs, 635–636
Flecainide, 230, 372
　effect on DFT of, 376, 380
Flecainide acetate, effect on DFT of, 375
Follow-up of ICD patients. See Patient follow-up
Foreign-body infection, 354
Fourth-generation ICDs, 113–114
Future directions in ICD development, 841–842, 845–870
　clinical applications, 851–856
　　adjunctive or alternative therapy, 854–855
　　atrial defibrillation, 854
　　improving total survival of ICD recipients, 851–852
　　prevention of SCD in high-risk populations, 852–854
　　secondary therapy with ICDs, 855–856
　elements of future ICD generators, 846–848
　evolution of lead systems, 848–850
　implant technique, 850–851
　technological developments, 854–865
　　ICD therapy in treatment of VT/VF, 863–865
　　improved tachycardia detection and monitoring, 856–862
　　tachycardia prevention, 862–863

Galvanic currents, interference of ICDs and PMs due to, 140–141
Gastrointestinal complications following ICD placement, 355, 360
Gated blood pool scan, 231

German Dilated Cardiomyopathy Study
   (GDCMS), 577–579
Glycopyrrolate, 326
Great arteries, transposition of, during childhood, 208

Halothane, 324
Hamburg Cardiac Arrest Study. See Cardiac Arrest Study of Hamburg (CASH)
Health Care Financing Administration (HCFA), 188–189
Heart transplantation. See Orthotopic heart transplantation (OHT)
Hematological disorders and malignancy, 260
Hematoma in generator pocket, postoperative, 342, 348–349
Hemodynamic stabilization technique, 63
Hepatitis, 354
High-energy shocks, 89
Historical development of ICDs, 279–280
   of the AICD, 173–186
      clinical results of therapy, 177–181, 183–184
      early patient implantation, 176–177
      FDA approach for marketing, 177
      improvement in design and device programmability, 181–182
      initial design and fabrication, 173–175
Holter monitoring, 231, 237
Home care for patients. See Patient and family teaching
Hybrid circuit technology of ICDs, 118
Hyperbaric oxygen chambers, interference of ICDs and PMs due to, 146
Hypertension, 328–329
Hypertrophic cardiomyopathy during childhood, 211–215
Hypoperfusion, 63
Hypotension, 63
   during ICD implantation, 327–328
Hypoxemia:
   due to endotracheal tube problems, 325–326
   during ICD implantation, 326–327

Ibuprofen, 336
ICD device-related complications following implantation, 354, 360–361
ICD devices index, 871–912
Idiopathic dilated cardiomyopathies during childhood, 210–211
Idiopathic ventricular fibrillation during childhood, 214–215

Implantable defibrillator shocks. See Shocks
Implantable spinal-cord stimulators, 145–146
Indications for the ICD, 187–194
   background, 187–189
   contraindications for implant, 191
   future indications, 191–192
   NASPE guidelines for implantation, 189–190
   use in patients with no inducible arrhythmias, 190–191
Indoleamines, 407
Indomethacin, 336
Infections in ICDs, 259, 495–504
   causative organisms, 498–499
   complications following ICD placement, 354, 360
   diagnosis, 499–500
   incidence of, 495–498
   prevention of, 501–503
   reuse of devices and, 500–501
   treatment, 500
Integration of ICD circuit components, 117–118
Intensive care and monitoring following ICD implantation, 331–332
Interactions between PMs and ICDs, 479–494
   ICD effects on permanent PMs, 483–485
   PM effects on ICDs, 479–483
   preventing adverse device-device interactions, 485–493
Intermediate-energy shocks, 89
Intermedics RES-Q (ICD device), 300–301
   epicardial pacing leads, 624
   European clinical experience with, 838–839
   patch leads, 612
   sensing, 307
Intermedics RES-Q models 101-01/101-01R, 640, 885–887
Intracardiac electrograms, 115
   storage of, 161, 164
Intraoperative testing of ICDs, 295–317
   DFT testing, 296–298
      equipment for, 298–301
      practical aspects of, 301–303
   device implantation and testing, 311–313
   elevated DFTs, 303–307
   in the operating room, 295–296
   pacing, 311
   sensing, 307–311
   troubleshooting, 311
Ionizing radiation, 141
   interference of ICDs and PMs due to, 145
   shielding CMOS circuitry from, 121

Ischemia colitis, 354
Isoflurane, 324

Ketamine, 322, 323
Ketoralac, 336

Lead systems, 607–633
  of the AngeMed Sentinel, 757–758
  complications following ICD placement, 360–361
  defibrillation leads, 607–622
    combining defibrillation-sense/pace leads, 625
    complications, 616–617
    nonthoracotomy lead systems, 617–622
    radiography for evaluation and trouble-shooting, 508–512
  future directions in development of, 629, 848–850
  lead signal evaluation, 626–628
  sense/pace leads, 622–626
    combined defibrillation-sense/pace leads, 625
    complications, 625–626
    endocardial leads, 624–625
    epicardial leads, 622–624
  unipolar system compared to nonthoracotomy transvenous system, 55–56
  of the Ventak devices, 663–664
    implantation and testing, 664–665
  See also DF nonthoracotomy lead system (Telectronics): Endotak nonthoracotomy lead system (CPI)
Left subcostal approach for ICD implantation, 286–288
  technique, 287–288
Left ventricular dysfunction, 558–561
Left ventricular reconstruction, 267–268
Lidocaine, 230, 335
  effect on DFT of, 375–379
Lifestyle changes, 270–271
  evaluation of quality of life, 598–599
Lithium/silver vanadium oxide (Li/SVO) chemistry of batteries, 125–126, 127, 128, 129, 130
Lithotripsy, interference of ICDs and PMs due to, 144–145
Liver function tests, 259
Local anesthetics for postoperative pain control, 335
Long-term cumulative data log, 160
Lorcainide, 372

Low-energy cardioversion (LEC), 89–98
  advantages of, 89–91
  combined use of antitachycardia pacing and, 72
  comparison with antitachycardia pacing, 95, 96
  definition of, 89
  disadvantages and limitations of, 95–96
  efficacy of, 91–95
    lead/waveform configuration, 92–93
    shock energy, 94
    tachycardia cycle length, 93–94
  guidelines for use of, 96–97

Magnesium deficiency, 259
Magnetic fields, 141
  ICD patient avoidance of, 400
  radiated, 140
Magnetic resonance imaging (MRI), 263, 519
  interference of ICDs and PMs due to, 144
Major depressive disorder (MDD), 410, 416
Malignant ventricular arrhythmias. *See* Ventricular fibrillation (VF); Ventricular tachycardia (VT)
Manic-depressive disorder, 417
Mathematical models of DFT, 35–39
Mechanisms of defibrillation, 10–21
  critical mass hypothesis, 13–16
  defibrillation waveforms, 18–19
  electrode systems, 19–21
  upper limit of vulnerability hypothesis, 16–18
Median sternotomy, 281–283
  technique, 282–283
Medicaid guidelines for ICD patients, 188–189
Medical diathermy, interference of ICDs and PMs due to, 145
Medical status of the ICD patient, preoperative assessment of, 259–260
Medicare guidelines for ICD patients, 188–189
Medication summary sheet for ICD patients, 396, 398
Medtronic pacemaker cardioverter-defibrillators (PCDs), 299, 305, 639, 683–694
  clinical performance of, 690–693
  endocardial defibrillation-sense/pace leads, 620
  European clinical experience with, 830–833
  follow-up procedures for, 430–432
  patch leads, 610
  system features, 683–690
Medtronic PCD models II and III, 308
Medtronic PCD model 7201, 640, 893–895

Index

Medtronic PCD model 7217B/D, 887–890
Medtronic PCD model 7219 (Jewel), 639, 890–893
Memory (data storage method), 113, 115, 155–159
  protection against memory errors, 119–120
Mepivacaine, 335
Metabolic abnormalities, 259
Metaproterenol, 326
Methohexital, 322, 323
Metoprolol, 192, 199, 229, 243–244
Mexiletine, 230, 372
  effect on DFT of, 375, 379
Microprocessor (data storage system), 113, 114–115, 154
Midazolam, 323
Mirowski, Dr. Michel, 173, 174
MODE (3-methyl-ODE), effect on DFT of, 375, 376
Monophasic waveforms, 296, 299
Morbidity of ICD implantation, 353, 682, 730–731
Moricizine, 230
Morphine, 323
Mortality of ICD implantation, 291–292, 353, 682, 730–731
Multicenter Automatic Defibrillation Implantation Trial (MADIT), 192, 244–245, 576–577
Multicenter Unsustained Tachycardia Trial (MUSTT), 192, 245, 575–576
Multiple-capture tachycardia terminiation methods (pacing strategy), 68–70
Multiple wandering wavelet hypothesis, 8–9
Muscle relaxants, 324
Mycobacterium chelonae infection, 497, 498
Myocardial depression, 81
Myocardial infarction:
  EP studies to assess risk of SCD after, 565–567
  following ICD placement, 354, 355–356
Myocardial ischemia:
  during ICD implantation, 328
  VF induced by, 1–4

Narcotics, 329
  as induction agents, 322, 323
  for postoperative pain management, 332–335
National database registry for ICD therapy (via ACC), 202
National Heart Lung and Blood Institute (NHLBI), 575, 579

[National Heart Lung and Blood Institute (NHLBI)]
  evaluation of ICD in survivors of cardiac arrest by, 192
Neostigmine, 324
Neurological impairment, 260
Neuromuscular blocking agents, 324
Neurotransmitters, role in SCD of, 406–407
Nitroglycerine, 328, 329
Nitroprusside, 329
Nitrous oxide, 324
Nonconversion problems, 437–439
Nondetection problems, 439–440
Non-EP cardiologist, 387–388
Noninducibility of arrhythmias,
  ICD use in patients with, 190–191, 238–239
Noninvasive programmed stimulation (NIPS), 635, 649–650
Nonsteroidal antiinflammatory drugs, 336
Nonthoracotomy defibrillation lead systems, 288–293, 617–622
  combined transvenous-subcutaneous/submuscular leads, 617
  compared to unipolar defibrillation system, 55–56
  complications and limitations, of, 622
  effect on ICD treatment, 201
  thoracoscopic lead systems, 622
  transvenous lead systems, 617–620
  See also DF nonthoracotomy lead system (Telectronics); Endotak nonthoracotomy lead system (CPI)
Nonthoracotomy ICD device placement, complications of, 362
North American Society of Pacing and Electrophysiology (NASPE) guidelines for ICD implantation, 189–190
Nuclear imaging, 518–519

Objections to use of ICDs, 55
Obsessive-compulsive disorders, 415
ODE (O-methyl encainide), effect on DFT of, 375, 376
One-lung anesthesia, 325–326
Open-circuit voltage (OCV) of a battery cell, 124–125
Optimal study (European study), 819–820, 822
Organisms causing ICD device infection, 498–499
Orthotopic heart transplantation (OHT), 585–593
  actuarial survival of patients after, 585

[Orthotopic heart transplantation (ORT)]
  contraindications to, 586
  future directions for, 591–592
  ICD as bridge to, 184, 270
  need for randomized data, 591–592
  population at risk, 586–587
  sudden death and congestive heart failure, 587
  therapeutic implications for, 587–589
  use of ICD in patients awaiting, 589–591
Overview of the ICD, 635–653
  antitachycardia pacing, 645–647
  bradycardia pacing, 645
  diagnostic capabilities, 650–651
  noninvasive programmed stimulation, 648–650
  sensing functions, 636–645
  shock therapy, 647–749

Pacemakers (PMs):
  antitachycardia, 242
  differences between ICDs and, 142–143
  interaction of Ventak devices with, 671
  See also Interactions between PMs and ICDs; Medtronic PCDs
Pace mapping, 269
Pacesetter-Siemens, 299, 307
Pacing, 113, 115–116
  bradycardia, 645
  defibrillation and adverse interactions, 76–80
  evaluating pacing threshold during intraoperative ICD testing, 311
  influence of antiarrhythmic drugs on, 382–383
  radiography for evaluation and troubleshooting, 505–508
  troubleshooting ventricular antitachycardia PMs and, 454–456
  See also Antitachycardia pacing (ATP)
Pain management, postoperative, 332–336
Pancuronium, 324
Panic, 414–415
Patch leads, 608, 612
Patch trials, 192, 244, 577
Patient and family teaching, 387–404
  assessing patient's understanding of ICD function, 402
  early postoperative period teaching, 395
  emergency contacts, 402
  implantation procedure, 394–395
    patient recovery procedure, 394
    preoperative preparation, 394

[Patient and family teaching]
  issues in patient care and teaching, 270–271, 351, 387–388
  predischarge teaching, 395–401
    discharge plan, 396, 397
    implantable defibrillator shocks, 399–400
    instructions for home care, 396
    medications and medication summary sheet, 396, 398
    patient precautions, 400–401
    patient's activity, 396–399
  preoperative teaching, 388–394
    introduction to the ICD, 391–393
    medical condition, 388–390
    obtaining formal consent, 393–394
    treatment options, 390–391
  support groups and activities for patient and family, 401
"Patient-controlled analgesia" (PCA), 333
Patient follow-up, 425–435
  ICD follow-up clinic, 426
  important follow-up issues, 434
  patients with ventricular antitachycardia pacing and ICDs, 448, 473
  social support, 433–434
  specific patient devices, 427–433
    CPI series, 429–430
    Medtronic, 430–432
    Telectronics, 432–433
    Ventritex, 430, 431
Pediatric ICD patients. See Children and adolescents
Pericarditis:
  following ICD placement, 354, 356–357
  postoperative, 342, 349
Phenytoin, effect on DFT of, 375
Pipercuronium, 324
Plastic film capacitors, 135
Pleural effusions, 354
Pneumonia, 354
Pneumothorax, 354
Postmyocardial Infarction Trial (FIRST-AID), 245
Postoperative care of the ICD patient, 341–352
  deep venous thrombophlebitis, 342, 350
  hematoma in generator pocket, 342, 348–349
  impact of third-generation devices on, 350–351
  impact of the transvenous devices, 350
  patient care issues, 351
  pericarditis, 342, 349
  postoperative routine, 341–344

Index

[Postoperative care of the ICD patient]
  pulmonary complications, 342, 348
  supraventricular tachycardia, 342, 344–346
  ventricular arrhythmias, 342, 346–348
Posttraumatic stress disorder, 409, 415
Power requirements, 113, 116–117
Predischarge teaching of the ICD patient, 395–401
  discharge plan, 396, 397
  implantable defibrillator shocks, 399–400
  instructions for home care, 396
  medications and medication summary sheet, 396, 398
  patient precautions, 400–401
  patient's activity, 396–399
Predischarge testing of the ICD, 367–369
  testing procedure, 368–369
Preoperative evaluation for ICD, 257–277
  cardiac evaluation, 261–263
  cardiac catheterization, 263, 264
  cardiovascular risks, 260–261
  EP studies, 264–266
  medical status of patient, 259–260
  preoperative evaluation for concomitant surgery, 266–271
Preoperative teaching for the ICD patient. *See* Patient and family teaching
Prilocaine, 335
Primary batteries, 125
Primary electrical diseases in childhood, 213–215
  idiopathic ventricular fibrillation, 214–215
  prolonged QT syndromes, 215
Proarrhythmia, 81
Procainamide, 230, 372
  effect on DFT of, 375, 376
Procaine, 335
Prolonged QT syndromes in childhood, 215
Propafenone, 192, 199–200, 229, 230, 243–244, 372
  effect on DFT of, 375, 377, 380
Propofol, 323
Propranolol, effect on DFT of, 375
Prostate carcinoma, 260
Protamine reaction, 354
Psychiatric aspects of the ICD, 405–423
  the EP study, 408–410
  experiencing the ICD, 411–419
  psychiatric management of malignant arrhythmia patients, 410
  psychiatric syndromes in the patient, 414–418

[Psychiatric aspects of the ICD]
  role of ANS and neurotransmitters, 406–407
  role of psychological stress, 407–408
Psychological adaptation to the ICD, 270–271
Psychotic disorders, 418
Pulmonary complications, postoperative, 342, 348, 354, 357–358
Pulse generators:
  implantation and testing of Ventak devices, 665–666
  radiography for evaluation and troubleshooting, 512–513

Quality of life, evaluation of, 598–599
Quinidine, 230, 372
  effect on DFT of, 374–375, 376
QT syndromes, prolonged, in childhood, 215

Radiated electromagnetic fields, effect on ICDs and PMs of, 140
Radiography, 505, 513
  in cardioverter/defibrillating lead system, 508–512
  in pulse generators, 512–513
  in sensing/pacing lead system, 505–508
Radiology of the ICD. *See* Computed tomography (CT); Echocardiography; Magnetic resonance imaging (MRI); Nuclear imaging; Radiography
Radionuclide ventriculography, 262
Random-access memory (RAM), 113, 115, 156–159
  comparison of operating power consumption in different RAM sizes, 168
Rate-sensing lead disruption, diagnosis of, 104
Read-only memory (ROM), 113, 115, 156–159
Renal insufficiency, 259
Reperfusion, VT induced by, 1–4
Research utility of data logging facility, 166
Resetting of ongoing tachycardia, 63–64
Revascularization, 266–267

SAMI study (European study), 819–820, 822
Scuba diving, 147
Secondary batteries, 125
Security systems, 147
Sense amplifier section, 113, 114
Sense/pace leads, 622–626
  combined defibrillation-sense/pace leads, 625
  complications of, 625–626
  endocardial leads, 624–625

[Sense/pace leads]
  epicardial leads, 622–624
  radiography for, 505–508
Sensing function, 636–645
  electrogram recordings in diagnosis of errors, 107–110
  evaluation during intraoperative ICD testing, 307–311
  problems with Endotak lead system, 789–790
  Siecure and, 744–745
  Telectronics Guardian 4202/4203 and, 308, 681–682
  Telectronics Guardian 4210/4211 and, 715–716, 730
  troubleshooting antitachycardia pacing systems and, 452–454
  Ventritex Cadence and, 307, 765–766
Sepsis, 354
Serratia species causing ICD device infection, 498, 499
Shocks, 63, 81
  asymptomatic, 441–442, 443
  defibrillation shock, 49–51
  predischarge teaching for ICD patient concerning, 399–400
Shock therapy, 647–649
Siecure (model 2120), 639, 733–754, 895–896
  administrative data, 749, 750
  arrhythmia identification, 736–739
  bradycardia support function, 733–735
  clinical experience, 751
  diagnostic telemetry, 747–748
  electrogram and event marker telemetry, 748
  EMI detection criteria and response, 745–747
  European clinical experience with, 839–840
  event counter telemetry, 749–751, 753
  event counters and other data storage, 749
  future developments, 751–752
  general characteristics, 733
  required rate samples, 739–740
  sensing of VT and VF, 744–745
  tachycardia confirmation, 740–742
  temporary mode, 748–749
  therapeutic options, 742–743
Signal-averaged electrocardiogram, 231, 261
Single-capture tachycardia termination methods (pacing strategy), 67–68
Sinus rhythm mapping, 269
Skin necrosis, 354
Slaved programmed electrical stimulation (PES), 635
  of the Ventak PRx, 704–705

Social support for the ICD patient, 433–434
Sotalol, 230, 372
  effect on DFT of, 375, 381–382
  d-Sotalol versus placebo/ICD study (European study), 819–820, 822
Staff nurse, 387–388
Standards for ICD and PM interference testing, 148
Staphylococcus aureus infection, 497, 498
Staphylococcus epidermidis infection, 497, 498
Stored ventricular electrogram analysis, 99–112
  abortive shock capability and, 107
  criteria for arrhythmia diagnosis using, 100–105
    atrial fibrillation, 103
    indeterminate, 104–105
    rate-sensing lead disruption, 104
    supraventricular tachycardia, 103–104
    VT, 100–102
  future directions, 110–111
  symptoms preceding ICD responses as index for ICD intervention, 99–100
  value in asymptomatic ICD therapy, 105–106
  value in diagnosis of logical sensing errors, 107–110
  value in studying the initiation of VT, 106
  in the Ventritex Cadence, 100
Stress, 407–408
  posttraumatic, 409, 415
Stun guns, 147
Subclavian vein thrombosis, 354, 358
Subendocardial resection, ICD implantation and, 267–268
Subthreshold stimulation, 62
Subxiphoid approach to ICD implantation, 285–286
  technique, 295–296
Succinylcholine, 324
Sudden cardiac death (SCD), 55
  amiodarone and, 188
  in childhood, 205–206
    cardiovascular diseases and SCD, 206–215
  congestive heart failure and, 587
  efficacy of ICD in, 195–197
  mortality rate for (U.S.), 187–188
  prediction and prevention of, 557–583
    in high-risk patients, 573–579
    risk strategies, 557–558
    tests to predict high risk, 558–573
  role of ANS and neurotransmitters in, 406–407
  VT/VF as mechanism for, 187

Index

Sufentanil, 323
Superior vena cava thrombosis, 354
Support groups for the ICD patient and family, 401, 433–434
Supraventricular tachyarrhythmias as limitation of low-energy cardioversion, 95–96
Supraventricular tachycardia:
   diagnosis using stored electrogram analysis, 103–104
   postoperative, 342, 344–346
Surface electrocardiogram, 261
Surgery:
   complications following ICD placement via thoracotomy, 353–355, 355–361
      cardiac complications, 354, 355–357
      gastrointestinal complications, 355, 360
      ICD device and lead complications, 360–361
      infection complications, 354, 360
      pulmonary complications, 354, 357–358
      vascular complications, 354, 358–360
   complications of nonthoracotomy ICD placement, 362
   preoperative evaluation for ICDs and concomitant surgery, 266–271
      aneurysmectomy, 267–268
      catheter mapping, 268–269
      ICD as bridge to heart transplantation, 270
      left ventricular reconstruction, 267–268
      revascularization, 266–267
      subendocardial resection, 267–268
      valvular surgery, 267
   surgical approach to ICD placement in young patients, 216
   techniques for ICD, 279–293
      anterolateral thoracotomy, 283–285
      bilateral anterior thoracotomy, 288–289
      general implantation considerations, 281
      historical perspective, 279–280
      left subcostal approach, 286–288
      median sternotomy, 281–283
      nonthoracotomy lead system, 289–293
      operative mortality, 291–292
      standard ICD system, 280
      subxiphoid approach, 285–286
      thoracoscopic implantation, 289, 290
      transdiaphragmatic implantation, 288
   for ventricular arrhythmias, 239–241
Survival and Ventricular Enlargement (SAVE) study, 588
Survival of ICD patients, 195–204
   effect on overall survival, 198–200

[Survival of ICD patients]
   efficacy of ICD in preventing sudden death, 195–197
   challenge to, 197
   improving total survival, 851–852
   reasons why available data may not support expanded use of ICDs, 200–202
Sympathetic nervous system (SNS), 406

Tachycardia. *See* Ventricular tachycardia (VT)
Teaching plan for the ICD patient, 388
Telectronics (ICD devices), 299, 897–909
   defibrillation (DF) nonthoracotomy lead system, 795–809
      acute human studies, 800–802
      animal studies, 798–800
      endocardial defibrillation lead system, 795–798, 802–808
   defibrillator patches, 609
   endocardial defibrillation/rate-sensing/pacing leads, 619
Telectronics Guardian model 4202/4203, 639, 676–682, 897–898
   clinical studies, 680–681
   engineering aspects of design, 675–676
   European clinical experience with, 834–837
   follow-up procedures for, 432–433
   implantation and intraoperative testing, 678–679
   programmable features and device function, 676–678
   sensing system, 308, 681–682
   telemetry, data storage, and noninvasive testing, 678–680
   troubleshooting, 680–681
Telectronics Guardian model II 4204, 641, 898–900
Telectronics Guardian model 4210/4211, 306, 308, 310, 641, 713–732, 900–904
   clinical studies, 727–731
   data storage, 724–725
   device function, 715–722
   engineering aspects of design, 713–715
   general characteristics, 713, 714
   implantation and device testing, 723–724
   system states and emergency function, 722–723
   troubleshooting, 726–727
Telectronics Guardian model ATP III 4215, 641, 904–907
Telectronics Guardian model ATP IV 4310, 907–909

Telemetry in the ICD, 636, 637–641
Tests to predict high risk of cardiovascular death, 558–573
  baroreflex sensitivity (BRS), 570–572
  combination of risk factors, 572
  EP studies after myocardial infarction, 565–567
  left ventricular dysfunction, 558–561
  randomized clinical trials to evaluate therapy, 573
  variability of RR intervals, 567–570
  ventricular arrhythmias, 561–565
Tetracaine, 335
Tetralogy of Fallot during childhood, 207
Thermal heating, interference of ICDs and PMs due to, 141
Thiopental, 322, 323
Third-generation ICDs, 201–202
  diagnostic capabilities, 650–651
  diagram of major component sections of, 113, 114
  European experience with, 832–840
    Intermedics Res-Q, 838–839
    Medtronic PCD, 830–833
    Siecure, 839–840
    Telectronics Guardian, 834–837
    Ventak defibrillators, 832–830
    Ventritex Cadence, 837–838
  postoperative impact of, 350–351
Thoracic nerve injury, 354
Thoracic surgeon, 295
Thoracoscopic implantation for the ICD, 289, 290
Thoracoscopic lead systems, 622
Tocainide, 230, 372
Torulopsis glabrata causing ICD device infection, 498, 499
Transcutaneous electrical nerve stimulation (TENS), interference of ICDs and PMs due to, 145–146
Transdermal fentanyl, 334
Transdiaphragmatic approach to ICD implantation, 288
Transposition of the great arteries during childhood, 208
Trauma, 354, 357
Triphasic waveforms, 19
Troubleshooting ICD system problems, 437–444
  antitachycardia pacing systems, 450–465
    effect of antiarrhythmic drugs, 464–465
    noninvasive EP study, 451–452
    pacing, 454–456

[Troubleshooting ICD system problems]
    sensing, 452–453
    tachycardia recognition, 456–459
    tachycardia termination, 459–464
  asymptomatic shocks, 441–442, 443
  intraoperative testing of the ICD, 311
  nonconversion, 437–439
  nondetection, 439–440
  Telectronics Guardian 4202/4203, 680–681
  Telectronics Guardian 4210/4211, 726–727
  Ventritex Cadence, 776

U-care registry (European study), 819–820, 820
Unipolar defibrillation, 55–60
  defibrillation threshold testing, 56–57
  lead system, 55–56, 57–58
United Network for Organ Sharing (UNOS), 586
U.S. Food and Drug Administration (FDA):
  approval for marketing of the ICD, 177
  standards for ICD and PM interference testing, 148
Upper limit of vulnerability hypothesis, 16–18, 46–48

Valvular surgery, ICP implantation and, 267
Vascular complications following ICD placement, 354, 358–360
Vasodilator Heart Failure Trial (V-HEFT), 587–588
Vecuronium, 324
Ventak (AICD device), 655–673
  clinical results and AICD statistics, 671
  electromagnetic interference/PM interaction, 668–671
  European clinical experience with, 823–830
  historical background, 655–656
  implantation and intraoperative testing, 664–666
  lead system, 663–664
  limitations, 672
  programming, 666–668
Ventak model 1500, 637
Ventak model 1510, 637
Ventak model 1520, 637
Ventak model 1550, 638, 656–661, 874–875
  arrhythmia detection, 656–660
  delivery of therapy, 660–661
  other device function, 661
  programmable and nonprogrammable parameters, 661
Ventak model 1555, 638, 662, 875–877
Ventak model P1600, 638, 662, 877–878

Index

Ventak model P2 1620/1625, 638, 662–663, 878–880
Ventak model PRx, 638, 695–711
  bradycardia pacing, 703
  clinical results, 709–710
  diagnostic data, 703–704
  European clinical experience with, 823–825
  mechanical specifications, 695, 696
  slaved programmed electrical stimulation, 704–709
  tachyarrhythmia detection, 697–700
  tachyarrhythmia therapy, 700–703
  tachyarrhythmia zones, 697, 698
Ventak model PRx II, 306
Ventak model PRx 1700/1705, 640, 880–882
Ventak model PRx II 1710/1715, 640, 882–885
Ventricular antitachycardia pacing with backup ICD:
  programming approach to, 445–449, 450
  troubleshooting pacing system, 450–465
  use of independent PMs and ICDs, 465–473
    implantation protocol, 466–470, 471, 472
    special problems during follow-up, 473
Ventricular arrhythmias:
  amiodarone for, 573–574
  postoperative, 342, 346–348
  surgery for, 239–241
  tests to predict high risk for SCD in, 561–565
Ventricular electrogram storage capabilities. *See* Stored ventricular electrogram analysis
Ventricular fibrillation (VF), 1, 187
  amiodarone efficacy tests for, 237–238
  catheter ablation techniques for, 241
  elevated defibrillation thresholds, 303–307
  ICD therapy for, 242–245, 575, 863–865
  idiopathic, 214–215
  initiation of, 1–8
    by electrical stimulus, 4–8
    by ischemia and reperfusion, 1–4
  maintenance of, 8–10
    degree of organization, 9
    frequency characteristics, 10
    multiple wandering wavelets, 8–9
  pharmacological therapy for, 229–237
  psychiatric management of, 410
  surgical therapy for, 239–241
  unipolar lead system for, 55–56
Ventricular premature complex (VPC) hypothesis, 557–558
Ventricular tachycardia (VT), 187
  amiodarone efficacy tests for, 237–238
  cardiac catheterization for, 263–264

[Ventricular tachycardia (VT)]
  catheter ablation techniques for, 241
  catheter mapping for, 268–269
  diagnosis using stored electrogram analysis, 100–102
  ICD therapy for, 242–245, 575, 863–865
  improved detection and monitoring of, 856–862
  low-energy cardioversion and cycle lengths, 93–94
  pharmacological therapy for, 229–237
  postoperative, 342, 346–348
  prevention of, 61–62, 862–863
  psychiatric management of, 410
  stored electrograms in studying initiation of, 106
  surgical therapy for, 239–241
  VT detection algorithms for Medtronic PCD, 687–690
Ventritex Cadence (tiered-therapy defibrillator), 229–300, 305, 763–777
  antitachycardia algorithms, 767
  backup pacing capabilities, 773
  clinical data on device performance, 774
  data storage and telemetry, 768–773
  defibrillation leads, 611
  European clinical experience with, 837–838
  general description, 763
  intraoperative testing and follow-up evaluation, 430, 431, 774–776
  noninvasive EP functions, 773
  noninvasive testing and troubleshooting, 776
  parameters of shock therapy, 767–768
  programmed device parameters, 763–765
  recognition algorithm, 766
  sensing system, 307, 765–766
  technical description, 773–774
  ventricular electrogram storage in, 100
Ventritex Cadence models V-100, V-100B, V-100C, 641, 909–912

Waveforms of defibrillation, 18–19
  biphasic, 18–19, 296
  monophasic, 296, 299
  triphasic, 19
Wolff-Parkinson-White syndrome, 31–32
Work environments, interference of ICDs and PMs due to, 147–148
Wound infection, 354

Young ICD patients. *See* Children and adolescents

About the Editors

N. A. MARK ESTES III is Director of the Cardiac Arrhythmia Service and the Cardiac Electrophysiology and Pacemaker Laboratory at the New England Medical Center and a Professor of Medicine at Tufts University School of Medicine, Boston, Massachusetts. The author or coauthor of over 100 original reports, reviews, and book chapters, Dr. Estes is an invited reviewer for numerous scientific journals. The President of the Massachusetts Electrophysiology Society, he is a Fellow of the American College of Cardiology; a Diplomate of the American Board of Internal Medicine in Cardiovascular Diseases, Medicine, and Clinical Cardiac Electrophysiology; and a member of the American Heart Association's Council on Clinical Cardiology and the North American Society of Pacing and Electrophysiology. Dr. Estes received the M.D. degree (1977) from the University of Cincinnati College of Medicine, Ohio.

ANTONIS S. MANOLIS is Codirector of the Cardiac Electrophysiology and Pacemaker Laboratory at the New England Medical Center and an Associate Professor of Medicine at Tufts University School of Medicine, Boston, Massachusetts. The author or coauthor of over 80 scientific publications, Dr. Manolis is a Fellow of both the American College of Cardiology and the European Society of Cardiology and a member of the North American Society of Pacing and Electrophysiology, the Athens Medical Association, and the Hellenic Society of Cardiology. He received the M.D. degree (1978) and the Sc.D. degree (1989) from Athens University School of Medicine, Greece.

PAUL J. WANG is Associate Director of the Cardiac Electrophysiology and Pacing Laboratory and Director of the Adult Heart Station at the New England Medical Center and an Assistant Professor of Medicine at Tufts University School of Medicine, Boston, Massachusetts. Dr. Wang is a Fellow of the American College of Cardiology and a Diplomate of the American Board of Internal Medicine in Clinical Cardiac Electrophysiology. He received the M.D. degree (1983) from the College of Physicians and Surgeons, Columbia University, New York, New York.